Rehabilitation Nursing

Process, Application, & Outcomes

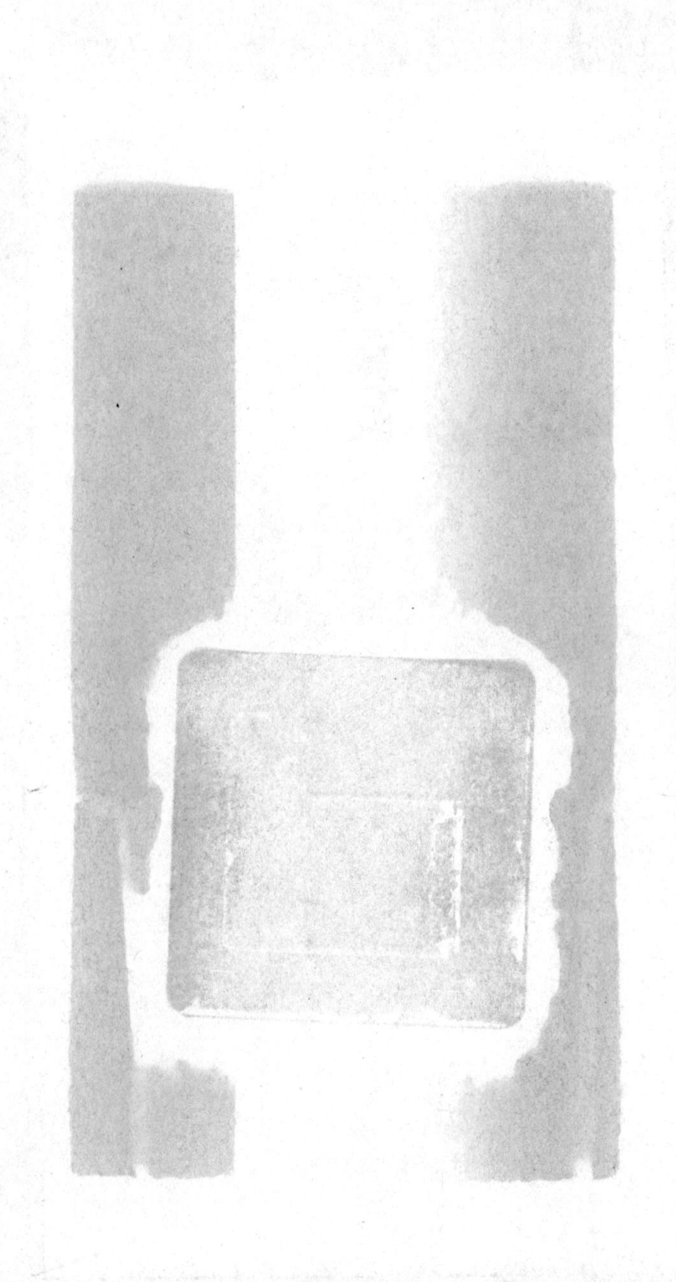

Rehabilitation Nursing

Process, Application, & Outcomes

Shirley P. Hoeman, PhD, MPH, RN, CRRN, CS
Health Systems Consultations, International
Naples, Maine

3rd Edition

With 247 illustrations

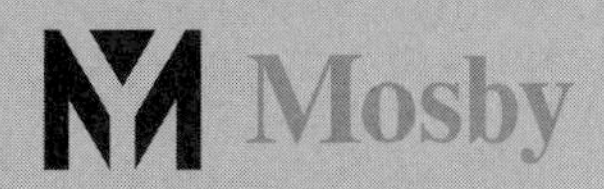

A Harcourt Health Sciences Company
St. Louis London Philadelphia Sydney Toronto

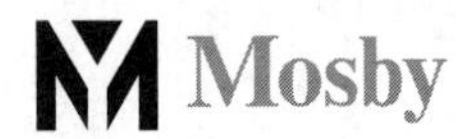

A Harcourt Health Sciences Company

Vice President, Nursing Editorial Director: Sally Schrefer
Senior Editor: Loren Wilson
Senior Developmental Editor: Nancy L. O'Brien
Project Manager: Deb Vogel
Production Editor: Deon Lee
Design Manager: Bill Drone
Cover Designer: Kathi Gosche
Cover Photographs: Charles Gupton/Corbis Stock Market *(top left),* Gabe Palmer/Corbis Stock Market *(top right),* Lori Adamski Peek/Stone *(bottom right)*

THIRD EDITION

NOTICE

Pharmacology is an ever-changing field. Standard safety precautions must be followed, but as new research and clinical experience broaden our knowledge, changes in treatment and drug therapy may become necessary or appropriate. Readers are advised to check the most current product information provided by the manufacturer of each drug to be administered to verify the recommended dose, the method and duration of administration, and contraindications. It is the responsibility of the licensed health care provider, relying on experience and knowledge of the patient, to determine dosages and the best treatment for each individual patient. Neither the publisher nor the editor assumes any liability for any injury and/or damage to persons or property arising from this publication.

Mosby, Inc.
A Harcourt Health Sciences Company
11830 Westline Industrial Drive
St. Louis, Missouri 63146

Printed in the United States of America

Library of Congress Cataloging-in-Publication Data

Rehabilitation nursing : process, application & outcomes / [edited by] Shirley P. Hoeman.—3rd ed.
p. ; cm.
Includes bibliographical references and index.
ISBN 0-323-01190-X
1. Rehabilitation nursing. I. Hoeman, Shirley P.
[DNLM: 1. Rehabilitation Nursing—methods. WY 150.5 R3453 2001]
RT120.R4 R423 2001
610.73′6--dc21

01 02 03 04 05 CL/MVY 9 8 7 6 5 4 3 2 1

To Denny

"Hear my cry, O God; attend to my prayer.
From the end of the earth I will cry to You,
when my heart is overwhelmed; lead me to the rock
that is higher than I."

Psalm 61:1-2

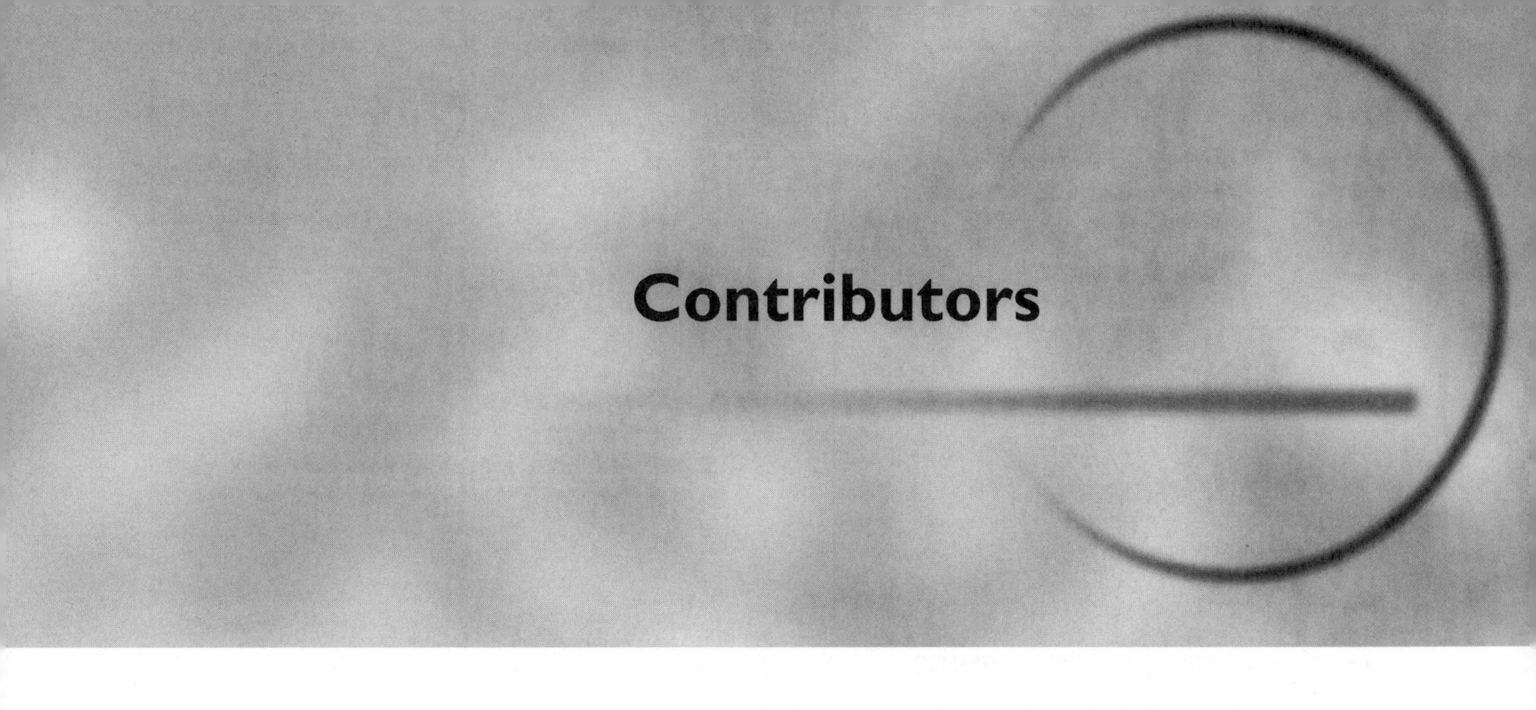

Contributors

Judith C. Allen, EdD, RN, CRRN
Nursing Education Coordinator
Kessler Institute for Rehabilitation
West Orange, New Jersey

Joan P. Alverzo, PhD(c), MSN, CRRN
Vice President, Clinical Support Services
Kessler Institute for Rehabilitation
West Orange, New Jersey

Jean M. Benjamin, MSN, RN, CRRN
Senior Consultant
Gill/Balsano Consulting
Atlanta, Georgia

Jean K. Berry, PhD, RN, CS
Clinical Assistant Professor, College of Nursing
University of Illinois at Chicago
Chicago, Illinois

Barbara J. Boss, PhD, RN, CFNP, CANP
Professor of Nursing
University of Mississippi
Jackson, Mississippi

Nicole Brandt, PharmD, CGP
Assistant Professor, Geriatric Pharmacotherapy
Deputy Director, Lamy Center on Drug Therapy and Aging
University of Maryland School of Pharmacy
Baltimore, Maryland

Linda Brewer, MSN, RN, CFNP, CACNP
Acute Care, Family Nurse Practitioner
Scott Regional Hospital
Morton, Mississippi

Lisa Cyr Buchanan, MS, RN, CRRN
Rehabilitation Clinical Nurse Specialist
The Maine Rehabilitation Center
Eastern Maine Medical Center
Bangor, Maine

Theresa Perfetta Cappello, PhD, RN, Ct.Hy
Associate Professor, School of Health Professions
Marymount University
Arlington, Virginia

Gloria T. Aubut Craven, MS, RN
Partner
Craven & Ober Policy Strategists, LLC
Boston, Massachusetts

Pamela M. Duchene, DNSc, RN, CRRN
Vice President, Patient Care Services
St. Joseph Hospital
Nashua, New Hampshire

Cindy Gatens, MN, RN, CRRN-A
Clinical Nurse Specialist
Dodd Hall/Rehabilitation
The Ohio State University Medical Center
Columbus, Ohio

Aloma R. Gender, MSN, RN, CRRN
Senior Vice President, Clinical Services
Good Shepherd Rehabilitation Hospital
Allentown, Pennsylvania

Carol A. Gleason, MM, RN, CRRN, CCM, LRC
Director of Resource Management
Shaughnessy Kaplan Rehabilitation Hospital
Salem, Massachusetts

Nancy H. Glenn-Molali, MSN, RN, CRRN
Rehabilitation Clinical Nurse Specialist
Private Practice
Havre de Grace, Maryland

Susan B. Greco, MSN, RN, CRRN
Director of Nursing
Touro Rehabilitation Center
New Orleans, Louisiana

A. René Hébert, MS, RN, CRRN-A
Clinical Instructor
Adult Health and Illness
The Ohio State University College of Nursing
Columbus, Ohio

Shirley P. Hoeman, PhD, MPH, RN, CRRN, CS
Health Systems Consultations, International
Naples, Maine

Diane Huber, PhD, RN, FAAN, CNAA
Associate Professor, College of Nursing
The University of Iowa
Iowa City, Iowa

Deirdre F. Jackson, MSN, APRN, CRRN
Director, Continuing Education and Staff Development
Children's Specialized Hospital
Mountainside, New Jersey

Joyce H. Johnson, PhD, MS, RN
Associate Professor, College of Nursing
University of Illinois at Chicago
Chicago, Illinois

Kelly M. M. Johnson, MSN, RN, CFNP, CRRN
Vice President, Patient Care Services
Craig Hospital
Englewood, Colorado

Margaret Kelly-Hayes, EdD, RN, CRRN, FAAN
Clinical Professor of Neurological Nursing
Boston University School of Medicine
Boston, Massachusetts

Deborah J. Konkle-Parker, MSN, FNP, ACRN
Nurse Practitioner, Division of Infectious Diseases
University of Mississippi Medical Center
Jackson, Mississippi

Patricia L. McCollom, MS, RN, CRRN, CDMS, CCM, CLCP
President and Nurse Consultant
LifeCare Economics and Management Consulting and Rehabilitation Services, Inc.
Ankeny, Iowa

Christina M. Mumma, PhD, RN, CRRN
Professor, School of Nursing
University of Alaska
Anchorage, Alaska

Leslie J. Neal, PhD, RNC, CRRN
Assistant Professor, School of Health Professions
Marymount University
Arlington, Virginia

Audrey Nelson, PhD, RN, FAAN
Associate Chief, Nursing Service for Research
James A. Haley VA Medical Center
Tampa, Florida

Grace Nolde-Lopez, MSN, RN, CWOCN, CRRN
Clinical Nurse Specialist
Craig Hospital
Englewood, Colorado

Rhonda S. Olson, MS, RN, CRRN
Rehabilitation Nurse Consultant
RS Consulting
Houston, Texas

Billie R. Phillips, PhD, RN, CDFS
Assistant Professor
Tennessee Wesleyan College
Fort Sanders School of Nursing
Athens, Tennessee

Marion A. Phipps, MS, RN, CRRN, FAAN
Rehabilitation Nurse Specialist
Beth Israel Deaconess Medical Center
Boston, Massachusetts

Marilyn Pires, MS, RN, CRRN-A
Rehabilitation Clinical Nurse Specialist
Rancho Los Amigos National Rehabilitation Center
Downey, California

Christy A. Price, MSN, RN, NP
Nephrology Nurse Practitioner
Nephrology Associates
Salt Lake City, Utah

Julie Pryor, CM, BA, MN, RN
Senior Lecturer in Rehabilitation Nursing
University of Western Sydney
Associate Director, Rehabilitation Nursing Research and Development Unit
Royal Rehabilitation Centre
Sydney, Australia

Maria B. Radwanski, MSN, RN, CS, CRRN
Gerontological Clinical Nurse Specialist
Private Practice
Reading, Pennsylvania

Gail Lynn Sims, MSN, RN, CRRN
Nurse Manager
TIRR Systems
Houston, Texas

Mary Ann Solimine, MLS, RN
Research Consultant
Westfield, New Jersey

Kim Vander Ploeg, MS, RN
Clinical Nurse Specialist
Pediatrics and Pediatric Intensive Care
Lutheran General Children's Hospital
Park Ridge, Illinois

Acknowledgments for Contributors to the First and Second Editions

Kay Lewis Abney, PhD, RN, CPNP

Denise B. Angst, DNSc, RN

Mila A. Aroskar, EdD, RN

Judith A. Behm, MSN, RN, CRRN

Rita J. Boucher, EdD, RN

Dorothy P. Byers, MS, RN

Marci Catanzaro, PhD, RN, CS

Sandra Chenelly, MS, RN

Susan L. Dean-Baar, PhD, RN, CRRN, FAAN

Sharon S. Dittmar, PhD, RN

Theresa P. Dulski, MS, RN,C

Susan M. Evans, MS, RN

Elizabeth Forbes, MSN, EdD, RN, FAAN

Mary Frances Gainer, EdD, RN

Kathy M. Graham, MS, RN

Cheryl Graham-Eason, MS, RN, CRRN

Margaret J. Griffiths, MSN, RN

Maureen Habel, MA, RN, CRRN

Denise Hanlon, MS, RN

Brenda P. Haughey, PhD, RN

Margaret M. Hens, MS, RN

Linda M. Janelli, EdD, MS, RN,C

Janet G. LaMantia, MA, RN, CRRN

Janet L. Larson, PhD, RN

Judith A. Laughlin, PhD, RN

Martha F. Markarian, MS, RN

Elizabeth A. Moody-Szymanski, MS, RN

Angela Moy, MSN, RN, CRRN

Mary Sue Niederpruem, MS, RN

Elizabeth C. Phelps, MS, RN

Josephine Ricci-Balich, MSN, RNC, CRRN

Dorothy Sager, RN, CRRN, CIRS, CCM

Joyce Santora, MS, RN

Yvonne Krall Scherer, EdD, RN

Jill A. Scott, MS, RN

Margie L. Scott, EdD, RN

Elizabeth L. Sharkey, MS, RN

Anaise Theuerkauf, BS, MEd, RN, CRRN, CCM

Margaret A. Umhauer, MS, RN

Barbara H. Warner, MS, RN

Barbara G. White, EdD, RN

Barbara Wisnom, MS, RN

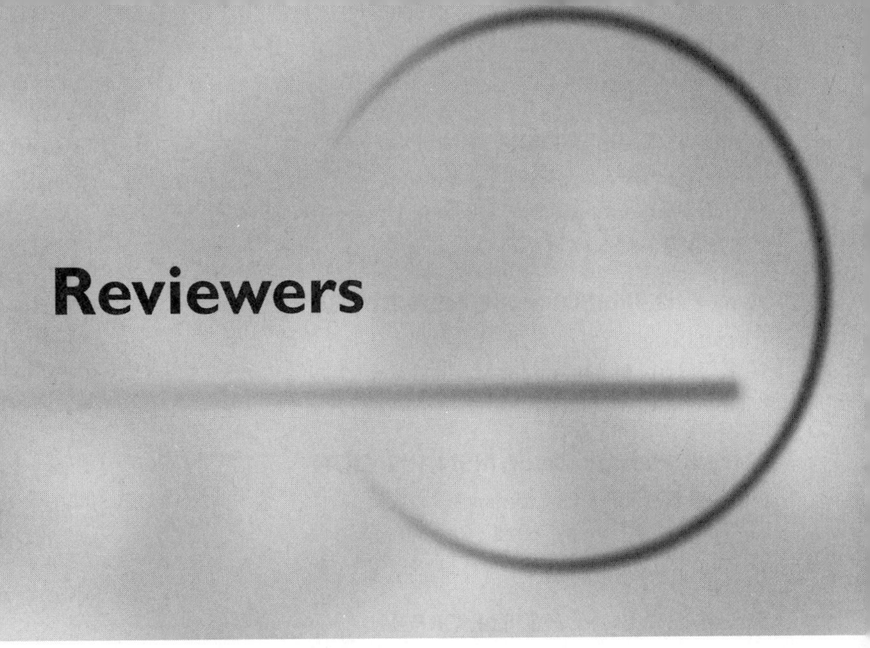

Reviewers

Jane H. Backer, DNS, RN
Associate Professor, School of Nursing
Indiana University
Indianapolis, Indiana

Barbara J. Boss, PhD, RN, CFNP, CANP
Professor of Nursing
University of Mississippi
Jackson, Mississippi

Carol Boswell, EdD, RN
Assistant Professor, School of Nursing
Texas Tech University Health Sciences Center
Odessa, Texas

Barbara Brillhart, PhD, RN, CRRN
Associate Professor, College of Nursing
Arizona State University
Tempe, Arizona

Teresa A. Bryan, BSN, MSN, RN, CRRN
Nurse Manager
Craig Hospital
Englewood, Colorado

Lisa Cyr Buchanan, MS, RN, CRRN
Rehabilitation Clinical Nurse Specialist
The Maine Rehabilitation Center
Bangor, Maine

Joanne Bullard, MN, APRN
Assistant Professor of Nursing
Our Lady of Holy Cross College
New Orleans, Louisiana

Nancy E. Dayhoff, EdD, RN
Clinical Nurse Specialist
CEO, Clinical Solutions, LLC
Columbus, Indiana

Paula DiBenedetto, MSN, RN
Instructor, Clinical Nursing
Texas Tech University Health Sciences Center
Lubbock, Texas

Pamela M. Duchene, DNSc, RN, CRRN
Vice President, Patient Care Services
St. Joseph Hospital
Nashua, New Hampshire

Kristen L. Easton, PhD(c), MS, RN, CRRN-A, CS
Assistant Professor of Nursing, Valparaiso University
Valparaiso, Indiana

Janet M. Farahmand, EdD, RN
Adjunct Professor of Nursing, Neumann College
Aston, Pennsylvania
Immaculata College
Immaculata, Pennsylvania

Mitzi A. Forbes, PhD, RN
Assistant Professor, School of Nursing
University of Wisconsin, Milwaukee
Milwaukee, Wisconsin

Judith K. Glann, MSN, RN, CCRN
Clinical Nurse Specialist, Cardiovascular/Critical Care
Lovelace Health Systems
Albuquerque, New Mexico

Nancy H. Glenn-Molali, MSN, RN, CRRN
Rehabilitation Clinical Nurse Specialist
Havre de Grace, Maryland

Cheryl Graham-Eason, PhD(c), MEd, MS, RN
Professor
Community College of Allegheny County
Adjunct Faculty, Carlow College
Pittsburgh, Pennsylvania

Philip A. Greiner, DNSc, RN
Associate Professor and Director
Health Promotion Center, Fairfield University
Fairfield, Connecticut

Amy E. Guilfoil-Dumont, MSN, RN, CCRN
Clinical Nurse Specialist
Holy Family Hospital and Medical Center
Methuen, Massachusetts

Mary E. Hanson-Zalot, MSN, RN, OCN
Clinical Resource Coordinator
University of Pennsylvania Hospital
Philadelphia, Pennsylvania

Susanne R. Hays, MS, RN, CRRN
Advanced Practice Nurse
Albuquerque, New Mexico

Dalice L. Hertzberg, MSN, RN, CRRN
Instructor
University of Colorado Health Sciences Center
Denver, Colorado

Cynthia S. Jacelon, PhD(c), RN, CRRN
Clinical Assistant Professor, School of Nursing
University of Massachusetts
Amherst, Massachusetts

Mary Ann Jacobs, MSN, RN, CRRN
Nurse Practitioner, Spinal Cord Injury
Jefferson Barracks VA Hospital
St. Louis, Missouri

Linda L. Kerby, BA, BSN, MA
Registered Nurse Consultant
Leawood, Kansas

Christina M. Mumma, PhD, RN, CRRN
Professor, School of Nursing
University of Alaska
Anchorage, Alaska

Sarah E. Newton, PhD, RN
Assistant Professor, School of Nursing
Oakland University
Rochester, Michigan

Maria E. Nowicki, PhD, RN
Director of Nursing
Mercy College of Northwest Ohio
Toledo, Ohio

Rhonda S. Olson, MS, RN, CRRN
Rehabilitation Nurse Consultant
RS Consulting
Houston, Texas

Phyllis Peterson, MN, RN
Assistant Professor, Division of Nursing
Our Lady of Holy Cross College
New Orleans, Louisiana

Mary L. Pickerell, BA, RN, CCM, CPUR
Nurse Review Specialist, Marriott International, Inc.
Washington, District of Columbia

Janet Johnson Prince, BSN, RN, CWOCN, CGRN
Clinical Nurse Manager, Endoscopy Unit Wound and Ostomy Management Services
St. Joseph Hospital
Nashua, New Hampshire

Patricia A. Quigley, PhD, ARNP, CRRN
Rehabilitation Clinical Nurse Specialist
James A. Haley Veteran's Hospital
Faculty, University of Phoenix
St. Petersburg, Florida

Terry Savan, BSN, MA, RN, CRNP, PA-C
Assistant Professor, PA Program
DeSales University
Center Valley, Pennsylvania

Mary R. Stange, MS, RN, CRRN
Clinical Nurse Specialist, Neuro Rehab
Drake Center
Cincinnati, Ohio

Teresa L. Cervantez Thompson, PhD, CRRN-A
Assistant Professor, School of Nursing
Oakland University
Rochester, Michigan

Karen L. Tomajan, MS, RNC, CRRN
Director, Clinical Education
Integris Health
Oklahoma City, Oklahoma

Mary Joe White, PhD, RN
Associate Professor of Nursing
University of Texas Health Sciences Center
Houston, Texas

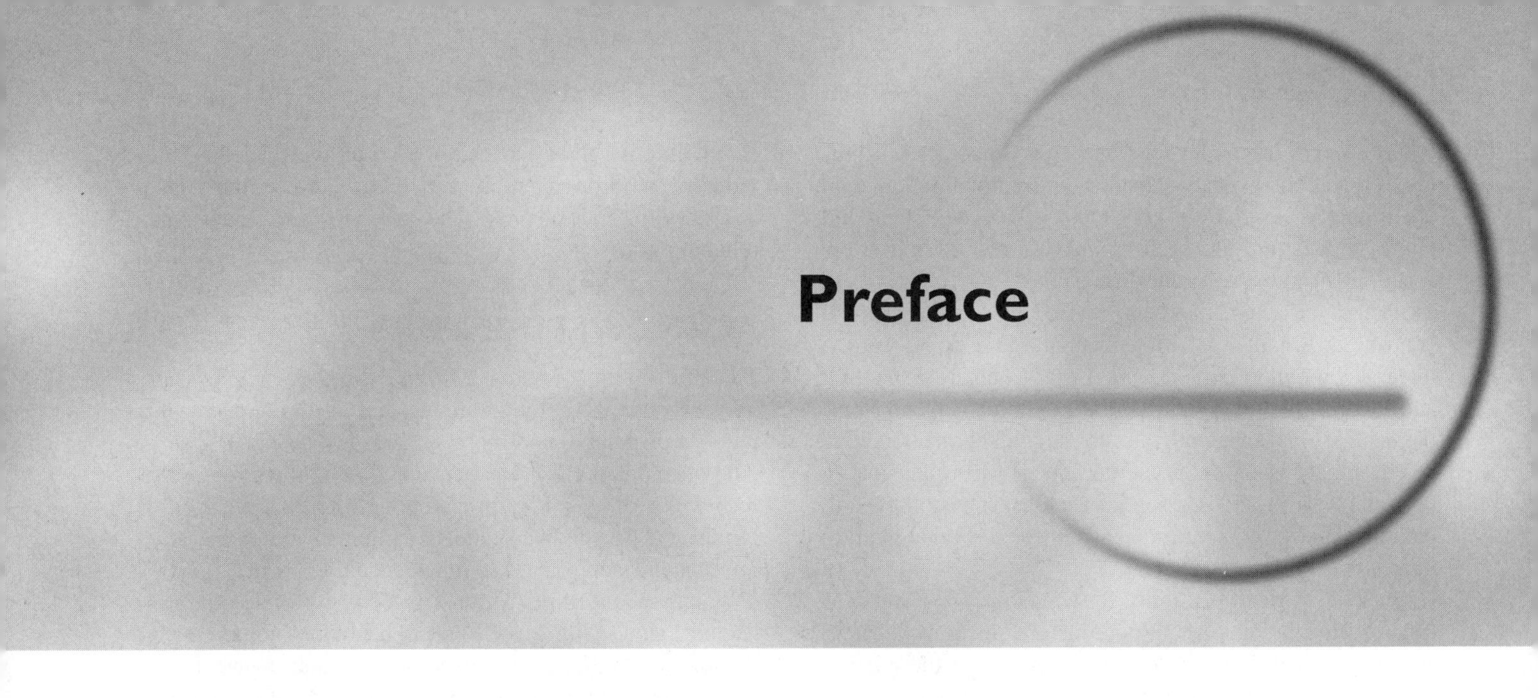

Preface

As editor of the third edition of *Rehabilitation Nursing,* I share with my contributors, all of whom are experts in the specialty, the conviction that principles found in rehabilitation nursing are essential components within all areas of professional practice. Rehabilitation nursing is essential in all levels of illness prevention, treatment, and restoration. Now as never before, few individuals elude the experiences of acuity, comorbidity, impairment, or chronicity as people live longer and survive formerly fatal illnesses and conditions. Individuals and families need competent, knowledgeable nurses to assist them in adjusting to their health situation and to achieve their optimal potential. When rehabilitation interventions are instituted early in primary and secondary levels of care, clients can experience improved satisfaction and quality of life. Rehabilitation nurses achieve this through employing high-level assessments of functional patterns, establishing mutual client and nursing goals for optimal levels of function, and using nursing actions that effect positive client outcomes, including independent function.

In this text we embrace the movement toward strengthening the team approach in community and international practice involving the client, family, and community. Overall, we seek to attain high levels of commitment, competence, caring, and compassion and to infuse these into rehabilitation nursing. The rehabilitation nursing system and techniques may change, but the intention of "making a difference" in someone's life never goes out of style.

The concept of change can scarcely be avoided when discussing health care coupled with entering a new century. The attributes and difficulties of change as it affects rehabilitation nursing practice and ultimately clients, families, and communities are discussed throughout this third edition. To understand and deal with changes in rehabilitation necessitates an appreciation of the history and premises upon which the specialty is based, as much as discerning new directions. Part of moving forward is to recognize where one began and to understand the purposes of action. Thus, in this third edition, we have endeavored to build a legacy and retain core elements and principles of rehabilitation nursing while instituting current information, incorporating findings from research or evidence-based studies, and presenting new areas of practice, including a strong prevention and community program.

Specifically, we have retained the peer review, scholarly approach, and overall themes relevant and essential to rehabilitation nursing. The conceptual framework continues to integrate Roper, Logan, and Tierney's nursing model with Gordon's Functional Health Patterns and Corbin and Strauss' chronic illness trajectory to emphasize the increased chronicity in client populations. Clinical chapters are organized according to the nursing process and use the most current Nursing Interventions Classifications and Nursing Outcomes Classifications, as well as initiatives for prevention and health promotion based on *Healthy People 2000/2010* objectives and consensus statements from the Agency for Healthcare Research and Quality. Beyond the discussion of rehabilitation models and theories (Chapter 2), content-specific theoretical concepts, legislation, and resources are introduced in appropriate chapters. For instance, the content in Chapter 29, Pediatric Rehabilitation, includes developmental theories, special needs legislation, and pediatric resources.

This text is organized into six sections. Section I, Foundations of Rehabilitation Nursing, contains chapters that address concepts and principles basic to rehabilitation nursing. These have all been completely revised. Chapter 1 delineates a history of rehabilitation, and Chapter 5 emphasizes rehabilitation research utilization.

Section II, Management for Client-Centered Programs, presents current information about quality and evaluation that is pertinent to rehabilitation and restorative care. All chapters reflect the multiple changes that have occurred within areas of case management, evaluation, and measures; standards are discussed for rehabilitation nursing management. The revised chapter on Movement and Functional Ability (Chapter 14) integrates content from movement science, exercise, and activities of daily living.

Section III, Principles for Improving Outcomes in Clinical Applications, contains chapters on improving individual client outcomes. Chapter 11, Outcome-Directed Client and Family Education, has been completely revised and offers function-specific client education guides. Chapter 12, Client and Family Coping, has been revised by an international contributor; Chapter 14, Movement and Functional Ability, integrates mobility content, and a new Chapter 13, Culture and Medical Systems: Conventional, Alternative, and Complementary Systems, contains current content on alternative health practices. Another new chapter, Neurophysiology (Chapter 15), provides essential anatomy, physiology, and pathophysiology content frequently needed by rehabilitation nurses.

Section IV, Health Patterns: Systems Functions, and Section V, Health Patterns: Psychosocial Functions, contain specific clinical practice content according to the nursing process. Muscle and Skeletal Function (Chapter 21) and Neuromuscular Rehabilitation (Chapter 22) have been reorganized into two chapters. Chapter 24, Sensations and Pain, reorganizes and integrates content on sensory function, sensation, and pain. Chapter 27 discusses Sleep and Recreation. The revised chapter on Spirituality (Chapter 28) makes an essential and unique contribution to rehabilitation nursing practice.

Section VI, Restoration and Rehabilitation: Special Populations, contains two new chapters on areas growing in importance to rehabilitation nursing practice: Chapter 34, Renal Rehabilitation, and Chapter 35, Cancer Rehabilitation. The Appendix outlines Pharmacology for Rehabilitation Nursing.

Features in this edition include increased focus on interventions and outcomes using NIC and NOC labels; content on illness, prevention, and community-based nursing; case studies, critical thinking exercises, and nursing resources, including sites on the World Wide Web. Personalized rehabilitation nursing experiences open each chapter.

Throughout this text, the focus is on the whole person, apart from the chronic, disabling, or developmental condition. In reality, some aspect of rehabilitation and restorative care will touch all of us sometime in our lives, whether individually or through family and friends. We will all need and hope to find a nurse who practices and understands rehabilitation.

ACKNOWLEDGMENTS

The third edition of *Rehabilitation Nursing* was possible only because of the commitment and encouragement of a number of people. Foremost, I thank my husband, Denny, who once again offered patience and solid direction as our lives were occupied by preparations for this edition. Our family and friends were understanding of the demands of my schedule and offered so much encouragement.

For a second time, a majority of my professional colleagues, along with several new contributors, joined me on the journey of preparing this edition. I thank them for their professional commitment and various levels of support and for helping me maintain a sense of humor. Pam Duchene, especially, assisted me with multiple situations, and many other contributors extended themselves to help and collaborate in finding solutions to problems. Whether sharing expertise and resources, responding to requests, or helping solve problems, we modeled the team approach we value in rehabilitation. The foreword by Dr. John Basmajian (my pater Armenian) speaks to the tribute due all rehabilitation nurses.

Finally, I thank the nursing editorial and production editing staff. Loren Wilson, Nancy O'Brien, Deon Lee, and others provided the editorial expertise to ensure all processes were completed and to guide this project toward a high level of quality. We all have worked to produce a third edition that is timely, scholarly, usable, and relevant.

I can speak for all in that we applaud in advance those nurses who study the processes in this book and apply the rehabilitation content in their professional practice to advance the specialty and to improve outcomes for clients worldwide.

Shirley P. Hoeman, PhD, MPH, RN, CRRN, CS
Naples, Maine

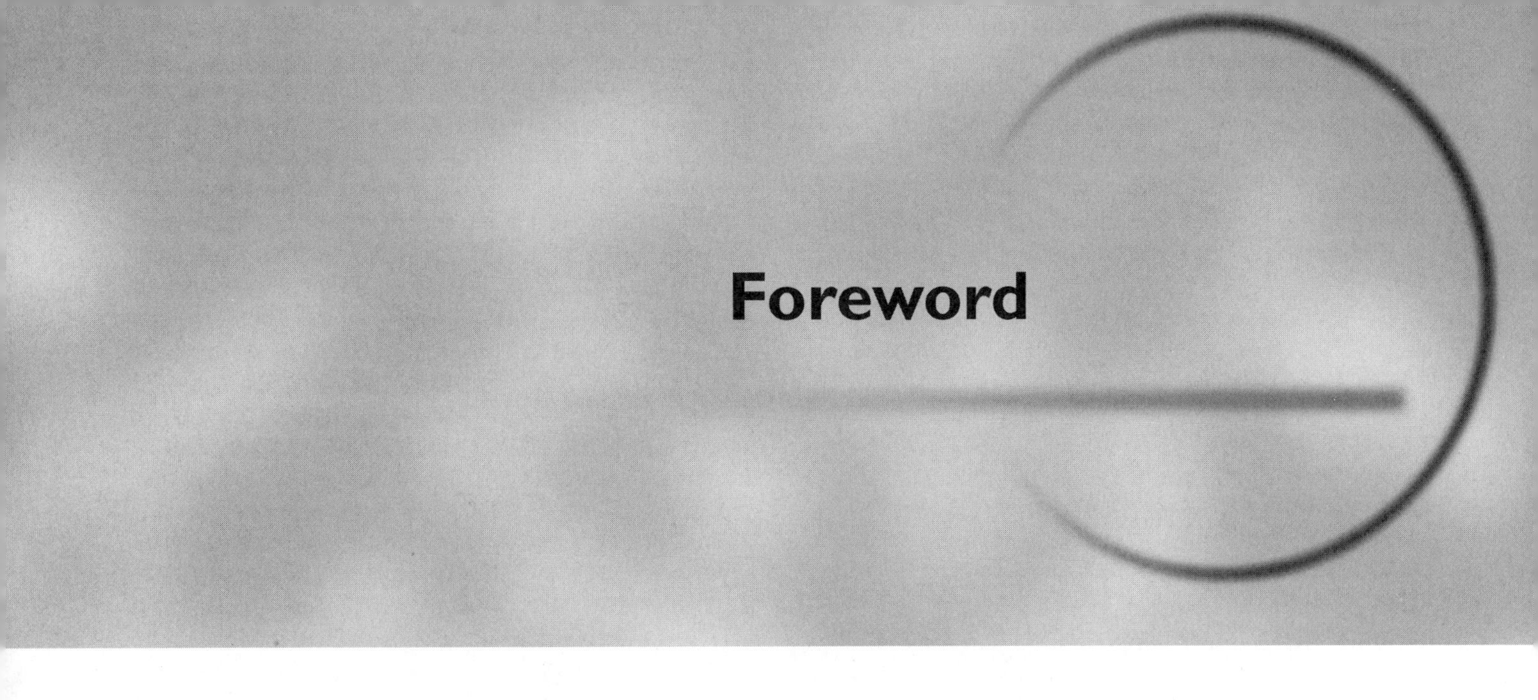

Foreword

How does one disguise a love letter that purports to be a foreword? Readers will see through my transparent attempts to remain "objective" about this book. They will become aware of my long-held conviction that fine rehabilitation nursing is the lifeblood of good-to-excellent rehabilitation care. Immersed as I have been with physicians, bioengineers, physical and occupational therapists, neuropsychologists, and other health workers and researchers, I have always proclaimed good rehabilitation nursing to be the central issue in restoring and stabilizing optimal healing.

First let us be clear: *healing care* is not synonymous with *health care.* Whereas, according to *Stedman's Medical Dictionary,* ed. 24, *health* is defined as "the state of the organism when it functions optimally without evidence of disease or abnormality," *healing* (of a person) is defined as "curing: restoring to health." These terms clearly describe two related but discrete entities.

In the latter half of the twentieth century, medicine and surgery, including medical rehabilitation, and a host of paramedical disciplines craved a new image. They glibly donned the modern garment of "health professions," but alas, this designation was simply a protective masquerade. They simply had reacted to the canard that they were concerned only with disease and injuries and not with health. Their critics claimed to be the custodians of that sacred vessel "health" but gradually found themselves taken over.

Both the learned professions and the manual trades are recognized by what they do or attempt to do as an occupation. On the one hand, specialization in the professions may result in subdivisions (e.g., cardiologists or orthopedists) in the medical field. On the other hand, tradesmen may get grouped together (e.g., building trades, airline employees, or civic servants). The observer is neither confused nor misled. However, to group all physicians, nurses, and therapists under the rubric of "health professions" is simply wrong. Most physicians and surgeons and other professionals related to them are rather bored with caring for the truly healthy even at the essential interface of prevention.

Of course, prevention of injury and ill health should be an important part of their daily work. However, in practice, it is often boring and unexciting even for family doctors. Of course, it is the first step in rehabilitation. Sadly, rehabilitation professionals tend to ignore active prevention of the very injuries and disease that eventually provide them with challenging jobs.

Fortunately, rehabilitation nurses are on hand (most of the time on a daily and hourly basis) to prevent aggravation of disabilities and organic diseases. However, funding restrictions in even the richest countries have hampered ideal conditions.

The tenets of this book will help to strengthen the foundations for the next generation. One can only hope and pray that administrators, officials, and politicians awake to the vital importance of rehabilitation nursing and its dedicated practitioners. On a personal basis, it is an honor for me to have had the opportunity to participate in its birth.

John V. Basmajian, OC, MD, LLD, FRCPC
Professor Emeritus, McMaster University
Hamilton, Ontario, Canada

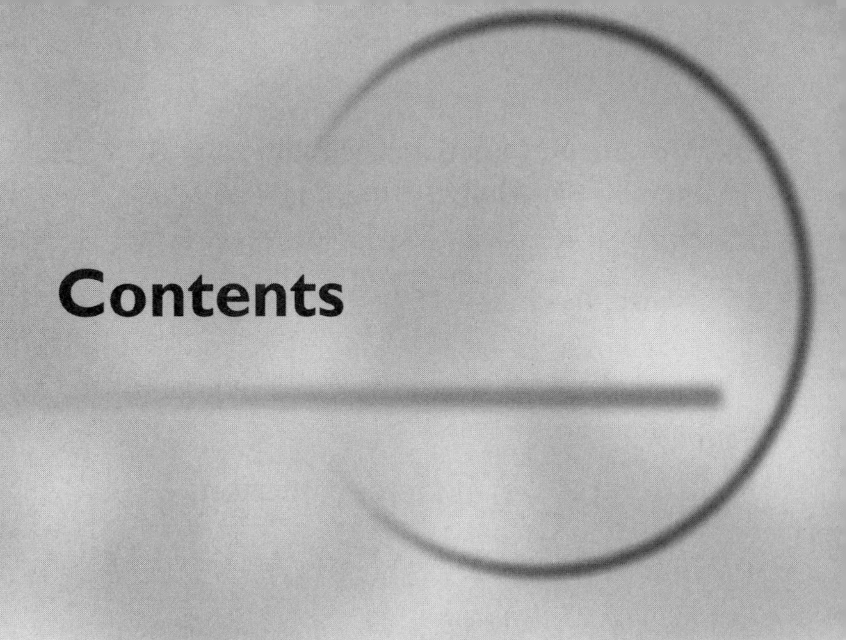

Contents

History, Issues, and Trends

1

Shirley P. Hoeman, PhD, RN, CRRN

It did not take long to hear stories about the ghost when I became Director of Nursing and Outpatient Services at Sister Kenny Rehabilitation Institute (KRI) in Minneapolis, Minnesota, in 1970. The ghost of Sister Kenny wearing her Australian outback hat still roamed the hallways. Those who had known Sister Kenny felt special, but none were so anointed as those who saw her apparition.

The nurses who worked at KRI had their own saga about the "polio years" and the patients who became part of their lives for months of care. It seemed they forgot no one. Warm memories flowed as they talked about their favorites, who often did not survive, and voiced regrets for being "unable to break through to the difficult ones." Administering care with their arms extended into the sleeves of the iron lung respirators and with feet straddling hoses and tubing was difficult and backbreaking; the equipment was cumbersome, and patient outcomes were unpredictable. Many nurses reading this book have never seen anything like the polio wards (Figure 1-1); those who have will never forget them.

Many of the nurses had served in the war (another source of stories), which perhaps prepared them for the uneven fight against disease and disability. They called one another by their last names—Miller, Schumacher, Brooks, Booth, and Haley, who was a pioneer of alternative therapeutics. Where the patients were concerned, the nurses were a team because they knew their roles, thrived on discipline, and scheduled time for their patients first. It seemed they knew every procedure, adapted equipment and wheelchairs to a patient's unique needs, and planned education precisely for the home environment and resources; they had seen and done it all without becoming cynical or losing faith.

A sense of camaraderie and challenge tinged their memories. They laughed when recalling how a ponderous, unmanageable, dark green rubber bladder, which served as a primitive waterbed, escaped full of water from the bed frame and rolled onto the floor, trapping several orderlies and a nurse under its weight. Fortunately no one was hurt, and they named the waterbed Harry (for Truman).

The nurses recounted the public fear of polio when the cause was unknown and before the vaccine. Many of the nurses rode public buses to work. However, if a nurse was in uniform or was seen coming from KRI, the bus more often than not would pass by without making the stop. The nurses changed clothes and slipped around to the bus stop on the block behind KRI. They lived with the realities of polio every day.

One of the nursing assistants who had been trained by Sister Kenny administered hot pack treatments to some patients. One day I had a terrible headache while at work, and she brought a Sister Kenny hot pack to my office. I cannot begin to describe the intense warmth generated deep into my muscles when that wool material was placed on my neck and shoulders. It was at once hot, moist, penetrating, and sublime. I understood many things, but still I did not see the ghost.

HISTORY AND REHABILITATION NURSING

Defining the Specialty

Rehabilitation is a specialty practice that was organized within professional nursing in 1964. From inception, rehabilitation nursing resonated with teachings of Nightingale (1859/1992); its principles underlie basic excellent nursing practice with respect for each individual's potential. "The physically handicapped person must be retrained to walk and to travel, to care for his daily needs, to use normal methods of transportation, to use ordinary toilet facilities, to apply and remove his own prosthetic appliances, and to communicate either orally or in writing. Too frequently these basic skills are overlooked" (Rusk, 1957, p. 11). Stryker (1977, p. 15) observed that rehabilitation nursing is "a creative process that begins with immediate preventive care in the first stage of accident or illness. It is continued through the restorative stage of care and involves adaptation of the whole being to a new life."

These distinctions dispute a persistent perception of rehabilitation as a third stage of health care, a kind of final resort. In 21st century definitions, the social construction of health has expanded to encompass improved quality of life and possibilities, as well as reduced morbidity and mortality. Core principles and practices of rehabilitation nursing are applicable at all levels of intervention, essential to quality care in all sectors of health, and foundational to other nursing specialties.

Formally, rehabilitation nursing is, "the diagnosis and treatment of human responses of individuals and groups to actual or potential health problems stemming from altered functional ability and altered lifestyle" (American Nurses Association [ANA] & Association of Rehabilitation Nurses [ARN], 1988, p. 4). In a world of aging populations, lengthened years of life, medical and technological advances, and global health, rehabilitation nurses are experts in preventing complications and averting further disability for their clients. Chronic conditions, associated with reduced life satisfaction and limited functional abilities, are often precur-

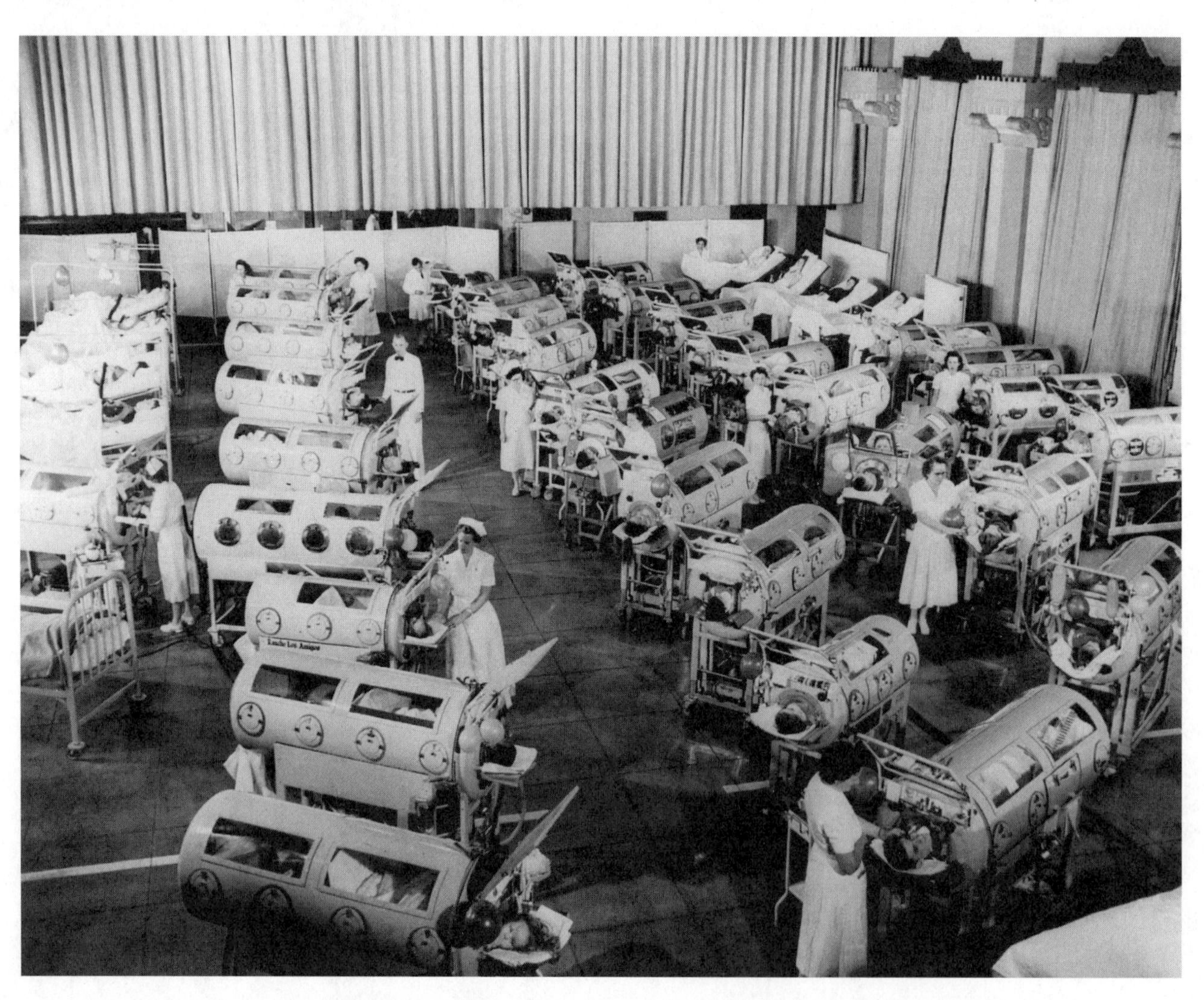

Figure 1-1 A polio ward during the epidemics of the 1950s. (Reproduced with permission of Rancho Los Amigos National Rehabilitation Center, Downey, CA.)

sors to disability. Indeed, a priority for rehabilitation nursing is to assist persons with disabilities or chronic conditions to achieve or maintain maximum functional abilities, optimal health and well-being, and effective coping with changes or alterations in their lives.

Rehabilitation nurses have experience enabling clients and families to become authorities and experts on their condition and situation and to negotiate mutual long- and short-range or lifelong goals. Their experience prepares them to examine ways the community and health systems can participate and include clients, as well as to ensure comprehensive primary care that has continuity with and support for rehabilitation goals. They are involved in assessment and innovations from prevention to incident or onset and provide continuity through optimal health restoration (Hoeman, 1999a).

Underlying Conceptual Frameworks

The primary conceptual frameworks for this book are adapted from a model for nursing that is based on a model for living (Roper, Logan, & Tierney, 1996) integrated with modifications of functional health patterns (Gordon, 2000). Both Roy's Adaptation Model (Roy & Andrews, 1980) and Orem's Self-Care Concepts (1989) are influential in rehabilitation nursing practice, whereas provisions of Corbin and Strauss' Chronic Illness Trajectory Framework (1992) are essential for aggregates with comorbid and chronic disabling conditions. Chapter 2 contains details on nursing theories essential to rehabilitation and their relationships with functional models of practice.

Neuman's Systems Model (1989), with levels of prevention and intervention, and Leininger's Transcultural Model (1988) address diversity in the population and the shift of services to community settings. Both Corbin and Strauss' (1992) and Neuman's models propose using the natural history of a condition and the situation of the person for making decisions about the appropriate type and level of interventions. Building on the classic work of Leavell and Clark (1965), integrating principles of epidemiology with levels of prevention for chronic, disabling conditions, prevention is shown to be as important in tertiary levels of intervention as in primary or secondary levels. Primary prevention is not the same as primary care, although the two share certain interventions. Table 1-1 shows levels of prevention across the levels of intervention and the benefits of early interventions.

Because health promotion and prevention are logical and essential components of care (Rusk & Taylor, 1965), it is necessary to place them firmly in rehabilitation nursing role functions. Leavell and Clark (1965) suggested that communities organize to meet needs of their members, a philosophy shared by rehabilitation center developers in the midtwentieth century and in need of revival today. The goals and objectives of *Healthy People 2010* (U.S. Department of Health and Human Services [USDHHS], 2000) include reducing disparities in access to health care and enabling persons to live healthy and functioning, as well as longer, lives. Clearly these goals target aggregates whose health outcomes are determined in the rehabilitation domain.

Rehabilitation nurses cannot rely on specific care plans standardized to medical diagnoses if they intend to practice at a level that will enable clients to achieve optimal outcomes. Individualized assessment and interventions are essential for the many with multiple conditions that are not only chronic and disabling but also increasingly complex, comorbid, or secondary stages of diseases. Lubkin (1995) identified the complexity built into the concept of chronicity and disability. A single client may have many chronic conditions, such as arthritis, progressive neuromuscular condi-

TABLE 1-1 Levels of Prevention as Interventions over the Natural Course of a Chronic Disease or Disability

Level of Prevention	Types of Interventions	Applications
Primary	Interventions: health promotion, education, and specific protections	Conducted before a condition or problem is clinically evident or at any stage to improve the situation and prevent further disability or complications
Secondary	Interventions for early diagnosis and treatment and to limit disability and impairments or control the disease processes	Screening or surveys, curative actions or treatments, halting of the disease process, and prevention of spread or complications after the disease has shown early signs or advanced
Tertiary	Interventions for restoration and rehabilitation toward optimal independence and function with quality of life, convalescence from acute or injury problems, and adaptation to impairments	Community, education, or vocation planning; self-care and ADL education; minimizing disability; primary prevention for whole persons, not a focus on disease or disablement

Adapted from Leavell, H.R., & Clark, E.G. (Eds.). (1965). *Preventive medicine for the doctor in his community* (3rd ed.). New York: McGraw-Hill.

TABLE 1-2 Historical Development of Ideas about Disability and Wellness

Theorist	Concepts	Overview
Goffman (1963)	Stigma, spoiled identity, passing for normal	Differences from the social norm become attached to the person as negative traits. Assimilating the stigma, the person reinforces the deviant negative image in personal "spoiled identity." Stigmatized persons learn to manipulate within the limited social acceptance; at best the difference is not readily visible, and they can "pass for normal" by hiding the disability.
Dembo (1969); Dembo, Leviton, & Wright (1975)	Spread theory, stigma; person devalued by attributes or status	A strong social perception of a person is assigned as if it were a characteristic of that person. The characteristic is then "spread" to represent the total perception of the person and even governs responses to the person. Even subtle perceptions of altered body state may be spread to ascribe (usually negative) traits to the person's attributes.
Wright (1983)	Social consciousness-raising about stigma, spread theory, labeling, and beyond; key concepts for enabling persons with disabilities to cope and hope in society and their own lives	Brought to attention concepts essential to understanding disability, instead of only focusing on medical diagnosis. Client rights advocated. Raised questions about underlying motives when using comparative standards based on culturally defined norms. Urged providers to examine their own concerns about personal health and status when working with persons who have chronic, disabling disorders. Extensive attention to helping children.
Safilios-Rothschild (1970)	Personal, social, and cultural levels of disability and rehabilitation; integrated spread, stigma, and perceptions of disability concepts	Created understanding about relationships between self-concept and body image that uphold several nursing diagnoses. A person's self-concept and response to a disability depend on values and emotions attached to the disability and, in turn, on the degree to which a disability affects a person's identity-influenced perception of body image. This response is reinforced by relationships with others in society, especially the able bodied. Social and cultural definitions and determinants of disability form an integral part of the person's self-concept and perception of self-value while assigning a social value. The levels are especially useful when a client enters the community after disability and social value is needed.
Maslow (1968)	Motivation, self-attainment of higher levels governed by Erikson's stage epigenesis (1968)	Hierarchy of human needs pyramid for client priorities and motivation. A person is motivated to prioritize and direct behavior toward meeting each successive layer of needs. Meeting needs reduces tension only until the next layer of need emerges; internal and external needs of all lower levels must be met before purposeful work occurs on higher levels.
Dunn (1959)	High-level wellness	An individual's maximum potential and holistic balance are integrated into a definition of health.
Eberst (1984)	Individuals have a wellness potential governed by genetic, social, and environmental factors—an ecological model; stress reduction is based on balance and synergy	Attention to balance within the whole is more productive for health than a focus on any one dimension. Wellness is a relative quality rather than a linear or polar medical model. There are many paths to health, but clients must be involved and take responsibilities. The model is depicted in a Rubik's Cube–like figure that supports the multidimensional and dynamic features of 6 interactive health dimensions: mental, physical, emotional, social, spiritual, and vocational.
Becker (1974)	Health belief model	Used extensively in rehabilitation and community nursing for program planning and client education. Although not rigorously tested, the model persists in the literature, as discussed in Chapter 11.
Bandura (1969)	Social learning	Many constructs of this theory underlie rehabilitation nursing interventions for clients with specific impairments, as discussed in Chapters 11 and 12.
Selye (1978), Lazarus (1999), Engel (1968), Lazarus & Folkman (1984)	Stress, coping, emotion, loss of control, helplessness	Observable steps in the "giving up–given up" complex are as follows: affect of giving up to helplessness or hopelessness; depreciated self-image; loss of gratification from life roles or relationships; sense of discontinuity among past, present, and future; and reactivation of memories of earlier periods of giving up. See Chapter 12 for details.
Lewin (1947); Lippitt, Watson, & Westley (1958)	Change theories; planned change, change agent role introduced	Change theory concepts appear in many theoretical models. The rehabilitation nurse change agent is an advocate who listens and learns about a client's values, lifestyle, goals, and preferences, ensuring that the person is fully informed and included in decision making whenever possible. Other actions are to identify barriers early on and to work with clients to reduce or overcome them and advocating for system changes.
Thomas (1966)	Disability, role theory	Building on Parsons' "sick role" for illness (1951), Thomas identifies 5 roles participated in by persons with disabilities. Although sequential, the occurrence, pattern, and steps vary with individuals.

tions, sensory impairments, or cardiopulmonary disease; consider the pitfalls of relying on medical diagnosis alone for that client.

Other assessments are important when disability and health status are defined within the perceptions of a particular culture (Chapter 13) or for clients who have developmental disabilities or unique and difficult problems that persist despite their not having a medical diagnostic label. However, rehabilitation nurses can manage these situations when using functional health systems assessment and interventions.

To date, no one unified model or combination of theories is adequate or sufficiently elegant to serve as the sole paradigm for practice of rehabilitation nursing; a repertoire to draw on may be necessary. Core theories, models, and concepts from a variety of disciplines contribute to a dynamic scientific knowledge base that can broaden the scope of rehabilitation nursing and benefit clients. Combining models with different ways of organizing and thinking is necessary to resolve the variety of problems and select efficacious treatment options. Conceptual frameworks from a variety of disciplines contributed over time to rehabilitation nursing's "ways of knowing" and are included in Table 1-2 to preserve the historical development of ideas. Contributors to chapters in this book present additional theories and discuss concepts related to the specific content of their chapters.

Box 1-1 Nursing Guidelines in the Late Nineteenth Century

Regarding Paralysis

"Paralysis is a symptom of other diseases that can occur gradually or suddenly. Generally, a first and partial attack is successfully treated. Friction, healthful living, digestible food, and electricity are common ways of domestic treatment. A physician is responsible for treating the cause. When long continued, great care must be taken that bedsores do not develop" (p. 96).

Regarding Bedsores

"When any part of the body is compressed for a long time, it loses its vitality; this would be the case even in health, but when a person is debilitated by disease, is paralyzed or wounded, and is obliged to remain in one position, the skin covering the points of the body that are pressed upon becomes congested and inflamed, and sometimes excoriated without any pain being felt so far by the patient, the lowered vitality of the part having to a certain extent deprived it of feeling" (p. 141). "The nurse intervened by daily examining the client for herself all the parts upon which pressure comes: the hip, the seat, the shoulders, elbows, heels, and so forth. It is not so much the severity, but the continuance that concerns. The client is to be kept clean and dry, placed on a waterbed, and bathed 3-4 times daily with spirits of wine or 2 grains of bi-chloride of mercury dissolved in wine" (p. 141).

Adapted from *A Handbook of Nursing*. (1879). New Haven, CT: U.S. Surgeon General's Office under direction of the Connecticut Training School for Nurses, State Hospital, New Haven.

REHABILITATION NURSING IN A SOCIOCULTURAL AND POLITICAL CONTEXT

Rehabilitation nurses cannot realize issues concerning what they know and how they think or about why they do things in certain ways without understanding the history and development of their profession within political and social contexts. Early nursing textbooks and guides hold clues about the origins of many practices. Although some interventions are best retired, nurses continue to battle many situations born over a century past. Consider the discussions on paralysis and bedsores in Box 1-1. Apart from Nightingale's work, this is one of the earliest descriptions of procedures for nurses, as well as for family members.

It is tempting to applaud achievements and progress in health care today without realizing that development began long ago. How we see ourselves as healers has developed and will continue in the context of our society and beliefs. The following section traces the sociocultural and political development of rehabilitation. Although not an exhaustive record, significant events in context contribute toward understanding how and why things are as they are and encourage thinking about consequences of actions. One cannot examine rehabilitation nursing apart from the entirety of rehabilitation. Likewise, a nation's health cannot be examined apart from the sociocultural and political context or other systems of a society and the world (Thomas, 1985; Starr, 1982).

Tired, Poor, and Civil War Torn (1750 to 1865)

Before the mid-1800s, most care of the sick or injured was performed by lay workers or untrained women at home or in religious settings. Being able to perform useful work was seen as part of recovery. It was 1752 before Benjamin Franklin and other Quakers began a hospital in Philadelphia and 1845 when Dorothea Dix reformed the custodial institutions for the mentally ill (Morrissey, 1951). During the Civil War, Clara Barton found the Union Army to be without support services or supply lines for distribution of basic goods and medical items in the field. Many wounded, loaded on trains without water, blankets, or hygiene, died needlessly; few trained nurses were available (Oates, 1994). However, in London, Nightingale began St. Thomas Hospital School for Nurses, and in Switzerland Dunant founded the International Red Cross in 1862, 15 years before the American Red Cross. Meanwhile, 30 million immigrants passed through Ellis Island between 1820 and 1910. Functional abilities and health status determined an immigrant's ability to work and enter the United States.

Social Consciousness and Reconstruction (1865 to 1914)

After the Civil War and emancipation, reconstruction was difficult; however, a new social consciousness led influential women to sponsor charitable organizations. The federal government created a market economy for "limb makers" by providing $15,000 toward artificial limbs for disabled soldiers and sailors who needed to work (Davis, 1973). In 1873 three schools of nursing in the United States used Nightingale's model: Massachusetts General Nurses' Training School in Boston, Bellevue Training School in New York City (Morrissey, 1951), and the Connecticut Training School in New Haven origins of the first nursing textbook in 1879. A decade later, in 1883, nursing curricula featured therapy with water, electricity, massage, as well as study of anatomy and physiology with other nursing topics (Young, 1989).

In 1892, the same year that sanitarium care emerged, Clara Weeks wrote a nursing manual that promoted massage and other muscle treatments. The American Orthopedic Association formed in 1887, and Ranch Los Amigos originated as a county poor farm. By 1893 community nurses worked with great autonomy in the New York settlement houses that preceded the Visiting Nurse Service (Morrissey, 1951). Identifying and classifying children who needed care and control of "contagious" diseases were priorities. Diarrhea was the most frequent cause of infant death; sanitation and living conditions were poor. In Europe, Nightingale penned the Pledge.

The turn of the century found immigrants again flooding the United States (Grun, 1975). Nurses provided community care, such as at the Children's Aid Society of New York City School for Crippled Children, with a focus on orthopedic and brace care (Young, 1989). Residential or specialized children's hospitals were established. The Children's Country Home in Westfield, New Jersey (Children's Specialized Hospital), and Blythesdale Children's Hospital in Valhalla, New York, are two of a group that remain operational. In 1900 the *American Journal of Nursing* began publication, targeting community nursing that encompassed physical and occupational therapy treatments. However, rehabilitation of a person with paraplegia was not part of medical or nursing expertise in 1904 (Morrissey, 1951). After the first great polio epidemic erupted in 1909, nurses began care for persons who had nervous system diseases at the New York Neurological Institute.

Women became social activists who protested harsh, hazardous labor conditions for children. Mary Wadley trained at Bellevue Training School for Nurses in 1907 and then began medical social service as a convalescent relief service. Bertha Wright and Mabel Weed led a women's social reform movement establishing the Baby Hospital in Oakland, California. Although male paternalism challenged their leadership, their work led to the Federal Children's Bureau (later part of the U.S. Public Health Service [USPHS]), where preventive health was a priority, and eventually to the Shepherd-Towner Act, which provided maternal and child health services (Nichols & Hammer, 1998). Efforts of the social reformers contributed to the basic Workmen's Compensation Laws drafted in 1911 in response to increased injuries to workers from occupational causes (Cioschi, 1993).

World War I and Professional Identities (1914 to 1929)

In 1914 events of World War I changed the world and created attention to rehabilitation. In nursing the National League for Nursing Education provided the first standard curriculum for schools of nursing in 1915. Nurses were in the forefront of public health services during the influenza pandemic of 1918 to 1920; 20 million persons died.

Patterned after the Belgian-French Ecole Joffre and funded by the Millbank family, the Red Cross Institute for Crippled and Disabled Men opened in New York City in 1917, to train disabled men for vocations (Gritzer & Arluke, 1985). The director, Douglas McMurtrie, coined the term *rehabilitation,* which replaced *physical reconstruction of the disabled,* and it was adopted by army hospitals. The 1918 Senate bill for vocational rehabilitation of servicemen legitimized it.

Large charitable foundations (Rockefeller, Carnegie, etc.) emerged along with private and religious organizations; sheltered workshops included Goodwill, the Rehabilitation Center for the Disabled, and Jewish Vocational Services. Local chapters, such as the National Society for Crippled Children and Adults, promoted rehabilitation centers in cities across the country in the 1920s (Morrissey, 1951).

When the Flexner Report publicized the poor state of medical education in 1910, medical education moved to universities (Braddom, 1988). However, professional roles and control of programs were issues within rehabilitation. During the war, physicians who practiced therapy methods (called *physical therapy physicians*) and physical therapy technicians (some were nurses) worked closely; at the war's end, the situation changed. In 1918, the American Medical Association lobbied the Surgeon General effectively for control of both medical and functional restoration through their leadership in the USPHS. With this movement, physical therapists were supervised by physicians for diagnosis and treatment, while retaining authority over their modalities. The physical therapy physicians struggled within their own profession, joining physical therapists in 1921 to form the American College of Physical Therapy (changed to the American *Congress* of Physical Therapy in 1930). This was a contentious but mutually beneficial association. Initially tied with the radiology groups, the physical therapists formed their own organization, the American Physical Therapy Association, in 1929, three years after physical therapy schools began at Northwestern University Medical School in Chicago (Young, 1989).

The USPHS gained control over programs to assist the 123,000 disabled veterans and established the first spinal treatment centers in the United States, modeled after those in Europe; one of these centers was Massachusetts General Hospital. The USPHS then began to recruit nurses, especially those who served as physical therapy technicians during the war, to work in veterans affairs (VA) hospitals assisting physicians with hydrotherapy, massage, and exercises. Some, like Marie Lotze, a nurse at Kosair Crippled Children's Hospital in Louisville, Kentucky, for 50 years, assisted orthopedic physicians (Zinner, 1990). Initially these nurses sought to manage therapy departments. Not wanting to lower standards of nursing training to do so, they concentrated instead on acute care (Young, 1989); however, they abandoned their heritage in the community.

In 1920 the Civilian Rehabilitation Act addressed persons with industrially acquired disabilities, and the Vocational Rehabilitation Act of 1920 transferred vocational rehabilitation from the Surgeon General to a non-physician-led federal department fostering multiple amendments over the years. The Vocational Rehabilitation Board retained control over civilian rehabilitation, and physical therapists established interdependent relationships with physicians. At first, occupational therapists moved into mental institutions and tuberculosis sanitariums. They organized in 1923 and applied their skills in sensory and cognitive areas as complements to physical therapy and vocational rehabilitation.

The Depression and the New Deal (1929 to 1939)

In 1935 Social Security gave civilians access to rehabilitation services formerly reserved for the military and veterans. This new market created competition between physical therapy physicians and others. The physical therapy physicians wanted supervision of therapists and thus to control the fee-for-service benefits. Physicians wanted to head physical therapy departments in hospitals so they could gain referrals, especially from orthopedic physicians. Therapists struggled for years to define their role and functions (Gritzer & Arluke, 1985). Elizabethtown Hospital and Rehabilitation Center, built to serve civilians in 1930, later served children in rehabilitation and remains in the Pennsylvania State University Hospital system.

The United States concentrated on domestic issues with President F. D. Roosevelt's New Deal prospects for social reform to combat the Depression. For the first time the federal government considered the health and education needs of children as a national interest. Nurses conducted early detection and treatment for children with potential or handicapping conditions and led health promotion, education, and prevention programs in schools, precursors of fitness programs.

Physical therapy, radiology, and physician organizations then changed names. The American College of Physical Therapy changed its name to the American *Congress* of Physical Therapy until 1945, when they reorganized as the American Congress of Rehabilitation Medicine (ACRM) (Cole, 1993). Physical therapy schools were approved in 1934 and in 1936. The American Medical Association endorsed the medical specialty of physical therapy physicians, establishing the American Academy of Physical Medicine and Rehabilitation (AAPM&R) in 1938. Their publication evolved to the *Archives of Physical Medicine and Rehabilitation.*

World War II Years (1939 to 1945)

World War II created a boon for rehabilitation. War manpower needs called attention to the health and fitness of the population. Despite the view of the United States as a young, healthy, and strong nation, 40% of those called for military service were rejected, or classified as 4F, because they could not meet the standard physical requirements for military service. Once enlisted, the most common reason for discharge from service was for neuropsychiatric problems (Kessler, 1970). The question of disability versus capability became more complex and critical to the national interest. The military demanded quantifiable explanations about what each person was able to do under what circumstances; whether a disability was permanent, continuous, or temporary; and so forth. Several repercussions of this trend were an awareness of a need to classify impairments and name the particular situation, information that later would be applied to vocational evaluations.

Dr. Henry Kessler's (1968) descriptions of his experiences in the field operating theater during World War II are illuminating in their rendering of the human destruction of war. He questions how as an orthopedic physician dedicated to rehabilitation he can be laboring to sever limbs from young soldiers, albeit to save their lives. But save their lives for what kind of life, he struggles to understand. At what point is an individual to be declared "unhealthy or unfit" and for what activities? How can negative labels be avoided, prejudicial social attitudes be contained, emotional factors associated with disability be managed, and the person reach peace in the situation and achieve productivity?

War injuries were the impetus for the VA hospitals and assistance programs. As young men experienced the realities and destruction of war and returned home with reduced functional abilities, they demanded to be accommodated into society. During the war, the rehabilitation model had combined care and cure. Survival improved because of antibiotics, better trauma care, and other advances that contributed to a revival of physical therapy modalities and rehabilitation nursing care on several fronts.

The Veterans Bureau and VA hospitals (headed by General Omar Bradley) solidified control over military rehabilitation via the Army Physical Medicine Consultants Division. Initially overwhelmed with the numbers of patients, the VA began programs of education, research, and clinical advances that established the influence of rehabilitation medicine in federal regulation and funding opportunities (Gritzer & Arluke, 1985).

Dr. Frank Krusen, in 1938, continued to promote the idea of the Society of Physical Therapy Physicians, in opposition to Dr. Howard Rusk, who wanted therapy within rehabilitation teams in the Army Air Corps Medical Corps (Cioschi, 1993). Rusk and Taylor (1965) presented the notion of "rehabilitation as the third or last phase of health care" to appease medical and surgical colleagues so they would include rehabilitation in the overall plan of care. This phrase was to haunt the specialty for years. When the value of early mobility prevailed over the prescription of bed rest for recuperation, rehabilitation gained another foothold in medical science, although therapy methods still were considered unconventional.

Private philanthropy funded the Baruch Committee to study the utility of physical modalities, to identify the medical education programs to best foster the specialty, and to contribute to disabled veterans. The committee recommended advancing the profession through teaching and research centers in cooperating universities, along with fellowship and residency programs (Cole, 1993). With Donald Covalt and George Deaver, Rusk joined the medical faculty at New York University Bellevue Hospital in 1945 and created the Department of Rehabilitation Medicine, precursor to the Rusk Institute.

The Vocational Rehabilitation Act of 1943 included vocational evaluation in rehabilitation services (Cioschi, 1993), and the Social Security Act amendments provided vocational rehabilitation and maintenance funds for persons with emotional problems or mental retardation. The Rusk Institute provided treatment for civilians, and parents became involved, promoting study of "mental deficiency," brain diseases, and retardation in children. Stroke, spinal cord injuries, back pain, spastic problems, and sequelae to traumatic injuries created another rehabilitation market. The Stoke Mandeville Center for Spinal Cord Injury Research in England used a team approach and included vocational rehabilitation and community integration programs; these were replicated in the United States by 1944.

Meanwhile, polio struck again, killing 1200 persons and leaving many with residual problems. The National Foundation for Infantile Paralysis (March of Dimes) formed in 1943. Centers, such as the Alfred I. duPont Institute for Pediatric Rehabilitation in Wilmington, Delaware, Rancho Los Amigos in California, and the Sister Kenny Rehabilitation Institute in Minneapolis, provided care (Figure 1-2). Before Sister (nurse) Kenny left Australia, she argued with physicians there over her methods for treating polio. She taught that muscle pain produced acute muscle spasms and that her special hot packs would relieve pain sufficiently for the person to perform range of motion exercises. Thus strength and mobility would be improved or retained, and paralysis, contractures, deformity, function, and pain would be prevented. Demonstrations of her techniques performed at the Mayo Clinic in Rochester, Minnesota, convinced many and led to the KRI and hallmark programs in rehabilitation nursing. Polio continued its devastation until the mid-1950s.

Wars, disasters, medical advances, social movements, and technology all influence ways of thinking in any era, and leaders emerge to stimulate change. For rehabilitation, events of the war years framed changes just as social consciousness movements at the turn of the nineteenth century mirrored nursing actions. Recall that Nightingale's work resulted from her experiences in the Crimean War and Wald's Settlement House was a response to the slum conditions in New York City (Backer, 1993). Mary Switzer has been heralded as the champion of government-funded programs of research and training in rehabilitation. During her decades as Director of the Federal Office of Vocational Rehabilitation (1950 to 1970), she began to include persons with disabilities in all levels of planning and laid the groundwork for the Independent Living Movement (Affeldt, 1988).

A need to address the social construction of disability was dawning. Although overall treatment of persons with disabilities was less harsh in the United States than in many places in the world, the language describing disability remained negative and derisive. When researchers traced legislation dealing with children who had special needs from 1903 to 1990, they found the language used to refer to the children changed with the changes in the social construction, which in turn was evident in legislative changes. No longer are words like *imbecile* or *cripple* used, nor are children classified as *trainable, educable,* or *minimally brain damaged* (Repetto & Hoeman, 1991).

In the next decades medical advances, antibiotics, and vaccines would prolong life, and soon everyone expected more from a longer life. With reduced mortality from infectious diseases or infection, there was increased opportunity to develop chronic diseases and experience disabling conditions. Automobile accidents and occupational hazards and accidents soon replaced armed conflict as major causes of disabilities. Questions arose about the role of rehabilitation. Can rehabilitation stand as a specialty that would be reimbursed for providing services to clients after stroke or for children with special needs? What are the limits of technology? Who will decide ethical and moral issues? Rehabilitation is at another crossroads (Hoeman, 1998).

Government Involvement (1946 to 1959)

The beginning of federal legislative involvement in rehabilitation was evident in 1946 with the Hill-Burton Act (Hospital Survey and Construction Act) and in 1954 with the Vocational Rehabilitation Act amendments of 1954 authorizing federal funds for research, training, and building of rehabilitation facilities. The National Mental Health Act and the Federal Security Agency (the Department of Health, Education, and Welfare in 1953) began also. The Office of Vocational Rehabilitation supported development of the rehabilitation centers that were staffed by physicians trained in physical medicine and rehabilitation under the 1958 Voca-

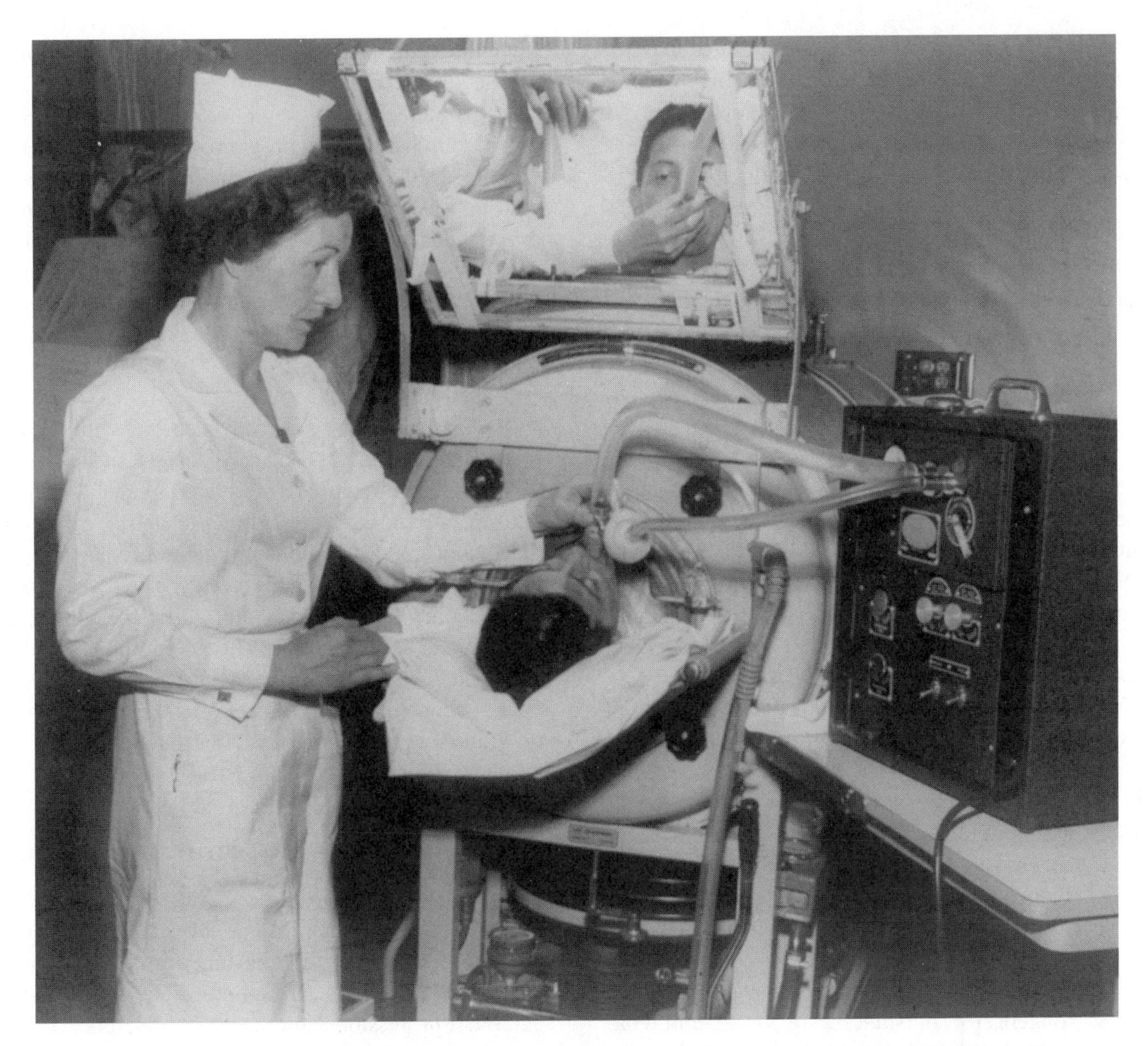

Figure 1-2 Until the mirror was added, a person in an iron lung could not see beyond its rim. When a film crew wanted to show the face of a young man in the ventilator, they realized this environmental barrier. The film crew supplied all those in the polio ward with mirrors. (Reproduced with permission of Rancho Los Amigos National Rehabilitation Center, Downey, CA.)

tional Rehabilitation Act. The 1950s found federal involvement in programs as diverse health, transportation, and communications for the stated purpose of building and protecting the nation's defense.

Another polio epidemic during 1952 brought 21,269 cases of acute polio (Martin, 1988). For every hospital admission, another 100 persons were admitted with subclinical polio. For persons with high levels of spinal or bulbar polio, the mortality rate was nearly 40%; many were children (McCourt & Novak, 1994). The National Foundation for Infantile Paralysis conducted the national March of Dimes campaign. Citizens, school children, and groups contributed dimes toward finding a cure, depositing their dimes into cardboard replicas of iron lungs that sat on the countertop of every pharmacy, grocery, and business place. Children in mechanical ventilators were displayed on the new medium of television, and everyone was afraid.

Research paid results in 1954, when Jonas Salk began administering his polio serum, and Enders and Weiler won the Nobel Prize for study of the poliomyelitis virus. By 1955 use of polio vaccine was widespread, so in 1961, 988 cases were reported; by 1967, fewer than 100 cases per year were reported, and between 1979 and 1983, only 12 cases per year were reported (Martin, 1988). The March of Dimes continued to support treatment and rehabilitation and educate health professionals. Attention to infectious disease control, including eradication of polio and smallpox, and to clean water and nutrition for children became global concerns.

Liberty Mutual Insurance Company hired the first rehabilitation insurance nurse, Harriet Lane, who worked at the company rehabilitation center in Boston. Alice Morrissey was nursing supervisor at Rusk Institute and Bellevue Medical Center and author of the first textbook on rehabilitation nursing in 1951. She identified nurses who performed the dual roles of provider and coordinator of care for persons with chronic or disabling conditions as rehabilitation nurses. Use of the term *activities of daily living* (ADLs), referring to self-care, ambulation, and hand activities, began at Rusk Institute (Young, 1989). Lena Plaisted, a nurse trained in physical therapy, directed the first graduate program in rehabilitation nursing at Boston University in 1956. She published *The Clinical Specialist in Rehabilitation* in 1969 (Cioschi, 1993).

Innovators such as Karl and Berta Bobath (who in 1958 founded the neurodevelopmental approach for treatment of persons with cerebral palsy or stroke) conflicted with physicians. Their experience was difficult, like that of Sister Kenny and others who had differences with the medical establishment model or suggested a team leader other than a physician.

Tears, Taxes, and the Moon (1960 to 1970)

Social concerns about the environment and quality of goods were fueled by events such as birth defects after use of thalidomide during pregnancy. Food additives were scrutinized; DDT was banned; and the federal government strengthened warranties on goods and services, began licensing and reviews, wrote more regulations, and began quality control through agencies.

Rehabilitation fared well in this turbulent decade. Harriet Lane, grounded in her work with rehabilitation clients from the insurance industry, developed specialized content for geriatric rehabilitation in the early 1960s and joined the rehabilitation nursing graduate program at Boston University (Cioschi, 1993). Barbara Madden (who established regional respiratory centers for the National Foundation for Infantile Paralysis) became director of nursing at Rancho Los Amigos Medical Center and began the first nursing graduate study residency program for rehabilitation specialization in 1965 (Fliedner & Rodgers, 1990). Nurses were so active in rehabilitation services that the ANA published "Guidelines for Practice of Nursing on the Rehabilitation Team: An Answer to a Growing Need."

The first regional rehabilitation research and training centers opened at the New York University Medical Center and at the Sister Kenny Institute in Minneapolis (affiliated with the University of Minnesota Medical School). The American Rehabilitation Foundation was established, and Krusen edited the first of many editions of the *Physical Medicine and Rehabilitation Handbook.*

The government accepted more responsibility for citizen's health as Congress passed medicare and medicaid legislation, the Workmen's Compensation and Rehabilitation Law, and Public Law (PL) 89-333, the Vocational Rehabilitation Act amendments of 1965. Within government, the Social and Rehabilitation Service (SRS) became a federal administrative department headed by experienced Mary Switzer. The Commission on Accreditation of Rehabilitation Facilities (CARF) formed in 1967 (Johnson, 1988).

Social change was visible with passage of PL 90-391, the Vocational Rehabilitation Act amendments of 1968. Deprivation of environmental, social, or cultural factors was considered handicapping and gave eligibility for services. National activities, such as the President's Committee on Employment of the Handicapped, attended to rehabilitation (Figure 1-3). Mental retardation and handicaps became civil rights issues, and the Independent Living Movement was launched.

Legislation, injury, and morbidity statistics created growth of rehabilitation programs and disciplines. Polio was no longer a threat, but injury and trauma from occupational and industrial accidents, automobile accidents, and leisure or sports accidents increased. Not only were incidences of head injury, spinal cord injury, and multiple traumas occurring in the general population, but with infectious disease control and medical advances, individuals began living longer and experienced problems related to conditions such as arthritis and stroke.

Rehabilitation nurses became central to holistic and comprehensive care across levels of care, especially to clients who survived infectious disease and trauma, once fatal conditions, only to develop chronic, disabling conditions. And they advocated for persons to attain optimal levels of function and independence with dignity. They taught ADLs, assessed home environments and workplaces, and prescribed wheelchairs and all types of home equipment and technology. They educated families and caregivers along with clients about managing their daily care and about special programs or procedures, and they made referrals to appropriate services or care (Hoeman, 1998).

Accountability and Community-Based Rehabilitation (1970 to 1980)

Demands for accountability affected businesses and corporations, products for the consumer, and government agencies; health care was not immune. The rehabilitation team and other professionals noticed that adherence to new criteria, computer data recording, and government reporting allowed less time for direct care and productivity. Dr. Carl Granger called on the AAPM&R to conduct outcome-based research. Private programs were developed to satisfy budding insurance programs and led to special interest groups in the AAPM&R (Granger, 1988).

Rehabilitation nursing established the ARN in 1974, led by Dagny Engle and the Rehabilitation Nursing Institute (RNI) in 1976. Specialized rehabilitation nursing courses were offered in major cities. Mary Ann Mikulic, a nurse with specialized rehabilitation experience in the VA hospitals, edited the *ARN Journal.* An ARN scholarship bears her name today (Cioschi, 1993). The second edition of Ruth Stryker's (1977) rehabilitation nursing text was published.

Issues and programs related to children with mental retardation had been assigned to various government bureaus, moving eventually to the Division of Maternal Child Health under Title V of the Social Security Act amendments. In 1962 President Kennedy created the National Institute of Child Health and Human Development and the President's Committee on Mental Retardation. This launched the University-Affiliated Facilities (UAFs), and in 1967 the Mental Retardation amendments (PL 91-170) extended UAF programs to research, training, physical education, and recreation. Beginning in 1970, the Developmental Disabili-

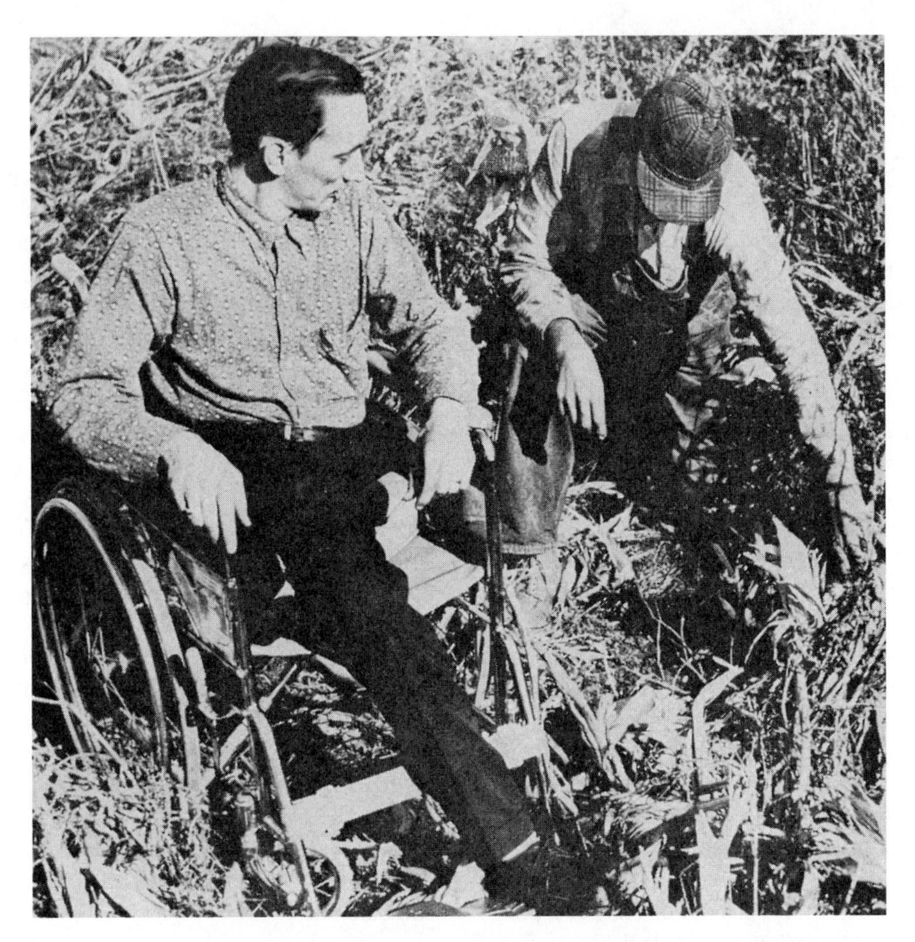

Figure 1-3 A federal crop insurance agent (Ronald C. Cutting) worked his wheelchair into cornfields as part of the President's Committee on Employment of the Handicapped in 1964. (From the President's Committee on Employment of the Handicapped [1964]. *Performance: The story of the handicapped* [Vol. XIV, No. 8, February] Washington, DC: U.S. Government Printing Office.)

ties Services and Construction Act defined mental, developmental, congenital, and related conditions.

The Developmental Disability Assistance and Bill of Rights (PL 94-103) provided persons with developmental disabilities the right to treatment, services, and habilitation according to each state plan. Earlier, developmental disabilities legislation included mental retardation, cerebral palsy, and epilepsy and related problems; now autism was included. All were defined functionally and categorically. The idea of writing individualized care plans and goals bolstered accountability and advocacy (Eberly, Eklund, & Simon, 1986).

The rehabilitation team discovered roles in the community when PL 94-142, the Education for All Handicapped Children Act, passed in 1975. Not only were all children to receive appropriate free education, regardless of disability, but they were to receive it in the least restrictive environment and with medically necessary services in both school and preschool settings; the concept of mainstreaming originated.

In 1972 disabled persons were incorporated into medicare coverage, and the federal government issued a host of specific guidelines for conducting inpatient rehabilitation services suitable for medicare reimbursement. Initial regulatory concerns were quality control; issues of fraudulent billing and proper services arose later. The Rehabilitation Act of 1973 provided protection against discrimination in the workplace and addressed barriers in the community. Persons severely injured and those with multiple or complex disabilities needed expert team care; the Model Systems for spinal cord injury and head trauma grew from this legislation. Team roles in the community were bolstered by medicare amendments authorizing care in Comprehensive Outpatient Rehabilitation Facilities (CORFS) (Ditunno, 1988). The Rehabilitation Act amendments of 1978 (PL 95-602) created the National Institute of Handicapped Research, provided comprehensive services for independent living, and promoted research (Verville, 1988).

New methods and approaches to managing and understanding disability and chronic conditions were introduced in the mid-to-late 1970s. Dr. John Basmajian (who wrote the foreword to this third edition) was a pioneer in rehabilitation research and education. Biofeedback interventions for paralysis, "psychosocial considerations in spinal cord injury, medical record keeping and team care, neuromuscular physiology, transcutaneous electrical nerve stimulation (TENS), and traditional clinical examination expertise" were significant advances (Granger, 1988, p. 31.)

Identity and Choices (1980 to 1990)

By 1981 the ARN offered a core curriculum in rehabilitation nursing and a second edition in 1987 (Mumma). In 1984 the ARN conducted the first national certification examination in rehabilitation nursing, followed by publication of *Rehabilitation Nursing Standards and Scope of Practice.* Rehabilitation nurses were most active in either insurance nursing or in rehabilitation facilities. By the mid-1980s rehabilitation nurse entrepreneurs founded consulting companies for assessment, case management, legal expertise, and related contracts. Martin, Holt, and Hicks (1981) published *Comprehensive Rehabilitation Nursing.* Eight years passed before Dittmar (1989) edited *Rehabilitation Nursing*; Hoeman (1996) edited the second edition.

Community-based agencies, including visiting nurse associations (VNAs), sought to capitalize on rehabilitation and restorative nursing. Physical therapists and speech-language pathologists flourished under medicare reimbursement, including contractual agreements with VNAs. Occupational therapists held contracts but did not gain independent reimbursement function from medicare until the mid-1980s, when the Health Care Finance Administration (HCFA) studied cost controls.

The International Year of Disabled Persons was proclaimed in 1981. Between 1980 and 1983, legislation such as PL 96-374 and PL 98-199, the Carl D. Perkins Vocational and Technical Education Act, and PL 98-524 ensured funding and other access to vocational educational services for persons with a wide range of disabilities and for those considered disadvantaged. Rehabilitation resources were tested by the needs of an aging population with increased prevalence of chronic, disabling conditions, aggregates of survivors, entitlements for children with disabilities, and poorly developed injury and disease prevention programs. The Hastings Institute examined the ethics of medical rehabilitation; their publications stirred public debate and challenged the moral beliefs of health professionals and the society.

The Rehabilitation Act amendments of 1986 (PL 99-506), the Technology-Related Assistance for Individuals with Disabilities Act of 1988 (related provisions were included in the 1975 Education for All Handicapped Children Act), and a later amendment in 1992 (PL 102-569) all provided assistive technology in some fashion. The Catastrophic Health Bill for the Elderly, to prevent poverty from catastrophic illness or trauma, and PL 99-457 for children at risk were enacted. Prevention of disabilities gained attention in 1986, when the National Council on Disability recommended that the Centers for Disease Control and Prevention (CDC) develop a program that used the public health expertise and systems. The Disabilities Prevention Program was launched in 1988. Accessible, affordable, appropriate, and acceptable care available for persons with disabilities from sources that were accountable was (and is) needed.

The World Health Organization (WHO) issued a supplement to the *International Classification of Diseases,* titled the *International Classification of Impairments, Disabilities, and Handicaps* (ICIDH). (Earlier Nagi [1965] developed a functional limitation framework with unclassified ADL content.) Although the ICIDH was adopted in a number of European countries, debates about internal consistency, arguments about connotations of words, and conflict from other frameworks remain. Pope and Tarlov's (1991) model of disability and preventive measures builds on those of the WHO and Nagi. Disability frameworks are discussed in Chapter 8.

The National Center for Medical Rehabilitation Research (NCMRR) at the National Institutes of Health (NIH) was proposed in the U.S. Senate in 1988 (Title V of S.2222) (Verville, 1988). Dorothy Gordon, a rehabilitation nurse served on the panel and the ARN, provided testimony (Hoeman, 1989). Within the decade, the NCMRR would claim institute status and engage in collaborative activities with other institutes.

The years between 1970 and 1990 were active for legislation for persons with disabilities and polarized relationships between rehabilitation and the federal government. Many in rehabilitation wanted decentralized federal services and proposed expanding both private and public sectors. Gains were recognition of unmet needs for rehabilitation in the community, increased international collaboration and service, and the beginning of funded research precisely for rehabilitation and outcomes.

Life Satisfaction, Holism, and Opening Research Options (1990 to 2000)

The last decade before a new century brought visibility to disability in the United States. Grassroots social actions and community planning began in the late 1950s and sprouted in 1990. The Americans with Disabilities Act (ADA) solidified social responses to needs of persons with disabilities. Not only were new populations of persons with chronic, disabling, or developmental disorders surviving, but they were entering the community in daily life, as well as in vocational pursuits. However, nursing manpower was short, and the HCFA pressured medicare funds to reduce costs, services, and lengths of stay in institutions. In an effort to advance a role for the "rehabilitationist," in 1993 the ACRM separated (as in 1968 to 1969) from the physicians of the AAPM&R.

Exposed to the goals of *Healthy People 2000,* the public began to vaguely appreciate a national agenda for preventive actions, including preventing disabilities, but cure was the desired outcome. The public did not raise expectations to live longer, better, and with more functional abilities and with disparities reduced. Public interest in alternative treatments fostered the Office of Alternative Medicine (OAM) in 1992, and its research centers for holistic approaches were established in 1995. The WHO Collaborative Centers in Traditional Medicine Research began in 1996.

Awareness of the hazards, injuries, and social effects of environment and occupation and the impact of culture and community grew. The interplay of medical advances and technology with public expectations for life satisfaction and quality influenced policy and practice. The Rehabilitation Act amendment of 1992 (PL 102-569) extended rehabilitation to those who were most severely disabled. Clients gained rights to participate in planning and for interdisciplinary team involvement, and persons from minority aggregates were given priority funding. The Family Leave Act of 1993 marked recognition of the challenges of caregiver and family roles.

Some rehabilitation professionals were concerned about quality and found ways to negotiate and participate with governmental agencies in matters of policy, research involvement, and funding. Others identified private resources as means to proceed without federal funding or to exercise research options apart from priorities set by the government.

The ARN published two journals, *Rehabilitation Nursing* and *Rehabilitation Nursing Research;* a third core curriculum (McCourt, 1993); an advanced practice core curriculum (Johnson, 1997); several specialty publications; and then a fourth core curriculum (Edwards, 2000). The ARN celebrated its 25th anniversary in 1999.

INTERNATIONAL REHABILITATION

International models influenced rehabilitation programs and thinking in the United States for many years. Facilities and schools were organized in the European manner to admit and treat persons with disabilities based on their specific disabilities (schools for the deaf or blind) and to remove them from the public. The medical model, isolation from the mainstream, and judgments about personal worth superseded any concerns for the social environment and construction of disabilities or individual empowerment (Groce, 1992).

After World War I a number of international programs emerged, the Red Cross Institute for the Crippled and Disabled in 1917 (the International Center for the Disabled today) and the International Society of Crippled Children in 1922 (Rehabilitation International today). The National Rehabilitation Organization began in 1923 with a heavy emphasis on vocational rehabilitation. World War II slowed international rehabilitation activities for a time. After the war, international organizations with interests in rehabilitation and rehabilitation physicians Rusk, Kessler, and Basmajian (Basmajian, 1993) traveled to collaborate with colleagues worldwide. The United Nations formed the Council of World Organizations Interested in the Handicapped (the International Council on Disability today) in 1953 (Groce, 1992) in an attempt to stimulate governments to recognize the needs of disabled persons. Governments began to recognize some responsibility for poor and disabled citizens but usually reserved resources for "worthy" persons, especially those who had potential to be "productive."

Rehabilitation physicians were interested in sharing information and learning about the technology and equipment being developed in Europe and the then Soviet Socialist Union countries, where political differences had impeded sharing scientific progress. Differing social and cultural definitions of disability affected how persons with disabilities were treated, but interest in international training and collaboration grew in centers such as the Rusk Institute of Physical Medicine and Rehabilitation and the Kessler Rehabilitation Institute. These activities synchronized with the new medical specialty of physical medicine and rehabilitation in 1947. Soon international exchanges flourished with conferences attended by academic faculty and education or service programs sponsored by nongovernment and voluntary agencies.

Switzer (Federal Office of Vocational Rehabilitation) was in a position to carry progressive program and social ideas forward. She enabled international rehabilitation funding for more than 500 researchers conducting projects in 14 countries under the International Rehabilitation Research and Demonstration Program (PL 83-840 and PL 86-610). By 1978 the National Institute on Disability and Rehabilitation Research (NIDRR) funded two projects to foster international linkages of persons and professionals with expertise in rehabilitation or disability studies by participating in short-term fellowships for study abroad. The International Exchange of Experts and Information in Rehabilitation (IEEIR) administered by the World Rehabilitation Fund was based on the East Coast, and the International Disability Exchanges and Studies Project (IDEAS) administered by the World Disability Institute (WDI) was on the West Coast.

In 1978 the WHO boosted community-based rehabilitation and primary care as international priorities. In 1992 the WHO joined with the World Bank to sponsor a study to identify and quantify health problems as they exist and to make projections about the cause and extent of mortality and disability through 2020. This is an effort to direct public health policy based on evidence. It was recognized that data about health outcomes of disease and injury that resulted in chronic, morbid, or disabling situations were not measured or collected in many parts of the world. Without data, these health areas were not included in planning or objectives for improving health outcomes (*Lancet* Editor, 1997). However, the impact of chronicity, disability, and related morbidity on the social, economic, and overall fiber of a society was tremendous.

Thus the Global Burden of Disease (GBD) was developed as a way of measuring the severity, incidence, duration, and prevalence of 107 diseases and injury conditions with corrections for regional differences. A standard unit of measurement, the disability-adjusted life year (DALY) was used to compare risk factors that influenced the problems. Prevention, control, and injury management were taken into account in the reports along with the socioeconomic, cultural, educational, and technological factors in a society (Murray & Lopez, 1997a, 1997b).

A Swiss study using DALYs to examine the relative importance of specific diseases and injuries to the general health of the population in Geneva revealed the value of morbidity as well as mortality data. Depression, ischemic heart disease, osteoarthritis, and alcohol abuse would have been omitted from health planning (Schopper et al., 2000). Clearly, chronic, disabling conditions have come to attention as major factors in the future of any country or region and have earned rehabilitation programs a place in the work of global health.

International Opportunities for Rehabilitation Nurses

Although eligible, rehabilitation nurses did not participate in the NIDRR projects. However, rehabilitation nurses were part of an interdisciplinary team sponsored by Project Hope to bring pediatric rehabilitation and education programs to (then Soviet) Armenia after the massive earthquake there in December 1988 (Hertzberg & Hoeman, 1991). One rehabilitation nurse served as a Fulbright Senior Scholar in Greece and in Jordan (Hoeman, 1992, 1999a). Opportunities exist to participate in multiple conferences and lead or join international delegations or to serve with mission programs. International nursing conferences are offered through the International Council of Nurses (ICN) and other professional organizations and are excellent opportunities for rehabilitation nurses to participate on the global scene. Volunteer service organizations have opportunities for international service according to their mission statements, funding, and needs of specific countries.

TRENDS IN REHABILITATION

Opening the Mind and Improving Outcomes (2000 and Beyond)

As rehabilitation nurses form partnership with clients, community agencies, and other health professionals, their goals remain consistent. Prevention of chronic, disabling, or developmental disorders; prevention of further disability or complications; promotion of optimal levels of freedom and independent function; reinforcement of effective coping and adaptation; and forming of therapeutic relationships never go out of style for rehabilitation nurses. Ideally the future holds more community and client involvement, improved clarity on ethical dilemmas, more international collaboration, improved outcomes, and stronger role clarity.

Disability Prevalence

Data collection, analysis, and tracking systems for managing information about the incidence and prevalence of chronic, disabling conditions are well under way across the world. However, the trend will be to enlarge the scope and capabilities or ability to interface data systems in multiple directions. One system in the United States is an ongoing national household survey, the National Health Interview Survey (NHIS), used for collecting data about health conditions and impairments related to disability. The survey definition of disability is "a limitation in social or other activity that is caused by a chronic mental or physical disorder, injury, or impairment." Congenital, acquired, or secondary deficits of psychical structure or function, sensory impairments, loss of limb, or problems in orthopedic or neuromuscular function all are impairments in the NHIS definition and are coded in a classification developed by the National Center for Health Statistics, a branch of the CDC. Diseases and injuries are coded using the WHO *International Classification of Diseases.* Although some persons report more than one condition, the implications of the data are clear, it is an extensive problem (National Center for Health Statistics, 2000).

Estimates are that 1 in 8 to 10 persons worldwide has some limitation severe enough to prohibit activity. Thirty-eight million persons in the United States report 61 million disabling conditions encompassing 42 million chronic conditions, 16.3 million impairments, 2 million mental health disorders, and 1 million other injuries. Injuries cause 13.4% of all disabling conditions, highlighting the need for increased preventive actions in rehabilitation nursing interventions. The 10 most common conditions that cause U.S. citizens to have limitations in activity are conditions within the domain of rehabilitation nursing practice. Heart disease leads at 13% of all conditions, orthopedic and arthritis-like conditions when combined are nearly 25%, and sensory impairments represent more than 5% (LaPlante, 1996). (Note: the data analysis from the latest survey will be available at http://www.cdc.gov/nchs/nhis.htm). The 1994 to 1995 National Interview Survey on Disability is available at www.socio.com.

Building Rehabilitation Nursing Roles

Rehabilitation nurses recognize the impact of context and social and physical environment. Understanding concepts from role theory is central to professional rehabilitation nursing practice. Role expectations, clarity, and boundaries must be understood, but more importantly the rehabilitation nurse must be able to communicate these to others on the team and in the community. Decision making, conflict resolution, team building among professional colleagues, and collaboration among various organizational departments or community providers are essential skills.

Trust and rapport, establishing and maintaining the therapeutic relationship with clients and families, are foundational to practice. Certainly, many conflicts in roles arise when caring for persons with chronic or terminal conditions, especially as more practice is conducted in the home and community. According to Thorne (1993) three intense stages precede trustworthiness in relationships. Initially, "blind trust" occurs during the first encounter because the professional has more information and power. Over time "disenchantment" sets in, especially when there is disagreement between parties or if the professional either errs or fails in some way to meet the client's expectation. Clients may become disenchanted when a hoped-for cure is not possible. Eventually, a third stage may emerge when the client needs the health system but vacillated in opposition, never achieving internal trust. Because providers intend for clients and families to participate in mutual goal setting and planning as comanagers of care, trust may never be gained or may not be retained; however, they all need one another. As a result, a "guarded alliance" is formed for all parties to survive the long relationship, but trust is fragile.

A rehabilitation nurse's role as an advocate and agent of change is to equalize power and reduce disparities for clients and families. They build partnerships with clients, families, and communities. Thus enabled, clients can know, envision, and evaluate options; plan mutual strategies and solutions; and identify the behaviors or actions to achieve the outcomes.

Rehabilitation nurses have clarified their roles on the team, frequently coordinating teams in the community. Common roles are educator, researcher, consultant, case manager, advocate, enabler/facilitator, expert practitioner, and team member. Rehabilitation nurses may be certified for both rehabilitation nursing (CRRN) and advanced practice (CRRN-A) and practice in emerging roles. For example, chapters in this book specify roles with special populations who require cardiac, pulmonary, renal, HIV, cancer, or burn care and attend to pediatric, adult or geriatric age groups. With advanced practice (APRN), roles are added, including administrator, international consultant, expert witness or legal consultant, advanced researcher, and performer of advanced practice functions. They practice in a growing variety of programs, agencies, residences, and centers. Key role functions for rehabilitation nurses are advocating and preventing the incidence of chronic or disabling conditions, managing complex health situations, intervening throughout the life span, perfecting advanced skills to improve client outcomes, forging partnerships with clients and communities, and meeting global health challenges. Not only agents of change but also adaptable to change, rehabilitation nurses historically have solid experiences in setting new directions for practice.

Trends and Rehabilitation Nursing Practice

Despite progress, ignorance persists about the proper introduction and institution of rehabilitation practices for a client. In part, the confusion stems from lack of understanding about differences between levels of prevention and levels of intervention and their relationship with the natural history of a chronic disease or disabling condition. As understanding about interrelationships among body, mind, and spirit became evident and the person regarded more holistically, it was easier for health providers to envision primary prevention occurring within levels of tertiary intervention. However, the business mentality in health continues to push thinking into narrow medical models without incorporating the social and cultural situation. Life satisfaction is compromised further when a person must add a classifiable, named disability or chronic condition to the cultural load. Twenty-seven years ago at the Smithsonian Institute exhibit on rehabilitation, Davis (1973, p. 5) noted, "From outright neglect, to pity, and sympathy, handicapped Americans have had to suffer doubly; once for their illnesses and again for the psychological, social, and economic rejection they subsequently experienced."

As the point of service has expanded to the community and beyond the institution, the team configuration necessarily has become fluid and more diverse and clients have become more interactive. Rehabilitation goals fit well with those to enable persons to live longer and better and to reduce disparities or inequality (Healthy People 2000, 2000). Stating goals and actualizing them are not the same process. Services organized according to population-based or aggregate needs with community involvement have been discussed for half a century. Changes in service needs, that is, for transportation, housing (independent and assisted living), shopping patterns, foods, pharmaceuticals, services, communication, and safety needs, are growing, especially for the aging population in most countries of the world.

Some trends that will emerge and impact rehabilitation nursing can be only imagined as this book is written. Others are visible by the "tips of their heads" and their impact or failure will be recorded. As Stryker (1977) observed in her classic, "the impact of rehabilitation programs is just beginning" (p. 11).

Trends predicted to be important for rehabilitation nurses and their clients are listed in Box 1-2.

Box 1-2 Trends in Rehabilitation: 2000 to 2006

- Attention to prevention and prevalence of disability, including injury
- Public expectation to have longer, healthy lives and involvement in choices
- New definitions of disability and new models
- National surveillance and monitoring systems
- National health policy for chronic, disabling disorders
- Medical advances and technology including biomedical electronics
- Changes in access to information and services and in client rights
- Scramble for roles in community-based practice
- Community partnerships, new models, and service delivery systems
- Ethical concerns and dilemmas including allocation of resources
- Genetics research and implications for treatment options; private or government attempts to "own" or patent genetic codes
- International global problems and collaborations, new configurations of regions
- Minority and ethnic group growth and population or economic shifts
- Alternative and complementary therapeutics mainstreamed; spirituality revived
- Professional role changes and challenges for rehabilitation nurses
- Workforce needs for professional nursing colliding with economic situations

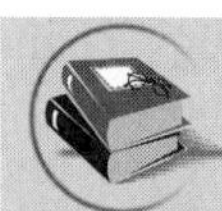

Case Studies ~ *Events That Shaped Nursing Rehabilitation*

Rehabilitation Centers

"American communities are waking up to the tremendous social and economic costs of disability as a major cause of dependency" (Switzer, 1957, p. v). "A community survey of the needs and a plan of operation are required in order to convince the local community leadership of the validity of a rehabilitation program and its purposes" (Lance & Landes, 1957, p. 206).

When exploring the past, we must pause before making pronouncements about the future. Health providers and administrators would find familiar themes should they read notes from the national movement to establish centers for rehabilitation services in the United States. Sponsored by health and government groups during the late 1950s and early 1960s, speakers at national conferences emphasized the "patient as a total person." They touted the benefits of a multidisciplinary team approach, coordinating and funding services, and value in ongoing evaluation and follow-up.

Rehabilitation leaders knew client participation and ADLs were important 50 years ago. They raised questions about the definition of disability and how to distinguish handicap from disability. An emphasis on vocational training and community living or placement underscored efforts between the rehabilitation program and resources from the person's community. What was clear then was that restoration of the person for effective living was a responsibility of the community (Speir, 1957, p. 58).

"Our greatest need is for a rehabilitation program for every community. Most of the rehabilitation problems of a community can be handled at that level if the philosophy of rehabilitation is present, and the resources of the community are utilized" (Covalt, 1957, p. 30). "Rehabilitation embodies the democratic ideals that each individual is unique, that each person has the right to participate in all aspects of life, and that each member of the community should contribute to society to the fullest extent of which he is capable. It (rehabilitation) is concerned with the physically disabled person as a human being who requires specialized help to realize his physical, social, emotional, and vocational potentials. It assumes an ideal goal—full development and utilization of abilities and maximum reduction of the effects of disabilities" (Roberts, 1957, p. 10).

In a new century, this seemingly natural connection of rehabilitation with community health and social action or service remains both conflicting and elusive.

Nursing within the Team Approach

Historically, rehabilitation nurses served as members of the multidisciplinary and interdisciplinary teams that are the hallmark of rehabilitation organizations. The character, roles, and composition of teams are discussed in detail in Chapter 2 and in the context of the community in Chapter 9. Originally the team was traditional, composed of the physician, nurse, therapists, social worker, psychologist, vocational or rehabilitation counselor, and other professionals according to the client's diagnosis and prognosis. The concept of team was highly regarded but hierarchical. In 1973 Rusk described the physician as "the captain of the team," who is aided by other professionals (Davis, 1973, p. 5).

The client was not a member of the team. In more than one rehabilitation institution great controversy arose when one person, usually a young adult with spinal cord injury, would ask to attend his evaluation conference. "Should he know what we say?" asked the team members of one another. "We're not sure all information is good for him." They reassured themselves, "We are all here for the patient, remember?"

An early rehabilitation textbook written by two physicians and a nurse at Contra Costa County Hospital and Fairmont Hospital of Alameda County, California, prepared for a multidisciplinary team audience. Authors stressed efficiency, economy, and continuity of care; maintenance of ADLs; and organization of care around what we recognize today as functional health patterns. Disabilities were classified as primary—those resulting from congenital disorders, disease processes, or injury—and as secondary, those arising from misuse or disuse syndromes. The community and the environment were considered in the plan of care with attention to individual differences (Hirschberg, Lewis, & Thomas, 1964).

Publications prepared by the nursing and physical therapy staff at Sister Kenny Institute in Minneapolis featured ADLs and are classic illustrations of technique and teamwork (Ellwood, 1964). Soon thereafter, the National League for Nursing published a series of programmed instruction on the "rehabilitative aspects of nurses," beginning with physical therapeutic nursing measures. The nurse is prominently featured, wearing her cap, as a member of the team (National League for Nursing, 1966).

Nurses in the 1960s were considered "coordinators of patient care," and they coordinated activities of other team members with patient care and families. They held key roles in preventing complications for patients after a medical event, such as stroke, or chronic condition, such as arthritis. Nurses helped patients learn ADLs as routines on the rehabilitation unit, practiced techniques of positioning and exercise for joint range of motion, and prescribed wheelchairs and adaptive equipment alongside physical therapists and under the physician's supervision.

Education to prepare the person and family to return home was essential. Patients and families practiced procedures with the nurses and then "returned demonstrations." Not only did clients have access to a special apartment within the rehabilitation facility where they could work with family members or attendants to practice what life would be like on their return home, they also spent several trial weekends at home before discharge from the unit. Time and resources were allocated for this important part of nursing education. Family and client education was documented as a modality, much as any therapy or medical procedure (Box 1-3).

From half a century ago comes guidance about the characteristics of a multidisciplinary team. The commentator sagely observed that professionals are not necessarily cooperative and may have vested interests. Team members were cautioned that they must have mutual respect and confidence in each other because "long education in a profession" often leads the individual to the conscious or unconscious assumption that treatment is centered in their particular profession. And finally, team members were reminded that a team exists for the patient, but patients must assist to the fullest extent of their capacity to achieve the goals established for them (Lance & Landes, 1957, p. 216).

Thus in the 1950s the patient and team were interrelated but not integrated; goals were set primarily by the team. Team roles have been modified, and the composition has changed. Not only

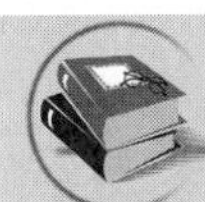

Case Studies ⁓ *Events That Shaped Nursing Rehabilitation—cont'd*

persons from the community, school, or religious affiliation are potential team members; practitioners of alternative health may be included. Importantly, the client, consumer, or person (changed from the *patient*) is a full member of the team and responsible for mutually setting goals with the team.

Nursing and rehabilitation have been integrated across levels of care and in multiple settings and along with other disciplines have incorporated new role functions. For example, therapists now work in the community with home care, long-term care, schools, outpatient satellite services, sports medicine clinics, and business-oriented independent clinics. Rehabilitation nurses who have advanced practice preparation or training in specialty roles are finding roles in special population services, such as cardiac, renal, or gerontology rehabilitation. Restorative care in home health care and schools; adult day care programs; organizations for arthritis, cancer, and multiple sclerosis; and orthopedics are other examples of specialized functions for rehabilitation nurses that often involve team roles.

Box 1-3 Family and Client Interviews: A Memory Note

A standing joke among the nursing staff was that the large bathrooms were the only spaces where family and clients could be gathered privately and "interviewed upon admission or given final instructions for exit home." Often family, client, and nurse sat on commodes surrounded by assorted wheelchairs, equipment, and supplies to conduct an education and demonstration session. One nurse complained that team members waited too long to decide on equipment ordered for the person returning home, including supplies such as catheters, padding, and wheelchair seat cushions. As a result, these items often arrived too late to give the family proper instructions. One nurse described herself "throwing all equipment, supplies, medications, and devices along with potted plants, clothing, photographs, and whatever else" onto the elevator with the departing client and family, barely managing to "toss everything inside the elevator before the doors closed." But the nurses were always available when the families would call for clarification about some procedure that same afternoon and for reassurance many times over the following weeks and months (Hoeman, 1972).

REFERENCES

Affeldt, J.E. (1988). The 1987 Mary E. Switzer Lecture: The tapestry of rehabilitation, its weavers and threads. *Journal of Allied Health, February,* 53-59.

American Nurses Association & Association of Rehabilitation Nurses. (1988). *Rehabilitation nursing: Scope of practice; process and outcome criteria for selected diagnoses.* Kansas City, MO: American Nurses Association.

Backer, B.A. (1993). Lillian Wald: Connecting caring with activism. *Nursing and Health Care, 14*(3), 122-129.

Bandura, A. (1969). *Principles of behavior modification.* New York: Holt, Rinehart, and Winston.

Basmajian, J.V. (1993). *I.O.U.: Adventures of a medical scientist.* Hamilton, Ontario, Canada: J&D Books.

Becker, M.H. (Ed.). (1974). *The health belief model and personal health behavior.* Thorofare, NJ: Slack.

Braddom, R.L. (1988). Medical education in the academy: Past, present, and a glimpse of the future. *Archives of Physical Medicine and Rehabilitation, 69,* 53-58.

Cioschi, H. (1993). The history of rehabilitation and rehabilitation nursing in the 20th century. In A.E. McCourt (Ed.), *The specialty practice of rehabilitation nursing: A core curriculum* (3rd ed., pp. 6-12). Glenview, IL: The Rehabilitation Nursing Foundation of the Association of Rehabilitation Nurses.

Cole, T.M. (1993). The greening of physiatry in a golden era of rehabilitation. The 25th Walter J. Zeiter Lecture. *Archives of Physical Medicine and Rehabilitation, 74,* 231-237.

Corbin, J.M., & Strauss, A. (1992). A nursing model for chronic illness management based on the trajectory framework. In P. Woog (Ed.), *The chronic illness trajectory framework: The Corbin and Strauss nursing model* (pp. 9-28). New York: Springer.

Covalt, D. (1957, February-March). Rehabilitation in war and peace. In *Rehabilitation Service Series No. 420. The planning of rehabilitation centers. Proceedings of the Institute on Rehabilitation Center Planning* (pp. 26-32). Washington, DC: U.S. Department of Health, Education, and Welfare.

Davis, A.B. (1973). *Triumph over disability: The development of rehabilitation medicine in the U.S.A.* Washington, DC: National Museum of History and Technology, Smithsonian Institution.

Dembo, T. (1969). Rehabilitation psychology and its immediate future: A problem of utilization of psychological knowledge. *Rehabilitation Psychology, 16,* 63-72.

Dembo, T., Leviton, G., & Wright, B. (1975). Adjustment to misfortune—A problem of social psychological rehabilitation. *Rehabilitation Psychology, 22,* 1-1000. (Original work published in 1948.)

Dittmar, S. (1989). *Rehabilitation Nursing.* St. Louis: Mosby.

Ditunno, J.F. (1988). Maturation of a specialty: The early 1980s. *Archives of Physical Medicine and Rehabilitation, 69,* 35-40.

Dunn, H.L. (1959). High level wellness for man and society. *American Journal of Public Health, 49,* 786-792.

Eberly, S., Eklund, E., & Simon, R. (Eds.). (1986). *Profiles in excellence: Twenty-five years of UAF accomplishment.* Silver Spring, MD: American Association of University Affiliated Programs for Persons with Developmental Disabilities.

Eberst, R.M. (1984). Defining health: A multidimensional model. *Journal of School Health, 54*(3), 99-104.

Edwards, P.A. (Ed.). (2000). *The specialty practice of rehabilitation nursing: A core curriculum* (4th ed.). Glenview, IL: Association of Rehabilitation Nurses.

Ellwood, P. (1964). *A handbook of rehabilitative nursing techniques in hemiplegia. Kenny Rehabilitation Institute.* Minneapolis, MN: Sister Elizabeth Kenny Foundation, Inc.

Engel, G.L. (1968). A life setting conducive to illness. *Annals of Internal Medicine, 69,* 293-300.

Erikson, E.H. (1968). *Identity, youth and crisis* (Chap. 3). New York: WW Norton.

Fliedner, C., & Rodgers, M. (1990). *Centennial Rancho Los Amigos Medical Center 1888-1988.* Downey, CA: Rancho Los Amigos Medical Center.

Goffman, E. (1963). *Stigma: Notes on the management of spoiled identity.* Englewood Cliffs, NJ: Prentice-Hall.

Gordon, M. (2000). *Manual of nursing diagnoses* (9th ed.). St. Louis: Mosby.

Granger, C.V. (1988). Breaking new ground: Academy growth from 1975 to 1979. *Archives of Physical Medicine and Rehabilitation, 69,* 30-34.

Gritzer, G., & Arluke, A. (1985). *The making of rehabilitation: A political economy of medical specialization, 1890-1980.* Berkeley and Los Angeles: University of California Press.

Groce, N. (1992). *The U.S. role in international disability activities: A history and a look toward the future.* Washington, DC: Rehabilitation International, World Institute on Disability, and World Rehabilitation Fund.

Grun, B. (1975). *The timetables of history: A horizontal linkage of people and events.* New York: Simon and Shuster.

Healthy People 2000. (accessed 2000). http://web.health.gov/healthypeople.

Hertzberg, D., & Hoeman, S.P. (1991, October). *Pediatric rehabilitation nursing in Armenia: An opportunity for change.* Presented at the 17th Annual Association of Rehabilitation Nurses Educational Conference, Kansas City, MO.

Hirschberg, G.G., Lewis, L., & Thomas, D. (1964). *Rehabilitation: A manual for the care of the disabled and elderly.* Philadelphia: JB Lippincott.

Hoeman, S.P. (1972). *Memories of Sister Kenny Rehabilitation Institute.* Personal files: unpublished notes.

Hoeman, S.P. (1989). *Testimony for a Rehabilitation Research Institute in the National Institutes of Health.* Representing the Association of Rehabilitation Nurses to the NIH Panel on Physical Medicine and Rehabilitation Research. Report of the Panel C-83-86 (November 20). Bethesda, MD: NIH.

Hoeman, S.P. (1992). *Community and rehabilitation nursing in Greece. Fulbright Senior Scholar award.* Washington, DC: International Exchange of Scholars.

Hoeman, S.P. (1998). Dynamics of rehabilitation nursing. In G. Goldstein, & S.R. Beers (Eds.), *Rehabilitation* (pp. 71–87). New York: Plenum Press.

Hoeman, S.P. (1999a). *Community and rehabilitation nursing in Jordan. Fulbright Senior Scholar award.* Washington, DC: International Exchange of Scholars.

Johnson, E.W. (1988). Struggle for identity: The turbulent 1960s. *Archives of Physical Medicine and Rehabilitation, 69,* 20-25.

Johnson, K.M.M. (Ed.). (1997). *Advanced practice nursing in rehabilitation: A core curriculum.* Glenview, IL: Association of Rehabilitation Nurses.

Kessler, H.H. (1968). *The knife is not enough.* New York: W.W. Norton.

Kessler, H.H. (1970). *Disability—Determination and evaluation.* Philadelphia: Lea & Febiger.

Lance, H.E., & Landes, R.H. (1957, February-March). Personnel recruitment, selection, and retention. In *Rehabilitation Service Series No. 420. The planning of rehabilitation centers. Proceedings of the Institute on Rehabilitation Center Planning* (pp. 205-216). Washington, DC: U.S. Department of Health, Education, and Welfare.

Lancet Editor. (1997). Editorial: From what will we die in 2020? *Lancet, 349*(9061), 1263.

LaPlante, M.P. (1996). Health conditions and impairments causing disability. *Disability Statistics Abstracts* (No. 16). San Francisco, CA: Disability Statistics Rehabilitation Research and Training Center, University of California, San Francisco, U.S. Department of Education, National Institute on Disability and Rehabilitation Research.

Lazarus, R.S. (1999). *Stress and emotion: A new synthesis.* New York: Springer.

Lazarus, R.S., & Folkman, S. (1984). *Stress, appraisal, and coping.* New York: Springer.

Leavell, H.R., & Clark, E.G. (Eds.). (1965). P*reventive medicine for the doctor in his community* (3rd ed.). New York: McGraw-Hill.

Leininger, M.M. (Ed.). (1988). *Care: The essence of nursing.* Detroit, MI: Wayne State University Press.

Lewin, K. (1947). Frontiers in group dynamics: Concept, methods, and reality in social science. *Human Relations, 1,* 5-41.

Lippitt, R., Watson, J., & Westley, B. (1958). *The dynamics of planned change.* New York. Harcourt, Brace, & World.

Lubkin, I.M. (1995). *Chronic illness: Impact and interventions.* 3rd edition. Boston: Jones & Bartlett.

Martin, G.M. (1988). Building on the framework: The Academy in the 1950s. *Archives of Physical Medicine and Rehabilitation, 69,* 15-19.

Martin, N., Holt, N.B., & Hicks, D. (1981). *Comprehensive rehabilitation nursing.* New York: McGraw-Hill.

Maslow, A.H. (1968). *Toward a psychology of being* (2nd ed.). Princeton, NJ: Van Nostrand Reinhold.

McCourt, A. (Ed.). (1993). *The specialty practice of rehabilitation nursing-A core curriculum* (3rd ed.). Glenview, IL: Rehabilitation Nursing Foundation.

McCourt, A.E., & Novak, S. (1994, September). *A history of the Association of Rehabilitation Nurses Association.* Presented at the Annual Educational Conference; Orlando, FL.

Morrissey, A.B. (1951). *Rehabilitation nursing.* New York: GP Putnam's Sons.

Mumma, C.M. (Ed.). (1987). *Rehabilitation nursing: Concepts for practice—A core curriculum* (2nd ed.). Evanston, IL: Rehabilitation Nursing Foundation.

Murray, C.J.L., & Lopez, A.D. (1997a). Regional patterns of disability-free life expectancy and disability-adjusted life expectancy: Global Burden of Disease study. *Lancet, 349,* 1347-1352.

Murray, C.J.L., & Lopez, A.D. (1997b). Global mortality, disability, and the contribution of risk factors: Global Burden of Disease study. *Lancet, 349,* 1436-1442.

Nagi, S.Z. (1965). Some conceptual issues in disability and rehabilitation. In M.B. Sussman (Ed.), *Sociology and rehabilitation.* Washington, DC: American Sociological Association.

National Center for Health Statistics. (accessed 2000). http://www.cdc.gov/nchs/. Atlanta: Centers for Disease Control and Prevention.

National League for Nursing. (1966). *Rehabilitative aspects of nursing.* New York: National League for Nursing.

Neuman, B. (1989). *The Neuman systems model.* (2nd ed.). East Norwalk, CT: Appleton & Lange.

Nichols, D.J., & Hammer, M.S. (1998). Case study of institution-building by Nurse Bertha Wright and colleagues. *Image—The Journal of Nursing Scholarship, 30*(4), 385-389.

Nightingale, F. (1859/1992). *Notes on nursing: What it is, and what it is not* (Commemorative edition). Philadelphia: JB Lippincott.

Oates, S.B. (1994). *A woman of valor: Clara Barton and the Civil War.* New York: Free Press.

Orem, D.M. (1989). Nursing concepts of practice (5th ed.). St. Louis: Mosby.

Parsons, T. (1951). *The social system.* New York: Free Press.

Pope, A.M., & Tarlov, A.R. (Eds.). (1991). *Disability in America: Toward a national agenda for prevention.* Washington, DC: Institute of Medicine, National Academy Press.

Repetto, M.A., & Hoeman, S.P. (1991). A legislative perspective on the school nurse and education for children with disabilities in New Jersey. *Journal of School Health, 61*(9), 388-391.

Roberts, D.W. (1957, February-March). Evolution of the rehabilitation center concept. In *Rehabilitation Service Series No. 420. The planning of rehabilitation centers. Proceedings of the Institute on Rehabilitation Center Planning* (pp. 1-17). Washington, DC: U.S. Department of Health, Education, and Welfare.

Roper, N., Logan, W.W., & Tierney, A.J. (1996). *The elements of nursing: A model for nursing based on a model of living* (4th ed.). Edinburgh: Churchill Livingstone.

Roy, S.C., & Andrews, H.A. (1991). The Roy adaptation model: The definitive statement. East Norwalk, CT: Appleton & Lange.

Rusk, H.A. (1957, February-March). International aspects of the rehabilitation center movement. In *Rehabilitation Service Series No. 420. The planning of rehabilitation centers. Proceedings of the Institute on Rehabilitation Center Planning* (pp. 11-25). Washington, DC: U.S. Department of Health, Education, and Welfare.

Rusk, H.A., & Taylor, E. (1965). Rehabilitation as a phase of preventive medicine. In H.R. Leavell & E.G. Clark (Eds.), *Preventive medicine for the doctor in his community* (3rd ed., pp. 474-494). New York: McGraw-Hill.

Safilios-Rothschild, C. (1970). *The sociology and social psychology of disability and rehabilitation.* New York: Random House.

Schopper, D., Pereira, J., Torres, A., Cuende, N., Alonso, M., Baylin, A., Ammon, C., & Rougemont, A. (2000). Estimating the burden of disease in one Swiss canton: What do disability adjusted life years (DALY) tell us? *International Journal of Epidemiology. 29*(5), 871-877.

Selye, H. (1978). *Stress of life.* New York: McGraw-Hill.

Speir, H.B. (1957, February-March). The measurement of rehabilitation needs in a community. In *Rehabilitation Service Series No. 420. The planning of rehabilitation centers. Proceedings of the Institute on Rehabilitation Center Planning* (pp. 47-59). Washington, DC: U.S. Department of Health, Education, and Welfare.

Starr, P. (1982). *The social transformation of American medicine.* New York: Basic Books.

Stryker, R. (1977). *Rehabilitative aspects of acute and chronic nursing care* (2nd ed.). Philadelphia: WB Saunders.

Switzer, M.E. (1957, February-March). Foreword. In *Rehabilitation Service Series No. 420. The planning of rehabilitation centers. Proceedings of the Institute on Rehabilitation Center Planning* (pp. v). Washington, DC: U.S. Department of Health, Education, and Welfare.

Thomas, E. (1966). Problems of disability from the perspective of role theory. *Journal of Health and Human Behavior,* 7-11.

Thomas, K.R. (1985). Rehabilitation services, training, and research: A political analysis. *Journal of Rehabilitation, Oct/Nov/Dec,* 17-21.

Thorne, S.E. (1993). *Negotiating health care: The social context of chronic illness.* Newbury Park, CA: Sage.

U.S. Department of Health and Human Services (USDHHS). (accessed 2000). Healthy People 2010: Conference edition. http://web.health.gov/healthypeople/document.

Verville, R.E. (1988). Fifty years of federal legislation and programs affecting the PM&R. *Archives of Physical Medicine and Rehabilitation, 69,* 64-68.

Wright, B. (1983). *Physical disability: A psychosocial approach.* New York: HarperCollins.

Young, M. (1989). A history of rehabilitation nursing: Fifteen years of making the difference. Skokie, IL: Association of Rehabilitation Nurses.

Zinner, N.L. (1990). Miss Marie recalls a half century of orthopaedic nursing. *Orthopedic Nursing, 9*(6), 33-35, 74.

BIBLIOGRAPHY

Groce, N.E. (1996). Rehabilitation in an historic perspective: the work of Bell Greve. *Journal of Rehabilitation, 62*(2), 7-10.

Hoeman, S.P. (1999b). Foreword. In J. Pryor (Ed.), *Rehabilitation—A vital nursing function* (pp. v-vii). Professional Development Series No. 11. Sydney, Australia: Royal College of Nursing, Australia.

Institute on Rehabilitation Center Planning. (1957, February-March). In *Rehabilitation Service Series No. 420. The planning of rehabilitation centers. Proceedings of the Institute on Rehabilitation Center Planning.* Washington, DC: U.S. Department of Health, Education, and Welfare.

Kottke, F.J., & Knapp, M.E. (1988). The development of physiatry before 1950. *Archives of Physical Medicine and Rehabilitation, 69,* 4-14.

Neal, L.J. (Ed.). (1998). *Rehabilitation nursing in the home health setting.* Glenview, IL. Association of Rehabilitation Nurses.

2 Theory and Practice Models for Rehabilitation Nursing

Christina M. Mumma, PhD, RN, CRRN
Audrey Nelson, PhD, RN, FAAN

An interview with a practicing nurse, Christine Hunt, RN, CRRN, revealed her view of the essence of rehabilitation nursing as "client and family teaching to facilitate independence and follow-through with the rehabilitation program toward the goal of sending persons home to live their lives." Ms. Hunt, a rehabilitation nurse for 14 years and certified since 1991, has worked for the past 12 years as an inpatient rehabilitation case manager. When asked about the changes in rehabilitation nursing during the past 12 years, Ms. Hunt replied, "The process of rehabilitation nursing hasn't really changed, but the nursing care delivery system has changed dramatically. Originally the unit functioned within a primary nursing model. About 5 years ago, for primarily economic reasons, the nursing care model was changed to one that used a mix of registered nurses and client care technicians (unlicensed personnel). That change resulted in moving registered nurses away from direct client care. The current nursing care model on the unit has incorporated differentiated nursing practice with a staff made up of both registered nurses and client care technicians. It has the potential to work well but has been difficult to implement effectively because of a low client census. My position (originally titled case manager *and now titled* clinical coordinator*) continues to involve a combination of screening patients before admission to the rehabilitation unit and discharge planning as patients prepare to leave the unit, as well as coordination of patient teaching done by the staff nurses."*

Ms. Hunt sees continued challenges to rehabilitation nursing practice because of limited resources. She further stated, "Limited resources have led rehabilitation nurses to having less time to complete essential teaching of clients and families. A key premise behind rehabilitation is teaching, and the teaching is not getting done as thoroughly as it could be. In the best of all rehabilitation worlds, there would be a return to primary nursing. Within a primary nursing model, teaching can be done while care is provided. Helping clients and families to help themselves takes time." The helping, teaching, and caring that are essential to the care of rehabilitation clients also require the continued commitment and compassion of rehabilitation nurses like Ms. Hunt.

The various theories and models developed by nursing, rehabilitation, and the social sciences, as well as models derived from practice, offer alternative foundations for rehabilitation nurses to use in providing care and when developing programs of service. The theoretical basis of care may be more implicit than explicit in the minds of many. Through interactions with hundreds of nurses regarding the theoretical basis of their practice, Mumma (2000) discovered that although they had difficulty articulating the foundations of care, their nursing practice was not atheoretical. Similar in-depth discussions with rehabilitation nurses revealed rich theoretical underpinnings and many principles highly consistent with major nursing theories and models.

This chapter presents theories and models from nursing and other disciplines that are relevant for rehabilitation nursing building on the works of Hoeman (1996) and McCourt (1993). The large, complex content is organized according to a now-classic framework developed by Donaldson and Crowley (1978). They identified three major concerns addressed through the essence or core of nursing. Concerns are with principles and laws that govern the life processes, well-being, and optimum functioning of human beings, sick or well; with the patterning of human behavior in interaction with the environment in critical life situations; and with the processes by which positive changes in health status are affected.

NURSING THEORIES AND MODELS FOR REHABILITATION PRACTICE

A number of frameworks useful to rehabilitation nursing have a primary focus that centers on life processes, well-being, and/or optimum functioning. These theoretical approaches address ways individuals function during health and illness. Of interest are grand theories of nursing developed by Orem (1995); Roper, Logan, and Tierney (1996); and Roy and Andrews (1991). Gordon's Functional Health Patterns (FHPs) (2000) and Corbin and Strauss' Chronic Illness Trajectory (1992) are essential frameworks for rehabilitation nursing practice.

Orem Self-Care Deficit Theory

The Orem (1995) Self-Care Deficit Theory for nursing is composed of three subtheories: the theory of self-care, the theory of self-care deficit, and the theory of the nursing system. Nursing care based on these theories provides assistance when clients cannot meet their own self-care demands. Self-Care Deficit Theory within rehabilitation nursing incorporates all of the types of nursing intervention described by Orem (1995): wholly compensatory, partly compensatory, and supportive-educative. The predominant method of assisting clients with disability and chronic illness within rehabilitation nursing is supportive-educative.

According to Davis and O'Connor (1999), Orem's theory lacks content for nonintervention. With a rehabilitation client, deliberate nonintervention may be an effective intervention when the nurse has expertise to know when to intervene and when to stand back. Another consideration for Orem's theory within rehabilitation nursing is a temporal component. Care for an individual recovering from an acute illness could be expected to move from wholly compensatory through partly compensatory to supportive-educative. However, a person with a severe disability or a chronic illness, who is dependent in areas of self-care, can become responsible for self-directing care. In this situation, all three of Orem's nursing systems would operate simultaneously.

The increase in prevalence of chronic conditions has led to nursing practice models for chronic illness. Burks (1999) described a nursing practice model based on the concept of intentional action, using the Orem (1995) Self-Care Deficit Theory as the conceptual framework. Key to successful implementation of this model is the need for rehabilitation nurses to relinquish control of the client and support the management skills of the client.

Roper Model for Living

Concepts from the Roper Model for Living (Roper et al., 1996) form part of the framework for this book. Roper et al. developed a Model for Living and a corresponding Model for Nursing. The major components are the activities of daily living (ADLs) (Table 2-1), which characterize the person. These ADLs represent all of the things persons do on a daily basis, and each is placed on a dependence-independence continuum. The multiple factors that have potential to influence ADLs are categorized as either biological, psychological, sociocultural, environmental, or politicoeconomic. Adding to the complexity of the model is the fact that all of the ADLs are interrelated and affect functioning of the whole person. For example, one individual with impaired mobility of the lower extremities may experience significant loss of interpersonal relationships, inability to dress independently, and difficulty accessing toilet facilities. Another person with a similar impairment and using a wheelchair for mobility may be independent in those same ADLs.

Roper et al. (1996) use the nursing process combined with the Activities of Living Model to achieve desired client outcomes. The emphasis on health teaching as a primary nursing tehnique is especially applicable for rehabilitation nursing practice. Nurses educate clients to prevent potential problems, alleviate actual problems, and cope effectively with problems that cannot be cured or solved. Individuality

TABLE 2-1 Roper's Activities of Living Model (1996) and Gordon's Functional Health Patterns (2000)

Activities of Living	Functional Health Patterns
Maintaining a safe environment	Health perception–health management pattern
Communicating	Cognitive-perceptual pattern Coping-stress-tolerance pattern Value-belief pattern
Breathing	Activity-exercise pattern
Eating and drinking	Nutritional-metabolic pattern
Eliminating	Elimination pattern
Personal cleansing and dressing	Activity-exercise pattern
Controlling body temperature	Nutritional-metabolic pattern
Mobilizing	Activity-exercise pattern
Working and playing	Activity-exercise pattern Self-perception–self-concept pattern Role-relationship pattern
Expressing sexuality	Sexuality-reproductive pattern Role-relationship pattern
Sleeping	Sleep-rest
Dying	Self-perception–self-concept pattern

From Gordon, M. (2000). *Manual of nursing diagnosis* (9th ed.). St. Louis: Mosby; and Roper, N., Logan, W., & Tierney, A. (1996). *The elements of nursing: A model for nursing based on a model of living* (4th ed.). Edinburgh: Churchill-Livingstone.

and active client participation are explicitly stated in applying the model, an attractive feature for rehabilitation nurses.

Roy Adaptation Model

With the Roy Adaptation Model (RAM) (Roy & Andrews, 1991), human beings are considered adaptive systems. Adaptation occurs within four adaptive modes: physiological, self-concept, interdependence, and role-function. When the need for adaptation exceeds the individual's current ability to adapt, the rehabilitation nurse intervenes by working within the client's adaptive modes to increase adaptation or by changing environmental stimuli to decrease the demands. This model is congruent with rehabilitation nursing and principles for working with clients as they make adaptations to disability or chronic illness.

Gordon Functional Health Patterns

Gordon (2000) developed the typology of FHPs primarily as a system for organizing assessment data. The FHPs are used in the care of individuals, families, and communities and evolve from client-environment interaction. Patterns are highly interrelated and are fully understood only within the context of the whole person. Not unique to rehabilitation nursing, the FHPs can be used to effectively organize assessment data from clients with disability and chronic illness. The FHPs, integrated with the Roper Activities of Living Model, form the organizing framework for this book.

Chronic Illness Trajectory

The Chronic Illness Trajectory framework developed by Corbin and Strauss (1992) has considerable utility within rehabilitation nursing practice. The trajectory framework proposes that disabling and chronic conditions have a predictable course over time that can be influenced or managed. Providers or clients themselves can attempt to produce outcomes that differ from the trajectory when they understand the nature of their condition. As a result, persons with disabilities or chronic disease can learn ways of managing limitations to participate as fully as possible in everyday activities.

Other Theories

The Theory of Culture Care

According to Leininger's Culture Care Theory (Reynolds & Leininger, 1993), health and illness experiences can be fully understood only within the context of culture. On the basis of this theory, the goal of nursing is to provide care that is congruent with the values, health beliefs, and lifestyles of different cultures. Culture care theory is highly applicable within rehabilitation nursing and can facilitate the provision of culturally competent care to clients living with disability or chronic illness.

Science of Unitary Human Beings

Rogers' (1990) Science of Unitary Human Beings was developed to provide a framework for wholistic nursing care. Within this framework, human beings are energy fields in constant interaction with environmental energy fields, both of which are infinite and irreducible. Nursing care within the science of unitary human beings involves recognition of patterns that emerge from person-environment interactions. Rogers' principles of homeodynamics guide nursing practice. These principles include resonancy, helicy, and integrality. Within rehabilitation nursing practice, the principles of homeodynamics can be used to assess patterns of interaction between individuals and their environments.

Social Learning Theory

Bandura (1986), a pioneer in behavior modification, found four factors that influence how children learn when observing others. A child attends to the situation, retains the observation, has a certain capacity to perform the action, and identifies rewards or punishments associated with performing the action. According to this theory, behavior change is based on the interaction between expectations about the outcomes resulting from engaging in a behavior and expectations about the ability to carry out the behavior. Application of social learning theory to rehabilitation nursing involves breaking behavior into small sequential steps to facilitate a client's confidence in performing new behaviors and transferring those new behaviors to a variety of situations. Whittemore (2000) describes the use of social learning theory in the development of strategies to facilitate lifestyle change for individuals with diabetes mellitus.

A Psychosocial Approach

Wright (1983), a pioneer in the study of concepts within the psychology of physical disability, raised social consciousness about a relationship between perceptions of disability and impressions about attributes of the person with disability. Wright's classic writings forced professionals to examine concerns about their own health and functional ability when working with persons with disabilities. Reflection and self-awareness remain critical components of rehabilitation nursing practice.

SPECIALIZED MODELS IN REHABILITATION

The development of rehabilitation specialty programs was in part shaped by the criteria set by the Rehabilitation Accreditation Commission (CARF). Although most rehabilitation care models attempt to address the unique needs of the persons they were designed to serve, the heterogeneity of the client population can make this a difficult process. Specialization is one way to address unique consumer needs because by targeting services to particular client groups, services to a more homogeneous population are restricted.

The Neal theory of home health nursing practice may

serve rehabilitation nurses. It evolved from research with practicing home health nurses, who defined home health nursing practice as a three-stage process leading to autonomy of practice. Nurses, regardless of their education or nursing experience, are initially dependent on beginning in-home health. *Dependence* refers to the need to rely on others to learn about both the logistical and clinical aspects of home health care. After approximately 6 months to 1 year, the nurse is moderately dependent. Although the length of time in each stage varies according to the individual, nurses are likely to move into stage 3 after 2 years of home health experience. However, nurses do not progress through the stages unless they are able to make adaptations to themselves and to their clients' situations to accommodate care needs. The theory differentiates nursing practice in home health from that in institutional settings, and it clearly supports that nurses must use adaptability to succeed in home care. The nurses unanimously agreed that the goal of home health nursing practice is to assist the client to be maximally independent through partnerships with clients and families, cooperation with the interdisciplinary team, and a philosophy of doing "with" the client, not "for" or "to" the client. Thus the theory demonstrates a congruity of home health nursing with rehabilitation nursing principles.

The advantages and disadvantages of specialization were illustrated in a survey of 114 facilities providing burn rehabilitation services. All of the facilities treated burns of similar severity and reported similar lengths of hospital stay and outpatient follow-up. Indicators of quality differed. Specialized burn facilities were more likely to have organized outpatient burn rehabilitation programs and scheduled outpatient clinics with staff trained in burn rehabilitation. They reported regular inpatient interdisciplinary conferences and structured educational activities (Cromes & Helm, 1992).

CLIENT-CENTERED MODELS

Client-centered care is the critical element of rehabilitation models. These models are referred to as "consumer driven" because they emphasize the needs, thoughts, feelings, and expectations of the client. Client-centered practice embraces a philosophy of respect and partnership between clients and providers that is essential to the development of an effective rehabilitation model. Gordon (1994) describes client-centered practice as an approach that consciously adopts the perspective of the clients, with careful consideration of what is important to each and how care is likely to affect them (Box 2-1).

Specialized services in rehabilitation that are client centered are organized under one of four program models. These are age or developmental level of the client, type of disability, social or cultural systems, or family systems.

Age or Developmental Level of the Client

Pediatric rehabilitation nursing goals related to comprehensive and holistic care are blended with creative strategies to address the unique developmental needs of children (Brothers, 1998). A normal, age-appropriate environment with opportunities for extended parent-child interaction is critical (Fuhrer, 1998). Radford (1998), a clinical nurse specialist in pediatric rehabilitation, discussed changes in attitudes underlying the care of children with chronic illness and disability and the emphasis on collaboration and partnership with parents. Chapter 29 discusses pediatric rehabilitation in detail. Rehabilitation services for adolescents address their critical development needs of independence, socialization, and sexuality education.

Box 2-1 Client-Centered Practice

Dimensions of Client-Centered Care

- Respect for client's values, preferences, and expressed needs
- Coordination and integration of care
- Information, communication, and education
- Physical comfort
- Emotional support, alleviation of fear and anxiety
- Involvement of family and friends
- Transition and continuity (Gordon, 1994)

Key Concepts

- Individual autonomy and choice
- Partnership
- Nurse and client responsibility
- Enablement
- Contextual congruence
- Accessibility
- Respect for diversity (Law, Baptiste, & Mills, 1995)

Geriatric rehabilitation nursing emphasizes discriminating evaluation and promotion of restorative function (Lander, 1996). Functionally impaired elderly clients perceived to be "at risk" for nursing home placement are targeted for inpatient geriatric assessment units. These programs encourage self-care and improved function to decrease nursing home placement and reduce mortality. One example is the Audiological Care Model, which describes the nurse's role in rehabilitation of age-related hearing loss in a dependent elderly client population (Tolson & Stephens, 1997).

Lorig et al. (1996) conducted a 6-month randomized trial comparing persons who participated in a geriatric rehabilitation education program with wait-list control subjects. Participants ($n = 1120$) were at least 40 years old, with a mean age of 64.7 years. Each had a physician-confirmed diagnosis of heart disease, lung disease, stroke, or arthritis. The education program was held in seven 2-hour sessions for small groups of clients with mixed diagnoses. The program presented information about techniques of managing cognitive symptoms, exercising, maintaining proper nutrition, using medications, managing fatigue and sleep disturbance, dealing with emotions or anger and depression, communicating with others including providers, using community resources, solving problems, and making decisions. No changes were made to participants' treatment regimens. Self-reported health status measures were for disability, fatigue, distress with health state, and limitations of social or role activities. Program participants, when compared with control subjects, demonstrated improvements in exercise, cognitive symptom management, communication with physicians, and health status.

Type of Disability

The Department of Veterans Affairs (VA) advocates comprehensive, coordinated care for homogeneous groups of clients on the basis of disability. Regional VA centers have been developed for treatment of spinal cord injury, traumatic brain injury, and rehabilitation of blind persons.

The National Institute on Disability and Rehabilitation Research (NIDRR) model systems program provides comprehensive care for persons with spinal cord injuries, including services for acute care, rehabilitation, community reintegration, and long-term follow-up (Zejdlik, 1999); significant outcomes have been reported. One disadvantage of disability-specific programs is that their central locations in urban areas often require clients to undergo treatment away from family and community. The programs are centered on a particular problem or disease and may not consider comorbidity or complexity of multiple chronic conditions. Without a holistic approach, treatment recommendations contradict one another or collide. For example, a person in a cardiac rehabilitation program may find compliance with the exercise prescription troublesome, if not impossible, because of painful arthritis of the knees or feet.

However, a community of caring or peer support often emerges because clients and families are exposed to others dealing with similar challenges. Although initially, prevention and control of complications are critical, reconditioning, retraining in ADLs, and viewing the client as a whole are critical features for specialty rehabilitation programs.

Social and Cultural Systems

Cultural diversity has implications for rehabilitation because outcomes, interactions, and responses to rehabilitation services are influenced by social and cultural factors. Studies to explore the unique culture that emerges in inpatient rehabilitation units help nurses appreciate the meaning and experiences of care in rehabilitation settings. Thompson (1990) described the culture from the perspective of the rehabilitation nurse, whereas Nelson (1990) examined it from the perspective of a client with a spinal cord injury. Culture and alternative care are discussed in Chapter 13.

A model integrating the rehabilitation team and community members into client-centered community rehabilitation described ways to bridge cultural barriers and improve access while being sensitive to competent culture care (Broughton & Lutner, 1995). The community and client become comanagers of care.

Stephenson, Yee, and Lisse (1997) examined the impact of the Arthritis Self-Help (ASH) program on African-Americans ($n = 26$) between 53 and 84 years of age. Activity and physical limitation, locus of control, life satisfaction, and self-efficacy for exercise and cognitive symptom management were key variables for assessing the effectiveness of the ASH program. Clients who completed the ASH program showed improvement in all variables except the self-efficacy measures. Further studies are needed to evaluate the role of self-efficacy for coping skills in this cultural group.

Family Systems

For treatment to be incorporated into daily life, full cooperation and commitment from the family are crucial. At times it is critical for the rehabilitation team to view the family, rather than the individual, as the client (Robinson, 1995). Models for family involvement in the rehabilitation process ultimately benefit the client. Identifying family needs and instituting short-term intervention at known crisis points in the rehabilitation process when family members are occupied with specific concerns are likely to be effective because attention is focused.

Ideally, long-term rehabilitation of a client is a joint team-family responsibility. Addressing the physical and emotional impact of care giving is a constant challenge for the rehabilitation nurse's role in identifying caregiver problems, helping them obtain assistance to continue the client's care at home. For example, Law et al. (1998) described the design and evaluation of a family-centered functional approach to therapy for children with cerebral palsy.

Rehabilitation nurses seek ways to involve clients and families as comanagers who participate as fully as possible in planning, implementing, and evaluating their care. Family systems theories are useful for rehabilitation nurses to understand family dynamics, including patterns of communication, interaction, power, and economics (Anderson, 2000). Chapter 12 discusses the family and rehabilitation.

Nurses promoting a scientific basis for family nursing propose an ecological model that covers the life-span development of all family members. This approach recognizes the complexity of variables that converge when family members of different sexes, generations, and developmental stages, as well as with different life experiences, interact with environmental structures and social systems.

The challenges of this convergence are evident in the example of a 50-year-old woman who has had a left-hemisphere stroke resulting in right body weakness and sensory loss as well as aphasia and dysphagia. She is returning home to a geographically remote North American setting after inpatient rehabilitation in an urban setting. She lives in a small home with her husband, three children, and one grandchild. Her successful reintegration into the community will depend to a large extent on involvement of her family and the entire small community in her continued rehabilitation.

Environment and Ecology

The context or environment within which individuals experience health and illness is prominent in theories and models that underlie rehabilitation nursing care. Environmentally focused theories and models include those created by Reynolds and Leininger (1993), Rogers (1990), Bandura (1986), and Wright (1983), and family and ecological systems describe the environments within which rehabilitation nurses practice (Pierce & Salter, 1997; Anderson, 2000).

Rehabilitation nursing program models, which can be thought of as emphasizing the environment within which human beings experience critical life situations, are those defined by the choice of setting. Rehabilitation takes place in many settings other than the traditional inpatient rehabilitation unit. In addition to these acute care facilities, rehabilitation nurses practice in long-term care settings, in community-based settings, and in clients' homes.

LEVELS OF INTERVENTION

Acute Rehabilitation Care

Since World War II, rehabilitation has been provided primarily in acute rehabilitation settings. Subacute rehabilitation units and a variety of community-based settings emerged as options in the 1990s. Given the shift from inpatient settings to delivery of rehabilitation services in the home and community-based settings, the combination of rehabilitation programs may look quite different in the near future.

Acute care rehabilitation settings have responded to changes within the economic and health care environments in a variety of innovative ways, such as utilization management systems. Issues include increased costs, lower reimbursement, length of stay, and staff morale. Rehabilitation nurses can have an impact on care in acute settings by ensuring that clients receive care to prevent complications that would disrupt or prohibit their performing well in rehabilitation. Basic principles of positioning and preserving skin integrity are essential for quality outcomes.

Phipps (1990) described her role as a rehabilitation nurse specialist in an acute care setting. She provided consultation throughout the hospital to assist primary care nurses to make client care decisions by giving expert opinion in collaboration with the nurse who requested the consultation.

Long-Term Care and Subacute Care

In 1993 less than 3% of rehabilitation nurses who responded to a job-analysis survey identified long-term care facilities as their practice setting (Habel, 1993). Accurate numbers of persons with chronic disability residing in long-term care facilities are difficult to determine. Certainly, elderly persons are overrepresented in institutional settings, with an estimated 4% to 5% living in institutions. An unknown number of younger persons with chronic disabilities reside in long-term care facilities (Administration on Aging, 2000).

Long-term care facilities generally provide a variety of rehabilitation services to clients with disabilities, not limited to rehabilitation nursing; rehabilitation medicine; and physical, occupational, and speech therapies. The scheduled number of hours of therapy per week compared with that in acute rehabilitation facilities is reduced. The overall rehabilitation goals are congruent with those in other settings: maximum independent functioning and quality of life.

Subacute rehabilitation emerged as a model in the 1990s. Clear, universally agreed-on definitions of subacute rehabilitation have not been established (Campbell & Case, 1999). Subacute rehabilitation facilities serve clients who require skilled medical and nursing care but not diagnostic or invasive procedures. Many subacute units admit persons whose medical treatment makes their participation in an acute rehabilitation program difficult or whose progress is too slow for participation in a regular rehabilitation program (Gill & Rovinsky, 1998). For example, a managed care model was described as a model for geriatric rehabilitation practice in subacute care, called *transitional care centers.* Transitional care centers were established in nursing homes and targeted residents who needed rehabilitation. The centers provided rehabilitative and geriatric evaluation services, which were less costly and had noted improvement in quality of care (Von Sternberg et al., 1997). A randomized controlled study of stroke rehabilitation within a subacute setting in Norway supported the benefits of this approach (Ronning & Guldvog, 1998).

Within subacute settings, the roles of the registered nurse are primarily planner, coordinator, and evaluator of client outcomes, as well as some direct-care provision. Much of the direct nursing care is provided by nursing assistants and licensed practical nurses (LPNs).

Inpatient settings that provide subacute and long-term rehabilitation services to clients with chronic disabilities and illnesses may be viewed in a number of different ways. For some clients these facilities may be an appropriate, cost-effective alternative to rehabilitation in a more acute setting. For other clients a subacute or long-term care setting may be one of several places of care and residence along their rehabilitation continuum of care. Others will be discharged to home from acute rehabilitation and later admitted to a subacute or long-term care facility.

Community Settings

The community, rather than the hospital or inpatient setting, has become a primary treatment setting in which many persons with disabilities manage their care and daily activities. The term *community-based rehabilitation* has been broadly defined and applied to a variety of programs and settings within which clients receive rehabilitation services. Community-based rehabilitation is discussed in detail in Chapter 9. Settings include outpatient clinics, day treatment programs, independent living centers, community reentry programs, and rural outreach programs.

A community-based rehabilitation model involves clients and families as copartners with professionals for the accomplishment of mutually established goals. The emphasis is on short-term, long-term, and even lifelong goals that lead to improvement in quality of life as defined within that client and family's context (Hoeman, 1992; Kaplan, 1999). Outpatient programs target client populations, such as cardiac rehabilitation centers that provide enhanced physiologic status, aerobic fitness, nutrition, and strengthening (Oldridge, 1997).

The rehabilitation literature includes a number of reports of rural communities that have successfully met the challenge of providing rehabilitation care in areas where resources are scarce. An innovative program was developed by the Rehabilitation Centre in Ottawa, Canada, to "take rehabilitation to the people" in rural Canada. Problems central to rural rehabilitation include limited access to the variety of services for individuals with disabilities, the number of persons who are elderly or have limited income, and time and money burdens of travel to centralized rehabilitation. Additionally a scarcity of professionals from specialty disciplines includes nurses, who make up the majority of direct-care providers in rural areas; they often lack specialized expertise in rehabilitation (Lavallee & Crupi, 1992).

A mobile interdisciplinary rehabilitation team, collaborative and dedicated to holistic practice, was developed to meet rehabilitation needs of clients in rural Ontario, Canada. Lavallee and Crupi (1992, p. 66) expect the mobile rehabilitation clinic to "help rural communities meet the challenges of tomorrow. It can do this because under the mobile clinic program the community as a whole becomes the client—a client for consultation, education, research, and advocacy interventions."

Home Care

Rehabilitation is increasingly being provided in home care settings (Moffa-Trotter & Anemaet, 1999). Home rehabilitation is generally viewed as a continuation of rehabilitation programs initiated in other settings, such as acute rehabilitation facilities, outpatient programs, and long-term care settings. Returning home is often one of the strongest desires for clients involved in inpatient rehabilitation programs. A measure of successful rehabilitation is the generalization or translation of skills to the natural setting—home. Home rehabilitation promotes client autonomy, independence, and community reintegration (Neal, 1998; Mayo, Wood-Dauphinee, & Cote, 2000). Community awareness of the availability and effectiveness of home health care is growing dramatically. There are essential differences between home care and hospital or rehabilitation facility care. Regardless of how "client friendly" inpatient units are designed to be, clients will quickly remind anyone listening that these settings are not home.

Technology is changing the way home health care is delivered, especially in remote areas of the country. Many disciplines have tested applications of telemedicine in their specialty areas. Telerehabilitation has emerged as a delivery model for providing rehabilitation services for persons who do not have ready access to comprehensive services. With videoconferencing and data acquisition technologies (Seelman, 1996), telerehabilitation has been used in physical therapy, pediatric and geriatric rehabilitation, rehabilitation outcomes (Garrett & Shapcott, 1998; Levine, 1996), and computer-based support groups.

Applications of telerehabilitation include providing the following: (1) comprehensive rehabilitation services to clients for whom transportation and disability limit access, (2) alternatives to on-site home evaluations, (3) a link between providers at remote sites to real-time consultation at a specialty hub, (4) support for clients and families transitioning to home by contact with rehabilitation staff, and (5) education programs among clinicians and rehabilitation experts (Cudney & Weinert, 2000).

A key element for successful rehabilitation outcomes is for each team member to develop a creative mind-set. "Creativity is generated when persons remove themselves from the 'ruts' of their training. Thus, staff are encouraged to utilize flexibility in their thinking processes in order to tap their own, along with the client's, potential" (Jaffe & Walsh, 1993, p. 41).

Several models for home health care are cited in the literature, including the Albrecht (1990) nursing model for home health care, a model supporting the congruence between rehabilitation principles and home health nursing practice (Neal, 1999), a model integrating case management and home health care (Aliotta & Andre, 1997), the Rice model for dynamic self-determination (Rice, 1994), the Neal model of home health nursing practice (Neal, 1998), and a conceptual framework for home health nursing (Coombs, 1984).

THERAPEUTIC PROCESSES

Other theories and models address the third major concern within the Donaldson and Crowley (1978) framework, the therapeutic processes and interventions designed to produce positive health outcomes for clients (individuals, families, and groups). Within rehabilitation nursing, this concern is expanded to acknowledge the importance of the rehabilitation team and the complexities of teamwork.

PROVIDER-CENTERED MODELS

The number and type of health care providers is integrally linked to the model of rehabilitation. Staffing needs in rural settings differ from those in suburban or urban areas. Reimbursement systems and third-party payers also shape the type of providers and thus the model of rehabilitation. Models that mainly focus on the role of the provider of care include primary care, case management, nurse-managed care, and independent practice/consultation.

Primary Care

A distinction in the nursing literature and within nursing practice exists between primary nursing as a care-delivery system within inpatient settings and primary care within ambulatory care settings (Shoenhofer, 1995). Primary nursing is discussed here, and primary care is discussed later in this chapter as part of independent practice. Primary nursing as a care-delivery system emerged more than 30 years ago as a response to fragmentation and depersonalization of team nursing. Under a team nursing model, a team leader (usually a registered nurse) supervises a variety of team members in the total care for assigned clients (Lyon, 1993). Members of the nursing team perform different care functions composing the clients' total care. A drawback of the team nursing model is that each client has multiple caregivers with no individual nurse clearly accountable for coordination of all care given.

An essential feature of primary nursing is the professional nurse's 24-hour responsibility for care provided to clients to whom that nurse is assigned (Lyon, 1993). A successful primary nursing system requires considerable communication and collaboration with the client and family, as well as with others involved in the care. Thus primary nursing continues to prove useful in settings where clients have chronic conditions (Jonsdottir, 1999).

Within inpatient rehabilitation settings, primary nursing has been modified in keeping with the interdisciplinary team approach to care. Acute rehabilitation settings that successfully use a primary nursing model have sufficient staff so that each primary nurse has accountability for care of a maximum of three clients at a time (Mumma, 2000). Financial constraints and decreased availability of registered nurses may alter primary nursing.

Case Management

Case management is a delivery model of comprehensive, client-centered, continuous care provided by a multidisciplinary team—a system and a process (Coile & Matthews, 1999). A rehabilitation nurse case manager who receives a referral for initial assessment while the client is in an acute rehabilitation setting may continue to provide follow-up for the client through outpatient and home settings. The concept and purposes of case management are highly congruent with rehabilitation philosophies and purposes. Individual client goals related to maximizing functional ability and quality of life are integral to both rehabilitation and case management. Case management is discussed in detail in Chapter 10.

Examples in the literature include provision of case management services for homeless individuals (Savarese & Weber, 1993), for persons cared for within a unit-based stroke program (Brown, 2000), for persons with Alzheimer's disease living in a rural setting (Schraeder, Shelton, Dworak, & Fraser, 1993), for children undergoing craniofacial reconstruction (Schryer, 1993), for persons with high cervical spinal injury (Hoeman & Winters, 1989), for elderly individuals at risk for institutionalization (Lyon, 1993), and for frail elderly persons living in the community (Guttman, 1999).

On the basis of the extent of discussion of case management in both the nursing literature and the rehabilitation literature, it is a care-delivery model whose popularity and usefulness will continue to grow. For many rehabilitation clients with complex health care needs, the most appropriate case management system may be a well-organized interdisciplinary team with a rehabilitation nurse as case manager. Although it is important to recognize the benefits of nursing case management, it is also important to develop valid, reliable measures of its effectiveness (Hale, 1995; Lee, Mackenzie, Dudley-Brown, & Chin, 1998).

Nurse-Managed Care

Managed care has in common with case management the goal of promoting cost-effective, high-quality care. Like case management, managed care emphasizes communication and coordination among members of the health care team. Critical pathways have been defined as process standards used as adjuncts to the client's plan of care. With the addition of expected outcomes to a critical pathway, client care can then be revised based on the difference between expected and actual process outcomes (Fox, Anderson, & McKinley, 1996).

Critical pathways and care maps graph a multidisciplinary care team's actions against a time line and describe the course of hospitalization for clients with similar problems and treatment plans as well as to determine costs for populations (Crummer & Carter, 1993). A rehabilitation clinical pathway was developed at the James A. Haley Veterans Hospital in Tampa, Florida, for clients' first admission for an initial stroke (Christian et al., 1994). This clinical pathway combines features of the critical pathway and the care map to provide a time line that includes expected outcomes on a weekly basis (Table 2-2).

Independent Practice

Opportunities abound for nurses prepared for advanced practice. In an increasingly complex health system and with mandates for the highest quality of care at the lowest cost, nurse practitioners and clinical specialists are in demand. Some nurse practitioners specialize in the care of clients with chronic illness and disability. With certification for advanced practice in rehabilitation nursing (CRRN-A), more rehabilitation nurses can be expected to practice with physiatrists or to enter private practices.

Text continued on p. 32

TABLE 2-2 Clinical Pathway; Stroke—Initial Rehabilitation, First Admission

Client Needs	Week 1	Week 2	Week 3	Week 4
Medical management (MD, RN, ARNP)	Medical problems, stroke risk factors, and appropriate treatment for these are identified; client is able to verbalize these. Client is able to participate in self-medication.	Client and family are able to verbalize medical problems and stroke risk factors. Client is able to participate in self-medication program.	Client completes self-medication program.	Client and family verbalize understanding of discharge instructions and medical follow-up.
Communication (ST, OT, RN)	Client is able to follow simple directions and simple conversation. Needs cueing 90% of time. FIM-1	Client is able to follow simple directions and simple conversation. Needs cueing 75% of time. FIM-2	Client is able to follow simple directions and simple conversation. Needs cueing 50% of time. FIM-3	Client is able to follow simple directions and simple conversation. Needs cueing less than 25% of time. FIM-4
	Client is able to respond to yes/no personal information questions. Needs cueing 75% of time. FIM-2	Client is able to communicate basic needs. Needs cueing less than 50% of time. FIM-3	Client is able to communicate basic needs. Needs cueing less than 25% of time. FIM-4	Client is able to communicate basic needs. Needs cueing less than 10% of time. FIM-5
Memory (ST, OT, RN, PT)	Client recognizes and remembers 25%-50% of time. Needs prompting more than 50% of the time. Client is able to indicate awareness of memory notebook. FIM-2	Client refers to environmental cues without verbal cue 50% of time. Refers to memory notebook 25% of time without cues. FIM-3	Client refers to environmental cues. Needs prompting less than 25% of time. Refers to memory notebook 50% of time without cues. Client requires cueing to initiate memory notebook entries 50% of time. FIM-3	Client refers to environmental cues. Needs prompting less than 10% of time. Makes entries in memory notebook. Client requires cues to initiate memory notebook entries less than 25% of time. FIM-4
Problem solving (ST, OT, RN, PT)	Client identifies that a routine problem exists and is able to initiate sequence to correct less than 50% of time. FIM-2	Client initiates sequence to self-correct problems 50%-75% of time. FIM-3	Client is able to self-correct problems 75%-90% of time. FIM-4	Client is able to self-correct problems 90% of time without assistance. FIM-5
Perception sensory/visual (OT, PT, RN)	Client initiates correct body positioning and alignment. Client initiates environment scanning.	Client maintains correct body position and scans environment without cues, compensating for deficits 50% of time.	Client maintains correct body position and alignment and scans environment, compensating for deficits 75% of time.	Client maintains correct body position and alignment and scans environment, compensating for deficits 90% of time.
ADL self-care deficits (OT, RN, KT)	Client performs self-care activities of feeding, bathing, personal grooming, and dressing undressing 25%-50% of time. FIM-2	Client performs self-care activities with adaptive equipment 50%-75% of time. FIM-3	Client performs self-care activities with adaptive equipment more than 75% of time. FIM-4	Client is able to perform self-care activities with setup and supervision, using adaptive equipment. FIM-5

Dysphasia Dietary (ST, OT, RN)	Client is able to indicate awareness of swallowing difficulty. Client receives adequate nutrition via appropriate mode (TF, GT, altered food/liquid consistency, po).	Client is able to demonstrate safe compensatory swallowing techniques with max to mod supervision.	Client is able to perform safe compensatory techniques with mod to min supervision.	Client is able to perform compensatory techniques in safe swallowing techniques.
Bowel Management Neurogenic Bowel (RN)	Client initiates verbalization of need to have bowel movement. Nursing initiates bowel management program. FIM-1	Client is continent of bowel with bowel care qod with suppository. FIM-4	Client is continent of bowel with diet supplement and/or stool softener. FIM-6	Client is continent of bowel with no accidents. FIM-7
Bladder Management Neurogenic Bladder (RN)	Client initiates verbalization of need to urinate. Nursing initiates bladder training program (DC/Foley catheter, initiate PVR, ICP). FIM-1	Client uses urinal for voiding with setup; uses EUD at night. Accidents occur less than one time per day. FIM-2	Client is continent, using toilet during waking hours. Uses urinal for night voiding only. FIM-6	Client is continent of bladder with no accidents. FIM-7
Mobility (PT, KT, OT, RN)	Client will demonstrate baseline abilities in bed and wc mobility. Requires assist in bed. FIM-2 Mobility 50%-70% of time, requires assist with wc mobility 25%-50% of time. FIM-2 Client is able to perform bed, wc, chair transfers with 50%-75% assist. FIM-2 Client is able to initiate pregait activities in the parallel bars. FIM-1	Client is able to reposition self in bed 25% of time. Client is independent in wc mobility for short distances on the ward and in physical therapy clinic. FIM-5 Requires 25% assist with long-distance wc mobility. FIM-2 Client is able to perform bed, wc, chair transfers with 25% assist. FIM-4 Client is able to perform tub/toilet transfers with 50%-75% assist. FIM-2	Client performs bed positioning with less than 10% assist. Client is independent in wc mobility on the ward and to/from therapies. FIM-6 Client performs bed, wc, chair transfers with less than 10% assist. FIM-4 Client performs tub/toilet transfers with less than 25% assist. FIM-4 Client ambulates distances of 50-100 ft with assistive device and contact guard. FIM-2	Client is independent in bed mobility. Client is independent in wc mobility in all terrains, inclines, curbs, and carpeting. FIM-6 Client is independent in bed, wc, chair transfers. FIM-7 Client performs tub/toilet transfers with less than 10% assist. FIM-4 Client ambulates independently a minimum of 150 ft with assistive device and/or orthosis. FIM-6

Adapted from Janet Christian, MSW; Cindy Ochipa, PhD, SP; Pat Quigley, PhD, RN; Camela Sciabara, RN; Steven Scott, DO; Susan Smith, OTR-L; Mary Jo Soscia, MPH, PT; Cathy Williams, CTRS; James A. Haley Veterans Hospital, Tampa, Florida, Physical Medicine and Rehabilitation Service. Used with permission.

MD, Medical doctor; *RN,* registered nurse; *ARNP,* advanced registered nurse practitioner; *ST,* speech therapist; *OT,* occupational therapist; *PT,* physical therapist; *FIM,* functional independence measure; *TF,* tube feeding; *GT,* gastrostomy tube; *DC,* dilation catheter; *PVR,* postvoiding residual; *ICP,* intermittent catheter program; *EUD,* urinary device; *mod,* moderate; *min,* minimal; *max,* minimum; *wc,* wheelchair.

Continued

TABLE 2-2 Clinical Pathway; Stroke—Initial Rehabilitation, First Admission—cont'd

Client Needs	Week 1	Week 2	Week 3	Week 4
Mobility—cont'd		Client is able to initiate gait activities with assistive device and human support outside the parallel bars. FIM-1	Client is an independent household ambulator. FIM-3	
Sexual Functioning (MD, RN, ARNP)	Client and spouse will identify sexual patterns before the stroke.	Client and spouse will understand common problems of stroke patients in sexual functioning.	Client and spouse can identify supportive resources and techniques to cope mentally and physically with sexual functioning after a stroke.	Client and spouse understand adaptive skills for sexual functioning.
Skin Integrity Potential Altered Skin Integrity Actual Impaired Skin Integrity (RN, PT, OT, ARNP)	Client and family initiate preventive skin program. Client initiates skin care program (includes preventive protocol).	Client and family are aware of risk factors for altered skin integrity. Client and family able to provide minimal assist with skin care strategies Skin integrity: healing.	Client and family are able to inspect skin with supervision. Client and family perform at least 50% of skin care strategies with cueing and supervision.	Client and family inspect and perform skin care without supervision. Client and family perform skin care without supervision.
Discharge Planning (SWS, PT, OT, ST, RN)	Client and family identify current social service needs. Client and family identify tentative discharge needs. Client and family present model of home environment.	Client and family are aware of discharge options. Client and family follow up on social service referrals (i.e., food stamps, public assistance).	Client and family finalize discharge plans (i.e., home, NHCU, HBHC, home health care agency, OP, other VA).	Client and family acknowledge discharge plans completed. Successful discharge accomplished and appropriate follow-up established.
Equipment (OT, PT, KT, RN, Prosthetics, ARNP)	Client receives initial assessment of ADL and functional status to determine basic equipment needs.	Client begins training in use of assistive devices/adaptive equipment. Client and family receive necessary equipment for use on therapeutic weekend pass; receive appropriate training in use of equipment.	Client equipment needs are adjusted according to changing status. Client and family demonstrate safe use of equipment 80% of time.	Client receives all necessary equipment for postdischarge use. Client and caregiver understand safe, effective use of all equipment.
Psychosocial Needs (SWS)	Client and family participate in interview with SWS to assess psychosocial needs. Primary caregiver is identified.	Client and family receive ongoing supportive therapeutic contact.	Client and family receive ongoing supportive therapeutic contact.	Client and family demonstrate improved coping/adjustment to lifestyle change. Continue to receive ongoing supportive therapeutic contact.
Leisure (RT)	Client and/or family participate in interview to assess leisure needs (quality of life).	Client and/or family indicate awareness of adapted leisure alternatives.	Client demonstrates adapted leisure involvement to be used upon discharge.	Client and/or family demonstrate knowledge of community resources for continued quality-of-life support.

Vocational (VRT)	Client and family participate in interview process to assess vocational status and potential. Client begins vocational evaluation if appropriate.	Client and family participate as needed in exploring/accessing community or government agencies for services. Client continues participation in vocational evaluation.	Client and family participate as needed in exploring/accessing community or government agencies for services. Client and family understand results of vocational evaluation.	Client and family are knowledgeable in services provided by community and government agencies, understand how to access these to apply for appropriate vocational and/or financial assistance, and participate in follow-through with recommendations for vocational or financial assistance.
Education (MD, RN, PT, OT, KT, ST, RT, VRT, SWS, ARNP)	Client and family are aware of needs regarding communicating, cognition and swallowing, exercises, needs, diet, equipment, home care, disease process, and stroke risk factors. Client and family learn unit routines.	Client and family begin participation in training program on the ward and in therapies. Begin return demonstration of care.	Client and family able to perform home exercise programs and compensatory techniques safely.	Client and family able to demonstrate knowledge of needs, diet, home care, exercises, and equipment use. Client and family receive and verbalize understanding of printed discharge instructions. Client and family are aware of follow-up plans and supportive resources.

Adapted from Janet Christian, MSW; Cindy Ochipa, PhD, SP; Pat Quigley, PhD, RN; Camela Sciabara, RN; Steven Scott, DO; Susan Smith, OTR-L; Mary Jo Soscia, MPH, PT; Cathy Williams, CTRS; James A. Haley Veterans Hospital, Tampa, Florida, Physical Medicine and Rehabilitation Service. Used with permission.

MD, Medical doctor; *RN,* registered nurse; *ARNP,* advanced registered nurse practitioner; *ST,* speech therapist; *OT,* occupational therapist; *PT,* physical therapist; *FIM,* functional independence measure; *TF,* tube feeding; *GT,* gastrostomy tube; *DC,* dilation catheter; *PVR,* postvoiding residual; *ICP,* intermittent catheter program; *EUD,* urinary device; *mod,* moderate; *min,* minimal; *max,* minimum; *wc,* wheelchair.

Shoenhofer (1995) emphasized the importance of providing primary health care from a nursing perspective and developing ways to empower communities. Nurse-to-nurse referral and consultations benefit provider and client alike. Collaborative practice between nurse practitioners and clinical nurse specialists can be the basis for excellent, cost-effective care, using the expertise of both roles for the benefit of clients (Conger & Craig, 1998). Opportunities for consultation and independent practice can be expected to expand considerably.

COLLABORATIVE PRACTICE MODELS

Treatment teams traditionally have been considered the best way to work with clients who have multiple complex rehabilitation needs. Coordinated, concurrent care from the onset of the disability through all phases of rehabilitation is critical to achieving the best results.

Teams vary in their structure, composition and configuration, and functions. Team functions deal with the way groups operate and the tasks they are to perform. Both structure and function factor in outcomes. The traditional rehabilitation team is composed of representatives from various disciplines united in purpose to improve rehabilitation outcomes for a client. Although the combination varies according to client needs and goals, team members typically include specialists in nursing; medicine; physical, occupational, recreational, and speech therapies; psychology; social work; dietetics; and orthotics. In rehabilitation the client and family are critical team members.

Multidisciplinary, interdisciplinary, and transdisciplinary teams differ in philosophy, structure, leadership, goal-setting practices, and goal-attainment strategies.

Multidisciplinary Teams

Multidisciplinary teams combine the efforts of various disciplines. Each discipline within a multidisciplinary team submits findings and recommendations, sets their own discipline-specific goals, and works within the discipline boundaries to achieve these goals independently. Discipline-specific progress in goal attainment is communicated directly or indirectly to the rest of the team. Thus the team's outcomes are the sum of each discipline's efforts (Dean & Geiringer, 1990). Effective communication between team members is viewed as the key to success (Figure 2-1).

Many rehabilitation professionals believe that the whole is greater than the sum of its parts, emphasizing the need for integrating the efforts of team members in a holistic manner. Physical, psychological, social, and spiritual goals for each individual cannot be fully met by isolating the goals and assigning responsibility to a specific discipline. Holistic care requires that each client be viewed as a whole, with the entire team working toward the attainment of all goals. Interdisciplinary and transdisciplinary teams are more likely than are multidisciplinary teams to strive to achieve comprehensive holistic care. These methods of team interaction (interdisciplinary and transdisciplinary) have been described as synergistic in that more comprehensive outcomes are produced than any one discipline alone would be able to accomplish (Dean & Geiringer, 1990).

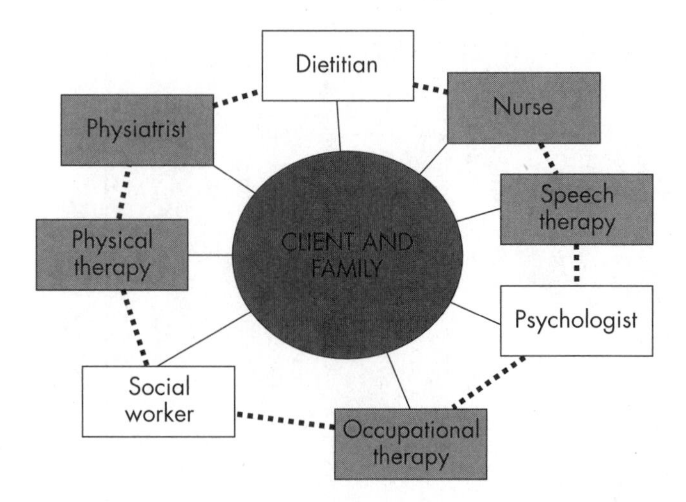

Figure 2-1 Multidisciplinary rehabilitation team, characterized by discipline-specific goals, clear boundaries between disciplines, and outcomes that are the sum of each discipline's efforts. Effective communication is the key to success for this type of team.

Interdisciplinary Teams

Collaboration replaces communication as the key to successful interdisciplinary teams. Although membership on an interdisciplinary team is quite similar to that on a multidisciplinary team, the way the disciplines function is different (Figure 2-2). Rather than each discipline identifying treatment goals, the team identifies goals and strives to avoid duplication or conflict in goals. Team members are involved in problem solving beyond the confines of their discipline. Once the team goals are identified, each discipline sets out to work toward goal attainment within the parameters of their discipline, collaborating when goals overlap discipline boundaries.

One obstacle to interdisciplinary efforts is that although each discipline is programmatically dedicated to the interdisciplinary team, organizationally they are aligned to their own discipline. To promote interdisciplinary team collaboration, some rehabilitation models have endorsed organizational changes to include a program director responsible for organizational leadership of several disciplines. Babicki and Miller-McIntyre (1992) described such a rehabilitation program model.

Transdisciplinary Teams

As resources shrink and client care demands grow, health care providers are looking for ways to accomplish goals effi-

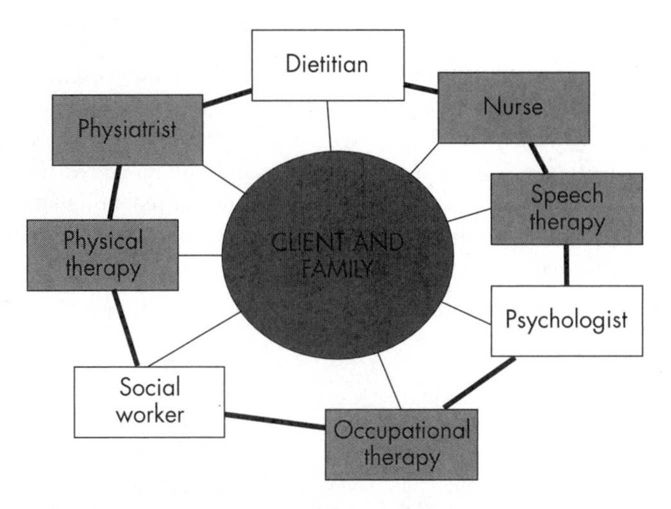

Figure 2-2 Interdisciplinary rehabilitation team. This type of team collaborates to identify client goals and is characterized by a combination of expanded problem solving beyond discipline boundaries and discipline-specific work toward goal attainment.

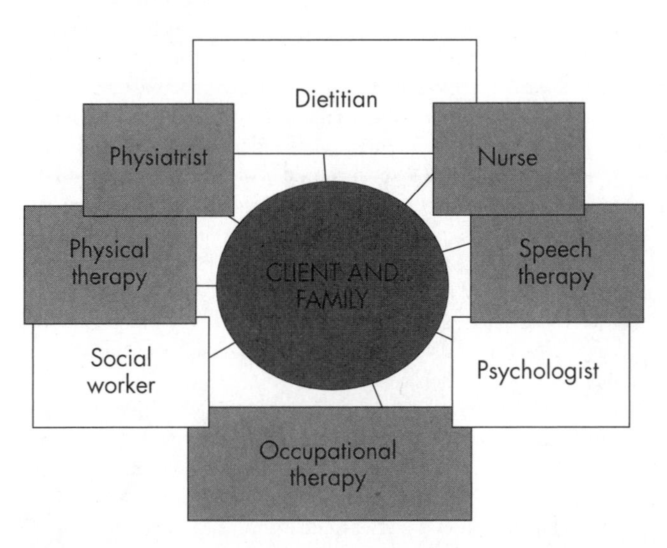

Figure 2-3 Transdisciplinary rehabilitation team, characterized by blurring of boundaries between disciplines, as well as implied cross-training and flexibility to minimize duplication of effort toward client goal attainment

ciently without jeopardizing quality. Transdisciplinary teams maximize the strengths of team members and minimize duplication in effort (Figure 2-3). One member of the team is selected to be the primary therapist (Diller, 1990). The identified primary therapist varies with each client, depending on the specific client needs. The other team members contribute information and advice through this identified primary therapist. In this way the team plans implementation to reduce joint collaboration when one team member can effectively accomplish the task, regardless of discipline. Transdisciplinary teamwork involves a certain amount of boundary blurring between disciplines and implies cross-training and flexibility in accomplishing tasks. Determining the range of capability of various team members is essential, and team members must be receptive and learn to cope with a wider domain of functioning. Hoeman (1993) described a transdisciplinary team model for the care of infants with special needs.

Future of Teams in Rehabilitation

The future use of teams in rehabilitation must begin with a critical analysis of the strengths and weaknesses of this approach to care delivery. Noted rehabilitation professionals have indicated that health care reform and the economic climate are working against the team approach (Diller, 1990; Schofield & Amodeo, 1999).

Major strengths of the team method of care delivery are that it is well established, promotes good communication and collaboration among disciplines, addresses comprehensive aspects of care, energizes staff, and views the client holistically (Gibbon, 1999; Wagner, 2000).

Weaknesses of the team approach may include cost, inefficiency, and reduction in time for direct client care. Rothberg (1981) stated that the team approach places psychological strain on staff. Problems related to role diffusion, ambiguity, status concerns, interpersonal conflicts, lack of commitment of some team members, and concerns regarding competency have been identified (Diller, 1990; Gibbon, 1999). From an operational standpoint, coordinated, cooperative, and goal-directed teamwork often is difficult to achieve.

Although the comprehensive treatment team has been viewed as the foundation of rehabilitation, Schofield and Amodeo (1999) questioned whether the team approach will erode in the face of economic constraints and health care reform. Accounts of third-party payers opting for a limited number of specific services, rather than paying for comprehensive care, are becoming more common. As health care reform continues to unfold, service delivery restructuring is already under way. Keith (1991) questioned the effectiveness of comprehensive treatment teams in rehabilitation, citing cost, inefficiency, and lack of research documenting the value of teams. He advocated the development of alternate treatment models, altering the configuration of teams to make them smaller, with access to consultation from other specialties, including the use of rehabilitation technicians to address the shortage of health care professionals. Although not everyone would agree with Keith's recommendations for the future, health care professionals clearly need to be creative and responsive to the changing health care environment.

SUMMARY

The nursing models and theories and rehabilitation-relevant models and theories from other disciplines described in this chapter, discussed within the framework of Donaldson and

Crowley's three major concerns (1978) for the discipline of nursing, provide organization for provision of rehabilitation nursing care. Whichever models or theories form the basis of care delivery in particular settings, services need to be integrated, comprehensive, and appropriate. Rehabilitation nurses—diverse in expertise, roles, and work settings—play a critical role in the effective use of models and theories for rehabilitation.

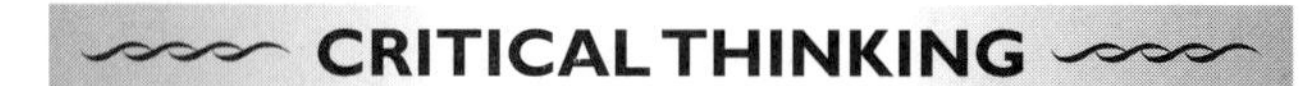

CRITICAL THINKING

1. How would the nurse's role differ within a transdisciplinary rehabilitation team compared with a multidisciplinary team?
2. Describe several strategies that can facilitate active involvement of the client and family in the rehabilitation program within an environmentally focused nursing practice model.

Case Study

Joe H., a 17-year-old high school senior, experienced a closed head injury (traumatic brain injury) about a month ago as a result of a motor vehicle accident. He was a passenger in an automobile driven by a friend who was giving Joe and several other friends a ride home from a party. Everyone had been drinking beer. Joe's friend ran a red light, and the car was struck on the driver's side. The driver was killed on impact. The other passengers experienced minor injuries and recovered sufficiently to return to school within a few days after the accident.

Joe was transported to the hospital by paramedics and was cared for in the intensive care unit for 3 days and in a medical-surgical unit for 2 weeks. Joe's brain injury was primarily to the right frontal and parietal lobes, with diffuse cortical impairment due to concussive forces. Joe also had a fractured right femur and left radius, which were both treated with internal fixation. During the second week in the medical-surgical unit, he was assessed by a nurse case manager from the acute rehabilitation facility to determine his care needs and his readiness for transfer to rehabilitation. He has now been in the acute rehabilitation facility for 13 days. On admission he was alert and agitated, with a short attention span and behavior that seemed inappropriate to the situation and was generally nonpurposeful. He is currently confused but nonagitated most of the time. He does become agitated by too much visual or auditory stimulation.

As Joe's cognition has improved, he has become depressed. He is increasingly aware of his deficits and is also grieving the death of his friend. Joe has many visitors; sometimes as many as five teenage friends come to see him. He is limited to one visitor at a time, for brief periods, to minimize agitation. His girlfriend and his mother stay with him for longer periods and assist with his rehabilitation program because they have a calming effect on him. Joe's parents are divorced, and Joe's father visits Joe only occasionally. On several of his visits, he became angry with Joe and told Joe to "shape up and start behaving." He also told Joe that the injury was Joe's own fault because he had been drinking at the party and should have known better than to get in a car with a driver who also had been drinking. The psychiatric clinical nurse specialist has set up several appointments with Joe's father, but he has not kept the appointments. He also said that he is too busy to meet with the rehabilitation team. Joe was visibly upset after his father's most recent visit and said that he did not want to see his dad for now. Joe's goal is to get home and back to school as soon as possible so he can graduate with his class.

Six weeks later, it is the decision of the rehabilitation team that Joe is ready for discharge from the acute rehabilitation facility. His case has been assessed by a nurse case manager who works with the insurance company that handles his health insurance. There has been little change in Joe's functional abilities in the past 2 weeks. He is able to walk with standby assistance and becomes unsteady after walking about 50 feet because of right lower extremity weakness. Joe is independent in dressing and undressing, needs standby assistance in the shower, and feeds himself. He has good urinary and bowel control. He continues to have cognitive problems, primarily distractibility, impaired problem solving, and impaired judgment. He is frustrated easily, with occasional angry outbursts. He wants to drive and to return to school. The team assessment is that he is not ready for school or driving yet, and it is also not safe for him to be left alone at home all day while his mother works.

Joe is discharged from the acute rehabilitation facility to a day treatment program within a long-term head trauma rehabilitation setting. He attends the program all day, Monday through Friday, and is home with his family at night and on weekends. As anticipated, Joe makes slow, steady progress in the day treatment program and is discharged from the program after 6 months. He then lives at home and attends outpatient therapy sessions for 2 to 3 hours, 3 days a week. He returns to the school the following semester and successfully completes high school. After graduation, he passes the driving test, and his parents give him a car for a graduation present. Currently he is taking community college courses and expects to move out of his mother's home within a year or so. In the opinion of the rehabilitation team, including Joe and his family, Joe's rehabilitation program was a success.

Joe's overall rehabilitation program included acute rehabilitation, day treatment at a long-term head trauma facility, and outpatient rehabilitation. The combination of services used by specific clients will vary based on client needs and preferences, client insurance coverage and financial resources, and available rehabilitation resources.

REFERENCES

Administration on Aging. (2000). *Profile of older Americans: 2000.* http://www.aoa.dhhs.gov/aoa/STATS/profile/.

Albrecht, M.N. (1990). The Albrecht nursing model for home health care: Implications for research, practice, and education. *Public Health Nursing, 7,* 118-126.

Aliotta, S. & Andre, J. (1997). Case management and home healthcare: an integrated model. *Home Healthcare Management & Practice, 9*(2), 1-2.

Anderson, K.H. (2000). The family health system approach to family systems nursing. *Journal of Family Nursing, 6*(2), 103-117.

Babicki, C., & Miller-McIntyre, K. (1992). A rehabilitation programmatic model: The clinical nurse specialist perspective. *Rehabilitation Nursing, 17,* 84-86.

Bandura, A. (1986). *Social foundations of thought and action: social cognitive theory.* Englewood Cliffs, NJ: Prentice-Hall.

Brothers, F.H. (1998). The rehabilitation home health nurse and pediatric clients. In L.J. Neal (Ed.), *Rehabilitation nursing in the home health setting* (pp. 175-186). Glenview, IL: Association of Rehabilitation Nurses.

Broughton, B., & Lutner, N. (1995). Chronic childhood illness: A nursing health-promotion model for rehabilitation in the community. *Rehabilitation Nursing, 20*(6), 318-322.

Brown, M.J. (2000). Stroke management: Beginnings. *Outcomes Management for Nursing Practice, 4*(1), 34-38.

Burks, K. (1999). A nursing practice model for chronic illness. *Rehabilitation Nursing, 24*(5), 197-200.

Campbell, I., & Case, C. (1999). Client management in the subacute unit. *Lippincott's Primary Care Practice. Long-Term Care, 3*(2), 231-241.

Christian, J., Ochipa, C., Quigley, P., Sciabara, C., Scott, S., Smith, S., Soscia, M.J., & Williams, C. (1994). *Clinical pathway: Stroke—Initial rehabilitation, first admission.* Tampa, FL: James A. Haley Veterans Hospital. Unpublished document.

Coile, R.C., & Matthews, P. (1999). Nursing case management in the millennium: Two perspectives. *Nursing Case Management, 4*(6), 244-254.

Conger, M., & Craig, C. (1998). Advanced nurse practice: A model for collaboration. *Nursing Case Management, 3*(3), 120-127.

Coombs, E. (1984). A conceptual framework for home nursing. *Journal of Advance Nursing, 9*(2), 157-163.

Corbin, J.M., & Strauss, A. (1992). A nursing model for chronic illness management based on the trajectory framework. In P. Woog (Ed.), *The chronic illness trajectory framework: The Corbin and Strauss nursing model* (pp. 9-28). New York: Springer.

Cromes, G.F., & Helm, P.A. (1992). The status of burn rehabilitation services in the United States: Results of a national survey. *Journal of Burn Care and Rehabilitation, 13,* 656-662.

Crummer, M.B., & Carter, V. (1993). Critical pathways—the pivotal tool. *Journal of Cardiovascular Nursing, 7,* 30-37.

Cudney, S.A., & Weinert, C. (2000). Computer-based support groups: Nursing in cyberspace. *Computers in Nursing, 18*(1), 35-43.

Davis, S., & O'Connor, S. (Eds). (1999). *Rehabilitation nursing: Foundations for practice.* London: Harcourt Brace.

Dean, B.Z., & Geiringer, S.R. (1990). Physiatric therapeutics. The rehabilitation team: Behavioral management Part 6. *Archives of Physical Medicine and Rehabilitation, 71*(Suppl. 4), 275-277.

Diller, L. (1990). Fostering the interdisciplinary team: Fostering research in a society in transition. *Archives of Physical Medicine and Rehabilitation, 71,* 275-278.

Donaldson, S.K., & Crowley, D.M. (1978). The discipline of nursing. *Nursing Outlook, 26*(2), 113-120.

Fox, S.W., Anderson, B.J., & McKinley, W.O. (1996). Case management and critical pathways: Links to quality care for persons with spinal cord injury. *American Rehabilitation, 22,* 20-26.

Fuhrer, M.J. (1998). The national center for medical rehabilitation research: Beyond infancy, looking toward maturity. *American Journal of Physical Medicine and Rehabilitation, 77*(5), 437-443.

Garrett, R., & Shapcott, N. (1998, November 26). *Applications of videoconferencing in rehabilitation.* Presented at the First South Australian Seminar on Technology for People with Disabilities (ARATA).

Gibbon, B. (1999). An investigation of interprofessional collaboration in stroke rehabilitation team conferences. *Journal of Clinical Nursing, 8*(3), 246-252.

Gill, H.S., & Rovinsky, M. (1998). Strategic implications of developing integrated levels of care. *Managed Care Quarterly, 6*(2), 21-30.

Gordon, M. (2000). *Manual of nursing diagnosis* (9th ed.). St. Louis: Mosby.

Gordon, S. (1994). Patient-driven system. *Critical Care Nurse, June,* 3-28.

Guttman, R. (1999). Case management of the frail elderly in the community. *Clinical Nurse Specialist, 13*(4), 174-178.

Habel, M. (1993). Rehabilitation nursing practice. In A.E. McCourt (Ed.), *The specialty practice of rehabilitation nursing: A core curriculum* (3rd ed., pp. 1-23). Skokie, IL: Rehabilitation Nursing Foundation.

Hale, C. (1995). Research issues in case management. *Nursing Standard, 9*(44), 29-32.

Hoeman, S. (1992). Community-based rehabilitation. *Holistic Nursing Practice, 6,* 32-41.

Hoeman, S. (1993). A research-based transdisciplinary team model for infants with special needs and their families. *Holistic Nursing Practice, 7,* 63-72.

Hoeman, S.P. (1996). Conceptual bases for rehabilitation nursing. In S.P. Hoeman (Ed.), *Rehabilitation Nursing* (2nd ed., pp. 3-20). St. Louis: Mosby.

Hoeman, S.P., & Winters, D.M. (1989). Theory-based case management: High cervical spinal cord injury. *Home Healthcare Nurse, 8,* 25-33.

Jaffe, K.B., & Walsh, P.A. (1993). The development of the specialty rehabilitation home care team: Supporting the creative thought process. *Holistic Nursing Practice, 7,* 36-41.

Jonsdottir, H. (1999). Outcomes of implementing primary nursing in the care of people with chronic lung diseases: The nurses' experience. *Journal of Nursing Management, 7*(4), 235-242.

Kaplan, L.C. (1999). Community-based disability services in the USA: A pediatric perspective. *Lancet, 354*(9180), 761-762.

Keith, R.A. (1991). The comprehensive treatment team in rehabilitation. *Archives of Physical Medicine and Rehabilitation, 72,* 269-274.

Lander, S. (1996). Motivation in geriatric rehabilitation. *Journal of the American Geriatrics Society, 44*(7), 891-892.

Lavallee, D.J., & Crupi, C.D. (1992). Rehabilitation takes to the road. *Holistic Nursing Practice, 6,* 60-66.

Law, M., Baptiste, S., & Mills, J. (1995). Client-centered practice: What does it mean and does it make a difference?

Law, M., Darrah, J., Pollack, N., King, G., Rosenbaum, P., Russell, D., Palisano, R., Harris, S., Armstrong, R., & Watt, J. (1998). Family-centered functional therapy for children with cerebral palsy: An emerging practice model. *Physical and Occupational Therapy in Pediatrics, 18*(1), 83-102.

Lee, D., Mackenzie, A., Dudley-Brown, S., & Chin, T. (1998). Case management: A review of the definitions and practices. *Journal of Advanced Nursing, 27*(5), 933-939.

Levine, K. (1996). Internet update. *OT Update, 1*(18), 14-15.

Lorig, K., Stewart, A., Ritter, P., Gonzalez, V., Laurent, D., & Lynch, J. (1996). *Outcomes measures for health education and other health care intervention.* Thousand Oaks, CA: Sage.

Lyon, J.C. (1993). Models of nursing care delivery and case management: Clarification of terms. *Nursing Economics, 11,* 163- 169.

Mayo, N.E., Wood-Dauphinee, S., & Cote, R. (2000). Prompt hospital discharge and home rehab is more beneficial for stroke patients. *Geriatrics, 55*(8), 60-61.

McCourt, A.E. (Ed.). (1993). *The specialty practice of rehabilitation nursing: A core curriculum* (3rd ed.). Skokie, IL: Rehabilitation Nursing Foundation.

Moffa-Trotter, M.E., & Anemaet, W.K. (1999). Cost effectiveness of home rehabilitation: A literature review. *Topics in Geriatric Rehabilitation, 14*(4), 1-33.

Mumma, C.M. (2000). *Personal notes on theory based practice.*

Neal, L. (1998). The Neal Model of home health nursing practice. In L.J. Neal (Ed.), *Rehabilitation nursing in the home health setting* (pp. 263-279). Glenview, IL: Association of Rehabilitation Nurses.

Neal, L. (1999). Research supporting the congruence between rehabilitation principles and home health nursing practice. *Rehabilitation Nursing, 24*(3), 115-121.

Nelson, A. (1990). Patients' perspectives of a spinal cord injury unit. *Journal of Spinal Cord Injury Nursing, 7* (3), 44-64.

Oldridge, N.B. (1997). Outcome assessment in cardiac rehabilitation: Health-related quality of life and economic evaluation. *Journal of Cardiopulmonary Rehabilitation, 17*(3), 179-194.

Orem, D. (1995). *Nursing concepts of practice* (5th ed.). St. Louis: Mosby.

Phipps, M. (1990). Rehabilitation nursing specialist practice in an acute care setting. *Nursing Administration Quarterly 14,* 12-16.

Pierce, L., & Salter, J. (1997). Family systems theory: A multicultural perspective. In K. Johnson (Ed.), *Advanced practice nursing in rehabilitation: A core curriculum* (pp. 42-50). Glenview, IL: Rehabilitation Nursing Foundation.

Radford, M.J. (1998). Clinical sidebar. *Image—The Journal of Nursing Scholarship, 30*(2), 177.

Reynolds, C.L., & Leininger, M.M. (1993). *Madeleine Leininger: Cultural care diversity and universality theory.* Newbury Park, CA: Sage.

Rice, R. (1994). Procedures in home care conceptual framework for nursing practice in the home: The Rice model for dynamic self-examination. *Home Healthcare Nurse, 12*(2), 51-53.

Robinson, C. (1995). Beyond dichotomies in the nursing of persons and families. *Image—The Journal of Nursing Scholarship, 27*(2), 116-120.

Rogers, M.E. (1990). Nursing: Science of unitary, irreducible human beings: Update 1990. In E. Barrett (Ed.), *Patterns of nursing theories in practice* (pp. 83-92). New York: National League for Nursing.

Ronning, O.M., & Guldvog, B. (1998). Outcome of subacute stroke rehabilitation: A randomized controlled trial. *Stroke, 29*(4), 779-784.

Roper, N., Logan, W., & Tierney, A. (1996). *The elements of nursing: A model for nursing based on a model of living* (4th ed.). Edinburgh: Churchill-Livingstone.

Rothberg, J. (1981). The rehabilitation team: Future directions. *Archives of Physical Medicine and Rehabilitation.* 62, 407-410.

Roy, C., Sr., & Andrews, H.A. (1991). *The Roy adaptation model: The definitive statement.* Norwalk, CT: Appleton & Lange.

Savarese, M., & Weber, C.M. (1993). Case management for persons who are homeless. *Journal of Case Management, 2,* 3-8.

Schoenhofer, S.O. (1995). Rethinking primary care: Connections to nursing. *Advances in Nursing Science, 17*(4), 12-21.

Schofield, R.F., & Amodeo, M. (1999). Interdisciplinary teams in health care and human services settings: Are they effective? *Health and Social Work, 24*(3), 210-219.

Schraeder, C., Shelton, P., Dworak, D., & Fraser, C. (1993). Alzheimer's disease: Case management in a rural setting. *Journal of Case Management, 2,* 26-31.

Schryer, N. (1993). Nursing case management for children undergoing craniofacial reconstruction. *Plastic Surgical Nursing, 13,* 17-28.

Seelman, K. (1996, October 30). *Rehabilitation engineering: Today's solutions, tomorrow's challenges.* Charleston, SC: Switzer Lecture Association of Schools of Allied Health Professions (ASAHP).

Stephenson, K., Yee, B., & Lisse, J. (1997). Adaptive coping skills for older African Americans with arthritis. *Topics in Geriatric Rehabilitation, 12,* 75-87.

Thompson, T.L.C. (1990). *A qualitative investigation of rehabilitation nursing in an inpatient rehabilitation unit using Leininger's theory.* Unpublished doctoral dissertation, Wayne State University, Detroit, MI.

Tolson, D., & Stephens, D. (1997). Age-related hearing loss in the dependent elderly population: A model for nursing care. *International Journal of Nursing Practice, 3,* 224-230.

Von Sternberg, T., Hepbern, K., Cibuzar, P., Convery, L., Dokken, B., Haefemeyer, J., Rettke, S., Ripley, J., Vosenau, V., Rothe, P., Schurle, D., & Won-Savage, R. (1997). Post-hospital sub-acute care: An example of a managed care model. *Journal of American Geriatrics Society, 45,* 87-91.

Wagner, E. (2000). The role of patient care teams in chronic illness management. *British Medical Journal, 320*(7234), 569-572.

Whittemore, R. (2000). Strategies to facilitate lifestyle change associated with diabetes mellitus. *Journal of Nursing Scholarship, 32*(3), 225-233.

Wright, B. (1983). *Physical disability: A psychosocial approach.* New York: HarperCollins.

Zejdlik, C.M. (Ed.). (1999). *Management of spinal cord injuries* (3rd ed.). Boston: Jones & Bartlett.

3 Legislation and Policy

Gloria T. Aubut Craven, MS, RN
Carol A. Gleason, MM, RN, CRRN, CCM, LRC

Nurses practicing in clinical settings often believe two things about government politics and policy: that they have no role in government and that they have no ability to effect changes in government. Contributors to this chapter challenged those assumptions in 1990 when approval of the Massachusetts Nurse Practice Act was pending in the state legislature. The result changed nursing practice throughout the Commonwealth of Massachusetts.

Studies have revealed that nurses have limited access to basic information about legislative issues affecting their practice. One in every 44 voters in Massachusetts is a nurse, a fact that could effect change. To inform nurses and stimulate political action, the contributors formed a new company and, from 1990 to 1995, published a monthly newsletter titled PLAN, Pertinent Legislation Affecting Nurses. *Former Speaker of the House Tip O'Neill endorsed the premier issue. The review of legislation informed nurses about pending legislation and how to influence laws to reflect nursing standards and philosophy.*

Under PLAN, *the contributors conducted annual research and educational seminars. One program was held during the time of the national debates on health financing and proposals for a single-payer system. The* PLAN *conference site was arranged in the historic, prestigious John F. Kennedy Library, and First Lady Hillary R. Clinton was invited to attend.*

On the conference day, the library was filled with, among others, delegations from the Board of Registration in Nursing and the Massachusetts Nurses Association, attorneys, and federal and state legislators. When the video screen, 2 stories high and 20 feet wide, dropped from the ceiling of the John F. Kennedy Library, it captured the attention and awe of all in the conference room. The First Lady addressed the conference through video brought by her representative, a federal nurse who served on the White House Task Force on Health Care Reform. Thus nurses working through PLAN *indelibly affected legislation for nursing practice in Massachusetts.*

Health care combines clinical skill, access to services, and reimbursement. Laws that govern nursing practice and care delivery dictate each component in part. Business trends and health economics also influence how care is delivered. This chapter is devoted to rehabilitation nurses' understanding of laws that affect rehabilitation clients and the impact of legislation and government actions on nursing practice. No area of practice is unaffected by law or regulation, and laws perform the following functions:

- Govern the scope of nursing practice
- Protect the registered nurse (RN) licensure title
- Define which services are provided, to whom, in which setting, and at what price
- Finance basic nursing education and nursing research
- Are the forum for ethical issues related to health care delivery dilemmas

Rehabilitation nursing practice is uniquely tied to law and regulation because rehabilitation grew from federal laws after both World Wars, when veterans returned home with disabilities. Disability definitions have broadened; however, laws that support a philosophy of adaptation to a disability have been enhanced only in the twentieth century.

This chapter clarifies regulations that rehabilitation nurses need to understand as client advocates, including laws that will affect practice in the early twenty-first century. Major legal aspects of rehabilitation law, financing laws and regulations, and legal-ethical issues that affect rehabilitation nursing practice are discussed. This chapter will integrate information about laws, regulations, and trends concerning delivery of care. Political activism is presented as a component of professional nursing practice.

REHABILITATION LAWS AND REGULATIONS: EFFECTS ON CLIENTS AND EMERGING ROLES FOR REHABILITATION NURSES

It is imperative for nurse advocates to understand both financing laws and disability laws. Examples of how major legislation affects clients are highlighted in the following discussion of legislation.

Funding Legislation

Major changes in health care delivery and health care financing began in 1983, when reimbursement mechanisms through medicare and medicaid were altered. Acute care hospitals received reimbursement according to a new formula under diagnosis-related groupings (DRGs), effectively abolishing traditional fee-for-service financing. Essentially, each admission is categorized by diagnosis, and hospitals are paid a fixed rate, regardless of the cost of care and the length of stay. For example, when a person is admitted with a diagnosis of cerebral vascular accident, whether the length of stay is 1 day or 2 months, the hospital receives a payment preauthorized for that diagnosis. The revenue incentive then is shifted to one of early discharge to offset the costs of those with complications or prolonged lengths of stay. This public policy, financing law, and trend has affected rehabilitation clients significantly, influencing both lengths of stay and discharge planning of all kinds.

Many health care systems and rehabilitation institutions are seeking ways to measure the actual costs of care. One such example is Class Act, the client classification system used by the Braintree Hospital Rehabilitation Network in Massachusetts. This activity-based resource-allocation system captures the unique characteristics of the rehabilitation client and reflects the required nursing care and the skill mix necessary to provide safe, efficient, and cost-effective care. "Charging for nursing services according to their actual consumption of the various types of nursing services, the hospital now uses the data generated by the activity based costing system in contract negotiations with insurance carriers and for management decisions concerning nursing work flow trends and staffing" (Crockett, DiBlasi, Flaherty, & Sampson, 1997, p. 298).

The health insurance industry changed mechanisms for payment of services to clients and providers. The traditional fee-for-service model, in which the consumer chose the provider and paid an annual deductible and medicare and private insurance companies were billed for services rendered, gave way to managed care as the predominant mechanism for reimbursement. Managed care offers payment at a preset premium and restricts consumers to a primary care physician (PCP) network, in which the PCPs act as gatekeepers for services. Usually services must be obtained at a designated facility, where rates have been established. Members who choose care elsewhere may be responsible for charges.

The most important legislation funding health care in the twentieth century was the Balanced Budget Act (BBA) of 1997. This legislation created a Prospective Payment System (PPS) that regulates payments to skilled nursing facilities (SNFs). To reduce the costs of health care, the government placed the risks of care delivery onto those who provide the services. Under PPS, the minimum data set (MDS) serves to determine a score in 1 of 44 resource utilization groups (RUGs). The RUG groups the clients according to care needs. Each RUG is assigned a payment rate. If use of services exceeds the RUG, the provider incurs a loss. Costs are all-inclusive and must be tracked carefully. MDS assessments are done on set schedules. The review of days 1 to 5 authorizes payment for client days 1 to 14. The review of days 11 to 14 seeks payment for days 15 to 30. The MDS assessment of days 21 to 29 covers payment for days 31 to 60. The MDS assessment of days 50 to 59 covers care rendered from days 61 to 90. The data from days 80 to 89 account for payment from days 91 to 100. Timely and accurate billing is one way to ensure payment of claims (Mariner Health Group, 1998).

Rehabilitation nursing knowledge is crucial in this planning process because predetermined care needs must be assessed and accurately recommended to ensure payment. Cost predictions and allocation of services are the responsibility of each team member, but the MDS nursing coordinator makes the final determination for payment. The purpose of PPS is client-focused, goal-oriented care. The enactment of the parameters of this financing law actually created a role for a well-versed nurse, whose specialty in rehabilitation could match the needs of clients with the financing of health care. This role is known as the rehabilitation MDS nurse coordinator. This position is crucial to the delivery of and financing for client care. In the last quarter of 1998, some SNFs were phased into the new reimbursement changes, as the PPS was first instituted. Most SNFs began documentation for PPS in January 1999. Rates were phased in at different levels and, at the time of this printing, continue to evolve.

The Interim Payment System (IPS) is part of the legislation and establishes a PPS for home health care using the Outcome and Assessment Information Set (OASIS). Acute rehabilitation hospitals will have PPS and some payment reductions. This will involve a 3-year phase-in project with a single payment based on a Functional Related Group (FRG), and as with the DRG, clients will be categorized by type. Two factors are key—the functional impairment classification based on diagnosis, such as the client with a traumatic brain injury, and the level of functional impairment. Another new coding system, the MDS for Postacute Care (MDS-PAC), will be used, and providers will obtain scores from evaluations during the admission process. Critical assessment of each client need is vital to receiving payment for services rendered. Data entry and collection are evaluated for time and accuracy; critical thinking, teaching, and planning times are reimbursed; and nursing care is a billable service, no longer part of room and board. Evaluations of this new system are in progress. Inclusion of nursing intensity for thinking and planning of care is important for rehabilitation nurses and clients because they will set the standards for future billable services. It is the first time that nursing staff actions have been included in the funding equations.

The Balanced Budget Refinement Act of 1999 was signed into law on November 29. The intention of this legislation was for financial relief to SNFs. Effective April 1, 2000, this bill allows SNFs to elect to bypass the transition to the PPS and be paid at the full federal rate. They also receive a temporary increase in payment for certain high-cost clients in 15 RUGs. These RUGs will have a 4% increase in fiscal years 2001 and 2002. Another provision is a short list of exclusions for certain ambulance services, prostheses, and chemotherapy drugs and some from consolidated billing, such as physician services.

Additionally the application of a 15% reduction in payment rates for home health services is delayed until a year after enactment of the implementation of home health PPS. The Act also created the State Children's Health Insurance Program (SCHIP), giving states an enhanced federal matching rate for covering uninsured children from low-income families in a separate state-run insurance program, a medicaid expansion, or a combination of the two. This program eliminated the program known as Aid to Families with Dependent Children (AFDC). The implication for rehabilitation nurses is a need to know individual state laws and program parameters. Many other changes in the Balanced Budget Refinement Act of 1999 (Public Law 106-113) can be reviewed in their entirety (www.HCFA.gov) to identify provisions that affect rehabilitation nursing practice.

Disability Laws

In addition to funding, rehabilitation nursing has been affected by passage of laws specific to disabled persons. The Americans with Disabilities Act of 1990 (ADA), one of the most important pieces of legislation in the latter half of the twentieth century, has become familiar throughout society, even to school children. In the United States children grow up with the societal changes that reinforce "justice" for all and greater acceptance of disability throughout the community.

Passage of the ADA has had micro and macro effects on the economy. The individual as a contributing member of the community with reasonable accommodation in the workplace is a key provision of this law. Employers often can comply with simple workstation redesigns, and increased awareness of cost savings can result in employment of persons with disabilities in a supportive environment. Enforcement includes the right to civil action when discrimination is based on disability, and some cases have been brought to trial. The ADA cannot answer questions for each situation but can provide a framework to assist in the decision-making process and hopefully ensure civil rights for all, but not without controversy. Coverage of the human immunodeficiency virus as a disability fueled many heated discussions during the legislative process, but its inclusion in the law offers protection today. Other arguments, such as drug and/or alcohol addiction or mental illness as a disability, continue to stir emotional controversy, especially because these conditions may be considered self-inflicted. Those who prepared the ADA hoped to educate the public about discrimination against persons with these types of condition and to increase awareness within the medical profession about conditions with an organic origin (Wikinson & Dresden, 1996).

The ADA was amended in 1999, creating the Ticket to Work and Self-Sufficiency Program. In the past, when disabled persons became gainfully employed, they risked the loss of vital health and social security benefits. The disincentive to work was real because the probability of a disability causing some changes in work productivity was real. In general, this new law guarantees that persons with disabilities may obtain vocational rehabilitation services, employment services, and other support services without risking the loss of other vital services provided those with disabilities, such as medicaid or social security disability insurance benefits. It encourages disabled persons to be gainfully employed, not be forced to live in poverty, and it ensures critical benefits packages.

The ADA is the beginning process for eliminating societal discrimination based on a disability. There may be overlaps between the ADA and individual state disability laws. Rehabilitation nurses should understand basic provision of the law and its impact on rehabilitation services and enhancing quality of life. Table 3-1 lists some of the basic provision of the ADA and its impact on nursing practice. Rehabilitation nurses need to monitor this law over time and be ready to use their unique knowledge to support amendments because future situations may warrant nursing interventions.

In addition to being involved with client-centered activities, rehabilitation nurses can advocate by serving on local disability commissions and developing relationships with elected officials to positively influence legislation for disabled persons. Nurses may run support groups, educate community groups with regard to disability, host cable channels on disability issues, and get involved in the causes of the Disabled American Veterans and the homeless, who are often disabled.

Other laws passed in the 1990s are pertinent to rehabilitation practice. In 1993 the basic premise of the Family and Medical Leave Act (FMLA) was to require employers with more than 50 employees to provide up to 12 weeks of unpaid job-protected leave for health-related problems of the employee or their family member. It is a critical law for rehabilitation nurses to understand because many families need this benefit to care for their loved one after a debilitating accident or illness.

In 1994 the Amendment and Technology Related Assistance for Individuals with Disabilities Act (Public Law 103-218) was passed, strengthening the 1988 law and providing grants to states to increase and promote available assistive technology. An example is the voice-activated computer. The

TABLE 3-1 Provisions of the ADA and the Impact on Disabled Persons

Provisions of the Law	Client Implications	Examples of Rehabilitation Nursing Interventions
Employment: ADA prevents discrimination in employment	Rehabilitation clients must be reasonably accommodated in the work site; focus is on ability and use of technological supports	Nurses coordinate an interdisciplinary team referral with an occupational or physical therapy evaluation for work site design Rehabilitation nurses provide educational services for employers regarding limits of the disability and how to accommodate for optimal client outcomes Team members may arrange for evaluation for computer-assisted technologies and grants for that equipment Nurses conduct and publish research findings on client outcomes related to ADA provisions
Public services	Access to public services provided by governmental agencies, such as public transportation via bus and rail and new-building and architectural accommodations	Rehabilitation nurses serve as consultants on building design and accommodations for local, state, and national governmental agencies Educate families and clients about special transportation and how to gain access Use credentials when writing to lawmakers and the media identifying deficiencies with accommodations or access
Public accommodations and services operated by public entities	This provision affects public accommodations in private existing business, commercial facilities, and public transportation offered in private existing businesses	Educate disabled persons about their rights to private accommodations in places such as bed and breakfast establishments, hotels, parks, entertainment centers, schools, convention centers, and shopping centers
Telecommunications	Adaptations for hearing and/or speech impairments must be provided; some public telephones must be wheelchair accessible	Educate families and clients about ways to accommodate personal telecommunications and technologies
Miscellaneous provisions	Allow future enhancement to ADA through state and local laws	Nurses become aware of local and state laws, which supersede ADA, and advocate for rehabilitation clients Nurses pursue ways of making accommodations of private health care buildings be accessible
Ticket to Work and Self-Sufficiency (1999 amendment)	Access to vocational and occupational rehabilitation services without loss of other benefits; opportunity for gainful employment without loss of disability benefits	Educate clients and families to access state rehabilitation commission and programs Educate client and family to availability of medicaid and other benefits Provide emotional support to diminish social isolation Encourage self-reliance and self-respect to promote healing

Health Insurance Portability Accountability Act (HIPAA) of 1996 was designed to protect the health insurance coverage for workers and families when a worker changes or loses a job. It is crucial if the wage earner has medical issues or has been involved in a catastrophic incident.

HEALTH CARE DELIVERY TRENDS AND ISSUES: NURSING SEQUELAE

The principles of economics involve the simple basics of human behavior: scarcity, choices, and how choices are made. Our society has unlimited wants. Because time and finances dictate purchasing power, individuals cannot have everything they want (Boyes & Melvin, 1994). Students of economics can predict why persons go through certain purchasing cycles to satisfy their self-interests and to yield satisfaction. Economists study these principles carefully because the BBA of 1997 sent health care economics into a tailspin. Controls, tightened to prevent waste and enforced to preserve social services, led to development of many economic-driven changes. Hospitals merged within shared catchment areas to form larger organizations or systems, which allowed them to condense services, with, for example, one hospital performing cardiac surgery and another specializing in trauma care. Hospital systems were able to purchase health care insurance at reduced rates because more persons needed coverage in a larger system, and purchasing power forced cost reductions from many suppliers. The hospital systems enhanced computer systems to accommodate mergers, Y2K technologies, and consolidated billing, expenses that were absorbed internally. But the high costs of mergers required a complementary increase in client census and led to staff downsizing and clashes of organizational cultures. Health care is big business, and rehabilitation nurses need to understand how economics play key roles in our daily practice.

Significant changes can be related directly to economic factors in health care. For example, nurses have voiced their concerns nationally about safety of client care when licensed professionals are replaced with unlicensed assistive personnel (UAP). The regulators of nursing in many states have mandated that nurses will be held accountable for all the care they deliver and direct irrespective of the environment in which the nurse works. Most hospitals and systems of care remain charitably immune. This means that there may be increased liability for any malpractice claim on the licensed professional nurse and not on the hospital or institution. Nurses are strongly advised to carry their own malpractice insurance. Concomitantly there are few laws and regulations that provide for mandating a safe environment in which the nurse can practice both competently and compassionately or that address how many clients a nurse can safely care for at any one time (although this is changing because of nurse activists). However, nursing data clearly indicate that the presence of a nurse dramatically increases a positive client outcome. In more than a dozen studies, hospitals that have a higher number of nurses per client have lower mortality rates. Hospitals with a higher ratio of nurses to clients have 6 fewer deaths per 1000 clients than hospitals with fewer RNs on staff (Hartz et al., 1989). Furthermore, according to a 1994 study of 244 hospitals, mortality rates were 5% lower in hospitals that employed more RNs relative to all other nursing staff. When these "magnet" hospitals were restudied in 2000, data remained the same. RNs identified magnet hospitals as good places to work because they were able to exercise professional judgment and quality care was valued in the hospital hierarchy (Aiken, 1994; Aiken, Havens, & Sloane, 2000).

Concerns of Professional Nursing

In every state, legislation trends are to require identification of the provider and license on name tags, to require that staffing ratios be published, to prohibit mandatory overtime policies, to enact nursing care data legislation, and to define what a nurse can and cannot delegate to UAP. Across the country many state nurse practice acts have been and will be redefined.

Decreased numbers of graduates indicate that the nursing shortage of the twenty-first century affects total numbers of nurses and specialty practices in all areas including rehabilitation. States may use legislative efforts, such as loan forgiveness programs for students choosing nursing (Shindul-Rothschild, Berry, & Long-Middleton, 1996).

The American Nurses Association (ANA) sponsored its national "Every Patient Deserves a Nurse" campaign. The ANA along with other specialty nursing organizations has attempted to educate the public that care provided by professional nurses is necessary to produce the best client outcomes (http://www.ana.org). Studies have corroborated the idea that the presence of a nurse is directly related to decreased morbidity and mortality.

The Occupational Safety and Health Administration (OSHA) is another resource for practice protection, such as legislation on the provision of safe needle-stick devices. New regulations concerning safety in the workplace to decrease worker's compensation claims and use of ergonomics to prevent back injuries are critical in rehabilitation.

Two key economic principles are supply and demand. The supply of physicians has decreased in areas providing care to the uninsured and in staffing general medical practices; many physicians flock to higher paying specialties. The aging population has caused a demand for care because elderly persons require more medical interventions (Boyes & Melvin, 1994), a global problem. As the number of elderly persons increases, so will their demands for social security benefits as a "right," and coverage of all health expenses will be expected. Demand for care will far outweigh the supply.

INVOLVEMENT IN POLITICS AND POLICY: A NURSING OBLIGATION

The monthly newsletter *PLAN* conducted a number of studies to determine the impact of nurses on the political process. In one study data from 271 participants from 16 states raised interesting issues. The central question was whether nurses who had greater access to legislative information were more active in the legislative process. Activity was measured in the number of times nurses visited, wrote, or spoke with their congressional or state lawmakers about any particular issue of concern. The average age of participants in an education program sponsored by *PLAN* was 45 years. They completed the questionnaire before the lecture. Participants were both subscribers and nonsubscribers to *PLAN*. Most were women (97%), and more than half (66%) had between 11 and 29 years of experience in nursing practice. Nearly one third completed baccalaureate education, and one fifth graduated from diploma nursing programs. Their areas of practice were diverse, ranging from school nursing and pediatrics to geriatrics, rehabilitation, and nursing education.

The nurses' interests in politics reflect those of the general population: 108 participants noted that their interest had peaked only during the last year due to the issues surrounding access to care, cost, and quality. Only 95 of those surveyed cited job security as a reason for interest. Readers of *PLAN* were slightly more active than other nurses in com-

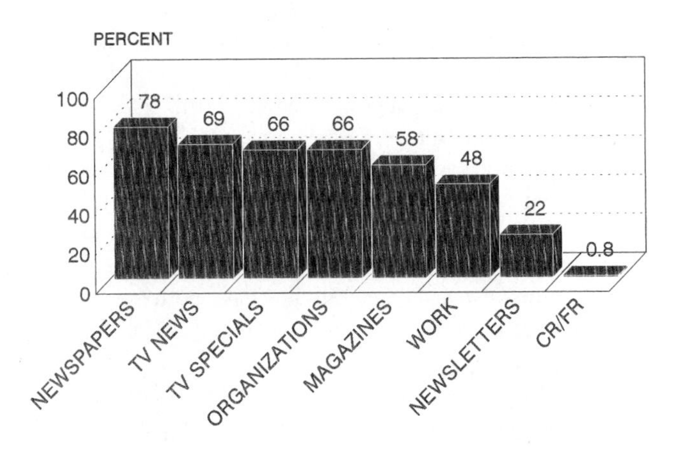

Figure 3-1 Sources of information. Does not include *Plan* as a source.

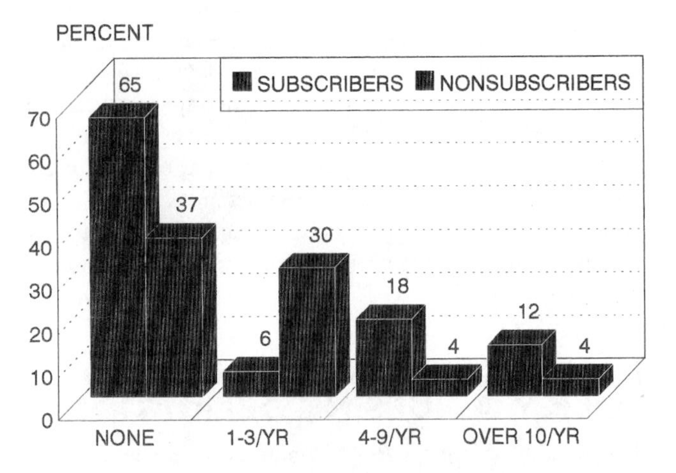

Figure 3-2 State contacts.

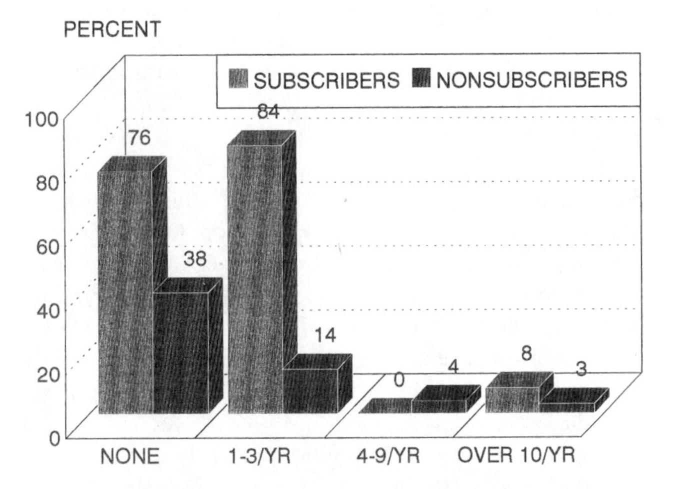

Figure 3-3 Congressional contacts.

municating with the legislators; however, the overall level of communication with legislators was extremely low. Of the 271 participants, 134 had never communicated with their state lawmakers, and 141 had never spoken with a member of their congressional delegation. Figure 3-1 reflects sources of information used by nurses. Data in Figure 3-2 quantify the numbers of contacts nurses have had with state lawmakers during the last 10 years. Figure 3-3 reflects the nurses' contacts with their individual congressional delegations.

The implication is for nurses to recognize a need to have access to information about the legislation that affects their practice, their clients, and their own health care. Nurses who learn how to put political knowledge into action can make a difference. Rehabilitation nurses have a professional obligation to know the laws and regulations that affect their practice and the standard of ethical practice that is common to all nurses, the ANA Code for Nurses (ANA, 1985). It is the basis of ethical decision making and the standard of nursing practice for all nurses in the United States, and it is the one recognized legal document on which a nurse's practice is judged in courts of law. Chapter 4 discusses ethical matters for rehabilitation nurses in more detail.

Laws and regulations that rehabilitation nurses are likely to be aware of at the state level include those directly related to nursing and those related to clients. Many state boards of nursing pass or seek to pass an interstate compact for licensure and discipline. Once in effect, an interstate agreement allows a nurse to practice across states with an original license in a state that is party to the agreement; it also allows discipline across states. This issue remains controversial because many in the nursing community continue to debate the language and what the compact should include and exclude. An unresolved controversy is with the language, "where nursing practice occurs." Does this mean where the nurse is (such as is the model for third-party billing and rehabilitation case management) or where the client is (the model proposed by the National Council of State Boards of Nursing)? This issue affects all professional nurses' practice. This impending law uniquely affects rehabilitation nurses because many whose practices are in telenursing, or even in certain types of consulting or case management, may hold a license only in the state of their residence, not in the state where they are directing nursing practice.

Legislation related to key nursing practice issues will also be witnessed in the new millennium. Issues such as staffing mixes, safe needle-stick devices, prevention of workplace violence, health care whistle-blowing, and managed care reforms to protect clients' rights are examples of legislative initiatives. Telenursing and telehealth and the increasing use of the Internet will change the dynamic of the nurse-client relationship, as well as regulations for nursing licensure. Examples of legislation that may have ethical implications include legislation related to the confidentiality of medical records and of genetic testing results, legislation to legalize marijuana and euthanasia, and legislation to prohibit selling genetic data.

RESOURCES

Resources for following the activities of state and national government are on the World Wide Web. Most state websites can be accessed on-line by using www.state.XX.us, with "XX" replaced by the two-letter postal code for the state (e.g., www.state.ma.us for Massachusetts). Other policy websites are the National Institutes of Health (www.nih.gov), the U.S. Department of Health and Human Services (www.dhhs.gov), and the National Library of Medicine (www.NLM.gov). Advocacy groups often advance a political agenda on their websites, and national organizations, such as the American Cancer Society (www.acs.org) or the National Coalition for Patients' Rights (www.nationalCPR.org), can be located on-line. The Internet is a source to learning how government affects practice and client outcomes.

SUMMARY

Rehabilitation nursing roles are evolving and emerging. Economics, systematic changes, and evolving laws and regulations shape professional practice and thus the client outcome. The legislative process presents an opportunity for rehabilitation nurses to share their expertise with local, state, and federal government agencies and legislators. Involvement can range from conducting programs related to unsafe or unhealthy behavior in schools to lobbying legislators to pass preventive legislation about seat belt use and smoking cessation. Rehabilitation nurses have unique knowledge and understanding of the long-term care needs of their clients with disabilities that position them to advocate for health care policy and reform (Craven & Gleason, 1993).

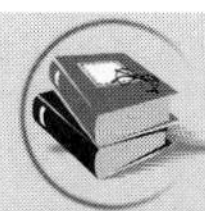

Case Study — *Successful Nursing Strategies That Influenced Legislation*

Nurses intervene at local, state, federal, and organizational levels to affect legislation from a professional perspective that has a direct impact on practice. Choose the issue that is a passionate one and for which you have concerns. *PASSION* is an acronym for *political action: social security in organized nursing* (Craven & Gleason, 1993). Political action is one mechanism to ensure laws are passed that are pertinent and appropriate to nursing practice. Table 3-2 illustrates nursing actions that have resulted in legislative actions because nurses demonstrated passion and concern for the outcome.

TABLE 3-2 Levels of Activism

Legislation: Actions Nurses Should Consider	Local Actions	State/Federal Actions	Organizational Actions
ADA	Seek appointment to city/town disability or housing commission(s) to secure community access	Monitor regulations to comply with ADA	Educate nursing organizations through publications about the provision of ADA and its relationship to nursing
Seat belt initiatives	Write articles for local newspaper or cable stations Speak as an expert for local police safety officers and programs in schools	Testify on pending seat belt legislation Identify self as expert to legislators—serve as resource	Work with League of Women Voters and/or emergency nursing organizations to educate public Become spokesperson for National Head Injury Foundation
Smoking prevention and cessation initiatives	Join local board of health smoking cessation efforts Apply for educational grants for smoking cessation and prevention Join efforts to ban smoking in restaurants and other public places	Support legislation that decreases smoking prevalence: tobacco tax, ingredient disclosure, ban on sales to minors Seek appointment on state tobacco settlement commission or board, which resulted from a national lawsuit against tobacco industry and created a 25-year funding stream from penalties into each state Advocate for spending on health care	Join American Cancer Society efforts and continued initiatives Encourage collaboration between American Cancer Society and national nursing organizations regarding smoking prevention efforts/programs

REFERENCES

Aiken, L. (1994) Lower medicare mortality among a set of hospitals known for good nursing care. *Medical Care 32(8), 771-87.*

Aiken, L. Havens, D., & Sloane, D. (2000). Original research: The magnet nursing services recognition program. *American Journal of Nursing, 100*(3), 26-36.

American Nurses Association. (1985). *Code for nurses with interpretive statements.* Washington, DC: Author.

Boyes, W., & Melvin, M. (1994). *Economics* (2nd ed.). Boston: Houghton Mifflin.

Craven, G., & Gleason, C. (1993). Passion for organized nursing. *PLAN, 3,* 32.

Crockett, M.J., DiBlasi, M., Flaherty, P., & Sampson, K. (1997). Activity based resource allocation: a system for predicting nursing costs. *Rehabilitation Nursing, 22*(6), 293-298, 302.

Hartz, A., Krakauer, H., Kuhn, E., Young, M., Jacobsen, S., Gay, G., Muenz, L., Katzoff, M., Bailey, R., & Rimm, A. (1989). Hospital characteristics and mortality rates. *New England Journal of Medicine, 321*(25), 1720-1725.

Mariner Health Group. (1998). *Getting to the mountain top: How to survive and thrive under PPS* (pp. 2-16) [Brochure]. New London, CT: Author.

Shindul-Rothschild, J., Berry, D., & Long-Middleton, E. (1996). Where have all the nurses gone? *American Journal of Nursing, 96*(11), 25-39.

Wilkinson, W., & Dresden, C. (1996). The Americans with Disabilities Act: an ethical perspective as the law develops. *NeuroRehabilitation, 6,* 145-160.

BIBLIOGRAPHY

Battistella, R. (2000). The future of employment-based health insurance. *Journal of Healthcare Management, 45*(1), 46-57.

DePender, W., & Idede-Chandler, W. (1990). An autopsy of an ethical dilemma. *Journal of Nursing Administration, 20,* 25-29.

Guinier, L. (1998). *Lift every voice: turning a civil rights setback into a new vision of social justice.* New York: Simon & Schuster.

Higgins, W. (2000). Ethical guidance in the era of managed care: an analysis of the American College of Healthcare Executives' code of ethics. *Journal of Healthcare Management, 45*(1), 32-42

McCourt, A.E. (1993). *The specialty practice of rehabilitation nursing: A core curriculum* (3rd ed.). Skokie, IL: The Rehabilitation Nursing Foundation of the Association of Rehabilitation Nurses.

Meier, E. (2000). Is unionization the answer for nurses and nursing? *Nursing Economics, 18*(1), 36-37.

Mullahy, C.M. (1998). *The case manager's handbook* (2nd ed., pp. 63-118). Gaithersburg, MD: Aspen.

Quinn, C., & Smith, M. (1987). *Ethical dimensions in the health professions.* Philadelphia: WB Saunders.

Riley, J.M. (1998). Wired on ethics. *Reflections, 32.*

Santos, S., & Cox, K. (2000). Workplace adjustment and intergenerational differences between matures, boomers, and Xers. *Nursing Economics, 18*(1), 7-13.

Ethical Matters in Rehabilitation

4

Shirley P. Hoeman, PhD, RN, CRRN
Pamela M. Duchene, PhD, RN, CRRN

On a hot summer afternoon, Effie C. suffered a cerebrovascular accident (CVA) involving the right hemisphere of her brain. She was admitted to a medical unit at the local hospital, and after 3 days her physician declared her medically stable and for rehabilitation. Effie had significant weakness of her left side but could speak clearly. On admission to rehabilitation, the speech pathologist evaluated her swallowing and found significant potential for aspiration of thin, thickened liquids and pureed foods. The speech pathologist recommended that she receive nothing by mouth pending further evaluation. Effie's nutritional needs were met through intravenous feedings, to which she protested loudly. She repeatedly requested liquids and food.

Two days later, the speech pathologist reported results of a modified barium swallow that supported the original conclusion. Effie's dysphagia was severe; she aspirated all types of liquid. The speech pathologist explained this result to Effie and to her family. A feeding tube was recommended to meet Effie's long-term nutritional needs, and she was advised to repeat the barium swallow before discharge. Effie refused the feeding tube and continued intravenous support. She demanded to be allowed to drink liquids, and her family expressed support of Effie's decision.

The team psychologist met with Effie and stated that her request for oral feeding could be linked to depression and suicidal ideations. She clearly showed signs of depression, refusing therapy, requesting that her door be closed, and spending her days in her room. Effie stated that if she were given food and fluids, she would feel more like participating in the rehabilitation program.

The team met and requested a consultation from the ethics committee of the hospital. The chairperson of the committee reviewed the case and met with Effie and her family to discuss the situation. Effie stated that if eating meant she might die, she would take the risk. Her family supported her decision.

The speech pathologist refused to continue treating Effie because she believed that Effie disregarded her recommendations. She advised the nurses that providing Effie with fluids and food would be causing her death.

The ethicist met with the nurses and reinforced that the decision to drink and eat was Effie's to make. She was competent and capable of making such decisions. Their role as rehabilitation nurses was to reinforce Effie's independence and to provide her the emotional support she needed during her hospitalization. Nurses who felt that the ethical conflict violated their own beliefs refused to provide care for Effie. Other nurses supported Effie's decision regarding food and fluid intake and worked with her during the remainder of her hospitalization.

Ethics commonly is defined as the social sense of what ought or ought not to be, a concern with what is agreed on to cause no harm and to do what is good. Ethics evolve from beliefs and values and thus have religious and cultural bases. Ethical behavior requires moral reasoning, problem solving, and decision making. Ideally, ethical actions can be justified against some agreement about proper behaviors in the group, such as professional codes or standards. True dilemma, the quandary of having no acceptable choices, is the paradoxical thorn in ethics. Dilemmas inherent in ethical situations or issues make regulation difficult, if not improbable, although ethical topics have been reflected in legislation. However, competing values, confusion about the issues, disagreement on moral questions, or true dilemmas regularly disrupt smooth pathways for ethics.

For years, the simple words of Hippocrates and Nightingale sufficed for ethics in health; certainly in rehabilitation ethical situations were not high-visibility areas. Whether insidious or not, unique and difficult ethical situations sometimes pose challenges for rehabilitation professionals. Global awareness and cultural diversity have thrust the values and practices of other health systems into the choices available in the United States. Advances in science, technology, and genetics result in decisions about situations and problems only imagined by a few scientists a generation ago. While seemingly reasserting their dominance, these scientific enterprises have become an ethical means to an end, usurping other arguments for justification. As noted many years ago by Eckenhoff (1981), rehabilitation developed to ease the uneasy situation created by advances in science. Because it is morally and ethically questionable to place a value on a life with a disability, rehabilitation provides a solution: achieving the biopsychosocial potential possible. Scientific advances never come without a price. The costs of implementing new advances in efforts to save lives and to promote quality care are staggering. Will rehabilitation become indispensable, or will it be necessary to ration the dollars available?

Uncharted Waters

In rehabilitation practice, increasing numbers of persons are survivors of formerly fatal conditions and are living longer lives with the assistance of medical and technological advances. Society has never encountered such medical wonders or challenged dilemmas of this nature concerning interventions and outcomes. In pioneer days individuals with disabilities and illnesses were "auctioned off" to the lowest bidder for care. The family of the individual would provide what they could to offset the expenses incurred. Many families could not afford or did not care to provide for their ill and disabled members. In these cases those with infirmities sometimes ended up in prisons or poor farms. The social reformer Dorthea Dix created awareness of the problem, and asylums were established. Asylums were replaced by state hospitals and then by rehabilitation and outpatient care. Never before has the burden of caregivers been as extensive as it is today. In fact, the burden of caregivers has been called an ethical question.

Rehabilitation nurses must have clear understanding of their own values and a premise for logical, critical thinking because personal ethics often differ from client beliefs, public rules, or professional codes. Even blind agreement with regulations is complex when outcomes are uncertain and engender ethical debates. The Baby Doe Regulations are an example of a situation that sparked heated debate. In 1983 a highly publicized case involved a baby, born with Down's syndrome and esophageal atresia, who was allowed by the parents, with the support of the hospital physicians and nurses, to die. In response to this case, legislation was enacted to prevent such an occurrence, based on the belief that discrimination occurred toward the baby because of the disability (Fost, 1999).

Compromise clauses appeared in 1984, only a year after initial Baby Doe Regulations required medical treatment for all infants. Subsequently treatment could be withheld if a newborn was in an irreversible coma or when there was no hope of survival, and interventions were not intended to prolong the dying process. The first legislation was based on ethical agreement about the sanctity of life, and the second was based on quality of life. However, there is no clear answer to questions such as who makes the decision and for which newborns is a decision made? Although outcomes cannot be predicted with any certainty, ethical differences in interpretation can and do exist among parents, health providers, advocates, and the courts (Cohen, Levin, & Powderly, 1987).

Rehabilitation nurses working in pediatrics encounter children who, because of the Baby Doe Regulations, received treatment as newborns and survived, often with multiple complex problems. The ethical question of uncertain outcomes and quality of life continues for these children.

SCOPE OF REHABILITATION CONCERNS

Throughout this book, rehabilitation and the specialty practice in nursing are shown as integral and essential across the levels of the health system. It follows that ethical principles emerge that are of concern to rehabilitation nursing regarding care throughout the health career of a client. Ethical principles in and of themselves cannot resolve many of the complexities, quandaries, and dilemmas found in the scope of rehabilitation. Values and expectations include ideas about what constitutes care. Consider the examples in the following section.

Levels of Intervention

Prevention is a key intervention level for rehabilitation nurses. For example, rehabilitation nurses spearheaded campaigns for prevention of spinal cord injury from diving accidents, for helmet laws to prevent head injury during bicycle and motorcycle accidents, and for education of elderly persons about home safety to prevent falls. Although it is possible to prevent injuries through the use of air bags in cars, helmets for bikes and scooters, and home evaluations, it is not possible to prevent injuries due to unhealthy lifestyle choices and noncompliance. Injury and chronic, disabling conditions due to unhealthy lifestyle choices (e.g., substance abuse, failure to monitor high blood pressure) are more taxing and frustrating concerns for rehabilitation nurses and other health care providers. Allocating resources to persons who have conditions that could have been prevented will become more contentious as resources and manpower dwindle.

In acute care, principles of rehabilitation nursing are used to prevent contractures, skin breakdown, and other problems of immobility, as well as to maximize independent functioning after total joint-replacement surgery. Rehabilitation nurses in specialty areas discussed in this book, such as cardiac, renal, burn, and cancer rehabilitation, have improved outcome for many clients. It is easy to justify the dollars spent for rehabilitation nursing care in such settings because rehabilitation nursing makes a difference in the length of recovery.

However, rehabilitation is not as readily available for many persons requiring what are considered tertiary levels of intervention. Highly ranked concerns are how resources are allocated, how goods and services are distributed for clients, and the rationale for finances awarded to support specialty programs. System criteria and requirements may make justifying benefits for older persons or those with comorbid and chronic conditions difficult, as opposed to rationing and restricting according to calculated benefits.

Selection Criteria

Furthermore, not all persons who become disabled or impaired have access to rehabilitation services. The initial hurdle is failure for many to consider rehabilitation; they or their provider have no understanding or experience in the specialty, and no one prepares a referral. Others, providers or family, simply have no confidence in outcomes from rehabilitation, they consider the person too old or severely disabled, or the person is unwilling. The ability to finance rehabilitation is a screening mechanism in itself; third-party reimbursement and criteria for coverage vary greatly. Some live outside the system, vulnerable, invisible, and marginal.

In fact, those who do receive rehabilitation must continue to demonstrate their potential, must meet the system requirements, and in some manner must participate. What truly is unique is the process the rehabilitation team uses, evaluating persons before selecting those who will be candidates for rehabilitation. The setting in which rehabilitation occurs is also selected before the individual's entry into the rehabilitation program. Although managed care has made an impact in directing clients away from acute rehabilitation programs and into subacute settings, the decision appears based more on age than on physical impairment, potential for recovery, and ability to participate.

Rehabilitation is considered strongly directed toward care, which is easily accomplished while expectations for cure remain low. Conflict can occur when clients and family hold hope for cure and providers promote rehabilitative themes, challenging advocacy. Certain themes are inherent in a rehabilitation world view. They include ideas about self-care, maximum independence, potential for education or vocation, caregiver involvement, and participation in the plan for care, especially when setting goals. "If you don't play, you can't stay," spouted one young man in a group meeting for those residing on the spinal cord injury unit. "But we can't do everything for everybody all of the time," the nurse and therapist lamented as though in chorus.

THEORETICAL BASES FOR ETHICAL PRACTICE

The four ethical theories presented in Table 4-1 encompass principles important for rehabilitation nurses to understand in making decisions. Table 4-2 illustrates how ethical principles relate to situations encountered in rehabilitation nursing practice or sphere of concern. The theories and principles presented are the result of centuries of thought and hypothesis. If one is in doubt that theories written more than 250 years ago can influence the way we think today, the works of Jeremy Bentham, founder of the utilitarian (happiness) theory, should be reviewed. This is the original theory of "if it feels good, do it" (Sweet, 1998). Although individuals may have defined values and beliefs, an understanding of ethical theories and principles is necessary to understand the society in which we live and practice.

Access

Access is a multidimensional word; indeed, it functions as both a verb and a noun, with the noun having extended connotations. Thus we refer to wheelchair or architectural access, access to goods and services, and access to the World Wide Web, and then we debate the accessibility of the same. The idea of access has become associated with the ability to obtain whatever the objective or to gain some right.

Persons with chronic, disabling conditions, among other aggregates, have made gains in the social construction of what "ought to" constitute proper accesses for them. The Americans with Disabilities Act, Patient Bills of Rights, and inclusion of children in education are examples of access-promoting legislation discussed elsewhere in this book. *Healthy People 2000* and *Healthy People 2010* list priority areas for reducing disparities in access to health goods and services (U.S. Department of Health and Human Services, 2000).

The media and public programs commonly feature positive images of persons with disabilities and highlight Special Olympics games. Certainly the open discussions of their chronic, disabling conditions by prominent individuals such as Christopher Reeve, Michael J. Fox, and Janet Reno have dented the wall of silence and invisibility. And a number of options, such as assisted living homes or group caregiver living arrangements, have served some needs.

Despite the encouragement, opportunities to obtain access to community and independent living and attendant care remain less than desirable for young adults with disabilities. Restricted benefits and reduced services, coupled with strict criteria for obtaining assistance in the home, have become limitations for older persons attempting to maintain their independent living. Of the 35 million disabled adults

TABLE 4-1 Ethical Theories for Practice

Theory	Description	Examples within Rehabilitation Nursing
Ethics of divine commands	Religious moralities: Right and wrong defined through divine commands (e.g., the Bible).	Many nurses believe that they have a calling to practice nursing. As such, their practice will be in line with their religious beliefs concerning right and wrong.
Ethics of selfishness	Egoism: Individuals define what is the ethical right for them. This is acceptable as long as the ethical right for oneself does not interfere with the ethical right for another.	Rehabilitation nurses have a responsibility to complete client education on the importance of pressure releases for position changes for the prevention of pressure ulcers. Clients choose whether to comply with the instructions. It is their right to choose, as long as the consequences of such actions (pressure ulcer) do not interfere with the rights of others (which could occur through preventable consumption of health care resources).
Ethics of duty and respect	Deontological theory: The science of "right." The theory specifies that there are definable principles of natural right associated with jurisprudence.	In rehabilitation nursing, the nurse has a responsibility to provide competent care in accordance with the nursing practice act. For example, it is right for nurses to administer medications and treatments in synchronization with physician orders. To violate this would be to fail the client in delivery of nursing care and to violate the ethic of duty.
Ethics of consequences	Utilitarian theory: Stipulates that principles or actions can be proved to be good. The best principles or actions are those resulting in good feelings. Also known as the happiness theory.	Rehabilitation leads to increased independence. This is good as long as independence is known to be good. For example, for many years rehabilitation specialists encouraged individuals with significant disabilities to walk without considering energy-conservation principles. Is walking "good" if the individual expends an excessive amount of energy in walking?

From Hinman, L. (1998). *Ethics: A pluralistic approach to moral theory* (2nd ed.). Fort Worth, TX: Harcourt, Brace.

eligible to vote, only 21 million actually register to vote. However, 20,000 or more polling sites are inaccessible for persons with disabilities (HalfthePlanet.org, 2000). Funds, services, manpower, and durable goods supplies diminish, whereas needs and demands escalate at all levels of care and stages of life. Access is not useful if the structure is empty. Such issues are important; Table 4-2 illustrates more about ethical principles applied to practice.

Family Responsibilities

More and more responsibility is placed on the family to care for its members. Recently society has paid more attention to the stress and burden on caregivers, recognizing that despite the love and dedication, it is a difficult and isolated role. Family and client coping are discussed in detail in Chapter 12. The Family Leave Act, company benefits with elder care programs, and lenient policies for workers who have family care responsibilities are helpful, but government and more funded programs will not be the answer. At some point programs and bureaucracies break down, they set limits and restrictions for care, and they take away individual rights because they give according to their own rules.

For example, the Children's Health Insurance Program is a national program funded in 1997 for $40 billion to be spent over the subsequent 10 years. Children whose family incomes are too high to qualify for medicaid and too low for private insurance were to receive assistance. However, 40 of the states will return their annual moneys unspent to the federal government because they have not used their allocations during the fiscal year. States report having difficulty implementing the program according to the rigid guidelines set by the federal government, not being able to find children who are eligible, and in some instances, finding fewer children needing the support in the improved economy of the time. In New Mexico, however, only 1000 of 30,000 uninsured children were eligible for the program (Associated Press, 2000).

Of course, barriers and obstacles to access must be removed, but ethically efforts must be purposeful to the targeted aggregate. Ultimately it is the community where the burden must be shared. The community has the foremost role and responsibility for rehabilitation of its members. In the United States many and varied resources are available. Access to the community is key, whether through churches, voluntary organizations, specialty associations, support groups, or others.

Advocacy

Advocacy is an acknowledged role for rehabilitation nurses. In many situations a nurse advocate can and has made enor-

TABLE 4-2 Relationship of Ethical Principles to Situations Encountered in Rehabilitation Nursing Practice or Sphere of Concern

Ethical Principle	Description	Examples
Autonomy	An individual's actions are independent from the actions and the will of others. Individuals have the ability to form their own perspectives on right, wrong, and values.	Rehabilitation nurses must acknowledge that individuals for whom they care have freedom regarding their bodies and actions. Nurses may provide education on wellness and health promotion, but compliance with programs cannot be forced. Clients have autonomy in their health care programs.
Nonmaleficence	The concept of doing no harm.	Rehabilitation nurses, like all health care practitioners, have a duty to do no harm to a client. To intentionally administer a lethal dose of medication to a client is an example of violation of the ethical principle of nonmaleficence. It is unthinkable for a nurse to intentionally harm a client.
Beneficence	The concept of doing good for another.	Nursing care is based on the concept of beneficence. Rehabilitation nurses intend to do good for others. The motivation that drives rehabilitation nurses to go the extra distance in care of their clients is an example of beneficence.
Advocacy	Loyalty: Championing the needs and interests of another.	Rehabilitation nurses are in an ideal position to advocate for their clients. Nurses often see clients on a 24-hour basis and have an awareness for and appreciation of client's abilities and energy levels that other disciplines may not. It is critical that such information be shared with team members in a way to advocate for the best plan for clients.
Veracity	Responsibility to speak the truth.	Nurses have an obligation to speak truthfully in all aspects of their role.
Financial responsibility (cost-benefit analysis)	Stewardship: Ensuring that there is sufficient benefit for the expense provided.	There is an ethical responsibility to meet the client's needs as well as possible while using as few resources as possible. For example, extending lengths of stay in hospitals, home health care, and subacute programs, when a client is capable of being discharged to a lesser level of care, is not in line with the nurse's financial responsibility for care.
Care	Providing for and meeting the needs of others for compassion, empathy, and good.	Care is a component of the rehabilitation nurse's role, regardless of the setting.
Sanctity of life	Value of life, right to life.	Rehabilitation nurses have an obligation to care for all clients, regardless of the extent of disability or potential for recovery, because all life is of value.
Quality of life	Condition of one's life, based on assessment of correlation between life and participation in valued activities and interests.	Quality of life is a frequent question for individuals with devastating disabilities and chronic illnesses. Rehabilitation nurses can assist individuals and families in reframing situations to find quality of life in remaining abilities.
Consent	Voluntary agreement with a procedure, process, or treatment.	The role of the rehabilitation nurse in informed consent is key. Because clients often confide in nurses, the rehabilitation nurse is in a position to validate understanding of a procedure, treatment, or course of therapy. As an advocate, the rehabilitation nurse supports the clients' abilities to make decisions and participate in their plans of care.
Confidentiality	Responsibility to keep information private.	Rehabilitation nurses are entrusted with substantial amounts of private information. Such information must be kept confidential, to be shared only as related to the nursing care and needs of the client.
Competence	The ability or legal right to make appropriate decisions.	The need for rehabilitation sometimes follows a disability or illness that affects the clarity the client's decision-making ability. This should not be confused with legal competence.
Values	Worthwhile or positive qualities held by an object or outcome. These should be chosen carefully but freely.	The question of the value of a life after a disability or chronic illness is sometimes placed in question. Rehabilitation nurses recognize the value of independence and of reframing prior values to achieve higher levels of life satisfaction.

From Ursery, D. (2000). *Principles of normative ethics.* Austin, TX: St. Edwards University; Madigan, T. (1997). Glossary: bioethics terms. In *Ethics Committee core curriculum.* Buffalo, NY: State University of New York at Buffalo; and National Reference Center for Bioethics Literature. (2000). *Bioethics Thesaurus 1999.* Washington, DC: Georgetown University.

mous differences in outcomes for clients with chronic, disabling disorders. Rehabilitation nurses educate clients and families to ensure that they know their rights, are fully informed and able to consent, and gain all benefits they are entitled to for their needs. At times, the legal system treats clients unjustly and perhaps unethically by, for example, restricting services.

Advocacy is a role that attempts to clarify the situation and broker the gap that may exist between ethics and the law. Clients in rehabilitation typically have complex, multidimensional, and lengthy problems. It is essential to clarify whether the problem involves ethics or regulations or other factors before moving to advocate. That is to say, avoid unnecessary dilemmas and complications by identifying the exact problem. Ethics are of broader scope than laws, but standards of practice and licensure are legal processes. Other advocacy actions important to the rehabilitation nurse are assisting clients in clarifying their values, resolving conflicts, solving problems effectively, and making decisions that leave them with satisfaction as well as quality of life. Advocacy themes are evident throughout discussions in this chapter.

Clarifying Values

Values are rooted in a person's culture, family, and beliefs and are moderated by experiences. Actions reflect values, but individuals are not always aware of the connections, especially when under duress from competing values. Identifying and clarifying values is a sequential process that involves the person choosing freely from alternatives, prizing or willingly accepting the choice, and acting or behaving in concert with the choice (Edge & Groves, 1994).

Moral reasoning develops through stages (Barger, 1998), with two stages at each level. First is the preconventional level, characterized by obedience and punishment and then by exchange and individualism. Second is the conventional level, which includes the good boy/girl, followed by the law and order stage. The postconventional level includes the stage of social contract, followed by progression to principled conscience. Although as with other stage theories, individuals may go backward and forward through the stages, overall, individuals should attain the sixth stage of principled conscience.

Autonomy

One ethical value proffered in rehabilitation is autonomy for the client. Persons with chronic, disabling conditions often must deal with the health system for extended periods. The nature of their situation or condition illustrates failure of the medicine to cure them and forces a model of care. Invasive, intensive, highly technological treatments may not be a client's choice. Not only are clients concerned about obtaining needed care, they also desire life satisfaction in daily living. Consider the difficulty in achieving intimacy in relationships apart from clinical discussions and caregiver scrutiny or the importance of inclusion, not just being mainstreamed, into schools. Consider the difficulty for clients living in managed housing or group homes with persons whom they did not know previously or being further segregated on selected blocks. Ethical dilemmas for a client's autonomy are predictable when a nurse attempts to serve as advocate as well as regulator or keeper of the system.

Client-centered, rather than system-driven, advocacy may include ensuring a client's right to autonomy in refusing a treatment or offering assertiveness training to clients who must deal with the system. Nurses are attuned to issues of confidentiality, anonymity, fully informed consent, and prevention of all aspects or threats of abuse and neglect. Likewise, they are exposed to applications of the OBRA Self-Determination Act of 1990, including advance directives, physical and chemical restraint policies, or guardianship and durable power of attorney issues. Many of these are compounded when a client is not able to function with autonomy or when that ability is in question.

Life Satisfaction

Safeguarding cultural or religious beliefs is an increasingly important advocacy action discussed further in Chapter 13. Competing values and ethical dilemmas are built into the meeting of alternative health systems, cultural experiences and expressions of health problems, and the conventional medical system that includes rehabilitation. Perhaps quality of life and life satisfaction issues fall most often within the varying belief systems and world views of individuals. These are difficult issues for the most dedicated advocate.

When catastrophic or progressive conditions occur, gathering information about a client's wishes, desires, and beliefs may be an ethical assessment. It may follow that a person's behaviors in life and stated beliefs or values are expressions or inferences of their intended meaning and thus become useful in making choices when the person cannot do so. In addition to the cultural assessment discussed in Chapter 13 and the steps in clarifying values, the advocate may learn the person's wishes about personal suffering or use of technology and medical interventions. Clients may talk about what constitutes quality and satisfaction in their lives and express opinions about decisions and who else should make them. Clients will have different perceptions about how their conditions place economic, emotional, or physical burdens on others.

Power in Relationships

Attaining and maintaining a therapeutic relationship grounded in trust is important for clients and providers. Honesty, active listening, cooperation, and shared responsibility for decisions and outcomes are effective actions in relationship building. One of the tripping stones in a relationship is power, especially when unevenly distributed. Nurses are well acquainted with roles that offer responsibility without sufficient authority and uneven power in team settings. The medical model maintains a dominant role in the social construction of disability; that is, medical diagnoses determine by definition or label who has what problem and whether something is to be done about it, or how much will be done and by whom. One cannot enter rehabilitation without meeting the criteria being selected.

However, power imbalance in the client-provider relationship is extensive and symbiotic. Without persons with chronic or disabling disorders, there would be no need for rehabilitation, providers, equipment manufacturers, or all of the others who interface with clients and families. As it stands, clients or their payment sources pay costs of rehabilitation and fees to providers. Providers attend conferences and obtain funding for research or provide care to clients in clinics and centers. Providers hold positions of prestige in society and gain a good income from their work. Clients are devalued in society and spend time and money in hope of improving their condition; they also often thank the providers (Gregory, 1997).

Changes in Practice Environment

Decisions about care of the client have always been the chief concern of nurses. Clearly, social changes as much as scientific advances alter the environment in which a nurse practices. For rehabilitation nurses, the implications are serious. Fifteen years ago, autonomy in rehabilitation was concerned with giving clients and families sufficient time and alternatives to enable them to deal with treatment decisions to stop rehabilitation services due to a lack of progress or an inability to restore physical or cognitive function. The team made decisions, and ideally the process involved a client or the family (Caplan, Callahan, & Haas, 1987).

Rehabilitation nurses must learn to consider the context of the social system (i.e., the political, legal, economic, educational, and microhealth situation) in understanding ethical situations, defining true dilemmas, and making judgments or decisions. In an environment created and constrained by business ventures, managed care is incompatible with autonomy and advocacy roles of nurses. Conflicted values about offering optimal levels of care as opposed to efficiency or cost measures quickly erode a therapeutic relationship.

VALUE OF THE PERSON

Few persons active in the workplace during the decade from 1980 to 1990 were not exposed to the management mantra of the "paradigm shift." And whether the shift meant moving into the new economy, postmodernism, or another realm, most agree that some things once believed to be permanently in place did, indeed, shift. However, when the shift involves proposed legislation that moves health providers away from the original tenet of "do no harm," the shift may become a landslide. Shifts from concern about risk versus benefits of a treatment or conflicts between conventional or alternative health practices become overshadowed in comparison. Managed care led to conflicts among members of the team as the need to "do more with less" called principles into question for some, but not all, team members. Self-determination, once deemed important for informed consent, is subject to legislation that stretches the ethical principle taut.

If social values dictate beliefs about self-determination and life satisfaction, persons with chronic, disabling disorders are at risk for promoted suicide even if they are not terminally ill. The hospice and palliative care programs of nursing are rejected in favor of aids to rapid death. The notion of dying as a life stage and a process is lost. The justification of resources being used for pain management, palliative care, family cohesiveness, and other support is open to challenge.

Self-determination legally permits clients to refuse unwanted treatment or to have full disclosure and information before consent, and suicide is not illegal. The national suicide rate is a concern for all persons. However, the shift and movement toward legislation that targets persons for approaches to suicide (legal ones) on the basis of their health status, age, or other attributes refute the ethical principles that self-determination was based on. Popular culture, such as the book *Tuesdays with Morrie,* and organizations, such as the Hemlock Society, have reduced quality-of-life issues to "having someone else wipe one's butt." Not Dead Yet, a grassroots disability rights group formed to oppose the movement to legalize assisted suicide and euthanasia, views the situation differently (Coleman, 2000). They propose that assisted suicide and euthanasia movements advocate legislation that would target persons with severe disabilities, whether their condition is terminal or not, and create a double standard for treatment and survival.

The American Nurses Association (ANA) statement on assisted suicide (ANA, 1994) does not support assisted suicide in any of its forms. Suicide, euthanasia, managed death, self-deliverance, or whatever name it is called—these are not nursing words. Assisted suicide in any variation for persons with disabilities is not a dilemma; it is a plan for devalued persons.

Moral Decision Making and Conflict Resolution

The ethical debates influencing rehabilitation nursing are significant and have the potential to affect the way in which nurses practice and the clients with whom they are able to work. Rehabilitation nurses have influence in determining the outcomes of ethical questions through moral decision making and conflict resolution. Moral decision making is the use of ethical principles to guide decision making through a rational course (Fieser, 2000). One process for conflict resolution that may be used for ethical dilemmas is included in Box 4-1.

PROFESSIONAL ADVOCACY

Rehabilitation nurses also have rights that must be protected. Recent practice issues range from unsafe staffing ratios to protections for whistle-blowers to violence against nurses in the workplace. No one should be forced or threatened to perform duties or actions that are against their moral beliefs. In many instances, nurses' rights need to be advanced and pro-

Box 4-1 Process of Conflict Resolution

1. Be sure the conflict or situation is an ethical dilemma (i.e., two morally correct courses of action are available and neither is an acceptable choice)
2. Assess the situation and collect available information or data
3. Clarify the type of problem and which moral issues or ethical principles are involved
4. Recognize the authorities being used to support components of the dilemma (i.e., cultural, legal, religious, or other)
5. Examine the alternatives and determine which are acceptable; then examine these
6. Understand the consequences
7. Decide on a course of action or intervention and engage it
8. Evaluate the process as well as the outcome
9. Discuss the entire resolution and assess any unfinished or unmet tasks; consider application in future dilemmas

tected. However, rehabilitation nurses also have a moral responsibility to professional standards, legal regulations, their employer, and their fellow team members. Many problems in the health system lend themselves to corrective action when reasonable actions are undertaken to demonstrate solutions.

The so-called "organizational culture," the underlying currents of how the mission statement and goals of the organization are handed down in daily practice, includes an ethical path or climate that affects professionals and care for clients. Ethical paths are evident in the way problems are handled, such as professional misconduct or errors, the perceived ability for staff to express opinions openly, and a sense of continuity in values from the top to the lower levels of the employee hierarchy. The organizational culture influences how providers make decisions or conduct moral reasoning during situations in which ethics are at question (Olson, 1995).

In a survey of hospital nursing administrators about ethical dilemmas they face in the workplace, issues concerning care of clients occurred most commonly. The conflicts arose between the moral obligation to the administrative (i.e., system) role and the standards of professional nursing practice. Maintaining staffing ratios and practice standards and allocating resources were ethical problem areas (Borawski, 1995).

With a national nurse shortage ahead, staffing will continue to be a difficult task, especially when nurses with experience in working with complex medical conditions are needed. Persons with disabilities are at risk. Nurses able to provide home care for children who rely on high technology are scarce already despite more children surviving and returning home. Home care agencies are closing or operating with large staff reductions across general nursing positions. Medicare restrictions of the 1997 Balanced Budget Act added to agency fiscal problems, and the burden on families increased; the impact is great on those who have disabilities (Sochalski & Patrician, 1998).

Ethics Committees

Every health organization benefits from an ethics committee composed of interdisciplinary professionals and consumer representatives. Accreditation organizations, such as the Joint Commission on Accreditation of Healthcare Facilities and the Commission on Accreditation of Rehabilitation Facilities (CARF), require an ethics committee for organizations to review questions and allegations within the organization (CARF, 2000). Potential ethical questions include, "Can program evaluation and monitoring of client outcomes realistically (read, ethically) serve as the basis for making decisions about allocating services to clients?" Leadership in establishing an ethics committee and ensuring proper representation is an example of an organizational advocacy role for rehabilitation nurses. Providers need to be involved with clients, their situations, and their decisions; however, providers should not be the sole determiners of allocation of scarce resources, such as when transplants, special drugs, or highly technological advances are at stake (May, 1995).

Research

Ethical considerations with rehabilitation research primarily focus around the issue of informed consent. Nurses often participate in collecting data for research conducted on client populations. An institutional review board review with full informed consent materials must be in place before any data collection, treatment interventions, or new product tests occur.

Two landmark events in human subject research have forever changed the way in which medical research is conducted. The Nuremberg Code was developed to prevent a reoccurrence of the medical experiments that occurred in Nazi Germany during World War II. The Nuremberg Code specifies 10 basic requirements for all medical experimentation (Box 4-2).

The Declaration of Helsinki further modified the specifications of the Nuremberg Code to protect human subjects participating in medical research. The Declaration of Helsinki, endorsed at the 18th World Medical Assembly (Helsinki, Finland, June 1964), reinforced that although research is important, it is the duty of the physician to safeguard health. The U.S. Department of Health and Human Services has guidelines for clinical research involving human subjects. Any rehabilitation nurse participating in a clinical trial or research initiative must be familiar with the basic requirements for research involving human subjects.

Codes of Ethics

Clients may express interest in euthanasia, assisted suicide, suicide, and related topics. Be clear that in these situations they are not presenting the rehabilitation nurse with an ethi-

Box 4-2 Nuremberg Code (Paraphrased)

1. Informed, voluntary consent of the subject is essential
2. The study must be expected to have a result that will be of benefit to others
3. The study must be based on an understanding of pathophysiology of the disease or problem or on prior animal studies
4. Suffering of subjects will be prevented during the study
5. Death or disability are not expected or predicted as a result of the study
6. The degree of risk does not outweigh the potential good to be gained
7. Subjects will be protected and safeguarded against problems that may occur during the study
8. Researchers will have the appropriate credentials to complete the research
9. Subjects may withdraw from studies if they cannot continue
10. Researchers will stop the study if at any time they deem it in the best interests of the subjects to discontinue the study

cal dilemma. Rather, these topics are legal issues and subject to the professional codes of practice.

However, no one code of ethics applies to rehabilitation as a specialty, despite the prevalence of chronic and disabling disorders treated at the tertiary level of care. Each professional discipline on the team maintains its own code of ethics. Many conflicts arise regarding the balance between the needs of clients with complex, severe disabilities and managing costs. Shortfalls in "manpower, money, and materials," the three Ms (Flax, 2000, p. 85), are tinder for conflicts among competing interests and ethical dilemmas. Statements related to ethics are found in standards for practice, state nursing practice acts, institution or agency policies and procedures, research ethics and reviews of research involving human subjects, vulnerable populations, and others. Each of the professional disciplines within the rehabilitation team has a professional code of ethics. For many of these disciplines, the code is posted on the Internet. Table 4-3 contains a listing of the disciplines with the websites for their codes of ethics.

TABLE 4-3 Websites for Codes of Ethics Prepared by Professional Specialty Organizations Relevant to Rehabilitation

Organization	Website for Code of Ethics
American Physical Therapy Association	http://www.apta.org/PT_Practice/ethics_pt/code_ethics
American Occupational Therapy Association	http://www.aota.org/members/area2/links/LINK03.asp
American Speech-Language-Hearing Association	http://www.asha.org/library/code_of_ethics.htm
American Therapeutic Recreation Association	http://www.recreationtherapy.com/rt.htm
American Academy of Physical Medicine and Rehabilitation	http://www.aapmr.org/about/codea.htm
American Nurses Association	http://www.nursingworld.org/ethics/ecode.htm (the 1985 Code for Nurses is currently available only through mail order and purchase; the AANA notes on their website that this is expected to change after July 2001)
International Council of Nurses	http://www.icn.ch/icncode.pdf

NURSING PROCESS

Assessment

Ask the client and family about values and beliefs important to them. In a trust relationship, this process will be easier and responses more reliable than when a client senses conflict or coercion.

The person who decides not to participate has in that regard made a choice; however, the nurse advocate ensures that the client has made a fully informed choice, and no penalties are assigned. The social construction of disability does influence beliefs and practices; however, nurses assess individuals first as part of but not equal to social or cultural models.

Assessment of children's values is a unique category that includes assessment of a child's development of moral reasoning; ability to understand the illness or disability; the severity, extent, and type of disability or condition; family or guardian involvement; and other subtle, complex factors. Children must be dealt with as children (Hays, 1991). The American Academy of Pediatrics (1996) has a statement about children's rights in care and treatment.

Value belief questions are about:

- Client and family self-ratings of life satisfaction and perceptions of quality of life
- Future goals or plans and being aware of bias for those who are not future oriented
- Involvement in community or other activities outside of self and self-care
- Support mechanisms, especially religious or spiritual
- Things that are considered important to do, such as rituals or family traditions

Nurse's Self-Assessment

Nurses bring their own values into a conflict or paradoxical situation. Clarifying personal values and identifying biases, as well as cultural differences, are preliminary to advocacy about values. Weis and Schank (2000) developed an instrument, the Nurses Professional Value Scale, intended for use in measuring professional nursing values and enhancing professional socialization. They found caregiving and activism to be the major factors. Caregiving included "providing care without prejudice" and "establishing standards as guides for daily nursing practice" (Weis & Schank, 2000, p. 203).

Nursing Diagnoses

Spiritual distress: Refer to Chapter 28 for discussion.

Decisional conflict: "This conflict occurs when the course of action forces choice among competing actions and involves risk, loss, and challenge to personal life values" (McCloskey & Bulechek, 2000, p. 726).

Related Factors

Social construction or beliefs about health, illness and disability, knowledge of the natural history of the disability, and full information concerning regimens and interventions are related factors. The person's coping and adaptation patterns and supports influence acceptance of the situation, and previous experiences with the system may alter acceptance. Difficulties arise when the person is not fully oriented, wavers among decisions, or breaks down in the process. Cultural differences are complex and make value clarification or mutual goal setting tenuous.

Nursing Interventions

Invoke codes of ethics and client rights and *Nursing's Agenda for Healthcare Reform* (ANA, 1992).

Educate client and family about the disease or disability, treatment options, and full disclosure.

Refer to community and other resources for assistance and support.

Offer therapeutic support or effective coping mechanisms, such as companion pets, humor, stress reduction and relaxation, music or art therapy, guided imagery, and so forth.

Use cognitive or behavioral therapy to improve thinking and communication.

Institute culture broker activities when indicated.

Refer for genetic counseling.

Help client to locate legal aid or assistance.

Encourage spiritual resources.

Use touch (if appropriate), time, and support from self as professional nurse.

Nursing Outcomes

Knowledge, fully informed, values clear

Consistent, logical information processing

Participation in health care decisions

Acceptance of health or disability status

ETHICAL ISSUES IN REHABILITATION NURSING

Already providers are confronted with issues that need resolution in areas where answers are not to be found readily and perhaps few responses are satisfactory. Many ethical issues of the next decade are applicable directly to rehabilitation nursing practice and populations. Important examples of ethical areas are listed below. Although not an all-inclusive list, most of these pose concerns for persons with impairments.

- Vulnerable populations, including children (May, 1995)
- The Human Genome Project and genetic engineering research (McPherson, 1995)
- Technology advances and death certification decisions
- Transplants, stem cell research, and other organ research
- Proposed legislation for assisted suicide and related movements

The ANA Code of Ethics clearly comes down on the side of clients and against assisted suicide. Rehabilitation nurses advocating for clients not only keep themselves knowledgeable but also ensure that other members of the team are aware of underlying, as well as overt, issues. They also advocate for ethical decision-making processes, including ethics committees with client representation, to be in place and for authority to operate with ethical quality standards.

INTERNET RESOURCES

American Academy of Pediatrics: http://www.aap.org.
Association of Programs for Rural Independent Living (APRIL): http://ruralinstitute.umt.edu/rtcrural/APRIL/Default/htm.
Disability Rights Education and Defense Fund (DREDF): http://www.dredf.org.
HalfthePlanet.org: http://www.halftheplanet.org.
Institute on Independent Living: http://www.independentliving.org.
Justice for All: http://www.jfanow.org.
National Council on Disability: http://www.ncd.gov/index.html.
National Council on Independent Living: http://www.ncil.org.
National Spinal Cord Injury Association: http://www.spinalcord.org.
Not Dead Yet: http://www.notdeadyet.org.
TASH—Disability Advocacy Worldwide: http://www.tash.org.
World Association of Persons with Disabilities (WAPD): http://www.wapd.org.
World Institute on Disability (WID): http://www.wid.org.

REFERENCES

American Academy of Pediatrics. Committee on Bioethics (1996). Ethics and the care of critically ill infants and children (RE9624) [Policy statement]. *Pediatrics, 98*(1), 149-152 (on-line at http://www.aap.org/policy/01460.html).

American Nurses Association. (1992). *Nursing's agenda for health care reform (PR-3 2/93R).* Washington, DC: Author.

American Nurses Association. (1994). *Position statement: Assisted suicide.* Washington, DC: Author.

Associated Press. (2000). Forty states to forfeit health care funds for poor children. CNN.com. September 24, News Report.

Barger, R. (1998). *A summary of Lawrence Kohlberg's stages of moral development.* Notre Dame, IN: University of Notre Dame.

Borawski, D.B. (1995). Ethical dilemmas for nurse administrators. *Journal of Nursing Administration, 25*(7/8), 60-62.

Caplan, A.L., Callahan, D., & Haas, J. (1987). *Ethical and policy issues in rehabilitation medicine* (Special supplement, August, pp. 1-19). Briarcliff Manor, NY: Hastings Center.

Cohen, C.B., Levin, B., & Powderly, K. (1987). The imperiled newborn: Section 1: A history of neonatal intensive care and decision making. *The Hastings Center Report 17*(6), 22-24.

Coleman, D. (2000). *Not Dead Yet website.* http://www.notdeadyet.org/docs/nydyopposed.html.

Commission on Accreditation of Rehabilitation Facilities. (2000). *Standards manual: Medical rehabilitation, July 2000–June 2001.* Tucson, AZ: Author.

Eckenhoff, E. (1981). The value of the disabled life. In N. Martin, N. Holt, & D. Hicks (Eds.), *Comprehensive rehabilitation nursing.* New York: McGraw-Hill.

Edge, R.S. & Groves, J.R. (1994). *The ethics of health care.* Albany, NY: Delmar Publishers.

Fieser, J. (2000). Moral rationalism. *The Internet Encyclopedia of Philosophy.* http://www.utm.edu.

Flax, H.J. (2000). The future of physical medicine and rehabilitation. *Archives of Physical Medicine and Rehabilitation, 79,* 79-86.

Fost, N. (1999). Decisions regarding treatment of seriously ill newborns. *Journal of the American Medical Association, 281*(17), 2041-2043.

Gregory, R.J. (1997). Definitions as power. *Disability and rehabilitation, 19*(11), 487-489.

HalfthePlanet.org. (2000). http://www.halftheplanet.org.

Hays, R.M. (1991). Health care ethics and pediatric rehabilitation. *Physical Medicine and Rehabilitation Clinics of North America, 2*(4), 743-763.

Madigan, T. (1997). Glossary: bioethics terms. In *Ethics Committee core curriculum.* Buffalo, NY: State University of New York at Buffalo.

May, C. (1995). Patient autonomy and the politics of professional relationships. *Journal of Advanced Nursing 21,* 83-87.

McCloskey, J.C., & Bulechek, G.M. (2000). *Nursing intervention classifications* (3rd ed.). St. Louis: Mosby.

McPherson, E.C. (1995). Ethical implications of the Human Genome Diversity Project. *Nursing Connections 8*(1), 36-43.

Olson, L. (1995). Ethical climates in health care organizations. *International Nursing Review, 42*(3), 85-90.

Sochalski, J., & Patrician, P. (1998, June 10). An overview of health care spending patterns in the United States: Using national data sources to explore trends in nursing services. Online Journal of Issues in Nursing. http://www.nursingworld.org/ojin/tpc6/tpc6_1.htm.

Sweet, W. (1998). Jeremy Bentham (1748-1832). *The Internet Encyclopedia of Philosophy.* http://www.utm.edu.

U.S. Department of Health and Human Services. (2000). *Healthy People 2010* (on-line edition). http://web.health.gov/healthypeople/document.

Weis, D. & Schank, M.J. (2000). An instrument to measure professional nursing values. *Journal of Nursing Scholarship 32*(2), 201-204.

5 Research-Based Rehabilitation Nursing Practice

Christina M. Mumma, PhD, RN, CRRN

Imagine that the year is 2099. The place? A freestanding rehabilitation center near Philadelphia. Haley Keller has been a certified rehabilitation registered nurse for the past 40 years and plans to work in rehabilitation nursing for at least 40 more years. The average life expectancy for women is now 135 years and climbing (125 years for men). This breakthrough is primarily due to the discovery of immune system-enhancing therapies that facilitate the human body's ability to fight almost all known diseases. Trauma is still a major health problem, so rehabilitation medicine and nursing are in high demand. Haley loves her work as a rehabilitation nurse and considers herself fortunate to be doing a job that is highly valued within both the local and global community. She has read the literature describing the history of rehabilitation nursing and realizes that nurses were not always held in high esteem. Haley is convinced that many of the positive changes within nursing in general and rehabilitation nursing in particular are due to the effects of a rich tradition of both qualitative and quantitative research conducted by rehabilitation nurses. She frequently retrieves the results of that research to assist her in providing research-based care. Haley can only imagine what rehabilitation nursing was like in "the old days," before the turn of the millennium, before nurses carried high-speed, hand-held computers with them at all times. It must have been difficult to wait hours or even days for the results of library searches! And it must have been especially difficult to have been a nurse back when nurses were expected to care for too many clients with too few resources. Haley is grateful to the many rehabilitation nurse researchers who consistently demonstrated the value of care provided by certified rehabilitation registered nurses working within highly integrated transdisciplinary rehabilitation teams. She and her clients are fortunate that rehabilitation nursing research clearly supports the importance of providing care that is based on a balance of technological competence and caring compassion. Research-based practice has become a reality.

The commitment to research within the discipline of nursing is well established (Burtt, 1999; Styles, 1995). The assumption that research is important within the specialty of rehabilitation nursing is evident by the inclusion of this chapter within a comprehensive rehabilitation nursing book. The integration of research within the practices of individual rehabilitation nurses may not be quite so evident. As a teacher of nursing research to undergraduate and graduate nursing students for the past 12 years, and before that as a presenter of nursing research workshops to practicing nurses, I have observed a wide range of enthusiasm about research as a basis for nursing practice. Regardless of the level of interest and enthusiasm I encounter at the beginning of a course or workshop, my goal is to facilitate a clear understanding of the importance of research to practice. Additionally, many students who initially had little interest in learning about research and research utilization have revealed that they enjoyed learning this content by the end of the course. Enthusiasm and passion about a topic really are contagious, and it is important for more and more nurses to realize the importance of research to nursing practice.

Because it is useful to put the present within the context of what has come before, this chapter begins with a historical overview of rehabilitation nursing research. Content is then provided relative to relationships among research, practice, and theory within rehabilitation nursing. Use of research findings to enhance clinical practice is then discussed. Finally trends for the future are explored.

HISTORY OF REHABILITATION NURSING RESEARCH

Assisting individuals of all ages and social and cultural groups to accomplish the tasks of daily living is a thread that can be identified in definitions of nursing beginning with Florence Nightingale (1860/1946) and continuing through the American Nurses Association (ANA) Social Policy Statement (ANA, 1995). Nightingale also set nursing on course for research through her detailed records of the effects of nursing actions on soldiers in the Crimean War. This history notwithstanding, rehabilitation nursing research has a short chronology. What we know today as rehabilitation had its roots after World War II. The professional organization the Association of Rehabilitation Nurses (ARN) was founded in 1974, and in 1976 the first research article was published in the *ARN Journal* (Steels, 1976).

Nursing research journals began in 1952 with *Nursing Research.* The first issue included an article on the adjustment of chronically ill older adults who were receiving home care (Mack, 1952). Nearly 10 years elapsed before a study more directly related to rehabilitation nursing described the development of an objective measure of decubitus ulcers (Verhonick, 1961). Forty years after the first nursing research journal, a journal devoted to rehabilitation nursing research, *Rehabilitation Nursing Research* (1992 to 1997), was published (Puetz, 1992).

The 1990s brought interest in the research role of the rehabilitation nurse (Langner & Wolf, 1996). Bachman (1990) urged nurses to work toward the goal of professional self-sufficiency by producing and using research. She noted that health care had become too complex for simple authoritarian solutions that are not scientifically based. The 1990s brought rapid, unprecedented changes in the way that health care is defined, delivered, and reimbursed. Health care reform and cost control continue to underlie discussion about providing health care to all Americans. The cost-benefit ratio of rehabilitation services will become increasingly important as health care systems evaluate what services will be provided, for whom, and under what circumstances. Rehabilitation nurse researchers will contrubute if they can demonstrate the effectiveness of public health policies to prevent and reduce disability from traumatic injuries, vascular insults to vital organs, and preventable causes of cancer. Rehabilitation nurses can have leadership roles in demonstrating the cost-effectiveness of rehabilitation nursing services during acute care rehabilitation and long-term care of those with chronic illnesses and disabilities. Clearly only those services demonstrated to be cost-effective in terms of shorter lengths of stay, decreased overall costs, and decreased utilization of expensive social and health services will be reimbursed under new health care systems. Research demonstrating that what rehabilitation nurses do makes a difference in client outcomes will be essential for those services to be included in health care reimbursement.

Rehabilitation nurses are making progress toward recognition as professionally self-sufficient and credible voices in demonstrating the value and cost-effectiveness of the services they provide and rehabilitation in general. The actual involvement of rehabilitation nurses in research has been explored only recently. Of the 8000 members of the ARN, only 186 (0.02%) responded to a survey included in the association newsletter about their involvement in research. Of those nurses responding, 41% reported that they had no involvement in research (Hoeman, Dayhoff, & Thompson, 1993). Why are so few involved? Perhaps the vast majority of nurses who claim rehabilitation as their specialty are not involved in research. Conceivably, many more are involved in some aspect of the research process, from generating researchable questions to critically analyzing published research reports for practice implications, but do not consider themselves researchers. Those who are actively involved in the research process may have neglected to respond to the survey. It is likely that such a survey conducted today would yield evidence of increased involvement in research.

Research has been praised and maligned among various groups of nurses. Some nurses believe that research is the only way we can improve the care of persons with disabilities, and others regard research as an ivory tower activity that has little relevance to enhancing the care that nurses provide. It is discouraging to confront the fact that, in the more than 50 years since modern rehabilitation began, so much more needs to be learned about the scientific basis to support the assumption that rehabilitation nursing care makes a difference in client outcomes. At the same time it is exciting to be a rehabilitation nurse today and to be in the forefront of developing research and theory-based practice.

RELATIONSHIPS AMONG PRACTICE, RESEARCH, AND THEORY

The value of rehabilitation nursing in the care of persons with disability and chronic illness is maximized through strong connections among practice, research, and theory. These connections require communication between rehabilitation nurses engaged in practice, research, and theory development.

The quality and effectiveness of the care that rehabilitation nurses deliver depend on research findings. Research is the process of posing an important, answerable question derived from practice and collecting and analyzing data to answer the question. Research based on rehabilitation nurses' experiences in clinical practice ensures that the outcome of the research will be relevant to the very essence of rehabilitation nursing: caring for individuals and groups with actual or potential health problems due to disability and chronic illness. Understanding which nursing actions under which conditions produce which client outcomes will allow rehabilitation nurses to provide care that can predictably accomplish desired outcomes.

The number of research reports with implications for rehabilitation nursing has increased markedly in recent years. A systematic approach to the development of a knowledge base for rehabilitation nursing practice is increasingly evident. One perspective on organizing and improving the research endeavor is to view research as a means toward developing theory to guide nursing practice. Rehabilitation nurses can expect to build a knowledge base through rigorous, scholarly, and systematic scrutiny of phenomena that influence practice.

Describing Phenomena

The purpose of theory is to describe, explain, and predict phenomena. Before we can propose a theory to guide practice, an understanding of the concepts involved in the theory is necessary. For example, practice based on a theory of helping individuals cope with disability is only possible if there is a clear understanding of the concepts of coping, client teaching, and outcome variables such as independence. The first stage of theory development therefore is based on the question "What is this?" This question can be answered in a number of ways, using either qualitative or quantitative research methods. Research at this level of theory development depends on literature review, open-ended questions, unstructured observations, and exploration of the phenomenon of interest in various settings.

Typically reports of research designed to answer the question "What is it?" fully identify and describe the phenomenon of interest. Descriptions may include a verbal description of a phenomenon; graphs; and reports of ranges, means, and standard deviations. The nursing and social science literature is replete with descriptions of phenomena. Many excellent studies have examined coping, adaptation, and the meaning of various disabilities and illnesses for the individual and for family members (Box 5-1). For example, Eakes, Burke, and Hainsworth (1998) described the inductively derived theory of chronic sorrow. This theory has been further validated through a series of qualitative studies of chronic illness and disability conducted by Eakes and colleagues within the Nursing Consortium for Research on Chronic Sorrow (Eakes, Burke, & Hainsworth, 1998).

In another example, a series of qualitative studies conducted during the past 11 years to describe the experience of living with multiple sclerosis (MS). The results of these studies indicate that individuals with MS strive to be as independent as possible for as long as possible and view living with MS in terms of losses and challenges and also as an opportunity for personal growth (Mumma, 2000).

Another approach to answer the question "What is this?" is concept analysis. Many concepts relevant to rehabilitation nursing practice have been described and analyzed, including loss (Robinson & McKenna, 1998), caring (Sourial, 1997), empathy (White, 1997), facilitation (Burrows, 1997), mutuality (Henson, 1997), hope (Kylma & Vehvilainen-Julkunen, 1997), social support (Langford, Bowsher, Maloney, & Lillis, 1997), family-centered care (Hutchfield, 1999), and vulnerability (Spiers, 2000).

Box 5-1 Research Example 1: Describing Phenomena

Pilkington, F.B. (1999). A qualitative study of life after stroke. *Journal of Neuroscience Nursing, 31*(6), 336-347.

This qualitative, descriptive study, based on Parse's human becoming theory, was conducted to increase knowledge about quality of life after stroke from the perspective of the person who experienced the stroke. Data collection involved 32 interviews with 13 participants, within 3 months after stroke onset. Data analysis revealed four themes representing participants' stroke experience: (1) suffering emerges amid unaccustomed restrictions and losses, (2) hopes for endurance mingle with dreams of new possibilities, (3) appreciation of the ordinary shifts perspectives, and (4) consoling relationships uplift the self. Interpreted on the basis of human becoming theory, the themes describe the experience of living with stroke and provide insights to enhance quality of care of persons who have had strokes.

Determining Relationships

Once concepts have been described and analyzed, the next step in making these studies applicable to practice is to determine how the concepts are related to one another. The researcher asks, "What is happening here?" Much of the rehabilitation-related nursing research has explored the relationship between concepts. For example, in lower limb amputations, increased age was associated with unfavorable outcomes in physical ability (Helm, Engel, Holm, Kristiansen, & Rosendahl, 1986). Younger adults were significantly better able than older adults to achieve independence in self-care and in bowel and bladder function (Penrod, Hegde, & Ditunna, 1990). Acorn and Bampton (1992) related loneliness in young and middle-aged adults in a long-term rehabilitation center to age and length of institutionalization and found that loneliness was more prevalent among those who had been admitted more recently but was unrelated to the age of the person.

Gender, on the other hand, has not been demonstrated to influence independence in physical activities; however, older and less educated women are disadvantaged in their access to rehabilitation resources (Ades, Waldmann, Polk, & Coflesky, 1992; Altman & Smith, 1990, 1992). In a phase II cardiac rehabilitation program, gender but not the demographic and diagnostic characteristics of participants was related to activity tolerance, anxiety, and efficacy in enduring exercise and activities of daily living (Schuster & Waldron, 1991).

In recent years, studies have been conducted to examine relationships among variables relevant to rehabilitation nursing practice. For example, Herbert and Gregor (1997) studied the relationship between quality of life and coping in a sample of 39 individuals with chronic obstructive pulmonary disease (COPD). The primary goal of another research study was to determine relationships among anxiety, self-efficacy, and selected psychosocial and physiological measures for clients with an implantable cardioverter defibrillator (Schuster, Phillips, Dillon, & Tomich, 1998). Other researchers examined relationships among control over daily life, the expectation of control, and caregiver burden in 30 spouse caregivers of older adults (Carlson & Keller, 1992), as well as the incidence and severity of pressure ulcers and injury and demographic characteristics of 125 adults with spinal cord injury (Carlson, King, Kirk, Temple, & Heinemann, 1992).

Research designed to determine the relationship among concepts uses more structured observations, asks more precise questions, and uses descriptive statistics to explain the connection among the concepts. Exploring the relationship among concepts is one step further along the continuum of establishing a theoretic base for rehabilitation nursing practice. Research at this level is the first step toward explaining how we might manipulate one factor to influence another factor. Descriptive statistics including correlations, *t* tests of group differences, and chi-square tests of independence are useful analytical strategies (Box 5-2).

Testing Relationships

After the phenomena are named and described and research has demonstrated that various phenomena are related, the next question that researchers ask is, "What will happen if . . . ?" This stage of theory development is probably the most important because it permits testing of relationships that were identified in the previous level of theory development. Factors believed to predict the relationships among the variables are stated and tested. Dille, Kirchhoff, Sullivan, and Larson (1993) used an experimental design to answer the question "What if vinyl urinary drainage bags are rinsed with dilute bleach?" Studies that ask the question "What will happen if . . . ?" are designed to impose maximum control over the concepts. The researchers randomly assigned the clients to the control and experimental groups. They measured urine colony counts weekly and evaluated the incidence of urinary tract infections between the two groups. They also assessed the aesthetic alterations and integrity of the bags and the inpatient cost of the two treatment conditions. They concluded that it was safe and cost-effective to reuse the bags for 4 weeks if they were decontaminated daily with sodium hypochlorite (household bleach).

Box 5-2 Research Example 2: Determining Relationships

Gallagher, M.S. (1998). Urogenital distress and the psychosocial impact of urinary incontinence on elderly women. *Rehabilitation Nursing, 23*(4), 192-197.

The purpose of this descriptive, correlational study, conceptually based on the Roy Adaptational Model, was to examine the possible relationship between urogenital distress and the psychosocial impact of urinary incontinence in elderly women. The sample consisted of 17 women older than 60 years who had urinary incontinence at least once per week. Results revealed a statistically significant relationship between urogenital distress and the psychosocial impact of urinary incontinence ($r = 0.673$, $P = 0.003$). These results support the need to assess elderly women for urinary incontinence and for the impact of urinary incontinence on their lives.

Venn, Taft, Carpentier, and Applebaugh (1992) tested four bowel-training protocols. A major finding of their study was that the clients in the morning bowel-training groups were significantly more successful than those in evening groups at establishing effective bowel regimens. Success was highest for those assigned to a bowel-training group whose time coincided with their previous pattern. They found no significant differences between scheduled and as-needed (prn) suppository use. Studies that test relationships are more challenging than studies at lower levels of theory development because they require the specification of necessary and sufficient conditions that will produce a desired outcome (Box 5-3).

Producing Situations

The ultimate question for rehabilitation nursing practice is, "How can we change the situation to bring about a desired outcome?" The last stage in theory development is goal oriented and situation producing and has been referred to as prescriptive theory. The question researchers ask is, "How can I make X happen?" Studies at this level often are referred to as *clinical trials,* in which researchers test the feasibility of a new treatment, determine the optimal use of a regimen or procedure, or compare the efficacy of two treatments or programs in achieving a desired outcome (Fetter et al., 1989). An example of this type of research is an experimental study conducted to determine the effects of nursing follow-up by an advanced practice nurse (APN) on coping strategies used by rehabilitation clients at and after discharge from inpatient rehabilitation (Easton, Rawl, Zemen, Kwiatkowski, & Burczyk, 1995). One hundred clients were randomly assigned to either the nursing follow-up (treat-

Box 5-3 Research Example 3: Testing Relationships

Stuifbergen, A., Seraphine, A., & Roberts, G. (2000). An explanatory model of health promotion and quality of life in chronic disabling conditions. *Nursing Research, 49*(3), 122-129.

The purpose of this study was to test an explanatory model of variables influencing health promotion and quality of life in persons living with the chronic disabling condition of multiple sclerosis (MS). The sample, 786 persons with MS, completed instruments measuring severity of illness-related impairment, barriers to health-promoting behaviors, resources, self-efficacy, acceptance, and perceived quality of life. Antecedent variables accounted for 58% of the variance in the frequency of health-promoting behaviors and 66% of the variance in perceived quality of life. The model supports the hypothesis that quality of life is based on complex interactions among contextual factors, antecedent variables, and health-promoting behaviors. The authors suggest the need for interventions to enhance social support, decrease barriers, and increase self-efficacy with the goal of improving health-promoting behaviors and quality of life.

ment) group or the no additional nursing follow-up (usual care) group. The authors stated that the treatment group reported significantly more effective and positive coping strategies than the usual care group.

A similarly designed study was conducted by Johnson and Pearson (2000) to examine the effectiveness of a structured education course on stroke survivors living in the community. The authors reported a positive effect of the course when comparing scores on three dependent variables—depression, hope, and coping—for the treatment group and the control group.

There are few cases in which a rehabilitation nursing intervention can be prescribed with confidence and assurance that the desired outcome will occur. Testing prescriptive theory requires that the findings be generalized beyond the specific situation. Prescriptive theory is dependent on an understanding of the mechanism of the variables studied. Rehabilitation nursing is building the knowledge basis for understanding the underlying mechanisms for nursing interventions, which precludes the conduct of situation-producing studies related to most rehabilitation nursing phenomena at this time. Studies that test theoretic relationships between concepts must be done first.

Outcomes Research

Outcomes research activities increased during the 1990s, partly in response to the high costs of health care (Kirchhoff & Rakel, 1999). The purpose of outcomes research is to document the effects or impact of a particular clinical program or intervention. Specific indicators selected as measures of client outcome depend on the purpose of the research and include such measures as infection rates, injury rates, client satisfaction with care, and number of nursing care hours provided per patient day. Additional outcome measures for rehabilitation facilities include functional health status, discharge to the community, rate of employment after rehabilitation, postdischarge medical complications, and hours of outpatient rehabilitation therapy (Kirchhoff & Rakel, 1999; Quigley, 1997).

ROLES OF NURSES IN CONDUCTING RESEARCH

Research often is thought of as something that is done by other disciplines or by nurses who have doctorates and are removed from clinical practice. Every rehabilitation nurse has an obligation to improve the rehabilitative care provided to those persons with actual or potential disabilities. Involvement in research is an essential element in the improvement of rehabilitation care. Nurses' involvement can range from generating questions from clinical practice to designing and implementing complex studies that answer the question "How can I make X happen?" Reading research reports and attending research conferences and then discussing with colleagues the relevance of the findings for clinical practice are ways of participating in rehabilitation nursing research. Learning more about the research process and collaborating with other members of a research team will also enhance the development of a scientific basis for rehabilitation nursing practice.

Mateo, Kirchhoff, and Schira (1999) discussed the development and refinement of research skills and elaborated on the guidelines set forth by the ANA (1989) for the investigative function of nurses. Nurses with associate degrees in nursing and nursing diplomas are a valuable asset in research because they raise questions about the effectiveness of nursing interventions and participate in data collection to answer these questions. As more research education is acquired, nurses become increasingly more involved in interpreting and evaluating research for practice, conducting investigations, and disseminating research findings (Table 5-1).

Rehabilitation nurses are part of a team that has as its goal returning individuals to their level of optimum function. Collaborative relationships between nurse clinicians and researchers are essential. Lindsey (1999) discussed this collaboration and emphasized the potential positive influence of nurses' involvement in research for developing nursing science and improving health outcomes. Nurses in clinical practice identify practice problems and reformulate these problems into research questions, critique research designs, evaluate the clinical feasibility of the research protocol, assist in implementing the research protocol, raise clinical questions relevant to data analyses, and interpret the results of the study from a clinical perspective.

Establish cluster groups with interest in specific methods or topics

Conduct multisite replication of studies or research utilization projects

TABLE 5-1 Research Responsibilities of Nurses

Preparation	Research Responsibilities
Associate degree and diploma	Collect data Identify researchable problems Appreciate value of research
Baccalaureate degree	Apply research findings to practice Share research findings Interpret and evaluate research for practice
Master's degree	Conduct investigations Facilitate access to clients Collaborate with other investigators Facilitate research Provide consultation Analyze and reformulate problems
Doctoral degree	Extend the scientific basis of practice Develop methods to measure nursing phenomena Provide leadership in research

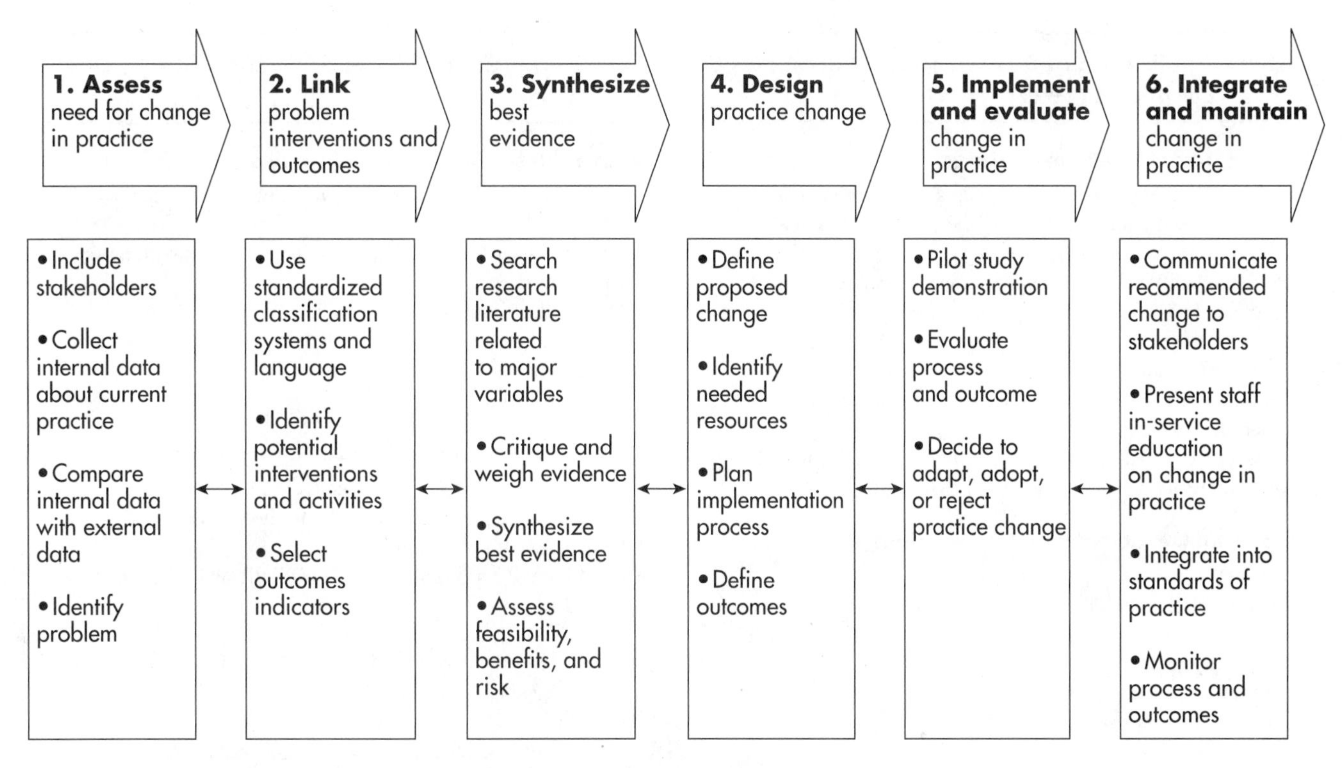

Figure 5-1 A model for evidence-based practice. (From Rosswurm, M.A., & Larrabee, J.H. [1999]. A model for change to evidence-based practice. *Image—Journal of Nursing Scholarship, 31*[4], 318.)

Use consultants to expand knowledge and skills
Broker networking opportunities for database and literature review systems (Hoeman, Dayhoff, & Thompson, 1993)

Using Research Findings

Not everyone needs to be involved in generating research findings. Every rehabilitation nurse, however, is obligated to use research findings appropriately to improve the care of clients with rehabilitation needs. Using research to guide practice has most recently been discussed within the context of evidence-based practice. The most effective evidence base combines clinical expertise with critical analysis of research results. Rosswurm and Larrabee (1999) included research utilization as a major component of their model for change to evidence-based practice (Figure 5-1). Their model is based in part on earlier research utilization models (Stetler, 1994; White, Leske, & Pearcy, 1995). The model was developed to guide practicing nurses through the process of changing to evidence-based practice. Within step 3 of the model (synthesis), results of both quantitative and qualitative research studies are critically analyzed. The best research evidence is then combined with clinical judgment and contextual evidence. The evidence rating scale was adapted from the rating scale used in research reviews within the Agency for Health Care Policy and Research (AHCPR), now the Agency for Health Research and Quality (AHRQ). A careful critique of the research is done that includes the problem studied, literature reviewed, setting and participants, design, instruments and measures, data analysis, and discussion and conclusions. The scientific and practice components of the research are analyzed at each phase of the critique.

Only if the study is found to have scientific merit are the fourth, fifth, and sixth steps of model application considered. In step 4 (design) a plan for pilot testing of the proposed change is developed for a particular clinical setting. Step 5 involves the implementation and evaluation of the change in practice, and in step 6 the change is integrated into practice, assuming the pilot study results support such integration (Rosswurm & Larrabee, 1999). The decision to apply the research to practice may confirm existing practice or require modifying or changing existing practice. Box 5-4 provides an example of application of the model to the care of clients with dysphagia.

Horsley, Crane, Crabtree, and Qood (1983) developed a model for research utilization called Conduct and Utilization of Research in Nursing (CURN). The CURN project identified six phases of the research utilization process that begin with identifying the nursing practice problem that needs a solution and assessing the research base for solving the problem. The research base is evaluated in relation to the identified practice problem, the organization's practices and values, and the potential costs and benefits of adopting the knowledge. Next the scientific merit of the knowledge base is examined. Finally a clinical trial of the innovation is conducted in the new setting, and a decision is made to reject, modify, or adopt the innovation.

Box 5-4 Application of Rosswurm and Larrabee's Evidence-Based Practice Model to Clients with Dysphagia (1999)

Step 1. Assess Need for a Change

- Discuss clinical problem of dysphagia with nurse managers, nurses, speech pathologists, and other rehabilitation team members
- Review quality assurance and risk management data on associated adverse events (primarily choking and dehydration)
- Assess nursing knowledge about dysphagia in clients with neurological and neuromuscular impairment
- Compare internal data with external data from similar rehabilitation settings
- Identify from findings the need to improve nursing staff knowledge and care of clients with dysphagia

Step 2. Link Problem with Interventions and Outcomes

- Link dysphagia with the appropriate Nursing Interventions Classification (NIC) interventions
- Include dysphagia management and aspiration prevention activities in nursing protocols
- Identify outcomes such as fluid intake levels, indicators of nutritional balance, and choking events

Step 3. Synthesize Best Evidence

- Review literature on dysphagia management
- Include nurses in critiquing research literature using worksheets
- Synthesize quantitative and qualitative research evidence
- Combine research evidence with clinical judgment and contextual data
- Assess system feasibility and benefits and risks of protocol to clients

Step 4. Design a Change in Practice

- Include nurses from pilot study units in drafting the evidence-based protocol
- Prepare forms for pilot study and its evaluation with input from unit nurses
- Identify tools for measuring outcomes such as fluid intake levels, indicators of nutritional balance, and choking events
- Educate all nurses on pilot study units in use of the evidence-based protocol

Step 5. Implement and Evaluate the Practice Change

- Implement pilot study on selected clinical units
- Monitor use of protocol throughout pilot study period
- Collect and analyze data
- Recommend adoption of protocol if indicated by pilot study results

Step 6. Integrate and Maintain the Practice Change

- Meet with staff nurses on pilot study units to review any revisions
- Present evidence-based protocol to hospital/agency-wide practice committees
- Communicate information to administration and collaborating practitioners
- Conduct in-service education for all nursing staff about the protocol
- Plan ongoing monitoring of outcomes on all units

Adapted from Rosswurm, M.A., & Larrabee, J.H. (1999). A model for change to evidence-based practice. *Image—Journal of Nursing Scholarship, 31*[4], 318.

The complexity of implementing planned change within an organization is exemplified by the attempt by Sparkman, Quigley, and McCarthy (1991) to implement the CURN model in a general medicine unit and in a rehabilitation unit. Their attempts to address the lack of collaboration between the physicians and nurses were thwarted because one unit used primary nursing, whereas the other used a team nursing approach, and there were differences in staffing patterns. High staff turnover rates, staffing shortages, administrative changes, and the differences in activity level between the units impeded their progress in implementing the proposed changes.

The many challenges to research utilization have been described in the nursing literature (Nicoll & Beyea, 1999; Retsas, 2000; Thompson, Bell, & Prevost, 1999). These challenges can be categorized as intrapersonal, interpersonal, and organizational. Some intrapersonal challenges or barriers to research utilization that have been identified include lack of interest or motivation to use research results, lack of knowledge about the research process, and resistance to change (Nicoll & Beyea, 1999; Retsas, 2000; Thompson, Bell, & Prevost, 1999). Interpersonal barriers include lack of collaboration between researchers and clinicians, research articles not written for clinicians, and lack of availability of consultants to assist clinicians to critically analyze research articles (Thompson, Bell, & Prevost, 1999). Factors within organizations or care systems have also been identified as barriers to research utilization and include lack of time and money allocated to research participation, lack of expectation for involvement in the research process, and lack of reward or positive reinforcement for research and research utilization (Retsas, 2000; Thompson, Bell, & Prevost, 1999). All of these challenges or barriers can be reframed as opportunities, and when present can facilitate the process of research utilization.

Conducting Research in the Clinical Arena

The clinical arena provides many opportunities and challenges. The opportunity to explore phenomena related to rehabilitation and to examine how various phenomena are related provides a basis for understanding practice. Further exploration ultimately can lead to confidence that prescriptions for nursing interventions will influence client outcomes in the expected direction. Unlike the laboratory, where circumstances can be tightly controlled, the clinical arena provides additional challenges related to its complexity and changeability.

Many excellent research textbooks are available to guide nurse researchers through the various stages of the research process, as well as the processes of reading and critically analyzing research reports (Burns & Grove, 1999; Fain, 1999; Mateo & Kirchhoff, 1999; Morse & Field, 1995; Norwood, 2000; Polit & Hungler, 1995). It is convenient to talk about the steps or stages of research, suggesting a linear sequence, whereas the actual process of engaging in research is more likely to involve moving back and forth between the various parts of the research process. For example, a researcher may identify a problem for study, formulate hypotheses, design the research, and then reformulate the problem as more information about what is known and the realities of the clinical situation are better understood.

CONCLUSIONS/PREDICTING THE FUTURE

There continue to be many questions about the effects of rehabilitation nursing practice. Rehabilitation nursing research has concentrated on describing the concepts of interest and exploring how these factors are related. Considerable work is needed to establish what the rehabilitation nurse does to bring about specific outcomes in persons requiring rehabilitation. The time is right for rehabilitation nurses to be proactive in developing a strong knowledge base for nursing practice and rehabilitation outcomes.

What will the future of rehabilitation nursing research bring? The changing health care climate with growing concerns about the spiraling cost of health care, an emphasis on cost-effectiveness of care, and an outcome-oriented society will continue to change significantly the rehabilitation nursing care environment into the future. The integration of practice, research, and theory will provide a knowledge base that will ensure that rehabilitation nurses are included in whatever configuration is taken by the future health care system. What exactly do rehabilitation nurses do to help clients achieve independence in physical activities? What nursing care measures are effective in decreasing complications of disability, such as urinary tract and respiratory infections and decubitus ulcers?

Rehabilitation nursing research will expand the qualitative description of living with chronic illness and disability from the perspective of persons with those experiences. Studies need to be critically reviewed, and theories that may explain the findings across studies need to be developed and tested. Studies that relate phenomena in such a way that predictions can be made of the outcome of selected client characteristics on rehabilitation are critical to the further development of the knowledge base for practice.

Research designs appropriate for small research samples will allow studies to build on one another. Single case studies can be conducted with small numbers of individuals and added to other cases, similarly studied, over time and at other sites. Multisite studies planned by nurses can evolve through the nurses who are employed by large health care corporations that operate multiple health care facilities. Members of the local chapters of the ARN are well placed to plan multisite studies.

The future will see an increased emphasis on interdisciplinary rehabilitation research, with nurses actively involved as members of the research team. These interdisciplinary research teams will be conducting much-needed research on innovative rehabilitation practice. There will be an increase in the development and implementation of research-based guidelines relevant to the care of persons with disability and chronic illness, such as *Multiple Sclerosis: Best Practices in Nursing Care* (Halper, 2000). Equally important will be interdisciplinary efforts toward evidence-based practice and research utilization within rehabilitation settings.

CRITICAL THINKING

1. Give one example of a clinical problem within rehabilitation nursing practice that would benefit from research.
2. List some possible strategies that could be used to overcome barriers to research utilization within rehabilitation settings.

REFERENCES

Acorn, S., & Bampton, E. (1992). Patients' loneliness: A challenge for rehabilitation nurses. *Rehabilitation Nursing, 17,* 22-25.

Ades, P.A., Waldmann, M.L., Polk, D.M., & Coflesky, J.T. (1992). Referral patterns and exercise response in the rehabilitation of female coronary patients aged greater than or equal to 62 years. *American Journal of Cardiology, 69,* 1422-1425.

Altman, B.M., & Smith, R.T. (1990). Rehabilitation service utilization models: Changes in the opportunity structure for disabled women. *International Journal of Rehabilitation Research, 12,* 149-156.

Altman, B.M., & Smith, R.T. (1992). Impact of rehabilitation on psychological distress: Gender differences. *International Journal of Rehabilitation Research, 15,* 75-81.

American Nurses Association (ANA). (1989). *Education for participation in nursing research.* Kansas City, MO: Author.

American Nurses Association (ANA). (1995). *ANA social policy statement.* Kansas City, MO: Author.

Bachman, C. (1990). Producing—and using—nursing research [Editorial]. *Rehabilitation Nursing, 15,* 176.

Burns, N.G., & Grove, S.K. (1999). *Understanding nursing research* (2nd ed.). Philadelphia: WB Saunders.

Burrows, D. (1997). Facilitation: A concept analysis. *Journal of Advanced Nursing, 25*(2), 396-404.

Burtt, K. (1999). Nursing research comes into its own. *American Journal of Nursing, 99*(1), 49-50.

Carlson, C.E., King, R.B., Kirk, P.M., Temple, R., & Heinemann, A. (1992). Incidence and correlates of pressure ulcer development after spinal cord injury. *Rehabilitation Nursing Research, 1*(1), 34-40.

Carlson, R., & Keller, M.L. (1992). Control over daily life and caregiver burden: Little things do count. *Rehabilitation Nursing Research, 1*(1), 6-13.

Dille, C.A., Kirchhoff, K.T., Sullivan, J.J., & Larson, E. (1993). Increasing the wearing time of vinyl urinary drainage bags by decontamination with bleach. *Archives of Physical Medicine and Rehabilitation, 74,* 431-437.

Eakes, G.G., Burke, M.L., & Hainsworth, M.A. (1998). Middle-range theory of chronic sorrow. *Image—The Journal of Nursing Scholarship, 30*(2), 179-184.

Easton, K.L., Rawl, S.M., Zemen, D., Kwiatkowski, S., & Burczyk, B. (1995). The effects of nursing follow-up on the coping strategies used by rehabilitation patients after discharge. *Rehabilitation Nursing Research, 4*(4), 119-127.

Fain, J.A. (1999). *Reading, understanding, and applying nursing research.* Philadelphia: FA Davis.

Fetter, M.S., Feetham, S.L., D'Apolito, K., Chaze, B.A., Fink, A., Frink, B.B., Houghart, M.K., & Rushton, C.H. (1989). Randomized clinical trials: Issues for researchers. *Nursing Research, 38,* 117-120.

Gallagher, M.S. (1998). Urogenital distress and the psychosocial impact of urinary incontinence on elderly women. *Rehabilitation Nursing, 23*(4), 192-197.

Halper, J. (2000). *Multiple sclerosis: Best practices in nursing care.* Columbia, MD: Medicalliance.

Helm, P., Engel, T., Holm, A., Kristiansen, V.B., & Rosendahl, S. (1986). Function after lower limb amputation. *Acta Orthopaedica Scandinavica, 57,* 154-157.

Henson, R.H. (1997). Analysis of the concept of mutuality. *Image—The Journal of Nursing Scholarship, 29*(1), 77-81.

Herbert, R., & Gregor, F. (1997). Quality of life and coping strategies of clients with COPD. *Rehabilitation Nursing, 22*(4), 182-187.

Hoeman, S.P., Dayhoff, N.E., & Thompson, T.C. (1993). The initial RNF research survey: Rehabilitation nursing research interests of ARN members. *Rehabilitation Nursing, 18,* 40-42.

Horsley J.A., Crane, J., Crabtree, K., & Qood, D.J. (1983). *Using research to improve nursing practice: A guide.* New York: Grune & Stratton.

Hutchfield, K. (1999). Family-centred care: A concept analysis. *Journal of Advanced Nursing, 29*(5), 1178-1187.

Johnson, J., & Pearson, V. (2000). The effects of a structured education course on stroke survivors living in the community. *Rehabilitation Nursing, 25*(2), 59-65.

Kirchhoff, K.T., & Rakel, B.A. (1999). Outcomes evaluation. In M.A. Mateo & K.T. Kirchhoff (Eds.), *Using and conducting nursing research in the clinical setting* (2nd ed., pp. 76-89). Philadelphia: WB Saunders.

Kylma, J., & Vehvilainen-Julkunen, K. (1997). Hope in nursing research: A meta-analysis of the ontological and epistemological foundations of research on hope. *Journal of Advanced Nursing, 25*(2), 364-371.

Langford, C., Bowsher, J., Maloney, J., & Lillis, P. (1997). Social support: A conceptual analysis. *Journal of Advanced Nursing, 25*(1), 95-100.

Langner, S.R., & Wolf, Z.R. (1996). Integrating research into acute care settings: Reflections of two nurse researchers. *Nursing Administration Quarterly, 20,* 41-52.

Lindsey, A. (1999). Integrating research and practice. In M.A. Mateo & K.T. Kirchhoff (Eds.), *Conducting and using nursing research in the clinical setting* (2nd ed., pp. 42-55). Philadelphia: WB Saunders.

Mack, M.J. (1952). The personal adjustment of chronically ill old people under home care. *Nursing Research, 1,* 9-31.

Mateo, M.A., & Kirchhoff, K.T. (Eds.). (1999). *Conducting and using nursing research in the clinical setting* (2nd ed.). Philadelphia: WB Saunders.

Mateo, M.A., Kirchhoff, K.T., & Schira, M.G. (1999). Research skill development. In M.A. Mateo & K.T. Kirchhoff (Eds.), *Conducting and using nursing research in the clinical setting* (2nd ed., pp. 64-74). Philadelphia: WB Saunders.

Morse, J., & Field, P. (1995). *Qualitative research methods for health professionals.* Thousand Oaks, CA: Sage.

Mumma, C. (2000). In process. Unpublished data on the experience of living with multiple sclerosis.

Nicoll, L.H., & Beyea, S.C. (1999). Research utilization. In Fain, J.A. (Ed.), *Reading, understanding and applying nursing research* (pp. 261-280). Philadelphia: FA Davis.

Nightingale, F. (1946). *Notes on nursing: What it is and what it is not.* Philadelphia: JB Lippincott.

Norwood, S.L. (2000). *Research strategies for advanced practice nurses.* Upper Saddle River, NJ: Prentice Hall Health.

Penrod, L.E., Hegde, S.K., & Ditunna, J.F., Jr. (1990). Age effect on prognosis for functional recovery in acute, traumatic central cord syndrome. *Archives of Physical Medicine and Rehabilitation, 71,* 963-968.

Pilkington, F.B. (1999). A qualitative study of life after stroke. *Journal of Neuroscience Nursing, 31*(6), 336-347.

Polit, D.F., & Hungler, B.P. (1995). *Nursing research: Principles and methods* (5th ed.). Philadelphia: JB Lippincott.

Puetz, B.E. (1992). Welcome to a new ARN publication [Editorial]. *Rehabilitation Nursing, 17, 56.*

Quigley, P. (1997). Program evaluation and measurement of outcomes. In Johnson, K. (Ed.). *Advanced practice nursing in rehabilitation: A core curriculum* (pp. 277-285). Glenview, IL: Association of Rehabilitation Nurses.

Retsas, A. (2000). Barriers to using research evidence in nursing practice. *Journal of Advanced Nursing, 31*(3), 599-606.

Robinson, D.S., & McKenna, H.P. (1998). Loss: An analysis of a concept of particular interest to nursing. *Journal of Advanced Nursing, 27*(4), 779-784.

Rosswurm, M.A., & Larrabee, J.H. (1999). A model for change to evidence-based practice. *Image—Journal of Nursing Scholarship, 31*(4), 317-322.

Schuster, P.M., Phillips, S., Dillon, D.L., & Tomich, P.L. (1998). The psychosocial and physiological experiences of patients with an implantable cardioverter defibrillator. *Rehabilitation Nursing, 23*(1), 30-37.

Schuster, P.M., & Waldron, J. (1991). Gender differences in cardiac rehabilitation patients. *Rehabilitation Nursing, 16,* 248-253.

Sourial, S. (1997). An analysis of caring. *Journal of Advanced Nursing, 26*(6), 1189-1192.

Sparkman, E.D., Quigley, P., & McCarthy, J. (1991). Putting research into practice. *Rehabilitation Nursing, 16,* 12-14.

Spiers, J. (2000). New perspectives on vulnerability using emic and etic approaches. *Journal of Advanced Nursing, 31*(3), 715-721.

Steels, M.M. (1976). Perceptual style and the adaptation of the aged to the hospital environment. *ARN Journal, 1,* 9-14.

Stetler, C.B. (1994). Refinement of the Stetler/Marram model for application of research findings to practice. *Nursing Outlook, 42*(1), 15-25.

Stuifbergen, A.K., Seraphine, A., & Roberts, G. (2000). An explanatory model of health promotion and quality of life in chronic disabling conditions. *Nursing Research, 49*(3), 122-129.

Styles, M.M. (1995). Nursing in the years to come. *World Health, 48*(Suppl. 5), 34-35.

Thompson, P.E., Bell, P., & Prevost, S. (1999). Overcoming barriers to research-based practice. *Medsurg Nursing, 8*(1), 59-64.

Venn, M.R., Taft, L., Carpentier, B., & Applebaugh, G. (1992). The influence of timing and suppository use on efficiency and effectiveness of bowel training after stroke. *Rehabilitation Nursing, 17,* 116-120.

Verhonick, P.J. (1961). Decubitus ulcer observations measured objectively. *Nursing Research, 10,* 211-218.

White, J.M., Leske, J.S., & Pearcy, J.M. (1995). Models and processes of research utilization. *Nursing Clinics of North America, 30*(3), 409-420.

White, S. (1997). Empathy: A literature review and concept analysis. *Journal of Clinical Nursing, 6*(4), 253-257.

6 Administration and Leadership

Aloma R. Gender, RN, MSN, CRRN
Jean M. Benjamin, MSN, RN, CRRN

After a year in rehabilitation nursing, where I discovered a "career" and not just a "job," I became evening charge nurse. Shortly after assuming my new role, I arrived on duty and was informed that a client had been admitted during the day shift with a spinal cord injury and brain injury due to gunshot wounds. The man, M, was 34 years old and worked in a convenience store, where he had been robbed and shot. He had a wife and two small children, a sister and a brother, and extremely supportive parents; all of them were present at his bedside when I made my rounds. I spent a great deal of time talking with the client and his family members. I gave them a tour of the unit and explained the therapy and nursing care that he would receive. I discussed the things that he and his family could expect to learn. Then I gave them some idea of what could be anticipated during his rehabilitation stay given his current physical condition. Each evening when his family visited, I spent time updating them on his progress and listening to their concerns.

Months later, M's sister told me that I had made a huge difference in their lives on that first day of admission. They had been frightened, and no one on the day shift had spoken much to them. They were in a panic state by the time the evening shift arrived. The time and consideration that I had shown when I walked into the room that first night had calmed them and helped them to see hope for the first time since his injury. M did extremely well and, although still confined to a wheelchair at discharge, was totally independent in his care.

Several years later, M's sister stopped by the unit. She told me that she was going into nursing because of me. She said that she had been impressed with the difference I had made not only in her brother's life but also in her family's life during her brother's rehabilitation stay. She wanted to make that same difference. I was astonished by her remarks because I had only been doing what I considered to be my job. I had not realized the impact that my actions had made in her life. She subsequently became a registered nurse and went on to obtain a master's degree in nursing.

I have thought about that family many times throughout my rehabilitation nursing and management career. Two things always come to mind that I share with new staff and with new leaders. The first lesson is how important it is as a charge nurse to spend time with newly admitted clients to calm their fears, to answer questions, and to help them acclimate to their new environment. It sets the stage for the entire rehabilitation stay and earns the client and family trust from the outset. The second lesson is to be the best leader and rehabilitation nurse that you can possibly be. You never know the kind of impact and far-reaching results you may have in the lives of others.

In medical rehabilitation the expectation is to produce high-quality, cost-effective, and client-centered care. Successes are measured by optimal functional outcomes, high client and staff satisfaction ratings, and cost-effective delivery of care. The responsibility to achieve these goals at a unit or work group level rests with the frontline nurse manager or supervisor (Fox, Fox, & Wells, 1999).

To cope with the complexity and the changes of today's health care environment, nurse managers must be skilled in both management and leadership techniques (Zenger, Ulrich, & Smallwood, 2000). In executing the manager role, the nurse maintains the work group or unit in a steady state, preserving morale, adhering to budget, and upholding policies and procedures. In a leadership role the nurse manager must be a visionary by anticipating future challenges, taking risks, introducing innovations, and motivating staff toward goal achievement (Manfredi, 1996). Peters' (1987) statement rings true: "The very essence of leadership is that you have a vision. It's got to be a vision you articulate clearly and forcefully on every occasion. You can't blow an uncertain trumpet" (p. 399).

Success in implementing the leadership role relies on without purposeful interaction with others. "The challenge is to be a light, not a judge; to be a model, not a critic" (Covey, 1992, p. 25). The leadership style that a nurse manager chooses ultimately affects the success of the organization (Perra, 2000). Developing leadership skills in oneself and in staff is foundational to achieving and maintaining high-quality care.

FACTORS ASSOCIATED WITH REHABILITATION NURSING MANAGEMENT AND LEADERSHIP

Expansion of Rehabilitation Nursing into Other Arenas

Public cost containment and pressures in the health care market have forced a shift in care delivery from high-cost acute care hospitals to lower cost ambulatory, community, and home-based settings (Buerhaus, 1998). This move is evident in rehabilitation environments where sites for care have shifted from comprehensive inpatient rehabilitation to day hospital, subacute rehabilitation, home health, and outpatient clinics. As the influence of managed care has increased, rehabilitation nurses have expanded into case manager roles with third-party payers. Recently, new venues for rehabilitation nurses have been appearing with adult day care services, assisted living, long-term acute care hospitals, and long-term care settings. Chapter 9 discusses community-based rehabilitation in detail.

Future Demand for Rehabilitation Services

The need for medical rehabilitation services is not disappearing. Rather, the demand for services will increase alongside population growth. The 200% increase in persons aged 85 years and older during the next 3 decades—from 4.3 million in 2000 to 8.5 million in 2030 (Coile, 1999)—will create increased demands for services (Buerhaus, 1998). Second, the prevalence and impact of more chronic illness will increase as the "baby boomers" age, until one third of all Americans will have a disability at some point (Williams, 2000).

A third reason for increased demand for health care, including rehabilitation services, is the continuous innovation in diagnostic, treatment, and monitoring technologies for all types of problems. In the past, improved technologies have led to the saving of lives that could not be saved before. The field of medical rehabilitation and the practice of rehabilitation nursing have benefited these survivors. And finally, as per capita incomes grow, the demand for health services keeps pace. Consumer movements in this country will continue to demand not only the best customer service and quality possible but also the most comprehensive range of services necessary to improve and maintain a functional lifestyle.

Local and National Demographics Related to Nursing as a Profession

The demand for nurses is expected to exceed the supply by 2010, until by 2015 there may be a deficit of 114,000 full-time registered nurse (RN) positions (American Health Consultants, 2000). Closer analysis of the data reveals that the average age of an RN is 44 years, only 5 years less than the mean retirement age for nurses of 49 years (Egger, 2000). The average age for new RN graduates is 31 years, leaving them with fewer years to work than the previous generation of graduates (American Health Consultants, 2000). The enrollment in nursing programs has been dropping since 1993, in part because of other college programs competing for students. Some majors have less stringent requirements than nursing; others simply promise graduates jobs in more lucrative fields. The turmoil in the health care industry and RNs' job dissatisfaction have created a negative image for entering into and remaining in the profession (Lucas, 1999).

On the other hand, the opportunities for a rehabilitation nurse leader have never been greater. Expansion of services into different arenas and demands for rehabilitation nursing services creates a challenge for nurses to provide outstanding leadership. They can develop high degrees of satisfaction, and retention among nursing staff can only result in high-quality care and satisfied clients.

FUNCTIONS OF A REHABILITATION NURSE MANAGER

The nurse manager role in rehabilitation has some unique functions beyond those traditionally expected from a front-line nursing manager. In 1994, while supporting the nurse manager's responsibilities, roles, and functions as defined in a 1992 document by the American Organization of Nurse Executives (AONE), the Association of Rehabilitation Nurses (ARN) added a supplement, a role description of the rehabilitation nurse manager. This section expands on those rehabilitation nurse manager functions.

Leadership

At the very heart of the nurse manager role is leadership. Fox, Fox, and Wells (1999) conducted a study to explore which nurse manager activity had the most positive impact on unit productivity levels. They found the leadership role to be most important. Manfredi (1996) stated that given the complex nature of the nurse manager's job, leadership skills are essential for survival. Several concepts make up the role of leader.

Vision/Goals

Leadership involves creating a vision or a mental image of a possible and desirable future state for the organization or unit (Manfredi, 1996). Nurse managers often carry a vision forward that has been set by the nurse executive, but nurse managers will also have personal vision for the unit. A vision must be articulated to those being led. In every activity, the nurse manager must be clear about the desired end state.

To create a vision, one must begin with the results desired and work back. Measurable, specific action steps are set to achieve the desired outcomes. Scorecards, often called "dashboards" or "balanced scorecards" can be developed to keep focus and motivation on progress toward goals (Figure 6-1). A leader should produce measurable results and ultimately leave behind a more robust, stronger organization than the one inherited. A leader with vision raises the bar on what an organization expects and helps employees seek ever loftier goals (Zenger, Ulrich, & Smallwood, 2000). Chapter 7 discusses quality management in detail.

Change

Leadership is about change. Leadership is not required to maintain the status quo. It is required to move an organization forward in a new direction or to a higher level of performance (Zenger, Ulrich, & Smallwood, 2000). In the past, companies wanted loyal employees. Today's organization calls for flexible employees who can adapt quickly, follow a new direction, and enjoy it again and again (Johnson, 1998). A nurse manager must be a change agent, able to cope with change, explain the rationale for change to the staff, and lead change.

Change theory concepts appear in many theoretical models; classic theories on planned change remain useful when a nurse manager intends to move an organization to a new "desired" state. Lewin (1947), is perhaps one of the easiest

Indicators		01 July-Sept	02 Oct-Dec	03 Jan-Mar	04 Apr-June	Targets	Benchmark
Patient satisfaction							
FIM: LOS efficiency							
D/C FIM score	Score: Target:						
FIM change	Score: Target:						
Community D/C %	Score: Target:						
Acute care D/C %	Score: Target:						
Medication error rate							
Restraint use Restraint days ÷ Patient days							
Nosocomial infection rate							
Percent occupancy							
Operating margin							
Cost per day							
Cost per stay							
Length of stay							
Nursing turnover rate							
Nursing vacancy rate							
Worked FTEs per adjusted occupied beds							

Figure 6-1 Quality scorecard. *FIM,* Functional Independence Measure. (Courtesy Good Shepherd Rehabilitation Hospital, Allentown, PA.)

theorists to use. Recognition of need to change triggers Lewin's "unfreezing" from the present situation. Moving toward a new level may involve resistance or environmental restraints, making the person vulnerable and affecting motivation for change and problem-solving abilities. When fit occurs between the change and a new idea or plan, "refreezing" begins. Changes are integrated into lifestyle, relationships, and behaviors, and a sense of closure signifies that the change is completed.

Interpersonal Skills/Emotional Intelligence

Leaders in health care are being charged with the responsibility of becoming more humanistic and with helping to meet staff's emotional needs, as well as helping them to develop better skill sets. When leaders fail, it is often because they lack expertise in the interpersonal side of management. In moving projects forward, the emotional aspect of issues often needs to be analyzed. Anticipating how workers will react to given situations and helping them deal with the emotional side of work-related issues are important skills. "Increasingly, successful leaders are recognized as those who lead with the heart" (Kerfoot, 1996, p. 59-60). Consumers want personalized attentive service. The expectation is for leaders to be more service directed, not only with the external customers, their clients, but with the internal customers as well, especially their staff (Kerfoot, 1996). The most effective leaders have a high degree of emotional intelligence, which can be learned (Goleman, 1998).

The components of emotional intelligence are as follows.

Self-Awareness. Leaders with emotional intelligence have a deep understanding of their own emotions, strengths, weaknesses, needs and drives. They are honest with themselves and others.

Self-Regulation. Persons high in emotional intelligence have control over their feelings and impulses. They self-regulate themselves and are able to create an environment of trust and fairness. Politics and in-fighting are sharply reduced.

Motivation. Emotionally intelligent leaders are driven to achieve for the sake of achievement, not for high salaries or a prestigious company. They have passion for their work, have unflagging energy to do things better, and are restless with the status quo.

Empathy. A leader must be able to sense and understand the viewpoints of every member of the team. An emotionally intelligent nurse manager thoughtfully considers employee's feelings when making decisions. This is important in retaining good talent.

Social Skill. Emotionally intelligent leaders have a wide circle of acquaintances and a knack for finding a common ground with many different types of employees. They work on the assumption that nothing important gets done alone (Goleman, 1998).

Coaching/Mentoring

Another role of a leader is to stimulate growth and development in others (Fox, Fox, & Wells, 1999). Everyone should be trained to lead. True leaders help employees perform better than they would have if the leader had not been there. The nurse manager determines what skills are needed in the staff to deliver the explicit results or outcomes for the unit (Zenger, Ulrich, & Smallwood, 2000). Training content is chosen to target competencies that staff members need for excellence in job performance. Training for irrelevant competencies is pointless and costly (Goleman, 1998). Educational and coaching plans are developed to move employees to a desired end point and should be linked with results.

The workplace has some of the elements of a family in that employees are looking for jobs where employees matter. They want to work *with* managers, not *for* them. Positive reinforcement, rather than fear and intimidation, is what will be successful in the new millennium. A motivational, rather than autocratic, style produces better results, not only in unit and client outcomes but also in low staff turnover and high employee morale (Eade, 1996).

An astute nurse manager will also realize that staff members vary in age and therefore in their expectations of the workplace. "Baby boomers" (born between 1946 and 1962) are workers who have corporate loyalty and generally expect to stay in the same institution for most of their work history. "Generation X" workers (born between 1963 and 1977), grew up in the information age. They learned how to think and communicate in a tidal wave of information (Tulgan, 1999). Generation X workers want meaning in their work and expect to have fun in the workplace. They want constant feedback and short-term rewards. Retirement plans tend not to be of high interest and they do not feel a strong sense of loyalty to their employers. They want honesty in their relationships with employers and are open to being shown potential career paths in organizations (Cole, 1999).

Persons born between 1977 and 1994 are called the "baby boomlet" or "generation next" workers. They compose 26% of the population, whereas the generation X workers compose only 16%. This group of workers is steeped in technology. They grew up in an age of great economic optimism. Money is an incentive, and they are more interested in being part of a team (Wellner, 1999). In coaching and developing staff and in providing an environment that will attract and keep rehabilitation nurses, the nurse manager needs to try to meet individual worker's needs and take into consideration what may be motivational factors for specific generations.

Clinical Nursing Practice and Client Care Delivery

The rehabilitation nurse manager is accountable for excellence in the clinical practice of rehabilitation nursing and the delivery of care on a selected unit or area with around-the-clock responsibility (American Hospital Association [AHA], 1992; Association of Rehabilitation Nurses [ARN], 1994). Expert clinical nursing practice is achieved only when nurses are willing to take steps toward the following excellence.

Rehabilitation Nursing Clinical Roles

The nurse manager supports the rehabilitation nursing staff in performing specific roles and empowers them to become more autonomous. The roles are client educator, caregiver, counselor, consultant, and client advocate (ARN, 1994). All structures, services, systems, and supports must be fully oriented to those the system serves. The rehabilitation nurse and the interdisciplinary team are the centerpiece of the point of service. The locus of control for resource use and decision making must be at this point of service.

Institutional and Professional Rehabilitation Nursing Values, Goals, and Objectives

The rehabilitation nurse manager promotes and translates institutional and professional rehabilitation nursing values, goals, and objectives to nursing staff and interdisciplinary team members (ARN, 1994).

To achieve collaborative practice, interdisciplinary team members must also be educated about the body of knowledge that is rehabilitation nursing. The nurse manager can promote this learning and ensure opportunities through new-employee orientation or education programs. Benner (2001) describes how nurses move from novice status to expert roles within the profession as they gain knowledge and experience and invest in their discipline.

Care Delivery System

To establish excellence in clinical practice, the nurse manager, along with the nurse executive, must first define the care delivery system (ARN, 1994) that will best meet client needs. Several models have been used successfully in rehabilitation settings.

Team Nursing. Team nursing uses an RN to supervise the clinical care of a large group of clients, usually 16 to 20 clients. The RN performs the professional tasks, and the direct client care is assigned to nursing assistants or licensed practical nurses.

Primary Nursing. The primary nurse model often uses an all-RN staff. Each nurse performs total client care for a group of clients, usually 4 to 5.

Modified Primary Nursing. The modified primary nursing model, or modular nursing model, uses a team of licensed and unlicensed nurses to work together in delivering client care. In this model licensed staff members perform direct client care as well as licensed procedures, working closely with a nursing assistant. Each staff member usually cares for 7 to 10 or 12 clients, more than with the primary nurse model.

Client-Focused or Program Model. The client-focused model of care can be overlaid on any of the above models and incorporates a more transdisciplinary model of care. Typically, all members of a team report to a single program director, coordinator, or product-line manager. Health care workers are cross-trained in several disciplines. A nursing assistant may work as a physical or occupational therapy aide and may perform phlebotomies. A housekeeper may be trained to assist with some client care activities, or respiratory therapists may be cross-trained to perform nursing tasks between treatments. A unit secretary may assist with medical record completion and admission paperwork. Usually, in this model universal duties are established that every member of the team, whether therapist or rehabilitation nurse, is able to perform, such as toileting, transfers, or answering phones and call lights.

The nurse manager must be involved in determining the best model for his or her setting to achieve the highest outcomes and satisfaction for the client and to meet budget costs. The model is then implemented and evaluated against targeted results. Chapter 2 contains more information on various types of models and theoretical bases for their use.

Standards of Practice and Competency Guidelines

The intent of the standards and guidelines of practice for rehabilitation nursing must be established in written policies and procedures. Staff nurses need to be educated in the practices and supervised to ensure competence. Client assignments are delegated according to the level of education, training, and competency of the personnel and according to state nursing practice acts. Education programs and delegation to off-hours supervisors, charge nurses, and staff fulfill requirements for the 24-hour supervision clause in the guidelines.

Standards of Care and Accreditation

The rehabilitation nurse manager is accountable for staying current on the content and intent of standards of care established by professional organizations such as the ARN and ANA. Also essential are regulations such as those by the Joint Commission on Accreditation of Health Care Organizations (JCAHO), by the Rehabilitation Accreditation Commission (CARF), and by government agencies such as medicare and medicaid. Nurse managers are able to determine the regulatory implications for a specific area or unit and to respond by promoting and ensuring compliance (ARN, 1994).

Strategies and Programs for Rehabilitation Nursing Care

The nurse manager is responsible for implementing strategies and programs for rehabilitation nursing care that are consistent with the facility or agency mission, vision, policies, goals, and objectives (ARN, 1994). All new programs are oriented to supporting positive client outcomes and satisfaction and should have targeted outcomes by which the success of the new venture can be evaluated. An example is a new pain assessment protocol used on admission and then on every shift. The tool measures a client's perception of pain as self-rated on a 10-point scale. The targeted outcome may be for clients to report higher satisfaction with nurses' pain management techniques.

Long-Range Plans, Unit Goals, and Objectives

With input from the nursing staff, physicians, administrative colleagues, and the nurse executive, nurse managers develop long-range plans for their areas that focus on the provision of high-quality, cost-effective care for the person with a disability. The plan for the nursing department is consistent with the strategic plan for the facility or agency (ARN, 1994).

The Nursing Process

The nurse manager will encourage use of the nursing process in multiple ways. The nursing process can be used to manage client care and ensure continuity from admission through discharge and return to family and community (ARN, 1994). It is useful to facilitate an interdisciplinary approach to care and documentation. The nursing process easily permits interdisciplinary assessments, diagnosis, collaborative client goal setting, client and family education, rehabilitation nursing and team interventions, and evaluation of progress toward goals.

Management Information Systems

Being proficient in the use of the institution's management information systems and understanding related policies and programs are increasingly essential functions of the rehabilitation nurse manager (AHA, 1992). Members of the nursing staff need education and training to become proficient in their use of the systems, and they often need assurance and confidence, as well as technical skills.

Participating in the design of a software program, such as a documentation system, or tailoring it to meet rehabilitation nursing and/or team needs may be a new role for nurse managers. They may need to research and write justifications for programs that improve rehabilitation nursing accuracy or efficiency in providing care. Examples are an automated medication-dispensing system or a program to schedule staffing.

A core competency for the nurse executive is to be able to create credible decision support systems, and input from the nurse manager is essential. Information systems to measure nursing workload, staffing, flexible budgeting, and client outcomes (e.g., software or other system programs) are needed to make clinical nursing decisions (Fralic & Denby, 2000).

Safe and Caring Environment

The environment must be maintained as a safe and caring place for clients, conducive to positive health teaching and health maintenance (AHA, 1992). A safe environment is one in which necessary equipment is ordered and kept in good repair, supplies are appropriate for client needs and readily available, environmental hazards are avoided, and systems are put in place to provide for accuracy with treatments. A caring environment is created when the nurse manager leads the staff in such a way that nurse satisfaction is positive and excellence in customer service results. Many rehabilitation facilities are adopting customer service models such as the Disney or Nordstrom department store approaches.

Aspects of a customer service model may include:

- Setting aggressive client satisfaction goals
- Establishing teams charged with improving key dimensions of client service
- Defining expected service behaviors for interactions between employees and clients

Instilling accountability by having nurse managers develop a monthly plan with goals and discrete action steps for improvement. Client satisfaction scores and individual comments are posted weekly for the client care unit. Executives make routine client rounds to observe service interventions and to speak with clients and staff. Service reprimands occur for violators of service expectations. Repeated violations result in counseling or termination.

Developing service recovery systems that include the nurse manager visiting all newly admitted clients to solicit concerns and complaints and working with staff to resolve problems on the spot. A fix-it fund is available, consisting of money for gift certificates, meal tickets, or flowers to correct problems and to acknowledge client inconvenience.

Hiring for service by aptitude through applicants undergoing multiple evaluations designed to assess service orientation (Health Care Advisory Board, 1999).

Collaborative Relationships

Because of the broad spectrum of problems and challenges that persons with severe disabilities or chronic illness present, treatment is organized around a team. Responsibility to help clients meet goals is an interdisciplinary effort rather than actions of a single discipline (Halstead et al., 1986). The nurse manager must therefore be able to forge collaborative relationships, be persuasive (Davidhizar & Eshleman, 1999), and facilitate collaborative work among professionals of various disciplines and cooperation with sometimes competing departmental agenda, all to deliver effective quality care (ARN, 1994).

Treatment team roles and functions are discussed throughout the book. The nurse manager supports the interdisciplinary team model, ensuring that care regimens are coordinated interdependently with all members of the team (ARN, 1994).

Critical paths or care maps are interdisciplinary tools that outline protocols for care and coordinate the team efforts in a predictable way (see Chapter 2). The interventions of each team member, as well as the client outcomes, are integrated into the care map. These tools help strengthen collaboration and teamwork because care delivery relies on mutually set goals and agreed upon outcomes, times, processes, and responsibilities (Bejciy-Spring, Neutzling, & Newton, 1994). A client's health progress can be plotted from admission to discharge, and the variances can be tracked on a care map. Interdisciplinary teaching plans (Figure 6-2) and discharge-planning forms are other useful tools.

Other role functions of the rehabilitation nurse manager include participating as members of interdisciplinary com-

Text continued on p. 78

Good Shepherd Rehabilitation Hospital **educational objectives** **patient/family educational tool** ☐CVA ☐Brain injury ☐General ☐SCI ☐Orthopedic ☐Other ____________	Addressograph											
Barriers to learning: ☐Aphasia ☐Cognitive ☐No barriers indicated ☐Physical ☐Language ☐Emotional/motivational ☐Visual/hearing ☐Perceptual ☐See comments **Learning preference key:** ☐Seeing/reading ☐Hearing ☐Demonstrating **Learner's educational level:** ☐None ☐Grade school ☐High school ☐College	Method	Learner	Learner readiness	Response	Method	Learner	Learner readiness	Response	Method	Learner	Learner readiness	Response
Objectives:												
A. Functional activities: 1. Demonstrates/instructs safe functional transfer techniques (date) Bed ________ Shower/Tub ________ Floor ________ Toilet ________ Sit to/from stand ________ Wheelchair ________ Car ________ Other ____________________ ☐Appropriate	Date: Initials:				Date: Initials:				Date: Initials:			
	Date: Initials:				Date: Initials:				Date: Initials:			
2. Demonstrates safe technique with functional ambulation ________ wheelchair ________ ☐Appropriate	Date: Initials:				Date: Initials:				Date: Initials:			
3. Demonstrates safe techniques with elevation Curb ________ Stairs ________ ☐Appropriate	Date: Initials:				Date: Initials:				Date: Initials:			
4. Demonstrates/instructs mat/bed mobility and positioning techniques ☐Appropriate	Date: Initials:				Date: Initials:				Date: Initials:			
5. Demonstrates/instructs caregiver in proper techniques for pressure relief ☐Appropriate	Date: Initials:				Date: Initials:				Date: Initials:			
6. Demonstrates/instructs caregiver in proper maintenance of wheelchair cushion ☐Appropriate	Date: Initials:				Date: Initials:				Date: Initials:			
7. Demonstrates/instructs caregiver in management of wheelchair and wheelchair parts ☐Appropriate	Date: Initials:				Date: Initials:				Date: Initials:			

Codes: *Refer to comment section (reassessments and problems or concerns).
Method: *V*, Verbal; *H*, hands on; *W*, written; *O*, observation; *A*, audio/visual;
Learner: *P*, patient; *S*, spouse; *O*, other (refer to comments);
Learning readiness: *E*, eager; *A*, acceptance; *N*, nonacceptance; *R*, refuses; *O*, other (describe in comments);
Response: *U*, understands and demonstrates competency; *G*, understands but requires guidance;
N, no understanding.
N or *R* responses require a reassessment or indicate barriers to learning.

Figure 6-2 Client/family education tool. (Courtesy Good Shepherd Rehabilitation Hospital, Allentown, PA.)

Continued

Objectives:	Method	Learner	Learner readiness	Response	Method	Learner	Learner readiness	Response	Method	Learner	Learner readiness	Response
8. Demonstrates ability to propel wheelchair on: level ________ curb ________ inclines ________ stairs ________ ☐Appropriate	Date: Initials:				Date: Initials:				Date: Initials:			
9. Participates in selection of wheelchair and options ☐Appropriate	Date: Initials:				Date: Initials:				Date: Initials:			
10. Demonstrates skill of appropriate upper/lower extremity positioning during functional activities ☐Appropriate	Date: Initials:				Date: Initials:				Date: Initials:			
11. Demonstrates carryover of appropriate techniques during ADLs and/or IADLs ☐Appropriate	Date: Initials:				Date: Initials:				Date: Initials:			
12. Demonstrates/instructs precautions during functional activities ☐Appropriate	Date: Initials:				Date: Initials:				Date: Initials:			
13. Demonstrates compensatory strategies for deficits during functional activities ☐Appropriate	Date: Initials:				Date: Initials:				Date: Initials:			
14. Identifies 1-2 areas of community accessibility for reintegration postdischarge ☐Appropriate	Date: Initials:				Date: Initials:				Date: Initials:			
15. Other: ☐Appropriate	Date: Initials:				Date: Initials:				Date: Initials:			
B. Communication/cognition: 1. Identifies impact of cognitive/perceptual impairments and utilizes appropriate compensatory strategies ☐Appropriate	Date: Initials:				Date: Initials:				Date: Initials:			
2. Explains and demonstrates techniques to maximize communication ☐Appropriate	Date: Initials:				Date: Initials:				Date: Initials:			
3. Defines receptive and expressive aphasia and demonstrates techniques to maximize communication ☐Appropriate	Date: Initials:				Date: Initials:				Date: Initials:			

Figure 6-2, cont'd Client/family education tool. (Courtesy Good Shepherd Rehabilitation Hospital, Allentown, PA.)

Objectives:	Method	Learner	Learner readiness	Response	Method	Learner	Learner readiness	Response	Method	Learner	Learner readiness	Response
4. Defines oral and verbal apraxia and demonstrates techniques to maximize communication ☐Appropriate	Date: Initials:				Date: Initials:				Date: Initials:			
5. Defines dysarthria and demonstrates techniques to maximize communication ☐Appropriate	Date: Initials:				Date: Initials:				Date: Initials:			
6. Other: ☐Appropriate	Date: Initials:				Date: Initials:				Date: Initials:			
C. Dysphagia: 1. Defines dysphagia and identifies signs/symptoms of aspiration ☐Appropriate	Date: Initials:				Date: Initials:				Date: Initials:			
2. Demonstrates use of safe swallowing strategies and diet texture modification ☐Appropriate	Date: Initials:				Date: Initials:				Date: Initials:			
3. Other: ☐Appropriate	Date: Initials:				Date: Initials:				Date: Initials:			
D. Adaptive technique/equipment: 1. Demonstrates use of adaptive and assistive devices ☐Appropriate	Date: Initials:				Date: Initials:				Date: Initials:			
2. Demonstrates proper care and use of bracing/splints/slings ☐Appropriate	Date: Initials:				Date: Initials:				Date: Initials:			
3. Verbalizes bracing/splint wear/care schedule ☐Appropriate	Date: Initials:				Date: Initials:				Date: Initials:			
4. Demonstrates use of adaptive devices and techniques for recreation skills ☐Appropriate	Date: Initials:				Date: Initials:				Date: Initials:			
5. Demonstrates ability or gives verbal direction to perform pin care, brace management, or collar management ☐Appropriate	Date: Initials:				Date: Initials:				Date: Initials:			

Figure 6-2, cont'd Client/family education tool.

Continued

Objectives:	Method	Learner	Learner readiness	Response	Method	Learner	Learner readiness	Response	Method	Learner	Learner readiness	Response
6. Other: ☐Appropriate	Date: Initials:				Date: Initials:				Date: Initials:			
E. Psychosocial reintegration: 1. Describes some of the major change in coping with altered social roles and activity pattern after hospitalization ☐Appropriate	Date: Initials:				Date: Initials:				Date: Initials:			
2. Identifies 1-2 community resources for leisure involvement/recreational activities for postdischarge ☐Appropriate	Date: Initials:				Date: Initials:				Date: Initials:			
3. Identifies community resources for continuum of care ☐Appropriate	Date: Initials:				Date: Initials:				Date: Initials:			
4. Identifies 1-2 recreational activities for involvement postdischarge ☐Appropriate	Date: Initials:				Date: Initials:				Date: Initials:			
5. Explains risk of alcohol/substance abuse and means of accessing treatment/support postdischarge ☐Appropriate	Date: Initials:				Date: Initials:				Date: Initials:			
6. Explains emotional and adjustment reactions that are experienced by the person and family/significant others ☐Appropriate	Date: Initials:				Date: Initials:				Date: Initials:			
7. Describes symptoms of postonset depression and means of getting help to cope ☐Appropriate	Date: Initials:				Date: Initials:				Date: Initials:			
8. Cites examples of changes in thinking and behavior that can occur as a consequence of disability ☐Appropriate	Date: Initials:				Date: Initials:				Date: Initials:			
9. Verbalizes understanding of sexuality issues postinjury ☐Appropriate	Date: Initials:				Date: Initials:				Date: Initials:			
10. Other: ☐Appropriate	Date: Initials:				Date: Initials:				Date: Initials:			

Figure 6-2, cont'd Client/family education tool. (Courtesy Good Shepherd Rehabilitation Hospital, Allentown, PA.)

Objectives:	Method	Learner	Learner readiness	Response	Method	Learner	Learner readiness	Response	Method	Learner	Learner readiness	Response
F. Risk management/prevention: 1. Verbalizes understanding of unit safety measures, including orientation to environment ☐Appropriate	Date: Initials:				Date: Initials:				Date: Initials:			
2. Verbalizes/demonstrates use of bowel program/elimination pattern, including ostomy care if applicable ☐Appropriate	Date: Initials:				Date: Initials:				Date: Initials:			
3. Demonstrates knowledge of bladder/elimination pattern; use of internal/external catheter ☐Appropriate	Date: Initials:				Date: Initials:				Date: Initials:			
4. Verbalizes appropriate use and management of medication ☐"Coumadin" booklet issued ☐Medications teaching reviewed and issued ☐Side effect ☐Appropriate	Date: Initials:				Date: Initials:				Date: Initials:			
5. Promotes skin integrity with developed awareness of signs and symptoms of infection ☐Appropriate	Date: Initials:				Date: Initials:				Date: Initials:			
6. Identifies methods to control edema ☐Appropriate	Date: Initials:				Date: Initials:				Date: Initials:			
7. Identifies methods and treatment to improve skin integrity, including foot care if diabetic. Identifies healthy stoma/peristomial skin if applicable ☐Appropriate	Date: Initials:				Date: Initials:				Date: Initials:			
8. Verbalizes/demonstrates knowledge of pain management ☐Appropriate	Date: Initials:				Date: Initials:				Date: Initials:			
9. Demonstrates appropriate energy conservation techniques ☐Appropriate	Date: Initials:				Date: Initials:				Date: Initials:			
10. Demonstrates appropriate joint protection techniques ☐Appropriate	Date: Initials:				Date: Initials:				Date: Initials:			
11. Verbalizes/demonstrates understanding of methods to increase home safety and accessibility ☐Appropriate	Date: Initials:				Date: Initials:				Date: Initials:			

Figure 6-2, cont'd Client/family education tool.

Continued

Objectives:	Method	Learner	Learner readiness	Response	Method	Learner	Learner readiness	Response	Method	Learner	Learner readiness	Response
12. Demonstrates proper SROM/PROM/AROM and home exercise program ☐Appropriate	Date: Initials:				Date: Initials:				Date: Initials:			
13. Learns stress management and stress reduction techniques ☐Appropriate	Date: Initials:				Date: Initials:				Date: Initials:			
14. Verbalizes understanding of discharge follow-up appointments (OT, PT, MD) and follow-up lab studies ☐Discharge teaching instructions given ☐Appropriate	Date: Initials:				Date: Initials:				Date: Initials:			
15. Verbalizes knowledge of basic principles of __________ diet ☐Appropriate	Date: Initials:				Date: Initials:				Date: Initials:			
16. Demonstrates ability to select items from patient menu according to prescribed diet ☐Appropriate	Date: Initials:				Date: Initials:				Date: Initials:			
17. Identifies basic spinal cord anatomy and physical abilities based on level of injury ☐Appropriate	Date: Initials:				Date: Initials:				Date: Initials:			
18. Demonstrates awareness of signs and symptoms of autonomic dysreflexia (AD) with ability to give verbal directions for interventions or treatment of AD ☐Appropriate	Date: Initials:				Date: Initials:				Date: Initials:			
19. Verbalizes knowledge of how to prevent medical complications, such as DVT, orthostatic hypotension, and poikilothermia, postinjury ☐Appropriate	Date: Initials:				Date: Initials:				Date: Initials:			
20. Verbalizes knowledge of spasticity and awareness of related problems with increase in spasms ☐Appropriate	Date: Initials:				Date: Initials:				Date: Initials:			
21. Identifies risk factors, prevention, and symptoms of disability ☐Appropriate	Date: Initials:				Date: Initials:				Date: Initials:			
22. Identifies disease process and course of recovery ☐Appropriate	Date: Initials:				Date: Initials:				Date: Initials:			

Figure 6-2, cont'd Client/family education tool. (Courtesy Good Shepherd Rehabilitation Hospital, Allentown, PA.)

Objectives:	Method	Learner	Learner readiness	Response	Method	Learner	Learner readiness	Response	Method	Learner	Learner readiness	Response
23. Demonstrates behavior management strategies ☐Appropriate	Date: Initials:				Date: Initials:				Date: Initials:			
24. Demonstrates/instructs appropriate oral health care ☐Appropriate	Date: Initials:				Date: Initials:				Date: Initials:			
25. Other: ☐Appropriate	Date: Initials:				Date: Initials:				Date: Initials:			
G. Pulmonary: 1. Understands use of oxygen therapy if indicated ☐Appropriate	Date: Initials:				Date: Initials:				Date: Initials:			
2. Understands rationale for and can demonstrate proper techniques in controlled breathing and coughing ☐Appropriate	Date: Initials:				Date: Initials:				Date: Initials:			
3. Understands how emotions affect respirations and can demonstrate proper relaxation breathing techniques ☐Appropriate	Date: Initials:				Date: Initials:				Date: Initials:			
4. Demonstrates the use of breathing techniques that will preserve energy conservation ☐Appropriate	Date: Initials:				Date: Initials:				Date: Initials:			
5. Demonstrates proper technique in performance of respiratory modality ☐Appropriate	Date: Initials:				Date: Initials:				Date: Initials:			
6. Is able to explain rationale for respiratory modality demonstrated ☐Appropriate	Date: Initials:				Date: Initials:				Date: Initials:			
H. Diabetes: 1. Verbalizes knowledge of hypoglycemia/hyperglycemia and measures to implement with either ☐Appropriate	Date: Initials:				Date: Initials:				Date: Initials:			
2. Identifies process and risk factors of diabetes ☐Appropriate	Date: Initials:				Date: Initials:				Date: Initials:			

Figure 6-2, cont'd Client/family education tool.

Continued

Objectives:	Method	Learner	Learner readiness	Response	Method	Learner	Learner readiness	Response	Method	Learner	Learner readiness	Response
3. Demonstrates independence with insulin administration (if applicable) and BS monitoring or is able to direct caregiver to do same ☐Appropriate	Date: Initials:				Date: Initials:				Date: Initials:			
I. Cardiac: 1. Develops understanding of angina/pain symptoms of MI and understands use of NTG ☐Appropriate	Date: Initials:				Date: Initials:				Date: Initials:			
J. Seizures: 1. Verbalizes knowledge of types and their manifestation and safety precautions related to seizure activity ☐Appropriate	Date: Initials:				Date: Initials:				Date: Initials:			
K. Preventative health: (circle) 1. Cholesterol/blood pressure/women's health/men's health/obesity/smoking/ foot care ☐Appropriate	Date: Initials:				Date: Initials:				Date: Initials:			
L. Other: 1. ☐Appropriate	Date: Initials:				Date: Initials:				Date: Initials:			
2. ☐Appropriate	Date: Initials:				Date: Initials:				Date: Initials:			
3. ☐Appropriate	Date: Initials:				Date: Initials:				Date: Initials:			
4. ☐Appropriate	Date: Initials:				Date: Initials:				Date: Initials:			

Comments: ______________________________

Figure 6-2, cont'd Client/family education tool. (Courtesy Good Shepherd Rehabilitation Hospital, Allentown, PA.)

mittees, in planning and in program development (ARN, 1994). The nurse manager in a rehabilitation setting can expect to meet routinely with directors of medical programs, various therapies, administrators, and other managers. A collaborative and collegial relationship reflects elements of mutual trust, respect, and support. Input from any and all parties is valued equally, and decisions are made after all perspectives are heard, including those of the client and family (Velianoff, Neely, & Hall, 1993; ARN, 1994).

Fiscal Management

Preparation of rehabilitation nurse managers for financial management is frequently on-the-job training combined with trial and error. Often the nurse manager's first exposure to fiscal management is preparing a budget or explaining variances. There are excellent texts specifically written to assist the nurse manager in fiscal management. The intent of this section is to provide descriptions of fiscal operations that a rehabilitation nurse manager can expect to perform.

Budget preparation and maintenance are the core of fiscal management for the nurse manager role (ARN, 1994). A budget is a fiscal plan for a designated period, usually 1 year. Budget preparation can be described as short-term fiscal strategic planning. Budget maintenance is the routine analysis of variances from the fiscal plan that may occur monthly, quarterly, or more often depending on the organization.

Three budget categories are revenue, expense, and capital. An operating budget is a combination of revenue and expense budgets.

Operating Budget

Revenue. The revenue budget projects income for a specific entity or area of responsibility. Although financial report forms vary between settings, typical contents include both current month and fiscal year-to-date information. Comparisons of actual income versus predicted income for the current month, and for the fiscal year to date, can be used to identify fiscal trends. Financial reports also often subdivide income by payer source. Review of the mix of payer sources and trends over time enables the nurse manager to evaluate implications of financial reimbursement. "Patient days" are the typical unit of fiscal measurement for inpatient settings. Multiplying dollars per patient day by anticipated patient days may project revenue. Client visits, procedures, and/or time increments may be used in the home health or clinic settings.

In a facility, the manager needs to note when the total number of patient days decreases while the admissions increase. This phenomenon may be due to shorter lengths of stay for clients. This may result in an increased workload for nursing staff, even though the average daily census is lower than previously experienced. Analyzing trends of admissions, patient days, and lengths of stay is an important activity in preparing and maintaining the budget. An inexperienced nurse manager may monitor and adjust expenses compulsively based on a fixed budget, while patient days and reimbursements fluctuate significantly above or below expectations, causing revenues and expenses to fluctuate also.

The experienced rehabilitation nurse manager uses the applicable unit of fiscal measurement—for example, patient days, visits, procedures, or other—to identify "break-even" points for the budget. These break-even points occur when revenues equal expenses. The nurse manager strives to increase revenues and decrease expenses while maintaining or improving effectiveness and efficiency of client outcomes. Payer sources vary in amount of reimbursement. The mix of clients by payer source affects revenue and therefore the number of patient days, visits, or procedures at which the break-even point occurs. As the rehabilitation nurse manager gains experience, comparison of diagnostic categories and related costs will be refined.

Expense

Personnel. The expense budget reflects the predictions of annual costs for area-defined expenses. Most costs in the expense budget for inpatient rehabilitation nursing areas are salaries, which include fringe benefits. Salaries frequently exceed 80% to 90% of the total expense budget. This fiscal effect is due to the labor-intensive aspects of rehabilitation and the need for rehabilitation nursing staff with specialized skills and knowledge.

The goal of the staffing function is to provide optimal quality care with the most economic staffing. Staffing in an inpatient setting is a process of determining and providing nursing staff to offer an effective number of nursing hours per patient day (HPPD), that is, the best mix of nursing staff with the correct distribution of personnel over the 24-hour day for 7 days a week. No one correct staffing configuration works for all rehabilitation units or outpatient settings (which may base staffing on the number of services or hours of service performed). A standard system of staffing based on research specific for rehabilitation needs does not exist. Differences in many variables, including client populations, physician practices, services available, acuity, and availability of various personnel levels make generic staffing approaches unrealistic. Rehabilitation nurse managers should retain input into whatever system is used to promote its appropriateness for their setting (ARN, 1999).

Acuity. Many variables affect staffing, but the primary variable is client acuity, a measure of each client's severity of illness and complexity related to the amount of nursing resources needed for care (Finkler & Kovner, 2000). Client classification systems are used by some facilities to quantify the number or mix of staff needed. A classification system typically divides clients into categories according to the intensity of care each one needs. In turn, the resulting acuity level indicates the mix and number of staff required. A client classification system must be valid and reliable in order for a manager to make realistic and accountable decisions about staffing.

Ter Maat (1993) found that 67% of the rehabilitation hospitals she surveyed used a system developed within the institution. A nationally established client classification system allows for comparisons of like institutions, but client diagnosis, age, and comorbidities may make comparisons difficult. Some rehabilitation units admit clients with orthopedic or chronic pain conditions where the acuity may be lower than for a unit admitting clients with mechanical ventilators after spinal cord injury or clients in coma management programs.

Administrators often are surprised to learn that the acuity and recommended HPPD are as high as in some step-down units. That clients need more time when guided or assisted through an activity than when full care is given by a caregiver is an underappreciated and unfamiliar concept. When an institution or agency develops or selects a client classification system, rehabilitation nurse managers ideally are key participants in decision making.

It is important when developing a system to represent quantifiable measures about the unique functions of rehabilitation nurses, such as their involvement in client education and prevention of complications. Time spent in performing multiple client transfers in and out of the wheelchair during the day, extensive wound management, and caring for cognitively impaired or combative clients are all unique to rehabilitation nursing and may need to be a part of a classification system, depending on the facility. Rehabilitation nurses also perform extensive assessments concerning client safety, adaptability, and access to community resources, as well as participating with community agencies and services in promoting continuity of care and preventing readmission to a facility. Sometimes these functions are not weighted as highly as technological interventions in classification systems that are nonspecific for rehabilitation.

Supplies/Services. The nonsalary budget includes supplies and services or direct expenses not related to employees. They are routine costs to nursing areas such as medical and nonmedical supplies. Communication and coordination with other departments are important when planning this part of the budget because budget plans in one department may affect what happens to rehabilitation nursing expenses. Expenses may be transferred to the nursing budget from other areas such as duplication, maintenance expenses, meals, or mattress-replacement costs.

The supplies/services budget accounts may yield opportunities to reduce expenses and improve client care at the same time. Although some cost-effective efforts may be small over the short-term, over time or in combination with others, positive results can be achieved. The rehabilitation nurse manager remains vigilant that rehabilitation needs are met in fiscal efforts. For example, individual trays for clients may be substituted for a cafeteria-style serving line in a rehabilitation facility. The intent is to reduce dietary employee full-time equivalents (FTEs) and preparation/wastage costs. The rehabilitation nurse manager ensures that the new procedure incorporates menu selection by clients and that the area where they eat retains the atmosphere of a dining room. In another instance, medications and equipment selected for bowel or bladder management protocols may have significant financial impact on the nursing department budget. These costs may be justified only if the protocols can be shown to improve client outcomes after the person reenters the community. The presence of large purchasing groups across the country may affect the manager's ability to individualize supplies to rehabilitation needs.

Becoming familiar with whether items used by clients are "charge" or "noncharge" and the costs for the items is essential to budgeting supplies. Items that are to be billed to clients are individual charges entered as each item is used. Noncharge items, such as disposable bedpans, must be limited to those situations that affect care because their costs can create deficits quickly. The manager can establish methods to avoid waste and monitor use of noncharge items. It is easy for an inexperienced manager to ask for an item to be added to the charge list, believing the cost will be covered by the person's payment source. In fact, many persons have a set per diem reimbursement rate, regardless of charges. Another subtle problem arises with charges that are lost to the billing process. When chargeable items are used for care or dispensed to the client but not billed correctly, the nursing budget usually must absorb the cost. The astute nurse manager knows meal and snack costs, linen charges, and similar facility-specific expenses.

The entire area of rehabilitation reimbursement is in the process of undergoing massive change because of the Balanced Budget Act of 1997. The implications are far reaching and fluctuating, but it has been determined that comprehensive inpatient rehabilitation reimbursement will involve functional-related groupings and be based on discharges.

Capital Budget

Capital budget covers equipment, building project costs, or larger items that cost more than a facility-specified amount but that have been planned as purchases for the fiscal year. Capital expense items are intended to be in use for a designated number of years. In planning capital expenditures, the rehabilitation nurse manager takes into account the feasibility of the item in meeting the special needs of rehabilitation clients. Examples include considering bed height conducive to transfer activities when buying new beds, installing effective safety-lock mechanisms on wheelchair shower chairs for persons who are physically or cognitively impaired, and obtaining dining room tables that have adjustable heights and that are able to accommodate wheelchair leg rests. Nurse managers often can justify a capital equipment purchase if it enhances rehabilitation activities, for example, installing a tub on the unit for clients to practice bathing when only showers are available or purchasing hydraulic lifts for safety and to help prevent back injuries in staff and families. Targeting specific amounts of money in a capital budget that can be allocated for new services or for replacing worn equipment or to buy specialized items for planned changes on units is within the fiscal planning responsibilities of the nurse manager.

Internal Fiscal Monitoring

The effective nurse manager uses internal monitoring to enhance fiscal control. Internal monitoring approaches vary among settings, but their purpose remains constant, to have current knowledge of the financial state of the area of accountability. Internal monitoring could include daily productivity measures (nursing HPPD, number of visits); monthly nursing labor and expense cost reports (including cost of overtime and supplemental staff from outside agencies); and linen, storeroom, or central supply utilization. Routinely evaluating lost charges with the staff develops their understanding of costs and resource allocation to encourage prudent use. Involving staff in identifying approaches to cost savings heightens their awareness of financial considerations and builds team "ownership" of responsibility. Monitoring the types of tests or procedures ordered is another extremely important way to reduce costs. For example, a follow-up chest x-ray film that is not critical to a client's rehabilitation care should be scheduled after discharge. Bringing staff into partnership for fiscal responsibility is a step in team building.

Prioritizing capital equipment purchases may also increase staff awareness of fiscal decision making. Often nursing staff members are unfamiliar with what a wheelchair shower chair, stretcher, or client lift costs. Knowing the cost of replacing seats for wheelchair shower chairs or slings for client lifts may encourage staff to take extra care with equipment and the benefits of maintenance. Staff meetings could include fiscal information related to monthly salary expense compared with budget, overtime use, storeroom charges, and other expenses. The rehabilitation nurse manager should share where there has been a significant variance between actual expenditures and the budgeted amount. Run charts or graphs may be helpful to demonstrate to staff the changes among expense accounts or lines from month to month and involve them in the process. Staff members may not recognize how costs in one area may reduce funds available in others when the expenses are not obviously related. A nurse manager may choose ways to monitor the budget, but there also may be internal monitoring requirements, such as a monthly budget variance report to the nurse manager's supervisor, explaining variances above or below expected utilization.

Many external factors have the potential to influence the budget. New regulatory expectations, such as the requirement by the Occupational Safety and Health Administration (OSHA) for the use of "safe needles" nationwide, have a fiscal impact because of the cost of supplies purchased and staff in-service programs. Third-party payment influences the fiscal bottom line because each payer has guidelines for which services, equipment, and supplies will be reimbursed. Financial "caps" to payment mean a designated number of visits, days, or procedures or a set dollar amount may not be exceeded. External controls, such as federal, state, or accreditation requirements may affect costs. Fiscal management is an intricate balance of ever-changing factors that enhance or adversely affect the budget bottom line. Vigilance and creativity are necessary if the rehabilitation nurse is to manage effectively and efficiently to maintain financial stability.

Quality Improvement

Employees want to do the best job that they are capable of doing. It is incumbent upon managers to create an environment where those closest to the client are able to adapt work processes and improve quality of care. Continuous quality improvement can help an organization meet or exceed customer expectations by encouraging employee participation in planning and implementing quality improvements. The nurse manager strives to create a work culture that is committed to continuous quality improvement and learning rather than simply correcting deficiencies or meeting current standards (Motwani, Klein, & Navitskas, 1999). Chapter 6 presents a comprehensive overview of the continuous quality improvement process.

According to ARN's (1994) role description, the rehabilitation nurse manager has three important functions in the quality process. The manager directs the unit's quality improvement program and continuously seeks to improve the quality of care, institutes practice changes based on evaluation, and supports interdisciplinary continuous quality improvement efforts to improve client care.

Direction of the Unit's Quality Improvement Program

The nurse manager must direct the unit or area's quality improvement program and continuously seek to improve the quality of care (ARN, 1994). The status quo cannot be the norm. Client care can be improved only when nurses and team members have both the desire and the authority to find better ways to do their jobs every day.

Priorities for performance improvement are typically set by the organization as a whole. Processes are then measured according to these priorities. Examples in rehabilitation are client satisfaction surveys and measurements of a client's functional outcomes on admission, at discharge, and at a predetermined point after discharge. The nurse manager, with the staff's input, may choose to measure other functional areas not identified as organizational priorities (Motwani, Klein, & Navitskas, 1999). Examples might be measuring a client's comprehension of teaching about medication regimens or skin care techniques, evaluating alternatives to restraints used by staff on a unit for persons with brain injury, or evaluating effectiveness and adequacy of pain control procedures for clients on an orthopedic unit.

Implementation of Practice Changes

Measuring processes or outcomes is meaningful only when results are evaluated to show areas in need of improvement or where gains have been made in training or program interventions. Evaluation requires examining data using appropriate statistical and analytical tools (Motwani, Klein, & Navitskas, 1999). Once changes that need to be made are identified, the nurse manager institutes changes in practice that directly relate to the need (ARN, 1994). The new practice or system then needs to be evaluated for stability and improvement over time.

Support of Interdisciplinary Continuous Quality Improvement

The interdisciplinary rehabilitation team members must take ownership for their work processes and for improved outcomes. The rehabilitation nurse manager supports interdisciplinary continuous quality improvement efforts (ARN, 1994) in which processes can be streamlined and made more efficient. Examples are the admission process, the system for client assessment and goal setting, client and family education, team conference formats, methods for establishing client goals, medication administration, and client scheduling. Communication among team members helps ensure consistency of care and follow-through 24 hours a day, 7 days a week. Quality improvement includes scrutinizing the steps of processes to identify those that can be eliminated to reduce errors or streamlined to improve flow of operations.

The rehabilitation nurse manager encourages staff members to become partners in improving the processes and outcomes. Staff members can identify concerns, become involved in endeavors to improve performance, assist with evaluating data, and implement changes. The manager who routinely shares data, recognizes teamwork, and celebrates with staff when changes lead to improved practice and outcomes also is building morale and staff development.

Nursing Staff Development

In collaboration with a clinical nurse specialist or an educator, the rehabilitation nurse manager ensures that licensed and unlicensed staff involved in providing direct care receive education and training (ARN, 1994). Four steps in defining content of the education program begin with identifying what resources are available to support or provide education. Educational resources may be manpower, such as the manager, nurses with experience or special expertise, clinical educators or faculty, other rehabilitation professionals, vendors of specialty items or adaptive equipment, and experts from community agencies or organizations, such as the Arthritis Foundation. Educational resources include books and journals, equipment or supply instructions, and audio cassettes or videotapes. Financial resources include funds for educational conferences or support for staff to obtain credentials.

The second step is to identify educational priorities related to the unique needs of clients, as well as for staff, for the facility, and for regulatory or accreditation requirements. The third step, educational needs assessment, can identify goals and objectives for staff development. Responses to a questionnaire or open discussions in staff meetings may yield information about learning needs that are important to staff. Outcome data and observations of clinical practice, as well as new programs or services, may also contribute to staff development goal achievement.

Without the fourth step of creating a supportive environment, education may be futile. The rehabilitation nurse manager serves as a role model to demonstrate continuous education through expectations and actions. By setting an example to enhance the value of ongoing education, the manager and staff are able to share ownership of an increase in knowledge and skills and the value of both. Chapter 11 contains information about all aspects of client and family education, including problem-specific teaching plans.

Staff Education

The nurse manager as role model, mentor, and coach provides opportunities for nursing staff to acquire clinical rehabilitation nursing skills and expertise (ARN, 1994). Staff education has three categories: orientation, in-service programs, and continuing education programs. Staff education processes address the learning needs of a variety of staff members, licensed and unlicensed, who work in the nurse manager's area of responsibility. Competency, both knowledge and skill, is an educational responsibility. Competency measurements must assess whether a staff member can apply specific knowledge and skills, not simply identify or list them. The rehabilitation nurse manager plans for staff to achieve competencies necessary for them to carry out their responsibilities in rehabilitation care. Excellent resources are available for teaching nursing assistants about restorative care in subacute, long-term care, and home settings (Hoeman, 1990; Tracey, 1999).

Orientation. Orientation is the process of transitioning a new staff member into a work area. Because rehabilitation nursing is not typically covered as an elective in most nursing programs, many new employees have no prior rehabilitation nursing experience. Without this experience, nurses and other staff members may need education about the unique "culture" of rehabilitation nursing, as well as information to clarify misconceptions they may have developed from lack of exposure to the specialty (Ruiz, 2000). Orientation is critical for transmitting rehabilitation nursing theory and concepts. The nurse manager sets a tone with current staff about the importance of orientation and the value of new employees. Following principles for teaching adult learners, the nurse manager intersperses classroom work with application opportunities. A preceptor or mentor program is often a good way to help new staff enter the field of rehabilitation nursing.

In-service Programs. In-service programs, a second category, help staff members keep current on new practices, procedures, products, or knowledge. In-service programs can be given in short blocks of time by lecture or discussion, mobile learning carts, posters or flyers, or self-learning study packets, to name a few methods. Creativity is essential to ensure that staff members receive ongoing education with their busy nursing practice schedule.

Continuing Education Programs. Continuing education programs are planned learning experiences for staff development beyond the basic nursing curriculum. Programs may include such diverse areas as advanced assessment parameters for a specific client population, growth and development of applications in rehabilitation, or exposure to ideas of rehabilitation nursing leaders. Ideally, continuing education programs will offer contact hours as continuing education units needed to maintain certification in the nursing specialty.

Typically there are more ideas for educational activities than there is time for staff members to attend or resources to provide them. Although educational activities are planned to meet staff development criteria, in reality they are offered within the context of a busy work area where client needs are priorities. When educational programs are interrupted continually or not attended, it becomes a quality issue and the manager intervenes.

Educational activities are evaluated to identify how well attendees learned and the effect of learning on client outcomes or clinical decision making. Evaluation is important on several levels. Results of evaluations will indicate how well the program was conducted and whether it was cost-effective. Another measure is participant's self-reports of their learning as a result of having attended the program. Over time, education programs are expected to influence changes in participants' behaviors or improve competencies in their professional practices. Only when educational evaluation data demonstrate results can programs be promoted as cost-effective and an appropriate use of resources.

Lifelong Education for Professional Nursing

It is appropriate for nurse managers to promote professional nursing responsibility for lifelong learning. With the rapid explosion of knowledge and technology in nursing, rehabilitation, and health care, it is impossible to maintain expertise in practice without actively pursuing ongoing learning.

The standards for professional nursing practice include a mandate to acquire and maintain current knowledge in nursing practice (ANA, 1991). Within this standard are criteria that address a nurse's responsibility for participating in ongoing educational activities related to clinical knowledge and professional issues, as well as in seeking experiences to maintain clinical skills and knowledge appropriate to the practice setting. The process that nurses use to meet this professional responsibility is similar to that used for client and family education. The assessment component requires the nurse to identify learning needs, readiness to learn, and the learning style that best supports acquisition of knowledge and skills. This requires the professional nurse to evaluate critically what knowledge and skills are needed. Once the assessment has been accomplished, the nurse develops a plan for achieving the desired learning. The plan includes specific goals and objectives, available resources, learning activities that will be used, and how evaluation of the plan will take place. Finally the plan is implemented and evaluated—an ongoing process.

Many strategies can be used to pursue lifelong professional learning. Continuing education programs are available in a variety of formats, such as seminars, workshops, or conferences offered on-site or by satellite transmission. Continuing education also is available in independent study modules or through various journals. Regularly reading and critiquing professional materials and books and discussing how to use research findings published in journal articles are popular activities of a staff journal club. Professional associations, health organizations, and government agencies sponsor resources available on the Internet, including health references and continuing education programs.

Learning needs may also be met when nurses participate in formal education programs to seek advanced preparation in the care of individuals with physical disabilities and chronic illnesses and to demonstrate excellence in the rehabilitation nursing specialty through CRRN certification (ARN, 1994). The CRRN is a generalist certification. Certain career goals or positions may lead nurses to complete an academic graduate program of study and seek advanced practice certification, the CRRN-A.

Education is an important component of rehabilitation nursing practice because it comprises a significant portion of what rehabilitation nurses do in providing quality care to individuals with disability and chronic illness. The nurse manager who seeks to maintain a competent staff will encourage staff to participate in educational opportunities; arrange for continuing education programs; inform staff about support for education and tuition; budget funds for educational activities, conferences, and professional literature; and reward and encourage staff members who attend continuing education programs.

Unlicensed Assistive Personnel/Multiskilled Workers

The preparation and ongoing education of unlicensed assistive personnel and multiskilled workers are areas in which the rehabilitation nurse manager may have significant impact. Although these two groups of workers have differing task assignments in the work area, both are involved in support of client care.

Unlicensed Assistive Personnel. The ARN position statement (ARN, 1995) addresses qualifications, scope of care at a basic and secondary level, and settings of care for unlicensed assistive personnel (UAPs). This document identifies UAPs' duties that occur in the rehabilitation area under the direction of an RN. UAPs have either received a nurse's aide certificate or completed at least 4 weeks of on-the-job training. UAPs provide care based on the client's plan of care and within demonstrated competencies.

Multiskilled Workers. The multiskilled worker is qualified to work in more than one task area. Multiskilled workers may perform technical tasks, such as phlebotomy or electrocardiograms, or may work in different settings, such as inpatient care units, rehabilitation clinics, or outpatient programs, at different times of the day or week.

Student Support

The nurse manager encourages an environment that supports nursing and allied health students as they learn rehabilitation skills (ARN, 1994). Nurse managers often interface with student nurses on their rotation for clinical or management experiences or when teaching rehabilitation principles to students as part of scheduled lectures.

There are three reasons that nurse managers should encourage students to have experiences in a rehabilitation facility, community agency, or other setting. First and foremost, experiences during basic education are opportunities to expose students to the specialty of rehabilitation nursing. Second, students who become interested in rehabilitation nursing may be recruited as staff. Third, when nursing students understand rehabilitation nursing principles and practices, regardless of their future areas of practice, they will be more likely to incorporate rehabilitation principles and practices into all areas of nursing, helping clients from onset of illness or injury throughout their care. The nurse manager shares student clinical objectives with faculty, students, and nursing staff so they can work together and enlist stronger support in achieving the objectives and enriching the student experience.

Alternatives to typical student experiences include providing follow-up for a client through the therapy schedule, following up on clients who have returned home, attending outpatient clinic appointments with clients, visiting community-based programs, and teaming with staff to learn about the rehabilitation care continuum. Students, staff, and faculty share their evaluations of the experiences.

Students from schools of allied health may have clinical rotations or internships on nursing units. The rehabilitation nurse manager can play an important role in their education and inform them about the roles and functions unique to rehabilitation nursing. Demonstrating knowledge and clinical skills in direct care, offering concise and insightful presentations during interdisciplinary staff meetings, and interacting collegially with both the students and their department representatives are team-building behaviors.

Principles and functions that nurses need to learn about the unique aspects of rehabilitation nursing include:

- Understanding the roles and functions of other disciplines that participate in rehabilitation teams and how those roles interface with rehabilitation care
- Applying the holistic approach to rehabilitation care that includes the client's family and environment
- Encouraging client and family involvement as part of the interdisciplinary team in care and lifelong care planning, with a focus on maximizing function, preventing complications, and maintaining optimal health
- Understanding the continuum of physical, psychosocial, and emotional adjustment to disability or chronic illness
- Incorporating knowledge of and adjustments to the client's home, work, educational and/or social environments, and support systems in the rehabilitation plan
- Encouraging and educating clients and families to learn to do for themselves and apply problem-solving techniques, rather than expecting the various health care providers to do care that the client is capable of completing
- Providing education, preventive interventions, and maintenance care as opposed to cure behaviors and even predicting needs beyond the immediate care setting
- Acknowledging the physical and emotional demands on staff inherent to the specialty practice of rehabilitation nursing

Human Resource Management

The rehabilitation nurse manager is on the front line to influence staff job satisfaction so that the objectives of the organization can be accomplished. As a frontline manager, the rehabilitation nurse manager is the individual primarily responsible for acquiring, developing, and retaining staff. A major function of the role is facilitating the work performance of a number of employees with a variety of preparation levels, experiences, and personal preferences. The rehabilitation nurse manager constantly seeks balance in providing a caring, nurturing environment with standardization of conditions so that the work is completed effectively and efficiently.

According to the ARN (1994), the rehabilitation nurse manager is accountable for the management of personnel functions of the nursing and support staff in the area or unit. The nurse manager seeks to recruit and retain an appropriate skill mix of qualified, competent, client-centered rehabilitation nursing personnel. The nurse manager is well served by investing time and effort to identify and obtain support through the organization's human resources or personnel department. Broad categories of supports from human resources are help with employment, compensation, benefits administration, and employee relations.

Employment

The rehabilitation nurse manager strives to recruit, interview, hire, and retain a skilled mix of qualified, competent, client-oriented personnel to deliver care and achieve the functional outcomes desired. With sparse exposure to rehabilitation, nurses may be unfamiliar with concepts unique to rehabilitation nursing. Recruiting staff for rehabilitation settings requires skill in communicating the satisfactions and frustrations of the specialty to those who may be unfamiliar with or misinformed about its rewards and demands. Nurses who prefer to concentrate on interpersonal interactions, teaching, counseling, supporting, and coordinating care across a continuum are well suited. Technology has changed the character of the client population entering rehabilitation; mechanical ventilation, cardiac, pulmonary, and burn rehabilitation have become subspecialties. Persons with significant disability, multiple diagnoses, or extensive complex medical needs are prevalent in many rehabilitation settings, and requirements for admission, levels of care, and lengths of stay have also changed.

The rehabilitation nurse manager is best served by giving a clear picture of each position and its performance expectations during the hiring process. The specific job description, the orientation process, ongoing development availability and expectations, performance evaluation time frames, hours of work, compensation and benefits, as well as employment and employee expectations should be clearly delineated and agreed on.

Human resource departments offer support to the manager's employment function by advertising positions, sponsoring career days or job fairs, arranging nursing school visits, and using other recruitment techniques. Human resources may be responsible for orientation to the organization and may screen applicants to provide background and reference checks, schedule physicals, extend employment offers, determine compensation, and assist with any relocation information or support.

Compensation

Compensation is typically supported through human resources, and the nurse manager works with human resource personnel to ensure that employees receive appropriate credit for previous experience or education. The nurse manager keeps human resources aware of local market trends, provides updates to job descriptions, and ensures that staff members are clearly aware of performance expectations and how they affect their compensation.

Benefits

Benefits are discussed separately, even though they are part of the overall compensation of an employee. The rehabilitation nurse manager becomes knowledgeable about all aspects of the benefits package available to employees. Employees often have questions regarding benefits, and the manager's ability to provide a rapid and accurate response may deescalate a potentially negative situation for the employee. Employees do not always equate the monetary equivalent of benefits as a substantial part of their compensation. The rehabilitation nurse manager uses actual dollar amounts to illustrate the worth of benefits as diverse as child care discounts; free parking; life, dental, or optical insurance; meal discounts; credit union membership; and a variety of elective and provided retirement plans, because this information may assist in recruitment and retention. Alternatively the nurse manager may work with human resources by identifying which benefits hold significant value for retaining employees, saving the high cost of turnover.

Employee Relations

Employee relations is a broad category that incorporates many aspects of interaction between the organization and employees. Interactions may be positive, such as employee recognition programs or activities such as picnics and banquets, or may cause concern, such as assisting employees with problems or addressing employees demonstrating negative performance and other behaviors.

Human resource personnel can help the rehabilitation nurse manager ascertain the appropriate assistance for an employee, interpret policies, and apply their provisions or expectations uniformly. Most organizations require managers to review planned disciplinary actions with human resources before meeting with an employee who has a grievance. Human resource personnel assist with grievance mechanisms and serve both employees and managers to achieve fair and equitable resolution to concerns or violation of the organization's rules and policies. The confidential nature of any employee disciplinary action or personal situation must be respected without exception. Even if an employee chooses to share information, the rehabilitation nurse manager must not do so.

The rehabilitation nurse manager can be proactive in creating a positive environment for employee relations, beginning with soliciting ideas from staff and sharing information in a timely manner. Nurse managers often vary their work hours or work different shifts to be in touch with issues that affect all staff members and resolve problems early on. Morale is enhanced and turnover rates reduced when employees and management are involved together in decision-making processes.

Advocacy

Advocacy for persons with disabilities is another role of the rehabilitation nurse manager (ARN, 1994). Advocacy may mean personal involvement and role modeling for nurses new to the specialty of rehabilitation nursing. Advocacy may take several directions. The rehabilitation nurse may advocate for clients through involvement in professional nursing organizations or interdisciplinary groups. Alternatively the manager may pursue advocacy by participating in and supporting national disability advocacy groups, such as the National Head Injury Foundation or the Spina Bifida Association of America. Chapter 4 discusses advocacy and ethical matters pertinent to rehabilitation.

The nurse manager may assist those with disabilities or chronic conditions through awareness programs or media promotions. In the community, the nurse may act by identifying barriers by an architectural review of public buildings, entertainment centers, churches, restaurants, and other areas where individuals with disabilities may want to go. Advocacy may be legislative, by selecting candidates to support, promoting causes with a positive impact for individuals with disabilities or chronic illnesses, and participating in telephone trees or mailings regarding advocacy issues to elected representatives. Chapter 3 provides discussion of political activism for rehabilitation nurses. The nurse manager, through example and organizational support, may introduce staff members to mechanisms of advocacy and encourage them to identify their own niche in supporting individuals with disabilities or chronic illnesses.

Research

The role of the rehabilitation nurse manager in research is to ensure that current rehabilitation research findings and rehabilitation nursing practices are incorporated into clinical practice and the delivery of care (ARN, 1994). Evidence-based research and consensus statements, such as those produced for poststroke rehabilitation, treatment of pressure ulcers, and urinary incontinence in adults by the Agency for Health Care Policy and Research (now the Agency for Quality Health Research), should be implemented in the clinical setting. Guidelines published by the Consortium for Spinal Cord Medicine on acute management of autonomic dysreflexia, neurogenic bowel management, and prevention of thromboembolism are other examples. As new research develops and is published, policies and procedures on delivering care must be updated. The nurse manager encourages staff to search for increasingly better methods of delivering care (Stetler et al., 1998).

A research-based professional practice model of care based on one of the nursing theories can also be used, depending on the setting. Chapter 2 provides discussion of theorists and functional models commonly used for practice in rehabilitation nursing.

Not all practice in a health profession is based on science. In some cases researchers have yet to accumulate a sufficient body of knowledge to dictate nursing practice in a given direction. In other cases "a different frame of reference provides the appropriate rationale for action" (Stetler et al., 1998, p. 47), such as ethical decision making.

The nurse manager should also support research activities and studies in the general field of rehabilitation as well as rehabilitation nursing (ARN, 1994). This support can be demonstrated by participation in actual studies, financial support to research, or response to surveys regarding practice that adds to the knowledge base.

IMPLICATIONS

The field of medical rehabilitation, while continuing to grow and expand into different settings, is facing a shrinking labor pool of nurses and a decrease in reimbursement for services. This is coupled with a vast movement in which consumers are demanding top-notch service or they will take their business elsewhere. Rehabilitation nurses and rehabilitation nurse leaders can make the difference in the new millennium that will be needed to provide high-quality, customer-focused, cost-efficient care.

Rehabilitation nurse managers must lead by instilling enthusiasm for their organization and its mission in everyone with whom they work. In an ideal world, a nurse manager who demonstrates true leadership skills and abilities will be able to direct the staff toward high employee morale, satisfied customers, and low turnover rates. Those who understand the goals and purpose of the unit are able to work together, are enthusiastic and mutually supportive, and have a sense of achievement and belonging. Furthermore, functional outcomes for their clients will improve and be sustained after discharge. In an ideal world, costs are kept below expenses and are in line with the budget. The nurse manager continually sets ever-higher targets in all of these areas and develops action plans with the staff on ways to reach targeted goals. Rehabilitation nurse leaders are at the forefront, poised to make a difference in the lives of those they serve.

> Think enthusiastically about everything;
> but especially about your job.
> If you do, you'll put a touch of glory in your life.
> If you love your job with enthusiasm, you'll shake it to pieces.
> You'll love it into greatness, you'll upgrade it,
> you'll fill it with prestige and power.
>
> —Norman Vincent Peale

CRITICAL THINKING

You are a staff nurse considering a management career in rehabilitation nursing. Identify from the chapter the rehabilitation nurse management roles in which you would need more education and training to assume a leadership role. Identify educational methods you might access or use to achieve the desired expertise.

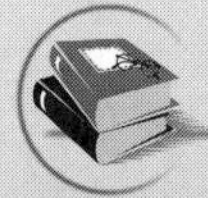

Case Study

The nurse manager on a 30-bed spinal cord injury and orthopedic unit has been receiving complaints about her evening charge nurse, M.P., for the past 3 months. The concerns brought forward by several nurses were that M.P. sat at the desk all evening and rarely left to make client rounds or to help the nurses with client care or answering call lights. They also stated that M.P. would disappear at times and was noticed making a lot of personal phone calls.

The nurse manager had spoken to M.P. about this and recorded it in her files as a verbal counseling. During the past 2 weeks, nearly all the evening staff expressed dissatisfaction with M.P., stating that the behavior was continuing. The nurses commented that they respected M.P.'s clinical skills and generally liked her but felt that her leadership and role modeling was poor.

The evening nurses were asked whether they would be comfortable meeting with the nurse manager and M.P. to discuss these issues openly. The nurses all agreed to the meeting. The nurse manager arranged the meeting the next day and informed M.P. of the purpose, which was to discuss charge nurse issues and expectations.

The nurse manager led the meeting. The staff nurses were open in telling M.P. what they liked and did not like about her actions. They stated that they respected her clinical skills but needed her to be more available as a resource to new staff or inexperienced nurses who need to improve their competency in rehabilitation skills. An example was given of a new nursing assistant who transferred a client incorrectly from the wheelchair to the bed. M.P.'s supervision and help were needed in this situation to ensure that neither the staff member nor the client encountered harm during the transfer. M.P.'s presence on the unit would have a positive impact on staff morale and on client satisfaction if care was supervised so that rehabilitation principles and practices were being followed.

M.P. listened constructively to the concerns, understood what they were saying, and agreed to make a change in behavior. The nurse manager reviewed the charge nurse shift routine with M.P., which called for making client rounds three times a shift, answering call lights, and helping out with client care, especially during the busy shift times. M.P. agreed to follow the guidelines. The expectations were outlined in an action plan for improvement, which M.P. signed. A follow-up meeting was scheduled in 2 weeks with the staff and M.P. to review progress.

The follow-up meeting was positive on both sides. The staff nurses felt that M.P. had made a definite change and that she was now part of their team and a leader with whom they could work positively and continue to respect. M.P. thanked the nurse manager for pointing out the issues and for helping her to further develop as a leader and to contribute to the success of the unit and institution.

REFERENCES

American Health Consultants. (2000). Staffing models: Nurse shortage spurs hunt for perfect ratios. *Healthcare Benchmarks, 7*(3), 13-17.

American Hospital Association. (1992). *Role and functions of the hospital nurse manager.* Chicago, IL: Author.

American Nurses Association. (1991). *Standards of clinical nursing practice.* Washington, DC: Author.

Association of Rehabilitation Nurses. (1994). *Rehabilitation nurse manager. Role description.* Skokie, IL: Author.

Association of Rehabilitation Nurses. (1995). *The role of unlicensed assistive personnel in the rehabilitation setting: Position statement.* Skokie, IL: Author.

Association of Rehabilitation Nurses. (1999). *Factors to consider in decisions about staffing in rehabilitation settings: Position statement.* Skokie, IL: Author.

Bejciy-Spring, S.M., Neutzling, E., & Newton, C. (1994). Nursing case management: Enhancing interdisciplinary care of the spinal cord injured patient. *SCI Nursing, 11*(3), 70-73.

Benner, P. (2001). From novice to expert: Excellence and power in nursing practice (Commemorative 1st ed.). Upper Saddle River, NJ: Prentice Hall.

Buerhaus, P.I. (1998). Is another RN shortage looming? *Nursing Outlook,* 46(3),103-108.

Coile, R.C. (1999). Nursing shortages: Ten strategies to becoming a "magnet hospital" for RN recruitment and retention. *Russ Coile's Health Trends, 11*(8), 1-7.

Cole, J. (1999). The art of wooing Gen Xers. *HR Focus,* November, 7-12.

Covey, S.R. (1992). *Principle-centered leadership.* New York: Simon & Schuster.

Davidhizar, R., & Eshleman, J. (1999). The friendly art of persuasion. *Health Care Manager, 18*(2), 41-46.

Eade, D.M. (1996). Motivational management. Developing leadership skills. *Clinician Reviews,* November/December, 115-125.

Egger, E. (2000). Nurse shortage worse than you think, but sensitivity may help retain nurses. *Health Care Strategic Management,* May, 16-18.

Finkler, S.A., & Kovner, C.T. (2000). *Financial management for nurse managers and executives.* 2nd ed. Philadelphia: WB Saunders.

Fox, R.T., Fox, D.H., & Wells, P.J. (1999). Performance of first-line management functions on productivity of hospital unit personnel. *Journal of Nursing Administration, 29*(9), 12-18.

Fralic, M.F., & Denby, C.B. (2000). Retooling the nurse executive for 21st century practice: Decision support systems. *Nursing Administration Quarterly, 24*(2), 19-28.

Goleman, D. (1998). *Working with emotional intelligence.* New York: Bantam.

Halstead, L.S., Rintala, D.H., Kanellos, M., Griffin, B., Higgins, L., Rheinecker, S., Whiteside, W., & Healy, J.E. (1986). The innovative rehabilitation team: An experiment in team building. *Archives of Physical Medicine and Rehabilitation, 67,* 357-361.

Health Care Advisory Board. (1999). *Hardwiring for service excellence.* Washington, DC: The Advisory Board Company.

Hoeman, S.P. (1990). Rehabilitation/restorative care in the community. St. Louis: Mosby.

Johnson, S. (1998). *Who moved my cheese?* New York: GP Putnam's Sons.

Kerfoot, K. (1996). Today's patient care unit manager. *Nursing Economics,14*(1), 59-61.

Lewin, K. (1947). Frontiers in group dynamics: Concept, methods, and reality in social science. *Human Relations, 1,* 5-41.

Lucas, D. (1999). National nursing shortage: PONL information for nursing leaders. *Pennsylvania Organization of Nurse Leaders Newsletter,* November/December, 3.

Manfredi, C.M. (1996). A descriptive study of nurse managers and leadership. *Western Journal of Nursing Research, 18*(3), 314-329.

Motwani, J., Klein, D., & Navitskas, S. (1999). Striving toward continuous quality improvement: A case study of Saint Mary's Hospital. *Health Care Manager, 18*(2), 33-40.

Perra, B.M. (2000). Leadership: The key to quality outcomes. *Nursing Administration Quarterly, 24*(2), 56-61.

Peters, T. (1987). Develop an inspiring vision. In *Thriving on chaos* (pp. 399-408). New York: Alfred A. Knopf.

Ruiz, M. (2000). Rehabilitation nursing: Another increasing shortage. Excellence in clinical practice. Indianapolis, IN: Sigma Theta Tau, International.

Stetler, C.B., Brunell, M., Giuliano, K.K., Morsi, D., Prince, L., & Newell-Stokes, V. (1998). Evidence-based practice and the role of nursing leadership. *Journal of Nursing Administration, 28*(7/8), 45-53.

Ter Maat, M. (1993). An appropriate nursing skill mix: Survey of acuity systems in rehabilitation hospitals. *Rehabilitation Nursing,18,* 244-248.

Tracey, C.A. (1999). *Restorative nursing. A training manual for nursing assistants.* Glenview, IL: Association of Rehabilitation Nurses.

Tulgan, B. (1999). Gen Xers: Will the workplace ever be the same? *Health Management Technology,* May, 8-9.

Velianoff, G.D., Neely, C., & Hall, S. (1993). Developmental levels of interdisciplinary collaborative practice committees. *Journal of Nursing Administration, 23*(7/8), 26-29.

Wellner, A. (1999). Get ready for generation next. *Training,* February 12, 44-48.

Williams, J. (2000). The new workforce. *Business Week,* March 20, 64-70.

Zenger, J., Ulrich, D., & Smallwood, N. (2000). The new leadership development. *Training & Development,* March, 22-27.

7 Quality: Indicators and Management

Pamela M. Duchene, DNSc, RN, CRRN

One Saturday, Sandy, a 50-year-old woman, had a stroke involving the left hemisphere of her brain and resulting in right-sided hemiplegia and mild dysphagia. Immediately after assessment in the emergency department, Sandy was admitted to acute care. Seeming to be medically stable 3 days later, she was transferred to the physical rehabilitation unit. It was a busy evening on the rehabilitation unit, with six admissions after 6 PM. The nurse admitting Sandy noted her indwelling catheter and explained, "The doctor will want that removed tonight." The doctor made rounds and ordered Sandy's catheter removed. It was around 10 PM before the nurse finally had time to remove the catheter, but she did it before the end of her shift. Two nurses scheduled for the night shift called in sick for work. The supervisor replaced 1 nurse, leaving a staff of 1 nurse unfamiliar with rehabilitation nursing and 2 nursing assistants for 18 clients, 6 of whom were new to the unit, including Sandy.

The night nurse usually worked acute care and thought it was great to be assigned to rehabilitation, where few clients were acutely ill. She had an extra cup of coffee, made her rounds casually, and did not awaken the sleeping Sandy for an assessment. Around 6 AM there was a loud noise from Sandy's room. All staff members rushed to Sandy's room and found her lying on the floor in obvious pain. She was holding her hip and had a large gash on her head where she had apparently struck the bedside stand when falling. Urine was everywhere. An x-ray film showed a right hip fracture, and Sandy returned to acute care for surgical intervention. Her family was livid and complained that it was negligence on the part of the rehabilitation nurses. Was it?

Georgette was a new nurse on the evening shift of a busy orthopedic rehabilitation unit. She was assigned eight clients and was assisted by a certified nursing assistant. Georgette was assigned a new admission, Ted, who had his left hip replaced 2 days previously. He arrived on the unit at 4:30 PM. His pain was under good control, his incision was clean, and the dressing was intact. Ted was more than 6 feet tall. The occupational therapist explained that she needed to leave on time today and did not have time to stay and meet Ted. She asked Georgette whether Ted appeared to need anything before she returned the next morning at 7 AM; she claimed that she would be able to take care of everything then. Georgette said that Ted was comfortable and that she would take care of whatever he needed. The physical therapist met Ted and was pleased with his healing and progress. She gave him clearance for non-weight-bearing activity on the left side but approved him for transfer to a wheelchair. She gave him a pillow for prevention of hip adduction.

Around 6 PM Georgette answered Ted's call light. He said he needed to use the bathroom, and given the clearance of his transfer status, Georgette said it should be no problem. She transferred him easily to the wheelchair and took him into the bathroom. As he lowered himself onto the toilet, a loud "pop" was heard, and he experienced sharp and severe pain in his left hip.

Georgette put on the emergency light and called for assistance. The physician was called, and Ted was taken to radiology on a cart, where initial films indicated a dislocation of his new hip. The surgeon arrived and manually manipulated the hip back into position. He requested a meeting with Georgette and the nursing supervisor. He stated that nursing incompetence had led to Ted's hip dislocation, and he wanted an apology from Georgette and recommended her dismissal from the nursing staff. Was it incompetence? Should Georgette have been terminated from employment on the rehabilitation unit?

Quality may be reflective of nursing competence, but more often is indicative of system function. In the first situation, with Sandy, a nurse without rehabilitation education and experience should not have been assigned as the only nurse for 18 clients, 30% of whom were new to the unit. According to the Commission on Accreditation of Rehabilitation Facilities (CARF, 2000, p. 94), a comprehensive integrated inpatient program provides for rehabilitation nursing services 24 hours a day, 7 days a week. The nurse assumed responsibility for a client population for whom she had not demonstrated competence or received education. An experienced rehabilitation nurse would have anticipated Sandy's response and would have aroused her to assess her urinary elimination status. The nurse was placed in an unsafe position by the nursing supervisor, who moved her from a medical unit to the rehabilitation unit. In answer to the original question, the family had a valid complaint. The nurse was not capable of providing care for 18 rehabilitation clients. Such a situation is not reflective of incompetence but of a lack of resources. The nurse was placed in a compromising position by the nursing supervisor.

In the second situation, the nurse was placed in a compromising position by the occupational therapist's failure to complete an assessment. Had she completed the initial evaluation, the occupational therapist would have identified that the client was at risk for hip dislocation because of the low height of the toilet, which for an individual more than 6 feet tall, placed the angle of the hip at less than 90 degrees. Rather than reflective of the nurse's level of competence as the surgeon assumed, the hip dislocation was indicative of a team communication failure. According to CARF (2000, p. 91), the interdisciplinary team needs to maintain consistent communication and integration at all times. The physical therapist completed her initial assessment, the occupational therapist deferred her assessment, and the nurse was not able to implement an integrated plan after the therapists left for the evening.

In both of the preceding cases, the clients served were affected by system failures. Such situations are not unique to or even rare in health care, as pointed out in a report by the Institute of Medicine (IOM) (Kohn, Corrigan, & Donaldson, 1999). According to the IOM report, there are between 44,000 and 98,000 deaths annually in the United States due to medical errors. If the clients had died, the two illustrations presented earlier would have been included in these numbers because both situations were preventable and occurred as a result of system failures. All efforts at rehabilitation are futile if client safety is not preserved.

When incidents such as those described above occur in succession on a rehabilitation unit, referring physicians and case managers are likely to say that the quality of care on the rehabilitation unit has declined. Unfortunately the initial response to such allegations is defensiveness and fault finding. Such a response is futile in correcting the underlying system issues. It is critical for client safety and for quality rehabilitation care that rehabilitation nurses comprehend ways to ensure effective system function.

This chapter will focus on the shift from traditional quality improvement strategies to the enhanced scrutiny of regulatory agencies and consumer advocacy groups to promote client safety in health care.

MEANING OF QUALITY

Quality is a matter of perception. What represents quality to one individual may not to another. For example, a complete head-to-toe nursing assessment is an indicator of quality to many acute care nurses. In rehabilitation, however, the focus of the assessment should be functional skills, independence, therapeutic teaching, and functional assessment. Neither perspective is entirely incorrect. Both are perceptions of quality care that are grounded in experience and education. From a consumer perspective, quality care may be more closely linked to how frequently the water pitcher is filled and how quickly the call light is answered, rather than with whether there is a head-to-toe assessment.

Defining quality health care is an arduous task. The Vice Presidential Planning Committee for the Forum for Health Care Quality Measurement and Reporting was initiated in June 1998 (Department of Health and Human Services for the Domestic Policy Council, 1998). The Forum was to be the means for measuring health care quality and would develop standardized measures and mandated data collection and reporting structures. The Forum would endorse core measures for standardized health care quality reporting. At the time this chapter was written, the Forum had identified quality indicators as including underuse, overuse, misuse, and variation in the use of health care services.

Underuse of Services

The Forum report identifies a key quality lapse as failure to provide services that are recognized as preventing complications, costs, and deaths. The focus within the Forum's report is acute care for clients with myocardial infarction, preventive eye care for clients with diabetes, and screening mammography and Papanicolaou tests for women. In rehabilitation, an equivalent example could be the individual who receives an above-the-knee amputation and is sent home without prosthetic training or gait training.

Overuse of Services

The Forum report discusses problems with overuse of antibiotics that add expense and may precipitate antibiotic-resistant strains of illness. An example in rehabilitation could be the unnecessary duplication of discipline evaluations. In many rehabilitation programs, clients are asked the same questions by each discipline because each has a specially designed form to meet their needs. Such evaluation systems waste the client's time as well as health care dollars that are better spent with interdisciplinary evaluations.

Misuse of Services

Unnecessary injuries and deaths, delayed diagnoses, and excess expense are all examples of the misuse of health care services. Both examples related earlier in the chapter indicate misuse of services. According to the Forum's report, 180,000 deaths annually can be attributed to errors in hospital care.

Medication errors fall within the category of misuse of services. In a landmark study Bates et al. (1995) found 28% of the adverse reactions to medications leading to injury were preventable. A follow-up study (Bates et al., 1997) placed the cost of preventable adverse medication events at a 700-bed tertiary care hospital at $2.8 million annually. These estimates, if applied to all hospitals within the nation, lead to an average of $2 billion worth of annual unnecessary expenses in treating the consequences of preventable adverse drug events.

Another complication of care categorized as misuse of service is pressure ulcer development. Findings from studies and consensus from panels of experts that one in four nursing home residents develops pressure ulcers, resulting in an estimated $1.3 billion annually worth of unnecessary expense, led the way for the Agency for Health Care Policy and Research (AHCPR) to develop clinical practice guidelines that address pressure ulcer risk identification, prevention, and treatment (AHCPR, 1995a, 1995b). In the Department of Veterans Affairs (VA), the incidence of pressure ulcers in their 140 long-term care facilities was 4.9% in 1990. Through the efforts of the VA Office of Quality Management, the VA system began a national focus on facility-specific pressure ulcer incidence (Berlowitz & Halpern, 1997). Through these efforts, the incidence declined to 3.1%, demonstrating that the problem is not inevitable but is correctable through an appropriate use of service and care.

Misuse of services may lead to a client's death. In their policy on reporting sentinel events, The Joint Commission on the Accreditation of Healthcare Organizations (JCAHO), encouraged self-reporting by organizations of errors or unanticipated events that resulted in a client's injury or death (JCAHO, 1998). In follow-up to any error resulting in injury or death, the JCAHO mandates an analysis of root cause. If facilities do not complete such activities and report to the JCAHO, the accreditation agency will place the organization on Accreditation Watch, designating that the facility is under close scrutiny by the JCAHO. Accreditation Watch status is publically disclosed during accreditation surveys.

Variation of Services

Differences in the health care practices throughout the United States are considered quality issues under the category of variation in services. The Forum found that clients in the northeastern United States are more likely to receive preventive care than are clients in western regions. This holds true for rehabilitation services as well. Clients in the Northeast are more likely to receive rehabilitation care after an orthopedic injury, stroke, or other neurological illness. Why this difference exists is unclear, but it likely stems from long-standing practice patterns.

The indicators of underuse, overuse, misuse, and variation in the use of health care services assist in the definition of quality health care. The IOM formed a committee in 1998 (Kohn, Corrigan, & Donaldson, 1999) to identify quality improvement strategies. The committee members identified quality as equated with client safety and error prevention. In health care, as illustrated in the opening examples, lapses in client safety and errors are frequently seen as the result of one person's failure to prevent injury or risk. Deming (1993) stated that quality improvement is possible only through correcting processes. It is critical that health care organizations adopt this strategy, rather than the traditional fallback of fault finding. Rehabilitation, like most areas within health care, is particularly susceptible to the temptation to try to assign blame when events do not go as planned.

For example, in one facility, a client was admitted who required a continuous infusion of morphine for control of pain related to sickle cell anemia. He had fractured a rib in a fall from a chair before admission, and his recovery had been prolonged due to a sickle cell crisis. As a result of the sickle cell disease and a lengthy hospitalization, he was debilitated and needed progressive, slow rehabilitation to return to the home environment. The day after admission he had respiratory depression caused by the morphine infusion. The nurse contacted the physician and received an order to hold the morphine infusion. He entered the client's room and turned off the intravenous (IV) pump connecting the morphine to the client's IV site. The pump remained in the room, with the IV morphine bag and a normal saline solution bag. The nurse flushed the heparin lock in the client's forearm, and he received bedside therapy for the remainder of the day. During the night, the client's status changed, and his output decreased. The night shift nurse contacted the physician, who ordered that a saline drip be initiated at 100 mL/hour to ensure hydration. The nurse entered the client's room at 2 AM as quietly as possible using a soft flashlight to avoid waking the client. She reconnected the IV fluid and turned the IV pump to the 100-mL rate and left the room. From 3 to 5 AM, the client slept with increased urine in the catheter bag. At 6 AM the nurse entered the room and noticed the client's respiratory rate was only 6 breaths/hour. She attempted to arouse him with difficulty. Assessing the situation, she noticed that the IV bag connected to the client was the morphine drip rather than the saline solution. In a panic, she quickly and appropriately disconnected the morphine and connected the saline solution, administered Narcan (kept at bedside for all clients receiving morphine infusions), called the nursing assistant to stay with the client, and left to contact the physician. The client began to regain consciousness. The physician was angry and requested the client be transferred to a unit that could "handle morphine infusions."

In this example, the problem within the system was multiple in nature. The IV morphine solution looked too similar to the saline solution. The morphine solution should not have been left at the bedside. A "hold" order is too confusing and needs parameters on how long the treatment should be held. A discontinue order would have been more appropriate. Finally, it is better to wake the person when providing a high-risk treatment (IV therapy) than to make an error. Assuming this error was only the result of one nurse's failure to double-check systems would allow the systems to remain in place that initially led to the error.

UNIVERSAL INDICATORS OF QUALITY

Other than looking at actual errors, what are the indicators of quality? As with the definition of quality, indicators of quality vary substantially from person to person. For example, in a letter to a chief executive nurse, a client complained that she had suffered a bruise on her upper arm due to the use of a thigh-sized cuff. To this person, the failure of the nurses to obtain a large cuff (which could, in fact, have actually been a thigh-sized cuff) was an indicator of poor quality. If the nurse had presented the large cuff as just a large cuff, rather than a thigh-sized cuff, the client may still have had a bruise but would not have seen it as a quality variation. (In this instance, the bruise was attributed to the client's use of Coumadin, rather than to an ill-fitted blood pressure cuff.)

Given the public and media demand for quality health care, several agencies have identified key indicators of quality. The AHCPR (1999a) published a system for consumers to quickly review the quality of health care systems. The AHCPR (1999a) writes that quality health care is "doing the right thing, at the right time, in the right way, for the right person—and having the best possible results." They advocate reviewing outcome measures, client satisfaction reports, accreditation reports, and clinical performance measures when making decisions on providers and health care systems. These methods continue to leave the interpretation of quality reports at the discretion of the consumer.

Many rehabilitation programs use the Functional Independence Measure (FIM) to assess client functional outcome from rehabilitation. Reports from the Uniform Data System FIM are not public information, but variables may be presented as components of the organization's program evaluation systems. Comparing rehabilitation facilities through the use of program evaluation systems is confusing to professionals and is likely to result in confusion of consumers as well. CARF (2000) requires that organizations disclose information on outcomes and accreditation status to consumers. Rehabilitation programs that are not CARF accredited may not comply with CARF standards, resulting in confusion for consumers. The question remaining unanswered is how to identify indicators of health care quality for rehabilitation.

COMMON HEALTH CARE INDICATORS OF QUALITY

Indicators of health care quality vary among regulatory groups, professional nursing associations, advocacy groups, and consumer groups. Application of the concepts of health care underuse, overuse, misuse, and variation is effective in assisting professionals and consumers in identifying quality rehabilitation programs. Beyond this general point, however, the amount of information and the number of opinions on health care quality are staggering. In this section regulatory perspectives, professional nursing perspectives, and advocacy group and consumer group perspectives on quality health care indicators will be addressed, with application to rehabilitation nursing.

Regulatory Perspectives

The Healthcare Research and Quality Act of 1999 authorized revision of the AHCPR into the Agency for Healthcare Research and Quality (AHRQ) to further accelerate the emphasis on health care quality and client safety. The Health Care Financing Administration (HCFA) is active in development of quality standards for programs that participate in medicare and medicaid reimbursement. HCFA controls quality violations by assessing fines and barring programs that violate quality from participation in medicare and medicaid reimbursement. One of the recent "conditions for participation" that the HCFA published (HCFA, 2000a) was the client rights requirement. This publication influences rehabilitation substantially. The condition of participation as published in 1999 requires all hospitals to promote client rights, including the right to be free from restraints. Failure to comply with the conditions of participation will jeopardize a facility's ability to receive medicare and medicaid funding. Compliance with these regulations requires nurses to change perspectives on the use of restraints. In rehabilitation settings the most common reason for use of a restraint device was client safety and to prevent harm to the person or to others. The change in regulation views the idea of a restraint as a safety device to be a violation of the client's right to be free of restraints. In this situation an agency of the government defines quality as no restraints, and nurses, physicians, and consumers of rehabilitation services must comply with the definition or work to change the regulation through involvement with policy formation.

Nursing Perspectives

Several organizations have defined indicators of quality nursing care. Much of the focus of the quality of nursing care has centered on the question of adequate nurse staffing. The AHCPR, the National Institute of Nursing Research (NINR), and the Division of Nursing of the Health Researches and Services Administration (HRSA) joined in the development of the Nurse Staffing and Quality of Care in Health Care Organizations Research Agenda (Department of Health and Human Services, 1996). The primary purpose of this joint workforce was follow-up to the IOM's Report (Wunderlich et al., 1996) and to identify relationships between care quality, staffing levels, and skill mix, with consideration for organizational variables. The research questions posed by this workforce are:

1. Identify the relationship between nursing care delivery, the organization, and client outcomes
2. Review the impact of the skill mix of nurses, including registered nurses, advanced practice nurses, and unlicensed assistive personnel, on client outcomes
3. Identify the impact of nursing care delivery and organizational variables on specific client outcomes, such as self-care
4. Review computer technology's impact on client outcomes
5. Assess methods of identifying cost-effective analyses for resource utilization and allocation
6. Identify nursing interventions that directly affect client issues and clinical care quality

Although there are no definitive answers to the above research questions, the agenda provides direction to areas that most closely aligned with the impact on quality client care through nursing services. From a rehabilitation perspective, it is of significance to note that the impact of nursing care and skill mix on client self-care is included in the agenda.

In an effort to place nursing quality variables in a standardized format, Lancaster and King (1999), proposed the use of a spider diagram (Figure 7-1). In this system, data from various sources are combined for decision-making purposes. This model provides an easy format for linking actual and potential quality variations with structure (workload measures and productivity), process (medication errors), and outcome (urinary tract infections, satisfaction) variables.

Research efforts directed toward client safety and quality outcomes have recently focused on nursing care components and staffing levels. The Woodhull study (Sieber, Powers, Baggs, Knapp, & Sileo, 1998) indicated that nurses were rarely mentioned in media coverage. In fact, Woodhull states that in more than 2000 health care articles, nurses were mentioned only 4% of the time. In light of such information, it is important to note that the recent attention given to nursing care and variables such as staffing levels is a positive reflection on the inherent value added by nursing care to client outcome.

Consumer Perspectives

According to a recent study in which 2006 adults were interviewed by telephone, most health care consumers in the United States believed that governmental regulation of health care quality was necessary. Specifically, most Ameri-

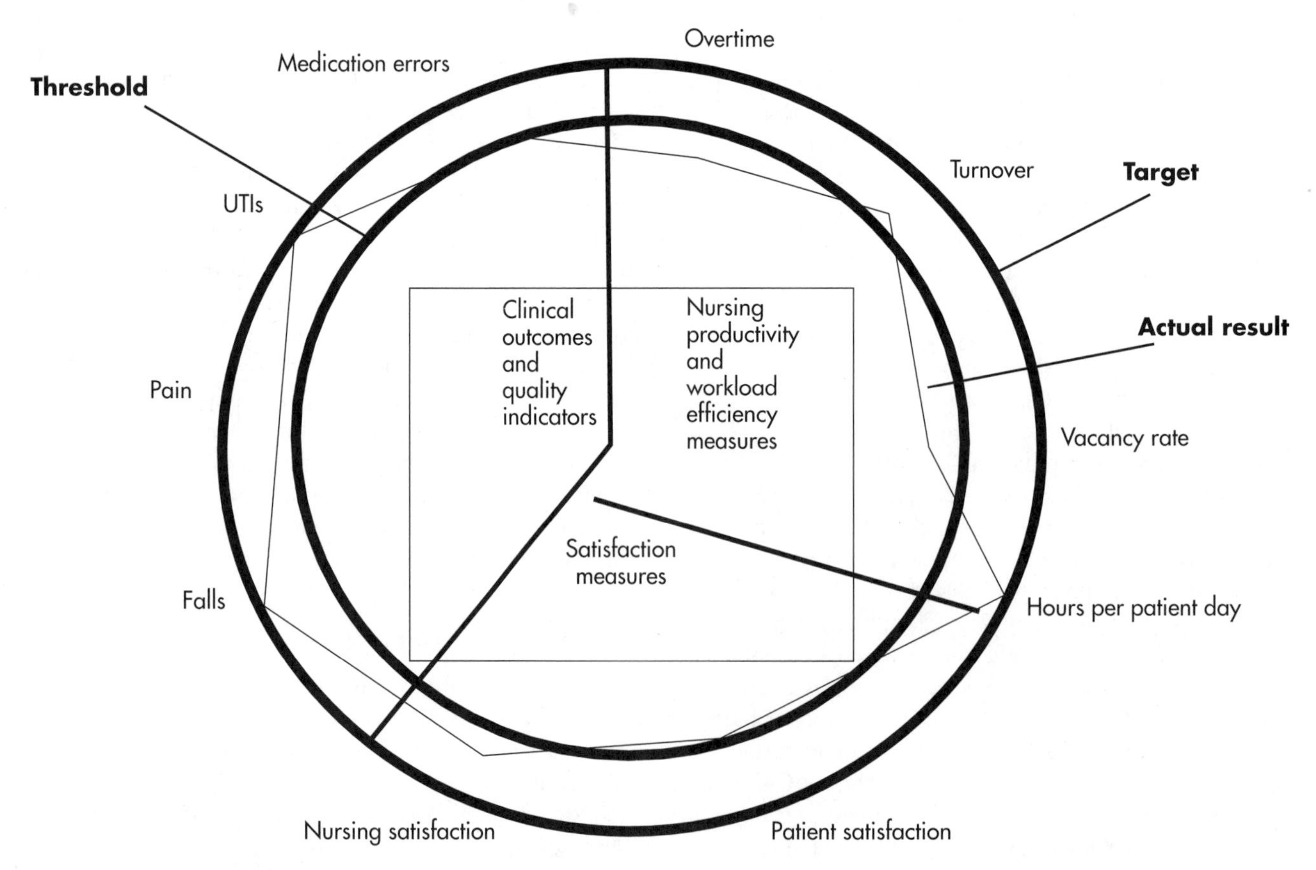

Figure 7-1 Spider diagram. *UTIs,* Urinary tract infections. (From Lancaster, D., King, A. [1999]. Spider diagram nursing quality report card: bringing all the pieces together. *Journal of Nursing Administration, 29*[7], 43.)

cans (88%) believed that quality information should be public and that the government should ensure a minimum quality standard. With respect to what defines the minimum quality standard, the report is nonspecific. According the report, consumers made health care decisions based on their knowledge of the physician and on referral from friends and colleagues. Consumer knowledge about nursing care quality was not identified as a core element of health care decision making (Kaiser Family Foundation, 1996).

Radwin (2000) completed a 3-year study of 22 clients with cancer. She followed their courses during the period and interviewed them to find out which components of nursing care made a difference to them. Participants in the study identified eight variables that they linked with quality client care (Box 7-1).

In rehabilitation, much of the impact of the work of all members of the interdisciplinary team is based on the recognition of the value of life with an impairment or disability. Rehabilitation nurses must keep the perspectives of their consumers in mind and understand their perspectives of quality nursing care variables. Some individuals with impairments hold the values of quality care listed in Box 7-2.

On an individual basis, nurses who hold these values will be perceived as providing quality nursing care. Nurses who disregard such values may provide timely care and service but may not achieve credibility with their clients with disabilities. In rehabilitation nursing, it is essential that clients perceive nurses as comprehending their value systems. This may be the key factor influencing the impact of nursing on client outcome. Individuals with impairments or disabilities, particularly those with chronic problems, must view practitioners as credible before adopting their advice and education. Because an essential element of rehabilitation nursing practice is client education, nurses must be aware of their attitudes toward individuals with disabilities. Before nurses complete education on preventive health care, they need to first demonstrate comprehension for the impact of the disability or chronic illness on the individual's lifestyle. As the saying goes, "People must know how much you care before they care how much you know."

Box 7-1 Variables Linked by Cancer Clients with Quality Client Care

1. Knowledge of nursing and health care
2. Client rapport
3. Inclusion of the client in decision making
4. Individualized treatment
5. Nurturing and caring
6. Prompt attention to needs
7. Continuity of care
8. Communication and coordination of care

From Radwin, L. (2000). Oncology patients' perceptions of quality nursing care. *Research in Nursing and Health, June 23*(3), 179-190.

Box 7-2 Values Held by Individuals with Disabilities Toward Health Care Providers

1. Tolerance for differences
2. Acceptance of interdependence on others
3. Tolerance of lack of resolution
4. Humor
5. Problem-solving skills
6. Creativity and flexibility for problem resolution
7. Future orientation
8. Attitudinal perceptiveness

Identification of Quality Indicators for Rehabilitation Nursing Practice

On the basis of the information presented, quality indicators for rehabilitation nursing practice parallel indicators for medical quality. Appendix 7A includes a listing of quality indicators for rehabilitation nursing practice.

Regardless of the indicators of quality identified, the demand is for controlling quality. It is critical that control of quality focus on a system perspective. Quality may be viewed as the integrity of a system, where system refers to "a set of interdependent elements interacting to achieve a common aim. The elements may be both human and nonhuman (equipment, technologies, etc.)" (Reason, 1990).

According to Senge (1990), quality requires that interrelationships, rather than specifics, be seen. Quality is dependent on the relationships between individuals and processes, with a need for oversight of change patterns.

MEASUREMENT OF QUALITY INDICATORS

Quality Must Be Measurable

According to George Lundberg, former editor of the *Journal of the American Medical Association,* "The single most important thing that American medicine . . . should do is define quality indicators and follow them" (Millenson, 1997). Certainly this is applicable to rehabilitation nursing. Once quality indicators are selected, measurement is critical. Indicators must be measurable, and measurements must be valid and reliable to be meaningful.

Consider the example of pain management. The JCAHO (1999a) identifies pain as a major health issue. The Comprehensive Accreditation for Hospitals incorporates the rights of clients to appropriate pain assessment and management in the standards on client rights and throughout the 1999 to 2000 *Comprehensive Accreditation Manual for Hospitals* (JCAHO, 1999c). The recognition of pain as a major health problem is long overdue. According to Dahl (1999) pain has been routinely undertreated because of a failure to assess and document pain. He claimed that a primary barrier to treatment of pain is that health care providers lack knowledge and skills for appropriate pain assessment and management. Campbell (1995), in his presidential address for the American Pain Society, stated, "Vital signs are taken seriously. If pain were assessed with the same zeal as other vital signs are, it would have a much better chance of being treated properly. We need to train doctors and nurses to treat pain as a vital sign. Quality care means that pain is measured and treated." Although there is widespread acceptance and endorsement of the need for assessment and management of pain, there is equally widespread disagreement on the tools for pain assessment.

Facilities across the country are implementing campaigns to recognize and treat pain, but the tools for pain assessment vary from facility to facility and even within programs and between practitioners. It is impossible to recognize the success of pain assessment and treatment campaigns if assessment systems are not standardized. Donabedian constructed a classic formula for medical quality that rests on three components: structure (the right equipment), process (the right procedure), and outcome (the right results) (Millenson, 1997). As applied to pain assessment, pain monitoring is the right procedure (process), but the tool must be standardized or monitoring outcome is worthless. If all practitioners in a system assess pain in a standardized manner, it is possible for one clinician to assess pain and provide a pain relief measure and for a second clinician to assess pain relief.

Measurement of quality is just one indicator to consider in rehabilitation nursing practice. With respect to establishing measurable indicators of rehabilitation nursing quality, suggested measures are listed in Appendix 7A.

Standardized Tools for Quality Measurement

Many different tools are available for measurement of quality that are applicable to rehabilitation.

Computerized Needs-Oriented Quality Measurement Evaluation System

The Computerized Needs-Oriented Quality Measurement Evaluation System (CONQUEST), established by the AHCPR (1999b), identifies quality of care as accessible, accountable, fair, effective, and safe. CONQUEST explains that quality of care is delivering the right care to the right client in the right way at the right time. CONQUEST provides a public-use, free software program for identification, comparison, evaluation, and selection of quality measures for clinical performance improvement. The CONQUEST program includes 1197 measures of clinical performances assembled as a tool for evaluation of health care quality. The program was developed collaboratively by the VA Department, HCFA, JCAHO, RAND Corporation, American Group Practice Association, United Health Care, and the National Committee for Quality Assurance. Many measures included in CONQUEST have been tested for reliability and validity and are ready for use by health care professionals, organizations, and third-party payers. CONQUEST is available on-line at http://www.ahcpr.gov/qual/conquest.htm.

Functional Independence Measure

Developed by the Uniform Data System for Medical Rehabilitation (UDS_{MR}), the FIM is used in facilities throughout the world. The current database is estimated at 2.5 million client records (U.B. Foundation Activities, 1999). The data obtained through FIM allow evaluation of rehabilitation service efficiency and efficacy. More information on FIM is available in Chapter 8 and on-line at http://www.udsmr.com.

Minimum Data Set

The Minimum Data Set (MDS) is a component of the Resident Assessment Instrument (RAI). Initiated in 1990 (Morris, Murphy, & Nonemaker, 1995), the RAI provides a means for integration of clinical data into regulatory support. The MDS is a standardized, regulated assessment database that is used by clinical staff members in long-term care to plan and organize the care that is provided. As of 1998, the MDS became the tool through which long-term care facilities receive their medicare reimbursement determination in the prospective payment system for long-term care. The MDS contains elements that are linked with quality of care (Rantz & Popejoy, 1998). Through this method, the HCFA identifies the quality indicators for all long-term care residents. Because the MDS is electronically submitted to state departments of public health, the HCFA is able to monitor the quality indicators for all long-term care residents throughout the country. The process is explained in Chapter 3. The MDS can be accessed through the HCFA website: http://www.HCFA.gov/medicaid/mds20.

MDS for Postacute Care

The MDS for Postacute Care (MDS-PAC) is a revision of the MDS for short-stay rehabilitation, intended for incorporation in the prospective payment system for rehabilitation hospitals and units (HCFA, 2000a). The MDS-PAC parallels the MDS in many respects, including the inclusion of quality indicators and in the determination of medicare reimbursement rates based on functional and acuity levels of the clients. The MDS-PAC can be accessed through a link from the HCFA website: http://www.HCFA.gov/medicaid/rehabpac.

SF-36

The Medical Outcomes Trust is a Massachusetts-based not-for-profit organization involved in the development and standardization of outcome measurement instruments for health care (Medical Outcomes Trust, 2000). The SF-36 is one of the instruments developed by the Medical Outcomes Trust and is a standardized instrument for assessment of health care outcomes. It contains 36 items that are reflective of health status and outcomes from the client's perspective. The instrument measures limitations in physical activities, usual role activities, body pain, health perceptions, vitality, limitations in social or usual role activities, and mental health. It can be administered by telephone, by computer, or in person. The SF-36 can be accessed at http://www.outcomes-trust.org/catalog/sf36.htm.

SF-12

Also developed by the Medical Outcomes Trust, the SF-12 is a shorter version of the SF-36 and contains only 12 items. As with the SF-36, the instrument provides an assessment of health care outcomes and is appropriate for repeated use with clients to measure the clients' perceptions of health status changes. The SF-12 can be accessed at http://www.outcomes-trust.org/catalog/sf12.htm.

Outcome and Assessment Information Set

The Outcome and Assessment Information Set (OASIS) is a comprehensive assessment system for adult home health clients. Developed by the HCFA and implemented in 1999, OASIS includes sociodemographic, environmental, support system, functional status, and health status information for adults receiving home health care. This tool is intended to provide the HCFA with quality and outcome information for home health clients throughout the nation (HCFA, 2000b). OASIS can be accessed at http://www.hcfa.gov/medicare/hsqb/oasis.

Standards

One method for assessing quality in a systematic manner is through comparison of actual practice with clearly defined standards. A standard is a norm for an agreed-on level of practice. JCAHO identifies standards that set maximum achievable performance expectations for areas that affect health care quality (JCAHO, 1999b). Standards do not explain or prescribe *how* to achieve compliance, but compliance must be clear to those reviewing practice: surveyors, consumers, and clinicians. Standards provide a direction for organizations, but leaders within the organization require vision to use the standards to achieve compliance.

In addition to the JCAHO, there are many other organizations that establish health care standards. The HCFA (1997) was formed in 1997 to provide administrative oversight of medicare and medicaid. The HCFA identifies health care quality standards for 228,200 facilities, including laboratories, nursing homes, hospitals, home health agencies, ambulatory surgery centers, and hospices. Through state inspection teams, the HCFA surveys health care suppliers and providers for compliance with federal health, safety, and quality standards of care. As with the JCAHO, the HCFA does not detail how to achieve compliance. Through their website (http://www.HCFA.gov) clinicians and providers can access the Sharing Innovations in Quality site.

Sharing Innovations in Quality is a project providing collaboration between the HCFA and state surveyors with professional, consumer, and industry representatives for health care. Creative ideas are collected and freely distributed throughout the country. One of the suggestions posted on the site is D'Youville Senior Care's (Lowell, Mass.) Green Leaf Program for fall prevention. The program uses green leaves that are posted on the wheelchairs, assistive devices, clothing, rooms, and records of residents who experience falls. The program provides fast visual cues to all staff members within the facility to focus fall preventive efforts on residents with high fall risks.

The JCAHO and HCFA publish standards for varied health care environments. CARF publishes standards specific to rehabilitation environments. Also known as CARF . . . The Rehabilitation Accreditation Commission, CARF began standard development for medical rehabilitation programs in 1966. It is a private, nonprofit, nongovernmental standard-setting agency (CARF, 2000). CARF brings third-party payers, consumers, advocacy group representatives, and providers together to determine standards. After standard identification, CARF sends draft standards to payer representatives, consumers, advocacy group representatives, and providers throughout the country for review. CARF standards are recognized on an international level as reflective of rehabilitation quality. CARF promotes outcome-driven, value-based programs for individuals with disabilities and chronic illnesses.

Compliance and Integrity

Beyond quality and standard attainment are issues with compliance and integrity. A top priority of the HCFA is the integrity of the medicare and medicaid programs (HCFA, 1999). The compliance and integrity efforts of the HCFA are directed toward paying the right providers the right amount for reasonable, necessary, covered services. During 1997, HCFA's antifraud efforts saved more than $7.5 billion. Operation Restore Trust, initiated in 1995, was a trial effort directed at investigating compliance and integrity issues. The project resulted in enhanced fraud detection and prevention. The savings generated through Operation Restore Trust, the widely publicized criminal investigation of some health care providers, and the HCFA's efforts to alert health care consumers to fraud, have resulted in consumer skepticism. In light of such issues, it is imperative that health care organizations work diligently to demonstrate quality initiatives, error prevention strategies, client safety efforts, and organizational integrity programs.

The Balanced Budget Act of 1997 targeted rehabilitation in long-term care, acute inpatient rehabilitation, and home health care as key areas for decreased spending (HCFA, 1999). It is the most significant legislation to affect rehabilitation since the inception of medicare and medicaid in 1965. Quality indicators are essential during this time of dramatic funding and reimbursement changes to monitor for changes in quality levels or change in rehabilitation outcomes. Diagnosis-related groups (DRGs) resulted in discharge of clients from acute care to rehabilitation settings after short acute care lengths of stay. Before DRG implementation, it was not unusual for clients recovering from total hip replacement to stay in the acute care setting for 2 weeks or more, after which they might receive rehabilitation. After DRGs, clients recuperating from total hip replacement might be transferred within a few days of surgery, or even just 1 day after surgery (Healthcare Advisory Board, 1999). Implementation of prospective payment for long-term care and for acute rehabilitation will result in dramatic changes for the rehabilitation process. Keeping track of outcome measures is necessary to ensure that clients continue to receive benefit from rehabilitation.

QUALITY DATA COLLECTION

Data collection processes typically involve client interviews, surveys, record reviews, and observations. Keys to obtaining usable, meaningful data include the following (George & Weimerskirch, 1998):

1. *Data are client focused.* For example, the FIM can be used to obtain client-focused data. A second example is use of the client's goals for rehabilitation. At the time of discharge from rehabilitation, did the client attain his or her goals? Another example is the use of client satisfaction information. Is the client satisfied with the information provided for client education, pain management, and overall care?
2. *Data are easy to collect.* Data collection systems that are long and complex will result in incomplete data or will require additional staff resources to complete. The FIM is successful as a data collection tool because of the ease with which clinicians can collect and report data. In collecting information on falls, for example, the information required should be as easy to document as possible. In an effort to make collection of information on medication errors as easy as possible, Kishwaukee Community Hospital initiated a specific error form for medication events. The form provided a simpler, more user-friendly approach to reporting medication errors, which resulted in an eightfold increase in medication error reports (Hume, 1999). This is a positive improvement because medication errors tend to be underreported. There is a fear of possible disciplinary action, legal consequences, or fault finding with the reporting of medication errors. Systems that promote medication error reporting create an opportunity for process improvement and correction of safety issues.
3. *Results are simple to communicate.* Results reported in graphs and charts are easy for readers to understand. Posting information in a visible location alerts all staff members, clients, and others of results of quality improvement initiatives. Program evaluation information, for example, on the percentage of individuals experiencing functional gains during rehabilitation, when posted on charts and graphs, can provide evidence of program quality.
4. *Managers and supervisors request, expect, and use the data.* Data need to be requested, expected, and used to be useful. Decision makers in the health care system need usable, reliable data for process improvement.
5. *Those closest to the process are involved in data collection and reporting.* Rehabilitation nurse managers should not learn at the performance improvement committee meeting about any problem with client satisfaction. This information should be provided to the managers before any committee meetings so that improvements may be discussed and actions identified.
6. *Data are used for process improvement, rather than for individual performance review.* Medication errors are underreported by as much as 95% because of a fear of punishment (Hume, 1999). The fastest way to sabotage a measurement system is to link data with evaluation (George & Weimerskirch, 1998). By viewing data with a system perspective, correction of problems and system issues can occur.
7. *Success is celebrated.* When goals are attained and improvements are noted, success should be celebrated. Recognition and celebration of quality improvements are as important as identifying problems. Identifying victories in problem resolution energizes staff members to focus on other identified issues.

QUALITY CONTROL AND IMPROVEMENT TOOLS

Benchmarking

Benchmarking is a tool used to identify best practices for specific indicators. In rehabilitation the incidence of rehabilitation-acquired pressure ulcers is an indicator that sometimes is used for benchmarking. Rehabilitation nurses within the organization use the information and strive to be better than average and to excel to best practice level.

Audits

Audits are a key method of quality of care assessment. Often, the only way to identify trends or issues is through a careful audit of records. In a recent quality issue, a rehabilitation program manager was concerned that four of the recent admissions to rehabilitation from acute care required transfer to intensive care within 24 hours of admission. On audit of the records, it was noted that each of the clients had been evaluated for admission more than 72 hours before transfer. In each case, a call before discharge from acute care services might have alerted the program manager to changes in status that would affect the individual's ability to safely participate in 3 hours or more of daily therapy. The issue was corrected through incorporating such screening calls.

Brainstorming

One technique that has been used for many years in looking at problem resolution to quality issues is brainstorming. The rules for brainstorming sessions are simple: members of the quality team suggest as many solutions and alternatives as possible without critique. During brainstorming sessions, participants gain momentum by contributing as many ideas as possible. All suggestions are written and evaluated at a later time.

Cause-and-Effect Diagramming

The cause-and-effect or "fish bone" diagram is a quality control tool (Figure 7-2). It is used for identification of causes of a quality problem and often is used in combination with a brainstorming session. A cause-and-effect diagram method identifies basic categories that can help reduce irrelevant discussion and complaints.

Check Sheets

A fundamental tool for quality control is a check sheet used for data collection (Figure 7-3). The check sheet provides a standardized method of systematically collecting and recording facts. Review of completed check sheets is done to analyze data, determine patterns, and arrive at conclusions.

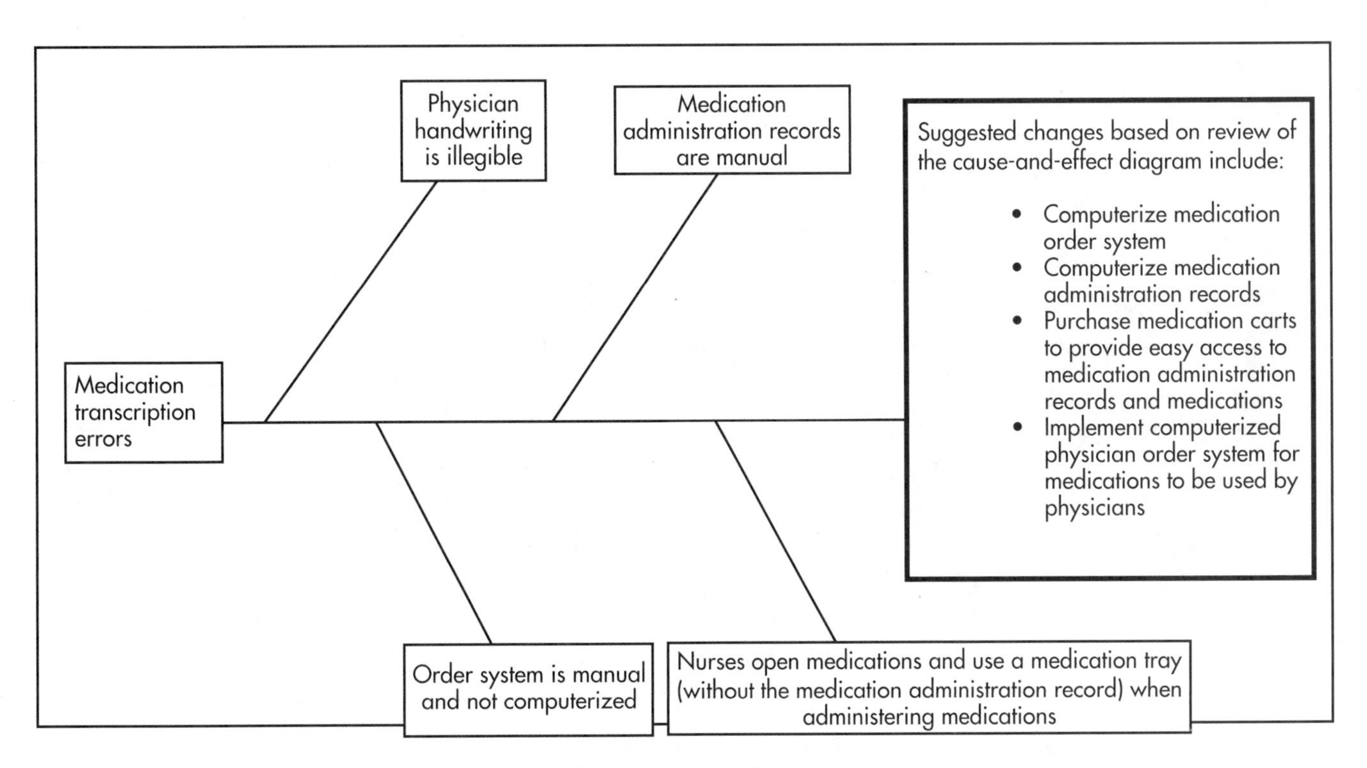

Figure 7-2 Cause-and-effect diagram.

Pain management audit	Pain assessed and documented on admission (1 = yes; 0 = no)	Pain assessed with every assessment of vital signs (No. of times pain/vital signs assessed)	Pain assessed before administration of analgesics (No. of times pain assessed/ analgesics administered)	Pain relief assessed after administration of analgesics (No. of times pain assessed/ analgesics administered)
MR #1234567	1	10/12	3/5	3/5
MR #2345678	1	5/13	3/3	2/3
MR #1345678	1	4/20	4/6	4/6
MR #3452345	1	20/24	4/7	3/7
MR #5899657	1	30/30	2/2	2/2
MR #0986389	0	3/3	1/1	0/1
Summary	5/6 = 83%	72/102 = 70.5%	17/24 = 71%	14/24 = 58%

Figure 7-3 Check sheet example.

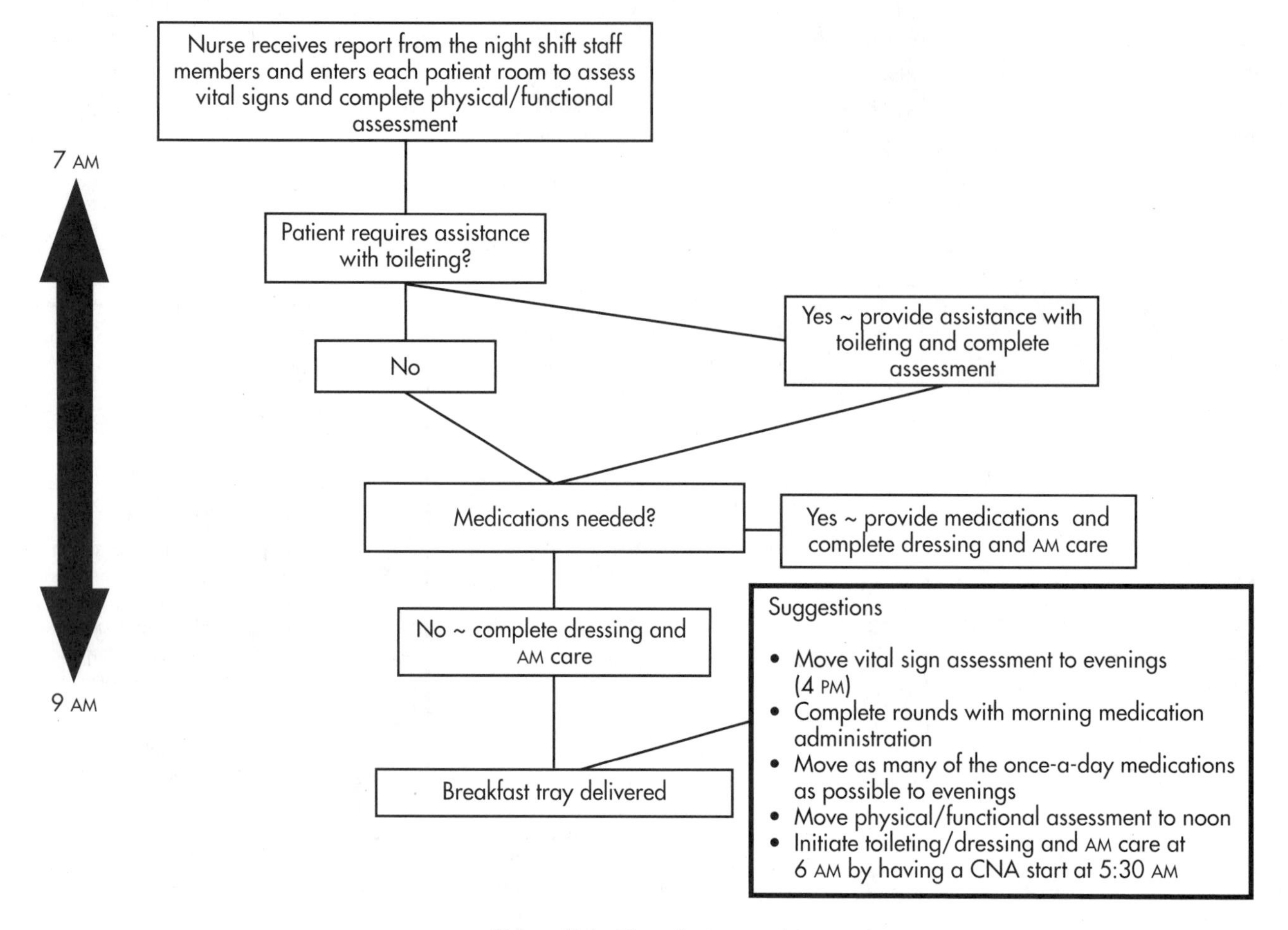

Figure 7-4 Flow chart example.

Flow Chart

With many quality control issues, it is difficult to determine why a problem exists. Flow charts document all steps included in a process from start to finish. Once the flow chart is complete, each step is reviewed for possible problems and opportunities for improvement (Figure 7-4).

Pareto Chart

Asserted in the Pareto principle is that 20% of the problems are responsible for 80% of the effects. Using a Pareto chart enables the user to focus on the primary issues or defects rather than trying to tackle all problems. A Pareto chart is created by listing (in descending order of frequency) all problems occurring in a process (Figure 7-5).

CAUTIONS WITH QUALITY IMPROVEMENT EFFORTS

Retrospective Versus Prospective Quality Reviews

One may complete quality reviews of processes and records either after the event is completed (retrospective) or as events are occurring (prospective). Retrospective reviews typically involve closed records and collected data and are relatively easy to complete. Such reviews require time for document perusal but do not necessitate extensive tracking systems because the individuals completing the review identify the files with appropriate information before the data collection period. In contrast, prospective reviews require tracking of information as it occurs. This can be difficult, particularly in inpatient settings, where there are three shifts of nurses spanning 24 hours of care. However, although retrospective reviews are sometimes easier to complete, the information gleaned may be less conclusive than those data collected through prospective reviews. Clinicians

Suggestions:

Because more than 80% of the causes of falls on the unit are attributed to urinary incontinence and equipment/clutter in the patient's room, the Pareto principle has nurses and team members focus on correcting those issues to reduce falls.

- Relocate equipment from room during HS care
- Complete rounds every hour
- Offer assistance for toileting on an every 2- to 3-hour schedule (as appropriate for each patient)

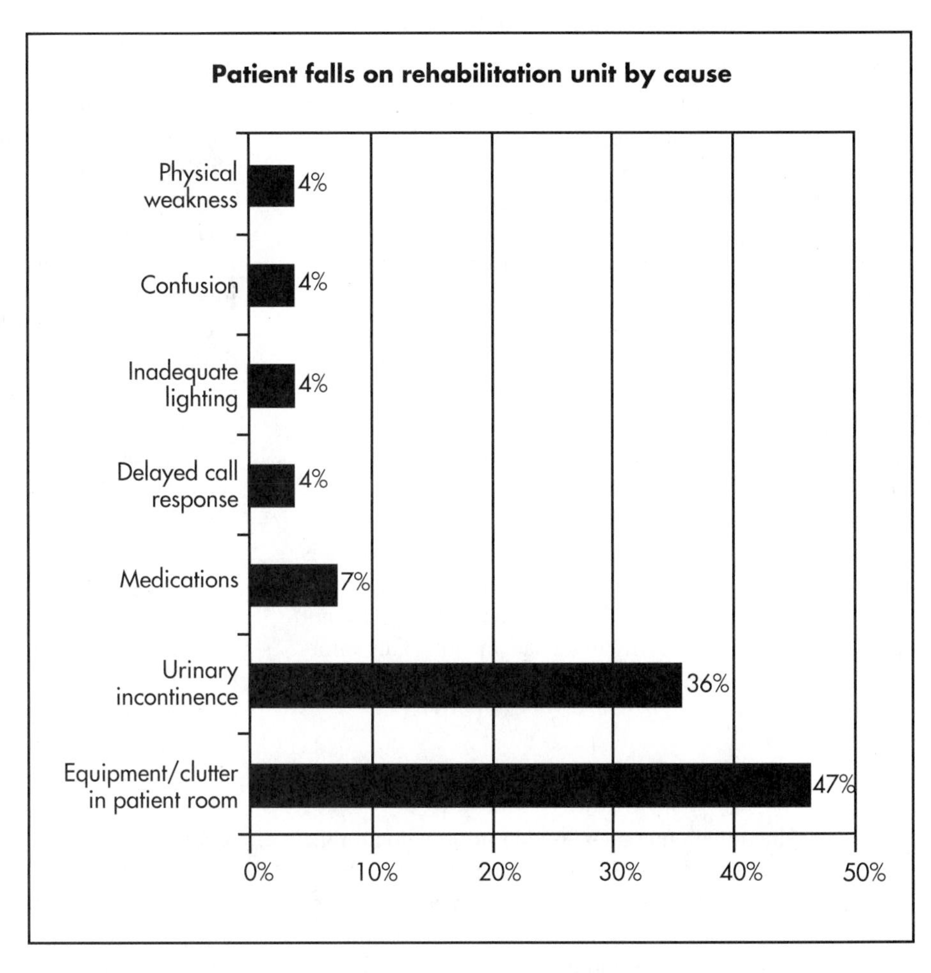

Figure 7-5 Pareto chart example.

find information through retrospective reviews that is easily detectable and "just waiting to be found." For example, identifying the incidence of documented complications to anticoagulation therapy through retrospective review would entail reviewing records for evidence of deep venous thrombosis, hematomas, and gastrointestinal bleeding. Such a review would not be difficult to complete. Taking a prospective look at the same issue, however, can result in a more comprehensive picture of the efficacy of anticoagulation therapy. As an example, in a prospective review of anticoagulation therapy, a data collection sheet would be developed through a team effort to identify as many components and contributing factors to complications with anticoagulation therapy as possible. The data collection sheets would be completed by members of the rehabilitation team and forwarded for analysis to the team leader or facilitator.

Costs

Although it is no longer accepted that higher quality is equated with higher cost, one must not assume that quality does not have a price. There are expenses associated with quality care. As an example, in a spinal injury program at a large freestanding rehabilitation hospital, the nurses place at-risk clients in specially designed pressure-relief boots. The boots cost about $150 for each boot, or $300 per pair. The incidence of rehabilitation hospital–acquired heel pressure ulcers is 0%. Although the cost is high, it is thousands of dollars less than the cost of time, care, and treatment associated with a pressure ulcer. It is sometimes necessary to spend a few dollars to save many.

OUTCOME ASSESSMENT

Most aspects of quality control and improvement apply to all health care programs; however, two additional methods—program evaluation and functional outcome measurement—are somewhat uncommon but key to the rehabilitation field. Program evaluation systems provide a holistic glimpse of the rehabilitation program. Functional outcome studies contribute the "so what?" data for rehabilitation or, in other words, provide substantiation that the rehabilitation expense results in functional gains.

Program Evaluation in Rehabilitation

Program evaluation systems are required in the standards of CARF. According to CARF (2000), a program evaluation system must have measures of effectiveness, efficiency, and participant satisfaction. Program evaluation systems include programmatic objectives, with thresholds for objective attainment. On a quarterly basis individuals measure attainment of the program evaluation objectives and determine needed actions and strategies.

Many organizations develop original program evaluation systems; however, there are some commercially available systems. The FIM of the UDS_{MR} is the most commonly used program evaluation system. The UDS_{MR} provides effectiveness measures of functional progress through the FIM. The UDS_{MR} provides efficiency measures by comparing charge and length of stay information for programs participating in the UDS_{MR} network. Because many rehabilitation programs are members of UDS_{MR}, the efficiency information is considered representative of the industry. The UDS_{MR} does not provide information on participant satisfaction. This information must be gathered by the organization to complete the program evaluation system.

Functional Outcome Studies

Studies on functional outcomes provide information on the essence of rehabilitation results. Although not every individual to enter a rehabilitation program will ambulate and return home, outcome studies give data on the probability of such occurrences. Outcome studies may link the individual's length of stay in a program with the cost and efficacy of the program. Review of such information should weigh the cost of the program against the benefit of the functional gain. At one time in rehabilitation (15 to 20 years ago), the criteria for continued treatment included continued progress, even if this progress was quite slight. However, in this age of health care reform, it is not acceptable to continue creating expense for functional gains that do not enhance the level of independence and lessen the dependence on the health care system.

Related to the legitimate concerns on the cost of rehabilitation and to the proliferation of rehabilitation programs and types of programs, functional outcomes from rehabilitation must be substantiated. In assessing outcomes from a rehabilitation program, one must consider the amount of experience with specific disability types and basic outcome quality indicators. Specifically the outcomes of clients with regard to quality of life, discharge disposition, and self-care independence should be appraised.

Outcome studies are not new to health care or to nursing. Perhaps the first individual to consider health care and nursing outcomes seriously was Florence Nightingale (Bull, 1992). The outcome measure by which she looked at success was mortality. After she began work with British soldiers, she found a 30% reduction in mortality levels within 6 months (Nutting, Dock, & Dock, 1907) through the incorporation of hand washing and promotion of infection control measures.

Specific outcomes for rehabilitation nursing practice have been documented in the literature. Baggerly and Di Blasi (1996) studied pressure sore prevention and management and the impact on program development, allocation of resources, and outcome evaluation. Rawl, Easton, Kwiatkowski, Zeme, and Burczyk (1998) reviewed the impact of an advanced practice rehabilitation nursing on follow-up for rehabilitation clients after discharge. They found that follow-up with the advanced practice nurse resulted in a significant decrease in anxiety levels and the number of calls to the rehabilitation unit. These studies are just two of many linking rehabilitation nursing care with a positive impact on functional outcomes and cost-effectiveness.

SUMMARY

Quality control and improvement have become an integral part of health care and rehabilitation nursing during the past two decades. As administrators and clinicians focus on defining quality and identifying customer satisfaction with services provided, standard-setting agencies such as the JCAHO work toward redefining the quality assessment process.

Issues with quality control have shifted to client safety, with an emphasis on outcomes and compliance with federally mandated standards. A primary challenge to clinicians is to transcend traditional departmental boundaries and work to refine processes. One current trend is to look at a 24-hour team for quality improvement (Carbonneau, 1999). In the 24-hour quality-improvement program, the key elements are captured through the acronym *FOCUS-PDCA:*

F ind a need for improvement
O rganize knowledgeable staff members into a team
C larify current information about the system
U nderstand causes of problems in the system
S elect methods for improvement and

P lan
D o
C heck
A ct

It is imperative in the current and future climates of financial exigencies that rehabilitation nurses constantly focus on doing more with less expense. Basic concepts of any quality control program include an organizational commitment to quality and client safety, a focus on client satisfaction, an empowerment of clinicians and staff members, a loss of department "territoriality" or specific links between quality threats or improvements and client outcome, and rewards for quality improvement. Rehabilitation nursing has made steps toward identifying positive outcomes of rehabilitation nursing on clients. But extensive work is needed in identifying and monitoring the outcome of rehabilitation nursing care.

CRITICAL THINKING

Unfortunately it is not unusual to hear rehabilitation nurses (or nurses from any clinical specialty) describe staffing situations where they feel their practice may be unsafe. What is meant by "unsafe" staffing? Identify four key characteristics of unsafe staffing levels and ways (excluding a numerical acuity system) of objectively quantifying safe levels of rehabilitation nursing care.

REFERENCES

Agency for Health Care Policy and Research. (1995a). *Pressure ulcers in adults: Prediction and prevention* (AHCPR Clinical Practice Guideline, No. 3, AHCPR Publication No. 92-0047). Rockville, MD: Author.

Agency for Health Care Policy and Research. (1995b). *Treatment of pressure ulcers.* (AHCPR Clinical Practice Guideline, No. 15, AHCPR Publication No. 95-0652). Rockville, MD: Author.

Agency for Health Care Policy and Research. (1999a). *A quick look at quality* (AHCPR Publication No. 99-0012). Rockville, MD: Author.

Agency for Health Care Policy and Research. (1999b). *Computerized Needs-Oriented Quality Measurement Evaluation System: CONQUEST 2.0* (AHCPR Publication No. 99-P001). Rockville, MD: Author.

American Nurses Association. (1999). Nursing—Sensitive quality indicators for acute care settings and ANA's safety and quality initiative (PR-28). Washington, DC: Author.

Baggerly, J., & Di Blasi, M. (1996). Pressure sores and pressure sore prevention in a rehabilitation setting: Building information for improving outcomes and allocating resources. *Rehabilitation Nursing, 21*(6), 321-325.

Bates, D.W., Cullen, D.J., Laird, N., Petersen, L.A., Small, S.D., Servi, D., Laffel G., Sweitzer, B.J., Shea, B.F., Hallisey, R., et al. (1995). Incidence of adverse drug events and potential adverse drug events: implications for prevention. *Journal of the American Medical Association 274,* 29-34.

Bates, D.W., Spell, N., Cullen, D.J., Burdick, E., Laird, N., Petersen, L.A., Small, S.D., Sweitzer, B.J., & Leape, L.L. (1997). The costs of adverse drug events in hospitalized patients. *Journal of the American Medical Association, 277,* 307-311.

Berlowitz, D., & Halpern, J. (1997). Evaluating and improving pressure ulcer care: The VA experience with administrative data. *Joint Commission Journal on Quality Improvement, 23*(8), 424-433.

Bull, M. (1992). Quality assurance: Professional accountability via continuous quality improvement. In C. Meisenheimer (Ed.), *Improving quality: A guide to effective programs* (pp. 3-20). Gaithersburg, MD: Aspen.

Campbell, J. (1995). *Presidential address to the American Pain Society.* November 11, 1995, Los Angeles, CA.

Carbonneau, C. (1999). Achieving faster quality improvement through the 24 hour team. *Journal for Healthcare Quality, 21*(4), 4-10.

CARF . . . The Rehabilitation Accreditation Commission. (2000). *2000 Medical rehabilitation standards manual.* Tucson, AZ: Author.

Dahl, J. (1999). New JCAHO standards focus on pain management. *Oncology Issues 14*(5), 27-28.

Deming, W.E. (1993). *Out of the crisis.* Cambridge, MA: Massachusetts Institute of Technology, Center for Advanced Engineering Study.

Department of Health and Human Services. (1996). Proposed research agenda. *Federal Register, 61*(220), 58194-58195.

Department of Health and Human Services for the Domestic Policy Council. (1998, June 17). *The challenge and potential for assuring quality health care for the 21st century* (Publication No. OM 98-0009). Washington, DC: Author.

George, S., & Weimerskirch, A. (1998). *Total quality management* (2nd ed.). New York: John Wiley and Sons.

Healthcare Advisory Board. (1999). *Joint camp.* Washington, DC: Author.

Health Care Financing Administration. (1997, April 20). Fighting fraud, waste, and abuse in medicare and medicaid. *Health Care Financing Administration fact sheet.* Baltimore, MD: Author.

Health Care Financing Administration. (1999). *HCFA's comprehensive plan for program integrity.* Washington, DC: HCFA Press.

Health Care Financing Administration. (2000a). *Inpatient rehabilitation facilities' prospective payment system.* Washington, DC: HCFA Press.

Health Care Financing Administration. (2000b). *OASIS overview.* Washington, DC: HCFA Press.

Hume, M. (Ed.). (1999). Changing hospital culture and systems reduces drug errors and adverse events. *Quality Letter for Healthcare Leaders, 11*(3), 2-9.

Joint Commission on Accreditation of Healthcare Organizations. (1998). *Sentinel event policy reference manual.* Chicago: Author.

Joint Commission on Accreditation of Healthcare Organizations (1999a, August 3). *Joint Commission focuses on pain management* [Press release]. Oakbrook Terrace, IL: Author.

Joint Commission on Accreditation of Healthcare Organizations. (1999b). *Joint Commission standards.* Chicago: Author.

Joint Commission on Accreditation of Healthcare Organizations. (1999c). *Comprehensive accreditation manual for hospitals: The official handbook (CAMH).* Oakbrook Terrace, IL: Author.

Kaiser Family Foundation. (1996). *Americans as health care consumers: the role of quality information: Highlights of a national survey* [Press release]. www.kff.org.

Kohn, L., Corrigan, J., & Donaldson, M. (Eds.). (1999). *To err is human: Building a safer health system.* Washington, DC: National Academy Press.

Lancaster, D., & King, A. (1999). The spider diagram nursing quality report card. *Journal of Nursing Administration, 29*(7), 43.

Medical Outcomes Trust. (2000). *The Trust home page.* Boston, MA: Medical Outcomes Trust.

Millenson, M. (1997). *Demanding medical excellence.* Chicago: University of Chicago Press.

Morris, J., Murphy, K., & Nonemaker, S. (1995). *Long term care facility resident assessment instrument (RAI) user's manual.* Washington, DC: Health Care Financing Administration.

Nutting, M., Dock, A., & Dock, L. (1907). *A history of nursing.* New York: GP Putnam's Sons.

Radwin, L. (2000). Oncology patients' perceptions of quality nursing care. *Research in Nursing and Health, June 23*(3), 179-190.

Rantz, M., & Popejoy, L. (1998). *Using MDS quality indicators to improve healthcare outcomes.* Gaithersburg, MD: Aspen.

Rawl, S., Easton, K., Kwiatkowski, S., Zeme, D., & Burczyk, B. (1998). Effectiveness of a nurse managed follow-up program for rehabilitation patients after discharge. *Rehabilitation Nursing, 23*(4), 204-209.

Reason, J. (1990). *Human error.* Cambridge: Cambridge University Press.

Senge, P. (1990). *The fifth discipline.* New York: Doubleday Currency.

Sieber, J., Powers, C., Baggs, J., Knapp, J., & Sileo, C. (1998). Missing in action: Nurses in the media. *American Journal of Nursing, 98*(12), 55.

U.B. Foundation Activities. (1999). *Uniform Data System for Medical Rehabilitation: Databases.* New York: Author.

Wunderlich, G.S., Sloan, F.A, & Davis, C.K. (1996). *Nursing staff in hospitals and nursing homes: Is it adequate?* Washington, DC: National Academy Press.

APPENDIX 7A

Application of Concepts: Nursing Report Card

Because of substantial pressures from regulatory and consumer groups and changes in health care delivery, nursing care is identified as a core factor in client safety, outcome, and care. The American Nurses Association (ANA) advocates recognition of key quality indexes for nursing within the nursing report card concept (ANA, 1999). The items identified by the ANA, in concert with items identified through the Institute of Medicine report on client safety, could be combined into the following system for rehabilitation nursing quality assessment.

Program Evaluation Application for the Rehabilitation Nursing Report Card

	Rehabilitation Nursing Quality Indicator	Measurable Definition	Goal	Actual Score	Weighting	Weighted Score
1	Nurse staffing skill mix including registered nurses, licensed practical nurses, nursing assistants, and unlicensed assistive personnel	Ratio of registered nurses to licensed practical nurses, nursing assistants, and unlicensed assistive personnel	Item not scored but used as demographic and descriptive information			
2	Total number of nursing care hours provided per patient day	Number of nursing personnel providing direct care multiplied by 8 hours/shift divided by the number of clients on the rehabilitation unit at midnight	Item not scored but used as demographic and descriptive information			
3	Pressure ulcers	Number of clients with stage I, II, III, or IV ulcers multiplied by 1000 divided by the number of patient days	<1%	2% = 50% of goal	10%	5%
4	Client falls	Number of clients with nonassisted falls multiplied by 1000 divided by the number of patient days	<1%	3% = 33% of goal	10%	3.3%
5	Medication errors	Number of medication errors divided by the number of dosages administered	<1%	0.5% = 200% of goal	10%	20%
6	Client satisfaction with pain management	Percentage of clients expressing satisfaction with pain management	>95%	98% = 103% of goal	10%	10.3%
7	Client satisfaction with client education information	Percentage of clients expressing satisfaction with education information received	>90%	88% = 98% of goal	10%	9.8%
8	Client satisfaction with rehabilitation nursing care	Percentage of clients expressing satisfaction with nursing care received	>92%	95% = 103% of goal	15%	15.45%
9	Nosocomial infection rate	Number of clients with confirmed infections multiplied by 1000 divided by the number of patient days	<1%	0.5% = 200% of goal	10%	20%
10	Nosocomial urinary tract infection rate	Number of clients with confirmed urinary tract infections multiplied by 1000 divided by the number of patient days	<1%	0.5% = 200% of goal	10%	20%
11	Nursing staff satisfaction	Percentage of nurses expressing satisfaction	>90%	85% = 94% of goal	15%	14.1%
Total Score					**100%**	**118%**

Action Plan

1. Evaluate pressure ulcer incidence to determine whether changes are needed in current pressure relief program. Provide an in-service consultation on skin management and pressure reduction. Monitor turn and repositioning schedules.
   Target date for completion: 30 days.
   Persons responsible: Nurse manager, charge nurses, clinical specialist.
2. Evaluate fall incidence. If linked with availability of fall alert devices, eliminate the problem by purchasing additional devices.

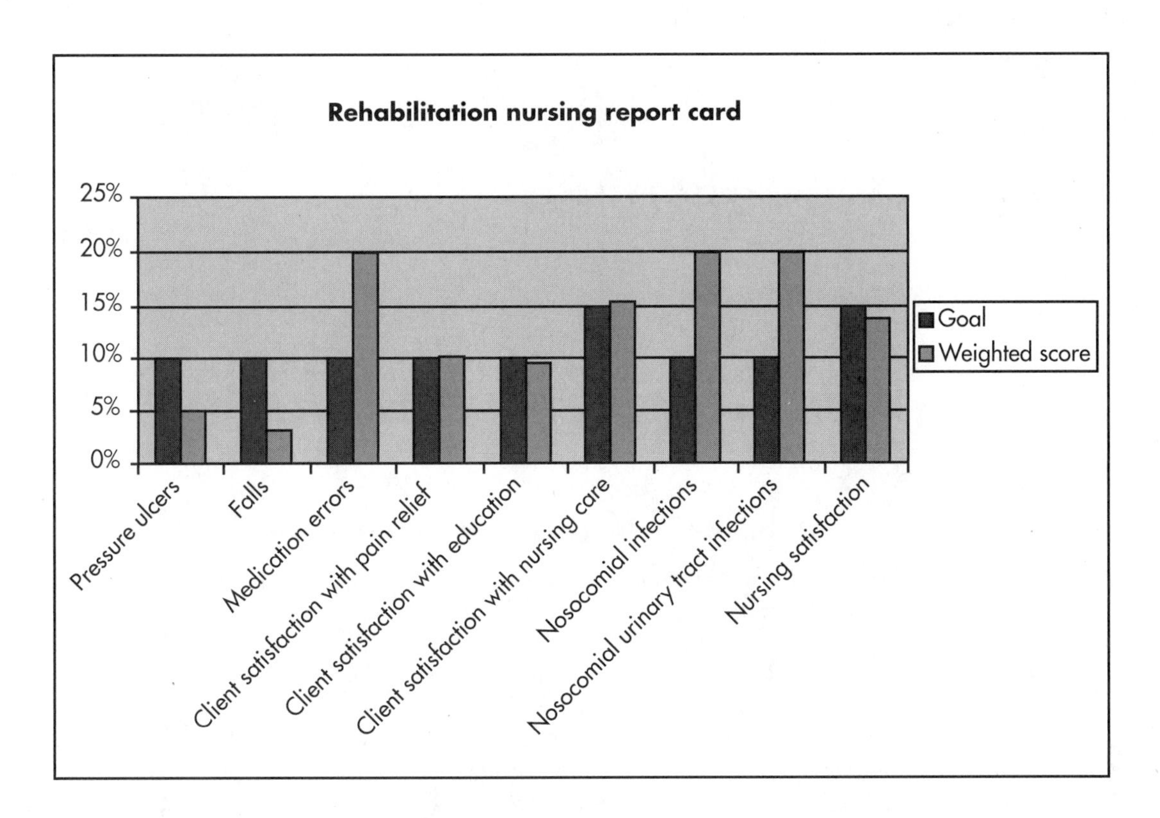

Target date for completion: 30 days.
Persons responsible: Nurse manager, charge nurses, clinical specialist.

3. Review medication error reporting because underreporting of errors is likely. Review incident reports to ensure that staff members are familiar with need for accurate and early reporting of medication errors.
   Target date for completion: 30 days.
   Persons responsible: Nurse manager, charge nurses, clinical specialist.
4. Review nursing satisfaction information. Are problems evident from review of satisfaction surveys? Is turnover below the goal?
   Target date for completion: 30 days.
   Persons responsible: Nurse manager, charge nurses, clinical specialist.

8 Evaluation and Outcome Measures

Margaret Kelly-Hayes, EdD, RN, CRRN, FAAN
Marion A. Phipps, RN, MS, CRRN, FAAN

John Baker was admitted to the rehabilitation hospital where I worked. He was in his mid-60s and had been quadriplegic since the age of 12 years. He was in the hospital for rehabilitation after a hip fracture.

At the time of his initial injury he was 12 years old, and no rehabilitation facilities were available to him. After his spine had been stabilized in an acute care hospital, John was sent home to the care of his large family. His bed was placed in the living room, and this space became the hub of family life and the setting of his rehabilitation. At first John stayed in bed, but over time he became more active. He was tutored at home and graduated from high school. He then went to college and began his own successful accounting firm from his parents' home. John was a gregarious man. He was knowledgeable and interested in a variety of topics. He had a special love of the opera and arranged frequent trips to New York with family and friends.

When we first met, he had many questions for me: What I was like as a person? How did I find joy in my work? What were my interests in life? John was quite stunned that I had never heard an opera. He asked me go to the library to check out tapes and soon gave me tickets to my first performance. John also wanted to ask about my philosophy of rehabilitation, and he wanted to talk about his. John believed his family's love and support had allowed him to develop self-confidence and enthusiasm for life. He believed his rehabilitation at home was successful because his family believed in him.

After his hip fracture John had many complications and setbacks. He told me that before this time he had never experienced sadness or depression. However, with these setbacks he had a period of severe depression. This came as a great surprise to him. He became quite knowledgeable on the subject of his depression. He told his caregivers that the source of this depression was the realization of his new limitations. In addition to the functional limitations of his disability, he now experienced those of aging and the complications of living with limited mobility for many years. John became our teacher. He reminded all who cared for him that the emotional response to disability is a very personal and individualized experience. No predictable patterns exist. John entered psychotherapy and found an enhanced level of understanding. Several years later John died, having come to peace with his life, his disability, and the burdens of aging.

The goals of rehabilitation are to improve function and promote independence and life satisfaction consistent with a person's impairment and environmental limitations (Johnston, Stineman, & Velozo, 1997). For rehabilitation nursing these goals are extended to include the client achieving and maintaining an acceptable quality of life, ensuring that specific needs are addressed, and promoting adaptation by clients and families to life changes while optimizing wellness (McCourt, 1993). The process by which these goals are met consists of comprehensive assessment and diagnosis, identification/description of expected client-centered outcomes, and planned interventions (ANA, 1998). With recent technological advances in rehabilitation, there is an increasing need to standardized the methods of assessment based on a conceptual framework. This includes the conceptualization and definition of disablement, reliable assessment of human performance, refinement of functional measures, and objective measurement of rehabilitation outcomes. In rehabilitation nursing these advances have strengthened the nursing process and form a major cornerstone of practice.

The determination of functional status is central to the planning and evaluation of restorative care. Integration of a person's health condition with functional performance and level of social support allows for the construction of a data set that profiles the whole individual. In an era of standardization in rehabilitation, evaluation using reliable and valid measures must be a part of the rehabilitation nursing process. Functional evaluation can be viewed as an extension of the traditional components of nursing assessment. Thus functional evaluation provides a framework for an orderly review of essential components deemed important to independent life. In some cases functional status may be as reliable in documenting overall health as knowing disease categories.

The concept of functional evaluation is an integral part of the rehabilitation nursing process. Nurses assess clients' capacities to meet their personal and rehabilitative goals. Rehabilitation nurses incorporate the results of assessment into client-centered care plans. This in turn has a direct influence on nursing diagnosis, nursing intervention, and nursing-specific outcome criteria. Today, nursing assessment of function, on the basis of validated and objective measures, contributes in a significant way to interdisciplinary evaluation and care planning.

Expansion of functional evaluation parameters has been guided by changes in the concept of disablement, the process of rehabilitation, and the populations being served. The incorporation of functional evaluation into the interdisciplinary process of rehabilitation provides a common denominator for the team effort, an essential component in rehabilitation. The rehabilitation team provides the collaborative effort, with each member accountable for his or her own profession-specific interventions. Regardless of the health condition of the client population being served, the rehabilitation team completes an interdisciplinary evaluation following discipline-specific assessments, develops mutually agreed-on goals, and initiates an intervention plan. Functional evaluation is an important component in each of these elements and is the responsibility of the nurse as well as other members of the rehabilitation team.

This chapter addresses functional evaluation primarily from a rehabilitation nursing perspective. The conceptual basis for disability is defined, and the terminology, purpose, and components of functional evaluation are described. Several specific assessment measures commonly used by rehabilitation professionals are described, along with their expected validity, reliability, and sensitivity. The types of instruments described in this chapter include measures of function, instrumental activities of daily living (ADLs), and quality-of-life measures. Because the status of the client does change over time, the type, frequency, and utilization of assessment need to reflect this dynamic. All of the presented instruments are appropriate for inclusion in a client-centered evaluation.

DISABILITY FRAMEWORK FOR EVALUATION

The focus of rehabilitation is to provide interventions to maximize function and to limit the impact of disability. The spheres of measurement to evaluate these interventions in rehabilitation have evolved from the conceptual framework of disablement. The term *disability* has been described as a physical or mental limitation within a social context, the gap between a person's capacity and the demands of the environment (Pope & Tarlov, 1991). Although by definition *disability* assumes interaction between the individual and the environment, it is frequently equated with separate and specific impairments. The relationship between severity of disability and independent living is apparent; however, many times the terms *impairment, disability,* and *handicap* are used interchangeably without consideration of their specific differences. These inconsistencies can pose obstacles to the appropriate use of terminology, correct measures specific to outcomes, and the evaluation of interventions.

The conceptual underpinnings for functional evaluation are based on the disablement models of Nagi (1965, 1969, 1976), Wood (1980), and the National Center for Medical Rehabilitation Research (NCMRR) (National Institutes of Health, 1993). Although each model has a different construct, a continuum from organ physiology to the whole person and the social context of disability is present in all of the models (Table 8-1). In Nagi's model of disablement (1976), three major potential consequences of active pathology or disease are impairment or physiologic abnormalities, functional limitations, and disability. Nagi defines disability as an inability to perform or a limitation in performing expected social roles. Disability occurs when conditions interfere with the performance of an individual in personally, socially, or culturally expected roles. In the NCMRR disablement model, limitations, disability, and social impact of disability are key variables. The NCMRR model describes the process an individual living with an impairment or disability may go through to achieve optimal environmental accommodation.

The World Health Organization (WHO, 1980) International Classification of Impairments, Disabilities, and Handicaps (ICIDH) is currently undergoing extensive revisions to reflect the evolution of the meaning of disablement. The new system will provide health outcomes in terms of body, person, and social function. One of the major changes in the model will be the elimination of the term *handicap* because of its negative connotation (WHO, 1999). As all disablement models evolve, the importance of social and environmental influences on health will continue to expand.

MEASUREMENT OF DISABILITY IN REHABILITATION

Applying disability theory and definitions to rehabilitation has been a difficult task because of the complexities in measurement of functional abilities and limitations. Some of the early work in this area was done in the 1980s. Colvez and Blanchet (1981) defined disability in terms of physical mobility, physical independence in basic activities, and ability to carry out normal activity. Later research expanded disability measures to include psychological status, communication ability, and ability to work (Charlton, Patrick, & Peach, 1983).

TABLE 8-1 Conceptual Models of Disability

WHO International Classification of Impairments, Disabilities, and Handicaps (1980)

"Disease"	Impairment	Disability	Handicap
Intrinsic pathology or disorder	Loss or abnormality of psychological, physiological, or anatomical structure or function at organ level	Restriction or lack of ability to perform an activity in a normal manner	Disadvantage due to impairment or disability that limits or prevents fulfillment of a normal role

Nagi Scheme (1965)

Active Pathology	Impairment	Functional Limitations	Disability
Interruption or interference with normal processes and efforts of the organism to regain normal state	Anatomical, physiological, mental, or emotional abnormalities or loss	Limitation in performance at the level of the whole organism or person	Limitation in performance of socially defined roles and tasks within a sociocultural and physical environment

NCMRR (NIH, 1993)

Pathology	Impairment	Functional Limitations	Disability	Societal Limitations
Any interruption of or interference with normal physiological and developmental processes or structures	Loss or abnormality at the organ or organ system level	Restriction or lack of ability to perform an action	Limitation in performance of tasks, activities, and roles	Restriction attributed to social policy or barriers

Summarized from World Health Organization. (1980). *International classification of impairments, disabilities, and handicaps (A manual of classification relating to consequences of disease)* (p. 23-43) Geneva: Author. Copyright 1980 by the World Health Organization.

The approach devised by Kane and Kane (1981) conceptualized health and disability as a hierarchical structure: the first level is general health or the absence of illness, the second level is basic performance of self-care and mobility activities that are critical for independence, and the third level is the ability to perform and maintain those complex activities and roles associated with a meaningful life. Kane and Kane's conceptualization of disability addresses the wide range of functional performances, from basic self-care to community reintegration. With a structural approach to disability, rehabilitation interventions are specific to treatment and outcome measures at each level.

Functional evaluation provides the information needed to assess and plan interventions and should include all parameters that affect "active life" functioning. Within the disablement model, functional evaluation should include the measurement of all domains that constitute independent life routinely assessed as part of the rehabilitation process. Today it is common in rehabilitation to use many assessment instruments to document impairments, basic ADLs, performance of instrumental ADLs, and quality-of-life parameters. The combination of these instruments provides the evaluation of critical components that make up independent active life. For rehabilitation nursing, assessment domains include physical, cognitive, affective, social, and quality-of-life measures (Gresham et al., 1995).

ASSESSMENT MEASURES: GENERAL CONSIDERATIONS

Information from assessment instruments is most commonly used to describe, evaluate, and/or predict outcome. Descriptive measures document the type and severity of impairments, functional limitations, or disabilities at a given time. Evaluative components measure clinically sensitive changes over time and treatment course. Predictive evaluation is used to establish goals and plan treatments. Ideally an assessment instrument should be practical, be simple to administer, and yield meaningful results.

The guiding principles for selecting a functional assessment instrument include validity, reliability, sensitivity to clinically important changes, and sensibility (Kane & Kane, 1981). These characteristics are defined as follows:

- *Validity.* Validity is the ability of an instrument to measure what it is intended to measure. An instrument's criterion validity is determined by comparing its results with a standard accepted within the field.
- *Reliability.* Interobserver reliability is the technique in which two individuals administer the same test to the same client and obtain similar results. Test-retest reliability refers to whether repeated use of a measure yields consistent results in the absence of a change in the client.
- *Sensitivity.* The sensitivity of an instrument is its ability to detect clinical change.

- *Sensibility.* Sensibility refers to whether it is a sensible tool that is applicable and easy to use.

Each assessment instrument should be able to measure disability, monitor progress, enhance communications, measure effectiveness of treatment, and determine the benefits of rehabilitation. Because assessment instruments are used repeatedly during the course of a person's rehabilitation, the data should be a reliable and valid measure of the disability being treated.

It is important to remember that the method of administration of the assessment instrument can influence the results obtained. Methodological differences in administration of the assessment tool and the type of populations being assessed are two sources for discrepancies in results. Often measures do not clearly differentiate between the presence of a functional impairment that makes an activity impossible to carry out and the actual performance of an activity. In a Framingham study of noninstitutionalized cohort members, performance of ADLs was shown to have an inherent cognitive component (Kelly-Hayes, Jette, Wolf, D'Agostino, & Odell, 1992). In his seminal work, Nagi (1965) documented that disability, unlike functional limitations, has a major social component. Because disability reflects performance within a sociocultural context, one could expect that daily performance would be strongly influenced by social as well as physical factors.

Assessment should determine daily performance, not the capacity to perform. Behavior that is executed in an ideal setting under controlled circumstances may not be an accurate measure of the extent of disability experienced in day-to-day life. Lack of motivation as well as environmental factors can impede the performance of certain activities conducted independently in the rehabilitation setting, but not when a person returns home. These factors need to be considered as part of any evaluation because of their influence on measurement.

Domains and Definition of Functional Assessment

Many assessment instruments are used to document the full range of domains affected by disability. These measures can be generic to rehabilitation in general or disease specific, depending on the intended use of the data. In general, most documentation of disability is determined with generic tools.

The general purposes of functional assessment in rehabilitation are to determine functional status, document the need for interventions and services, devise a treatment plan, and assess and monitor progress. A measure of physical functioning can be derived from many different combinations of items. One of the earliest definitions of functional assessment, defined by Lawton (1972), describes objective measurement in a variety of areas such as physical health, emotional status, and quality of self- maintenance. Granger et al. (1995) stated that functional assessment is a method for describing abilities and limitations to measure an individual's use of a variety of skills included in performing tasks necessary to daily living, leisure activities, vocational pursuits, social interactions, and other required behaviors. Quantitative measurements across multidimensional function areas are apparent in both definitions, demonstrating that assessment is not unidimensional but rather evolves along with the underlying philosophy of rehabilitation.

Within the domain of measurement of function, there is considerable agreement that self-care and mobility are central to rehabilitation. This focus of self-care and mobility, however, does not adequately describe the actual range of interventions necessary for an independent life. Although functional skills are important parameters in reducing dependence on others, the repertoire of behaviors required to lead a meaningful life is obviously much broader. Most rehabilitation programs incorporate measures of cognitive, emotional, perceptual, social, and vocational functioning. Rehabilitation nurses are involved in assessment of all of these areas.

Assessment Measures Beyond the Rehabilitation Setting

Long-term care and home health agencies have followed a different progression in the measurement of outcomes after the onset of disability. In both settings extensive assessment and care planning for all clients are required by law. For long-term care, the Minimum Data Set (MDS), a 300-item instrument that documents ADLs, continence, communication, behavior, and cognition is completed for each resident. Validity (Lawton et al., 1998) and interrater reliability have been demonstrated when administered by trained assessors (Hawes, Phillips, Mor, Fries, & Morris, 1992; Hawes et al., 1995; Casten, Lawton, Parmelee, & Kleban, 1998). With the growth of rehabilitative services in nursing homes, rehabilitation clients are being assessed routinely using the MDS, without supplement from more standardized evaluation instruments.

For home health agencies, the Outcome and Assessment Information Set (OASIS) is used to assess status within the community setting (Crisler, Campbell, & Shaughnessy, 1997). The OASIS instrument data items include sociodemographic information, environment, support system, health status, and physical function. Both of these data sets are used primarily for planning care. In a comparison study between the Functional Independence Measure (FIM), the MDS, and the OASIS, many of the same items collected were similar; however, many were significantly different (Warren & Currie, 1998). Although the MDS and the OASIS instruments are effective for planning, thus far they have not been submitted to the rigorous study for validity, reliability, sensitivity, and sensibility that the instruments in more traditional rehabilitation settings have been (Snowden et al., 1999; Williams, Li, Fries, & Warren, 1997).

SELECTED DISABILITY SCALES

Functional assessment and evaluation instruments are designed to capture domains and constellation of domains involved in an independent life. The framework represent impairments, disability, and social limitations. The following section and Table 8-2 describe validated scales that have met the accepted criteria for reliability, validity, and sensitivity to change. Each has descriptive and evaluative properties in the clinical setting. The utility of these instruments is that they provide a description of overall functioning and can be appropriately used to follow broad measures of a clinical course. These instruments expand across disease categories and physical impairments to address the resultant disability targeted by rehabilitation efforts. Although other outcome measures are available, the instruments presented here were chosen because of the extensive testing and validation in the rehabilitation field.

Measures of ADLs and Functional Assessment

ADLs refer to those basic skills that one must possess to care for oneself independently. ADL skills usually include assessment of self-care (eating, dressing, bathing, grooming, etc.), transfers, continence, and in most cases locomotion. These activities are hierarchical, from basic functions such as eating to higher level functions like stair climbing. Ability is judged by observing actual performance, rather than capacity, which is the highest level of function often demonstrated in an artificial setting such as in therapy. Although many functional assessment instruments have been developed for use in rehabilitation, currently the most widely applied scales are the Barthel Index (Mahoney & Barthel, 1965) and the FIM.

The Barthel Index is the most commonly administered outcome measure worldwide and in clinical trials. It is a weighted scoring system that measures basic activities of ability in mobility, self-care, and continence. With a score ranging from 0 to 100, a score of 100 indicates complete independence in all 10 domains measured, and 0 indicates complete dependence in all 10 domains. To be considered independent, the client does not require human assistance in any of the measured activities.

The FIM (*Guide,* 1997) was designed to document severity of disability and the outcomes of rehabilitation in a uniform and reliable method. As seen in Figure 8-1, the FIM is an 18-item assessment that measures self-care, sphincter management, transfers, locomotion, communication, and social cognition. Using a seven-level scoring system, an FIM score ranges from a maximum score of 126 points, representing complete independence in all performance areas, to a minimum score of 18, representing dependence in all areas evaluated. The conceptual basis for the scale is that the level of disability should indicate the burden of care or the cost to the individual or society for that person not to be functionally independent (Granger et al., 1995). One of its unique strengths is the ability to measure communication and social cognition. The measure is used to establish criteria for admission, discharge, and maintenance of rehabilitation gains. The instrument can be administered by those who practice rehabilitation and who have been certified in its administration.

Measures of Instrumental ADLs

Beyond the basic performance of ADLs, the ability to accomplish certain activities that make independent living possible are the instrumental ADL measures. Activities include a variety of tasks, including using a telephone, shopping, preparing meals, and managing money. These skills are often part of rehabilitation retraining but are difficult to evaluate until the individual returns home. Instrumental ADL scales may be rated by either an interviewer or by the individual, depending on the disability and circumstances. These scales can often be invalid or insensitive to change unless directly rated and do not take into account safety as a feature of performance. Instrumental ADL tools listed here are the Older American Resources and Services Scale (OARS) (Duke University, 1978) and the Philadelphia Geriatric Center Instrumental Role Maintenance Scale (PGC) (Lawton, 1972).

Cognition and Mood Assessment

Cognitive status evaluation should be an integral part of the rehabilitation assessment. The ability to acquire and retain new information, the underpinning of the rehabilitation process, can be obtained by observation of the client's interactions, responses to questions, and general knowledge. In addition, incorporation of a mental status test as part of the assessment process can serve as a guide in planning outcome goals and identifying those at risk for difficulty in adapting to disability. The Mini-Mental State Examination (MMSE) (Folstein & McHugh, 1975) has been widely used in a variety of populations and is well validated, reliable, and brief.

Affect is a powerful determinant of successful rehabilitation. Depressive symptoms can often be exacerbated by loss of physical well-being and independence. In some conditions such as stroke, depression actually may be a feature of the disease. Berkman et al. (1986) studied the association between depression and functional disability in elderly persons. They found that depression varied by health characteristics, with individuals having major functional disabilities demonstrating higher levels of depression. If not recognized and treated, depression can have a profound negative impact on all rehabilitation efforts. The CES-D scale (Radloff, 1977) is one of the most widely used measures for screening depression.

Quality-of-Life Measures

Quality-of-life measures capture a wide range of capabilities, symptoms, and psychosocial characteristics that describe function and satisfaction with life. Components of

TABLE 8-2 Selected Measures of Disability

Scale	Description and Type of Scale	Reliability, Validity, Sensitivity	Time and Administration	Comments
Measures of Activities of Daily Living				
Barthel Index (Mahoney & Barthel, 1965)	Ordinal scale with scores from 0 (totally dependent) to 100 (independent); 10 weighted items: feeding, bathing, grooming, dressing, bladder control, bowel control, toileting, chair/bed transfer, mobility, and stair climbing.	Well-documented reliability and validity; not sensitive to minor changes at higher levels of ADL functioning.	Clinician observation; <20 minutes. Appropriate for screening, formal assessment, monitoring, maintenance, and clinical trials.	Widely established measure for disability; excellent reliability and validity.
FIM (Granger et al., 1986; *Guide,* 1997)	Ordinal scale with 18 items, 7-level scale with scores running from 18 to 126. Areas of evaluation include feeding, self-care, sphincter control, mobility, locomotion, communication, and social cognition.	Well-documented reliability and validity; able to detect minor changes with 7 levels; physical and cognitive components able to detect increments of change.	Clinician observation; <40 minutes. Appropriate for screening, formal assessment, monitoring, maintenance, and program evaluation.	Widely accepted in rehabilitation; broad measure of ADL and social cognition. Standardized interobserver reliability by certification of clinicians.
Measures of Instrumental Activities of Daily Living				
OARS: I-ADL (Duke University, 1978)	Multidimensional assessment tool containing 105 questions in 5 domains: social resources, economic resources, mental health, physical health, and ADL.	Documented reliability and validity.	Interviewer; >20 minutes. Appropriate for monitoring in community.	Measures broad base of information necessary for independent living; complex domains assessed.
PGC I-ADLs (Lawton, 1972)	Guttman Scale; questions on use of telephone, walking, shopping, food preparation, housekeeping, laundry, public transportation, and medicine.	Documented reliability and validity.	Interviewer; <30 minutes. Appropriate for monitoring in community.	Measures broad base of information necessary for independent living.
Cognitive Status				
Mini-Mental State Exam (Folstein & McHugh, 1975)	Measures 7 domains including orientation, registration, calculation, recall, language, and visual construction.	Documented reliability and validity; sensitive to change.	Interviewer; <15 minutes. Appropriate for cognitive screening.	Several functions with summed scores; education considerations.
Assessment of Affective Disorders				
CES-D Scale (Radloff, 1977)	Measures severity of depressive symptom; 20 items.	Documented validity and reliability; sensitive to change.	Self-rating or interviewer; <15 minutes. Appropriate for depression screening.	Brief, easily administered, and effective for screening possible depression.
Measures of Quality of Life				
MOS 36-Item Short Form Survey (Ware & Sherbourne, 1992)	Assesses 8 health domains including physical and social activities, mental health, general health perceptions, vitality, and discomfort.	Documented validity and reliability.	Interviewer, in person or over phone; <30 minutes. Appropriate for monitoring in community.	All items are well standardized; widely used in community.
SIP Scale (Bergner et al., 1981)	Subscales evaluating ambulation, self-care, emotions, communications, alertness, habits, home and recreation, vocation, and social interactions.	Documented validity and reliability; sensitive to change.	Interviewer, in person or over phone; <30 minutes. Appropriate for monitoring in community.	Comprehensive evaluation; behavior rather than subjective health items; focus on community life.

MOS, Medical Outcome Study; *SIP,* Sickness Impact Profile; *OARS,* Older American Resources and Services; *PGC,* Philadelphia Geriatric Center Morals Scale; *I-ADLs,* instrumental activities of daily living.

FIM Instrument

Levels		
	7 Complete independence (timely, safely) 6 Modified independence (device)	**No helper**
	Modified dependence 5 Supervision (subject = 100%+) 4 Minimal assist (subject = 75%+) 3 Moderate assist (subject = 50%+) **Complete dependence** 2 Maximal assist (subject = 25%+) 1 Total assist (subject = <25%+)	**Helper**

	Admission	Discharge	Follow-up
Self-care			
A. Eating			
B. Grooming			
C. Bathing			
D. Dressing—upper body			
E. Dressing—lower body			
F. Toileting			
Sphincter control			
G. Bladder management			
H. Bowel management			
Transfers			
I. Bed, chair, wheelchair			
J. Toilet			
K. Tub, shower			
Locomotion			
L. Walk/wheelchair	W Walk C Wheelchair B Both	W Walk C Wheelchair B Both	W Walk C Wheelchair B Both
M. Stairs			
Motor subtotal score			
Communication			
N. Comprehension	A Auditory V Visual B Both	A Auditory V Visual B Both	A Auditory V Visual B Both
O. Expression	V Vocal N Nonvocal B Both	V Vocal N Nonvocal B Both	V Vocal N Nonvocal B Both
Social cognition			
P. Social interaction			
Q. Problem solving			
R. Memory			
Cognitive subtotal score			
Total FIM score			

Note: Leave no blanks. Enter 1 if patient not testable due to risk.

Figure 8-1 The Functional Independence Measure (FIM) instrument. (Copyright © 1997 Uniform Data System for Medical Rehabilitation, a division of UB Foundation Activities. Reprinted with the permission of UDS_{MR}, University at Buffalo, 232 Parker Hall, 3435 Main St., Buffalo, NY 14214.)

quality of life include social roles and interactions, functional performance, intellectual functioning, perceptions, and subjective health. Indicators can include standards of living and general satisfaction with life. Although there is controversy over the measurement of quality of life, it is a strong indicator of successful rehabilitation. Several measures have been developed, but few of these have been as well validated as the Medical Outcome Study (MOS) 36-Item Short-Form Survey (Ware & Sherbourne, 1992) and the SIP (Bergner, Bobbitt, Carter, & Gilson, 1981) scales.

Timing of Assessment for Rehabilitation Clients

As stated earlier, the systematic assessment of disability is the major means of describing, monitoring, and evaluating specific interventions essential at each stage of the recovery process (Figure 8-2). Equally important is assessing an individual at the appropriate times along the rehabilitation continuum. Assessment should initially take place at the first clinical contact, usually at the time of admission to an inpatient facility, an outpatient facility, or a rehabilitation program in the community. Often the first examination is a screening for impairments and disability related to the condition for treatment. This assessment can be used to validate the appropriateness of the referral, formulate treatment goals, confirm the management plan, and provide a baseline for monitoring change. The client's progress should then be assessed at periodic intervals during rehabilitation. Assessment should include a baseline and then a subset of the baseline, which are particular targets of intervention. Well-established, reliable measures are essential to achieving valid comparisons among clients with similar problems.

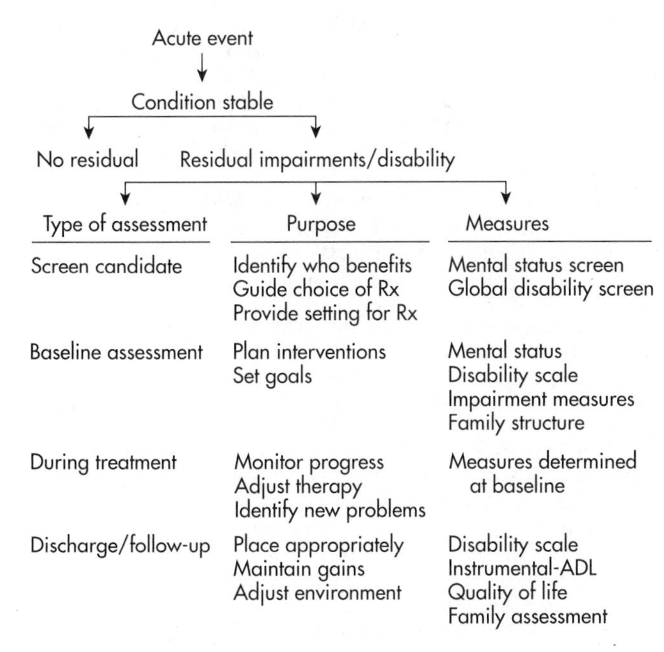

Figure 8-2. Stages of assessment.

After discharge from rehabilitation, assessment is useful to monitor adaptation to the community and for maintenance of functional gains made during rehabilitation.

APPLICATIONS OF FUNCTIONAL EVALUATION IN PRACTICE AND RESEARCH

The main purposes of functional evaluation in rehabilitation in general (Dittmar & Gresham, 1997) and for rehabilitation nursing specifically (Dittmar, 1984) have been identified. These include systematic identification of functional limitations requiring preventive, maintenance, and restorative actions; documentation of feedback about progression toward goal achievement; allocation of resources; coordination of care and facilitation of placement decisions; provision of objective data with which to analyze costs, benefits, and quality of care; and assistance for accreditation bodies, program evaluation, and third-party payers.

The specialty practice of rehabilitation nursing is founded on the belief that rehabilitation is a process of restoring and maintaining a client's optimal health—physiological, emotional, vocational, and social. More poetically, Lena Plaisted, a rehabilitation nursing pioneer, stated that "rehabilitation nursing is nursing with an awareness of the patient's tomorrow and the relationship between what does and what does not happen today and the tomorrows that follow" (McCourt, 1993, p. 13). Rehabilitation nurses help individuals and families adapt to life changes that have been caused by illness and disability.

Rehabilitation nursing is, by its nature, a relationship-based practice. To be effective in this work, the nurse must have a connection with the client, the family, nursing colleagues, and those in other disciplines. This connection is formed through knowing the client and family, possessing a strong basis in rehabilitation nursing science and knowledge, and having a deep understanding of the contributions made by all members of the care team.

Knowing the client begins with an initial assessment. The 1998 ANA Standards of Clinical Nursing Practice (ANA, 1998) describe criteria within the standard for nursing assessment. These criteria include using appropriate assessment techniques and instruments and having data that are documented and in a retrievable form (ANA, 1998). Functional assessment instruments, used as part of overall client assessment, can serve as an important part of the initial assessment and meet the criteria described in this standard. This baseline information, if well documented and retrievable, provides the nurse with a rich source of data to examine the client's status at one time and to measure changes that occur. For example, in older adults functional decline not only may occur with aging but also may reflect a variety of health problems (Shelkey & Wallace, 1998).

From this initial assessment, the rehabilitation nurse can identify client diagnosis and expected outcomes. Functional assessment can be used as a vehicle to identify client risk factors. Bourie, Phipps, Mckay, Goldsmith, and Safran (1999) used an adapted Katz Index of Independence in Activities of Daily Living as part of a "risk to fall" alert in an on-line nursing assessment. In this alert, individuals who need help ambulating, transferring, and/or toileting are identified as "at risk to fall."

Assessment data provide the nurse with the means to evaluate client progress toward the attainment of outcomes (ANA, 1998). Use of functional assessment as part of this evaluation provides the nurse with a universal language to communicate to other nurses and other health care professionals. This is particularly important in a health care era, when clients and families move rapidly between settings of care and providers of health care services.

This evaluative approach is a valuable tool in nursing research. Nurse-sensitive measures of acuity and the need for nursing care must include some measure of functional status in populations of clients being served in particular settings of care. Dependence in self-care and toileting requires that an individual client have more assistance and more attention to the prevention of iatrogenic complications. Measurement of functional status has been described as an important tool in the rehabilitation and rehabilitation nursing literature. Recent studies have highlighted the critical nature of the relationship between functional status and illness for hospitalized elderly persons (Sager et al., 1996; Landefeld et al., 1995). Changes in functional status in elderly persons may in fact serve as a marker of quality hospital care.

As Virginia Henderson (Halloren, 1995) so eloquently taught nurses, knowing the client and family provides the nurse with the tools to help them in their journey through illness, recovery, and adaptation, or to find a comfortable and peaceful death. Knowing the client and measuring the impact of nursing interventions are best accomplished through continual assessment of the client over time. Evaluating the impact of interventions on populations of individuals requires measurement at particular times. Assessment of functional ability is vital to planning nursing care of each person as well as in evaluating nursing approaches to populations of clients.

REFERENCES

American Nurses Association. (1998). *Standards of clinical nursing practice* (2nd ed.). Washington, DC: American Nurses Publishing.

Bergner, M., Bobbitt, R.A., Carter, W.B., & Gilson, B.S. (1981). The sickness impact profile: development and final revision of a health status measure. *Med Care, 19,* 787-805.

Berkman, L.F., Berkman, C.S., Kasl, S., Freeman, D.H., Jr., Leo, L., Ostfeld, A.M., Coroni-Huntley, J., & Brody, J.A. (1986). Depressive symptoms in relation to physical health and functioning in the elderly. *American Journal of Epidemiology, 124,* 372-388.

Bourie, P., Phipps, M., Mckay, M., Goldsmith, D., & Safran, C. (1999). Risk alerts in on-line nursing assessment. *Proceedings of the American Medical Informatics Association.* Fall symposium.

Casten, R., Lawton, M.P., Parmelee, P.A., & Kleban, M.H. (1998). Psychometric characteristics of the minimum data set I: confirmatory factor analysis. *Journal of the American Geriatrics Society, 46*(6), 726-35.

Charlton, J.R.H., Patrick, D.L., & Peach, H. (1983). Use of multivariate measures of disability in health surveys. *Journal of Epidemiology and Community Health,* 37, 296-304.

Colvez, A., & Blanchet, M. (1981). Disability trends in the United States population 1966-76: Analysis of reported causes. *American Journal of Public Health,* 71, 464-470.

Crisler, K.S., Campbell, B., & Shaughnessy, P.W. (1997). *OASIS basics center for health services and policy research.* Winter No. 3.

Dittmar, S. (1984). Functional assessment in nursing. In C. Granger & G. Gresham (Eds.), *Functional assessment in rehabilitation medicine* (pp. 194-209). Baltimore, MD: Williams & Wilkins.

Dittmar, S., & Gresham, G.E. (1997). *Functional assessment and outcome measures for the rehabilitation health professional.* Gaithersburg, MD: Aspen.

Duke University Center for the Study of Aging and Human Development. (1978). *Multidimensional functional assessment: the OARS methodology.* Durham, NC: Duke University.

Folstein, M.F., & McHugh, P. (1975). Mini-Mental State: A practical method for grading the cognitive state of patients for the clinician. *Journal of Psychiatric Report, 12,* 189-198.

Granger, C., Kelly-Hayes, M., Johnston, M., Deutsch, A., Braum, S., & Fiedler, R. (1995). Quality and outcome measures for medical rehabilitation. In R. Braddom (Ed.), *Textbook of physical medicine and rehabilitation* (pp. 239-254). Philadelphia: WB Saunders.

Granger, C.V., Hamilton, B.B., & Sherwin, F.S. (1997). *Guide for the use of the uniform data set for medical rehabilitation* (version 5.1). Buffalo, NY: Uniform Data System for Medical Rehabilitation Project Office.

Gresham, G.E., Duncan, P.W., Stason, W.B., Adams, H.P., Adelman, A.M., Alexander, D.N., Bishop, D.S., Diller, L., Donaldson, N.E., Granger, C.V., Holland, A.L., Kelly-Hayes, M., McDowell, F.H., Myers, L., Phipps, M.A., Roth, E.J., Siebens, H.C., Tarvin, G.A., & Trombly, C.A. (1995, May). *Post-stroke rehabilitation* (Clinical Practice Guideline, No. 16, AHCPR Publication No. 95-0662). Rockville, MD: U.S. Department of Health and Human Services, Public Health Service, Agency for Health Care Policy and Research.

Guide for the uniform data set for medical rehabilitation (including the FIM™ instrument) (Version 5.1). (1997). Buffalo, NY: State University of New York at Buffalo.

Halloren, E. (Ed.). (1995). *A Virginia Henderson reader.* Excellence in nursing. New York: Springer.

Hawes, C., Morris, J.N., Phillips, C.D., Mor, V., Fries, B.E., & Nonemaker, S. (1995). Reliability estimates for the minimum data set for nursing home resident assessment and care screening (MDS). *Gerontologist, 35*(2), 172-8.

Hawes, C., Phillips, C.D., Mor, V., Fries, B.E., & Morris, J.N. (1992). MDS data should be used for research. *Gerontologist, 32*(4), 563-4.

Johnston, M.V., Stineman, M., & Velozo, C.A. (1997). Outcomes research in medical rehabilitation. Foundations from the past and directions for the future. In M. Fuhrer (Ed.), *Assessing medical rehabilitation practices. The promise of outcomes research.* Baltimore, MD: PH Brookes.

Kane, R.A., & Kane, R.L. (1981). *Assessing the elderly: A practical guide to measuring.* Lexington, MA: Lexington Books.

Kelly-Hayes, M., Jette, A., Wolf, P.A., D'Agostino, R., & Odell, P. (1992). Functional limitations and disability among elders in the Framingham study. *American Journal of Physical Rehabilitation, 82,* 841-845.

Landefeld, C.S., Palmer, R.M., Kresevic, D.M., Fortinsky, R.H., & Kowal, J. (1995). A randomized trial of care in a hospital medical unit especially designed to improve the functional outcomes of acutely ill older patients. *New England Journal of Medicine, 332*(20), 1338-44.

Lawton, M.P. (1972). Assessing the competence of older people. In D. Kent, R. Kastenbaum, & S. Sherwood (Eds.), *Research planning and action for the elderly.* New York: Behavioral Publications.

Lawton, M.P., Casten, R., Parmelee, P.A., Van Haitsma, K., Corn, J., & Kleban, M.H. (1998). Psychometric characteristics of the minimum data set II: validity. *Journal of the American Geriatrics Society, 46*(6), 736-44.

Mahoney, F.I., & Barthel, D. (1965). Functional evaluation: the Barthel Index. *Maryland State Medical Journal, 14,* 56-61.

McCourt, A. (1993). *Rehabilitation nursing: Concepts and practice—A core curriculum* (3rd ed.). Skokie, IL: Rehabilitation Nursing Foundation.

Nagi, S.Z. (1965). Disability concepts revisited. In M.B. Sussman (Ed.), *Sociology and rehabilitation* (pp. 100-113). Washington, DC: American Sociological Association.

Nagi, S.Z. (1969). *Disability and rehabilitation: legal, clinical and measurement.* Columbus, OH: Ohio State University Press.

Nagi, S.Z. (1976). An epidemiology of disability among adults in the United States. *Milbank Memorial Fund Quarterly, 54,* 439-467.

National Institutes of Health, National Institute of Child Health and Human Development. (1993). *Research plan for the National Center for Medical Rehabilitation Research* (U.S. Department of Health and Human Services, Public Health Service (NIH) publication No. 93-3509). Rockville, MD: National Institutes of Health,

Pope, A.M., & Tarlov, A.R. (1991). *Disability in America: Toward a national agenda for prevention.* Washington, DC: National Academy Press.

Radloff, S.L. (1977). The CES-D scale: A self-report depression scale for research in the general population. *Applied Psychological Measurements, 1,* 385-401.

Sager, M.A., Rudberg, M.A., Jalaluddin, M., Franke, T., Inouye, S.K., Landefeld, C.S., Siebens, H., & Winograd, C.H. (1996). Hospital admission risk profile (HARP): Identifying older patients at risk for functional decline following acute medical illness and hospitalization. *Journal of the American Geriatrics Society, 44(3),* 251-7.

Shelkey, M., & Wallace, M. (1998). Katz index of independence on activities of daily living ADL. In *Best practices in nursing care of older adults* (Vol. 1, No. 2). New York: Hartford Institute for Geriatric Nursing.

Snowden, M., McCormick, W., Russo, J., Srebnik, D., Comtois, K., Bowen, J., Teri, L., & Larson, EB. (1999). Validity and responsiveness of the Minimum Data Set. *Journal of the American Geriatrics Society, 47*(8), 1000-4.

Ware, J.E., Jr., & Sherbourne, C.D. (1992). The MOS 36-item short form survey (SF-36). I. Conceptual framework and item selection. *Medical Care, 30,* 473-483.

Warren, R.L., & Currie, G.A. (1998). Comparing OASIS, FIM™ and MDS in assessing disability. *Home Care Provider, 3*(1), 47-50.

Williams, B.C., Li, Y., Fries, B.E., & Warren, RL. (1997). Predicting patient scores between the functional independence measure and the minimum data set: development and performance of a FIM™-MDS "crosswalk." *Archives of Physical Medicine and Rehabilitation, 78*(1), 48-54.

Wood, P.H.N. (1980). The language of disablement: A glossary relating to disease and its consequence. *International Rehabilitation Medicine, 2,* 86-92.

World Health Organization. (1980). *International classification of impairments, disabilities, and handicaps (ICDIDH).* Geneva: Author.

World Health Organization. (1999). *ICIDH-2: International classification of functioning and disability, beta-2 draft, short version.* Geneva: Author.

9 Community-Based Rehabilitation

Lisa Cyr Buchanan, MS, RN, C, CRRN
Leslie Jean Neal, PhD, RN, C, CRRN

"He is in denial about his spinal cord injury." These were the words of the inpatient rehabilitation team. My new client was a 65-year-old man who had just fallen from his camp roof and sustained a C5-C6 spinal cord injury (SCI). He was being discharged to the community to live at home with his 72-year-old wife. His primary caregiver would be his daughter-in-law during the initial community reentry phase. I went to the home with a preconceived notion about John's denial. What I learned from this client and his wife over the course of the next 9 years cannot be captured on paper; it is a matter of the heart. John and Martha taught me about hope, spirituality, love, and devotion. The attitudes we exhibit can have an insidious beginning. I went to the home with a bias, an attitude. John was not in denial. His spirituality led him to believe that the Lord might heal him some day. John never complained or asked why this had happened to him. John's hope and spirituality gave him a deep inner strength that manifested itself in his demeanor, his outlook on life, and his ability to cope with the catastrophic event that changed his and his wife's lives forever. Martha was by his side at all times, despite her own health problems. She lovingly fed him three meals a day, went without sleep to meet his personal care or medical needs, maintained their home, and learned about multiple procedures required to keep John at home. Martha's devotion was the key to John's being able to remain at home, along with intense emotional and physical support from family and friends. John and Martha received support services through a home health agency, but these services were intermittent. Before he died from a hospital-acquired infection, John stated "I have done more for Christ in this wheelchair than when I was walking." This was a profound statement. These experiences as a rehabilitation nurse cannot and should not be quantified. The profound impact this client and his family had on my life cannot be measured. However, I am convinced that rehabilitation nurses receive great rewards for taking the time to care, to understand, and to love clients. These rewards are beneficial to the clients entrusted to the care of rehabilitation nurses in the future.

Scientific and technological advances, a growing and aging world population, violence, and participation in leisure activities have created a milieu in which more individuals of all ages are living with chronic disabling conditions. In the year 2000, 34 million (13%) Americans were older than 65 years (Taylor, Resick, D'Antonio, & Carroll, 1997). Changes in eligibility and state funding for nursing home care and reimbursement for home health services, shorter lengths of hospital stay, and fewer hospital beds have resulted in many clients leaving hospitals with complex health care needs. These issues are coupled with decreased access to primary health care services, a paucity of rehabilitation services for individuals younger than 60 years, and a general dearth of rehabilitation services in the community (Adams, 1998; Hickey, Ouimette, & Venegoni, 1996; Smith, 1997).

All societies face a rising cost of health care services. Traditionally focused on diagnosis and treatment of disease, providers treated clients within institutional walls (Hickey et al., 1996). The global challenge is how to increase access, reduce costs, allocate scarce resources, and prevent primary and secondary disabilities.

It is imperative to address ways to improve health for all and develop models that meet the complex health care needs of communities, not only the needs of providers. A thorough assessment of individual community needs, beyond funds and mandates, precedes developing programs or providing health care and rehabilitation services. Full vision addresses community needs in developing and developed countries.

Smith (1997, pp. 108-109) states, "Health for all requires the engagement of communities . . . every community, no matter how disadvantaged, has assets." Conducting needs assessments, involving formal and informal community leaders, and training caregivers at the grass roots level will promote successful community-based rehabilitation (CBR) programs (Smith, 1997). Peat (1991a, p. 162) states, "The focus of CBR is determined by the community it serves."

The *Healthy People 2000/2010* initiative includes goals and objectives in the categories of health promotion, health protection, and prevention services (U.S. Department of Health and Human Services [USDHHS], 2000). *Rural Health: A Vision for 2010* establishes a plan for providing health care services to all communities through integrating care, promoting safe environments, integrating culturally appropriate care, and creating partnerships between communities (Federal Office of Rural Health Policy and NRHA, 1998). Legislation mandates can ensure access to programs and services.

OVERVIEW OF COMMUNITY-BASED PRACTICE

The World Health Organization (WHO) conceptualized CBR in 1978 (Lysack & Kaufert, 1994). The genesis of the CBR model and the independent living program (ILP) movement (Table 9-1 and Box 9-1) were based on the recognition that the traditional rehabilitation models were ineffective in meeting the plethora of problems associated with disability. The CBR model is aligned with the national agenda for health care reform in that there is a focus on prevention and taking responsibility for one's own health. Nursing practice models have shifted to integrate the principles of CBR with the health of entire communities (Adams, 1998; Nolan & Nolan, 1998; Rawl, Easton, Kwiatkowski, Zemen, & Burczyk, 1998).

Partnerships

The core of CBR programs is population-based, community focus. A CBR program will be inherently different from the next because its design incorporates the unique attributes, needs, and resources of a particular community. An effective CBR model will incorporate collaboration and planning between community, the person, providers, and family. CBR services are set in noninstitutional arenas where services are sparse or access is limited for persons with disabilities (Peat, 1991a).

Rehabilitation is an integral part of the WHO model of primary care for all nations and is foundational to the goals of the *Healthy People 2000* and *Healthy People 2010* initiatives. Peat (1991a) states that "while illness is the concern of the health professional, the effect of the illness is the real problem to the individual." Hence, there is a need to educate clients, family members, caregivers, and communities about the principles of CBR, the resources available in a community, how to access services, and how to train and use community workers.

New paradigms for health care led to new partners for delivery of services. Changes produced restructuring of institutions providing services, redesigning who provides care according to staff mix ratios, reengineering the processes used to provide client care (Hickey et al., 1996), and attempting to incorporate the concept of prevention. By fostering new alliances, institutions can combine resources with communities and capitalize on their combined strengths, resources, and assets. Individuals and communities need the appropriate tools, knowledge, technology, and impetus to empower them to take charge of their own health care. Sharing knowledge with communities promotes their health and empowerment and creates partnerships in which they require more of the expertise available from health profession-

TABLE 9-1 Components of Independent Living Programs and Community-Based Rehabilitation

Independent Living	International Community-Based Rehabilitation
Established during the 1960s in the United States	Established by WHO during 1978 at the Alma-Ata Conference
Focus: Develop independence in self-care	Focus: Prevent disabilities
Goal: Decrease barriers to access	Goal: Reach a large number of persons
Target: Individuals	Target: Entire communities
Control: Individual consumers with disabilities	Control: Create partnerships
Political: Small number of persons making decisions for others ("elite")	Political: Leaders may be privileged in developing countries ("elite")
Self-help and problem solving	Take responsibility for own health
Reduce environmental barriers	Reduce dependency on professionals
Eliminate discrimination	Cultural sensitivity
Peer counseling	Incorporate volunteers, consumer leaders
Consumer advocacy	Cost-effective approaches
Increased power base of consumers	Professionals may have greater power base in developing countries

Adapted from Lysack, C., & Kaufert, J. (1994). Comparing the origins and ideologies of the independent living movement and community based rehabilitation. *International Journal of Rehabilitation Research, 17*(3), 231-240.

Box 9-1 Basic Principles of Community-Based Rehabilitation

- Cultivate positive attitudes and behaviors toward those with disability
- Enable persons with disability to live and function independently in the community by eliminating barriers
- Empower persons with disability to access appropriate community resources
- Promote development of self-help skills and ownership of self-responsibility for health
- Provide recipients of health care services and lay workers in the community with knowledge about prevention, healthy behaviors, and rehabilitation
- Provide health care services in the community

Adapted from Peat, M. (1991). Community based rehabilitation—Development and structure: Part 1. *Clinical Rehabilitation, 5,* 161-166.

Box 9-2 Community-Based Rehabilitation Practice Knowledge and Skill Base

- Adult learning principles
- Advocacy
- Case management
- Change theory
- Cognitive/behavioral models
- Communication skills
- Conflict resolution
- Counseling
- Cultural competence
- Detailed knowledge of anatomy and physiology
- Disability management
- Early intervention
- Educator
- Environmental influences
- Family systems theories
- Group dynamics
- Health promotion, prevention
- Legislative mandates
- Management of chronic illness
- Negotiation between competing groups
- Normalization
- Research and application to practice
- Service delivery systems
- Sexuality: Counseling and interventions
- Spiritual awareness, support
- Systems theory
- Theoretical framework for clinical practice

als. Partnerships can generate the power necessary to implement changes in the delivery of services to communities and, in turn, enable institutions, communities, all levels of health care providers, and clients to become efficient and effective in their quest for comprehensive health care services (Smith, 1997).

While rehabilitation providers often focus on treating the illness and attaining functional gains, adjustment to illness or disability is the primary concern of the client and family. The trajectory of the disability loses its focus—how will life change for this client? When providers step back from medical management to rehabilitation, a clearer picture emerges of what clients and communities need for community reintegration. No medical model can prevent disabling conditions, slow the pace of disability, or change the aging population. Ideally, CBR nursing practice with prevention and education based on the national initiatives may improve outcomes for many rehabilitation clients.

Much of CBR practice is rehabilitation nursing applied to the home, especially encouraging optimal functional independence and self-care as clients' goals (Neal, 1999a). Ideally clients are involved in discharge planning, controlling their environments, and becoming responsible for their health maintenance plan and lifestyle behaviors. The community health nurse views the community as a whole and fosters collaboration and communication among all providers. Operating within the environment where the client lives, nurses should work with (not for) clients, regard their priorities, and provide quality care.

Scope of Practice

Practitioners in CBR nursing define a scope of practice, develop a comprehensive knowledge base, and develop an extensive clinical skill base that relies on core knowledge from public health. The core includes, but is not limited to, epidemiology; population-based care, growth, and development; spiritual beliefs; sanitation of the environment; study of communicable diseases; disease prevention; impact of community values; and biological, physical, and behavioral sciences (Tinkham & Voorhies, 1977).

Rehabilitation community health nurses are registered nurses with specialty training and experience in rehabilitation; they practice a variety of role functions in different community settings. For instance, they provide direct care to clients with (increasing) high acuity within their homes or offer education and consultation with some direct care to clients in clinics, schools, or parishes. Roles include staff nurses, educators, administrators, and advanced practice nurses (APNs) in specialty areas of practice, such as incontinence, wound management, cardiac rehabilitation, and the like. Box 9-2 contains a list of skills and knowledge expected of the rehabilitation community health nurse, roles that extend beyond providing direct care to individuals. Excellent skills in communication, negotiation, and interviewing are essential because community health nurses regularly help individuals and groups to think critically and solve problems (Bramadat, Chalmers, & Andrusyszyn, 1996).

The ability to manage care and other health care professionals while prioritizing and economizing is particularly valuable in the community because nurses coordinate care delivery, as well as professional and ancillary services in the home. Practice in the community enables rehabilitation nurses to expand their knowledge base, to try new and innovative methods for accomplishing goals, and to be flexible because every community is unique and dynamic.

Rehabilitation nurses who visit clients' homes encounter a new environment with each client. Plans and services that a rehabilitation nurse coordinates from any institution or community setting always take the client's home environment and resources into account. Data about home and vocational environments are used in planning or implementing care and evaluating a client's outcomes.

THEORETICAL FRAMEWORKS OF CBR

Rehabilitation nursing in the community relies on an eclectic combination of theoretical frameworks. Orem provides frameworks for delivering care to clients to maximize independence and self-care. Roy's work is useful to understand how the rehabilitation community health nurse supports the adaptation of the client to disability, chronic illness, or an otherwise altered lifestyle. Neuman's Systems Model is used in CBR because it is based on holism and a systems approach (Haggart, 1993) as the client in the community interacts with multiple systems. Neal's research (1999b) deals specifically with home health nurses but can be generalized to other community health nurses. Nolan and Nolan (1998) describe a model of rehabilitation practice and specify skills needed for the rehabilitation nursing role to be more comprehensive than it is presumed to be currently.

Nolan and Nolan (1998) suggest that rehabilitation nurses need specific skills (Table 9-2) to practice within the recommended model. They intend that their model will "more closely align professional practice with the needs of chronically ill and disabled persons and their carers" (p. 526). Theorists are discussed further in Chapter 2.

THE COMMUNITY AS THE CLIENT

What is the community? As early as 1977, Tinkham and Voorhies stated that the community could be viewed in the context of a place, the persons who reside there, and a social system. The community as a place encompasses the environment, availability of housing, transportation, health care providers, geographic location, resources, and access to community buildings. The social system includes the patterns of communication and interactions between the residents, cultural and spiritual patterns, societal attitudes, leadership style of those in power, and how the individual systems within the community interact to carry out the major functions of the community. Nurses must be adept at assessing all of the subsystems that influence each entire community system.

Residents of a community will experience health problems as individuals or as a members of one or more aggregates. "The community, therefore, is in reality not buildings, organizations, or a geographic area. It is people—people who are transmitters of value systems and culture, of attitudes toward health and illness, and who vary in myriad ways as to ethnicity, social class, education, religion, and health" (Tinkham & Voorhies, 1977, p. 195). Twenty-five years later, providers find themselves at the same place, working on many of the same issues, and challenged to identify high-risk populations and develop comprehensive plans for population-based health care. In *Healthy People 2010,* "individual health is closely linked to community health—the health of the community and environment in which indi-

TABLE 9-2 Indicative Areas of Knowledge and Skills Necessary for Fulfilling a Variety of Potential Nursing Roles in Rehabilitation

Role	Knowledge/Skills
Assessment of physical condition, delivery of skilled care, and prevention of secondary complications	Detailed physiology and related anatomy and pathology of relevant conditions (e.g., stroke, multiple sclerosis); knowledge of normal physiology and a range of therapeutic interventions; knowledge of a range of measurement indexes and their operational bases
Education/counseling	Detailed knowledge of adult learning and counseling theory, group facilitation, processes, etc.; ability to assess readiness, capacity, and motivation to learn; assessment of preferred learning style
Psychosocial interventions	Ability to assess mood state; understanding of a range of theoretical areas, particularly stress theory; ability to assess appropriateness of coping styles and modify accordingly; use of cognitive behavioral models
Family carers	Detailed knowledge of family systems theories; ability to assess family dynamics
Sexuality	Ability to address sexuality on an individual basis; knowledge and skill in counseling and intervention techniques relevant to identified need
Coordinating role, liaison, and facilitating transitions through the health care system	Detailed knowledge of multidisciplinary working; high level of communication skills, diplomacy, assertiveness; knowledge of service delivery systems

From Nolan, M., & Nolan, J. (1998). Rehabilitation: Scope for improvement in current practice. *British Journal of Nursing, 7*(9), 522-526.

viduals live, work, and play . . . community health is profoundly affected by the collective behaviors, attitudes, and beliefs of everyone who lives in the community" (USDHHS, 2000, p. 3).

CBR incorporates the concepts of populations at risk and population-based care and comprehensive assessments of communities. Rehabilitation nurses already bring expert clinical performance and extensive experience in providing in-depth education to other health providers, clients, and families, as well as how to function as a core member of a team and to cultivate a spirit of self-help and self-responsibility within groups. Not only does experience improve a nurse's expert care to clients, but it also improves the ability to assess and comprehend the intricate workings of a community. Nurses in CBR can identify obstacles to public health and address solutions to complex health issues.

Milieu

CBR nursing is practiced within the context of the client's environment, culture, and geographic location. The rehabilitation community health nurse considers the impact of these variables in planning for CBR services. The credibility of rehabilitation nurses in a CBR practice setting extends beyond clinical expertise, as they practice on clients' turfs. Families have multiple health care, social, economic, and psychological needs and seek expertise to articulate solutions and provide support. Exhausted caregivers need respite care. Children living in inner cities and rural areas may have limited access to primary care because of financial or geographic constraints. Violence and abuse are major health care issues in the nation. How are rehabilitation nurses to help? Rehabilitation nurses' clinical knowledge and skills must join with a passion for understanding, caring, and assisting clients to be as healthy as they can be.

The Environment

In this chapter, *environment* refers not only to the physical setting in which the client lives, works, and functions but also to the dynamics of family and other support systems that might affect the client's ability to function independently. The client's financial status, ability to obtain nutrition and medicine, capability of receiving spiritual care, and own psychosocial state all are influential elements of the environment.

It is not uncommon for the nurse to focus on changing the environment while neglecting to view clients in the context of their environment. The focus perhaps should be to assess how the nurse might assist the client to make adaptations to function more optimally within the current environment. The person who is chronically ill or disabled is affected significantly not only by the home environment but also by every physical environment encountered. Barriers to access abound and are discussed in detail later in this chapter.

Culture

"Although influenced by education, life experience, and creative thought, culture is the lens through which we see everything. Whether client or nurse, our views, decisions, and actions are seen through our own particular cultural lens" (Narayan, 1997, p. 664).

The term *culture* refers not only to ethnicity or ancestry but also to customs observed by a particular individual or within a family. Rehabilitation community health nurses view the client within the context of the client's culture and attempt to avoid introducing bias into their care. The client's home has its own culture, whereas the vocational setting may have a very different culture. The rehabilitation community health nurse is a guest at either site and is therefore expected to respect the cultural values therein.

Culture often presents and predisposes to barriers to health care. Language differences often interrupt smooth communication. Health as a priority and the definition and influence of community related to health behavior may vary significantly among cultures. For example, the Vietnamese view the meaning of *community* differently than do persons from the United States (Lang & Torres, 1998) or Germany or Puerto Rico.

The acceptance of particular attitudes and behaviors, such as spousal abuse, may be at odds with American views (Perry, Shams, & DeLeon, 1998) and therefore must be approached with sensitivity. Attitudes and behaviors significantly influence adherence to plans of care because clients must accept the need for a change and understand that the change will make them feel better.

The rehabilitation community health nurse performs a cultural assessment that includes customs; verbal and nonverbal means of communication; the client's perception of the problem; and the diet, medications, and psychosocial status of the client. The nurse determines who makes decisions for the client (if not the client), relevant sick-role behaviors, and the client's community resources (Narayan, 1997).

Some community health organizations make efficient use of lay community health workers recruited from within the community to assist in identifying health needs and to ensuring access to care. The lay workers assist professionals and clients in overcoming barriers to care from language or culture (May, Mendelson, & Ferketich, 1995).

Geographic Location

Both urban and rural populations can have limited access to health care. Urban populations, while being close to centers for health care delivery commonly experience financial and cultural barriers to care. One study found that financial barriers to health care persist despite the availability of hospitals and clinics (Kiefe & Hyman, 1996). The approximately 40 million persons in this country who are "uninsured", as well as the millions more who are underinsured, depend on combinations of programs that remain inadequate to meet health care needs (Glick, 1999).

In rural areas, fewer residents translates into fewer opportunities to socialize, lack of transportation for access to health care (Puskar, Tusaie-Mumford, Sereika, & Lamb, 1999; Puskar, Tusaie-Mumford, & Boneysteele, 1996), and shortages of health care providers (Mason, Coates, & Millette, 1997).

A prevailing attitude among many rural residents is that health relates to functional ability, not to symptoms. Consequently they tend not to seek assistance until they can no longer be productive or until they must rely on those within the community to compensate for functional loss (Mason et al., 1997). Rehabilitation community health nurses take advantage of social activities and other informal opportunities that arise within the rural community to offer health teaching. Also, the extended family is considered influential in the client's health care and is approached by the nurse during meaningful interactions (Mason et al., 1997). Rural surgeons are more likely than urban surgeons to treat clients who have gastroenterologic diseases, and rural physicians care for more elderly clients than do urban physicians. Likewise, obstetrician-gynecologists working in rural settings are more likely to treat ailments outside of their specialty, such as diabetes and hypertension, than their urban counterparts (Baldwin, Rosenblatt, & Schneeweiss, 1999). According to Bushy (1998, p. 66), "there are regional variations in health status but, in general, compared with urban, rural Americans have higher rates of: (i) infant and maternal morbidity; (ii) chronic illnesses . . ., (iii) certain occupational health problems . . ., and (iv) mental illness and stress-related diseases."

Special Populations

Mentally Ill Clients

The trend toward community reentry for those with mental illness continues, as many legislative mandates attempt to ensure access to community services for those with severe mental illness. Wadhwa & Lavizzo-Mourey (1999, pp. 414-415) state, "comprehensive, community care, compared with inpatient hospitalization, resulted in similar or better outcomes, reduced severity of symptoms, improved functioning more quickly, and was preferred by patients." Kuno, Rothbard, and Sands (1999) report that providing intense community support services to those with severe mental illness does reduce the incidence of institutionalization.

Persons with a combination of cognitive and physical disabilities have needs that challenge attempts at community reintegration. A comprehensive assessment of cognitive and physical abilities is imperative because providers tend to focus on obvious disabilities and neglect more subtle impairments when planning for community reentry. Rehabilitation nurses may consult with interdisciplinary team colleagues often when planning community reentry for persons with multiple disabilities because managing the complexity expertise requires more than one professional discipline, and conditions may be rare and unique.

Pediatric Clients

Many infants and children have physical and mental disabilities (Ramey & Ramey, 1998). In the United States about 15% of children are born with manifest or latent disabilities that will result in delays (Fugate & Fugate, 1996). Glascoe (1999, p. 24) found that "Half of all children with disabilities are not identified before school entrance, precluding their participation in early intervention programs with known value in reducing high school dropout rates, increasing employment, delaying child-bearing, and reducing criminal behavior."

Geriatric Clients

Health care reform is being pushed in part by the demographic trends in our nation. One fifth of the population in the United States will be older than 65 years by the mid-twenty-first century, and the population older than 85 years will experience the most growth (Klein, Kita, Fish, Sinkus, & Jensen, 1997; Resnick & Daly, 1998). These trends will have economic, medical, and social consequences. In fact, there are rapidly increasing numbers of persons living in the community who will require some type of rehabilitation services for the rest of their lives. In a milieu of decreasing resources, managed care, and increasing numbers of those requiring community resources, rehabilitation nurses and other allied health professionals must become skilled at ensuring successful community reentry and become politically active to ensure that services to persons with disabilities are continued.

Older adults make up the largest population of clients in the community. Because of their high incidence of functional impairments and effects on their quality of life, the expertise of rehabilitation community health nurses is essential to quality care (Barker, Mitteness, & Muller, 1998). One fifth of elderly Americans cannot independently perform at least one basic activity of daily living (National Center for Health Statistics, 2000).

A study comparing client and physician perceptions of functional ability for elderly clients found physicians were "far more likely to underestimate impairment than to overestimate it, i.e., clinicians were likely to think their patients more capable than the patients reported themselves to be" (Barker et al., 1998, p. 31). This finding illustrates that functional assessment must be conducted accurately and as part of a comprehensive assessment if clients are to achieve optimal well-being.

It follows that a physician who underestimates a client's functional ability would not order home visits or too few visits to assist the client to maximal independence within the home. Reimbursement for essential home health services would then be reduced or eliminated. Rehabilitation nurses can influence changes in this situation because they are skilled at assessing functional ability, can accurately predict the composition of the interdisciplinary team needed to meet the client's needs, and are respected by physicians for their specialized knowledge.

Other obstacles for elderly populations are their inability to access transportation and income status and unavailability of services (Elnitsky & Alexy, 1998). Additionally, older adults tend to have a higher incidence of mental health problems (15%-25%) than that found in the general population, impairments that can interfere with functional ability (Farran, Horton-Deutsch, Loukissa, & Johnson, 1998).

They also use more over-the-counter medications. Polypharmacy increases the risk of medication mismanagement and, consequently, adverse effects (DeBrew, Barba, & Tesh, 1998), some of which can be related to altered functional ability. A medication assessment provides essential information when formulating a comprehensive picture of the client's status and potential for independence and self-care. The rehabilitation community health nurse assesses a client's physical environment and ability to navigate the environment, leave the home, and obtain and finance health care and nutrition, as well as the psychosocial status and support systems in the environmental context.

Multiple issues affect definitions of CBR nursing practice. The knowledge base and skills required of a rehabilitation nurse will vary with the setting, the characteristics and needs of the community, and the types of impairment or disability. A review of the issues and critical needs of clients, families, and communities contributes to development of innovative and appropriate practice models, especially when the need is for comprehensive care plans across the life span.

Box 9-3 Community Resources

Community Resources Available and/or Needed

- Home health care services
- Attendant care
- Transportation
- Support services/groups
- Support from family/friends/clergy
- Disability-related information
- Respite care
- Outpatient rehabilitation services
- Contingency plan if caregiver is ill or unavailable
- School services
- Early intervention services
- Partnerships
- Employee assistance program
- Supported employment
- Volunteer helpers
- Church and church groups
- Local chapters of national organizations
- Rescue squad and fire department
- Planned recreation
- Providers of alternative therapies
- Legal services
- Adult day care
- Specialized care centers
- Assisted living
- Senior centers and programs
- Pharmacy to special order
- Equipment, supplies, and oxygen vendors
- Special camps

Client/Caregiver Knowledge Base

- Caregiver training for direct care needs
- Emergency services
- Financial resources
- Health care resources
- Equipment care and repair
- Infection control procedures

Home Evaluation

Access to Community Environment

Home Pass Assessment before Discharge

COMMUNITY REINTEGRATION

The term *community reintegration* is poorly defined in the literature. It has been given a barrage of meanings, hence confusing the issue. However, a concise definition is vital for the purpose of research. Dijkers (1999, p. 39) defines community reintegration as referring to some aspect of:

- Being part of the mainstream of family and community life
- Living independently
- Discharging the roles and responsibilities that are considered normal for someone of a specific age, sex, and culture
- Being an active and contributing member of one's social group and of society as a whole

Discharge Planning

Many challenges face providers, clients, and families in planning for the transition from an acute rehabilitation facility to the community (Myers, 1997). Rehabilitation nurses and skillful discharge planning can be instrumental in successful community reintegration. The term *discharge planning* is used in different ways, but the process is the same; it begins when a client is admitted to an institution. The process is aided when nurses have in-depth knowledge about the resources available in a community for the client's reintegration. Providers can develop and maintain a list of community resources (Box 9-3) that is validated and updated regularly. This is one tool for discharge planners who struggle to arrange proper comprehensive services within a short time when a client is leaving the institution.

The time just before discharge from an acute hospitalization is critical and involves intense discharge planning efforts if community reintegration is to be successful. Older adults are at risk for failure, especially when preadmission factors such as previous functional status are not included in the plan. In fact, the Health Care Financing Administration (HCFA) may contribute to failure with the lengthy documentation required before authorizing home health services (Hall & Oskvig, 1998).

Thorough discharge planning considers the home and community environment early in the process. For example, any home modifications must be planned so they can be completed quickly. The team will not have the luxury of postponing a discharge because of incomplete home modifications.

Shortened lengths of stay may have generated more efficiency within programs. However, some providers believe that clients are denied the crucial time required adjusting to a catastrophic event or life-changing illness. The client and family are often grieving while attempting to adjust to role changes, provide personal care, coordinate services and finances, and manage the overall impact of the situation on the family unit. The rehabilitation community health nurse coordinates evaluations from many members of the interdisciplinary team to promote a successful community reintegration.

Renegotiating Roles

The challenge, then, is to assist persons with physical and/or mental impairments to reestablish previous roles as desired, develop new roles, adapt to the impact of the disability (persons never *accept* disabilities, and providers should delete this notion from their vocabularies), provide support and education for caregivers, and provide the client and family with the skills and knowledge necessary for successful community reintegration. Certain populations of clients are at high risk for failure to reintegrate into the community unless they receive intense follow-up support services (Glascoe, 1999; Kuno et al., 1999; Mueser, Bond, Drake, & Resnick, 1998; U.S. Agency for Health Care Policy and Research, 1996; van der Sluis, Eisma, Groothoff, & ten Duis, 1998), including education. Populations at risk include elderly clients; infants and young children with physical or developmental disabilities; and individuals with psychiatric disabilities, acquired traumatic brain injury, autism, and physical disabilities. Education, including written materials that can be used after discharge, are related to clients' successful community reintegration. The shock of the situation, such as after a stroke, may distract clients and families from absorbing education provided during rehabilitation (Watson & Quinn, 1998).

Strategies

Comprehensive discharge planning can help prevent re-admissions to hospitals. Implementing client and caregiver involvement in the planning process for community reintegration; using home passes, intensive home assessment, extensive client/caregiver teaching; and coordinating and securing community resources and services before discharge from an institution will contribute to successful community reintegration. The rehabilitation nurse has a vital role in identifying individual, family, and community needs; developing a knowledge base about the availability of community resources and services; developing methods for accessing services; and planning for ongoing evaluations in the community to ensure that the services are adequately meeting changes in needs. These strategies will facilitate successful community reintegration and prevent hospital readmissions or institutionalization.

Discharge planning includes education about preventing complications or further disability and promoting healthy lifestyles and behaviors. Developing partnerships in the community and a thorough assessment of client and community needs and resources, access to health services, and barriers to community reintegration are essential components and areas where rehabilitation nurses can be instrumental in improving outcomes.

Barriers to Community Reintegration

Multiple barriers to receiving health care prevent or affect clients' reintegration, especially when they have chronic or disabling conditions. One barrier to receiving home health care occurs when the client is unqualified because of ineligibility to receive services. Each person who receives home health care must satisfy requirements, such as being homebound or medically stable. If caring for a client in the home imposes "an undue administrative or financial burden" (Kennedy, 1999, p. 7) on the home health agency (e.g., because of lack of reimbursement), the agency may refuse to provide care. No legislation, including the Americans with Disabilities Act (ADA), rules that an agency must provide care if doing so overly taxes the agency's resources. Another barrier to care is a client's need for a service (e.g., psychiatric nursing) not available within the agency or if the agency personnel are not trained or equipped to treat the condition (Kennedy, 1999).

As noted earlier, cultural or attitudinal prejudices and socioeconomic status are other potential obstacles to community reintegration. Transportation, attendant care, employment, housing, caregiver concerns, and reimbursement practices are barriers discussed in the following sections.

Transportation

Transportation can make the difference between community reintegration and institutionalization for the many clients. The ADA of 1990 required that public transportation be accessible. Rehabilitation community health nurses are advocates for accessible, affordable transportation for their clients. Some forms of public transportation still have specific criteria for access, for example, through levying extra or special charges or requirements, such as an attendant to accompany clients during the ride.

Attendant Care

Many adults with disabilities or chronic illnesses live at home and function independently or with minimal assistance. However, there are others for whom an attendant may make the difference between being able to live at home and go to school or work and becoming institutionalized. Attendants' training, qualifications, and functions vary according to the client's needs, financial status, preferences, and insurance coverage. A number of persons with disabilities are ineligible for attendant programs or are not covered by certain programs for the extended hours of care they require, leaving responsibilities of caregiving with family members or friends. At a recent conference, family members of clients with chronic diseases discussed their needs for attendant care. They identified the need for flexible nurses and aides, attendants who could provide caregivers respite, and attendants and other caregivers who could develop a relationship with the client and family that went beyond paying for a professional service. They expected the attendant to be able to communicate with the client and family, display a positive attitude, and be knowledgeable about community resources (National Association for Home Care, 1999).

"Cluster care" is a relatively new program first instituted in New York City. This program "enables an elderly person to use an aide for a minimum number of hours because the aide is shared with others who require assistance and who live in the same building or nearby" (Rosengarten, Milburn, & Ryan, 1996, p. 640). This program is less expensive than other methods for obtaining attendant or personal care while providing time to fulfill the client's needs.

Housing

Insufficient housing is a barrier for many persons in the community, and especially for those with impairments or disabilities. They lack affordable, accessible or federally funded housing options and encounter housing discrimination.

> People with disabilities are treated unfairly in many community-based housing programs. Forcing a person to participate in a program simply because he or she is a tenant is discriminatory and many advocacy groups are questioning the legality of he practice. People with disabilities must be able to choose where they wish to live and the services they need (Tamley, 1999, p. 6).

The individual's ability to make decisions about housing is severely hampered by the government view that everyone with a similar diagnosis has the same needs for services and that affordability and access can be acquired only by mandating that they have their living arrangements set up for them (Table 9-3). Rehabilitation community health nurses can serve as advocates for clients seeking fair and accessible housing in their communities.

Caregiver Concerns

Family members, congregations, and neighbors are increasingly burdened with providing care for persons they care about who reside in community settings. This is due largely to the tendency to discharge clients "quicker and sicker." Additionally reimbursement for long-term care is often insufficient, especially if a facility with adequate staffing and a small staff-to-client ratio is desired. During a time when extended family rarely reside in the same town and family members commonly work full-time while caring for elderly parents and young children, it is not uncommon for disabled and chronically ill persons to be attended by professional caregivers and hired companions.

Often a family caregiver's social/interpersonal, physical, psychological, and financial circumstances are influenced by the caregiving role. Inadequate sleep and fewer opportunities for social interaction, as well as a changed relationship with the person being cared for, compromise the caregivers quality of life (Canam & Acorn, 1999).

Unfortunately issues related to the person for whom care is being provided often are overridden by the multiple concerns and issues confronting the caregiver. Caregivers may experience emotional problems, changes in there own health, stress-related alterations, and guilt. The health of the caregivers is threatened because of their own health problems, fatigue, and inadequate attention to their own health care needs (Holicky, 1996).

TABLE 9-3 Housing Options for Disabled Persons

Type	Description
Congregate	Segregated community living developed for individuals with mobility impairments
Residential	Support services shared by a group of persons with disabilities living in proximity; services managed by others
Independent living center	Persons with disabilities assisted with housing referral, attendant referral, attendant training, advocacy, equipment repair, and other services; services not managed in a single setting
Institution	Person receives individualized care according to nursing care plan 24 hours/day
Boarding home	Private or state run; person usually required to perform own personal care and must demonstrate ability to be mobile in environment with or without assistive device
Supervised environmental living facility	Supervised apartment program for chronically mentally ill persons; provides comprehensive, supportive, and rehabilitative services to promote community reentry
Integrated housing: private residence or rental	Independent living; may receive support services from the community such as home health care, attendant care
Group home	Supervised living environment; persons with similar disabilities live together
Assisted living	Persons have their own rooms within a building or complex but are offered services such as meals, medication, personal care, and screening services; persons are unable to live alone without some supervision

Violence and Abuse

Women, children, individuals with disabilities, and elderly persons are at risk for abuse and violent assaults (Children's Defense Fund, 1999; Draucker & Madsen, 1999; Krug, Dahlberg, Rosenberg, & Hammond, 1998; USDHHS, 1991a, 2000). Concurrently individuals may use substance abuse as a means of coping with a disability. Violence and abuse are national issues. "Alcohol and illicit drug use are associated with child and spousal abuse; sexually transmitted diseases, including HIV infection; teen pregnancy; school failure; motor vehicle crashes; escalation of health care costs; low worker productivity; and homelessness" (USDHHS, 2000, p. 20). Public policies, emigration of populations to other neighborhoods, and housing overcrowding lead to degradation of communities (Wallace & Wallace, 1998). Substance abuse, unemployment, and psychosocial stress can precipitate violence in the workplace or community (Drury, 1999).

Nurses are at risk for violent attacks in the workplace (Carroll & Morin, 1998). Increased violence in the workplace prompted the Occupational Health and Safety Administration (OSHA) to mandate that employers protect their employees (Gates, Fitzwater, & Meyer, 1999). The social, economic, and psychological effects of workplace violence can be damaging to the employee and employer. Employers are obligated to protect the health and safety of their employees. Rehabilitation nurses must be cognizant of the risk factors for violence and abuse in any community setting and report incidents according to agency policies and OSHA guidelines. Recognition is the first step toward ensuring safe communities and workplace environments.

Reimbursement Practices

Community-based nursing practice has undergone major change, especially with regard to home health care. Reimbursement for home health services has changed along with government regulations for clients qualifying for and receiving home health services. New mandates for methods of measuring and ensuring quality services have resulted more than 2500 home health agencies closing since 1997 and the loss of many home health care jobs across the nation (St. Pierre & Dombi, 1999).

Nurses working in community settings visit approximately eight clients per day. Now with clients being discharged from the hospital with an increasingly high level of acuity after short stays, the community nurse also must provide care at levels that were the responsibility of the hospital staff and in the same number of visits per day.

Managed care limited the numbers of allowable home health visits significantly. Services are further restricted due to perceived need or the particular policy. Some insurance companies do not cover occupational therapy or medical social work services in the home. However, many managed care companies have loosened their restrictions, and this is partially attributable to replacing non–health-care professional case managers with nurses. Restrictions have forced home health professionals to become more efficient with visits. A positive effect is maximizing the care provided per visit. However, care for the elderly, those who require more time to learn, or clients with chronic, disabling conditions can be short-changed with this increased efficiency.

The Health Plan Employer Data Set (HEDIS) defined outcomes to provide a standard of quality for managed care companies despite community differences. However, health care needs and issues do vary among communities, and managed care organizations must be responsive to the specific demographics and needs of the community. "Ultimately, success depends on establishing and maintaining effective business relationships with integrated delivery systems . . . . Alliances, mergers, and partnerships are being forged to provide greater economies of scale, efficient use of resources and greater negotiating power" (Doniger, 1998, p. 18).

Managed care, medicare, and medicaid typically rely on homebound status (i.e., the client cannot leave the home without great difficulty or the assistance of another person) as the main criterion for care. Nursing documentation must indicate that there are skilled needs in the home and that the client cannot easily access other health care options (such as an outpatient clinic) to receive care. The payer readily refuses to reimburse for care without confirming need.

Medicare recognizes "restorative" care as a skill. However, whereas physical therapy, occupational therapy, and speech therapy are reimbursable services, rehabilitation nursing is subsumed by nursing and is not recognized as a specialty. This, incidentally, is the case with most nursing specialties offered in home health. Managed care does provide opportunities to plan for healthy communities, it does not guarantee that the community's health will improve. Managed medicaid does not guarantee care to the poor (Doniger, 1998), nor does managed medicare.

Changes in Home Health That Affect Health Care Delivery

In 1999 the HCFA mandated the collection of outcome data by home health organizations regardless of the client's payer. The collection tool is called the Outcome and Assessment Information Set (OASIS). All nurses and therapists are required to collect OASIS data on every client they admit to home health services. These data are then coded and transmitted to the HCFA. Agencies receive feedback regarding the aggregated data, and this information is then used for quality improvement.

The OASIS, in its longest form, is 79 questions. It is administered in some form on admission to service, on discharge, when the client is due for recertification, and when the client resumes care after an inpatient stay midservice. Most of the questions are related to functional ability despite the inadequate knowledge of the generalist nurse regarding assessment of functional ability. Other questions include inquiries regarding client demographics, wound status, and pain management. It typically takes an experienced nurse 1 to 1.5 hours to complete the full-length OASIS. The Outcomes Based Quality Improvement (OBQI) program mandated by the HCFA is also relatively new to home health. It is based on indicators chosen as foci (by each agency) when reviewing OASIS data.

INTERVENTIONS

Thus far, this chapter has provided the reader with an explanation of the need for CBR, the role of the rehabilitation community health nurse in CBR, the influences on the care of community-based clients, and barriers to care. The next section describes interventions by the rehabilitation community health nurse used to provide CBR.

Teams

Case management is discussed extensively in Chapter 10. The focus here is to briefly discuss how the rehabilitation team can facilitate reintegration into the community for the client with a disability. It is paramount for all rehabilitation teams to be experts at identifying the multiplicity of factors that may facilitate or impede successful community reintegration. The changing demographics of our nation's population create a milieu in which rehabilitation teams must be astute and thorough in planning for community services for populations such as elderly clients. Clinical nurse specialists, hospital discharge teams, and British hospital-to-home programs have proved to be efficacious in reducing readmissions, increasing the quality of life, and improving specific outcomes (Coast, Inglis, & Frankel, 1996; Houston & Luquire, 1997; Richards et al., 1998; Shepperd et al., 1998; Urden, 1999). However, continued study by Shepperd, Harwood, Gray, Vessey, and Morgan (1998) found some hospital-to-home programs that purport to reduce costs are actually shifting costs and do not actually reduce the total cost of health care services.

Outcomes for clients and families improve through interdisciplinary collaboration between professionals in the institution and the community (Saks, 1998; Urden, 1999). Ideally the client and family are at the center of the team regardless of the environment (e.g., hospital, home, transitional living). Core players should include the client, family, physician, registered nurse, physical therapist, occupational therapist, speech therapist, social worker, clergy, psychologist, and nutritionist when available and appropriate. The team may include these traditional healers as well as providers of alternative complementary services (e.g., acupuncturist). In the transition to the community, the team is expanded and may include the school nurse, rescue squad, department of human services, and neighbors. The nurse may be the builder of these unique teams. The reimbursement structure may dictate the types of teams formulated. Reimbursement is more lucrative for interdisciplinary teams versus transdisciplinary teams. In underserved areas (rural or city) there may be too few professionals and or there may be an increased cost generated for team meetings. These factors may prevent the team from meeting formally. Team members will need to be creative in collaborating and communicating and in planning, implementing, and evaluating client care.

The goal of the team is the same whether in the institution or in the community: to work collaboratively in meeting the physical, emotional, social, vocational, cultural, spiritual, and economic needs of clients, caregivers, and family members in the community. Adams (1998) states that clients' goals usually focus on functioning in the community instead of improving their ability to participate in their own activities of daily living. Community rehabilitation may be more motivating for clients and families than institutional care.

It is vital to have reliable and qualified team members. Rehabilitation nurses often coordinate and facilitate the team process (Box 9-4). The complexity of care provided to clients in the community warrants an expert level of functioning by all team members. Health care professionals must be adept at identifying barriers; facilitating the strengths of the client, family, and community; procuring services; and empowering clients and their support systems through education and the acquisition of skills. These skills will promote successful community reintegration.

Box 9-4 Team Building

- Interdisciplinary model
- Leader chosen based on communication skills, ability to resolve conflict, and clinical expertise
- Unity within group promotes establishing specific goals
- Group process facilitates cohesiveness between members
- Collaboration provides direction in developing comprehensive client care plans
- Change process implemented when required to enhance team functioning
- Role clarity established

Attendant Care

Funding sources for attendant care may be obtained through a variety of programs. The client will be required to meet eligibility requirements specific to each program. Some of these programs include: medicare, medicaid, worker's compensation, private health care insurance, health maintenance organizations (HMOs), Veterans Affairs benefits, preferred provider organizations, and auto liability policies. It is imperative that rehabilitation professionals assist clients and caregivers to identify individual needs relative to attendant care requirements—specific tasks requiring assistance, number of hours per day—and to obtain the resources required to promote independent community living.

In the wake of managed care changes in the medicare/medicaid eligibility for home health care and other services, it is a challenge for case managers and discharge planners to obtain the needed resources for clients and caregivers. Case managers must be proactive and current about regulations and guidelines.

Independent Living Programs

The Rehabilitation Act Amendments of 1992 and 1993 revised the funding process for the Centers for Independent Living in an attempt to increase access to rehabilitation services for persons with severe disabilities (Weber, 1994). These centers are to be based in the community, nonprofit, and managed by persons with disabilities. Any residential programs were to be closed by 1994. ILPs mandated by the Rehabilitation Act Amendments strive to embody the philosophy of the early models: to provide client advocacy, promote community reintegration and participation, be consumer based, provide a range of services above and beyond housing, and serve persons with a variety of disabilities (Peat, 1991a, 1991b; Weber, 1994). Factors influencing the choices individuals make regarding community living are listed in Box 9-5.

Effective ILPs are proactive, rather than reactive, when identifying and eliminating social, environmental, and economic barriers in the community. Trained, available, and knowledgeable staff to work with persons as they reenter their homes and communities, but control and management is by the consumers.

Employment and Education

Return to work after a disabling event depends on variables that include the type and severity of injury; employer bias; the client's age, sex, culture, control over environment, educational level, and previous work habits; employer conflict; availability of disability benefits; and job accommodations provided by the employer (Baldwin, Johnson, & Butler, 1996; Blanck & Pransky, 1999; Braveman, 1999; Garcy, Mayer, & Gatchel, 1996; Teasell & Harth, 1996).

Disabilities in the workplace can cause payroll expenses to be as high as 8% for employers (Strosahl & Johnson, 1998) and in hundreds of billions of dollars for worker's compensation claims (Lipow, 1997.) Hence, many employers have developed work site disability management programs to facilitate return to manage employee injuries, to address the complex issues surrounding disabilities, and to stem the tide of rising cost of disabilities. CBR nurses are active in case management to ensure that programs are in place and are meeting the needs of persons with disabilities who want to return to the workforce.

Box 9-5 Factors Influencing Choices of Community Living Alternatives

- Financial resources
- Type of disability
- Geographic location
- Availability and need for social support systems
- Need for skill acquisition and training
- Availability of attendant care in the community
- Availability and affordability of transportation services
- Ability to manage own finances
- Ability to hire, train, and supervise attendants
- Access to primary care providers and health care facilities

The Americans with Disability Act of 1990 was enacted to prevent employers from discriminating against those with disabilities. The Rehabilitation Act Amendments of 1992 and 1993 were enacted to enhance vocational outcomes of those with severe disabilities. Some sources state that there remains a paucity of educational and employment opportunities for this population (Collins, Bybee, & Mowbray, 1998; Wall, Niemczura, & Rosenthal, 1998).

Despite mandates, lack of funding may negate access to services, especially for those who require long-term services (Pennel & Johnson, 1997). This is borne out in part by the increasing numbers of applications for the Social Security Administration's Disability Insurance (SSDI) program (Hennessey & Muller, 1995).

Health care providers, policy makers, and taxpayers have examined findings from cost-benefit studies to ascertain whether vocational interventions demonstrate stated outcomes. Unfortunately, many studies lack consensus in design and methodology, preventing generalization of the outcomes (Rogers, 1997; Rogers, Sciarappa, MacDonald-Wilson, & Danley, 1995). Concurrently job placement efforts demonstrate a positive impact on return to work, but only 2% of beneficiaries received these services (Hennessey & Muller, 1995).

Employee Assistance Programs

The genesis of employee assistance programs (EAPs) was to provide substance abuse treatment, then broadened to services for employees who were experiencing stress due to family, work, finances, or disabilities (Talbot, 1998). Cohen, Gard, and Heffernan (1998) found the magnitude of employees' personal problems was far greater than it had been 20 years ago. The field of EAPs has expanded, "total national enrollment in EAPs grew from 27 million persons in 1994 to 39 million in 1997, a 45 percent increase" (Talbot, 1998, p. 550). Although the productivity of workers is reduced during personal crises, research about the cost-effectiveness of EAPs is sparse. Until more is known, it may be more cost-effective to provide comprehensive EAP services to reduce the costs of lost time and worker inefficiency (Cohen et al., 1998).

Different types of EAPs have emerged during the past several years. Employers should look for EAPs that provide comprehensive services to employees in an effort to promote customer satisfaction, reduce recidivism, and control costs. Cohen et al. (1998, pp. 48-51) provide the following recommendations for such models: there should be gatekeeper services related to behavioral health benefits; EAP staff should have a minimum of a master's degree with experience in a mental health–related field and be state licensed; EAP services must be available 7 days per week, 24 hours a day, for emergency situations; an EAP vendor should be committed to quality assurance and should aim to ensure client satisfaction for services provided; case management should advocate the use of the least restrictive forms of care whenever possible; confidentiality must be ensured; thorough examination should be performed because in the absence of a comprehensive assessment, concomitant difficulties would remain unaddressed and their costs unchecked; collaboration with managers should be encouraged; and the program should serve as a prevention tool for employees and their family members.

Major competition in this new market of EAPs occurs as employers opt to contract for EAP services. The expertise required in managing health care benefits, federal mandates, and employee retention and productivity all create a milieu where employers must provide comprehensive, cost-effective EAP services.

Supported Employment

The 1992 and 1993 amendments to the Rehabilitation Act of 1973 were designed to encourage an increase in the development of supportive employment programs for those with physical and psychiatric disabilities. The Rehabilitation Act also now allows for the provision of services under the vocational rehabilitation program rather than solely under Title VI . Despite the mandates contained within the Rehabilitation Act and the recent amendments, there is a dearth of programs designed for persons with severe disabilities, for whom the program was originally designed (Weber, 1994). In the amendments to the Rehabilitation Act of 1973, the components of supported employment must include the following: integrated work settings, competitive employment, services for persons with severe disabilities, ongoing support services (e.g., job training, job development), and extended support services to facilitate a client's ability to remain in the employment arena (Goodall, Lawyer, & Wehman, 1994; Weber, 1994).

Supported employment programs have demonstrated successful outcomes for clients with traumatic brain injury (TBI) (Goodall et al., 1994) and they go beyond simply providing employment opportunities (West, 1995). Clients are employed in worthwhile jobs that promote job retention. One study demonstrated benefits of supported employment for clients with psychiatric disabilities that could not be easily quantified. Benefits include the ability to increase earnings, a decreased use of expensive mental health services, increased employment rate, and increased employment in integrated settings. More research is needed to demonstrate a positive cost-benefit ratio (Rogers et al., 1995).

The literature has demonstrated that access to educational programs can be beneficial for persons with psychiatric disabilities and may promote employability. A psychiatric disability does not preclude an individual from wanting to pursue higher education. This study also demonstrated that these outcomes were more efficacious for participants (versus nonparticipants) who were part of this study's supported education program (Collins et al., 1998). This lends credence to the premise of the Rehabilitation Act Amendments of 1992 and 1993 that those with severe disabilities can reach the goal of employment when the they are the recipients of the necessary support services (Goodall et al., 1994).

Disability Management

The cost of managing work place disabilities is increasing . Corporations have recognized the need to provide disability management programs in an effort to reduce the costs of worker's compensation and disability while concurrently improving employee benefits (Shrey, 1996). The ADA of 1990 mandates that persons with disabilities (as defined by the law) have equal rights to employment by prohibiting discrimination, requiring accommodations in the workplace, and providing a means to resolve conflict (Blanck & Pransky, 1999).

In a new direction, disability management services are being provided in the workplace (the community) where the employer maintains involvement and control over many aspects of the disability management plan. The control is taken away from rehabilitation professionals at community-based clinics. Employer involvement is paramount to the success of the program. There are multiple components of an effective disability management program at the work site (Box 9-6).

The effectiveness of the ADA of 1990 has been challenged by many because of the lack of reliable and valid methods to encapsulate the data required for measuring outcomes. Other sources maintain that corporations that are proactive in integrating comprehensive disability management programs in the workplace will reduce employee recidivism, increase satisfaction, decrease worker's compen-

Box 9-6 Components of a Disability Management Program

- Team approach including the primary care physician
- Restoration of function, not a focus on cure
- Definitions of *disabling* and *early return to work* provided for the employee
- Empathy provided
- Early return-to-work program
- Role identification of employer, employee, case managers, and health care providers
- Job accommodations (may be temporary)
- Safety programs
- Functional goals for return to work established
- Psychosocial reactions and functioning through use of EAPs established

Adapted from Lipow, V.A. (1997). Disability management strategies. *Rehabilitation Management: The Interdisciplinary Journal of Rehabilitation, 10*(1), 32, 34, 36; and Strosahl, K., & Johnson, P. (1998). The new direction in disability management: Tactical teamwork. *Business & Health, 16*(12), 21-24.

sation costs, decrease the incidence of injury, and increase productivity (Lipow, 1997; Shrey, 1996).

Vocational Rehabilitation

Over the years a number of legislative mandates have addressed the vocational rehabilitation services needed for persons with disabilities. Initially the Smith-Fess Act of 1920 mandated vocational training opportunities for those with disabilities. Later the Vocational Rehabilitation Act Amendments of 1954 and 1965 expanded services for those with mental disabilities, as well as awarding federal grants for the development of statewide service delivery systems. The Social Security Act Amendments (1954 and 1972) established permanent vocational rehabilitation programs. The Rehabilitation Act of 1973 mandated that vocational services be made more available to individuals with severe disabilities. The Rehabilitation, Comprehensive Services, and Developmental Disabilities Amendments of 1978 provided federal funding for vocational services that included counseling, case management, physical rehabilitation services, therapeutic treatment, equipment, and employment programs (Rubin & Roessler, 1983).

The 1992 and 1993 amendments to the Rehabilitation Act had multiple purposes: to increase access to services for those with severe disabilities and minorities, expand the scope of rehabilitation services, promote supportive employment under the umbrella of vocational rehabilitation services, provide independent living services, mandate personnel development to counteract the shortage of qualified personnel, expand the role of consumer involvement, and delineate process and procedure for provider accountability for outcomes (Pennell & Johnson, 1997; Weber, 1994).

The primary foci of any vocational rehabilitation program are gainful employment for persons with disabilities and management by the consumers who use them. Services may include making vehicle and home modifications, meeting transportation requirements, assessing the job market, providing supportive employment, providing job training and job placement, recommending reasonable accommodations at the workplace, and educating employers (Goodall et al., 1994; Pennell & Johnson, 1997; Weber, 1994).

High unemployment rates continue for those with disabilities; approximately 15 million persons in the United States have severe disabilities, and nearly 75% of them are unemployed (Wall et al., 1998, p. 39). This number exists despite findings that vocational rehabilitation services do have a positive impact on employees' desire and success in returning to work (Hennessey & Muller, 1995). The challenge is for states to find and allocate funds to implement the services as mandated by the 1973 Rehabilitation Act Amendments of 1992 and 1993.

One model for clients with TBIs that embraces vocational rehabilitation with supportive employment targeting persons with severe disabilities, especially those who are economically disadvantaged. The combination of individualized return-to-work incentives, job coaches, work restructuring, performance evaluations, collaboration between vocational rehabilitation staff and program staff, and employer and community involvement have led to the overall success of the program (Wall et al., 1998). This model needs to be evaluated for application to other programs that operate from a community base.

Rehabilitation professionals have a professional obligation to assist persons with disabilities to obtain vocational services when appropriate. Inherent in this process is implementing client advocacy to eliminate the disparities that continue to exist and educating employers about the federal mandates relative to vocational rehabilitation and supportive employment services.

Early Intervention

The entire process of early intervention is family centered. A thorough assessment leads to comprehensive planning and intervention that will meet the complex needs of infants and children. This assessment must identify the strengths, resources, preferences, and coping strategies of the entire family. The family, as possible, sets the goals and make decisions about the services.

Early intervention programs have demonstrated effectiveness in improving cognitive and developmental functioning in infants and children (Berlin, Brooks-Gunn, McCarton, & McCormick, 1998; Ramey & Ramey, 1998) when early identification is combined with prompt referrals. Teamwork, collaboration, and use of standards for assessment will facilitate the effectiveness of early intervention programs (Bagnato & Neisworth, 1999).

The literature is replete in its discussion of the best methods for identifying issues affected by a disability (Gresham & MacMillan, 1998). Asking parents to describe the impact of the developmental, psychosocial, and familial issues cited provides evidence about developmental problems in infants and children. Parental concerns and professional expertise are the combination necessary to identify early on infants and children who are at risk for developmental delays and physical and mental disabilities and to intervene effectively. Rehabilitation community health nurses; physical, occupational, and speech therapists; special education teachers; and social workers are key team members who work with other professionals in the community. They conduct comprehensive assessments, educate parents and caregivers, perform program evaluation, and serve as advocates.

Legislation authorizing early intervention services for infants and toddlers is found in Part H of the Individuals with Disability Education Act (IDEA) (1986, 1991). The benefits to families are: family-centered care, community-based services, comprehensive program planning, individualized care plans, development of standards of practice for nurses, multidisciplinary approach to care, involvement of parents in planning and implementation phases, and a timeline for identification, referral, and assessment (Fugate & Fugate, 1996; Pokorni, 1997; Saunders, 1995). Home health professionals, case managers, and teachers in schools or day care centers have major roles to play in implementing early intervention services. Chapter 29 contains other information about pediatric rehabilitation services.

Intervention Programs: Educational, Institutional, and Community Agency Collaboration

Leaders in community health nursing are seeking ways to advance models of practice to meet changing needs and to keep pace with the evolving health care delivery system while preserving the integrity of professional nursing practice. Three examples of innovative models are presented in Table 9-4.

OUTCOMES, EVALUATION, AND RESEARCH

The current focus of health care delivery is on evidenced-based practice, measurement of outcomes in the community and in clinical practice, development of models for specific populations of clients, and program evaluation (Baldwin et al., 1996; Macpherson, Jerrom, Lott, & Ryce, 1999; Saks, 1998; Stilwell, Stilwell, Hawley, & Davies, 1998; Thommessen, Bautz-Holter, & Laake, 1999; Urden, 1999; van der Sluis et al., 1998; Wadhwa & Lavizzo-Mourey, 1999). Legislators, consumers, and payers are demanding efficiency, effectiveness, and accountability from providers. Striving to meet the public health goals of health promotion, health protection, and preventive services of the *Healthy People 2010* initiative goes hand in hand with developing valid and reliable instruments for measuring clinical outcomes in CBR practice settings.

Wadhwa & Lavizzo-Mourey (1999) reviewed 24 articles describing the effects of innovative health care delivery models in three areas: multidisciplinary teams, case management, and home care. The models provided services to clients who were terminally ill or those with mental illness. Most models operated for a short time, which may have contributed to their failure to demonstrate positive functional outcomes. Although most studies cited client satisfaction, they did not weigh the costs against effectiveness of different models. Many studies were not blinded and did not distinguish well between conventional care and innovative strategies. Evidence-based practice models of health care delivery require careful scrutiny because they must demonstrate research-based clinical outcomes and improved quality. The research must contain a standard outcome measure, use control groups, and assess cost-benefit relationships (Wadhwa & Lavizzo-Mourey, 1999).

Stilwell et al. (1998) developed a model for their study in the United Kingdom using the Community Outcome Scale. It was developed to acknowledge individual priorities by measuring the impact of problems on community outcome and act as a measure of community response. It also would discriminate between impairments and disabilities on the one hand and handicap on the other (p. 522). The scale is intended to incorporate a community focus rather than identifying problems of individuals.

EVIDENCE-BASED PRACTICE

To maximize outcomes of the quality and cost-effectiveness of health care delivery, skills in critical thinking and methods based on evidence are essential. Research that has clinical relevance combined with clinical expertise and client preference leads to effective and individualized quality care. Rosswurm and Larrabee (1999) developed a model that is useful for CBR evidence-based practice and research, and in Chapter 5, the model is applied to clinical practice with a client who has dysphagia. The following steps are from the model:

1. Assess need for change in practice
2. Link problem, interventions, and outcomes
3. Synthesize best evidence
4. Design practice change
5. Implement and evaluate change in practice
6. Integrate and maintain change in practice

The OASIS and OBQI programs are examples of current efforts by the home health industry and the federal government to collect data and design quality improvement measures based on the data. "It is easy to underestimate the extent to which organizational and cultural barriers limit the effectiveness of research-based evaluation, particularly in areas where the standard model of clinical trials of precisely defined interventions cannot be applied" (Dawson & Heyman, 1997, p. 255). It is particularly difficult "to evaluate services if the evaluation is not medically man-

TABLE 9-4 Intervention Programs

Educational	Institutional	Agency and Institutional Collaboration
Advanced graduate diploma in community nursing practice (Getzlaf, 1996) Registered nurse-to-bachelor's of science in nursing program of study (Merrow et al., 1998): Integrating home/community concepts with rehabilitation principles Associate/bachelor's degree in nursing: Medical-surgical nursing of the chronically ill using a rehabilitation approach (Neal, 2000)	Nurse-managed centers (Watson, 1996): Services provided by advanced practice nurses and nursing students to vulnerable populations in the community Community health advocate (CHA) (Rodney et al., 1998): Outreach workers who bridge the gap between community peers and health care professionals; CHA speaks the same language and is part of the same culture as community members	Medical school and home health agency collaboration (Engelke et al., 1998): Medical students provide home health visits to clients in the community who have complex needs Medical schools and schools of nursing send out teams of medical students and nursing students

aged, and involves nonspecific, multidisciplinary interventions . . ." (p. 256) . Nurses find a rich source of researchable issues and problems in their community practice. The broad range of uncontrolled variables makes research within the community setting challenging and interesting. Research initiatives may come from the agency or the community, or the nurse may identify research questions from clinical practice. Rehabilitation community health nurses, for example, may form research questions centered on improving outcomes for persons with chronic illnesses, impairments, or disabling conditions and altered levels of functional abilities. They may examine the effectiveness of interventions designed to assist clients to manage their own care.

CONCLUSION

The rehabilitation community health nurse is a vital player in CBR. Within the community, the rehabilitation nurse offers a perspective that differs from that of nurses who practice within institutional settings and builds on public health nursing principles. The roles of the rehabilitation community health nurse are varied, and the potential for creativity is almost limitless. Whether assisting clients with community reintegration, forming partnerships with clients and community, identifying resources to maximize clients' independence, promoting the nation's primary initiatives, or participating in research, rehabilitation community health nurse roles are likely to expand as more clients receive care in community settings.

CRITICAL THINKING

Mr. Q returns home after a below-the-knee amputation of his left leg. He has type 1 diabetes with severe atherosclerotic vascular disease. He is concerned about being able to afford his medicine, and you observe that there is not much food in his refrigerator. English is his second language, and he has no family in the area. Prioritize his needs, design a teaching plan that addresses his problems, and propose interventions that will help keep Mr. Q at home. Be sure to include the use of community resources and justify their involvement.

Case Study

Mr. B is a 46-year-old man who sustained a T11 spinal cord injury (SCI) as a result of a fall from a tree at his home. Mr. B has a long history of alcohol and drug abuse, risk-taking behaviors (reports he has had a combination of 25 motorcycle and motor vehicle accidents in his lifetime), and more recently has suffered from depression. He feels (and Mrs. B confirms) that his antidepressant medication has not been helpful. Mr. B has hepatitis B and C. Mr. B was incarcerated for 3 years for smuggling cocaine and was released 2 years ago. Mr. B has been free from alcohol and drug use since his release from prison. Mr. B has a wife and two teenage children. Mrs. B works for an agency that requires she be gone overnight from Monday at 8 AM until Wednesday at 2 PM. The teenage children both attend high school and are involved in many activities.

Because he has managed care insurance coverage, Mr. B was discharged to his home before the modifications were completed. A ramp was built and doorways replaced, but there was no access to his bathroom or the second floor. His family converted the dining room into a bedroom for Mr. B. He must wear his thoracic lumbar sacral orthosis (TLSO) brace for another 2 months. Home health services are provided for 2 to 3 weeks. Mr. B has had difficulties with the initial transition to the community.

Elimination Pattern: Urinary Retention

Mr. B is on an intermittent catheterization program (ICP) every 6 hours. He learned how to use a clean technique during his acute rehabilitation stay but has required antibiotics for urinary tract infections (UTIs). Mr. B is unable to reach his bathroom to empty his own urinal and does not measure intake and output at home. He had catheterization volumes above 500 ml four to five times per week during his acute rehabilitation stay. Mr. B's wife has not performed the catheterization procedure.

Goals:
Client will:
1. Identify and report signs and symptoms of a UTI
2. Demonstrate knowledge about the purpose, action, and side effects of medications
3. Have catheterization volumes of less than 500 ml
4. Demonstrate knowledge of managing fluid intake to regulate bladder volumes
5. Demonstrate knowledge about preventing UTIs

Interventions:
1. Teach regarding prevention of UTIs, medications (purpose, action, side effects), and signs and symptoms of a UTI
2. Instruct client to avoid fluids that act as irritants, are diuretics, or cause an increase in the pH of urine
3. Demonstrate clean, intermittent catheterization technique and have client's wife provide return demonstration
4. Instruct client to monitor intake, output, and catheterization volumes for the first 2 to 3 weeks

Bowel Incontinence

Mr. B was in acute rehabilitation for 2.5 weeks. He takes docusate sodium (Colace) 100 mg three times per day and psyllium hydrophilic mucilloid (Metamucil) 1 packet every day at bedtime. Mr. B has a morning program (his premorbid pattern) and uses only digital stimulation and a custom-made adaptive device. He has hard stools and difficulty completing his hygiene independently after an occasional accident. He is alone for some time.

Goals:
Client will:
1. Have a bowel movement every day while on the commode and without accidents

Continued

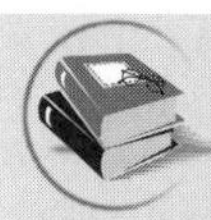

Case Study—cont'd

2. Demonstrate knowledge of factors promoting bowel continence: timing of program; nutritional intake; digital stimulation technique, frequency of use, managing with adaptive equipment; exercise; fluid intake; and effects of medications
3. Manage own hygiene

Interventions:
1. Teach about techniques to promote bowel continence: digital stimulation; fluid intake and balance intake with catheterization volumes; use of exercise to facilitate evacuation, such as range-of-motion exercises, forward bends, and Valsalva maneuver; and nutritional intake
2. Teach about managing own hygiene: keep TLSO on, use skin inspection mirror, elevate head of bed, have hygiene equipment within reach, use adaptive equipment from the occupational therapist for attaching washcloths, do hygiene independently each time, and ask for help only if absolutely necessary

Family Coping: Potential for Growth

Mr. B and his wife have had marital problems and no sexual relations for 2 years. Mrs. B has no desires, and she wants to get Mr. B settled at home and then reevaluate their marriage; they have had marital counseling previously. However, Mrs. B is not ready for Mr. B come home, and their children have mixed feelings about Mr. B's parenting, which they describe as his "barking" orders at them. Mrs. B says she is comfortable telling him when his communication style is inappropriate. The family dynamics and the disability are overwhelming. Mrs. B states, "I really wanted everything to be done before he came home. It would have made make things a lot easier."

Goals:

Mr. B and the family will:
1. Express feelings and emotions freely
2. Demonstrate knowledge about psychosocial adjustment to a spinal cord injury
3. Seek professional assistance when required

Interventions:
1. Evaluate impact of disability on family roles and facilitate client/family description of changes in roles for each family member
2. Teach client and family about the grieving process, psychosocial adjustment after an SCI, methods to use for communicating appropriately with family members and others, constructive outlets for feelings of frustration and anger
3. Encourage social and community activities
4. Encourage client to foster relationship with Mr. C, a 39-year-old man who lives in Mr. B's community and who visited the client twice during Mr. B's rehabilitation admission
5. Assist client and family to identify available support systems and counseling options

Altered Role Performance: Change in Physical Capacity to Resume Role

Mr. B (except while incarcerated) was employed for less than a year as a painter at a local paper mill. His employer has agreed to pay his salary for 6 months; he has no short or long-term disability insurance. Mr. B built a home and maintained the building and grounds. He considers selling his home and building one that is accessible. He wants to return to work.

Goals:

Mr. B will:
1. Identify specific changes in roles that have been affected by the disability
2. Demonstrate the ability to perform family role behaviors
3. Return to work and perform work role behaviors

Interventions:
1. Provide family support
2. Initiate referral for vocational rehabilitation
3. Encourage participation in social and community activities
4. Initiate referral to advocacy group for peer support and counseling
5. Evaluate employment and job retraining opportunities in current employment situation

Altered Sexuality Patterns

Mr. and Mrs. B had no sexual relations for 2 years before the SCI. and marital discord for years. Mr. B promised his sister before she died that he would stay with his wife for the children. Mrs. B states that she is not interested in having a sexual relationship and plans to wait until the family has adjusted to Mr. B's return home and then work on their marriage. Both are amenable to seeking counseling again. Mr. B says one issue is his wife's body image, Mrs. B has concerns about intimacy with discord. She wants to renew marriage vows if they decide to continue their relationship. Mr. B received extensive teaching and counseling regarding sexuality while in rehabilitation.

Goals:

Mr. and Mrs. B. will:
1. Express positive psychosocial adjustment to the life change caused by the disability
2. Identify issues causing marital discord

Interventions:
1. Facilitate client/wife participation in a support group
2. Arrange for marital counseling
3. Provide sexual counseling
4. Teach regarding sexual functioning and sexuality after an SCI

Nursing Care Plan for a Client with a Lower Motor Neuron Spinal Cord Injury

Nursing Diagnosis	Plan/Interventions	Expected Outcomes
Decreased cardiac output r/t immobility	Perform ROM of lower extremities at least every 8 hr	No deep venous thrombosis or pulmonary emboli*
Impaired skin integrity r/t immobility and poor tissue perfusion	Inspect all areas of skin (particularly over bony prominences) every day, instruct client to perform seat pushups every 15 minutes, teach client about adequate nutritional intake, maintain hygiene of skin, teach client/family about risk of pressure ulcers	Skin will remain intact, no pressure ulcers
Constipation	Auscultate bowel sounds at each visit, note nausea and vomiting, begin bowel program that includes suppositories every other day and stool softeners; teach client and wife about adequate food and food intake, including bulk and fiber, encourage exercise (ROM) to facilitate evacuation	Established bowel program, bowel movement every day or every other day
Urinary retention r/t injury and limited fluid intake	Teach client/family intermittent catheterization (to be done every 6 hr), teach client/family to maintain intake and output records, encourage fluid intake (2-4 L/day), teach client/family about signs/symptoms of UTI	No urinary retention, able to perform self-catheterization
Impaired physical mobility r/t spinal cord injury	Assess motor and sensory function at each visit, teach family and client to perform passive ROM on lower extremities, teach use of splints and orthoses to prevent contractures	No complications of immobility
Altered nutrition: less than body requirements r/t increased metabolic demand	Encourage high-protein, high-carbohydrate, high-calorie diet with high bulk; weigh client at each visit (weekly)	Weight loss <10 lb
Risk for injury r/t sensory deficit	Assess environment for potential safety hazards, teach client/family to anticipate possible threats to safety within the home and community settings	No injuries
Altered family processes r/t change in the functional ability of a family member	Assess dynamics of family and roles and responsibilities of family members, encourage open communication and discussion of long-term planning, encourage understanding of each family member's feelings by other family members, assist in design of plan to meet the client's needs, include client and family in team approach to meeting the needs of the family	Family makes maximum use of individual and collective strengths to adapt to altered lifestyle
Risk for ineffective individual family coping r/t loss of control	Assess for inability to accept diagnosis/prognosis, provide support and acceptance of client's feelings, assist with problem solving, encourage use of support systems to solve problems, offer accurate information and answer questions honestly, teach positive coping behaviors and behavioral techniques to reduce stress	Client expresses ability to cope
Body image disturbance r/t paralysis	Encourage client to discuss feelings about altered body image, allow client to grieve losses, foster social interaction with others, encourage family members to support client, refer for counseling as appropriate	Client verbalizes feelings about self and adaptation to altered body image

r/t, Related to; *ROM,* range-of-motion exercises.
*Consortium for Spinal Cord Medicine (1997).

REFERENCES

Adams, J. (1998). Community rehabilitation collaboration: Working with the voluntary sector to facilitate home rehabilitation. *British Journal of Occupational Therapy, 61*(10), 465-466.

Bagnato, S.J., Neisworth, J.T. (1999). Collaboration and teamwork in assessment for early intervention. *Child and Adolescent Psychiatric Clinics of North America, 8*(2), 347-363.

Baldwin, L., Rosenblatt, R.A., & Schneeweiss, R. (1999). Rural and urban physicians: Does the content of Medicare practices differ? *Journal of Rural Health, 15* (2), 240-251.

Baldwin, M.L., Johnson, W.G., & Butler, R.J. (1996). The error of using returns-to-work to measure the outcomes of health care. *American Journal of Industrial Medicine, 29*(6), 632-641.

Barker, J.C., Mitteness, L.S., & Muller, H.B. (1998). Older home health care patients and their physicians: Assessment of functional ability. *Home Health Care Services Quarterly, 17*(2), 21-39.

Berlin, L.J., Brooks-Gunn, J., McCarton, C., & McCormick, M.C. (1998). The effectiveness of early intervention: Examining risk factors and pathways to enhanced development. *Preventive Medicine, 27,* 238-245.

Blanck, P.D., & Pransky, G. (1999). Workers with disabilities. *Occupational Medicine, 14*(3), 581-593.

Bramadat, I.J., Chalmers, K., & Andrusyszyn, S. (1996). Knowledge, skills and experiences for community health nursing practice: The perceptions of community nurses, administrators and educators. *Journal of Advanced Nursing, 24*(6), 1224-1233.

Braveman, B. (1999). The model of human occupation and prediction of return to work: A review of related empirical research. *Work: A Journal of Prevention, Assessment and Rehabilitation, 12*(1), 13-23.

Bushy, A. (1998). Rural nursing in the United States: Where do we stand as we enter a new millennium? *Australian Journal of Rural Health, 6*(2), 65-71.

Canam, C., & Acorn, S. (1999). Quality of life for family caregivers of people with chronic health problems. *Rehabilitation Nursing, 24*(5), 192-196.

Carroll, V., & Morin, K.H. (1998). Workplace violence affects one-third of nurses. *American Nurse, 30*(5), 15.

Children's Defense Fund (1999). *The state of America's children yearbook.* Washington, DC: Author.

Coast, J., Inglis, A., & Frankel, S. (1996). Alternatives to hospital care: What are they and who should decide? *British Medical Journal, 312*(7024), 162-166.

Cohen, G.S., Gard, L.H., & Heffernan, W.R. (1998). Employee assistance programs: A preventive, cost-effective benefit. *Journal of Health Care Finance, 24*(3), 45-53.

Collins, M.E., Bybee, D., & Mowbray, C.T. (1998). Effectiveness of supported education for individuals with psychiatric disabilities: Results from an experimental study. *Community Mental Health Journal, 34*(6), 595-613.

Consortium for Spinal Cord Medicine. (1997). *Prevention of thromboembolism in SCI.* Washington, DC: Author.

Dawson, P., & Heyman, B. (1997). Evaluating community health services: Conflict and controversy. *Health and Social Care in the Community,* 5(4), 255-260.

DeBrew, J.K., Barba, B., & Tesh, A.S. (1998). Assessing medication knowledge and practices of older adults. *Home Healthcare Nurse, 16*(10), 686-691.

Dijkers, M. (1999). Community integration: Conceptual issues and measurement approaches in rehabilitation research. *Journal of Rehabilitation Outcomes Measurement, 3*(1), 39-49.

Doniger, A.S. (1998). Enlisting managed care organizations to participate in community health improvement. *Journal of Public Health Management and Practice, 4*(1), vii-viii.

Draucker, C.B., & Madsen, C. (1999). Women dwelling with violence. *Image, 31*(4), 327-332.

Drury, T. (1999). How to defuse a walking time bomb. *Nursing Management, 30*(5), 58, 59-61.

Elnitsky, C., & Alexy, B. (1998). Identifying health status and health risks of older rural residents. *Journal of Community Health Nursing, 15*(2), 61-75.

Engelke, M. K., Britton, B.P., Burhans, L., & Hall, S. (1998). Is there a doctor in the house? *Home Care Provider,* 3(5), 260-265.

Farran, C.J., Horton-Deutsch, S.L., Loukissa, D., & Johnson, L. (1998). Psychiatric home care of elderly persons with depression: Unmet caregiver needs. *Home Health Care Services Quarterly, 16*(4), 57-73.

Federal Office of Rural Health Policy and National Rural Health Association. (1998, January). *Rural health: A vision for 2010.* Rockville, MD, and Kansas City, MO: Authors.

Fugate, D.L., & Fugate, J.M. (1996). Putting the marketing plan to work: Practical suggestions for early intervention programs. *Infants and Young Children, 8*(4), 70-79.

Garcy, P., Mayer, T., & Gatchel, R.J. (1996). Recurrent or new injury outcomes after return to work in chronic disabling spinal disorders. *Spine, 21*(8), 952-959.

Gates, D.M., Fitzwater, E., & Meyer, U. (1999). Violence against caregivers in nursing homes: Expected, tolerated, and accepted. *Journal of Gerontological Nursing, 25*(4), 12-22.

Getzlaf, B.A. (1996). Advanced community nursing practice: Athabasca University meets the challenge of primary care. *Alberta Association of Registered Nurses Newsletter,* 52(11), 12.

Glascoe, F.P. (1999). Using parents' concerns to detect and address developmental and behavioral problems. *Journal of the Society of Pediatric Nurses, 4*(1), 24-35.

Glick, D.F. (1999). Advanced practice community health nursing in community nursing centers: A holistic approach to the community as client. *Holistic Nursing Practice, 13*(4), 1.

Goodall, P., Lawyer, H.L., & Wehman, P. (1994). Vocational rehabilitation and traumatic brain injury: A legislative and public policy perspective. *Journal of Head Trauma Rehabilitation, 9*(2), 61-81.

Gresham, F.M., & MacMillan, D.L. (1998). Early intervention project: Can its claims be substantiated and its effects replicated? *Journal of Autism and Developmental Disorders, 28*(1), 5-13.

Haggart, M. (1993). A critical analysis of Neuman's systems model in relation to public health nursing. *Journal of Advanced Nursing, 18*(2), 1917-1922.

Hall, W.J., & Oskvig, R.O. (1998). Transition care: Hospital to home. *Clinics in Geriatric Medicine, 14*(4), 799-812.

Hennessey, J.C., & Muller, L.S. (1995). The effect of vocational rehabilitation and work incentives on helping the disabled-worker beneficiary back to work. *Social Security Bulletin, 58*(1), 15-28.

Hickey, J.V., Ouimette, R.M., & Venegoni, S.L. (1996). *Advanced practice nursing: Changing roles and clinical applications.* Philadelphia: JB Lippincott.

Holicky, R. (1996). Caring for the caregivers: The hidden victims of illness and disability. *Rehabilitation Nursing, 21*(5), 247-252.

Houston, S., & Luquire, R. (1997). Advanced practice nurse as outcomes manager. *Advanced Practice Nursing Quarterly, 3*(2), 1-9.

Kennedy, E.M. (1999). Home care and the ADA: Do limitations on coverage violate the law? *Caring, XVIII*(6), 6-11.

Kiefe, C.I., & Hyman, D.J. (1996). Do public clinic systems provide health care access for the urban poor? A cross-sectional survey. *Journal of Community Health, 21*(1), 61-70.

Klein, G.L., Kita, K., Fish, J., Sinkus, B., & Jensen, G.L. (1997). Nutrition and health for older persons in rural America: A managed care model. *Journal of the American Dietetic Association, 97*(8), 885-888.

Krug, E.G., Dahlberg, L.L., Rosenberg, M.L., & Hammond, W.R. (1998). America: Where kids are getting killed. *Journal of Pediatrics, 132*(5), 751-755.

Kuno, E., Rothbard, A.B., & Sands, R.G. (1999). Service components of case management which reduce inpatient care use for persons with serious mental illness. *Community Mental Health Journal, 35*(2), 153-167.

Lang, P., & Torres, M. I. (1998). Vietnamese perceptions of community and health: Implications of the practice of community health education. *International Quarterly of Community Health Education, 17*(4), 389-404.

Lipow, V.A. (1997). Disability management strategies. *Rehabilitation Management: The Interdisciplinary Journal of Rehabilitation, 10*(1), 32, 34, 36.

Lysack, C., & Kaufert, J. (1994). Comparing the origins and ideologies of the independent living movement and community based rehabilitation. *International Journal of Rehabilitation Research, 17*(3), 231-240.

Macpherson, R., Jerrom, B., Lott, G., & Ryce, M. (1999). The outcome of clinical goal setting in a mental health rehabilitation service. A model for evaluating clinical effectiveness. *Journal of Mental Health, 8*(1), 95-102.

Mason, G., Coates, J., & Millette, B. (1997). Immunizations and rural health: Considerations for nurse practitioners. *Clinical Excellence for Nurse Practitioners, 1*(7), 428-436.

May, K.M., Mendelson, C., & Ferketich, S. (1995). Community empowerment in rural health care. *Public Health Nursing, 12*(1), 25-30.

Merrow, S.L., Edwards, P.A., & Schultz, P.S. (1998). Home care and rehabilitation nursing: A winning combination. *Nurse Educator, 23*(4), 21, 34.

Mueser, K.T., Bond, G.R., Drake, R.E., & Resnick, S.G. (1998). Models of community care for severe mental illness: A review of research on case management. *Schizophrenia Bulletin, 24*(1), 37-74.

Myers, C.S. (1997). Discharge planning: Juggling administrative, financial, and family pressure to achieve length-of-stay goals. *Rehab Management, 10*(6), 58, 60-61.

Narayan, M. (1997). Cultural assessment in home healthcare. *Home Healthcare Nurse, 15*(10), 663-670.

National Association for Home Care. (1999). Caregiving: Into the minds and hearts of family caregivers. *Caring, XVIII*(7), 34.

National Center for Health Statistics (2000). http://www.cdc.gov/nchs/.

Neal, L.J. (1999a). Research supporting the congruence between rehabilitation principles and home health nursing practice. *Rehabilitation Nursing, 24*(3), 115-121.

Neal, L.J. (1999b). The Neal theory: Implications for practice and administration. *Home Healthcare Nurse, 17*(3), 181-187.

Neal, L.J. (2000). The "R" word and the new millennium. *Home Healthcare Nurse, 18*(1), 35-37.

Nolan, M., & Nolan, J. (1998). Rehabilitation: Scope for improvement in current practice. *British Journal of Nursing, 7*(9), 522-526.

Peat, M. (1991a). Community based rehabilitation—development and structure: Part 1. *Clinical Rehabilitation, 5,* 161-166.

Peat, M. (1991b). Community based rehabilitation—development and structure: Part 2. *Clinical Rehabilitation, 5,* 231-239.

Pennell, F.E., & Johnson, J. (1997). Legal and civil rights aspects of vocational rehabilitation. *Physical Medicine and Rehabilitation Clinics of North America, 8*(2), 245-261.

Perry, C.M., Shams, M., & DeLeon, C.C. (1998). Voices from an Afghan community. *Journal of Cultural Diversity, 5*(4), 127-131.

Pokorni, J.L. (1997). Promoting the overall development of infants and young children receiving home health services. *Pediatric Nursing, 23*(2), 187-190.

Puskar, K., Tusaie-Mumford, K., & Boneysteele, G. (1996). Rurality and advanced practiced nurses. *The Journal of Multicultural Nursing and Health, 2*(4), 43-47.

Puskar, K.R., Tusaie-Mumford, K., Sereika, S., & Lamb, J. (1999). Health concerns and risk behaviors of rural adolescents. *Journal Of Community Health Nursing, 16*(2), 109-119.

Ramey, C.T., & Ramey, S.L. (1998). Prevention of intellectual disabilities: Early interventions to improve cognitive development. *Preventive Medicine, 27,* 224-232.

Rawl, S.M., Easton, K.L., Kwiatkowski, S., Zemen, D., & Burczyk, B. (1998). Effectiveness of a nurse-managed follow-up program for rehabilitation patients after discharge. *Rehabilitation Nursing, 23*(4), 204-209.

Resnick, B., & Daly, M. (1998). Predictors of functional ability in geriatric rehabilitation patients. *Rehabilitation Nursing, 23*(1), 21-29.

Richards, S.H., Coast, J., Gunnell, D.J., Peters, T.J., Pounsford, J., & Darlow, M. (1998). Randomised controlled trial comparing effectiveness and acceptability of an early discharge hospital at home scheme with acute hospital care. *British Medical Journal, 316*(7147), 1796-1801.

Rodney, M., Clasen, C., Goldman, G., Markert, T., & Deane, D. (1998). Three evaluation methods of a community health advocate program. *Journal Of Community Health, 23*(5), 371-381.

Rogers, E.S. (1997). Cost-benefit studies in vocational services. *Psychiatric Rehabilitation Journal, 20*(3), 25-33.

Rogers, E.S., Sciarappa, K., MacDonald-Wilson, K., & Danley, K. (1995). A benefit-cost analysis of a supported employment model for persons with psychiatric disabilities. *Evaluation and Program Planning, 18*(2), 105-115.

Rosengarten, L., Milburn, F., & Ryan, M.C. (1996). Helping home care aides work with newly dependent elderly in a cluster care setting. *Home Healthcare Nurse, 14*(8), 638-646.

Rosswurm, M.A., & Larrabee, J.H. (1999). A model for change to evidence-based practice. *Image, 31*(4), 317-322.

Rubin, S.E., & Roessler, R.T. (1983). *Foundations of the vocational rehabilitation process* (2nd ed.). Austin, TX: PRO-ED.

Saks, N.P. (1998). Developing an integrated model for outcomes management. *Advanced Practice Nursing Quarterly, 4*(1), 27-32.

Saunders, E.J. (1995). Services for infants and toddlers with disabilities: IDEA, Part H. *Health & Social Work, 20*(1), 39-45.

Shepperd, S., Harwood, D., Gray, A., Vessey, M., & Morgan, P. (1998). Randomised controlled trial comparing hospital at home care with inpatient hospital care. II: Cost minimisation analysis. *British Medical Journal, 316*(7147), 1791-1796.

Shepperd, S., Harwood, Jenkinson, C., Gray, A., Vessey, M., & Morgan, P. (1998). Randomised controlled trial comparing hospital at home care with inpatient hospital care. I: Three month follow up of health outcomes. *British Medical Journal, 316*(7147), 1786-1791.

Shrey, D.E. (1996). Disability management in industry: The new paradigm in injured worker rehabilitation. *Disability and Rehabilitation, 18*(8), 408-414.

Smith, G.R. (1997). Creating community power in health care. *International Nursing Review, 44*(4), 105-109.

St. Pierre, M., & Dombi, W.A. (1999). Home health PPS: New payment system, new hope. *Caring, XIX*(1), 6-11.

Stilwell, P., Stilwell, J., Hawley, C., & Davies, C. (1998). Measuring outcome in community-based rehabilitation services for people who have suffered traumatic brain injury: The community outcome scale. *Clinical Rehabilitation, 12*(6), 521-531.

Strosahl, K., & Johnson, P. (1998). The new direction in disability management: Tactical teamwork. *Business & Health, 16*(12), 21-24.

Talbot, J.A. (Ed.). (1998). Rapidly growing employee assistance programs face major changes, more intense competition. *Psychiatric Services, 49*(4), 550-551.

Tamley, K. (1999). Fair play on the housing front. *Caring, XVIII*(7), 6-8.

Taylor, C. A., Resick, L., D'Antonio, J. A., & Carroll, T. (1997). The advanced practice nurse role in implementing and evaluating two nurse-managed wellness clinics: Lessons learned about structure, process, and outcomes. *Advanced Practice Nursing Quarterly,* 3(2), 36-45.

Teasell, R.W., & Harth, M. (1996). Functional restoration: Returning patients with chronic low back pain to work—revolution or fad? *Spine, 21*(7), 844-847.

Thommessen, B., Bautz-Holter, E., & Laake, K. (1999). Predictors of outcome of rehabilitation of elderly stroke patients in a geriatric ward. *Clinical Rehabilitation, 13*(2), 123-128.

Tinkham, C.W., & Voorhies, E.F. (1977). Community health nursing: Evolution and process (2nd ed.). New York: Appleton-Century-Crofts.

Urden, L.D. (1999). Outcome evaluation: An essential component for CNS practice. *Clinical Nurse Specialist, 13*(1), 39-46.

U.S. Agency for Health Care Policy and Research. (1996). Poststroke rehabilitation: Assessment, referral, and patient management. *Topics in Stroke Rehabilitation, 3*(2), 1-26.

U.S. Department of Health and Human Services. (1991a). *Healthy children 2000: National health promotion and disease prevention objectives related to mothers, infants, children, adolescents, and youth* (DHHS Publication No. HRSA-M-CH 91-2). Washington, DC: U.S. Government Printing Office.

U.S. Department of Health and Human Services. (2000). *Healthy people 2010: Conference edition* [On-line]. Available at: http://web.health.gov/healthypeople/document.

van der Sluis, C.K., Eisma, W.H., Groothoff, J.W., & ten Duis, H.J. (1998). Long-term physical, psychological and social consequences of severe injuries. *Injury, 29*(4), 281-285.

Wadhwa, S., & Lavizzo-Mourey, R. (1999). Do innovative models of health care delivery improve quality of care for selected vulnerable populations? A systematic review. *Journal on Quality Improvement, 25*(8), 408-421.

Wall, J.R., Niemczura, J.G., & Rosenthal, M. (1998). Community-based training and employment: An effective program for persons with traumatic brain injury. *NeuroRehabilitation, 10,* 39-49.

Wallace, D., & Wallace, R. (1998). Scales of geography, time, and population: The study of violence as a public health problem. *American Journal of Public Health, 88*(12), 1853-1858.

Watson, L.D. & Quinn, D.A. (1998). Stages of stroke: A model for stroke rehabilitation. *British Journal of Nursing, 7*(11), 631-640.

Watson, L.J. (1996). A national profile of nursing centers: Arenas for advanced practice. *Nurse Practitioner, 21*(3), 77-81.

Weber, M.C. (1994). Towards access, accountability, procedural regularity and participation: The Rehabilitation Act Amendments of 1992 and 1993. *Journal of Rehabilitation, 60*(3), 21-25.

West, M.D. (1995). Aspects of the workplace and return to work for persons with brain injury in supported employment. *Brain Injury, 9*(3), 301-313.

BIBLIOGRAPHY

Abraham, R., & Fallon, P.J. (1997). Caring for the community: Development of the advanced practice nurse role. *Clinical Nurse Specialist, 11*(5), 224-230.

American Nurses Association. (1985). *The scope of practice of the primary health care nurse practitioner.* Kansas City, MO: Author.

Baker, E.L., Melton, R.J., Stange, P.V., Fields, M.L., Koplan, J.P., Guerra, F.A., & Satcher, D. (1994). Health reform and the health of the public. *Journal of the American Medical Association, 272,* (16), 1276-1282.

Neal, L.J. (1995a). The rehabilitation nurse in the home setting: treating chronic wounds as a disability. *Rehabilitation Nursing, 20*(5), 261-264.

Neal, L.J. (1995b). The rehabilitation nursing team in the home healthcare setting. *Rehabilitation Nursing, 20,* 32-36.

Neal, L.J. (1998). *Rehabilitation nursing in the home health setting.* Glenview, IL: Association of Rehabilitation Nurses.

Neal, L.J. (1999c). Neal theory of home health nursing practice. *Image, 31*(3), 251.

Nolan, M., & Nolan, J. (1998). Stroke 2: Expanding the nurse's role in stroke rehabilitation. *British Journal of Nursing, 7*(7), 388-392.

SmithBattle, L., Diekemper, M., & Drake, M.A. (1999). Articulating the culture and tradition of community health nursing. *Public Health Nursing, 16*(3), 215-222.

U.S. Department of Health and Human Services. (1991b). *Healthy people 2000: National health promotion and disease prevention objectives* (DHHS Publication No. PHS 91-50212). Washington, DC: U.S. Government Printing Office.

Case Management 10

Patricia L. McCollom, RN, MS, CRRN, CDMS, CCM, CLCP
Diane Huber, PhD, RN, FAAN, CNAA

"You were our guardian angel! You seemed to know what we needed, when we needed it, and how to get it. You were the one who taught us what we needed to learn and at what pace! When we first met, we had no idea what a case manager was or how you could possibly help. Our son had a brain injury and nothing could make that better. But you helped make sure he was well taken care of and that we always were informed. You helped us to survive this ordeal!"

Mr. and Mrs. ES, August 1999

Case management has emerged as a key strategy and an innovative approach to improving client care within a rapidly changing health care delivery system. Fueled by pressures of rising costs and the spread of managed care, case management was adopted as a way to manage risk and coordinate care services. Providing a framework for planning, implementing, and evaluating care, case management is an effective tool for dealing with the increasing complexity, fragmentation, and constraints of the delivery of health services. It has been defined and developed by the multidisciplinary professional organization that represents case management professionals, the Case Management Society of America (CMSA), which was founded in 1990 and grew throughout that decade.

Case management is not a profession in itself, but rather a functional area of practice within one's profession, with various and complex transdisciplinary relationships. Case management processes benefit clients, families, communities, providers, and payers by assisting individuals with chronic illness, injury, or disability to reach their potential for independence and to gain satisfaction with quality of life. Case management also benefits populations when optimum health outcomes are attained by a group through the use of strategies such as close follow-up, continuous teaching and reinforcement, systematic therapeutic adjustments, and linkage and advocacy.

The processes of case management contribute to a new focus within health care, consumer involvement, which emphasizes the goals of prevention and health. The role of client advocate facilitates individual and family involvement in self-care and health-related autonomy. Research findings have confirmed the contribution of nurse case managers to positive health outcomes such as achieving near-normal control of blood sugar levels in persons with diabetes (Aubert et al., 1998). Shifting from a medical model of diagnosis/treatment/cure, case management offers a method of forging partnerships within the community and among clients, families, and providers to improve the quality of service and access to care. This new focus has evolved as a result of the growth of managed care, the beginning of restructuring of the U.S. health care system, the need for economic accountability, and the pressure for measurements of the results of care and treatment or outcomes.

ORIGINS OF CASE MANAGEMENT

Case management began in the late 1800s and early 1900s with nurses and social workers who were interested in care of the urban poor and in coordinating community services. Models of social casework spread into nursing and social work practice in the early 1900s in settlement houses and public health programs. Early disciplines using case management were nursing, social work, and psychiatry. Case management was further developed in the 1960s in the insurance industry and in the 1970s in social work, health maintenance organizations (HMOs), long-term care, and mental health arenas. In the 1980s case management diffused into acute care hospital nursing and became popularized as nursing case management (Cesta, Tahan, & Fink, 1998). By the 1990s, case management had spread into most health care, insurance, and social services settings. In the 1990s, *case management* became the term of choice as the concept of *cost control* was implemented.

Legislation has been one driving force for case management, especially in rehabilitation. By the 1940s, legislation for the disabled began to affect the public sector, resulting in the insurance industry assuming a more proactive role in addressing rising health care costs. The Vocational Rehabilitation Act of 1943, which funded professional training and research for persons with disabilities, served to establish vocational case management. This area of case management was strengthened by the Workers' Compensation Rehabilitation Law of 1960, the Rehabilitation Act of 1973, and subsequent amendments.

The insurance industry was one major driver in the development, implementation, and application of case management principles (Siefker, Garrett, Van Genderen, & Weis, 1998). In 1945 Liberty Mutual Insurance began hiring nurses to coordinate care and assist injured workers to return to work. In 1970 the Insurance Company of North America began the first private-sector rehabilitation company, International Rehabilitation Associates. Nurses and vocational rehabilitation counselors were hired to coordinate care and to create long-term plans to address the needs of persons with disabilities. Crawford and Company, at the time the largest insurance-adjusting company, followed into this field. By the mid-1970s, thousands of smaller companies had been spawned from these pioneers.

As the insurance industry contributed to the growth and development of case management outside the traditional boundaries of health care delivery systems, within health care facilities, especially hospitals, the effects of cost control and external influences on care delivery became apparent. Nursing case management within acute care hospitals was introduced in 1985, to allow a mechanism for evaluating care and containing costs (Cohen & Cesta, 1997). Models of hospital-based case management promoted outcome-based care, the use of standardized tools such as critical pathways, and the integration of clinical and community services. The goal was to support the quality and consistency of care across the continuum of service delivery.

DEFINITIONS

The definition of case management varies depending on the area and discipline of practice. The CMSA, an international, nonprofit, multidisciplinary society of case management professionals, promotes professional development of health care case management practitioners in various settings and has defined case management and developed standards of practice, including ethical guidelines. In 1995 the CMSA Board of Directors approved and published the following definition: "Case management is a collaborative process which assesses, plans, implements, coordinates, monitors and evaluates options and services to meet an individual's health needs through communication and available resources to promote quality cost-effective outcomes" (CMSA, 1995, p. 8). This definition is considered by CMSA as the foundation for their standards of practice. The group sees case managers as the advocate and link among clients, providers, and payers. The CMSA definition is widely referred to as the definition of case management because this is generated by the professional organization for case management practice.

TABLE 10-1 Comparison of Two Case Management Definitions

CMSA (1995)	Cohen & Cesta (1997)
Case Management	**Case Management**
• Is a process	• Is an approach
• Is collaborative	• Supports autonomous practice of nursing
• Communicates across continuum	• Integrates clinical services
• Promotes cost-effective care	• Places internal controls on resources used for care
• Considers service options in the community	• Limits or may limit service options to a system
• Facilitates outcomes	• Facilitates outcomes

Alternative definitions abound, usually associated with the model of case management used or a specific practice discipline. For example, Cohen and Cesta (1997, p. 5) suggested that "nursing case management is an approach that focuses on the coordination, integration, and direct delivery of client services and places internal controls on the resources used for care. Such management emphasizes early assessment and intervention, comprehensive care planning, and inclusive service system referrals."

Although the multiple definitions of case management have commonalities, certain distinctions between the definitions of case management practice can be identified. These disparities support the need for ongoing dialogue regarding continuing evolution of the practice and the role and function of case management (Table 10-1). This is especially true in the field of nursing, where the definitions of case management have widely diverged between a process and a care delivery system, and between the fields of nursing and social work, where the issue of cost containment responsibilities has created a rift.

MODELS OF CASE MANAGEMENT

As health care has continued to transform, the need for case management has grown in a variety of practice settings. Promoted by managed care initiatives, case management has evolved from the prominence of the catastrophic and worker's compensation focus by independent case managers to the growth of jobs within facilities and specific to organizations and populations. Case managers from numerous disciplines now work in private practice, corporations, insur-

Box 10-1 Outcomes of Case Management Plan

- Mutually agreed-on plan with client/family
- Goal identification
- Defined resources and alternatives
- Health and wellness promotion emphasized

ance companies, managed care organizations, HMOs, clinics, and physician practice groups. Case managers work in hospitals, long-term care facilities, specialty care facilities, and public/community settings. Those practicing facility-based case management may be involved with disease management, critical pathways for care, variance analysis, and outcomes management. Data gathering and analysis are specialized functions in a complex care environment that serve as a key case management foundation and become the means for decision making and improvement of care.

Case managers serve diverse populations that are in need of medical, vocational, psychosocial, and other coordinated care. For example, the disease management of persons with congestive heart failure or diabetes may be the focus of case managers who are nurses. The case management of persons needing substance abuse treatment may be the focus of case managers who are social workers. The practice in all settings and models involves involving the consumer/family, coordinating and linking the availability of resources and services, and developing a mutually agreed-on plan to achieve goals promoting health, well-being, and satisfaction with health care services (Box 10-1).

The CMSA (1995) developed a triangle model to depict the triad of case management (clients, providers, payers) and the role functions encompassed by case management practice. These components of case management practice are client identification, assessment, planning, resource identification, resource linkage, coordination, and evaluation.

COMPONENTS OF CASE MANAGEMENT PRACTICE

Client Identification

Case managers identify individuals or groups appropriate for intervention. Specification of the criteria signaling the need for case management services is based on the relationship between diagnosis, complications, potential cost, and geographic availability of needed resources.

Assessment

Case managers conduct a comprehensive, objective evaluation of an individual's status, including psychosocial and functional assessment, and of the epidemiological characteristics of a population. Box 10-2 represents a listing of categories necessary for case management assessment focused on the individual.

Box 10-2 Case Management Assessment Categories

Health Status

- History
- Review of systems
- Current status
- Medications (include pharmacist)
- Nutritional status
- Eating habits
- Height
- Weight

Functional Skills

- Self-care
- Cognition
- Communication
- Behavior
- Mobility
- Elimination
- Safety
- Community involvement

Psychosocial Status

- Family/friends
- Client/family values
- Community support
- Mood/affect
- Coping mechanisms
- Stressors
- Substance use/abuse
- Sleep patterns

Environment

- Architectural barriers
- Geographic barriers
- Health hazards
- Need for modification
- Transportation

Financial Status

- Income
- Assets
- Monthly costs
- Insurance
- Guardian/conservator
- Power of attorney
- Living will

Planning

Case management plans identify long- and short-term needs and methods for meeting the client's needs. The plan is mutually agreed on and considers available resources to achieve goals.

Resource Identification

Case managers research and assess various financial and community resources available to assist in meeting clients' and families' needs. The identification of community resources is an ongoing activity because of the dynamic nature of public and private agencies, their diversity, and the intensive need to link and coordinate among agencies.

Resource Linkage

Case managers define methods of linking clients and resources within case management plans. This involves the development of relationships and networking with community agencies and services, as well as communication with the client/family.

Coordination

The case manager acts as a pivotal point for communication, monitoring actual services delivered and conducting follow-up for the implementation of the case management plan. This component of case management distinguishes the practice from other health care practices and requires extensive documentation and direct involvement in service delivery.

Evaluation

Case management practice demands a measurement of the outcomes of care, including the client's response to care and services, as well as the quality of care and services. This process requires continuous monitoring and the autonomous ability to proactively make decisions regarding alterations to the case management plan that individualize it, customize it, and flex to meet dynamic challenges.

STANDARDS OF PRACTICE

Standards of professional practice are designed by a profession to (1) define the parameters of the practice, (2) provide a basis for evaluation of practice, (3) stimulate the development of the practice, and (4) encourage research to validate the practice. CMSA (1995) developed and published standards of professional practice for case managers.

Although case management is an interdisciplinary field, it is estimated that 70% of professionals who are identified as case managers actually are nurses by professional training (Chan, Leahy, McMahon, Mirch, & DeVinney, 1999). This represents an interesting professional phenomenon because nurses are accountable for practice as described by the American Nurses Association (ANA, 1995). Thus nurses who are case managers are accountable for nursing practice standards (for nursing) and case management practice standards (for case management). Because the CMSA standards of practice (1995) clearly outline practice and performance standards expected from case managers, nurses who are case managers need to be knowledgeable about both sets of standards.

For rehabilitation practice, the Association of Rehabilitation Nurses also has published standards of rehabilitation nurse practice (1994) with the associated documents *Standards and Scope of Practice for Rehabilitation Nursing Practice* and *Conceptual Framework for Rehabilitation Nursing Practice.* Thus a nurse practicing in rehabilitation case management has three layers of practice for which there are definitions and standards of practice for accountability: basic nursing practice, the scope of case management, and the practice of rehabilitation nursing. These publications all define process and declare professional responsibility for acting in the client's best interest, assuming responsibility for care delivery, and practicing with accountability and advocacy. The components of case management practice presented here are consistent with current published standards of practice in nursing and rehabilitation.

CASE MANAGEMENT PROCESS

The case management process is a series of activities applied to the management of client care. The case management process emphasizes a systematic approach to client care delivery and management of health care resources (Tahan, 1999). As a result of application of the components of case management within the parameters of standards of practice, four major processes of case management are identified:

1. Care coordination
2. Quality management
3. Outcomes management
4. Cost management

Care Coordination

In all practice settings, the case manager is the coordinator of the work of the care team. This coordinator role encompasses both clinical and financial accountability.

From a clinical perspective, the case manager coordinates and collaborates to meet needs and achieve goals that are outlined in the plan of care. Coordination activities include provision of day-to-day care, discharge planning, client/family education, and movement through the health system into appropriate follow-up services within the community, thus promoting community reentry.

The coordinated clinical activities represent a foundation for financial coordination. Coordination of necessary care results in cost-efficiency, elimination of duplication, and decreased fragmentation of services, which save money by streamlining and increasing efficiency. Ongoing coordination of care and services also supports early intervention to avoid problems and complications. The case manager is in the position to act to change the plan of care, to avoid delays in treatment or discharge, and to access appropriate services. The advantage of case management services is highlighted in the next section.

Example of Case Management Services

Case managers involved in a capitated elder care program that spanned the health care continuum from inpatient facilities to outpatient community-based programs implemented a new protocol for health status evaluation. Eager to improve the quality of client health and prevent inpatient stays, case managers enrolled their clients in the new program. Subsequently funding for the project was lost in a budget reforecast. With the administrative staff, the case managers then worked to continue the project by developing a clinic approach to the health status evaluation of clients and by reaching out to collaborate on the project with local parish nurses who provided client monitoring. By assuming accountability for the well-being of their clients, these case managers devised a creative, collaborative solution to a problem arising from budgetary constraints.

Quality Management

The term *quality* has evolved over time to a broader meaning. Quality now includes aspects of the availability and accessibility of care, improvement in the health of an individual, the level of community reentry, and the client/family's perceived satisfaction with services. Case management affects quality in health care primarily through the process of care coordination. Case management processes require continuous monitoring of care, services, and outcomes, focused on individuals or groups. The case manager is in a unique position to carry out these processes over the course of care, therefore promoting necessary and timely care, treatment, and services.

In case management, quality management is both a concurrent and a retrospective process (Cohen, 1996). Concurrently, case managers continually evaluate care and response and then intervene when the plan of care requires adjustment. This is a critical monitoring function that promotes consistency and positive, durable outcomes. Retrospectively the case manager is able to identify problem areas, process limits, and feasible options for improved care/services. The important synthesis and surveillance elements of case management services relate directly to cost-effective outcomes. This is illustrated in the next section.

Example of Cost-Effective Outcomes

A managed care plan determines that a client with severe osteoporosis should not be approved for nontraditional pain management treatment but is willing to continue reimbursement for narcotic administration and the surgical implantation of a morphine pump. The client feels little benefit from the narcotic and requests assistance. A case manager discusses other options for pain management that are under consideration by the individual and gathers data to objectively evaluate options, which are provided to the managed care plan. The outcome is approval for the nontraditional treatment, which is successful.

Cost Management

Managed costs are clearly an outcome of case management. Case managers purchase, negotiate, and coordinate care and services, resulting in effective use of resources. Within the processes of case management, there is the opportunity for creativity and development of nontraditional options to meet client needs. Such flexibility is necessary for achieving cost-effectiveness. In general, positive cost management results from care coordination by eliminating duplication of services and decreasing fragmentation. The outcome of case management, simply stated, is use of available funding and resources in the client's best interest. This simple goal is explained in the next section.

Example of Cost Management

Nurses working in a rehabilitation facility note that clients receiving benefits from a specific plan are not receiving durable medical equipment from local providers, but instead a mail-order provider has been approved. The nurses' options are to accept the plan's restrictive approval or to gather data demonstrating the effect this decision is having on their clients. The nurses gather data on repair costs, parts availability, and service. They include data about services in rural communities and the impact of downtime on clients when equipment has to be sent in for servicing. Their concern for the clients' well-being results in a change by the payer to authorize local provider approval.

Outcomes Management

Outcomes are defined as the results obtained from the efforts directed toward accomplishing a goal (Huber & Oermann, 1997). Outcomes management focuses on the results of the delivery of health care to individuals and groups, based on specific measurements.

Outcomes management combines care coordination, quality, and cost management processes into a systematic research effort to improve clinical practice and care provision and to reduce costs. Emphasizing quality, outcomes management programs recognize the importance of accurate data collection and analysis and move case management into the arena of research-based practice. Research efforts to create a national database for outcomes in health care are under way. Such information will guide professionals, health care systems, and case managers in decision making and evaluation processes.

Outcomes measurement is the foundation for outcomes management. Measurement of outcomes serves to assist professionals to achieve goals, internally, externally, or with specific individuals or groups. Key data elements in all sectors include trends, history, clinical decisions, and the identification of patterns of interest.

Categories for the measurement of client outcomes are physiological, psychosocial, functional, behavioral, knowledge, home functioning, family strain, safety, symptom control, quality of life, goal attainment, client satisfaction, utilization of service, and nursing diagnosis resolution (Marek, 1997). These categories may be easily applied by case management practitioners to clarify and specify the results of interventions for individuals and groups.

CASE MANAGEMENT AND REHABILITATION NURSING

The concept of case management practice is readily adapted to rehabilitation nursing. A coordinated effort among all care providers and across disciplines correlates with the long accepted model of the rehabilitation team. There are two additional members of the team: (1) the payer source, approving or denying services; and (2) the community, providing alternate resources.

Case management enhances client and family involvement because long- and short-term needs must be identified for both to attain the objective of the appropriate use of available resources. With the increased communication inherent in case management, the client and family have greater knowledge about care, services, and options. Energies may then be directed to urgent health issues and direct rehabilitation efforts.

ISSUES IN CASE MANAGEMENT

The system of health care delivery in the United States is in dire need of ongoing reform. Change has been occurring at a rapid pace, and challenges stand before us to meet the needs of a new practice environment. The challenges for case management are those that exist for nursing as well. However, because case management practice is carried out in various settings by various professionals and with various expectations associated with the role, the future of case management will depend on the ability of this transdisciplinary group to come to a consensus about definition, goals, purposes, and outcomes. Agreement about the fundamentals of case management practice creates a foundation for moving forward with progress toward resolving other practice issue dilemmas, such as certification, accreditation, accountability, and answers to legal and ethical dilemmas.

Certification

Certification is a nationally recognized method for documenting individuals' abilities to serve the needs of their client/clients, based on a predetermined set of criteria outlining required education and experience. Typically certification is voluntary. However, professional disciplines may view certification as a major method for ensuring individual practitioners' competence. As a result, jobs may require certification as a condition of employment to present quality criteria outcomes and provide a marketing or negotiating advantage.

Certified Care Manager

The certification process to obtain the designation *Certified Case Manager* is administered by the Commission for Case Manager Certification. As of January 2000, more than 20,000 practitioners have been certified through this process, which includes passing an examination. The examination is research based and reflects the transdisciplinary practice of case management.

The American Nurses Credentialing Center (ANCC) also has developed a certification for nurse case managers. Focused on facility-based practice, the application criteria include a minimum of a bachelor's degree in nursing (ANCC, 1998).

The National Rehabilitation Counseling Association's Professional Standards Committee investigated the need for accountability among rehabilitation counselors and case manager service providers in the 1960s. The Commission on Rehabilitation Counselor Certification was established in 1974 and administered the first Certified Rehabilitation Counselor (CRC) examination in 1976 (May, Turner, Taylor, & Rubin, 2000).

Accreditation

Accreditation is the process of a critical review of a program, service, facility, or health system by comparison to national standards that have been approved by peers within the field.

Two accreditation processes exist for case management facilities or agencies. The Commission on Accreditation of Rehabilitation Facilities (CARF) developed standards for medical rehabilitation case management that were implemented July 1, 1999. CARF believes that case management is an integral part of rehabilitation care. Coordination, communication, and advocacy are primary themes within the CARF standards. The American Health Care Commission/Utilization Review Accreditation Commission (URAC) developed standards as an accreditation process in 1998, designed to promote innovation and best practice in the case management industry. Convening multiple professional groups to develop standards, the goal was to create a case management system for health care organizations that promotes a level of structure and processes to further improve client care quality (D'Andrea & Hamill, 1999).

Implications for Practice

The nature of the role of case management in any practice setting is complex and difficult. Case managers may have the responsibility to approve care or deny services, to coordinate community resources and justify expenditures, to implement clinical pathways and design research methods, and to find ways to meet clients' needs and affect outcomes. Case managers are accountable to professional groups, to one another, to payers, and to those entrusted to their care. This integrated role in health care creates multiple legal and ethical considerations for case management practice.

Legal issues within case management practice are only beginning to emerge. The concepts of liability and accountability for outcomes of care appear to be the basis for potential litigation involving case managers. Negligent referral is another area for potential litigation. Case management programs with clear documentation of action and consistency with standards and practice guidelines will be better able to respond to legal action and demonstrate that they meet the standard of care.

Ethical issues face case management practitioners on a daily basis. When the element of cost control/containment enters the practice dialogue, there is an inherent ethical dilemma with the case manager's advocate role. As a case manager, does one have the moral right to deny care, speed discharge, or inform a payer about the client's substance abuse? When case management is practiced by professionals, the guiding principles must be advocacy, acting in the client's best interest, and proper use of existing resources.

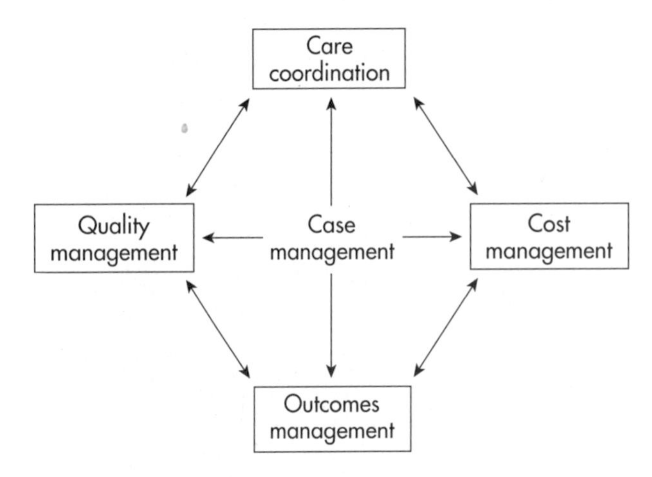

Figure 10-1 Case management as an integrated process.

SUMMARY

Case management has emerged as a key strategy and innovative approach to improving client care within a rapidly changing health care delivery system. Future demands for case management are unlimited and will grow as definitions of practice are refined and new roles for case managers are developed.

Case management practice is evident in multiple practice settings; however, case managers are bonded by consistency in components of practice and process (Figure 10-1). Case management is an integrated process of care coordination, cost management, quality management, and outcomes management. Increased awareness of case management outcomes will prompt tremendous growth in the specialty, particularly in the areas of long-term care, aging, and chronic disease case management. The continuing evolution of case management is projected to be a critical link that contributes to enhancement of quality of care, promotion of research-based problem solving, and the facilitation of cost-effective health care outcomes.

CRITICAL THINKING

1. JS has experienced a significant closed head injury, resulting in a persistent vegetative state. The family has chosen to modify their home and provide care for their son at home. Discuss the case manager's role in accessing resources and assisting the family to provide quality care.
2. Discuss three goals for rehabilitation care for JS.
3. Identify the case manager's role in each of the following areas: relationship with the family, interaction with the payer, and identification of community resources.
4. List three nursing diagnoses that will affect implementation of the case management plan.

Case Study

Through review of the process of case management flow diagram (Figure 10-2), the process of case management may be viewed as a method for the organization of care, a tool for evaluation of services, and a framework for resource allocation. An application of these concepts can be used to analyze the following case study report.

Initial Assessment

JS was observed and his family interviewed for assessment purposes on January 10, 2000.

Date of injury: December 29, 1999

Medical diagnosis: Status post severe head injury; emergency and intensive care treatment completed at Comprehensive Medical Center, Chicago, Illinois. Coma is noted in medical records as 10 days. Acute rehabilitation was initiated and is in process.

Current Status

Age: 17 years
Sex: Male
Marital status: Single
Living relatives: Father, mother, brother, paternal grandparents
Role in family: Older child
Occupation: Student
Recreational interest: School sports; participated in football, music

Continued

Case Study—cont'd

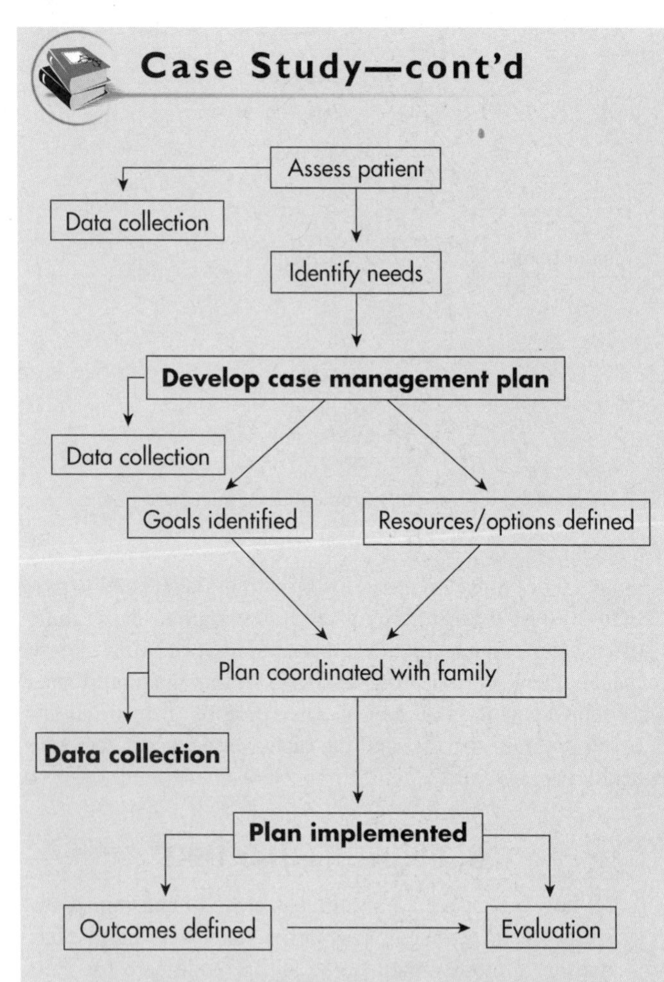

Figure 10-2 Process of case management flow diagram.

Housing: Requires total care for his health, wellness, and safety. He is maintained at QC Rehabilitation Center, participating in post acute brain injury treatment.

JS responds inconsistently to verbal, visual, and environmental stimuli. He participates in a full rehabilitation program daily. He is wheelchair dependent for mobility with full assistance required for transfer; the right side of his body is nonfunctional with hypertonicity of the right upper extremity. Physical therapy promotes sitting balance, range of motion, and walking with adaptive devices (with two-person assistance). Daily psychological therapy focuses on verbal and visual stimulation; visual perception cannot be assessed at this time. Speech therapy focuses on consistent use of a voice output communication aid.

JS experiences generalized seizures one to two times daily; continuous drooling was noted from the right side of the mouth. Skin breakdown at the coccyx and right hip was noted. JS is dependent in mobility, dressing, and personal hygiene. He is independent in oral intake with prompting and adaptive equipment. A gastrostomy tube for feeding was placed January 3, 2000.

Health History

JS had the usual childhood diseases, fractured his left wrist in June of 1997, is allergic to house dust and molds, and completed desensitization in October of 1992.

Current Medications

As noted on chart.

Education

One semester tenth grade.

Work History

Not applicable.

Family Status

JS's parents have been actively involved in all facets of their son's care. His mother has resigned from work as a legal secretary to participate in care. Both parents have participated in brain injury education programs provided by the facility; they are attending the Head Injury Association support group weekly. JS's father is employed as a regional supervisor for sales of farm equipment (annual salary, $48,000); health and accident coverage is Blue Cross/Blue Shield of Illinois. JS has $2000 in a savings account. Because of his personal savings, he has been declared ineligible for Supplemental Security Income (SSI) medicare funding.

Medical Records Reviewed

Comprehensive medical center: (1) records of emergency care, (2) Consultation reports, (3) operative reports, and (4) discharge report to QC Rehabilitation Center.

Additional Information

A meeting was held January 11, 2000, with the following in attendance: J. Jerry, MD; K. Olson, speech therapist; T. Davis, PhD, psychologist; M. Goode, MSW, social worker; and T. Strong, PT. The following needs were discussed: (1) further evaluation of uncontrolled seizures, (2) assistance to family for home modifications, and (3) clarification of insurance benefits.

REFERENCES

American Nurses Association. (1995). *Nursing's social policy statement.* Washington, DC: Author.

American Nurses Credentialing Center. (1998). *Nursing case management catalog.* Washington, DC: Author.

Association of Rehabilitation Nurses. (1994). *Standards and scope of rehabilitation nursing practice.* Chicago, IL: Author.

Aubert, R.E., Herman, W.H., Waters J., Moore, W., Sutton, D., Peterson, B.L., Bailey, C.M., & Koplan, J.P. (1998). Nurse case management to improve glycemic control in diabetic patients in a health maintenance organization. *Annals of Internal Medicine, 129*(8), 605-612.

Case Management Society of America. (1995). *CMSA standards of practice for case management.* Little Rock, AR: Author.

Cesta, T.G., Tahan, H.A., & Fink, L.F. (1998). *The case manager's survival guide.* St. Louis: Mosby.

Chan, F., Leahy, M.J., McMahon, B.T., Mirch, M., & DeVinney, D. (1999). Foundational knowledge and major practice domains of case management. *Journal of Care Management, 5*(1), 10-30.

Cohen, E., & Cesta, T. (1997). *Nursing case management: From concept to evaluation* (2nd ed.). St. Louis: Mosby.

Cohen, E.L. (1996). *Nurse case management in the 21st century.* St. Louis: Mosby.

D'Andrea, G., Hamill, T. (1999). Case Management Organization accreditation under way. *The Case Manager, 10*(1), 53-61.
Huber, D., Oermann, M. (1997). New horizons. *Outcomes Management for Nursing Practice, 1*(1), 1-2.
Marek, K. (1997). Measuring the effectiveness of nursing care. *Outcomes Management for Nursing Practice, 1*(1), 8-11.
May, V.R., III, Turner, T.N., Taylor, D.W., & Rubin, S.E. (2000). The life care planning process and certification: current trends in health care management, Part 1. *Journal of Care Management, 6*(1), 38-48.
Siefker, J.M., Garrett, M.B., Van Genderen, A., & Weis, M.J. (1998). *Fundamentals of case management: guidelines for practicing case managers.* St. Louis: Mosby.
Tahan, H.A. (1999). Clarifying case management: What is in a label? *Nursing Case Management, 4*(6), 268-278.

BIBLIOGRAPHY

Hosack, K. (1998). The value of case management in catastrophic injury rehabilitation and long term management. *Journal of Care Management, 4*(3), 58-67.
Huston, C. (1999). Outcomes measurement in healthcare: New imperatives for professional nursing practice. *Nursing Case Management, 4*(4), 188-195.
Jacox, A., Bausell, B.R., & Mahrenholz, D.M. (1997). Patient satisfaction with nursing care in hospitals. *Outcomes Management for Nursing Practice, 1*(1), 20-28.
Luquire, R., & Houston, S. (1997). Outcomes management: getting started. *Outcomes Management for Nursing Practice, 1*(1), 5-7.
Mass, S., & Johnson, B. (1998). Case management and clinical guidelines. *Journal of Care Management, Nov* (Special ed.), 18-25.
McPheeters, M., & Lohr, K.N. (1999). Evidenced based practice and nursing: commentary. *Outcomes Management for Nursing Practice, 3*(3), 99-101.
Mullahy, C., & Brick, L. (1997). *The case management source book: a guide to designing and implementing a centralized case management system.* New York: McGraw-Hill.
Wayman, C. (1999). Hospital-based nursing case management: Role clarification. *Nursing Case Management, 4*(5), 236-241.

11 Outcome-Directed Client and Family Education

Judith C. Allen, EdD, RN, CRRN

The day Mr. Rainne and his wife left for home was a proud day for the staff of the spinal cord injury (SCI) unit. Almost 6 months to the day, Mr. Rainne had been working at his home in a rural area, when a bullet came out of the woods behind his home. The bullet went through a window, striking him in the neck as he sat at his desk. He has a diagnosis of C1-C2 tetraplegia.

Mr. Rainne and his wife faced many problems both physically and emotionally. Their shared goal was for him to return home and be with their children. Mrs. Rainne would provide most of his care. The determination and devotion of this couple inspired the nursing staff to do everything in their power to help them achieve their goal.

The rehabilitation team worked with Mr. and Mrs. Rainne to develop a teaching plan. The plan began with simple tasks and built to the more complex as the couple became more comfortable with learning. Many changes resulted from the spinal cord injury he sustained, and a great deal of learning was necessary to perform the care and make adjustments. Slowly and steadily Mr. Rainne and his family became accomplished in directing and providing the care he needed to resume his life at home.

A date was set, and discharge planning was coordinated with community agencies in the Rainnes' home region, including the care plan for home and all the necessary equipment. Finally, with assurances from the staff that they could telephone the SCI unit any time with questions, the couple left for home confident they were prepared to move to the next phase in their lives. Of course, this was not the end of their story, but it is the chapter in their lives about how education programs make a difference and help with setting new beginnings in the best manner possible.

Client education is a central component of the specialty practice of rehabilitation nursing; an essential part of an effective rehabilitative plan. The focus of education in rehabilitation is helping individuals learn to live with a disability in their own environment. Success is evident in the individual's ability to incorporate adaptive behavior into a preferred lifestyle. The education process fosters self-care by helping the individual or family acquire new information, develop new skills, competently apply knowledge and skill to functional activities, develop adaptive behaviors to manage the illness or impairment, and prevent further disability (Diehl, 1989).

Previous education processes focused on the information given to clients. Clients who practiced what they were taught were assumed to have learned, and evaluation of learner outcomes was inconsistent. Those who did not follow treatment advice or practice self-care risked being labeled *noncompliant;* minimal effort was expended to determine why instructions were not followed. For a myriad of reasons, clients are not always receptive to information about their condition, treatments, care, and prevention. Client education has shifted from teaching to client learning, specifically to measurable learning outcomes and observable behavior change. The shift parallels a growing consumer movement in health care wherein the consumer has access to information and may wish to participate in health care decisions.

Individuals have access through ever-expanding technology to a wide range of information on health. Television advertisements promote prescription medications, as well as over-the-counter drugs and remedies; news programs and talk shows regularly feature segments on health care. Newspaper and magazine articles on health and illness detail the latest research reports and newest treatments or technological advances. Individuals enter the health care system already familiar with resources for information. The health educator today needs to do much more than give information to the client.

A more organized and effective approach to client education with emphasis on learning means paying attention to the various factors that influence client learning. Providers are challenged to develop role functions that facilitate client learning and find ways to involve the person in decisions. Recognizing the social and economic costs when clients do not adhere to instructions or do not follow their treatment regimens is an impetus to change. Involving clients in decisions about learning processes and fitting education content with their lifestyle requires innovative change on the part of the educator. The underlying philosophy in rehabilitation is to enable clients to learn how to be as independent as possible and fits well with increased decision making and the teaching-learning process in rehabilitation. The focus of this chapter is education of the client and family about rehabilitation and restorative care. Practical information for teaching content for specific deficits will assist nurse educators in planning and delivering effective education and improving client outcomes.

CLIENT EDUCATION

Client education, client teaching, and *client instruction* are familiar terms; however, they are not interchangeable. Client teaching implies imparting knowledge, the transfer of knowledge from the teacher to the learner. Client education implies planned activities designed to change clients' health behaviors or health status (Lorig, 1992). However, before client education can be effective, learning must take place. Learning involves more than just the transfer of knowledge; learning is evident in a change in behavior, a new or improved skill, and the learner's attitude.

Before the 1980s client education was conducted and evaluated according to outcomes set by the provider, apart from what the learner actually learned. As changes such as Diagnostic Related Groups (DRGs), and managed care swept through health care, client outcomes became important. Client education became a process in which the educator and the client work together to build the knowledge, skills, and outlook to manage health adaptations needed when illness or disability occurs. Client education requires assessment of the client's knowledge, skills, and attitudes over time. It is participatory education designed to empower learners, whether they be individuals, the family, or the community, with knowledge to control their own care and have control over their own lives (Rankin & Stallings, 1996). A provider today supplies professional expertise and correct information but concentrates on fostering learning and changes in behavior that will improve outcomes.

Although cost-effective in one area, clients' reduced lengths of stay are barriers to education and learning. Providers must identify priorities and streamline the education process. Clients come to rehabilitation earlier in their recovery, although often sicker, having less education provided while in acute care. The rehabilitation nurse often finds that teaching about acute and comorbid conditions that are high-priority items carried over from inpatient settings reduces opportunity for learning about rehabilitation skills and coping.

The rehabilitation team may be left to concentrate on three or four priority learning goals because too much learning activity attempted in a short time results in a client who is confused and frustrated. Ideally education for learning goals can be planned so teaching is carried over into community settings. Provider responsibilities are to prepare referrals that include solid information and resources. Resources must be correct, current, appropriate for the person, and transferable to other settings. The system changes in both inpatient and community settings create a situation in which blocks of time may not be available for education. The rehabilitation professional must make the most of every moment with the client and the family. Each contact with the client and family becomes a "teachable moment," and all interactions help the them learn new skills and incorporate adaptive behavior into their lifestyles.

Accreditation Standards and Client Education

Renewed emphasis on client and family education began in 1993 when the Joint Commission on the Accreditation of Healthcare Organizations (JCAHO) incorporated a section for client education standards into their guidelines. The JCAHO (2000) has continued to refine the standards addressing client-family education with the stated goal of improving client health care outcomes by promoting healthy behaviors and involving clients in care and care decisions (Box 11-1).

In addition, The Commission on Accreditation of Rehabilitation Facilities (CARF) also addresses education in its standards. Standards for the Rehabilitation Process for the People Served state:

- It is the right of the individual that the program provide sufficient information to facilitate decision making
- The organization communicates all information to persons served in a form, manner, and language that can be understood by them and respects their rights and dignity

In the standard for programs, the program must provide a multifaceted education effort that is:

- Organized
- Goal-directed
- Appropriate to the needs of the persons and families served (CARF, 2000)

The accreditation standards depict client education as an interactive, outcome-oriented process that is a primary responsibility of hospitals. Continued emphasis placed on client and family education by accreditation organizations has helped support client education that in the past has struggled for resources and recognition. The rehabilitation nursing philosophy of helping clients, families, or communities

Box 11-1 Standards for Patient-Family Education

- Assess the educational needs and abilities and learning readiness of patients and families
- Assess the cultural and religious practices that may affect learning, motivation, and barriers to learning
- Assess school-age children's and adolescent's schooling needs
- Educate patients about the safe and effective use of medications and medical equipment
- Educate patients about potential drug-food interactions and provide counseling on nutrition and modified diets
- Educate patients about rehabilitation techniques to help them adapt or function more independently in their environment
- Inform and teach patients that pain management is part of treatment
- Inform patients about access to additional community resources
- Inform patients about obtaining any needed care after discharge
- Inform patient and family of their responsibilities related to the patient care and give them the knowledge and skills necessary
- Assist and encourage the patient to take responsibility for basic personal hygiene and provide personal care education if needed
- View patient education as a joint process
- Provide the patient with discharge instructions and communicate instructions to the person or organization responsible for the patient's continuing care
- Access resources available for an organized, planned patient and family educational process
- View patient and family education as a collaborative interdisciplinary process

Adapted from Joint Commission on Accreditation of Health Care Organizations. (2000). *Comprehensive manual for hospitals.* Oakbrook, IL: Author.

learn to be as independent as possible also recognizes the central role of client education in nursing practice. This chapter reviews the following theories that underlie education and principles that apply to the process of client-centered education in rehabilitation nursing:

- The client is an active participant in the education process
- The client's individual needs are assessed
- A trusting relationship between client and educator facilitates the education process
- The education process enhances the client's knowledge, skill, and decision making
- Emotional support of the client is an integral part of the education
- Monitoring and evaluation of client's response and outcomes are ongoing

CONCEPTUAL FOUNDATIONS OF CLIENT EDUCATION

Models and theories to guide practice and research and to organize behavior in rehabilitation nursing are discussed in Chapter 2. Theories and models especially pertinent to client education are discussed in the following section and in Table 11-1.

Health Belief Model

The health belief model (HBM) from the social sciences has been used commonly to measure components of client education. It is helpful for understanding the client's perception of the disease or impairment and how clients make decisions to use health care services including health education. In client education the HBM has been used to assess what is needed for behavior change and thus aid in the logical construction of an education plan. According to the HBM, individuals will be more receptive to education when:

- They believe they are personally at risk
- The risk is serious enough to affect their lives
- They believe the benefits of action outweigh the barriers to action
- They are confident they can perform the action

Useful teaching strategies based on the HBM include helping the person to acknowledge risks and that the risks are serious, helping the person to recognize ways to reduce risks and that benefits occur when risks are reduced, and showing options for lowering barriers to behavior change (Becker, 1974).

Self-Efficacy Theory

The self-efficacy theory (Bandura, 1997), a social learning theory, considers the role of individuals' confidence in their ability to perform a needed behavior. A person with low self-efficacy would be less likely to change behavior than a person with high self-efficacy. Educators use this principle to develop education interventions that build confidence so that clients can accomplish the desired health care behavior (Robinson-Smith, Johnston, & Allen, 2000). Factors that help build confidence include (1) the person initially perceiving that the task is doable; (2) the person learning to break down a task, especially if complex, into small, sequential parts that are easier to perform; (3) the person repeating the task or behavior; and (4) the educator recognizing or reinforcing performance of the task. A teaching plan would begin with building confidence in the person's own ability, perhaps by pointing out things he or she has done successfully, with praise and encouragement at each step.

Locus of Control

Locus of control is a social psychology theory useful in client education. Individuals' beliefs about how much con-

TABLE 11-1 Education and Behavioral Models and Theories

Theory	Theorist	Summary	Application
Health belief model	Hochbaum	Framework developed to predict a person's health behaviors and understand a person's motivation and decision making in seeking health services	Assess what is needed for behavioral change; aid in selection of content and sequencing of material
Self-efficacy model	Bandura	A social learning theory that looks at the role of a person's confidence in learning a new health behavior	Plan education to build a person's confidence; break tasks into small, doable parts and give learner recognition and reinforcement
Locus of control theory	Wollston	An individual's belief about whether behavior results in outcomes; persons who believe they are in control of their health status are more likely to change behavior than those who believe forces outside themselves are in control	Be helpful in planning educational approach; point out action that can be taken to reach goal
Cognitive dissonance theory	Festinger, Lewin	A high level of discomfort is motivation for change; individuals act to reduce the discomfort	Plan education to foster discomfort with present behavior; when change occurs, work to keep dissonance low
Adult learning theory	Knowles	Adults are self-directed learners who are concerned with managing and solving their own problems; adults are active learners who bring life experiences to the learning situation and for whom internal motivators are stronger than external motivators	Teacher takes role of facilitator of learning, and learner takes active role in developing goal and objectives of learning; learning should be problem centered with opportunity for application

trol they have over their own health and about whether their behavior influences life outcomes will affect their receptivity to education. Those with an internal locus of control believe their own actions influence outcomes and are thus more likely to change behavior to influence health. Persons with an external locus of control believe that external forces, fate, God, or authority figures influence outcomes. When an external locus of control stems from a cultural belief, clients are less likely to change their behaviors. Locus of control can be evaluated during an educational needs assessment. In developing a teaching plan, clients with an internal locus of control will be receptive; for those with external locus of control, the educator can suggest actions to reach a certain goal without focusing on client responsibility.

Cognitive Dissonance Theory

This social theory (Festinger, 1957) is useful in identifying motivators that can influence behavior change through education. Cognitive dissonance is the sense of discomfort individuals feel when what they do differs from what they believe. It forms a discomfort zone, and they try to reduce the discomfort. For instance Susie may be overweight; she knows it is unhealthy and feels uncomfortable being overweight. The discomfort she feels may make her receptive to information on healthy eating and take steps to change her eating behaviors. Educators can use any dissonance on the client's part to motivate behavior change.

Developmental Theory

The development level is an important factor in the delivery of education to the rehabilitation client. Development frameworks such as those of Erickson, Piaget, and Duvall, which are taught in nursing education programs as basis for assessment and intervention, are also useful in preparing age-appropriate teaching plans. Teaching-learning strategies for specific age groups are discussed later in this chapter. Ecological frameworks (Bronfenbrenner, 1989) help the nurse educator understand the multiple determinants that influence development, the dynamic nature of development, and its influence on client learning. Thus such factors as personal characteristics and demographics may influence learning.

Adult Learning Theory

The dominant theory used for adult learning originally was outlined by Knowles (1984). His model of adult learning is based on five key assumptions:

- The adult learner is a self-directed learner
- The adult learner brings both a greater quantity and a greater quality of life experiences to the learning situa-

tion, which results in a need for highly individualized learning plans
- Adults are ready to learn when they experience a need to know something in order to perform more effectively in some aspect of their lives
- Adult learners have a life-centered, task-centered, or problem-centered orientation to learning
- Adult learners are highly motivated by internal motivators, such as self-esteem, recognition, better quality of life, and greater self-confidence; an external motivator such as a better job or salary does influence adult learning, but not as strongly as an internal motivator

Applying the principles of adult learning, the educator practices the roles of facilitator of learning, designer of the learning processes, and manager of procedures. Several elements have been identified in designing a learning experience for the adult learner. Because most rehabilitation clients are adult learners, experiences are designed to be problem centered, and the learner helps develop objectives. The education plan provides opportunities for applying learning, and the learner also shares in evaluating learning. Using these elements and the key assumptions of the theory, the rehabilitation nurse can develop individualized and meaningful learning experiences with clients.

Full use of the adult learning principles requires learners who are willing to take responsibility for directing their own learning and are comfortable in this role. This condition may not always exist because of the client's previous experience with education, because of their response to their illness or disability, or because of a cognitive or related impairment. Pratt (1988) proposed a framework for examining teaching-learning situations based on the degree of direction and support needed by the learner. Educational situations are placed into one of four categories according to the amount of support and direction needed by the learner. In one instance, learners need both direction and support because they lack both competence in the content and commitment or confidence in their ability to learn the information. In a second category, learners need direction in mastering the content but need less support because of confidence or commitment that the new information can be mastered. In a third category, learners need support but can be fairly self-directed in determining content needs and require less direction. In the fourth category, learners are at least moderately capable of providing their own direction and support. In the last two categories the teaching-learning process is a more learner-directed approach because of the lower need for direction.

The categorical approach supports the principles of adult learning but allows for the reality that in some situations learners may be unable or unwilling to assume responsibility for their own learning. It allows the rehabilitation nurse to assess with the client the specific teaching-learning needs. A plan is then developed that draws on the expertise of the rehabilitation nurse in content areas that the client might be totally unfamiliar with, such as bowel and bladder programs. The plan also can be individualized to provide the appropriate level of support depending on the level of commitment and confidence expressed by the client or family.

THE CLIENT EDUCATOR

Because client education has always been an integral part of their practice, rehabilitation nurses need to recognize and develop knowledge and skill in this area. It is often assumed that anyone with a health care background can conduct client education. However, client education is a complex process that involves knowledge, skills, and qualities that need to be learned and developed. Some member of the rehabilitation team and other health professionals have received little or no formal training to prepare them to conduct client education. As nurses work together with the various members of the rehabilitation team, they are coordinating, developing, and sharing skills of client education.

Benner's Model

Nurses have been introduced to the client education role in their basic programs with an introduction to teaching-learning theories and opportunities to develop teaching plans for individuals and groups. Benner's model of moving from novice to expert can be applied in client education, as in professional continuing development and practice (Benner, 1985, 2001). Benner describes the four developmental phases a nurse passes through to reach the level of *expert.* In the first phase the advanced beginner masters technical skills and learns to organize care. At this stage the nurse *depends on a preceptor* to provide teaching and coaching in situations, manages situations by rules and procedures, and learns from situations. Second, nurses at the *competent* stage of nursing practice begin to see patterns and recognize relationships, wish to limit the unexpected, and engage in deliberate planning and goal setting. The nurse begins to see the client and family in new ways and to personalize care. At the third level, the *proficient* nurse recognizes patterns and sees changing relevance. This nurse can streamline practice, redefine priorities, and break the rules if it benefits the client. Finally, the *expert* nurse shows an excellent clinical understanding of the whole situation and is comfortable in changing situations. Attending to the context as well as to the environment, experts make excellent mentors for nurses in the competent and proficient stages.

Benner's model is useful in acknowledging the developmental needs of rehabilitation nurses in becoming expert client educators. Clinical judgment and intuition are needed to streamline teaching, establish priorities, provide culturally sensitive care, and engage clients and families. The nurse learns these skills through mentorship and the experience and reflection of passing through these developmental milestones (Rankin & Stallings, 1996). The novice nurse moving into client education needs guidance and practice in developing educator skills. In applying Benner's model, novices or nurses new to rehabilitation may not have orga-

TABLE 11-2 Critical Thinking in Patient Education

Attributes of Critical Thinking	Critical Thinking in Patient Education
Entails purposeful, outcome-directed thinking	Outcome that should result from the teaching
Is driven by patient, family, and community needs	Assessment and priority of learning needs based on patient, family, and community
Is based on principles of nursing process and scientific method	Knowledge needed to address learning needs
Is guided by professional standards and ethical code	Guide by ethical standards
Requires strategies that maximize individual strengths and compensate for problems created by individual differences	Strategies to overcome barriers to learning and patient variables
Constant reevaluation, self-correction, and striving to improve	Evaluation, correction

Adapted from Alfaro-LeFevre, R. (1999). *Critical thinking in nursing: a practical approach* (2nd ed.). Philadelphia: WB Saunders.

nized their knowledge and experience to the unique needs of clients and families. They lack experiences to adapt teaching to clients who have a wide range of impairments and chronic conditions. For example, the nurse new to rehabilitation or the beginning practitioner may not recognize that learning styles of persons with right or left hemiplegia differ and how to adapt teaching. Staff members are not equally skilled, and nurse managers need to make efforts to improve and expand competencies in the educator role.

In a study examining barriers to client teaching, nurses stated that they lacked the skills needed for teaching (Boswell, Pichert, Lorenz, & Schlundt, 1990). Continuing education, staff in-service programs, self-study through the literature, and mentoring are ways nurses augment their skills for effective client education.

The Effective Client Educator

Knowledge of the subject is paramount to teaching. The insecure teacher may impart inadequate, inaccurate information or no information at all. Although no one can expect to be expert in all areas; it is a professional responsibility to keep abreast of new information related to the population served. In the same manner, not everyone is comfortable teaching all topics; someone with more expertise or who is comfortable discussing the topic may better serve clients. For example, sexuality education is important for many clients in rehabilitation. A nurse who has the knowledge, expertise, and comfort is a solid choice for client education on the topic. Qualities of an effective educator are as follows:

- Has knowledge of the subject and is comfortable with the topic
- Thinks critically
- Communicates effectively
- Is aware of own attitudes and values
- Respects the learner
- Creates a caring environment
- Includes the client as a participant
- Monitors and evaluates the education process

The ability to think critically is crucial in assessing needs, making plans, solving problems, and conducting client education. The educator must identify clearly what must be learned and initiate a timely, effective teaching plan. Ultimately the nurse is responsible for assessing what the client must know, establishing priorities, and initiating a plan that draws on the person's strengths (Table 11-2).

All aspects of communication will influence the teaching-learning process. The educator is an active listener who communicates not only with words but also with the eyes, gestures, body language, and voice inflection. Barriers to communication may be ones own feelings, the language, or environmental distractions. Choose words carefully; simple, factual information that is to the point is most effective. Words that match the person's education and occupation may be better understood. An effective educator recognizes client and family concerns; has empathy, patience, and sensitivity to the person's mood; and allows sufficient time to encourage and address concerns. Attitudes and values may be subtle, so put aside any assumptions or stereotypes. Respect client wishes and incorporate them, as far as possible, into the teaching plan.

TEACHING THE LEARNING PROCESS IN REHABILITATION

The familiar steps of the nursing process apply to client education. Evaluation is ongoing to track and quickly spot problems. Documentation is added as a step for the education process (Figure 11-1).

Assessment

Assessment of the client's educational needs begins the educational process. Assessment yields basic data for a teaching plan: learner needs, what is already known, client and family readiness to learn and learning style, what the client wants and needs to learn, and factors that affect learning. Assessment provides opportunity to develop rapport with the client and to start building a helping relationship (Pestonjee, 2000) and is an ongoing process beyond the first encounter. Assessment topics include client and family readiness to learn, their motivation, cog-

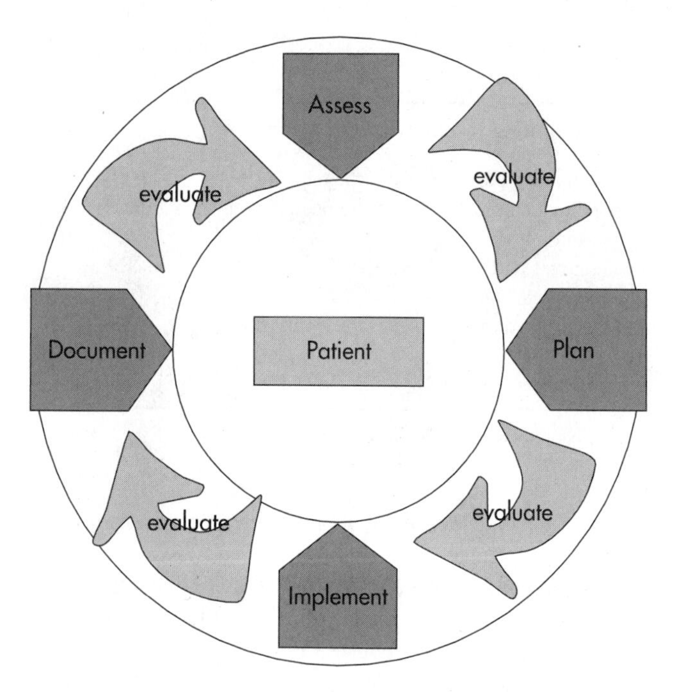

Figure 11-1 Model of client education.

nitive ability, and development level. Other learner variables include:

- Age
- Sex
- Occupation
- Culture
- Language
- Literacy
- Educational level
- Motivation
- Belief system
- Self-concept
- Access to caregivers
- Potential to teach others

Identifying Learning Needs

Learning needs are identified in various ways mentioned by the client, family, a team member, or other person associated with the client. Needs may be obvious through direct request or during assessment. The assessment of learning needs should begin at admission and continue throughout the client's stay. Four categories of problems affect learning needs. In the first instance clients have limitations resulting from the present situation or a previous illness or impairment. The rehabilitation nurse assesses present and past function, mobility, transfer activities, dressing, eating, elimination, and personal hygiene. Questions such as "Which hand do you use in eating?" or "Do you need any type of assistance walking?" or "Does your apartment building have an elevator?" will provide clues.

How clients understand the course of illnesses or disability, how they view relationships, and their lifestyle preferences are all important to education. For example, does the client who has had an amputation understand the relationship between peripheral vascular disease and smoking? Does the client comprehend the relationship between heart disease and decreased endurance after stroke? An individual's knowledge level may not relate to the length of time with an impairment or illness because their knowledge about the condition may be incomplete or obsolete.

The second category deals with social needs. How has the impairment compromised the client's life roles? For example, if the client was the sole financial support of the family before the disability, major adjustment problems for the client and family will relate to finances and plans for the future. Other factors include the type of living arrangement, whether the client owns or rents a home or apartment, who else will live with or help with the client, whether the client is married, whether there are children in the home, and whether the environment is accessible and safe.

The third category encompasses psychological needs. Anxiety and depression are two emotions that influence learning. Clients may feel overwhelmed by a sense of hopelessness, even by grief, despair, and discouragement, as they realize the changes imposed on their lives by disease or disability. Instilling hope and dispelling hopelessness are part of client education. A client and family may resist, using psychological defense mechanisms, denial, rationalization, or humor to protect them from the reality of the situation. The defense of humor can be used to avoid reality; making jokes keeps reality at bay and is a way to cover up anxiety. The distress imposed by the illness or disability and the protective mechanisms used may indicate a referral for psychological counseling and influence the client's ability to participate in learning. For example, a person who experiences denial about the consequence of spinal cord injury may not accept loss of function and may be unwilling to learn about a bowel program.

The fourth category focuses on vocational problems, unemployment, or loss of job-related skills. Vocational counseling and training may be needed. Obviously the nurse educator will not attend to all educational needs but will advocate for clients to ensure they reach their potential and lend support to what other team members teach.

Assessing Readiness to Learn

Readiness to learn is defined here as the capability to expend energy and focus attention for a given purpose. The definition contains three elements necessary for learning. First, clients must be physiologically capable of participating in a learning experience. Second, the purpose of the learning experience must be such that intellectually clients find it relevant to their needs. Third, the purpose has emotional appeal so clients are willing to participate actively, which can influence the motivation to learn. Although readiness has been a basic principle of teaching and learning, in today's health care environment the nurse educator is working within a limited time frame. A client may not have reached the stage of readiness for education before discharge. The responsible educator begins the education process during the person's admission, provides critical "survival skills" at discharge, and communicates an education plan to family and community providers to continue after discharge.

The physiological capacity to learn depends on more than just neuromuscular functioning; any limitations, old or new, that impair a client's capacity to learn are significant. Immediate basic needs such as relief from pain, anxiety, or the need to void, or limitations such as joint stiffness from arthritis, sensory deficits, or decreased cardiac reserve, take priority over learning. The physiological capacity for learning needed skills may not have been reestablished during the shortened stays in rehabilitation. For example, a young man with paraplegia spends 5 days in acute care and then spends 2 weeks on the rehabilitation unit. This may not allow sufficient time to resolve the spinal shock resulting from the trauma to the spinal cord before he is sent home. His physiological capacity for any learning is poor. His bowel and bladder program will not be established and will need continued adjustment at home. As spinal shock resolves, he may experience new situations or problems, such as spasticity, while at home. Clients and their families need information to anticipate needs and resources for continued learning at home.

Emotional readiness to participate actively in the learning process is enhanced by positive life experiences, beliefs, and values. Helplessness, hopelessness, and negative beliefs about the disease process or injury or unpleasant past experiences are barriers as well as clues to the client's stage of adaptation to any actual or perceived loss. Common reactions for those who are anxious or in denial are to "not hear" what they are told; they may even deny later that the information was ever presented. Incorporating strategies such as repetition and reenforcement into teaching when a client has a great deal of anxiety or denial may help transmit the information.

At times, clients' cognitive abilities to learn and remember are not sufficient for them to understand the relevance of new knowledge and skills to future well-being or for them to learn and remember the information. Assessment of cognitive and intellectual ability includes information about orientation, attention span, concentration, perception, and memory (Redman, 1996).

Sensitivity to the needs of the family must begin immediately on the person's admission to the nurse's care. How well family members adapt and their readiness to participate actively in the learning process are significant in a client's rehabilitation potential. Families with close relationships before the onset of injury or disability are more likely to have positive attitudes and display supportive behavior enhancing the client's rehabilitation and prospect for returning home. Conversely, in families where hostility, alienation, or other negative attitudes prevail, the support system is likely to be less effective. Another important factor is how the learner feels toward the family member designated as the "backup" learner; compatibility facilitates carryover of learning. The family member should realize they back up the client and provide assistance only with activities the client is unable to perform. The family member's potential to understand and follow through with learning influences their supportive behavior. Providing information about the illness and impairment and the recovery process enhances family participation. The perceptions and concerns of the family, not only those about the physical care but also those in other areas, are important.

Weeks (1995) found the number one educational "want" of family caregivers was to normalize the daily routine of the disabled adult within the bounds of the impairment. Much family anxiety can be anticipated and allayed through continuous and open communication, leaving the family with more energy to support the client and to participate in the education process.

Assessing Learning Style

The success of the teaching-learning process is influenced by how well the nurse educator uses a variety of methods to tailor the learning experience with client preferences. Preferences are influenced by previous learning experiences or styles. Some learn by doing; others are visual or auditory learners. Visual learners use written materials or watch demonstrations or videotapes. Auditory learners can learn by listening to an explanation or an audiotape presentation. Some clients need to conceptualize the whole picture, whereas others find that overwhelming; they master individual pieces until the whole picture emerges. In a visual and technical world, clients may prefer computer modalities. Clients may know how they learn best, so ask them. Assess their learning style to select materials and strategies best suited.

Challenge of Clients with Low Literary Skills

One in five Americans is functionally illiterate and cannot benefit from simple booklets or handouts. Illiteracy is an invisible impairment that is not apparent in appearance or speech, that is unrelated to economic status, and that is not restricted to immigrants. Lack of literacy skills does not mean lack of intelligence. These persons are not easily identified because they have learned to cope with and hide their limitations from others, and health providers treat them unawares everyday. Details of ways to design programs that present effective education for persons who are functionally illiterate are available (Doak, Doak, & Root, 1996) and personal assistance is offered through groups such as the Literacy Volunteers of America. Following are some tips for teaching clients with low literacy skills:

- Give short, direct, specific messages
- Use pictures, illustrations, and graphics, along with words
- Break information down into basic points
- Teach sequentially, step by step
- Use examples of real-life situations
- Ask client to restate
- Ask client to demonstrate
- Review frequently

Learner Characteristics

Developmental Level. Most rehabilitation client education is directed toward the adult learner. Clients who are younger or older benefit from education processes that consider learner characteristics.

Teaching Children. Teaching and learning programs for children take into account the child's growth and development, as well as the cognitive level or chronological age. Information from school reports and developmental assessments detail the learning potential and special needs of a child. Children are included in decisions about learning as appropriate; however, the fact remains that the parents will oversee the child's care. The educator works to establish rapport with both the child and the parents and to ensure positive educational outcomes for the child. Learning readiness and the quality of the parent-child relationship are important assessments. Sensitivity to child-rearing practices and cultural issues also plays a role in planning effective education for the pediatric client, and family involvement is essential.

Children have short attention spans, so material is presented best in limited amounts over short periods. Affection and praise support and nurture the child during the educational sessions. Children learn through play and active participation that help them assimilate the material. It is through play that the child integrates new information. Play is the major vehicle for children to learn about their disease or impairment and care. Excellent play therapy and teaching programs are available; most involve the family and the interdisciplinary team approach. Evaluation of the education process for children uses information about achievement of developmental tasks, chronological age, neurological function, and specific skills needed for learning (Table 11-3). Chapter 29 discusses pediatric rehabilitation in detail.

Teaching Adolescents. Adolescents are in a time of transition, and their learning needs are wide and varied. Although education includes the family, the focus of teaching is on the adolescent because adolescents are independent and control outcomes of education. Adolescents are capable of abstract thought and logical reasoning. In the process of forming their own identity and emancipating themselves from their parents, they develop a sense of invulnerability. An attitude of "it won't happen to me" often leads them into risk-taking behaviors. Peer groups are strong influences. They are adapting to a changing body and become preoccupied with body image and appearance. In teaching the adolescent client, consider the following:

- Adolescents need to assert their independence; they may rebel against authority figures
- A guidance approach to learning works better than lecturing

TABLE 11-3 Teaching Children

Development/Cognitive Level	Approach to Teaching
Birth to 2 Years	Make child feel as secure as possible
Starts by not being able to differentiate self from environment	Use direct teaching toward parents
Learns actions have effects on objects	Use age-appropriate toys and games
Begins to make associations	Use safety precautions with activities
	Give older infants a chance to hold and manipulate objects
Preschool: 2-6 Years	Be careful with explanations because the child will take what is said quite literally and will not generalize
Cognitively concrete and literal	Keep explanations simple and matter of fact
Unable to generalize	Allow manipulation of safe equipment
Egocentric	Reassure no one is to blame for their condition or pain (may think they are to blame)
Thinks objects have life or human characteristics	Use play and simple picture books
	Use dolls and puppets in play situations
	Use rhymes and rhythms to instill patterns
	Differentiate between chronological age and developmental age
	Pay attention to patterns of growth
	Observe safety precautions for child
School Age: 7-12 Years	Use drawings and models in learning
Concrete but more realistic and objective cognitive development	Relate child's care to experiences of other children
Understands cause and effect and can use deductive reasoning	Use films, models, computer-assisted instruction, and group activities
Is able to compare objects and experiences	Use child's interest in science to explain condition and care
Is able to understand another's point of view	Use principles of sequential learning
	Break tasks into small, sequential units
	Teach with the intent that the child will perform his or her own care or self-direct care
	Keep fun in learning
	Encourage independence and praise accomplishments
	Observe safety precautions

Adapted from Rankin, S., & Stallings, K. (1996). *Patient education: Issues, principles, practice.* (3rd ed., p. 304) Philadelphia: JB Lippincott.

- Honesty and trust are important when working with adolescents
- Adolescents may have less knowledge about their bodies than is assumed
- The importance of the peer group should be used through group learning
- Body image is important to adolescents

Teaching Older Adults. Learning by elderly persons may be affected by multiple factors. Sensory impairments, altered cognitive processes, fatigue, comfort such as with seating or position, frequent toileting, room temperature, type or amount of medication, and nutritional requirements all may interfere with learning. Intergenerational language, acronyms, jargon, or even speaking too rapidly may become barriers to learning. The educator should not attribute loss of competence and slowness simply to age. Although some persons experience difficulty with understanding complex sentences and drawing inferences as they age, other factors, such as visual deficits, may be involved. Older clients learn effectively when educational programs are tailored to their unique needs; for instance, material written in large type helps those with diminished vision. Older persons may feel intimidation when faced with large learning modules, tests, or quizzes or anxiety with a program modeled after a school routine. Teaching strategies for elderly clients include:

- Present the material at a slower pace
- Present smaller amounts of information at a time
- Speak in a low tone of voice because elderly persons hear low tones better than high-pitched sounds
- Allow time for integration and assimilation of conceptual material; be concrete rather than abstract
- Repeat information frequently
- Reinforce oral presentation with audiovisual material
- Use written examples
- Use examples and analogies
- Decrease outside stimuli
- Use group experiences to improve older persons' problem-solving abilities
- Remember that elderly clients are cautious and do not make changes easily

Culture and Language. Cultural factors have a profound effect on client education. The realization that the United States is a mixture of many cultures necessitates a culturally sensitive approach. Providing culturally relevant client education requires an understanding and application of transcultural concepts, including understanding cultural needs, understanding the cultural context of the client and family, using culturally sensitive strategies, and using resources from a variety of cultural subsystems in the community. The variety of cultures in most countries today makes it difficult for the health care provider to be knowledgeable about all groups. Therefore a cultural component belongs in every assessment. References on cultural groups, including Internet sites, and local representatives from various backgrounds can be resources for the education and rehabilitation staff.

Diversity brings a bewildering array of languages. Language barriers result in confusion, frustration, and misunderstanding for both clients and providers. A client who speaks a different language is a significant challenge for the health educator, and solutions must match the situation. Services of an interpreter are preferable to those of a translator. Interpreters are trained to interpret accurate meaning of words and phrases in addition to word-by-word translations, from health care terms into the client's language and vice versa. A translator may not have fluency in both languages, may lose cultural meanings in the translation, or may be unaware of medical or health-related words. Family members are least desirable as translators because they may filter what the educator is telling the client or edit what the client is saying to the educator; the role especially may be difficult when the condition is serious.

Most health care facilities have lists of interpreters and translators for various languages. In the community, local government and libraries may have lists of volunteers, AT&T has a translator service available over the telephone at a charge, translation specialists are listed in the telephone yellow pages, and others have websites. Written materials and videos about specific conditions and treatments are available in a variety of languages. Pharmaceutical and other medical-related companies supply information about their products in several languages. For example, consumer product information about warfarin sodium (Coumadin) is published in 51 languages.

Planning and Implementation

Planning learning experiences involves developing goals and objectives, identifying learning activities, developing content, and identifying resources. After an initial assessment the nurse and client work to set mutually agreed-on learning goals and objectives they both believe to be achievable (Box 11-2). Goals direct educator and learner toward expected behavioral changes and to measure learning outcomes. Learning objectives are specific behaviors related to the goals. A learner who does not understand clearly that achieving objectives leads to achieving goals may have difficulty. If, for example, Mr. Parsons does not connect the objective "apply a molded ankle foot orthotic (MAFO)" with his goal of "ambulate independently," he may not value or learn how to apply the MAFO. He may expect that someone else will apply the MAFO for him.

Box 11-2 Example of Goal and Objective

Goal: The desired outcome of learning (e.g., maintain intact skin)

Objective: Specific statement related to goal that describes in more detail the behavior that will be performed to meet the goal (e.g., weight shift every 30 minutes when seated in wheelchair)

Families have major roles in identifying goals and objectives. Their involvement or lack thereof influences success or failure. Family involvement in planning the learning experiences enhances the client's potential for rehabilitation and helps ensure that the goals are realistic. Learning goals and objectives may outnumber the time available in the rehabilitation facility. Setting priorities is difficult when faced with multiple learning needs; the focus is on meeting needs that are critical to the person's basic survival. Goals of client and family education in rehabilitation include:

- Achieving survival skills
- Recognizing problems/complications
- Making decisions
- Adapting to disability
- Integrating the disability

In the hierarchy of human needs basic survival needs must be met first (Box 11-3).

Time is a major consideration in developing a teaching plan. Clients may not have overcome physiological or psychological barriers or may feel overloaded with learning materials and frustrated by the lack of time to practice skills. Educators feel the stress of limited time and energy, especially when a client's discharge date is imminent. Identify what the client and family consider important to learn before discharge in order to be safe at home, including the medication regimen and how to recognize problems or complications. A person recovering from stroke may place priority on mastering self-toileting skills before discharge over progressing from a walker to ambulating without an assistive device. Clients' concerns are potential barriers to learning. For example, with a fear of needles, a client may not reach a goal to self-administer enoxaparin sodium (Lovenox). Clients may set their own limits. The person who will not give up smoking can concentrate on reducing other risk factors.

In an ideal world seamless communication of the education plan moves from the inpatient setting to the community setting, whether the outpatient clinic, the home, the physician's office, or the support group. To overcome the lack of continuity, teaching plans and outcomes can be sent along with discharge records to clinics or home health care agencies. Clients can be instructed to call help lines, where they can talk with familiar staff for advice and help.

A teaching plan includes appropriate learning domains, instructional methods, and resources for the client and the goals of learning (Table 11-4). Educators divide behaviors into three domains: cognitive, dealing with intellectual abilities; affective, dealing with feelings, attitudes, and values; and psychomotor, dealing with motor skills. Each domain is further divided into a ranked taxonomy. The cognitive and psychomotor domains are ordered by the complexity of the behavior, and the affective domain progresses from awareness to internalization of behavior. The taxonomies guide development of learning objectives and selection of appropriate learning methods. Teaching about a medication regimen is in the cognitive domain. Behavioral objectives progress from naming the medications to explaining their actions and to adjusting for drug-food interaction. In teaching a motor skill, behaviors progress from observing the task to practicing with guidance, to practicing independently, and finally to mastery of the task.

A teaching plan is based on the behavioral domain best suited to learning and in light of any impairment in that domain. Not every client needs or is able to learn in all domains. Learning about a medication is cognitive, and preparing and giving an insulin injection uses cognitive and

Box 11-3 Hierarchy of Basic Needs for the Rehabilitation Client

Physiological and Safety Needs

- Management of pain
- Administration of medications and treatments
- Recognition of health problems, complications, and what to do about them (e.g., autonomic dysreflexia)
- Management of bowel and bladder
- Maintenance of skin integrity
- Safe transfer

Safety and Security Needs

- Effective communication
- Access, use, and maintenance of adaptive supportive equipment
- Safe environment
- Adequate housing
- Ability to work and earn
- Prevention of abuse
- Financial resources to meet basic needs for housing, food, medication, etc.

Love and Belonging Needs

- Maintenance of family and social roles
- Adaptation to peer group
- Need to feel lovable and worthwhile despite illness or disability

Esteem and Recognition Needs

- Maintenance of self-care
- Control of own life and choices
- Dignity and privacy
- Recognition as a valued individual
- Ability to deal with lack of respect or ill use on job or in family

Self-Actualization

- Ability to meet developmental milestones
- Success through own definition of what is desirable

Adapted from Rankin, S., & Stallings, K. (1996). *Patient education, issues, principles, practice* (3rd ed., p. 159). Philadelphia: JB Lippincott.

TABLE 11-4 Behavior Domain and Learning Activity

Domain	Definition	Teaching-Learning Method
Cognitive	Knowledge, intellectual skills	Lecture, discussion, printed materials, independent study, demonstration, tests, simulation; Learning facts, information
Psychomotor	Perform physical skills within limits of disability	Demonstration, practice, simulation, role-playing
Affective	Attitudes, values, feelings	Discussion, role-playing, simulation

psychomotor domains. Rehabilitation needs often involve all domains, such as a client with paraplegia acquiring knowledge, skills, and attitudes to prevent skin breakdown.

Instructional Methods and Instructional Resources

The teaching format can be conducted for individuals, groups, or a combination of these to accomplish learning objectives. In rehabilitation, clients with similar disabilities gather in groups to learn about their condition or disease and their care. In groups clients share information and experiences and provide support for one another. Families learn about the impairment and ways of providing care and form their own support group to share adjustments or ask questions of those who have related problems. Although run by clients or families, support groups may be sponsored by the health care facility, a local or national organization, or community agencies. These groups recognize the benefits of mutual support in adjustment to chronic disease and management of disabling conditions.

One-to-one, or individual, teaching is a reliable format for continued assessment and psychomotor training, such as insulin injection or self-catheterization. It provides a setting for sharing confidential information and problems and overcoming barriers such as culture, anxiety, or low literacy. Often the initial teaching format, it is flexible and allows for feedback and unstructured moments. Individual teaching may reinforce information and skills learned in groups. A topic, such as skin care, is discussed in the group, but individual learning needs are followed up on a one-to-one basis.

Although individual teaching plans continue in use, education is incorporated into care maps and critical pathways that guide the sequence and timing of a client's progress. Care maps and critical pathways with an education component have been developed for various diseases and conditions; they prescribe approaches and combine individual, group, and self-directed learning. Clients and families are taught from standardized content tailored to optimize individual situations and reduce barriers to the learning process. Education is linked with client outcomes at specific points and designed for efficiency and quality while reducing length of stay.

Selecting Learning Activities

Learning can be an enjoyable experience, and a variety of learning activities can make learning interesting, challenging, and effective for both the teacher and the learner (Rankin & Stallings, 1996). The learning activity matches the objective and the learner's functional and cognitive abilities (Table 11-5).

The rehabilitation environment provides learners with opportunities to practice new behaviors with the support and encouragement of the staff. An overnight or weekend pass to home gives the client and family a chance to try skills or behaviors, test themselves, and review areas of perceived difficulty with the team. An independent-living center in the facility serves the same purpose as a client and family try out behaviors, identify successes or problems, and overcome barriers with the staff on call.

The Internet as a Resource in Client Education

The Internet has changed the way we obtain information and documents and how we communicate. Literature searches, full-text professional articles, current research, practice guidelines, and chat rooms are available. Consumers are sensitized to health care issues and educational material. Materials are available from government sites, national nonprofit organizations for specific diseases, drug companies, websites for physicians, and clients' personal websites. Searching for client education or a condition, such as diabetes or stroke, with a major search engine will elicit a multitude of websites for review. Professional journal articles discuss websites helpful in practice and client education. So much information is on the World Wide Web that guidebooks are published for health information on the Internet. One survey found that in a 12-month period as many as 70 million persons searched the Internet for health information. As clients become more informed and involved in their care, they expect closer participation with health providers.

The problem may not be finding information on the Internet but rather locating accurate and high-quality resources; clients need help to evaluate health information. Rehabilitation nurses need to research reliable Internet sites for the populations they serve and prepare to discuss information on the sites with clients as necessary (Box 11-4). The Health on the Net (HON) Foundation, an international organization,

TABLE 11-5 Learning Activities

Learning Activity	Uses and Advantages
Lecture	Most often used method in transmitting information. Effective in teaching cognitive information. More effective when used with discussions. Enhanced by handouts and visual aids; presented at the level of the patient's understanding; should be limited in length.
Demonstration	Useful for cognitive and psychomotor learning. Can be presented in person or by video; used to teach skills; return demonstration and repetition needed.
Group discussion	Requires 2 or more persons; actively involves learner; promotes understanding and application of knowledge and development of positive attitudes.
Role-playing and return demonstration	Practicing and doing. Help learner apply knowledge. Help patients recognize and solve problem situations. Helpful in teaching affective behaviors.
Tests	Demonstrate learner's progress in cognitive and psychomotor objectives. Introduced as a positive learning tool and used to reinforce learning. May cause anxiety in some learners.
Printed material (pamphlets and information sheets)	Most common teaching tools; used to enhance participative learning; contents appropriate for patient's language and educational level; review information in writing with patient. Provide a reference when the patient goes home.
Games and simulations	Involve the patient in teaching and learning. Introduce information and offer practice in simulated situations; incorporate problem solving. Can take a course of action and look at consequences in a nonthreatening way.
Computer-assisted learning and programmed instruction	Self-paced, self-directed learning. Many commercial products available. Factors in use: motivation, readiness, literacy level, visual and hearing ability, language, and physical or cognitive impairment. Older adults may not be familiar with use. Nurse should introduce materials and then follow-up the learning.
Slides and transparencies	Help learner focus thoughts; pictures can attract and maintain viewer's interest; visual images can promote understanding and encourage discussion. Use to bring out main points.
Audiotapes	Small, inexpensive, and easy to use; commercial tapes available on many health-related topics; can be teacher made and tailored to individual patient. Taped segments should be short—interest flags after about 5 minutes; well suited to patients with vision loss.
Videotapes	Can teach cognitive, psychomotor, and affect behaviors; present life situations that promote understanding and problem solving. Choose videotapes that are appropriate to learner; run no longer than 20 min; introduce and follow with a discussion. Can be shown over in-house television system with follow-up by staff.

developed a set of principles aimed at "unifying the practice of providing medical and health information on the web." In 1996 the HON Code of Conduct was published on the Internet as a guide to help standardize the quality of health information. Sites that display the HON logo agree to adhere to the code voluntarily (Wald, 2000). Health professionals use the Internet and e-mail to communicate with clients and colleagues to share research findings, give information such as appointment reminders, and answer questions. E-mail, customized newsletters, client reminders, and the like are new modalities in education. The Internet's potential for improving communication between clients and providers and providing access to information helps clients use information to improve their health.

Documentation of Education

Maintaining a record of client education is imperative. Records not only inform colleagues of education plans and progress but are also major components of accreditation review and health maintenance organization (HMO) standards. Documentation enhances continuity in the education process. A well-planned program requires coordination of teaching plans and materials, institutional policies and goals, and a plan for referral to outside agencies.

Educators document what was taught in the teaching plan and what the client learned as client outcomes. The teaching plan and the client's progress in meeting the goals and objectives are part of the permanent client record conveyed to all members of the interdisciplinary team to maintained continuity and avoid duplications. It also provides a legal record of teaching and learning for reimbursement. Documentation in client education should cover all aspects of client education, including:

- Special needs of the client
- Client's learning needs, styles, and readiness
- Client's current knowledge
- Learning objectives and goals as determined by the client, family, and educator
- Information taught
- Teaching methods used
- Objective reports of client responses to teaching
- Evaluation of learning and how that learning was evaluated

Box 11-4 Sample of Internet Health Care Resources

When typing the topic for a search, connect the words of a multiword topic with + (e.g., +patient+education, +spinal+cord+injury, +physical+rehabilitation)

Information from Pharmaceutical Companies

Name of company.com (Pfizer.com; park-davis.com; lily.com)

Search Engines

Yahoo.com
NorthernLight.com
AltaVista.com
Infoseek.com
Lycos.com
Dogpile.com

Professional Sites

Worldwide Nurse: www.wwnurse.com
Springhouse: www.springnet.com
Clinweb: www.ohsu.edu.cliniweb/
Health Web: http://healthweb.org
BioMedNet: www.biometnet.com
Medscape: www.medscape.com

Consumer Health Sites

National Institutes of Health: www.search.info.nih.gov
Healthfinder: www.healthfinder.gov
Medicare website: www.medicare.gov (get information on medicare coverage)
New York Online Access to Health (NOAH): www.cuny.edu
Health Oasis (Mayo Clinic): www.mayohealth.org
Wellness Web: www.wellweb.com
Achoo Health Care Online: www.achoo.com
Health AtoZ: www.healthatoz.com
Diabetes Organization: www.diabetes.org

Other Health-Related Sites

American National Heart Association
National Stroke Association
National Rehabilitation Information Center: www.naric.com
Rehab Central: www.rehabcentral.com (sources of equipment, forms, etc.)
Heart: www.cardio.net
Sources of low-cost prescriptions: www.institute-dc.org
Forum One: www.forumone.com

Evaluation in Client Education

Evaluation is as essential in the teaching process as in the nursing process. Too often evaluation is forgotten or neglected, time is not allocated, learning is not documented, and client learning outcomes, especially behavioral changes, are difficult to evaluate. Evaluation completes the circle back to assessment to determine further education needs throughout each stage of the learning process. Feedback at each stage helps the educator adjust information, methods, and materials to optimize learning, a continuous process. The nurse educator can refer to the information in the Nursing Interventions Classification (NIC) (McCloskey & Bulechek, 2000) and the Nursing Outcomes Classification (NOC) (Johnson, Maas, & Moorhead, 2000) for nursing interventions and outcomes in education domains. Education outcomes are useful to evaluate knowledge. For example, the outcomes for teaching the safe use of medications match client outcomes of the medication regimen. Although rehabilitation-specific nursing interventions and outcomes have not yet been delineated, teaching plans, care maps, and critical pathways incorporate NOC nursing outcomes plus other evaluations of client and family learning. However, if the client's learning goal is a change in behavior, it is more difficult to measure over the long-term than knowledge attainment. A client and family may demonstrate understanding of information and perform the skill successfully, but not transfer the behavior to the home and community. Do persons with diabetes follow their diet at home? Does the client make changes to reduce risk factors after stroke? Does the young man with paraplegia do everything he knows to prevent skin breakdown? Follow-up visits at clinics and physician's offices or telephone calls help in following up on education programs through client's self-reports of knowledge, skills, and attitudes. This remains an area for continuing work because these means do not offer consistent evaluation of behavior change as an end product of learning. Is it sufficient for the educator to assume learning has occurred if clients have a low rate of complications or readmissions? A challenge to client educators is to answer the question of how to evaluate learning as behavior change.

THE REHABILITATION NURSE AND COMMUNITY EDUCATION

Clients are returning to the community from both acute care and rehabilitation facilities with unmet continuing rehabilitation requirements and need for community-based support, including health promotion and prevention of further disability or complications. Ensuring continuation of rehabilitation and supporting the client and family are ongoing concerns. The rehabilitation nurse has a role in facilitating clients' integration into the community and aiding them to connect with persons, groups, and services that can assist them. Knowing the community services available is central to preparing clients for home and developing a teaching plan that can continue after discharge. Being aware of agencies and support groups in their community helps clients leave for home and community better prepared for resuming independence.

An educator may develop reciprocal relationships with agencies and groups. For example, volunteering to teach rehabilitation skills, such as safe transfers, through a church or community group introduces better care to the community. The result is safer care and helpful association with groups that could benefit others, including support for family caregivers. Other continuing education programs might deal with the prevention of chronic disease or care for persons with specific impairments. Resources for client education in the community are as follows:

- National organizations for special disease conditions (American Heart Association, American Cancer Society, etc.)
- Local health departments
- County and city hospitals with free clinics
- Government-sponsored clinics
- United Way
- National Jewish Federation
- Local churches and parish groups
- Internet consumer health sites and health-related chat rooms
- Hospital websites

Health promotion activities in the community help reduce risk factors and the burden of chronic illness. They also facilitate the independence and well-being of individuals and groups. Community health education may be local, regional, national, or global and cross all age, social, cultural, and economic groups. Education may take place in schools, community centers, churches, the workplace, and storefront clinics, anywhere in the community accessible to target groups. Telecommunications is another technology area that is becoming adaptable to client education. Interactive telecommunication by video screen connecting the health facility to satellite centers and to clients' homes would allow for ongoing education, monitoring, and evaluation.

Box 11-5 Two Programs to Reduce High-Risk Behavior and Violence

Think First

Think First is a nationwide program that teaches school children how to prevent spinal cord injuries (SCIs) from vehicular, sports, and diving accidents. Local chapters teach school children how to protect themselves from the consequences of SCI. The program trains young SCI patients as presenters of the program, and these peer presenters share their stories with the audience. The program has found wide acceptance in the schools.

Rise Above It

A youth outreach program, Rise Above It, was a direct response to the increasing number of severe SCIs resulting from violence in the urban areas of New Jersey. The program targets the school-age population and uses peer presenters and presenters with SCIs caused by violence. A curriculum of 10 lessons teaches skills to help students deal with anger and prevent violence. The Rise Above It program has been so well accepted that the Newark Board of Education made it part of the health science curriculum for grades 7 through 12.

Box 11-6 Teaching Tips: Clients with Motor Deficits

- When assistive or adaptive devices are necessary, allow sufficient time for the client to become familiar with the equipment
- Include demonstration with instructions whenever teaching a task
- All staff teaching the client a task or skill should use the same teaching plan, methods, and terminology
- When the need to adapt a skill or task arises, elicit suggestions from the client or family
- When the client experiences difficulty, take over the task (step) and have the patient move on to the next task
- Do not push the client to the point of frustration or failure; assume responsibility for the task and have the client return to it later

TABLE 11-6 Teaching Tips: Clients with Sensory-Perceptual Deficits

Deficit	Teaching Tip
Deficit in one or more sensory areas (vision, hearing, touch)	Engage intact senses in teaching
Neglect/visual field cuts	Identify area of intact vision and direct teaching methods accordingly
Short attention span/inability to focus or maintain attention	Use short teaching segments, vary topics to hold interest and keep engaged, break learning into small segments, alternate cognitive and psychomotor domains, engage all intact senses
Impaired directional concepts	In teaching, use environmental cues rather than directional; say "pull your slacks toward your waist" rather than "pull your slacks up"
Altered perception of body part or position	Patient may respond better to gestures indicating the part rather than words; touch the body part when teaching the patient to dress or move a part
Apraxia (inability to perform a previously learned action)	Give instructions that refer to a goal rather than a specific action; say "get dressed" rather than "put your arm into your shirt sleeve"
Agnosia (unable to recognize familiar objects and symbols by means of senses)	Use alternate senses to help the client recognize object or symbol; if the client cannot recognize an object by sight, he or she may know it by touch

A national initiative to improve the health of the nation, *Healthy People 2010* establishes priorities for health promotion, prevention, and health protection services. The overall goals are to help individuals change negative health behaviors, eliminate unequal access to health care, and rid the nation of many of the essentially preventable chronic conditions that are costly in terms of lives and dollars. The rehabilitation community can claim special involvement in addressing some of the goals of *Healthy People 2010* that have relevance. One such example is the reduction of violence and other risk-taking behaviors that lead to injury and disability. Educational programs that target high-risk populations and elicit changes in behaviors that contribute to injury and disability are services rehabilitation nurses can offer to the community (Box 11-5).

COMMON CHALLENGES IN CLIENT EDUCATION IN REHABILITATION

Much of the teaching that occurs in rehabilitation is focused specifically on accommodating the cognitive, sensory-perceptual, and motor impairments resulting from an impairment, disability, or chronic condition. Members of the rehabilitation team collaborate to identify the specific strategies that will work best for each client. A few of the commonly occurring problems and teaching strategies to accommodate impairment in these areas are presented in Table 11-6 and Boxes 11-6 and 11-7. Detailed information on intervention and approaches to treating cognitive, sensory-perceptual, and motor impairments is found in other chapters in this book. Safety is a key consideration in all teaching-learning activities, whether in a health care facility or in the community.

CHALLENGES FOR CLIENT EDUCATION

Emphasis on cost containment and efficacy in rehabilitation is increasing pressure on and scrutiny of client education. The introduction of the prospective payment system (PPS) to acute rehabilitation is expected to affect length of stay and, in turn, further streamline client education with critical pathways and care maps. Critical thinking questions may be asked about client education. Can client education improve health status, reduce complications, and reduce readmission to hospitals? If so, how can these educational outcomes be demonstrated? How will the changing responsibilities within the rehabilitation team that may accompany PPS affect client education? Will rehabilitation team members with many additional demands placed on them give client education a low priority?

Who will pay for client education? Presently it is budgeted as a part of the cost of care in many agencies. If client education were viewed as an invaluable component of health care, would it not be a separate cost center and be reimbursable? These questions represent issues and trends affecting client education in the changing rehabilitation environment and point out the need for further study. The JCAHO (2000) standards stipulate that a health facility must designate resources in their budget for client and family education. All the points raised here and in other forums testify to the dynamic nature of client education and the challenges it presents to the rehabilitation nurse.

Box 11-7 Teaching Tips: Client with Cerebral Damage (Associated with Stroke or Traumatic Brain Injury)

Right Hemisphere Damage (Associated Left Hemiplegia)

- Difficulty with broad concepts; teach specific information, be concrete, direct
- Accompany all visual material with verbal cues due to visual-motor impairment and loss of visual memory
- Short attention span; teach in short segments, vary topics, tasks
- Break tasks into small parts
- Eliminate distractions
- Identify any visual field loss and adjust teaching accordingly
- Lacks insight and judgment; use continuous reinforcement
- Quick to say he/she understands whether does or does not: use frequent reinforcement, evaluation, and redirection
- Use positive aspects of impulsivity such as willingness to try new things
- Does not learn from mistakes
- Inability to follow through; monitor, remind
- May lack awareness of limitations
- Performance may not improve

Left Hemisphere Damage (Associated Right Hemiplegia)

- Make use of visual learning methods
- Behaviors to be learned should be demonstrated step by step, encouraging imitation
- Will learn by observing others
- Unable to communicate effectively
- Able to pick up ideas of conversation through body language, tone of voice, and facial expression; use gestures, pantomime
- May assume that the person comprehends much more than able to indicate
- Able to synthesize parts of a task
- Learns from mistakes
- Cautious and unorganized when approaching an unfamiliar situation
- Give lots of feedback
- Has normal attention span
- Set up learning experiences to ensure success
- Underestimates ability; give encouragement

Subject: ____________________
Client/learner: ____________________ Learner #2: ____________________
Language spoken: ____________________ Able to read ☐ yes ☐ no Language read: ____________________

Assessment	Date	Yes	No	Comments
1. Does client have a disability that will affect diabetic management?				
2. Does client have a disability that will affect teaching/learning?				
3. Is client on insulin?				
4. Is client on oral hypoglycemic medications?				
5. Has client had previous diabetic teaching?				When? Where?
6. Can client demonstrate the following?				
a. Monitor blood glucose				
b. Describe type(s) of insulin used				
c. Prepare insulin for administration				
d. Administer insulin				
e. Describe site rotation				
f. Apply sick day rules				
7. Is client a candidate for teaching?				
8. Nutrition assessment and diet teaching				Clinical dietitian?
9. Does client need home health care follow-up?				

Topic	**Adaption for disability**	**Teaching code**	**Learning code**	**Date/initial**
Self-administration of insulin	Use one-handed technique or use paralyzed hand to stabilize equipment			
Given and reviewed printed materials	Consider adaptations for vision impairment			
Type(s) of insulin	Provide frequent reinforcement, short sessions; be concrete			
Preparation of insulin for injection	Break down into discrete steps; use insulin pen with disposable cartridge; use magnifiers and syringe stabilizers			
Insulin injection	Use verbal cues with a demonstration			
Site rotation	Repeat, reinforce; use pictures, diagrams			
Blood glucose monitoring	Utilize trial lancets for ease of use			
Frequency and range	Repeat, reinforce			
Care and use of glucometer	If visual impairment, use glucometer with audio cueing; use 2-person quality check			
Signs and symptoms of hypoglycemia and hyperglycemia	Use short teaching segments, evaluate frequently, reinforce; post visual charts, encourage Med-Alert bracelet use			
Treatment of hypoglycemia and hyperglycemia	Use easy-open liquid or paste concentrates; teach to open; use visual reminder of sick day rules			
Foot and skin care	If altered sensation, teach safety			

Teaching code: A, Questions answered; B, verbal information given; C, written information given; D, audiovisual teaching aid; E, skill demonstrated.
Learning code: A, Needs further instruction; B, verbalizes understanding; C, can direct others; D, returns demonstration with help; E, returns demonstration independently; F, refuses information.

Figure 11-2 Teaching plan. Diabetes management for client with stroke (left hemiplegia).

REHABILITATION TEACHING PLAN

The rehabilitation nurse has responsibility to teach clients about managing comorbid conditions, procedures, and medication regimens. Teaching plans for clients must be adjusted to take into consideration any limitations and challenges presented by the specific impairment or disability. The teaching plan in Figure 11-2 is one example of how a teaching plan designed for managing a chronic disease can be adapted to meet the unique learning needs of a person who has a disability.

CRITICAL THINKING

With computer and Internet technologies to access information, how will client educators ensure that clients receive relevant and accurate information or communication?

REFERENCES

Bandura, A. (1997). Self-efficacy. New York: WH Freeman.

Becker, M.H. (Ed.). (1974). *The health belief model and personal health behavior.* Thorofare, NJ: Slack.

Benner, P. (1985). *From beginner to expert: Excellence and power in clinical nursing practice.* Reading, MA: Addison-Wesley.

Benner, P. (2001). *From novice to expert.* Commemorative 1st ed). Upper Saddle River, NJ: Prentice Hall.

Boswell, E., Pichert, J., Lorenz, R., & Schlundt, D. (1990). Training health care professionals to enhance their patient teaching skills. *Journal of Nursing Staff Development, 6*(5), 233-239.

Bronfenbrenner, U. (1989). Ecological systems theory, *Annuals of Child Development* 6, 187-249.

Commission on Accreditation of Rehabilitation Facilities. (2000). *The 2000 standards manual.* Tuscon, AZ: Author.

Diehl, L.N. (1989). Client and family learning in the rehabilitation setting. *Nursing Clinics of North America, 24,* 257-264.

Doak, C., Doak, L., & Root, J. (1996). *Teaching patients with low literacy skills* (2nd ed.). Philadelphia: JB Lippincott.

Festinger, L. (1957). *Theory of cognitive dissonance.* Stanford, CA: Stanford University Press.

Johnson, M., Maas, M., & Moorhead, S. (2000). *Nursing outcomes classification (NOC)* (2nd ed.). St. Louis: Mosby.

Joint Commission on Accreditation of Hospitals. (2000). Comprehensive accreditation manual for hospitals. Oakbrook, IL: Author.

Knowles, M. (1984). *Andragogy in action.* San Francisco: Jossey-Bass.

Lorig, K. (1992). *Patient education: a practical approach.* St. Louis: Mosby.

Pestonjee, S. (2000). *Nurses handbook of patient education.* Springhouse, PA: Springhouse.

McCloskey, J., & Bulechek, G. (2000). *Nursing interventions classifications.* St. Louis: Mosby.

Pratt, D.D. (1988). Andragogy as a relational construct. *Adult Education Quarterly, 38,*160-181.

Rankin, S., & Stallings, K. (1996). *Patient education, issues, principles, practice* (3rd ed.). Philadelphia: JB Lippincott.

Redman, B. (1996). *The process of patient education* (8th ed.). St. Louis: Mosby.

Robinson-Smith, G., Johnston, M., & Allen, J. (2000). Self-care efficacy, quality of life and depression after stroke. *Archives of Physical Medicine and Rehabilitation,* 81, 460-464.

Wald, A. (2000). *Internet's impact on nurse-patient relationship.* Long Island, NY: Nursing Spectrum.

Wallston, K., Wallston, B., & DeVellis, R. (1978). Development of the multidimensional health locus of control (MHLC) scales. *Health Education Monographs, 6*(2), 160-170.

Weeks, S. (1995). What are the educational needs of prospective family caregivers of the newly disabled adults? *Rehabilitation Nursing, 20*(5), 256-260.

BIBLIOGRAPHY

Alfaro-LeFevre, R. (1999). *Critical thinking in nursing* (2nd ed.). Philadelphia: WB Saunders.

Chachkes, E., & Christ, G. (1996). Cross cultural issues in patient education. *Patient Education and Counseling, 27,* 13-21.

CoumaCare. (2000). *Multilingual support for patient on coumadin therapy.* Wilmington, DE: DuPont Pharma.

Iacono, J., & Campbell, A. *Patient and family education: The compliance guide to the JCAHO standards* (2nd ed.). Marblehead, MA: Opus Communication.

Geissler, E. (1994). *Pocket guide to cultural assessment.* St. Louis: Mosby.

Maynard, A. (1999). Preparing readable patient education handouts. *Journal for Nurses in Staff Development, 15*(1), 11-18.

McLennan, M., Starko, G., & Pain, K. (1996). Rehabilitation learning needs: Patient and family perceptions. *patient education and counseling, 27,* 191-199.

Price, J., & Cordell, B. (1996). Cultural diversity and patient teaching. *Journal of Continuing Education in Nursing, 25*(4), 163-166.

12 Client and Family Coping

Julie Pryor, RN, CM, BA, MN

Jenny, a young mother, was admitted to my ward fully dependent on nursing staff for all of her care after an intracranial hemorrhage. She was immobile, incontinent, and could not communicate verbally. Her significant physical deficits were clearly visible. For those who stopped to look beyond her bodily dysfunctions, her suffering could only be imagined. Many years of clinical experience did not prepare me for this person's refusal to accept my attempts to establish a therapeutic relationship. Establishing rapport took on new dimensions as I struggled to interpret Jenny's preferred style of coping with her situation.

Coping is central to the experience of being human. It is a process that is entered into in response to the everyday experiences of individuals striving to maximize their quality of life and satisfaction with life. When wellness required for optimal quality of life is disrupted by an episode of illness (Morse & Johnson, 1991), the immediate effects and the life consequences are central to nursing.

Coping is defined as "constantly changing cognitive and behavioral efforts to manage specific external and/or internal demands that are appraised as taxing or exceeding the resources of the person" (Lazarus & Folkman, 1984, p. 141). This definition provides a clear distinction between coping and the stresses and strains of bodily homeostasis that Cannon (1914, 1935) explained. Lazarus and Folkman (1984) found that coping is a process, with an emphasis being placed on *efforts to manage* rather than *outcomes and mastery* and that "coping is a powerful mediator of the emotional outcome of a stressful encounter" (Lazarus, 1999, p. 121).

A rehabilitation nurse who would optimize health processes and outcomes for clients and families must understand the body of knowledge related to coping. This chapter introduces concepts and theories relating to how clients and their families cope, especially with interruptions in health. These theories are applied to rehabilitation nursing practice by relating the nursing process to the coping-stress-tolerance functional health pattern with the aim of developing an understanding of how individuals cope.

CONCEPTS AND THEORIES

Foundation Concepts

The concepts of wellness, comfort, stress, adversity, emotions, and self-efficacy are foundational to understanding how persons cope with interruptions in health.

Wellness

Wellness is "a state of harmony, energy, positive productivity, and well-being in an individual's mind, body, emotions and spirit" (Jones & Kilpatrick, 1996, p. 259). Wellness is about person-in-environment functioning, including relationships with family, the community, society as a whole, and the physical environment. Although illness can disrupt wellness (a state of optimal comfort [Morse & Johnson, 1991]), even persons who have a chronic, disabling, or developmental disorder can achieve wellness.

Comfort

Comfort is the state of having met basic human needs for ease ("a state of calm or contentment"), relief ("the experience of a patient who has had a specific need met"), and transcendence ("the state in which one rises above problem or pain") (Kolcaba, 1991, p. 239). Comfort, however, is always relative. "Comfort has no meaning without discomfort, nor comfortable without uncomfortable" (Morse, Bottorff, & Hutchinson, 1995, p. 14). There are physical, social, psychospiritual, and environmental contexts of client comfort (Kolcaba, 1991); it can be given and received. Kolcaba (1995, p. 123) concludes that "comfort is holistic, complex, individualized, dynamic, immediate, and measurable."

Stress

Our understanding of stress began with the physical body, and now is related to the total person. Cannon (1914/1935) wrote about how affective states activated parts of the body. Pelletier (1977) adds that people experience a fight-or-flight response, but may not have options to fight or run from sources of stress, or these options may not be socially acceptable. Thus the physiological stress response continues and is detrimental to health.

Selye (1976, p. 55), built on Cannon's work. He defined stress as "the nonspecific response of the body to any demand," i.e., the general adaptation syndrome (GAS), a specific response pattern of the body to nonspecific noxious stimuli. Lazarus (1999, p. 46) explains that the GAS is not only triggered by physically noxious stimuli but may also be "brought about by psychological harms and threats."

Lazarus and Folkman (1984, p. 19) were instrumental in extending the concept of stress, taking into account the roles of personal characteristics and the environment in creating a stressful situation. "Psychological stress is neither solely in the environment itself nor just the result of personality characteristics, but depends on a particular kind of person-environment relationship" (Lazarus, 1999, p. 29). Lazarus (1999) distinguishes three types of psychological stress: harm/loss, threat, and challenge. Harm/loss relates to something that has already happened; threat relates to harm or loss that is yet to happen; and challenge relates to difficulties that can be overcome.

Types of Stress/Stressors. Various types of stress have been categorized. Pelletier (1977) noted acute and chronic stress could occur with chronic, disabling, or developmental disorders. Elliott and Eisdorfer (1982) described four broad types of stressors: (1) acute, time-limited stressors (e.g., having sutures removed or awaiting pathology results); (2) stressor sequences (e.g., relearning how to toilet safely with a recently acquired hemiplegia); (3) chronic intermittent stressors (e.g., hemodialysis for a person who experiences frequent complications); and (4) chronic stressors (e.g., parenting a child with spina bifida).

Stressors associated with life events are discrete, observable events followed by a well-defined set of subevents, and an end point. Chronic stressors may start slowly, continue, and be open-ended. Forms of chronic stress include threats, demands, structural constraints, complexity, uncertainty, conflict, restriction of choice, underreward, and resource deprivation (Wheaton, 1997).

Adversity

"Adversity is anything that threatens or seems to threaten one's self or what one considers integral to one's self (Vash, 1994, p. 3). Adversity is serious stress, "any stimulus that evokes avoidance behavior, negative emotion, or conscious thoughts of repudiation might be termed 'adverse'" (p. 5).

Emotions

"Coping is an integral part of the process of emotional arousal" (Lazarus, 1999, p. 37). Stress, emotion, and coping form one conceptual unit: when there is stress, there is emotion. "Each emotion has a different scenario or story about an ongoing relationship with the environment" (Lazarus, 1999, p. 34).

Self-Efficacy

Bandura's work, applied with health promotion and lifestyle changes, is relevant to coping. Persons who believe they are capable of effective coping with particular situations or stressors have a sense of control; the reverse is also true.

Self-efficacy, self-concept, and self-esteem all differ. *Self-concept* is a composite view of self. *Self-esteem* relates to self-worth. *Self-efficacy* refers to "beliefs in one's capabilities to organize and execute the course of action required to produce given attainments" (Bandura, 1997, p. 3) and is a major basis for action. Self-concept is the cognitive view of self, self-esteem is the affective view (Seigley, 1999).

Rehabilitation nurses promote development of self-efficacy in clients and families. The beliefs of a group about their shared capabilities for action (Bandura's [1997] collective efficacy) is applicable to family units.

Enduring and Suffering

Enduring and suffering exist on a continuum in the response to illness or injury but differ in nature and purpose. Enduring is about holding on: "It is a condition in which the individual expends extraordinary amounts of energy 'holding oneself together.' When enduring, the individual is relatively devoid of emotion [and] is focused on the immediate present" (Dewar & Morse, 1995, p. 959). Individuals usually do not have a choice about the situations they have to endure (Morse & Carter, 1995), such as enduring a life-threatening event. Enduring is fostered when nurses understand how clients and families suffer and facilitate effective coping processes early in the chronic illness trajectory.

Suffering, on the other hand, "refers to the emotional response to the loss. Suffering requires reflection, a looking back, an evaluation of the immensity of loss. . . . Suffering is work, an all-consuming endeavor that one must experience to work through the event" (Morse & Carter, 1995, p. 40). Rodgers and Cowles (1997, p. 1048) note that suffering is "an individualized, subjective, and complex experience that involves the assignment of an intensely negative meaning to an event or a perceived threat." Suffering is undertaken intentionally when one feels strong enough to do so. Clients and families who are suffering are likely to be encountered by rehabilitation nurses.

Failure to endure, or the unbearable aspects of illness, are both intrapersonal and interpersonal (Dewar & Morse, 1995) (Box 12-1).

How Persons Cope

Human beings are continually interacting with their environments and coping by responding to their interpretations. Several schools of thought offer explanations. Symbolic interactionism and the early work of Lazarus and Folkman (1984) on stress, appraisal, and coping are useful frameworks for understanding coping. Box 12-2 provides a summary of theories about how persons cope in general and with interruptions in health.

Symbolic Interactionism

Symbolic interactionism is based on the premise that "human beings act towards things on the basis of the meaning that the things have for them" and that "the meaning of such things is derived from, or arises out of, the social interaction that one has with one's fellows" (Blumer, 1969, p. 2). It is a process that forms human conducts and not only an expression or a means to an end. Symbolic interactionism can explain interactions between clients and nurses or between clients and their families.

Nonsymbolic interaction, direct response without interpretation, differs from the appraisal before action in symbolic interaction (Blumer, 1969) .

Stress, Appraisal, and Coping

Psychological stress cannot be adequately explained by simply focusing on either the nature or the relative size of the stimulus or stressor or on the characteristics that make one

Box 12-1 Unbearable Aspects of Illness

Intrapersonal

- Pain for which the person is unprepared or that is unanticipated, unexplained, or irretractable
- Physical damage associated with a loss of former self
- Recurrence of symptoms after cure is believed to have happened
- Loss of function and dependency
- Loss of control
- Isolation
- Confronting reality
- Uncertainty

Interpersonal

- Not believed or listened to by caregivers
- Being treated as an object
- Being made to feel a burden
- Caregiver insensitivity
- Disregard from significant others
- Burdening significant others
- Causing grief to significant others

Data from Dewar, A.L., & Morse, J.M. (1995). Unbearable incidents: failure to endure the experience of illness. *Journal of Advanced Nursing, 22*, 957-964.

Box 12-2 Summary of Coping Theories

How Persons Cope

- Symbolic interactionism (Blumer, 1969)
- Stress, appraisal, and coping (Lazarus & Folkman, 1984; Lazarus, 1999)
- Making meaning as coping (Thompson, 1991; Barnard, 1985; Park & Folkman, 1997)
- Stress, appraisal and emotions (Folkman, 1997; Lazarus, 1991; Lazarus, 1999)

How Persons Cope with Interruptions to Health

Clients

- Sick role (Parsons, 1951)
- Stage theory of grief and loss (Kubler-Ross, 1969; Teel, 1991; Martin, 1994)
- Coping with life-threatening illness (Doka, 1995)
- Loss of self in chronic illness (Charmaz, 1983, 1987, 1995)
- Reactions to disability (Antonak & Livneh, 1991; Antonak et al., 1993)
- Psychosocial adaptation to chronic illness and disability (Livneh & Antonak, 1997)
- Salutogenic model of health (Antonovsky, 1972, 1979, 1996)
- Responding to threats to self (Morse & Johnson, 1991; Morse, 1992; Morse et al., 1994, 1995; Morse, 1997; Dewar & Morse, 1995; Morse & Carter, 1995, 1996)
- Chronic sorrow (Olshansky, 1966; Teel, 1991; Eakes et al., 1998)

Families

- Sick role (Parsons, 1951)
- Stage theory of grief and loss (Kubler-Ross, 1969; Teel, 1991; Martin, 1994)
- Salutogenic model of health (Antonovsky, 1972, 1979, 1996)
- Responding to threats to self (Morse & Johnson, 1991; Morse, 1992; Morse et al., 1994, 1995; Morse, 1997; Dewar & Morse, 1995; Morse & Carter, 1995, 1996)
- Chronic sorrow (Olshansky, 1966; Teel, 1991; Eakes et al., 1998)
- Family adaptation (McCubbin et al., 1993)
- Families' explanations of childhood chronic conditions (Garwick et al., 1999)
- Caregiver coping as chronic stress (Gignac & Gottlieb, 1997)

person more vulnerable than another to a particular stimulus. The cognitive appraisal process—"the meaning constructed by a person about what is happening" (Lazarus, 1999, p. 55)—differs among persons and groups. To understand variations "we must take into account the cognitive processes that intervene between the encounter and the reaction, and the factors that affect the nature of this mediation" (p. 23).

Lazarus and Folkman (1984) described three types of cognitive appraisal: primary, secondary, and reappraisal. In later work, Lazarus (1999) added gaining a benefit from the encounter as another dimension to primary appraisal. The nature of each type of cognitive appraisal is outlined in Box 12-3.

Appraising is an active process that can be accomplished by deliberate and largely conscious or intuitive, automatic, and unconscious evaluating "whether or not what is happening is relevant to one's values, beliefs about self and world, and situational intentions" (Lazarus, 1999, p. 75). Goal commitment, the strongest influence, "implies that a person will strive hard to attain the goal, despite discouragement or adversity" (p. 76). As has been found during previous experiences with the same kind of problem, a slight cue can provoke the stress reaction and associated coping process.

Acknowledging that appraisal takes place within a context, Lazarus (1999) discusses environmental and personal variables that will influence a person's reaction through the appraisal process. Environmental variables consist of demands, constraints, opportunity, and culture (Box 12-4). The personal variables are goal and goal hierarchies, beliefs about self and the world, and personal resources (Box 12-5).

The process of coping described by Lazarus and Folkman (1984) has three main features: observation and assessment of what the person actually thinks or does; examination of the context; and coping as a process that shifts as the relationship of the person to his or her environment changes. These changes trigger reappraisal and subsequent coping efforts. Lazarus (1999) notes that *no universally effective or ineffective coping strategy exists,* and the study of what the person thinks and does at each stage of the coping process must also include examination of the context in which it takes place.

The function of coping is related to the purpose of a particular strategy and not the outcome of that strategy. Thus emotion-focused coping aims to reduce the emotional distress, or conversely, to temporarily increase emotional distress for a particular purpose. Examples of emotion-focused coping are cognitive reappraisal of the situation to be less significant, selective attention or avoidance, and distraction. Self-deception is a potential risk associated with this type of coping (Lazarus & Folkman, 1984).

Problem-focused forms of coping are similar to, but broader than, strategies used for problem solving. They are "often directed at defining the problem, generating alternative solutions, weighing the alternatives in terms of their costs and benefits, choosing among them, and acting" (Lazarus & Folkman, 1984, p. 152). Problem-focused forms

Box 12-3 Types of Cognitive Appraisal

Primary Appraisal

- Judgment of an encounter as irrelevant, benign-positive, or stressful
- Stressful appraisals may pose harm/loss, threat, challenge, or benefit
  - Harm/loss refers to damage already sustained
  - Threat refers to anticipated losses or harms
  - Challenges are events that are possible to master
  - Benefit may be gained from the encounter

Secondary Appraisal

- Judgment of what might and can be done
- Considers options and evaluates the consequences of each option

Reappraisal

- A changed appraisal in response to new information

Data from Lazarus, R.S., & Folkman, S. (1984). *Stress, appraisal, and coping.* New York: Springer Publishing; and Lazarus, R. (1999). *Stress and emotion: A new synthesis.* New York: Springer.

Box 12-4 Environmental Variables

Demands

- Pressure to behave a certain way
- Pressure to possess socially correct attitudes

Constraints

- Pressure not to do certain things
- May be associated with punishment

Opportunity

- Arises from fortunate timing
- May depend on wisdom to see the opportunity

Culture

- Cultural differences have potential to affect stress, coping, and emotion in individuals
- Reality of multiethnic and multicultural societies challenges previous generalizations about culture

Data from Lazarus, R. (1999). *Stress and emotion: A new synthesis.* New York: Springer.

Box 12-5 Personal Variables

Goals and Goal Hierarchies

- Goals provide motivation
- Emotions result from evaluation of the fate of one's goals
- Relative value of the goal and the probability and cost of attainment determine choice of goal and emotions

Beliefs about Self and World

- Shape our expectations about what might happen and what we hope for

Personal Resources

- Include intelligence, money, social skills, education, supportive family and friends, physical attractiveness, health and energy, and sanguinity

Data from Lazarus, R. (1999). *Stress and emotion: A new synthesis.* New York: Springer.

may be directed at the self as well as the environment, and may occur with emotion-focused coping.

Meaning-Making as Coping

Persons seek to maintain a sense that life is meaningful (Thompson, 1991). When meaning is lost it may be a source of stress. The work of Park and Folkman (1997) highlights the importance of reappraisal, which follows primary and secondary appraisal.

Building on an understanding of meaning as a perception of significance, Park and Folkman (1997, p. 116) explain two types of meaning—global and situational. "Global meaning encompasses a person's enduring beliefs and valued goals." Situational meaning "is formed in the interaction between a person's global meaning and the circumstances of the particular person-environment transaction."

Global meaning includes beliefs about order as well as the person's life goals and purpose. The notion of order includes beliefs about the world, beliefs about self, and beliefs about the self in the world. Global meaning is built through experiences across the person's life span and is reported as possessing three attributes: stability, optimistic bias, and personal relevance.

Situational meaning is reported as having three major components (Park & Folkman, 1997): appraisal of meaning, search for meaning, and meaning as outcome. These are explained in Box 12-6.

Situational meaning, the search for meaning, and meaning as outcome were common themes in Folkman's (1997) longitudinal study of carers of partners who are dying, with 99.5% of the 1794 persons interviewed reporting positive meaningful events during their experiences of caregiving or bereavement. On the basis of these findings, Folkman (1997) supported an alternative outcome of coping (i.e., positive emotion).

Box 12-6 Situational Meaning

Appraisal of Meaning

- Primary appraisal
- Secondary appraisal
- Comparison of appraised meaning with global meaning

Search for Meaning

- Reappraisal of meaning
- Functions of reappraisal
  - To transform the appraised meaning
  - To modify the appraised meaning
  - To modify relevant beliefs and goals
  - To decrease threat of the event
- Changing appraised meaning
  - Changing appraised meaning of attributes (e.g., reasons why it happened, why it happened to me, responsibility)
  - Perception of benefits
- Changing global meaning
  - Revising beliefs
  - Revising goals

Meaning as Outcome

- Enduring changes in global meaning (e.g., changes in philosophical or religious beliefs)
- Personal growth
- Not all meaning-related outcomes are positive

Data from Park, C.L., & Folkman, S. (1997). Meaning in the context of stress and coping. *Review of General Psychology, 1*(2), 115-144.

Stress, Appraisal, and Emotions

Folkman's (1997) model demonstrates that emotions flow from our appraisal of what is happening. "The arousal of emotions actually depends on reason and follows clear rules" (Lazarus, 1999, p. 86). Our evaluation of what is happening (based on what is known, competing goals, and hierarchy of goals) determines our emotional reaction to it.

Thus it is extremely difficult to understand others' evaluation of a situation or event. Their response may appear irrational to others, but rational for that person based on what is known or able to be known. Lazarus (1999) attributes failure of reason to four common causes of erroneous judgments:

- Having a disorder that involves damage to the brain
- Lacking knowledge
- Not paying attention to the right things
- Experiencing denial

Lazarus (1999) proposes a cognitive-motivational-relational theory of emotions as a propositional understanding of how emotions work, listing 15 emotions, each with a different appraisal process and a core relational theme. For example, the core relational theme for anger is "a demeaning offense against me and mine" (Lazarus, 1991, p. 122).

How Persons Cope with Interruptions in Health

Knowledge about how a person copes with interruptions in health enriches nurses' abilities to understand the experiences of their clients and families.

Understanding of the complexity of how persons cope has grown over the past 5 decades. More recently, nursing research has begun to scrutinize the usefulness of coping theories for clinical nursing practice.

The Sick Role

Parsons (1951) introduced the notion of "being sick" as constituting a social role rather than just a natural phenomenon that happened to individuals. He also alluded to acceptable and unacceptable motives of those who adopt or choose to stay in the sick role. For him coping with interruptions to health was at both an individual and a social system level. Although Parson's work has been replaced, many clients and families may uphold the expectations associated with Parson's sick role.

Stage Models of Grief and Loss

Stage models offer explanations about adjustment to grief and loss. Kubler-Ross' (1969) classic study found that persons grieve in stages: initial shock with anxiety and disbelief, denial and avoidance, anger accompanied by guilt and shame, realization of permanence of loss and depression, and finally resolution with relief. The stage model has been used extensively by rehabilitation professionals to assess and intervene with clients and their families, based on the belief that a person was to move sequentially and in a timely manner through the stages and then signal acceptance.

Stage models may explain loss without death. Martin (1994) applied Parke's phases of grief to the family of a head-injured client as they moved from a state of alarm through searching behaviors, mitigation, anger and guilt, and on to the development of a new identity. "The grieving process is said to be successfully completed once the individual is able to recall the loss without the intense pain experienced during the initial period" (p. 136).

Despite their popularity, stage models of grief and loss have been seriously challenged. Stage models suggest that a normal response is time limited, and failure to progress through the various phases is abnormal (Teel, 1991); it is a continual experience (especially chronic sorrow) for clients with chronic, disabling problems and their families. Lindgren, Burke, Hainsworth, and Eakes (1992) suggest that the term *chronic sorrow* describes this experience of dealing with loss.

Box 12-7 General Tasks of Coping with Life-Threatening Illness

- Responding to the physical fact of the disease
- Taking steps to cope with the reality of disease
- Preserving self-concept and relationships with others in the face of disease
- Dealing with affective, existential, and spiritual issues created or reactivated by the disease

From Doka, K.J. (1995). Coping with life-threatening illness: a task model. *OMEGA, 32*(2), 117.

Box 12-8 Tasks of Recovery from Life-Threatening Illness

- Dealing with psychological, social, physical, spiritual and financial after-effects of illness
- Coping with fears and anxieties about reoccurrence
- Examining life and lifestyle issues and reconstructing one's life
- Redefining relationships with caregivers

From Doka, K.J. (1995). Coping with life-threatening illness: a task model. *OMEGA, 32*(2), 117.

Coping with Life-Threatening Illness: A Task Model

Doka (1995) critiqued Kubler-Ross and argued for a new model to help understand the experiences of individuals with life-threatening illness. A framework outlines the phases and tasks of life-threatening illness from prediagnostic to acute; chronic; and terminal, which may become a recovery phase.

The tasks associated with life-threatening illness are described generally as well as specifically for each of the phases. The general tasks of coping with life-threatening illness are listed in Box 12-7.

See Doka (1995, p. 118, Table 1) for the complete list of the specific tasks associated with the acute, chronic, and terminal phases. The tasks of recovery are listed in Box 12-8.

Loss of Self in Chronic Illness

Physical consequences of chronic illness are recognized more readily than loss of self. Charmaz (1983) has noted that Western health care systems treat acute illness, while chronic illness "results in spiralling consequences such as loss of productive function, financial crises, family strain, stigma, and a restricted existence" (p. 169). She explains that sources of suffering are complex: for example, being discredited may lead to a more restricted life

Box 12-9 Characteristics of Identity Levels

The supernormal self assumes:
- Success values
- Social acceleration
- Struggle in a competitive world

The restored self assumes:
- Return to former life
- Current situation is normal after serious illness

A contingent personal identity is:
- Defined as questionable
- Perhaps possible in the future
- Associated with possible failure

A salvaged self:
- Attempts to see self as positive
- Attempts to present self to others most favorably
- Is associated with adverse circumstances
- Holds little hope of realizing typical adult identities

Data from Charmaz, K. (1987). Struggling for a self: Identity levels of the chronically ill. *Sociology of Health Care, 6,* 283-321.

and, consequently, limited opportunities to construct a valued self. The values of individualism and independence discredit a restricted and often homebound life focused on the illness. Recurrent discrediting leads chronically ill clients to perceive themselves as permanent failures and as burdens.

In their struggle for identity, chronically ill clients prefer to construct their lives to find motivation apart from their illnesses. On the basis of data from 85 in-depth interviews with chronically ill persons, Charmaz (1987) created a hierarchy of identities listed in Box 12-9.

The concept of identity is related to the person's vision of future self; failure to regain a valued identity is viewed as a failure of self.

Subsequently, Charmaz (1995) conducted 115 intensive interviews with 55 adults with serious, intrusive chronic illnesses and found that adapting (accommodating the physical losses by altering self and life) is *one* mode of living with loss of bodily function or impairment. Not everyone adapts; adaptation may be a recurring theme down through the levels of identity.

Three major stages were found in adapting to impairment: (1) experiencing an altered body; (2) assessing one's altered body, appearance to self and others, and the context of life; and (3) surrendering to the sick body (Charmaz, 1995).

"Other ways of living with illness include ignoring it, minimizing it, struggling against it, reconciling self to it, and embracing it" (p. 657); differing from resigning to it, being overtaken by the illness, or giving up, surrender is about a new unity between the self and the body.

Reactions to Disability

Antonak and Livneh (1991) analyzed the responses of 118 persons with acquired disability to the Reactions to Impairments and Disability Inventory (RIDI) and found sets of adapted and non-adapted psychosocial reactions to disability. Denial was an independent reaction.

Acknowledgment is about the person's "intellectual recognition of the permanency of the condition and its future implications. *Adjustment* entails further assimilation, affectively and behaviorally, of the ramifications of the disability" (Antonak & Livneh, 1991, p. 21). They suggest that depression, internalized anger, anxiety, and externalized anger are prerequisites to adaptation; however, these reactions do not occur in any particular sequence and are independent of each other. To this they add, "experiencing shock is apparently prerequisite to experiencing depression and internalized anger" (p. 21) and that shock, anxiety, and externalized anger appear to be experienced concurrently.

Antonak, Livneh, and Antonak (1993) reviewed research on the psychosocial adjustment of persons with traumatic brain injury (TBI) and found many methodological problems. Further research is needed.

Psychosocial Adaptation to Chronic Illness and Disability

Livneh and Antonak (1997) extended their earlier work through a comprehensive review of literature relating to the psychosocial adaptation to traumatic or sudden-onset disabilities, disease-related health disorders, sensory impairments, and neurological and neuromuscular disabilities. They found four classes of variables associated with psychosocial adaptation:

Class 1: Variables associated with the disability itself

Class 2: Variables associated with sociodemographic characteristics of the individual

Class 3: Variables associated with personality attributes of the individual

Class 4: Variables associated with characteristics of the physical and social environment

These variables are incorporated into their model (Figure 12-1), which depicts psychosocial adaptation status as well as the psychosocial adaptation process.

The Salutogenic Model of Health

Antonovsky (1996) developed the salutogenic model of health as an alternative view to pathogenesis by considering the total being as contributing to health maintenance, and health breakdown rather than disease having a purely external cause. *Breakdown* as a substitute term for disease situates health on the *health ease/disease continuum,* with low breakdown referring to the healthy end of the continuum. He describes four dimensions of breakdown (pain, functional limitation, prognostic implication, and action implication) and suggests that an individual's health can be profiled by scoring each of these dimensions (Antonovsky, 1972/1979).

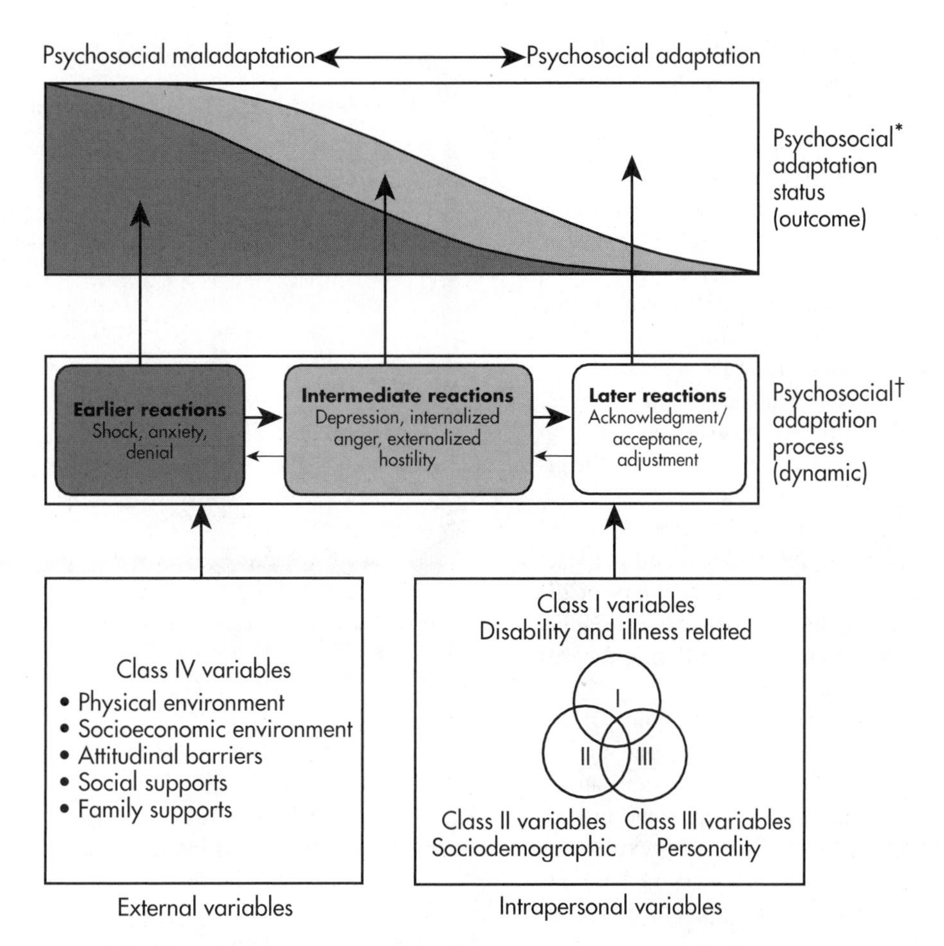

*Psychosocial adaptation status is an assessed outcome that ranges from unsuccessful or maladaptive functioning (dominance of earlier reactions such as anxiety, denial, depression, or anger) to successful or adaptive functioning (dominance of later reactions such as acknowledgment or acceptance, and behaviors reflecting adjustment such as those indicating positive self-esteem, adaptive coping, self-efficacy, and personal mastery)

†Psychosocial adaptation process can be viewed both *internally*, indicating a transition through psychosocial experiences and reactions in a phaselike process that is uniquely defined for each person, and *externally*, indicating a dynamic congruence or balance between the person's attributes, skills, and resources and environmental or community demands and requirements

Figure 12-1 A model of psychosocial adaptation to chronic illness and disability. (From Livneh, H., & Antonak, R.F. [1997]. *Psychosocial adaptation to chronic illness and disability.* Gaithersburg, MD: Aspen.)

The core concept of the model, *sense of coherence,* is thought to be closely related to a person's health. This concept is not about being in control; it is perceptual, having both cognitive and affective components. Antonovsky (1979) outlines psychological, social-structural, and cultural-historical sources of the sense of coherence and has developed a questionnaire to measure this concept (Antonovsky, 1987). The sense of coherence is "a generalized orientation towards the world which perceives it, on a continuum, as comprehensible, manageable and meaningful" (Antonovsky, 1996).

When confronted with a stressor, the person with a strong sense of coherence will (1) wish to or be motivated to cope (meaningfulness), (2) believe that the challenge is understood (comprehensibility), and (3) believe that resources to cope are available (manageability) (Antonovsky, 1996). "The strength of one's sense of coherence is determined by three types of life experience: consistency, underload-overload balance and participation in socially valued decision-making" (p. 15).

Life experiences shape the sense of coherence and that generalized resistance resources (GRRs) provide the person with sets of meaningful life experiences. A strong sense of coherence mobilizes the GRRs and specific resistance resources (SRRs) available to a person. Ubiquitous stressors create a state of tension that is managed by the GRRs and SRRs. Successful management of tension strengthens the sense of coherence and maintains the person's position on the health ease/disease continuum; when unsuccessful, a person is closer to the breakdown or disease end of the continuum at that time.

Responding to Threats to Self

Morse (1997) presented a comprehensive theory that incorporates human responses to acute illness, chronic illness, and injury. Despite differences in the onset and prognosis, "the pattern of responses to a threat to the integrity of the self has remarkable commonalities" (p. 28).

The model provides valuable insights into strategies clients employ as they move through each of the 5 stages: maintaining vigilance, enduring to survive, enduring to live, striving to restore self, and learning to live with the altered self.

Enduring and suffering exist on a continuum in the response to illness or injury but differ in nature and purpose. Enduring, associated with physical pain after injury or illness, continues once the physiological crisis passes. Enduring for survival shifts to enduring to live; suffering focuses on the implications of the event.

When clients' conditions improve to the point of acknowledging the illness or injury and recognizing the effects, the struggle of mourning what was lost and an altered future begins from release of fixation on the present and permits anticipation of a future. They may experience sudden, overwhelming emotion as they work to heal, resolve suffering, and make sense of the experience (Morse, 1997).

> Suffering is work, an all-consuming endeavor that one must experience to work through the event. Furthermore, suffering demands that horror be relived again and again, for in this process of reviewing the horror is recontextualized, revalued, resorted, and eventually resolved (Morse & Carter, 1995, p. 40).

Chronic Sorrow

The concept of chronic sorrow has been developed into a midrange theory with breadth of application to both single and group loss events. Olshansky (1966) developed the concept while counseling families with mentally retarded children. "Almost all families with mentally defective children experience what I call 'chronic sorrow,' which I feel is an understandable, non-neurotic response to a tragic fact. The sorrow is chronic and lasts as long as the child lives" (p. 21). Recurrent sorrow for the potential person is a response to loss that is continually redefined as new situations arise and as a trigger for sadness across the life span. The family experiences recurrent sadness when expected developmental milestones are not achieved (Lindgren, Burke, Hainsworth, & Eakes, 1992). Chronic sorrow may occur in persons with multiple sclerosis and their caregivers, and may be associated with many losses of the elderly (e.g., partner, friends, home, and good health).

Disparity is a key component of the process in the chronic sorrow model (Figure 12-2) (Eakes, Burke & Hainsworth, 1998). It is relevant for individuals experiencing losses as well as their family caregivers.

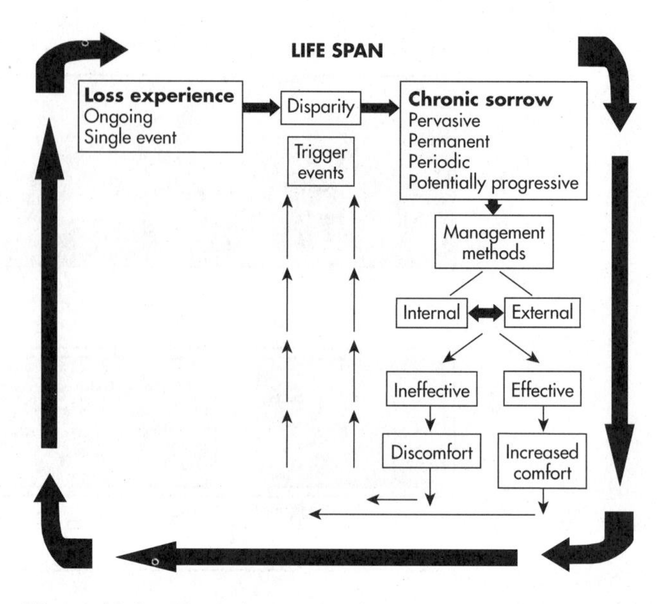

Figure 12-2 Theoretical model of chronic sorrow. (From Eakes, G.G., Burke, M.L., & Hainsworth, M.A. [1998]. Middle-range theory of chronic sorrow. *Image—Journal of Nursing Scholarship, 30*[2], 179-184.)

Family Adaptation

Families have a variety of structures including nuclear and extended families, single-parent, blended, gay/lesbian, and communal; and recently "empty-nest and return-to-the-nest syndromes" when young adults leave the parental home but return after a time (Youngblood, 1999, p. 135).

McCubbin, Thompson, Thompson, & McCubbin's work on family coping (1993) explains how the family's pattern of functioning is shaped by their appraisal of the situation. This appraisal takes place on three levels (Box 12-10).

A family schema and paradigm, influenced by the individual schema of the adult family members, develops over time and guides family behavior and interpretation of phenomena. The paradigm upheld may be questioned when crisis threatens its congruity and coherence. Family adaptation is complex.

> The roller-coaster course of adaptation is made difficult by the very nature of family systems that strive to achieve congruency among all levels of appraisal; congruency in paradigms among family members; congruency between the family's schema, paradigms, and the pattern of behavior families adopt to adapt to the situation; and a complementarity among coping strategies taken by family members (McCubbin et al., 1993, p. 249).

Chelsa (1999), using the McCubbin and McCubbin model of family stress, adjustment, and adaptation as a theoretical framework, studied how couples manage non–insulin-dependent diabetes. Central to their experience were the practical knowledge and skills required to live with and

Box 12-10 Levels of Family Appraisal

Level 1: Family's definition of the stressor or crisis precipitating event and its severity
Level 2: Family's paradigm or appraisal of the crisis situation (the family's appraisal that takes into account the stressor, community stigma, friends' reactions, extended family's reactions, social norms, husband's reaction, spouse's reaction, and their future expectations)
Level 3: Family's schemata or world view (shaped by the family's values, shared beliefs, goals, expectations, and priorities)

Data from McCubbin, H.I., Thompson, E.A., Thompson, A.I., & McCubbin, M.A. (1993). Family schema, paradigms, and paradigm shifts: Components and processes of appraisal in family adaptation to crises. In A.P. Turnbull, J.M. Patterson, S.K. Behr, D.L. Murphy, J.G. Marquis, & M.J. Blue-Banning (Eds.), *Cognitive coping, families, and disability* (p. 240). Baltimore: Paul H Brookes.

Box 12-11 Classes of Caregiver Coping

- Meaning-making
- Positive framing
- Avoidance/escape
- Emotional expression
- Optimistic future expectancies
- Pessimistic future expectancies
- Verbal symptom management
- Acceptance
- Wishful thinking
- Vigilance
- Emotional inhibition
- Humor
- Help seeking
- Behavioral symptom management

Data from Gignac, M.A.M., & Gottlieb, B.H. (1997). Changes in coping with chronic stress: The role of caregivers' appraisals of coping efficacy. In B.H. Gottlieb (Ed.), *Coping with chronic stress* (pp. 245-267). New York: Plenum Press.

manage the disease. The concept of attunement (i.e., skills in knowing and responding to the other person's concerns about diabetes) was elaborated. Two patterns of skill development emerged. First, some couples worked as a team to learn about the disease and make lifestyle changes. Alternatively, those with diabetes retained the knowledge about the disease and managed it independently; their partners were dissatisfied with their exclusion. Neither pattern proved better.

Caregiver Coping as Chronic Stress

Effective coping strategies are essential to manage the chronic stressors and demands of caregiving that are typically repetitive, persistent, and long-term, and may involve chronic sorrow.

Short-term coping strategies may prove ineffective over time, a role not predicted, anticipated, or believed. Reappraisal triggers alternative coping strategies as long-term coping becomes apparent. Caregivers' ongoing coping appraisal may alter the coping process and their perception of the situation or their care ability.

Content analysis of narrative accounts of coping from 91 caregivers yielded 14 classes of coping (Gignac & Gottlieb, 1997) as listed in Box 12-11.

Caregivers' appraisals of their coping fell into four categories: efficacious coping outcomes, nonefficacious coping outcomes, means/ends insights, and strategic planning. Caregivers appraised coping classes of symptom management, avoidance/escape, and help seeking that were aimed at problem solving and regulating and shaping the social interactions as effective. Emotional expression/inhibition and meaning making were frequently appraised as inefficacious. Caregivers reported not hiding their emotions. Caregivers' self-efficacy and feedback about the effectiveness of their actions are reflected in their appraisal (Gignac & Gottlieb, 1997).

Families' Explanations of Childhood Chronic Conditions

Families construct and share meanings about the stressful situation and the family identity and their world view that affect how they respond to stressful situations. Investigating culturally sensitive Hispanic-American, African-American, and European-American family explanations of their school-aged children's chronic illness or disability, researchers studied 63 families with children between 5 and 12 years of age who had chronic physical impairments. The explanations were categorized as biomedical explanations, environmental explanations, traditional beliefs, fatalistic beliefs, absence of known causes, or personal attribution (Garwick, Kohrman, Titus, Wolman, & Blum, 1999).

Biomedical explanations included genetic and prenatal factors, premature birth and physiological explanations, and trauma. Environmental explanations included cold air, dust, and cigarette smoke. Traditional explanations included spiritual and religious beliefs, folk beliefs, and a family curse. Fatalistic beliefs (high among Hispanic-Americans) included random and predetermined events. Personal attribution included caregiver blaming self or questioning personal responsibility for the child's condition (Garwick et al., 1999).

Once an understanding of how the condition came about was established, family resilience was associated with more effective coping for all explanations, except with caregiver blame.

Factors Influencing Appraisal and the Coping Process

Some persons cope better than others. Both personal and environmental factors influence appraisal of an event or situation and the response to that appraisal.

With a chronic, disabling, or developmental disorder, the physical, social, temporal, and economic environment in which the event takes place influence how the person and others associated with the person are affected, either directly or through the consequences of the event. Earlier in the chapter, variables in the disorder itself, the individual, and the physical and social environment were identified as influencing the appraisal of stress and the coping process. Characteristics of a sense of self-efficacy, hardiness, hope, learned resourcefulness, optimism, and coherence help persons resist the effects of stress (Lazarus, 1999). Uncertainty features throughout the coping literature.

Understanding these concepts helps rehabilitation nurses assist clients and families to appraise and respond to stress effectively. Identifying and assessing these characteristics in clients and families and planning interventions to strengthen them are skills. The concepts are discussed in the following section.

Hardiness

Hardiness, a constellation of stress-resistant tendencies, has been debated as a mediator between stress and adjustments. A long-standing view held hardiness to have three key dimensions: commitment, control, and challenge. Persons who exhibited commitment were actively involved in their own lives and expressed a sense of purpose or direction. Those who believed they could influence, perhaps not prevent, the way events in their life progressed were seen as having control, rather than feeling powerless. Similar to an internal locus of control, they viewed challenge as stimulating and necessary and as opportunity for personal growth or skills development (Kobasa, Maddi, & Kahn, 1982; Kobasa, Maddi, & Zola, 1983).

What is termed *hardiness* may influence how events are cognitively appraised and how coping occurs, thus enabling a person to effectively resist health threats arising from stressors. It would follow that persons with hardiness predictably resist illness, whereas persons who are vulnerable (i.e., have low hardiness) may have lowered resistance to stressors and increased health problems (Pollock, 1986, 1989).

Hardiness is a motivating factor for persons who exhibit strong psychosocial adjustment and problem-solving skills. Families who had a child with a developmental disability were able to maintain effective family coping, social networks, self-appraised satisfaction, and family integration when they had strong hardiness attributes (Failla & Jones, 1991).

Resilience, an ability to defuse a potential stressor into a nonstressor event, may be due in part to an ability to recover rapidly, or "bounce back." Those who view change as opportunity while valuing commitment and enjoying challenge, along with a sense of humor, tend to "bounce back" from loss or failure (Kobasa, 1979; Kobasa et al., 1983). They seek change and thrive on it (Orr & Westman, 1990).

Three themes in family life combine to breed hardiness in children: (1) children who receive interest, encouragement, and acceptance from the parents "come to view self and the world as interesting and worthwhile" (Maddi & Kobasa, 1991, p. 246); (2) children sense they can influence their environments when they have mastered tasks with moderate difficulty; and (3) children learn to appraise change as challenge, not chaos, when their parents see change as "interesting and developmentally valuable" (p. 248) and communicate this to their children. Not related to socioeconomic status, once hardiness has developed, children take it into their adult lives.

Hope

Rees and Joslyn (1998) explain that hope can be generalized to mean that things will improve, or it can be a specific client goal (e.g., being able to walk again). The opposite of despair, hope can be a coping strategy, an emotion, a feeling, a conviction or experience, or a personal attribute. In a study of 77 clients with spinal cord injuries, higher levels of hope were associated with higher levels of social support and self-esteem (Piazza et al., 1991).

Morse and Doberneck (1995) explored hope with clients awaiting heart transplant, clients with spinal cord injuries, breast cancer survivors, and breast-feeding mothers returning to work. The data revealed seven conceptual components of hope: realistic initial assessment of threat or predicament, envisioning of alternatives and setting of goals, bracing for negative outcomes, realistic assessment of personal resources and external conditions/resources, solicitation of mutually supportive relationships, continuous evaluation for signs that reinforce the selected goals, and determination to endure.

Learned Resourcefulness

Learned resourcefulness is a personality repertoire consisting of beliefs as well as self-control skills and behaviors that make a positive contribution to a person's health (Rosenbaum, 1990). This effect is twofold: "(a) coping with the physical discomforts that are caused either by illness or by painful medical procedures and (b) adoption of and adherence to health behaviors" (p. 17).

Persons who are highly resourceful use redressive self-control strategies to cope with physical discomfort. These consist of behaviors to regulate the internal responses, such as emotions, pain, and thought, to restore homeostasis (Rosenbaum, 1990). Reformative self-control is used to guide behavior change (e.g., smoking cessation, diet modification, and maintenance of an exercise program).

Optimism

Optimism is associated with the expectation of a good outcome as optimists make the best of whatever situation. They are more likely to use problem-focused coping strategies because they expect a positive change. Pessimists, preoccupied with their emotions, try to deny the reality of the stressor and may give up (Scheier & Carver, 1987).

Downe-Wamboldt and Melanson (1998) found older persons with arthritis used optimistic coping strategies when the stressor was appraised as a challenge, and this enhanced psychological well-being.

Uncertainty

Uncertainty, the inability to determine the meaning of illness-related events, occurs in situations where the decision maker is unable to assign definite values to objects and events and/or is unable to accurately predict outcomes because sufficient cues are lacking (Mishel, 1990, p. 256).

According to uncertainty theory, the two appraisal processes used are inference and illusion. On the basis of previous similar situations, an individual's inferences may appraise the uncertainty as an opportunity or as a danger. Illusion facilitates the construction of a positive outlook (Mishel, 1990). Conscious illusion may have value as an effective coping strategy, not a defense mechanism when a belief in one's own ability serves as the catalyst for effective responses to a stressor (Brown, 1993).

Uncertainty about progress and outcome in chronic, disabling, or developmental disorders is a troublesome but familiar concept in rehabilitation. Bailey and Nielsen (1993) studied the experience of 23 women with rheumatoid arthritis living with continual uncertainty. Women who perceived high levels of uncertainty concerning immobility, pain, or impaired functional abilities after rheumatoid arthritis may appraise uncertainty as danger. If correct, an appraisal of danger would increase anxiety, fear, physiological responses, and ineffective coping behaviors.

Certainty and predictability are valued in Western cultures where persons are uncomfortable with not knowing what to expect and with not knowing how to influence what is expected. Preferred thinking is linear, organized, controlled, and precise. Valued traits are self-efficacy, control, goal direction, and time management, whereas not knowing when or how is less acceptable. Thus when clients face chronic, disabling, or developmental disorders that have uncertain outcomes, they initially want to know how to cure the problem to counteract system breakdown. When chaotic rhythms (Mishel, 1990) are used to illustrate the nature of uncertainty, clients may be able to shift their paradigms to think in terms of possibilities, diversity, randomness, or nonlinear relationships.

Uncertainty as a concept has gained international interest. Nyhlin (1990) used a qualitative approach to learn how persons who had diabetes mellitus accompanied by severe complications dealt with uncertainty of outcome. Basic coping strategies used by clients were normalizing their lives, explaining events in their lives to make sense of the situation, coming to terms with their changing status, accepting increased dependence on the health care system, and adjusting while "keeping going" despite uncertainty and related barriers. Overall these persons managed well within their limitations.

An unexpected but important finding was that some uncertainty was introduced needlessly into clients' lives by policies or routines embedded in the health system. Attention to the uniqueness of each client's entire system, rather than illness alone, was suggested for improving coping effectiveness.

For clients recovering from lower limb fracture, uncertainty persisted past the initial trauma, through the hospitalization, and continued after discharge (Griffiths & Jordan, 1998). For these clients the uncertainty was associated with pain, insufficient information from health professionals, concerns about the effectiveness of the treatment, fear of falling, and concerns about making the injury worse. "They coped with this period of uncertainty by positive attempts to gain control over their situations, guided by an over-riding desire to 'return to normal'" (Griffiths & Jordan, 1998, p. 1276).

The quality of information available to a person has been associated with uncertainty by Babrow, Kasch, and Ford (1998). Lack of clarity, concerns about accuracy, concerns about completeness, the volume of information, ambiguity and inconsistency of information, applicability of the information, and lack of confidence in the source of the information were associated with evaluations about the quality of information. Rehabilitation nurses can, and should, address all these issues.

Coping and Emotions across the Life Span

Decades of research studies report the importance of understanding the changing patterns of coping across the life span associated with age and sex. Individuals can be readily categorized into various stage-related life trajectories that depict the typical experiences and stressors for that group. However, Lazarus (1996) warns that what has been observed in these studies is largely governed by time and culture. He suggests that a more useful way of looking at this problem is to consider the influence of the changing life context on coping and argues that we should take a more individualized and concrete approach to the exploration of how persons cope as they age.

Nonetheless, it is worthwhile to note some examples of work that has been done. These will help extend our understanding of coping for various groups across the life span, while we keep in mind that generalizations and stereotyping should be avoided.

Neonates

Field (1991) suggests that stress and coping probably start at conception, since fetal stress can be reduced by reducing maternal anxiety during pregnancy. Nonnutritive sucking on a pacifier and natural stroking of the infant were demonstrated to reduce neonatal intensive care unit stressors.

Infants and Young Children

Infants who display distress, as with crying or fussing, are presumed to be experiencing stress. Infants cannot communicate the detail of their appraisal to others in any other way than by behavioral evidence of physical, psychological, or environmental discomfort. We can sometimes infer the nature or source of that discomfort; however, overprotection may prevent opportunities to learn coping. Overexposure of infants to stress is undesirable (Karraker & Lake, 1991).

Very young infants, including those of very low birth weight, who were born prematurely, or are medically fragile, may be at increased risk of overexposure. Hoeman (1992) notes that stimulation that benefits the uncompromised infant (e.g., from light, sound, changing clothes, or being held) may be stressful for a premature or very low birth weight infant. Their families may experience chronic sorrow and uncertainty about the future for their infant, themselves, and their other children.

Adolescence

Rehabilitation nurses work with adolescents as clients and as family members. Coping with chronic, disabling, or developmental disorders occurs within the adolescent context, a flurry of physical and psychosocial changes. Psychosocial development enables adolescents to expand their world view to encompass global issues and plan for their future, while leaving them vulnerable to stressors over which they have no sense of control.

A major life event, buildup of multiple stressors, or world events stretch the coping resources of adolescents. Technology, illicit substances, freedom of expression, multiple career choices, public violence, and confrontation of moral values are stressors. Concerns for the preservation of the environment, high-technology wars, and natural disasters are greater stressors to adolescents than commonly realized. Adolescents may be reluctant to share their concerns or hopes with persons other than their peers. Personalized stressors may have undesirable consequences.

Suicide, the ultimate expression of hopelessness, is a global concern for adolescents and is correlated with stressors from chronic conditions and life events (Greene, Werner, & Walker, 1992). Holistic assessment focuses on the individual and developmental stage, not on the disease or disability; some ineffective coping behaviors are due to illness or disability.

To add complexity, symptoms or complications of chronic conditions may progress, diminish, or reappear along with varying changes (Keller & Nicolls, 1990). Chapters 4 and 28 contain additional information about clients and suicide.

It follows that there would be differences in how those in adolescent substages use coping skills to participate in care, manage their care, and learn about their condition. However, in practice, these discriminations may not be clear without careful assessment. In a study examining how preadolescents and adolescents cope with insulin-dependent diabetes mellitus, younger persons displayed more overt verbal behaviors such as yelling and arguing. Older adolescents, who had a wider range of freedom, began avoidance behaviors associated with poor internal control such as smoking, drinking alcohol, or staying away from home. Some adolescents may have acquired traumatic injuries as a result of previous ineffective coping with stressors and now face stressors from the disability (Grey, Cameron, & Thurber, 1991).

Hertzberg (1999) explains that rebellion in adolescents with chronic or disabling conditions may take the form of rebellion against medical regimens as well as parental authority. Particularly at risk are adolescents with spina bifida or spinal cord injury who are prone to urinary tract infections, pressure areas, and incontinence as a result of poor self-care behaviors.

Adolescents who had cystic fibrosis and their parents offered projections about the adolescent's life plans. Regardless of uncertainty about progression of the cystic fibrosis, adolescents projected plans significantly farther ahead, possibly due to an emerging self-identity. Adolescents and families worked through the illness at differing paces, but each group's responses were consistent with trajectory patterns for chronic illness (Yarcheski, 1988).

Transitions

Transitions between various levels of services—whether early intervention into preschool or, for adolescents, into university or vocational training programs—signal adjustment to a new stage. As persons with disabilities develop, they may have difficulty locating health professionals who will manage their care. For example, a child may visit a developmental pediatrician and work with an interdisciplinary team until reaching adolescence or young adulthood. Then "too old" for the pediatric team, they find adult or family practitioners are neither trained nor comfortable providing their care. The system becomes another source of stressors.

Coping strategies are needed on multiple levels when clients may themselves be caring for aging parents, supporting their young adult children and perhaps grandchildren, as well as negotiating their own health status. As they near the midpoint in their lives, additional chronic or disabling conditions may emerge. For example, persons with chronic conditions such as fibromyalgia or complications from untreated Lyme disease, or those who seek restorative care after cancer surgery or require specialized care skills for renal or burn care, must develop coping strategies for consequences of conditions with little-known trajectories.

Young Women

Gramling, Lambert, and Pursley-Crotteau (1998) found women aged 25 to 35 years used similar coping strategies. However, a developmental transition experienced around the age of 30 years resulted in "an ability to make accurate assessment concerning the nature of the problem and her coping abilities" (p. 1089), structured by life experience.

Older Persons

The growing aging population may be challenged with comorbidity, reemerging syndromes, or sequela diseases, and experience unique stressors.

Consider those who survived poliomyelitis in childhood only to develop postpolio syndrome as adults. Whatever coping strategies they used during and after the initial manifestation of the disease may now be threatened. Stress arises from potential loss of functional ability and independence, role changes, relationship strains, economic hardship, or worsening of symptoms. The person not only ages but ages with sequelae to a disabling condition that was thought to be arrested.

Although aging is associated with inevitable social, physical, and psychological decay (Lazarus, 1996), "successful aging depends on the acquisition of attitudes and coping processes that permit an aging person, despite increasing deficits or the threat of them, to remain independent, productive, and socially active for as long as possible" (Lazarus, 1998, p. 122). Older persons do not share a universal experience of hopelessness and despair. Lazarus (1996) proposes the focus on age be removed and be replaced with a focus on changes in coping that occur in response to the changing social, physical, and psychological contexts of life.

Older Mothers of Dependent Adults

Krauss and Seltzer (1993) studied the coping strategies of older mothers of adults with retardation. In a longitudinal study of 462 American families with mothers at least 55 years old, Krauss and Selter (1993) found that the use of adaptive coping strategies was much more common than the use of maladaptive strategies. Adaptive strategies used by the mothers included acceptance, positive reinterpretation, and growth, turning to religion and planning.

Family Life Cycle

Newby (1996) explained that families usually experience a life cycle featuring periods of family closeness and family distancing. Chronic disease, with its uncertainty and role changes, may pull families closer. This pull, however, may conflict with the current family cycle and lead to increased stress.

APPLICATION OF THEORY TO REHABILITATION NURSING PRACTICE

Assessment

Assessment relative to coping with chronic, disabling, or developmental disorders determines the client's and family members' needs and directs the nursing response. Many and varied needs require nurses to monitor the client and family, plan nursing interventions, refer to the team or community resources, and form mutual creative solutions.

Triage is appropriate when certain aspects of a client's situation are clearly associated with unbearable distress. Prioritizing interventions to facilitate clients' comfort (physical, social, psychospiritual, or environmental) may enable them to participate in the rehabilitation program and life in general.

Assessment of effectiveness in coping is a complex, multidimensional process that encompasses cognitive, affective, and psychomotor domains. Developing rapport and trust with the client and family who are experiencing times of great vulnerability takes time. A comprehensive database for each client includes and values information about preferences, goals and hopes, frustrations and fears. Especially important for clients with cognitive and communication impairments, the life before the current situation has purposes in relation to the functional health pattern of coping-stress tolerance. Knowledge of the client's previous lifestyle:

- Tells us about the client's likes and dislikes and preferred activities.
- Helps us to consider the possible consequences of the current situation for the client's life.
- Alludes to concerns that the client may have but is not verbalizing.
- Uncovers details of unresolved conflicts of concern to the client.
- Provides information about important roles, activities, persons, or pets that can be used by the nurse to establish links for clients about what is happening now and for the rest of their lives.
- Provides valuable cues to be used when exploring the consequences of the current situation and planning for discharge and the future

The history of the current situation may provide insight into the client's knowledge about the condition, prognosis, and management, while details of the acute situation and its management may explain client or family responses. Assessment incorporates the primary and secondary appraisals described by Lazarus and Folkman (1984):

- Has the client appraised the event/situation as a harm or loss, a threat, a challenge, or a benefit?
- What has the client decided might or can be done about the event/situation?
- What personal and environmental variables are relevant?
- What meanings have been associated with the situation by the client?
- What emotions is the client been experiencing?
- What problem-focused coping efforts has the client put in place?
- What emotion-focused coping efforts has the client put in place?
- Does the client believe he or she is capable of coping with the current situation?
- Does the client evaluate his or her coping strategies as effective?

For us to understand how the current situation came about, the client or family member needs to tell us. Reliving the event may itself be stressful for the client or family member. This should not necessarily be viewed as a negative experience, in light of Park and Folkman's (1997) work on reappraisal and meaning-making. Persons seek to make sense of what is happening and search for meaning by reappraising the situation and its significance. Providing an opportunity for the client and family to tell their stories may be therapeutic.

Using a variety of sources (e.g., eyewitness accounts, newspaper articles, and medical reports) to reconstruct the event will enhance the completeness and accuracy and assist the client or family to gain a more complete understanding of the event.

The assessment of coping needs to be informed by an accurate interpretation of the emotions experienced by the individual. Lazarus' (1991) core relational themes for each emotion can be used as a framework to interpret emotions from the stories of clients and their families (Lazarus, 1991, p. 122).

The needs of individuals and groups will be many and varied. To meet these, rehabilitation nurses need to approach their role with a genuine desire to understand individual perspectives and experiences and a commitment to respect the individuals. Listen to everything you are told and interpret what you see. Every piece of information helps to piece together a picture of the complex situation faced by a client and/or family and to identify the coping strategies chosen in response to that situation.

Assessment of Coping Effectiveness in the Individual

History and Subjective Data. A history is used to assess a clients' effectiveness in coping, including insight into their appraisal of stressors, underlying meanings, emotions, and ways of coping. The following section contains suggestions and sample queries for eliciting subjective data about coping effectiveness during the course of therapeutic conversation between nurse and client or family.

Suggestions

- An interview may include questions to elicit a client's descriptions of beliefs about health and illness, potential causes of the condition, remedies that have been tried, what will help, who can or should help improve things, and how long before relief is expected.
- Parents or significant caregivers may report data for infants or persons with impaired communication or cognition. However, ascertain reliability of the person's report and validate with other assessment data from the individual, family, or social system.
- Select a model for assessment or combine several. Begin by asking clients about their perceptions of what are personal stressors, what strategies they use in coping, and what emotions they are experiencing.
- What is the developmental stage, both individual and family? Draw a health and social genogram to depict family patterns, identify resources, or pinpoint difficulties with adjustments during life transitions, events, or happenings.

Sample Queries

- Sample queries include the following. What was the nature and extent of the loss? What does this situation or event mean to you? Have you or your family or friends experienced similar events before? If so, what did you do? Are these resolved, recurrent, or unresolved? How does your family handle stressful events or situations?
- Who was or is involved or affected? What is your role in this event? What do you think you are able to do about it?
- What has changed specifically due to this loss or event? For example, ask about changes in lifestyle, role relationships, health, self-perception including body image, occupation, functional independence, social system, quality of life, behavioral patterns, financial status, attitude or world view, and vocation or education.
- If you could change three things now, what would they be and why were these selected? What do they mean to you?
- Describe what is stressful to you. How would you describe your feelings; are you anxious or fearful? Do you feel helpless or hopeless? How would you describe the way you typically handle stressful situations or deal with loss? (After the client responds ask about the use of alcohol or controlled substances; other addictive responses such as food or sexual activity; diversional activities; exercise; and emotive behaviors such as crying, anger, acting out, and leaving/withdrawal.) Do you engage in these behaviors now?
- What do you think will happen as a result of this stress or this event? What are your major concerns other than this stressor?
- Do you have a lot of daily hassles? How do you respond to annoyances? What is most important to you at this time?
- How will this event affect your worth as an individual; who else will be affected by this?
- Why do you think this event happened? Are you or someone else able to control what is happening, or is there anything that can be done to change things? What kind of control do you believe you have over what happens?
- Do you believe you know enough about what has occurred? Are you uncertain about any aspect of the situation or your condition? Where do you go for help and for information? Has this event affected your ability to make decisions or the way in which you make decisions? Have others questioned your decisions more than usual; what do they propose you to do?
- How have you and/or your family managed? What have you tried? Who or what is helpful to you? What do you think will be helpful to you now? Are there things you believe you should not do or things you must do?
- What will be the greatest difficulty for you since this stress or event has occurred? How would you have described another person with your (condition or injury) before your now being in this situation? Are you concerned about how

others will view or respond to you, who may reject you, or what others may say about you? What would you call someone like yourself?

- Will you be able to follow the medical and health care plan? Can you perform or direct your own care? Do you have a caregiver or attendant? Do you have questions about your condition or care plan? What do you envision for your future (next day, week, or year, as appropriate)?
- Do you have pain? Since the event have you experienced difficulty or changes in patterns of sleeping; eating; grooming; handling sexuality; working; concentrating; communicating; performing self-care skills; or dealing with emotions, thoughts, physical functions or sensations, or other feelings?
- What are environmental stressors or barriers for you?
- What are your specific strengths and resources? Examples include family, pets, sense of humor, sense of control and self-determination, religious faith, education, income or employment, living arrangement, assistive devices or equipment, interests or hobbies, service agency supports, an acceptable caregiver, other social supports, and personal goals with hope.

Objective Data. Objective data obtained by examination, observation, inspection, and direct report are correlated with subjective, psychosocial data.

- Verify medications, health products, or therapeutic items.
- Elicit the person's description and definition, or denial, of the stressor event. Note whether the person is able to describe concerns in present sense, use proactive approaches, or verbalize need for assistance. Assess whether the person is able to depict the situation and roles of self and others accurately.
- Observe affect; alertness and mood; or nonverbal signs such as crying, lack of eye contact (unless culturally inappropriate), withdrawal responses, irritability or anger, inappropriate behavior, nervous manifestations (e.g., picking, twitching, or tapping), or signs of socioemotional deprivation. A child may sleep, suck the hands or toys, avoid response, or engage self in play; attempt several observations apart from clinical examination, such as in the playroom or with other children while in the waiting area. For older clients ensure that they are not tired or hungry from traveling, waiting, or needing medications before assessment.
- Inspect physical appearance for poor grooming or hygiene, bruises, cuts, hair pulling, or other nervous self-inflicted injuries; assess for abuse or neglect by others. Observe gums and mucosa for biting lesions.
- Assess self-destructive manifestations such as weight gain or loss, eating disorders, substance abuse, changes in health maintenance, or self-reported actions.
- Measure weight, vital signs, and blood pressure.
- Conduct a review of systems referring to the following list of signs or symptoms that have been associated with ineffective coping responses; this list is not exhaustive. All signs or symptoms are evaluated in the context of the whole person and family.

Physical Data Regarding Effective Coping. Possible physical manifestations of stressors are racing pulse, palpitations, dizziness or fainting, shortness of breath, hyperventilation, nausea, indigestion, "burping," refluxlike symptoms, burning sensations, changes in tongue or mucosa, difficulty swallowing, constipation, diarrhea, irritable bowel signs, urinary frequency, localized itching, headache, pain or geographic pain, "nervous twitches," fatigue, neck ache, posture, grinding or clenching teeth, or skin eruptions.

Acute episodes such as strep throat have been found to follow stressful events; chronic conditions such as arthritis or lupus may be exacerbated with stress.

Evaluate sensory manifestations such as ability to concentrate, memory loss, confusion, changes in speech patterns, changes in communication style or amount, depressive reactions, pain or discomfort, altered hearing, or visual disturbances. Compare assessment with data about location, severity, duration, and type of injury or impairment.

Inspect injured area, altered or impaired body part, or functional disability. Concurrently assess the client's perception of body image and whether the client looks at his or her body or withdraws, verbal comments, and destructive or inappropriate mood swings.

Assessment of Coping Effectiveness in Family Systems

An early assessment of the family is essential to effective coping, growth, and future goal setting. Family genograms with psychosocial entries, assessment of open versus closed boundaries, identified problems or concerns, and recent loss or change provide important family data. Although rehabilitation nurses commonly work one-on-one with a client, the nursing process and outcome must be based on each person as a part of a family, social network, and community system. All family members experience some degree of risk when the system is threatened by illness or disability. This is especially critical when the client is a child.

Most families experience multiple stressors from various sectors of their lives. Stressors may occur simultaneously; family members develop at different stages, hold unique appraisals, and have personal response times and coping styles. Few families analyze their management style, patterns of communication or action, or coping strategies in preparation for a crisis event. In fact, it may be difficult for a family under great stress to identify and mobilize their resources and strengths. Families may be dysfunctional before the stressor event at hand or overwhelmed by the situation. Criteria indicating a family system has maladjusted coping behaviors include regular neglect (even denial) of client's care, family duties, or responsibilities. Communication among family members may exhibit irritability, resentment, criticism, and frequent arguments. Physical symptoms, anxiety, emotional responses, and feelings of being overwhelmed may occur for any family member (Power, 1985).

Many older adults return to the community after a stay in a hospital or rehabilitation facility with functional or cognitive impairments that require them to live with family members. Family systems may become dysfunctional when family members become caretakers for an older family member who has a disability or chronic condition and are overburdened with responsibility or lack caring warmth. They may lack knowledge about the client's care, condition, or resources. Some caregivers may deny their own health needs or delay seeking care. Unresolved conflicts may emerge, overshadowing care decisions and excluding the client from decision making (Kemp, 1986). Ideally, rehabilitation nurses will forge collegial relationships with community health nurses or serve as consultants in the community. In these roles nurses can use results of home assessments and family system evaluations as a basis for working with clients to develop preventive interventions and plans to improve outcome for clients and families.

Other signals may alert a nurse that an individual family member (or system) may collapse or is breaking down. Several or many of the indicators listed in Box 12-12 may appear.

Caregiver Coping

The role of caregiver may be a chronic stressor. The demands are typically repetitive, persistent, and long-term. In addition, the caregiver is commonly in a close relationship with the recipient of care and may be experiencing chronic sorrow. To make their situation manageable, caregivers must use effective coping strategies.

When the role of caregiver was first undertaken, the long-term nature of the role may not have been predicted, anticipated, or believed. Coping strategies that were chosen for their short-term effectiveness may quickly become ineffective as time passes. The process of coping outlined earlier from the work of Lazarus and Folkman (1984) depicts a cycle of repetitions of cognitive and/or behavioral efforts followed by reappraisal. Reappraisal becomes the trigger for the choice of alternative coping strategies, especially as the long-term and demanding nature of the role becomes apparent. Gignac and Gottlieb (1997) highlight the importance of ongoing coping appraisal by the caregiver. These appraisals may alter the coping process, their perception of the situation, or their perception about their own ability as a caregiver.

Box 12-12 Indicators of Potential Individual Breakdown

- Chronic fatigue
- Anger leading to cynical, sarcastic, or irritable behavior
- Impatience and exhaustion
- Anxiety and fears bordering on paranoia
- Disturbed sleep and rest patterns
- Distress in role relationships
- Illness and accidents or injuries
- Maladaptive behaviors such as depression, substance abuse, avoidance or isolation, inattention to personal care, or eating disorder
- Potential for suicide
- Depleted or inaccessible resources
- Perception of few options

Warning

The nursing assessment assumes that the appropriateness and effectiveness of coping undertaken by individuals, families, or communities can actually be assessed by a person other than the individual. Accurate assessment may not always be possible.

The particular problem-focused or emotion-focused strategies are assessed to determine whether they have been used to achieve the function for which they were chosen: that is, aimed at managing harms, threats, and challenges (problem focused); or managing the emotional reaction to the harm or threat (emotion focused). Neither are defined as outcomes (Lazarus, 1996).

The three types of outcomes of coping that have been identified are long-term in nature—"functioning in work and social living, morale or life satisfaction, and somatic health" (Lazarus & Folkman 1984, p. 181). During assessment, the rehabilitation nurse interprets a person's coping history based on the identified long-term outcomes of coping and evaluates the person's responses to the current stress or stressors (associated with the chronic, disabling, or developmental disorder). These data determine the appropriate nursing diagnoses and response.

Development of Assessment Skills

Working with clients and their families as they experience chronic, disabling, or developmental disorders, nurses develop a generic understanding of the impact of these disorders on their lives. Many differences exist in the extent to which individuals appraise a situation as taxing in relation to their resources. An equally wide range of human responses to stress and adversity are governed by expectations related to sex, age, religion, ethnicity, or culture. Many are simply individual differences.

To help nurses gain a deeper appreciation of these differences, a number of alternative sources complement scientific writings. For instance, reading biographical and autobiographical accounts of experiences of disability and illness (written from the perspective of persons of persons living with them) helps in understanding human responses to chronic, disabling, or developmental disorders.

Nursing Diagnoses

Nursing diagnoses are identified after interpretation of the assessment data that may take additional time to collect for a comprehensive database. This is particularly relevant in the coping-stress-tolerance functional health pattern, where the time-intensive processes of developing rapport and trust are key to information sharing.

The nursing diagnoses chosen are those identified by Gordon (2000) for the functional health pattern of coping-stress-tolerance. Nursing diagnoses relevant to the *client* are outlined in Box 12-13; nursing diagnoses relevant to the *family* are in Box 12-14; and nursing diagnoses relevant to the community are in Box 12-15.

Once the nursing diagnoses have been identified appropriate nursing outcomes and the intervention required to achieve those outcomes need to be selected. A selection of the nursing diagnoses identified by Gordon (2000) for the coping-stress-tolerance health pattern have been matched to the nursing outcomes and nursing interventions presented by Johnson, Maas, and Moorhead (2000) and McCloskey and Bulechek (2000). These are presented in Table 12-1.

Goal Setting

Mutual goal setting is a foundation stone of successful rehabilitation. The purpose of rehabilitation goals is to guide the rehabilitation process. Rehabilitation is a process experienced and owned by clients (Pryor, 1999a), and when clients own their rehabilitation goals, they are much more likely to perceive that they have the capabilities to achieve those goals and strive toward them.

Client participation in the rehabilitation process should be facilitated through the establishment of a partnership between the rehabilitation nurse and the client. Goal setting is an ideal vehicle for the establishment of that partnership. The goals must be relevant to the client as well as the domains of expertise of the rehabilitation professionals.

Broad goals that may enhance goal setting and guide rehabilitation nursing practice include maximizing self-determination, restoring function, and optimizing lifestyle choices (Pryor, 1999b).

Client goals are usually linked to what matters to them. Lambert (1999) tells how a young man clearly articulated his need to deal with his loss following an above-knee amputation before he learned amputation care. In a review of the literature on clients' experiences of stroke, Hafsteinsdottir and Grypdonck (1997, p. 585) concluded that "the stroke patient often has clear goals for himself in relation to functional abilities, against which he measures all success and forward progress in his rehabilitation." Rehabilitation nurses need to clearly relate the steps on the way with the client's personal goals, especially since the steps on the way are often the health provider's focus. Mutual goal setting may provide opportunity to explain the roles of rehabilitation team members and how each contribute toward achieving the client's goals (Kirkevold, 1997).

All the client's goals may influence the effectiveness of the chosen coping strategies. Rehabilitation goals must be achievable; those the client perceives as unrealistic may act as deterrents to client participation and become stressors. Goal setting may be a vehicle for fostering hope and harnessing motivation.

Recall that self-efficacy is considered to have a positive effect on a person's ability to cope with stressors (Lazarus, 1999) and that children will develop a sense that they can influence their environments when the tasks they have encountered have been mastered with moderate difficulty (Maddi & Kobasa, 1991). When clients perceive they have a good chance of achieving their goals, they are more likely to achieve them.

The importance of the relationship between rehabilitation nurses and their clients cannot be overstressed because goal setting is about negotiation (Jones, O'Neill, Waterman, & Webb, 1997; Keatinge, 1998). Community nurses in one study demonstrated that goal setting is "a matter of balancing the realistic with the desired, the professional view with the lay view, and the objective plan with subjective motivation" (Lawler, Dowswell, Hearn, Forster, & Young, 1999, p. 408).

Goals should facilitate the ability of families or individuals to:

- Activate strengths and resources
- Remove barriers to effective coping
- Establish health maintenance and safety programs
- Identify and resolve issues
- Gain access or referral to resources, services, and activities that promote independence
- Prevent further disability or complications
- Rectify knowledge deficits and enhance capabilities
- Be involved and empowered in planning and decision-making processes
- Use culturally, developmentally, and personally appropriate intervention methods
- Develop coping responses/behaviors that lead to improved health outcomes

Nursing Outcomes

The ongoing work of the Iowa Outcomes Project is evidence that rehabilitation nurses must continue to demonstrate that they make a difference to the process and outcome of rehabilitation for their clients and their families. The identification of desired outcomes helps us clarify our goals and focus our efforts.

Outcomes from Johnson et al. (2000) that are relevant for the coping-stress-tolerance functional health pattern are many and varied. For the individual the relevant outcomes include the level 2 classes of psychological well-being; psychosocial adaptation; self-control; social interaction; health and life quality; and symptom status. For the family, relevant outcomes can be found in the level two classes of family caregiver status, family member health status, and family well-being under the domain of family health. The domain of community health is also relevant for rehabilitation nursing.

Table 12-1 includes a selection of nursing outcomes related to coping.

Box 12-13 Nursing Diagnoses Relevant for the Client

Ineffective Coping (Individual)

Diagnostic Cues

- Reports presence of life stress or problems (specify)
- Reports feeling anxious, apprehensive, fearful, angry, and/or depressed
- Expresses inability to cope or ask for help
- Uses defense mechanisms ineffectively or inappropriately (forms of coping impede adaptive behavior [see Avoidance Coping, Denial])

Defensive Coping

Diagnostic Cues

One or more of the following:

- Denial of obvious problems or weaknesses
- Projection of blame or responsibility
- Rationalization of failures
- Hypersensitivity to a slight or criticism
- Grandiosity

Impaired Adjustment

Defining Characteristics

- Disability or health status requiring change in lifestyle
- Failure to take actions that would prevent further health problems
- Demonstration of nonacceptance of health status change
- Failure to achieve optimal sense of control

Risk for Posttrauma Syndrome

Risk Factors

- Nonsupportive environment
- Inadequate social support
- Survivor's role in the event
- Exaggerated sense of responsibility
- Perception of event
- Duration of event
- Occupation (police, fire, rescue, corrections, emergency room staff, mental health provider)
- Displacement from home
- Diminished ego strength

Avoidance Coping (Not to Be Confused with Hope or Adaptive Denial)

Diagnostic Cues

- Perceives threat to health, self-image, values, lifestyle, or relationships
- Minimizes, ignores, or forgets information after clear communication or observation
- Mislabels events
- Does not use problem solving, information seeking, and incorporation of new information into future planning

Ineffective Denial or Denial

Diagnostic Cues

Unable to admit impact of disease or event on life pattern as manifested by one or more of the following:

- Delays seeking or refuses health care to the detriment of health; does not admit fear of death or invalidism; displaces fear of impact of the condition; has unrealistic plans
- Selectively integrates information
- Does not perceive danger or personal relevance of symptoms; minimizes symptoms or event

Support System Deficit

Defining Characteristics

One or more of the following:

- Lack of one or more persons who communicate positive regard about personal worth and competence
- Insufficient or absent social network to provide instrumental assistance (e.g., transportation, household tasks)
- Lack or unavailability of a confidant

Posttrauma Syndrome

Defining Characteristics

Reaction

- Intrusive thoughts
- Detachment
- Psychogenic amnesia
- Hypervigilance
- Substance abuse
- Compulsive behavior
- Avoidance
- Alienation
- Shame
- Guilt
- Grief
- Hopelessness
- Denial, repression

Emotional/cognitive

- Sadness
- Depression
- Anxiety, fear
- Horror
- Anger, rage, aggression
- Irritability
- Panic attacks
- Difficulty concentrating
- Flashbacks
- Exaggerated startle response

Physical

- Gastric irritability
- Neurosensory irritability, palpitations
- Headaches
- Enuresis (in children)

Sleep

- Intrusive dreams
- Nightmares

Box 12-14 Nursing Diagnoses Relevant for the Family

Compromised Family Coping

Diagnostic Cues

Client or another person expresses concern or complaint about significant other's response to client's health problem and one or more of the following:

- Significant person displays protective behavior disproportionate (too little or too much) to client's abilities or need for autonomy
- Significant person describes preoccupation with personal reactions (e.g., fear, guilt, anticipatory grief, anxiety) to client's illness, disability, or other situational or developmental crises
- Significant person describes or confirms inadequate understanding of knowledge base that interferes with effective assistive or supportive behaviors (specify)
- Significant person withdraws or enters into limited or temporary personal communication with client at time of need
- Significant person attempts assistive or supportive behaviors with less than satisfactory results

High-Risk Populations

- 24-Hour home care
- Home care with periodic health crises
- History of family life stresses

Disabled Family Coping

Diagnostic Cues

- Neglectful care of client in regard to basic human needs and/or illness treatment

And one or more of the following:

- Distortion of reality regarding client's health problem, including extreme denial about existence or severity (see also Denial)
- Intolerance
- Rejection
- Abandonment
- Desertion
- Performance of usual routines, disregarding client's needs
- Psychosomaticism
- Expression of client's signs of illness
- Decisions and actions by family that are detrimental to economic or social well-being
- Agitation, depression, aggression, hostility
- Impaired restructuring of a meaningful life for self, impaired individuation, prolonged overconcern for client
- Neglectful relationships with other family members
- Client's development of helpless, inactive dependence

High-Risk Populations

- 24-Hour home care
- History of family life stresses
- Home care with periodic health crises

Family Coping: Potential for Growth

Defining Characteristics

- Family member is moving in direction of health-promoting and enriching lifestyle that:
  —Supports and monitors maturational processes
  —Audits and negotiates treatment programs
  —Generally chooses experiences that optimize wellness
- Individual expresses interest in making contact on a one-to-one basis or on a mutual-aid group basis with another person who has experienced a similar situation
- Family member attempts to describe growth impact of crises on own values, priorities, goals, or relationships

Data from Gordon, M. (2000). *Manual of nursing diagnosis* (9th ed.). St. Louis: Mosby.

Nursing Interventions

Nursing inventions in the coping-stress-tolerance functional health pattern have two purposes: the promotion of effective appraisal and coping and the prevention of ineffective appraisal and coping. These are relevant to most of the 28 focal areas in the United States *Healthy People 2010* initiative that established national goals for health (*Healthy People* website, 2000).

Rehabilitation nurses are in an ideal position in their everyday client-nurse interactions to promote physical activity and fitness; a healthy diet; mental health; the safe use of food and drugs; and the reduction of unintentional injury, suicide, and violence. When health has been interrupted and clients are expending efforts toward rehabilitation, it is an opportune time to raise all aspects of health promotion. When focused on their current health breakdown, most clients appreciate the time taken to explain how they can contribute to their future health status. Rehabilitation nurses can address issues relevant to reducing the risk factors of many diseases, for example, diabetes, heart disease, and stroke.

Prevention and Monitoring of Stress and Coping

Prevention of health breakdown in general, and ineffective coping in specific, are integral components of the nursing response relating to the coping-stress-tolerance functional health pattern. Although nursing diagnoses are useful in the identification of problems, relying solely on nursing diagnoses may mean that the rehabilitation nurse's vital contribution to prevention is overlooked.

Accurate identification of the environment or resources needed by clients to support their coping efforts enables the rehabilitation nurse to support the client through considerations such as:

- The number of clients in one room
- Choice of roommates

Box 12-15 Nursing Diagnoses Relevant for the Community

Ineffective Community Coping

Defining Characteristics

- Community does not meet its own expectations
- Deficits in community participation
- Excessive community conflicts
- Expressed vulnerability
- Expressed community powerlessness
- High illness rate
- Stressors perceived as excessive
- Increased social problems (e.g., homicides, vandalism, arson, terrorism, robbery, infanticide, abuse, divorce, unemployment, poverty, militancy, mental illness)

Readiness for Enhanced Community Coping

Defining Characteristics

- Deficits in one or more characteristics that indicate effective coping
- Active planning by community for predicted stressors
- Active problem solving by community when faced with issues
- Agreement that community is responsible for stress management
- Positive communication among community members
- Positive communication between community and/or aggregates and larger community
- Programs available for recreation and relaxation
- Resources sufficient for managing stressors

Data from Gordon, M. (2000). *Manual of nursing diagnosis* (9th ed.). St. Louis: Mosby.

- Choice of preferred recreational, leisure, or social activities
- Peer support programs
- Family participation in therapy program
- Increasing flexibility in routines and protocols to facilitate involvement of family or friends
- Availability of quiet rooms as well as noisy social areas

Ongoing monitoring of the responses of the client and family members to the current situation will aid the early identification of increasing or overwhelming stress and appropriate interventions. In addition, when clients and their families know someone is monitoring their progress, their ability to cope may be enhanced. In a study of the effectiveness of nursing follow-up of rehabilitation clients after discharge, the treatment group had a higher prevalence of optimistic coping scores on the Jalowiec Coping Scale (Easton, Rawl, Zemen, Kwiatkowski, & Burczyk, 1995). The transition to home of this group was managed by an experienced rehabilitation nurse, and it was suggested that the higher scores "could be attributable to the security they felt in knowing that someone with specialized skills who was familiar to them would be there to assist" (p. 126).

In addition, the provision of timely information to clients has been demonstrated to reduce distress during health care procedures. Clark (1997) found clients who received concrete objective information before a procedure had fewer negative emotions commonly associated with procedures. Concrete objective information included the procedural steps, physical sensations, spatial information, and temporal information.

Promotion of Effective Appraisal and Coping

The nursing interventions identified in this section have been drawn from the Iowa Interventions Project (McCloskey & Bulechek, 2000). They are suggestive of some of the nursing interventions that may be chosen in response to a comprehensive assessment and the nursing diagnoses identified for an individual client or family member, family unit, or community. Individual nursing interventions commonly work to both prevent and promote.

Interventions for the coping-stress-tolerance functional health pattern would most likely be chosen from the level 2 classes of behavior therapy, cognitive therapy, communication enhancement, coping assistance, client education, psychological comfort promotion, crisis management, and risk management for the client. Many of these interventions will also be relevant for members of the client's family. In addition, the level 2 class of intervention, life span care, particularly targets the family. The community is targeted under community health promotion and community risk management. Table 12-1 includes a selection of nursing interventions relevant to coping.

Nursing interventions for cognitive restructuring, coping enhancement, hope instillation, touch, complex relationship building, and milieu therapy are discussed below. Because nursing interventions intended to enhance coping often are interrelated, self-awareness enhancement, goal setting, humor, emotional support, self-esteem enhancement, learning facilitation, active listening, and music therapy are incorporated in the discussion. (Italic type has been used to highlight these terms in the following sections.) In other chapters, spirituality and complementary therapies also are related.

Cognitive Restructuring. Cognitive restructuring is defined as "challenging a patient to alter distorted thought patterns and view self and the world more realistically" (McCloskey & Bulechek, 2000, p. 219).

When the primary appraisal of an encounter is determined as a harm/loss or threat (Lazarus & Folkman, 1984), a client may be unable to consider other possibilities. Similarly, during secondary appraisal, when a person considers that little or nothing can be done, a feeling of hopelessness may dominate the person's world view. Cognitive restructuring may be used in these instances to introduce to the client alternative ways of appraising the stressor and their

TABLE 12-1 Selected Nursing Diagnoses, Nursing Outcomes, and Nursing Interventions

Nursing Diagnosis	Nursing Outcomes Classification (NOC)	Nursing Intervention Classification (NIC)
Ineffective coping (individual)	Coping Hope Identity Self-esteem Depression level Will to live Acceptance health status Psychological adjustment: Life change Aggression control Anxiety control Fear control	Cognitive restructuring Self-awareness enhancement Mutual goal setting Coping enhancement Hope instillation Touch Milieu therapy Decision-making support Self-esteem enhancement Anger control assistance Emotional support Music therapy
Defensive coping	Acceptance of health status Coping Grief resolution Psychological adjustment: Life change Distorted thought control Mood equilibrium	Self-awareness enhancement Cognitive restructuring Coping enhancement Emotional support Active listening
Avoidance coping	Acceptance health status Coping Grief resolution Pain: Psychological response Psychological adjustment: Life change Anxiety control Depression control Distorted thought control	Coping enhancement Learning readiness enhancement Self-awareness enhancement Active listening Cognitive restructuring Learning facilitation Emotional support
Support system deficit	Loneliness Role performance Social interaction skills Social involvement Social support	Touch Complex relationship building Milieu therapy Self-awareness enhancement Support system enhancement Socialization enhancement
Family coping: Potential for growth	Caregiver life disruption Caregiver stressors Caregiver emotional health Caregiver well-being Family coping	Learning readiness enhancement Self-awareness enhancement Cognitive restructuring Learning facilitation Coping enhancement Emotional support Decision-making support

Data from Johnson, M., Maas, M.L., & Moorhead, S. (2000). *Nursing outcomes classification (NOC)* (2nd ed.). St. Louis: Mosby; McCloskey, J.C., & Bulechek, G.M. (2000). *Nursing interventions classification (NIC)* (3rd ed.). St. Louis: Mosby; and North American Nursing Diagnosis Association. (2001). *Nursing diagnosis: definitions and classification 2001-2002* (4th ed.). Philadelphia: Author.

ability to respond. This may mean reframing the stressor as a challenge and reviewing previous episodes of effective coping.

Newbold (1996) discusses the use of cognitive restructuring as an important nursing intervention to combat arthritis-helplessness in persons with rheumatoid arthritis. He suggests that nurses can help clients: (1) to recognize irrational beliefs they have about themselves by asking the clients to provide evidence to support their claims and verifying them with another source, (2) to produce statements of belief in self that help combat helplessness, and (3) to sustain positive behaviors over time.

Coping Enhancement. Coping enhancement is defined as "assisting a patient to adapt to perceived stressors, changes, or threats that interfere with meeting life demands and roles" (McCloskey & Bulechek, 2000, p. 234).

Nursing initiatives aimed at coping enhancement can be applied at the single client or family level and at a program level. At the client level, cognitive restructuring and motivation are easily identifiable components of coping enhancement. McCloskey and Bulechek (2000) include motivation under *self-awareness enhancement.*

Motivation is commonly associated with effective rehabilitation outcomes, and nurses are in the ideal position to positively influence client motivation. Brillhart and Johnson (1997) asked 12 persons with spinal cord injury how rehabilitation nurses helped motivate them. Five domains were identified as associated with motivation and coping. These were independence, education, socialization, *self-esteem,* and realization. Nurses were noted as making a positive contribution to these clients through *learning facilitation,* by treating them as individuals, by creating a comfortable environment in the rehabilitation ward, and by using a matter-of-fact approach to elimination.

Using a series of interviews with five women with an average age of 87 years in a rehabilitation ward, Resnick (1996) identified factors that increased motivation as well as factors that decreased motivation. Having *goals,* the use of *humor* by the staff, experiencing a sense of being cared for, being encouraged, believing in the staff and rehabilitation, and experiencing "power with" interactions with the staff were noted as promoting motivation. The provision of encouragement is one aspect of *emotional support* (McCloskey & Bulechek, 2000).

The factors that acted as demotivators included a client's beliefs about the necessity or appropriateness of rehabilitation, domination, and their responses to domination (Resnick, 1996). Domination was reported to take several forms. These included domination by physical force by others, domination by one's own body, domination by brainwashing from staff as well as from family, and domination by the rules and regulations of the rehabilitation setting. In response to these factors the women felt hopeless, devalued, voiceless, and fearful. Rehabilitation nurses must carefully monitor the cultural practices of rehabilitation to avoid these demotivators.

At the program level nurses have introduced a variety of initiatives demonstrated to enhance coping. When former rehabilitation clients continued to seek support from the inpatient rehabilitation team through ongoing phone contact, a formal nurse-managed follow-up program was begun. Using a randomized control trial, Rawl, Easton, Kwiatkowski, Zemen, and Burczyk (1998) implemented a follow-up program consisting of visits and telephone consultations. Although on discharge the anxiety scores of the two groups were similar, four months after discharge the 49 clients in the treatment group experienced significantly less anxiety.

Hope Instillation. Hope instillation is defined as "facilitation of the development of a positive outlook in a given situation" (McCloskey & Bulechek, 2000, p. 379).

Rehabilitation nurses interact with clients who experience feelings of fear, uncertainty, and loss of body control on a daily basis. Nurses contribute to the development of a positive outlook in a variety of ways. Hafsteinsdottir and Grypdonck (1997) linked the fostering of hope with the provision of information and emotional support after stroke.

Hope instillation needs to address the individual situation of the client. Rees and Joslyn (1998) noted that nurses can improve a client's level of hope by encouraging small successes, emphasizing potential rather than limitations, and providing encouragement to develop a sense of the possible. These findings are supported by a study of Australian rehabilitation nurses (Pryor & Smith, 2000). Empowerment can also be an important mechanism for instilling hope.

Uncertainty is a form of chronic stress (Wheaton, 1997) that needs to be addressed to develop a positive outlook. In a study by Close and Procter (1999) uncertainty was expressed by both clients and their carers after stroke. These clients "proactively, without explicit guidance, [built] supportive relationships and gain[ed] knowledge and information from those around" to counteract the uncertainty (p. 141). These findings clearly demonstrate client self-assessment and motivation to meet identified needs. Furthermore, clients and their families are not passive recipients of care awaiting their fate. Rehabilitation nurses must encourage client participation in rehabilitation.

Empowerment is "a process between a nurse and client designed to assist the client to develop proactive healthy behaviors" (Ellis-Stoll & Popkess-Vawter, 1998). The defining characteristics of empowerment are the acquisition of individualized knowledge of the client, *active listening,* and mutual participation by both the client and the nurse.

Our objectives in providing encouragement are "to help individuals identify consequences of their decisions, define purpose, spur vitality, overcome free-floating anxiety, and try new ways of living, rather then those that would otherwise maintain dependency" (Beck, 1994, p. 9). Encouraging clients in care of self (i.e., care that goes beyond physical care) is an essential component of rehabilitation nursing (Singleton, 2000). The nurses in this study used the development of client-nurse relationships as a vehicle to provide encouragement, and they manipulated their time to facilitate more communication with their clients.

Nurses have also focused on self-efficacy to encourage the client to have a positive outlook. Brown and Conn (1995) demonstrated that self-efficacy is a good predictor of walking in clients after coronary artery bypass surgery. They suggested that nurses could enhance self-efficacy by providing feedback to their clients about normal and abnormal physiological responses as they walked. On-the-spot feedback helps the client form an accurate evaluation of progress and set realistic goals. They also suggested that the nurses use a telephone follow-up service to continue the provision of feedback after discharge.

Touch. Touch is defined as "providing comfort and communication through purposeful tactile contact" (McCloskey & Bulechek, 2000, p. 669).

Once again, nursing initiatives involving touch need to be individually constructed and negotiated between the nurse and the client. Like empowerment, they need to be informed by knowledge of the individual client or family member.

Touch is associated with the provision of comfort. The nine themes of discomfort described by Morse, Bottorff, and Hutchinson (1994) provide a valuable framework for understanding the client's discomfort and developing comfort interventions. By determining the origins of discomfort (i.e., from the diseased body, the disobedient body, the vulnerable body, the violated body, the enduring body, the resigned body, the deceiving body, the betraying body, and/or the betraying mind, the rehabilitation nurse can best determine whether and how touch may provide comfort.

The difference between instrumental touch and affective touch has been demonstrated in a study by Caris-Verhallen, Kerkstra, and Bensing (1999). Instrumental touch is associated with a task undertaken by the nurse, and affective touch is spontaneous and not associated with a task. From 165 nursing encounters with elderly residents of a nursing home, they found that affective touch was associated with 40% of the encounters. These interventions were deliberate, but they were not time-consuming. They accounted for only about 1.5% of the total observation time. Rehabilitation nurses should incorporate individualized affective touch interventions into their everyday interactions with their clients.

Touch, however, is not always appropriate. Davidhizar and Giger (1997, p. 203) note that, "while touch has been described as the most important of all the senses, the astute health care professional must be cognizant of times when touch is not appropriate and when touch may distract from the development of a therapeutic and helpful relationship." Clients may hold negative interpretations of touch. Nurses are advised to be alert for clients' personal values concerning touch during interactions and modify their approach accordingly. A client's age, gender, and social or cultural affiliation affect the response to touch. Some persons may fear contracting disease through touch or be offended (Davidhizar & Giger, 1997).

Complex Relationship Building. Complex relationship building is defined as "establishing a therapeutic relationship with a patient who has difficulty interacting with others" (McCloskey & Bulechek, 2000, p. 227).

The client who appears isolated and alone is not an unusual phenomenon. Many clients feel no one can understand their situation. Emotions take over, and the ability to develop rapport with others is compromised by the overwhelming nature of the stressors. These clients are sometimes labeled difficult or unpopular.

Avoidance has been used by some nurses to manage difficult client behavior (Carveth, 1995), but this response is not uniform. In Carveth's study of 52 nurses, communication difficulties featured strongly in the list of difficult client characteristics. The findings of this study suggest that some nurses may have spent time trying to resolve the problems. Johnson & Webb (1995) also found evidence that although nurses label clients as unpopular for a variety of reasons, these labels are not predictive of care. Furthermore, their study indicated that these labels can be renegotiated.

Several studies have demonstrated the importance of the client-nurse relationship. Lo (1999) studied adherence to health regimens of persons with insulin-dependent diabetes. Although the study demonstrated that less stress seemed to facilitate the following of health regimens, the findings also indicated that the quality of rapport with their health professionals is crucial to client adherence. Mutual goal setting and care planning were identified as features of quality rapport.

The literature exposes a concern about clients who do not follow the advice of health professionals and health promotion campaigns, but further exploration of an individual's coping processes may reveal the complexity of the lived experience of compliance or adherence. Wichowski and Kubsch (1997) suggest that by not following recommended regimens, some adults may be able to avoid acknowledging their chronic illnesses. On the other hand, children who have had their disorders since birth or a young age are more likely to accept their health status as normal.

Denial, Lazarus (1999) points out, may be an effective coping strategy in some circumstances. "When nothing can be done to alter the illness or prevent further harm, denial may be beneficial" (p. 111). One teenager used denial effectively to avoid the reality of being having paraplegia by deciding to stay in bed for a day. In bed his deficits were not so visible. To the observer, he did not appear to have paraplegia.

Complex relationship building may be a slow process. Nurses must begin by ensuring realistic self-awareness of their own attitudes towards the client and proceed to develop rapport and trust by listening in a nonjudgmental and unhurried manner.

Milieu Therapy. Milieu therapy is defined as "use of people, resources, and events in the patient's immediate environment to promote optimal psychosocial functioning" (McCloskey & Bulechek, 2000, p. 456).

The creation of a physical and social environment that is rehabilitative for a particular individual is a complex undertaking in the inpatient setting. The creation of a rehabilitative milieu has been discussed by Pryor (2000) as a mechanism by which rehabilitation nurses can enhance the rehabilitation process for their clients. This will have a positive flow-on for the psychosocial well-being of clients and their families. The main ingredients that contribute to the rehabilitation process were identified as factors associated with the participants, the activities and the setting. Many of these, in particular ward routines, can be manipulated to enhance their effectiveness. Most importantly, the preservation of an individual client's identity has been identified as an important aspect of the rehabilitation process.

Kirkevold (1997) notes that nurses need to provide a context conducive to rehabilitation. She describes the integrative function of nursing, which is an important aspect of ensuring that rehabilitation is extended beyond the input of therapists. Ward atmosphere, a subset of the rehabilitative milieu, is heavily influenced by nurses (Waters, 1986). Clients notice that the rehabilitation setting has a different atmosphere from acute care settings. Clients value *humor* and *encouragement* in their interactions with rehabilitation nurses.

The resources available for the continuation of rehabilitation by clients and their families play a significant part in milieu therapy. There is some evidence of this in the literature. Newall, Wood, Hewer, & Tinson (1997) report a kitchen, computer room, and coffee shop were provided as initiatives to increase client participation in the activities of daily living beyond the therapy areas. An accessible cafe and breakfast buffet were used similarly in another rehabilitation facility (Weeks & Feuer, 1998).

Music, noise, and human voice in the nurse-client environment are the focus of work by Pope (1995). Beyond the formal *music therapy* interventions advocated by Wiens, Reimer, and Guyn (1999), Pope notes that it is each individual's perception of sound that matters. Rehabilitation nurses themselves create sound, as well as intentionally introduce sound in the form of music to their clients' environments. This can be done more therapeutically if nurses learn to interpret client's responses to sound in its various forms. One client's therapy may be another client's torment.

CRITICAL THINKING

As a rehabilitation nurse case manager, you have two families who are caring for clients in the home. During the past 2 months, the behavior of the clients has changed, and both families have asked you to assess their home care situation. Discuss how you would assess the two situations with the outcome of effective coping in mind. What are potential interventions and caregiver roles and responsibilities?

Family 1. The first family consists of a husband and wife (both 52 years old) and three young adults, one of whom is graduating from college this year; the other two have recently entered the workforce. The client is the husband's mother, aged 77 years, who has lived with the family for 4 years, since her husband's death. Although physically able to perform activities of daily living, she has become progressively unattentive to personal care and has poor nutritional intake. Last week she refused to leave her room and slept in a chair, never changing her clothing or showering. The family is concerned and wonders what is happening to the grandmother. They also state that they feel their plans to travel, now that their children are on their own, must be curtailed.

Family 2. Martha, 7 months old, was born with multiple congenital deficits that are complex medical problems. Martha's room at home looks more like a pediatric intensive care unit than a home nursery. The family consists of parents, both aged 34 years, and twin boys aged 4 years. Care for Martha requires so much time and energy that the mother has quit her job, even though she was able to work from home, and canceled all of her outside activities. The parents have not had time away from Martha since she was born. They worry that the twins are not receiving the attention they need, but they are too tired from being up three times every night to care for Martha. Some outside help has been provided for night duty, but six home health care aides have cycled through the home during the first 10 weeks of help; although they qualified for a registered nurse, none was available. They do not know how long they can maintain this pace and support their family needs.

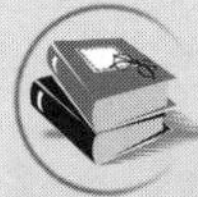

Case Study

At the beginning of the chapter, the story of Jenny, a young mother who suffered an intracranial hemorrhage, provides a rich case study to demonstrate the application of the nursing process to the coping-stress-tolerance functional health pattern.

Jenny is a 30-year-old woman who had been a healthy, active woman, a wife, and mother of 2-year-old Tess. Two weeks before we met, Jenny suddenly collapsed at home. An intracranial hemorrhage was diagnosed.

On admission to the rehabilitation service, the extent of Jenny's dependence became clearer. She was dependent on nursing staff for all her personal care needs and activities of daily living. Unable to turn over in the bed, she was incontinent of urine and feces, had difficulty communicating, was unable to swallow safely, and she experienced a right-sided hemiplegia.

Reading Jenny's history revealed a tragic story. Jenny was overseas with her husband, Tran, at the time of her collapse. Tran had taken the overseas posting to extend his experience in the company and increase his chances of a promotion. Jenny was pregnant with her second child when she suffered the hemorrhage. The baby died in utero and was delivered by caesarian section. The baby was of 6 months' gestation and was yet to be buried when she was admitted to the rehabilitation facility. The funeral and burial had been delayed to allow Jenny time to recover sufficiently to attend.

Jenny's rehabilitation commenced with planning her baby's funeral. While Tran made all the arrangements, the rehabilitation nurses worked with Jenny to ensure her wishes were understood by those involved.

As Jenny's communication improved, her anger became apparent to all who came near her. She was extremely frustrated by her deficits and commonly lashed out physically at the nurses. Her verbalizations also included swearing and abuse. Jenny did not talk about the baby she had lost or about her family. She expressed anger about her situation and a determination to fight.

All my efforts to comfort Jenny were repelled. Jenny did not want to be touched. She would tolerate instrumental touch, but af-

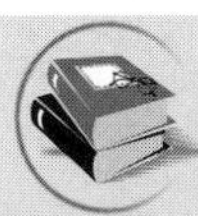

Case Study—cont'd

fective touch was unacceptable. She did not want to celebrate her successes, and she did not want to socialize. She wanted to regain her independence and get out of the hospital.

Appearance was important to Jenny, but in her current situation a satisfactory body image was unattainable. She gave up. She started to eat junk food, gain weight, and smoke.

Once Jenny had relearned her self-care skills, she began to relearn the skills she would need to resume her role as primary carer of her young daughter. With enormous determination and self-efficacy, Jenny learned how to dress and groom Tess. She also renegotiated her parenting role with Tran.

Jenny demonstrated a degree of hardiness and determination seldom seen. She battled on against enormous adversity and periods of intense loneliness and despair. I never connected with Jenny, but she taught me many things about rehabilitation nursing. The most painful was my experience as spectator of extreme human suffering—forbidden to touch and comfort. The most privileged was the role of learner as Jenny showed us all how she confronted her unbearable situation with determination and honesty.

The nursing diagnoses, desired outcomes, and nursing interventions for the stress-coping-tolerance functional health pattern for Jenny and her family are outlined below.

Cues	Nursing Diagnosis	Desired Outcomes	Nursing Interventions
No risk factors or warning signs of hemorrhage No opportunity to prepare for stressor Stressors appraised as harm and loss No previous experience with major stressors in life Impaired communication Self-care deficit Inability to meet role expectations as mother and wife Angry verbal outbursts associated with dependence on nursing staff Abuse of chemical agents perception of no control	Ineffective coping (individual)	Jenny sustains a will to live Jenny maintains hope Jenny copes with her stressors effectively Jenny achieves mood equilibrium Jenny regains a positive body image Jenny commences the journey of grief resolution Jenny develops appropriate and effective social interaction skills Jenny increases her social involvement with family and friends Jenny controls her own abusive behaviors Jenny's suffering and anguish reduce over time Jenny experiences increasing levels of psychological comfort	Grief work facilitation Cognitive restructuring Coping enhancement Active listening Hope instillation Body image enhancement Role enhancement Emotional support Self-esteem enhancement Mutual goal setting Complex relationship building Health education Learning readiness facilitation Learning facilitation Socialization enhancement
Primary support unable to sufficient, effective support and comfort Limited interaction between Jenny and her family Tran expresses little insight into Jenny's psychosocial needs Jenny's mother has chronic health problems that prevent her from visiting frequently and caring for Tess	Compromised family coping	Family uses effective coping strategies Family is able to meet Jenny's support needs Family integrity is maintained Family participates in decision making and provision of care Tran maintains a satisfactory level of well-being Tran positively appraises own abilities as caregiver Tran and Jenny develop a positive relationship in the roles of carer and care recipient	Active listening Grief work facilitation Role enhancement Emotional support Caregiver support Family integrity promotion Family involvement promotion Family process maintenance Family support Hope instillation Health education

REFERENCES

Antonak, R.F., & Livneh, H. (1991). A hierarchy of reactions to disability. *International Journal of Rehabilitation Research, 14,* 13-24.

Antonak, R.F., Livneh, H., & Antonak, C. (1993). A review of research on psychosocial adjustment to impairment in persons with traumatic brain injury. *Journal of Head Trauma Rehabilitation, 8*(4), 87-100.

Antonovsky, A. (1972). Breakdown: A needed fourth step in the conceptual armamentarium of modern medicine. *Social Science and Medicine, 6,* 537-544.

Antonovsky, A. (1979). *Health, stress and coping.* San Francisco: Jossey-Bass.

Antonovsky, A. (1987). *Unraveling the mystery of health: How people manage stress and stay well.* San Francisco: Jossey-Bass.

Antonovsky, A. (1996). The salutogenic model as a theory to guide health promotion. *Health Promotion International, 11*(1), 11-18.

Babrow, A.S., Kasch, C. R., & Ford, L.A. (1998). The many meanings of uncertainty in illness: Towards a systematic accounting. *Health Communication, 10*(1), 1-23.

Bailey, J.M., & Nielsen, B.I. (1993). Uncertainty and appraisal of uncertainty in women with rheumatoid arthritis. *Orthopedic Nursing, 12,* 63-67.

Bandura, A. (1997). *Self-efficacy: The exercise of control.* New York: WH Freeman.

Barnard, D. (1985). Psychosomatic medicine and the problem of meaning. *Bulletin of the Menninger Clinic, 4*(1), 10-28.

Beck, R.J. (1994). Encouragement as a vehicle to empowerment in counseling: An existential perspective. *Journal of Rehabilitation, July/August/September,* 6-11.

Blumer, H. (1969). *Symbolic interactionism: Perspective and method.* Berkeley: University of California Press.

Brillhart, B., & Johnson, K. (1997). Motivation and the coping process of adults with disabilities: A qualitative study. *Rehabilitation Nursing, 22*(5), 249-256.

Brown, J.D. (1993). Coping with stress: The beneficial role of positive illusion. In A.P. Turnbull, J.M. Patterson, S.K. Behr, D.L. Murphy, J.G. Marquis, & M.J. Blue-Banning (Eds.), *Cognitive coping, families, and disability* (pp. 123-133). Baltimore: Paul H Brookes.

Brown, S.K., & Conn, V.S. (1995). The relationship between self-efficacy and walking in the rehabilitation of postoperative CABG patients. *Rehabilitation Nursing Research, 4*(2), 64-71.

Cannon, W.B. (1914). The interrelations of emotions as suggested by recent physiological researches. *American Journal of Psychology, 25,* 256-282.

Cannon, W.B. (1935). Stresses and strains of homeostasis. *The American Journal of the Medical Sciences, 189*(1), 1-14.

Caris-Verhallen, W.M.C.M., Kerkstra, A., & Bensing, J.M. (1999). Nonverbal behaviour in nurse-elderly patient communication. *Journal of Advanced Nursing, 29*(4), 808-818.

Carveth, J.A. (1995). Perceived patient deviance and avoidance by nurses. *Nursing Research, 44,* 3173-3178.

Charmaz, K. (1983). Loss of self: A fundamental form of suffering in the chronically ill. *Sociology of Health and Illness, 5*(2), 168-195.

Charmaz, K. (1987). Struggling for a self: Identity levels of the chronically ill. *Sociology of Health Care, 6,* 283-321.

Charmaz, K. (1995). The body, identity and self: Adapting to impairment. *The Sociology Quarterly, 36*(4), 657-680.

Chelsa, C.A. (1999). Becoming resilient: Skill development in couples living with non-insulin diabetes. In H.I. McCubbin, E.A. Thompson, A.I. Thompson, & J.A. Futrell (Eds.), *The dynamics of resilient families* (pp. 99-133). Thousand Oaks, CA: Sage.

Clark, C.R. (1997). Creating information messages for reducing patient distress during health care procedures. *Patient Education and Counseling, 30,* 247-255.

Close, H., & Procter, S. (1999). Coping strategies used by hospitalized stroke patients: Implications for continuity and management of care. *Journal of Advanced Nursing, 29*(1), 138-144.

Davidhizar, R., & Giger, J.N. (1997). When touch is *not* the best approach. *Journal of Clinical Nursing, 6,* 203-206.

Dewar, A.L., & Morse, J.M. (1995). Unbearable incidents: Failure to endure the experience of illness. *Journal of Advanced Nursing, 22,* 957-964.

Doka, K.J. (1995). Coping with life-threatening illness: A task model. *OMEGA, 32*(2), 111-122.

Downe-Wambolt, B.L., & Melanson, P.M. (1998). A causal model of coping and well-being in elderly people with arthritis. *Journal of Advanced Nursing, 27*(6), 1109-1116.

Eakes, G.G., Burke, M.L., & Hainsworth, M.A. (1998). Middle-range theory of chronic sorrow. *Image—Journal of Nursing Scholarship, 30*(2), 179-184.

Easton, K.L., Rawl, S.M., Zemen, D., Kwiatkowski, S., & Burczyk, B. (1995). The effects of nursing follow-up on the coping strategies used by rehabilitation patients after discharge. *Rehabilitation Nursing Research, 4*(4), 119-127.

Elliott, G.R., & Eisdorfer, C. (1982). *Stress and human health: Analysis and implications of research.* New York: Springer.

Ellis-Stoll, C.C., & Popkess-Vawter, S. (1998). A concept analysis on the process of empowerment. *Advances in Nursing Science, 21*(2), 62-68.

Failla, S., & Jones, C.J. (1991). Families of children with developmental disabilities: An examination of family hardiness. *Research in Nursing and Health, 14,* 41-50.

Field, T. (1991). Stress and coping from pregnancy through the postnatal period. In E.M. Cummings, A.L. Greene, & K.H. Karraker (Eds.), *Life-span developmental psychology: Perspectives on stress and coping* (pp. 45-59). Hillsdale, NJ: Lawrence Erlbaum Associates.

Folkman, S. (1997). Positive psychological states and coping with severe stress. *Social Science Medicine, 45*(8), 1207-1221.

Garwick, A.W., Kohrman, C.H., Titus, J.C., Wolman, C., & Blum, R.W. (1999). Variations in families' explanations of childhood chronic conditions: A cross-cultural perspective. In H.I. McCubbin, E.A. Thompson, A.I. Thompson, & J.A. Futrell (Eds.), *The dynamics of resilient families* (pp. 165-198). Thousand Oaks, CA: Sage.

Gignac, M.A.M., & Gottlieb, B.H. (1997). Changes in coping with chronic stress: The role of caregivers' appraisals of coping efficacy. In B.H. Gottlieb (Ed.), *Coping with chronic stress* (pp. 245-267). New York: Plenum Press.

Gordon, M. (2000). *Manual of nursing diagnosis* (9th ed.). St. Louis: Mosby.

Gramling, L.F., Lambert, V.A., & Pursley-Crotteau, S. (1998). Coping in young women: Theoretical retroduction. *Journal of Advanced Nursing, 28*(5), 1082-1091.

Greene, J.W., Werner, M.J., & Walker, L.S. (1992). Stress and the modern adolescent. *Adolescent Medicine: State of the Art Reviews, 3,* 13-28.

Grey, M., Cameron, M.E., & Thurber, F.W. (1991). Coping and adaptation in children with diabetes. *Nursing Research, 40,* 144-149.

Griffiths, H., & Jordan, S. (1998). Thinking of the future and walking back to normal: An exploratory study of patients' experiences during recovery from lower limb fracture. *Journal of Advanced Nursing, 28*(6), 1276-1288.

Hafsteinsdottir, T.B., & Grypdonck, M. (1997). Being a stroke patient: A review of the literature. *Journal of Advanced Nursing, 26,* 580-588.

Healthy People 2010. (accessed 2000). http://www.health.gov/healthypeople/

Heller, T. (1993). Self-efficacy coping, active involvement, and caregiver well-being throughout the life course among families of persons with mental retardation. In A.P. Turnbull, J.M. Patterson, S.K. Behr, D.L. Murphy, J.G. Marquis, & M.J. Blue-Banning (Eds.), *Cognitive coping, families, and disability* (pp. 195-206). Baltimore: Paul H Brookes.

Hertzberg, D.L. (1999). Child growth, development, and maturation. In P.A. Edwards, D.L. Hertzberg, S.R. Hays, & N.M. Youngblood (Eds.), *Pediatric rehabilitation nursing* (pp. 144-198). Philadelphia: WB Saunders.

Hoeman, S.P. (Ed.). (1992). *The parent infant project manual for professionals and parents.* Morristown, NJ: U.S. Department of Energy.

Johnson, M., Maas, M., & Moorhead, S. (2000). *Nursing outcomes classification (NOC)* (2nd ed.). St. Louis: Mosby.

Johnson, M., & Webb, C. (1995). Rediscovering unpopular patients: The concept of social justice. *Journal of Advanced Nursing, 21,* 466-475.

Jones, G.C., & Kilpatrick, A.C. (1996). Wellness theory: A discussion and application to clients with disabilities. *Families in Society: The Journal of Contemporary Human Services, 77*(5), 259-268.

Jones, M., O'Neill, P., Waterman, H., & Webb, C. (1997). Building a relationship: Communication and relationships between staff and stroke patients on a rehabilitation ward. *Journal of Advanced Nursing, 26,* 101-110.

Karraker, K.H., & Lake, M. (1991). Normative stress and coping processes in infancy. In E.M. Cummings, A.L. Greene, & K.H. Karraker (Eds.), *Life-span developmental psychology: Perspectives on stress and coping* (pp. 85-108). Hillsdale, NJ: Lawrence Erlbaum Associates.

Keatinge, D. (1998). Negotiated care—Fundamental to nursing practice. *Collegian, 5, 36-42.*

Keller, C. & Nicolls, R. (1990). Coping strategies of chronically ill adolescents and their parents. *Issues in Comprehensive Pediatric Nursing, 13,* 73-80.

Kemp, B. (1986). Psychosocial and mental health issues in rehabilitation of older persons. In S.J. Brody & G.E. Ruff (Eds.), *Aging and rehabilitation: Advances in the state of the art.* (pp. 122-158). New York: Springer.

Kirkevold, M. (1997). The role of nursing in the rehabilitation of acute stroke patients: Towards a unified theoretical perspective. *Advances in Nursing Science, 19*(4), 55-64.

Kobasa, S.C. (1979). Stressful life events, personality, and health: An inquiry into hardiness. *Journal of Personality and Social Psychology, 37,* 1-11.

Kobasa, S.C., Maddi, S.R., & Kahn, S. (1982). Hardiness and health: A prospective study. *Journal of Personality and Social Psychology, 42,* 168-172.

Kobasa, S.C., Maddi, S.R., & Zola, M.A. (1983). Type A and hardiness. *Journal of Behavioral Medicine, 6,* 41-51.

Kolcaba, K.Y. (1991). A taxonomic structure for the concept of comfort. *Image—Journal of Nursing Scholarship, 23*(4), 237-240.

Kolcaba, K.Y. (1995). Comfort as process and product, merged in holistic nursing art. *Journal of Holistic Nursing, 13*(2), 117-131.

Krauss, M.W., & Seltzer, M.M. (1993). Coping strategies among older mothers of adults with mental retardation: A life-span developmental perspective. In A.P. Turnbull, J.M. Patterson, S.K. Behr, D.L. Murphy, J.G. Marquis, & M.J. Blue-Banning (Eds.), *Cognitive coping, families, and disability* (pp. 173-182). Baltimore: Paul H Brookes.

Kubler-Ross, E. (1969). *On death and dying.* New York: MacMillan.

Lambert, J. (1999). Meeting the emotional needs of a patient. *Rehabilitation Nursing, 24*(4), 141-142.

Lawler, J., Dowswell, G., Hearn, J., Forster, A., & Young, J. (1999). Recovering from stroke: A qualitative investigation of the role of goal setting in late stroke recovery. *Journal of Advanced Nursing, 30*(2), 401-409.

Lazarus, R. (1991). *Emotion and adaptation.* New York: Oxford University Press.

Lazarus, R. (1999). *Stress and emotion: A new synthesis.* New York: Springer.

Lazarus, R.S. (1996). The role of coping in the emotions and how coping changes over the life course. In C. Magai & S.H. McFadden (Eds.), *Handbook of emotion, adult development, and aging* (pp. 289-306). San Diego: Academic Press.

Lazarus, R.S. (1998). Coping with aging: Individuality as a key to understanding. In I.H. Nordhus, G.R. VandenBos, S. Berg, & P. Fromholt (Eds.), *Clinical geropsychology* (pp. 109-127). Washington, DC: American Psychological Association.

Lazarus, R.S., & Folkman, S. (1984). *Stress, appraisal, and coping.* New York: Springer.

Lindgren, C.L., Burke, M.L., Hainsworth, M.A., & Eakes, G.G. (1992). Chronic sorrow: A lifespan concept. *Scholarly Inquiry for Nursing Practice: An International Journal, 6*(1), 27-40.

Livneh, H., & Antonak, R.F. (1997). *Psychosocial adaptation to chronic illness and disability.* Gaithersburg, MD: Aspen.

Lo, R. (1999). Correlates of expected success at adherence to health regimens of people with IDDM. *Journal of Advanced Nursing, 30*(2), 418-424.

Maddi, S.R., & Kobasa, S.C. (1991). The development of hardiness. In A. Monat & R.S. Lazarus (Eds.), *Stress and coping: An anthology* (pp. 245-257). New York: Columbia University Press.

Martin, K.M. (1994). Loss without death: A dilemma for the head-injured patient's family. *Journal of Neuroscience Nursing, 26*(3), 134-139.

McCloskey, J.C., & Bulechek, G.M. (2000). *Nursing interventions classification (NIC)* (3rd ed.). St. Louis: Mosby.

McCubbin, H.I., Thompson, E.A., Thompson, A.I., & McCubbin, M.A. (1993). Family schema, paradigms, and paradigm shifts: Components and processes of appraisal in family adaptation to crises. In A.P. Turnbull, J.M. Patterson, S.K. Behr, D.L. Murphy, J.G. Marquis, & M.J. Blue-Banning (Eds.), *Cognitive coping, families, and disability* (pp. 239-255). Baltimore: Paul H Brookes.

Mishel, M.H. (1990). Reconceptualization of the uncertainty in illness theory. *Image—Journal of Nursing Scholarship, 22*(4), 256-262.

Morse, J.M. (1992). Comfort: The refocusing of nursing care. *Clinical Nursing Research, 1*(1), 91-106.

Morse, J.M. (1997). Responding to threats to integrity of self. *Advances in Nursing Science, 19*(4), 21-36.

Morse, J.M., Bottorff, J.L., & Hutchinson, S. (1994). The phenomenology of comfort. *Journal of Advanced Nursing, 20,* 189-195.

Morse, J.M., Bottorff, J.L., & Hutchinson, S. (1995). The paradox of comfort. *Nursing Research, 44*(1), 14-19.

Morse, J.M., & Carter, B.J. (1995). Strategies of enduring and the suffering of loss: Modes of comfort used by a resilient survivor. *Holistic Nursing Practice, 9*(3), 38-52.

Morse, J.M., & Carter, B. (1996). The essence of enduring and expressions of suffering: The reformation of self. *Scholarly Inquiry for Nursing Practice: An International Journal, 10*(1), 43-60.

Morse, J.M., & Doberneck, B. (1995). Delineating the concept of hope. *Image—Journal of Nursing Scholarship, 27*(4), 277-285.

Morse, J.M., & Johnson, J.L. (1991). Towards a theory of illness: The illness-constellation model. In J.M. Morse, J.L. Johnson (Eds.), *The illness experience: Dimensions of suffering* (pp. 315-342). Newbury Park, CA: Sage.

Newall, J.T., Wood, V.A., Hewer, R.L., & Tinson, D.J. (1997). Development of a neurological rehabilitation environment: An observational study. *Clinical Rehabilitation, 11,* 146-155.

Newbold, D. (1996). Coping with rheumatoid arthritis: How can specialist nurses influence it and promote better outcomes? *Journal of Clinical Nursing, 5*(6), 373-380.

Newby, N.M. (1996). Chronic illness and the family life-cycle. *Journal of Advanced Nursing, 23,* 786-791.

Nyhlin, K.T. (1990). Diabetic patients facing long-term complications: Coping with uncertainty. *Journal of Advanced Nursing, 15,* 1021-1029.

Olshansky, S. (1966). Parent responses to a mentally defective child. *Mental Retardation, 5*(4), 21-23.

Orr, E., & Westman, M. (1990). Does hardiness moderate stress, and how? A review. In M. Rosenbaum (Ed.), *Learned resourcefulness: On coping, self-control, and adaptive behavior.* New York: Springer.

Park, C.L., & Folkman, S. (1997). Meaning in the context of stress and coping. *Review of General Psychology, 1*(2), 115-144.

Parsons, T. (1951). *The social system.* New York: The Free Press.

Pelletier, K.R. (1977). *Mind as healer, mind as slayer.* London: George Allen & Unwin.

Piazza, D., Holcombe, J., Foote, A., Paul, P., Love, S., & Daffin, P. (1991). Hope, social support and self esteem of patients with spinal cord injury. *Journal of Neuroscience Nursing, 23*(4), 224-230.

Pollock, S. (1986). Human responses to chronic illness: Physiologic and psychological adaptation. *Nursing Research, 35,* 90-95.

Pollock, S.E. (1989). The hardiness characteristic: A motivating factor in adaptation. *Advances in Nursing Science, 11,* 53-62.

Pope, D.S. (1995). Music, noise, and the human voice in the nurse-patient environment. *Image—Journal of Nursing Scholarship, 27*(4), 291-296.

Power, P.W. (1985). Family coping behaviors in chronic illness: A rehabilitation perspective. *Rehabilitation Literature, 46,* 78-83.

Pryor, J. (1999a). Nursing and rehabilitation. In J. Pryor (Ed.), *Rehabilitation: A vital nursing function* (pp. 1-13). Deakin, ACT, Australia: Royal College of Nursing Australia.

Pryor, J. (1999b). Goals and focus. In J. Pryor (Ed.), *Rehabilitation: A vital nursing function* (pp. 79-96). Deakin, ACT, Australia: Royal College of Nursing Australia.

Pryor, J. (2000). Creating a rehabilitative milieu. *Rehabilitation Nursing, 25*(4), 141-144.

Pryor, J., & Smith, C. (2000). *A framework for the specialty practice of rehabilitation nursing.* Rehabilitation Nursing Research and Development Unit Monograph Series, No 4. Sydney, Australia: Royal Rehabilitation Centre Sydney.

Rawl, S.M., Easton, K.L., Kwiatkowski, S., Zemen, D., & Burczyk, B. (1998). Effectiveness of a nurse-managed follow-up program for rehabilitation patients after discharge. *Rehabilitation Nursing, 23*(4), 204-209.

Rees, C., & Joslyn, S. (1998). The importance of hope. *Nursing Standard, 12*(41), 34-35.

Resnik, B. (1996). Motivation in geriatric rehabilitation. *Image—Journal of Nursing Scholarship, 28*(1), 41-45.

Rodgers, B.L., & Cowles, K.V. (1997). A conceptual foundation for human suffering in nursing care and research. *Journal of Advanced Nursing, 25,* 1048-1053.

Rosenbaum, M. (1990). The role of learned resourcefulness in the self-control of health behavior. In M. Rosenbaum (Ed.), *Learned resourcefulness: On coping skills, self-control, and adaptive behavior* (pp. 3-30). New York: Springer.

Scheier, M.F., & Carver, C.S. (1987). Dispositional optimism and physical well-being: The influence of generalized outcomes expectancies on health. *Journal of Personality, 55*(2), 169-210.

Seigley, L.A. (1999). Self-esteem and health behavior: Theoretical and empirical links. *Nursing Outlook, 47*(2), 74-77.

Selye, H. (1976). *The stress of life.* New York: McGraw-Hill.

Singleton, J.K. (2000). Nurses' perspectives of encouraging clients' care-of-self in a short-term rehabilitation unit within a long-term care facility. *Rehabilitation Nursing, 25*(1), 23-30, 35.

Teel, C.S. (1991). Chronic sorrow: Analysis of the concept. *Journal of Advanced Nursing, 16,* 1311-1319.

Thompson, S.C. (1991). The search for meaning following stroke. *Basic and Applied Psychology, 12*(1), 81-96.

Vash, C. (1994). *Personality and adversity: Psychospiritual aspects of rehabilitation.* New York: Springer.

Waters, K. (1986). The role of nursing in rehabilitation. *CARE—Science and Practice, 5*(3), 17-21.

Weeks, S.K., & Feuer, T.E. (1998). The rehab cafe and breakfast buffet. *Rehabilitation Nursing, 23*(1), 46.

Wheaton, B. (1997). The nature of chronic stress. In B.H. Gottlieb (Ed.), *Coping with chronic stress.* New York: Plenum Press.

Wichowski, H.C., & Kubsch, S.M. (1997). The relationship of self-perception of illness and compliance with health regimens. *Journal of Advanced Nursing, 25,* 548-553.

Wiens, M.E., Reimer, M.A. & Guyn, H.L. (1999). Music therapy as a treatment method for improving respiratory muscle strength in patients with advanced multiple sclerosis: A pilot study. *Rehabilitation Nursing, 24*(2), 74-80.

Yarcheski, A. (1988). Uncertainty in illness and the future. *Western Journal of Nursing Research, 10,* 410-413.

Youngblood, N.M. (1999). Family-centred care. In P.A. Edwards, D.L. Hertzberg, S.R. Hays, & N.M. Youngblood (Eds.), *Pediatric rehabilitation nursing* (pp. 129-143). Philadelphia: WB Saunders.

Culture and Medical Systems: Conventional, Alternative, and Complementary Health Patterns

13

Shirley P. Hoeman, PhD, MPH, RN, CRRN
Theresa Perfetta Cappello, RN, PhD

A friend invited me to attend her last yoga class for the season. Students would demonstrate their yoga postures and share food and fun. Molly, who was around 30 years old, demonstrated a bridge. With her feet flat on the floor, she bent backwards and touched the floor with both hands. I was impressed. I noticed that Molly had a portable medication pump with tubing protruding from her gym pants. Curious, I asked about the pump, and Molly said, "This is for my pulmonary hypertension. It is most often a life-threatening disease, but since I am on some medication and have learned to control the stress in my life through yoga and meditation, I don't worry about it any more. My life is a lot better now, and I take time for myself even better than before my diagnosis. It's all about who you are and what you think, not what you have."

The purposes of this chapter are to acquaint the rehabilitation nurse with some ways that cultural factors influence health assessment, interventions, and outcomes and to explain the relevance of alternative medical systems and complementary therapeutics in rehabilitation nursing practice. Certainly this is not an exhaustive discussion because these topics are addressed in full textbooks. The viewpoint is toward holism in nursing offered from an anthropological approach; it is not intended to be a presentation of holistic nursing per se. A goal is to provide information and access to information that will enable rehabilitation nurses to make informed and critical decisions about cultural, alternative, and complementary beliefs and practices.

CULTURE AND WORLDVIEWS

Historical Development

From tribal times, healing was ascribed to selected persons who knew how to use magic, herbs, and rituals properly and to connect with a spiritual domain. Most enduring of primitive healer-spiritual roles is the shaman, whose interactions with the spiritual world empowered healing. Throughout Egyptian eras, classical Greco-Roman years, Celtic Druid times, and Oriental medicine, healers were affiliated with temples and aligned with appropriate gods. Hippocrates was a student of the priest-physicians of the Greek demigod Aesculapius, and the Indo-Asian concepts of Ayurvedic medicine are attributed to Dhanvantari, patron of physicians in India. As Christianity spread throughout the Western world monks, nuns, and religious layworkers tended to the sick, disabled, and poor in response to their spiritual calling. Residing in monasteries, many monks and nuns became recognized for apothecary knowledge and skills with herbal concoctions. Even the Arabic physicians, with their emphasis on mathematical and scientific approaches, incorporated a spiritual component about health (Keegan, 1994). Chapter 28 discusses holism in another vein, establishing the relationship between spirituality and healing.

Despite varying success with cure or even palliative care, all of these healers held holistic views supporting elementary concepts of prevention and health maintenance. They envisioned an individual life force, knew a need to maintain balance or harmony, and attempted to align the natural world with spiritual forces. Certainly cultures and societies had specific requirements, taboos, beliefs, and practices. However, body, mind, spirit, and their interaction with the natural and supernatural environments influenced health and healing.

Culture, Health, and Disability

Health is an underlying system of society along with education, legislation, religion, family, economics, and so forth.

The World Health Organization (WHO) promotes a global definition of holistic health and a system of community-based rehabilitation, and it offers a classification system to distinguish among severity and levels of impairment, handicap, or disability. However, health or illness, modes of care and caring, and identities of practitioners are defined, understood, and communicated, and the behaviors are carried out, within the boundaries of the culture.

Each society assigns meaning to what constitutes health or illness; defines roles and actions for persons who are well, ill, or impaired; and sets expectations for the person and responsibilities of family and society. Micozzi (1996, p. 31) describes "healthcare as cultural modeling." Culture not only teaches under what circumstances and symptoms a person becomes ill or disabled but also provides a social construction of the situation (Box 13-1).

Box 13-1 Social Construction of Illness

Social construction means that cultures or societies use their systems to define and prescribe:

- How and why illness or disability occurred
- What should be done about it
- Who should perform healing
- Which interventions should be used
- How the person and others are to respond to and perform roles
- What meaning is given to the illness or disability
- What is the cost (financial, social, and otherwise)
- What should be the outcome

Members of the culture know these ways; although social meanings are powerful, it is essential to remember that they do not prevent individuals from constructing their own meanings

Culture and Symptoms

Zborowski's (1958) landmark study, which found that culturally prescribed responses to pain differed among clients from three sociocultural groups, opened the door to research in culture and health. Another classic work by Parsons (1951) affirmed that illness behavior is prescribed and defined culturally. In fact, persons' descriptions of their condition and the appropriate cause, treatment, and expected outcomes are products of cultural explanatory models (Kleinman, Eisenberg, & Good, 1978).

Symptoms and names of some diseases may be recognized and understood only within a particular culture. The fact that a disease or syndrome is not listed in the materia medica does not mean that it does not exist; it simply does not have diagnostic labeling for conventional medicine. The importance of how language is used when describing symptoms or providing renditions of subjective experiences or reporting health status has been devalued and underrated in conventional medicine. With interest in bioethnographic research and growth of population diversity, "culture bound" symptoms and syndromes, such as susto, empacho, falling down disease, or spiritual curses, and treatment theories, such as hot-cold theory (Harwood, 1971), have been well established in the literature.

However, studies have not affixed labels to Western culture–bound symptoms. These may be diseases resulting from human activity in the environment or resulting from medical diagnostic procedures or interventions (Hudson, 1987). Iatrogenic problems, especially medical errors or acquired infections, have been in the public eye. Other diseases may be born of responses to civilization and technological advances, such as heart disease or problems resulting from stress, obesity, anorexia, repetitive motion, or even sick-building syndrome. Hudson lists diseases resulting from cultural lifestyles or behaviors such as trichinosis from eating pork that is cooked insufficiently, lung cancer and emphysema from using tobacco, and hookworm from not wearing shoes. Violence as a way of life or problem solving often results in disability or premature death.

While leading a delegation to the People's Republic of China, I was bemused to learn that the Chinese consider attention-deficit hyperactivity disorder (ADHD) as a Western condition that is not acknowledged in the Orient (Hoeman, 1992). Similarly practitioners in Asian, Hispanic, and African cultures are astounded at the inability of Western medical practitioners to diagnose or treat based on a person's psychosocial or spiritual symptoms.

Two common complaints about conventional medicine from clients of other cultures are the short time allotted for the visit and the number of questions asked of the client by the physician or nurse. Alternative and traditional healers tend to spend more time with clients and thus allow information about the person to emerge. Typically the person expects the healer to use special skills, apply therapeutic techniques, provide herbal or other remedies, or form connections with the nonphysical world to identify the person's problem. Then the healer states what is needed for restoring balance and returning to health (Box 13-2).

SOCIAL CONSTRUCTION OF DISABILITY

Persons with impairment or disability have been treated unequally for centuries, their conditions being considered as punishment for wrongdoing; due to a curse; or less often, as an insight, blessing, or call to a special role function in the society. The surviving member of Jonathan's household in the Bible was a youth saved because of his deformed lower limbs, and Caesar was subject to epileptic seizures. Negative traits were attributed to the personality of many literary characters with deformities or disabilities, from Richard III to the Hunchback of Notre Dame.

During the Modern Period, persons with disability were viewed as a deviation from the intact person and were subject to ridicule or debasement and devalued. Deformity, often associated with being a fool, frequently was a target of

Box 13-2 Defining Conventional and Complementary/Alternative Medicine

Conventional (biomedical, traditional, contemporary, and allopathic) medicine: The dominant philosophical paradigm of medicine in the Western developed world. This scientific, reductionist method of medicine is taught in all U.S. medical schools. Rehabilitation is a specialty within conventional medicine.

Complementary/alternative medicine (CAM): A broad range of nonallopathic healing practices primarily stemming from Eastern medical philosophy and spiritual traditions of many cultures. Western conventional medicine does not commonly use, accept, study, understand, or make available CAM therapies. Until recently, CAM therapies were not found in U.S. medical school curricula and generally not recognized by third-party payers in the United States. However, many medical schools have developed courses, and reimbursement for selected modalities has become more common. CAM therapies are considered holistic, considering the physical, mental, emotional, and spiritual aspects of each person.

The terms *complementary* and *alternative* often are used interchangeably. However, *alternative medicine* refers to a system of treatments that replace conventional medical practices, whereas *complementary medicine* refers to a system of treatments that enhance, support, or supplement conventional medicine.

cruel humor among adults, as well as children (Cassell, 1985). Only recently in the United States and other developed nations have ideas about quality of life and life satisfaction provoked legislation, such as the Americans with Disabilities Act and school education acts.

In the professional culture of rehabilitation nursing, a holistic mind-body-spirit view extends beyond mere survival with intact physical abilities as outcome criteria. The love of family members and their role in a community is neither one-dimensional nor linear (Hoeman & Nordin, 2001). Holism takes into account what Sobel (1979) identified as nonmedical determinants of health, that is, genetic, behavioral, and physical and psychosocial environmental factors. He envisioned an integrated approach, a synthesis of conventional science and alternate systems of healing. The mutual approach of provider or healer and client are factors also.

Ethnocentrism, or the tendency to gauge situations and filter experiences through one's own, usually thought to be superior, cultural point of view, is a typical response. Not only do providers bring their own cultural backgrounds to the therapeutic encounter, but they also come with the extensive beliefs and practices of the culture of conventional medicine. Leininger's (1978) chapter depicts medicine and nursing as two tribes and satirizes many behaviors inherent in their professional cultures. Current research by Fadiman (1997) effectively illustrates how cultural dissonance prevailed in a Hmong family's encounter with conventional medicine despite highly competent practice by caring professionals. In this ethnographic account, everyone was good and tried hard, everyone shared the same desired outcome for the child, and everyone was willing to do what had to be done so far as he or she could understand and envision. Still the cultural cues were misconstrued as nonadherence or simply dismissed as irrelevant to the medical diagnostics. The family did not trust the physicians wholeheartedly because they continued to believe in the spirit world. Both groups continued to talk and act in vacillation with each other, relying on data but without real understanding, and solutions were lost.

Simply gathering information is not equal to understanding the cultural meaning. Haddad and Hoeman (2000) explain the significance for the nurse to learn about the history of a client's culture and how events have shaped beliefs and practices within the context of the culture. Paul's classic anthology of case studies (1955) demonstrates repeatedly that culture is a system larger than the sum of its parts. In one encounter a Peruvian village woman confronts health workers whose attempts to have her boil contaminated water raise argument. She reasons that any microbes would drown themselves in the water and that if these invisible organisms exist at all, they must have come "stuck on" from other sources. She questions why she should worry about minuscule, invisible animals, the microbes, when there are real threats of cold, hunger, and poverty (Wellin, 1955). Nurse healers know that interpersonal trust and mutual faith in the intervention are essential because the healer and client "behold one another through different kinds of cultural glasses" and "sickness is as much a moral as a physical crisis" (p. 107).

Cultures determine their own construction for chronic conditions, impairment, and disability and how the situation will be managed within the social system. However, social or cultural construction is not the same as reality for those who have the strength of moral absolutes. Individuals can and do rise above social constructions of relativism and negative designations within their own awareness, but this is difficult. Rehabilitation nurses are advocates to forestall certain ways of thinking, even when subtle or unaware, that contribute to social language and meanings to devalue and disable those who have impairments. Zola (1991, p. 11), examining his work and himself as a person with postpolio syndrome, comments on the difference between language describing the person "confined to a wheelchair" and a person "using the wheelchair."

DOMINANT ROLE OF CONVENTIONAL MEDICINE

Accusations launched from the Flexner Report (1910) revealed much about the unsubstantiated scientific basis and unequal quality of conventional medical practice in the early 1900s. Findings stimulated university-based medical education and enabled medical advances flowing from World War II. Since then, the undisputed cultural model of health care in the United States has been what is now called conventional, that is, the Western medical or allopathic model. Conventional medical system ways of knowing are its means for determining whether something is scientific, as opposed to unscientific. Until recently the body was viewed mechanistically, as a machine, and dealt with apart from the mind and spirit. Based on cartesian concepts, positivism, objectivism, and reductionism (Micozzi, 1996) and augmented by advances in pharmaceutics, technology, and surgery, the dominant political and economic power of conventional medicine as a cultural system is unparalleled (Starr, 1982). Practitioners are indoctrinated into the culture of the system and adhere to the professional roles and standards of practice.

Thus practitioners of conventional medicine found it easy to disregard other health systems and interventions as illogical and unproven, effectively excluding them from legitimate status and, importantly, from the reimbursement process. Conventional medicine flourished and dominated, its blatant paternalism abetted by consumer expectations for cures and technological solutions. Initiatives for preventive care and self-care were discarded in lieu of fantastic and expensive procedures, equipment, and technology that promised more cures. Ironically, rehabilitation medicine itself was considered alternative and struggled for acceptance as a specialty by conventional medicine before World War II.

Erosion of Trust in Medical Diagnosis and Care

Reliance on treatments and technology interfered with the interpersonal relationship between health professionals and clients, dismantling the worth of the family physician, house calls, and bedside manner. Some clients blamed themselves when drugs or surgical interventions did not resolve their conditions. Ziporyn (1992) discusses the miserable status of the person who lives with multiple symptoms for which conventional medicine cannot assign a disease or condition. Even an unwelcome diagnosis, such as multiple sclerosis or muscular dystrophy, assigns meaning and validates the person's suffering situation. Once suffering is given a name, the person can move toward the process of dealing within constraints of the condition and, just as important, is able to realize that the symptoms are real and the feelings are legitimate. For clients with chronic, disabling conditions, a diagnosis may hold the risk of becoming the definition of their person. Conventional medicine regards the mind and the body as if on separate planes to the point of providers excluding subjective history and intuition born of experience.

Functional Health Patterns as Advocacy

However, rehabilitation nurses understand that chronic conditions and comorbidity cannot be fit into a single diagnostic label and that the responses and reserves of an individual cannot be cataloged. They recognize the exquisite fine-tuning needed to identify a person's optimal abilities, eke out every possibility, and then minimize problems. Rehabilitation nurses examine functional patterns to assess a client's multiple strengths and unique deficits, such as those that might follow a stroke. Interventions are specific to each client beyond the scope of the diagnosis. This is superior because no single medical diagnosis can encompass an individual's whole situation when the goal is to restore or maintain optimal levels of function on all fronts. The disease or disability does not exist on its own and is not representative of the person. In part, this rationale justifies use of functional health patterns for the holistic conceptual framework of this book.

Self-Healing

Another relationship exists with self-care nursing principles wherein clients and their families have a great deal of responsibility for directing and conducting their health care. In the realm of *psychoneuroimmunology* (PNI), a term signifying a body of research that examines mind-body connections, cognitive, emotional, and psychological factors are found to influence the body's immune system, that is, these factors can effect self-healing. In Eisenberg (1997) found that 58% of alternative therapies used were for health promotion or disease prevention. This interest combined with an emphasis on the body's ability to heal itself and correct imbalance makes alternative therapies and remedies enticing options for persons with previously incurable chronic or disabling conditions.

Persons with chronic, disabling conditions are among those who choose to inform themselves and manage many aspects of their own health care. Complementary therapies, used in conjunction with conventional medicine, may enable clients to access a variety of modes of treatment and exercise their greatest potential for healing (Maley, 1997). No one discipline or single approach is prepared to manage the complexity of chronic, disabling conditions. Thus inquiry must be conducted into what Waksman (1994, p. 16), in his analysis of PNI relationships with multiple sclerosis, calls "the full, appropriate context" (i.e., within multidimensional frameworks).

Health Seeking

Many of the complex problems encountered by persons with chronic, disabling, or developmental disorders remain out of reach of conventional medical cures. Clients and families learn about optional treatments through the World Wide Web and other news sources, and they recognize that allopathic medicine and technology will not resolve all problems. They seek improved quality in their lives and no longer believe that medical science alone will provide it. Paternalism is rejected, and individual's have more confidence in seeking health care alternatives (Jonas, 1998).

Clients' assessments of quality of care may be related to their satisfaction with social interaction with the health professional (Reid, Wang, Young, & Awiphan, 1999; Callahan, Bertakis, & Azari, 2000). Equally important is the lack of culturally relevant tools or ways to measure client outcomes or satisfaction. The fact that a person is participating in a rehabilitation program indicates some degree of experience with the medical system (Hoeman, 1989). However, it remains unclear whether satisfaction or rating of quality of care is influenced by cultural factors including values, perceptions, expectations, mode of expressing agreement or concerns, use of alternative therapies, or other reasons (Murray-Garcia, Selby, Schmittdiel, Grumbach, & Quesenberry, 2000).

Other research findings support reliability and validity of self-report measures of impairment and disability. Researchers found that homeless persons, including many with chronic disabling conditions, would seek care when referral mechanisms were in place and when they believed their situation was serious (Gelberg, Andersen, & Leake, 2000). On the other hand, skepticism about the worth of Western medicine to the point of indulging in risky behavior or placing excessive trust in untested remedies, may lead to early death with certain conditions (Fiscella, Franks, Clancy, Doescher, & Banthin, 1999).

Diversity and Utilization

Diversity is a growing reality that extends beyond cultural lines to encompass persons who are vulnerable, marginalized, refugees, and immigrants, or marked by socioeconomic class (Meleis, Isenberg, Koerner, Lacey, & Stern, 1995). Falling into thinking about stereotypical categories is unwise in any arena. In particular, intraethnic diversity is often overlooked or underestimated by providers eager to become culturally sensitive (Hoeman, 1996).

Education, experiences or acculturation, occupation, and economic status do influence how closely a person or family adheres to the traditional medical beliefs and practices of a culture. When asked about folk or traditional practices, persons with higher education and socioeconomic status tended to deny use or state they knew about them but did not partake of them. These persons reported use of conventional medical pharmacology, surgery, and technology (Hoeman, 1998). Because folk and traditional practices are not always the same as complementary practices, similar personal factors (i.e., more education and economic success) have been associated with use of therapies, such as acupuncture, that are alternative or complementary to conventional medicine (Hufford, 1995).

Increasingly clients use alternative and conventional medicine in conjunction with one another, albeit in a variety of ways. Conventional medicine may be the last resort when other culturally prescribed or alternative treatments fail; clients may also switch between treatment programs. Some persons rely on a cadre of spiritual, alternative, and allopathic practitioners, or they may devise their own version and combinations, adding other interventions.

Prevalence of Alternative Therapies

New awareness among consumers about options in selecting health care emerged from rapidly changing demographics and global influences. Not only do individuals travel across the world, but also the population of the United States has diversified so that health beliefs, practices, and practitioners from multiple cultures are evident in the social mainstream.

The World Wide Web has created a means to homogenize cultural differences. The virtual community does not recognize differences in skin color, weight, clothing, wealth, religion, accent, and so forth. List serves, chat rooms, news groups, and discussion groups allow individuals to share common interests. Support groups for persons with all kinds of illness are on-line via the Internet. Cyberspace provides a moratorium from reality and a forum for individuality (Kelly & Fitzsimons, 2000).

Consumers have access to information, globalization and travel, and resources (Austin, 1997), as well as the willingness to expend personal funds for services (Eisenberg et al., 1998). Some clients are designing their own programs of health care. The number of persons in the United States using alternative therapies has increased from 33.8% to 42.1% of the population in the 8 years since the landmark study by Eisenberg et al. (1993). In 1997 clients personally paid $27 million and made 629 million visits to alternative practitioners, an increase of 200 million visits in 7 years.

Nearly 62% of clients who use alternative therapies or healers do not inform their physician despite 42% of the alternative therapy being sought for specific treatment of an existing health condition (Eisenberg et al., 1997). A community nursing study found older rural women to be uninformed about the safety and efficacy of alternative products, therapies, or practitioners, and they did not tell their physicians about using them (Johnson, 1999). Providers do not ask clients about their use of alternative treatments or fail to understand what they hear. Inability to cure is the negative benchmark for conventional medicine, whereas care, prevention of further disability, and maintenance of function are left begging. This is a major breakdown in the interpersonal and therapeutic relationship and the basis for erosion of trust. Certainly *Healthy People 2010* data document socioeconomic and ethnic disparities that exist in health care quality and access (U.S. Department of Health and Human Services, 2000).

Failure of conventional medicine to produce the now expected cure for many conditions has encouraged consumers to seek alternatives, especially in our aging global population. Similarly persons of all ages who have survived formerly fatal conditions only to continue battle with multiple complex problems seek relief in any form. Hope is strong for finding cures for cancer, arthritis, multiple sclerosis, Alzheimer's disease, and Parkinson's disease and for progress toward relieving chronic back pain and other painful conditions and restoring nerve function for spinal cord injury and other nerve-related conditions. Meanwhile, clients continue to struggle and suffer and seek solutions.

As more alternative therapies are accepted as mainstream practices, critical thinking demands having an understanding of how of their conceptual bases differ from those of conventional medicine. Nurses are familiar with clients who hold health beliefs and practices and who rely on remedies from folk, family, or other lay sources or religious healing. Other persons call on specific practitioners from particular cultural origins.

NURSE AS HEALER

Nurses share philosophies about caring, holism, and healing with healers from many alternative systems. With one foot in the conventional cure model of medicine and the other in nursing's holism healing model, nurses can serve as bridges or brokers between systems (Engebretson, 1996), and more importantly, they can build the trusting and therapeutic relationships with clients that are so fragile in this new century.

Nursing is unique in that while operating under the scientific banner, its practitioners understand healing as the art of making whole and holistic health as process and outcome. Nurses have practiced holism for centuries and have used many healing practices to complement mechanistic medical procedures. For example, modalities such as touch and massage; hot and cold applications; combinations of nutrition, hygiene, and exercise; the relaxation response; a therapeutic relationship; stress management; pain management; environmental manipulation; therapeutic touch; and others clearly are within the historical purview of nursing practice.

"Complementary therapeutics are of particular interest to rehabilitation nurses because many of the techniques are holistic, maximize (clients') independence in terms of care and function, and are within the boundaries and scope of rehabilitation nursing practice" (Hoeman, 1997, p. 64).

In the twenty-first century, nurses are practitioners of alternative and complementary care while bringing understanding of cellular and organic disease, movement theory, and pharmaceutical and technological advances; nurses subscribe to holism and value the therapeutic relationship. In addition, each nurse brings combined personal, familial, and cultural history into the therapeutic relationship. They know that physical and mechanical principles explain only a portion of a person's health.

CLASSIFICATIONS OF ALTERNATIVE MEDICINE

The following classifications are according to the National Center for Complementary and Alternative Medicine (NCCAM), although other versions and groupings of categories exist and some disagree; however, at this time the NCCAM is the major source of funding and research (NCCAM, 2000).

Traditional Medical Systems

Traditional medicine has been portrayed erroneously as a type of folk or lay healing. Certainly from the viewpoint of conventional medicine, the differences are difficult to comprehend. Thinking of the body in terms of meridians or types, study of the flow of energy or concerns with restoring balance are not concepts currently accepted by conventional medicine. Conventional medicine does not discern that lack of balance or restricted flow of energy (*chi, prahna,* and others) leads to illness. However, traditional Chinese medicine has been practiced for more than 2000 years, and practitioners of Chinese traditional medicine engage in programs of study that are longer and more intensive than those of their Western physician counterparts. Traditional medical systems are complete systems that include conceptual frameworks, practice guidelines, standards for practitioners, and detailed pharmacopoeia. Usually traditional systems are best understood from worldviews of the particular cultures or regions where they have been practiced for centuries.

Although conventional medicine relies on newtonian physics—dealing with structures larger than molecules, essentially at the cellular level—many traditional medical systems are more closely aligned with quantum physics and electromagnetic concepts that deal with subatom, minuscule phenomena. A comparison has been made between conventional medicine's view of the person as a machine (biomechanical) and the traditional view of person as a garden (holographic) (Bienfield & Korngold, 1995).

The major traditional medical systems are listed briefly. Attempting to provide description of any one system would be comparable to discussing the conventional medical system. However, rehabilitation nurses use alternative interventions complementary to conventional professional practice and need to understand the source, theoretical base, and context of therapeutics.

Traditional Chinese or Oriental medicine deals with balance and imbalance of the vital energy called *qi (chi)* and with *yin* and *yang.* It is a complex system that has ancient origins dating to 206 BC. Acupuncture is the intervention most familiar in the West; herbal preparations, *qi gong,* special types of massage, moxibustion, and proper attention to diet, exercise, and rest are important therapeutics.

A great deal of rehabilitation research is centered on learning about the benefits of traditional Chinese medicine. Acupuncture has been reported as effective in reducing pain due to joint problems such as osteoarthritis, low back pain, and tennis elbow. An important benefit of acupuncture has been reduced intensity of pain in persons with spinal cord injury (Wong & Rapson, 1999).

India's traditional medical system, *Ayurveda,* has gained popular attention in the West as a "science of life." *Prahna* is an essential energy flow, and diet, massage, herbal preparations, fresh air, and sunshine are prescribed according to individual body types. Programs of exercise (yoga), meditation, and a form of controlled breathing place emphasis on maintaining or restoring harmony and connection among the body, mind, spirit, and environment. Traditional and *Maharishi* are two approaches to *Ayurveda.*

Homeopathy gained a popular following in the West during the mid-nineteenth century, which diminished by the early 1920s, and it continues to gain a following wherever or whenever persons place an emphasis on the body's capacity for self-healing. A large pharmacopeia includes many remedies prepared from herbal and plant sources, minerals, and some animal secretions or venom. The Law of Similars, which holds that a condition could be cured by inducing a mild form of a like condition, was further developed from the notion that every illness has its own remedy within itself (Jacobs & Moskowitz, 1996). Small doses of potentially toxic remedies, often involving several preparations to be taken in a certain order, time, and dose, are used to stimulate the body's self-healing mechanisms against illness.

Curanderismo is a traditional healing system found in Puerto Rican, Mexican, Latin-American, and related cultures. Many culturally specific diagnoses and treatments are used, and syncretism with some Catholic Church practices may occur. Theoretically, illness classifications encompass natural or biomedical diseases, as well as supernatural conditions. One or both types can emerge when a person has a disease, whether it is alcoholism, cancer, diabetes, or nerves. Supernatural conditions may result from evil spirits, spells placed by an angry or jealous person, or other spiritual agents.

Curandismo, the healers, use and integrate conventional medicine treatments, beliefs, and medications for natural illnesses. Prayers, incantations, use of objects or animals, rituals, and altered consciousness states are common interventions in conjunction with conventional medicine (Sobel, 1979; Krippner, 1995). In a recent study, Mexican Americans who are at high risk for adult-onset diabetes mellitus reasoned that prayer and herbal remedies, when used in conjunction with conventional medical treatments, enhanced the power of the insulin (Hunt, Arar, & Akana, 2000).

Naturopathic medicine is another system that focuses on prevention of disease and restoration of health and is less concerned with treatments. The rationale incorporates the philosophy that the body has potential for healing itself when one lives within the laws of nature. Thus it follows that naturopathic practitioners rely on noninvasive remedies of nutrition, herbal preparations, and counseling, especially about prevention and lifestyle. In addition, ultrasound, electric therapies, soft tissue and spinal manipulations, acupuncture, multiple types of hydrotherapy, and pharmacology are used. Practitioners study premedicine as a biological science and then study for 4 years incorporating conventional medicine curricula and naturopathic therapeutics. Naturopathic physicians are accredited and licensed under the Council on Naturopathic Medical Education (CNME) (Pizzorno, 1996).

Other traditional medical systems are found in cultures of Native American, Middle-Eastern, African, Aboriginal, Tibetan, and Central and South American peoples (NCCAM, 2000).

Mind-Body Interventions

As discussed earlier, PNI is a framework for research of the body-mind connection using biological measures of outcome. Research supports the mind-body pathway's influence on the immune system. Simplistically the higher cognitive and limbic (emotional) centers of the brain affect health and healing via the autonomic nervous system and neuroendocrine body-mind pathways to the immune system (Waitkins in Micozzi, 1996, pp. 58-9). This is a category where some nurses have conducted client and family education and counseling. Complementary therapies activate brain-immune pathways to improve well-being. To this end, nurses incorporate interventions such as prayer, relaxation, meditation, group sessions, guided imagery and visualization, hypnotherapy, reframing and cognitive or behavior modification, pet therapy, humor, and support groups into practice. Table 13-1 provides short descriptions of selected complementary alternative modalities of interest to nurses.

Examples of studies in the mind-body category include effectiveness of movement therapies, such as yoga, *t'ai chi,* and dance therapy. *T'ai chi* has been found not only to promote relaxation and movement but also to reduce pain and improve mood (Peck, 1998). It may improve strength and balance, thus helping prevent falls in elderly persons (Wolf et al., 1996; Lumsden, Baccala, & Martire, 1998). Initial results indicate that dynamic exercise has promise for improving muscle strength and aerobic capacity. More research is needed to determine its potential with joint mobility (Van den Ende, Vliet Vlieland, Munneke, & Hazes, 1999).

The benefits of pet ownership continue to grow. In a yearlong study of older persons (mean age 73 years) who were living independently, those who had pet companionship had higher ratings for activities of daily living (ADLs) and were better able to withstand crisis situations irrespective of their social support. In rehabilitation, pets have provided assistance as well as companionship. Equine or hippotherapy is therapeutic horseback riding. The motion of the horse in movement helps clients to develop muscle strength, control, and balance. Furthermore, riders of all ages gain a sense of confidence, self-image, and access to the larger world from the saddle.

Related therapies, such as music, art, and dance, influence the brain hemisphere responses and cognitive processes in positive ways. Used in conjunction with relaxation and visualization or guided imagery, these therapies have potential for improving outcomes for clients. Journal writing is a favorite technique used in conjunction with these therapies. Smyth, Stone, Hurewitz, and Kaell (1999) used journal writing about experiences that were emotionally stressful as a means to reduce symptoms for clients with diseases, such as rheumatoid arthritis and asthma, thought to be exacerbated by stress. After writing for a third of a year, nearly half the clients experienced clinically relevant improvements. These therapies are discussed in Chapter 28 also. Nurses do participate in other techniques complementary to mind-body concepts (i.e., hypnosis, psychotherapy, and biofeedback) but only with special training.

TABLE 13-1 Selected Complementary Alternative Modalities

Type	Description
Therapies	
Mind-body interventions	Interventions based on the recognition that the mind and body are integrated and therefore influence each other for purposes of healing.
Biofeedback	A procedure to alter or change a physiologic function such as brain waves while external monitoring provides feedback. Freeman and Lawless (2001) present studies using biofeedback for tension headaches, pain management, migraine headaches, and cardiovascular disease.
Hypnotherapy	Use of a state of heightened awareness that alters subjective feelings or creates expectancy so the person is more likely to follow suggestions posed by the therapist or through autosuggestion. Hypnotherapy is useful in the removal of warts; pain reduction including chronic pain; and treatment of irritable bowel syndrome, asthma, and pregnancy-induced nausea. It can also help shorten postoperative hospital stays (Freeman & Lawless, 2001).
Imagery and visualization	Sensory input into the use of the imagination and thoughts and feelings as inner representation of one's experience and fantasies. Imagery is the essence of dreams, daydreams, memories, reminiscence, plans, and possibilities. Guided imagery, or goal-directed imagery, can produce physiological changes within the body. Imagery is useful in pain control; treatment of eczema, acne, and breast cancer; and modulation of immune function (Freeman & Lawless, 2001).
Meditation	Used for thousands of years in many parts of the world, meditation involves blocking out nonessential thoughts while focusing on the present, thereby calming the mind. Types of meditation include concentrative, mindfulness, and transcendental. Studies described in Freeman and Lawless (2001) confirm that meditation is useful in controlling cholesterol, hypertension, epilepsy, chronic pain, and addictive behaviors.
Progressive relaxation	The practice of purposefully relaxing the skeletal muscles of the body. Progressive relaxation has been useful in controlling chemotherapy-induced nausea and anxiety, hypertension, painful epileptic seizures, anxiety, and depression (Freeman & Lawless, 2001). Benson (1996) was a pioneer in promoting the benefits of the relaxation response.
Energetic therapy	Healing therapies based on the existence of a universal life force or energy. Therapies unblock the flow of energy or use energy for healing purposes (Nurse's handbook, 1998).
Acupuncture	An ancient Chinese system of healing, acupuncture involves the insertion of fine needles at specific points on the body to unblock *Qi,* or energy, that circulates throughout the body along pathways called *meridians.* The NCCAM reports the efficacy of acupuncture in the treatment of knee osteoarthritis, fibromyalgia, and back pain (NCCAM, 2000).
Magnet therapy	According to Eliopoulos (1999), magnets generate controlled magnetic fields that accelerate healing by attracting and repelling charged particles in the blood. Magnets also stimulate the nervous system to block pain sensations. There are no definitive studies on the use of magnets; however, magnets have been used for arthritic pain, headaches, circulatory problems, and sleep disorders.
Therapeutic touch (noncontact)	Developed by Dolores Krieger in the 1970s, this is a method of moving the hands over the body to balance the body's energy, or *Qi.* The goal of therapeutic touch, according to Krieger, is to restore the harmony and balance of the body, mind, and spirit by bringing an individual into alignment with the universal energy that sustains all life. Turner, Clark, Gauthier, and Williams (1998) documented the efficacy of therapeutic touch on pain, wound healing, and anxiety in patients with burn injuries. Other studies reported benefits of wound healing, decreased fever and inflammation, reduced postoperative pain, and easier breathing in patients with asthma (Nurse's handbook, 1998). Villaire (1999) describes the benefits of touch therapy after coronary artery bypass surgery.
Transcutaneous electronic nerve stimulation (TENS)	TENS devices block pain by directing a stimulating electronic current to local nerves. TENS has been used for chronic and acute pain and postsurgical pain (Nurse's handbook, 1998).
Reiki	This therapy involves the transfer of universal energy, *Qi,* through a trained Reiki master to achieve balance of mind and body. This ancient Eastern practice involves "laying on of hands for healing" (Rivera, 1999). Used in a wide range of diagnoses, a controlled study on the treatment of stroke is currently under way (Spencer & Jacobs, 1999).
Manual therapy	Musculoskeletal adjustments that involve the application of pressure that relieves pathological pressure on nerves or reduces blocked energy channels of the body (Nurse's handbook, 1998).
Acupressure	Acupuncture without needles, this technique involves firm finger pressure over acupuncture points to relieve symptoms. No definitive studies were found regarding the efficacy of acupressure. Proponents believe it has illness-resistant benefits by sustaining the immune system response (Decker, 1999).

TABLE 13-1 Selected Complementary Alternative Modalities—cont'd

Type	Description
Therapies—cont'd	
Alexander technique	The use of proper body posture, especially the head, neck, and trunk, to facilitate health and prevent injury. It may be useful in the treatment of chronic conditions of the head, neck, and back; myalgia; and breathing problems and the prevention of repetitive stress injuries (Nurse's handbook, 1998).
Massage therapy	The intentional manipulation of the soft tissues of the body, modern massage can be traced to P. H. Ling, a Swedish physician. According to Gertrude Beard at Northwestern University (Nurse's handbook, 1998), massage increases blood flow to muscles, therefore promoting relaxation and pain relief; sedates the nervous system; increases peristalsis; increases lymphatic circulation; and decreases scar tissue, adhesions, and fibrosis due to injury and immobilization (Nurse's handbook, 1998).
Reflexology	The practice of applying pressure to specific points on the feet and sometimes hands to restore balance and energy flow in the body and enhance health. The exact mechanism of action is unknown. The intent of reflexology is to mitigate symptoms. No definitive studies on the use of reflexology were found; however, it has been used for diarrhea, constipation, asthma, chronic pain, psoriasis, and fatigue among others (Decker, 1999).
Rolfing	The manipulation of connective tissue in order to reverse misalignment and allow the body to move appropriately. The practitioner applies pressure to soften and lengthen fascia. Antidotal evidence suggests that changes during rolfing are long-lasting (Decker, 1999).
Trager method	A gentle body work that involves stretching and rocking the body to loosen stiff joints and muscles. Developed by Milton Trager, this technique uses movement to produce pleasurable sensations and deep relaxation. Trager used this technique for patients with multiple sclerosis, muscular dystrophy, and polio. No research evidence could be found; however, proponents of this method claim improved function in those with asthma and emphysema (Nurse's handbook, 1998).
Botanicals	
Aloe	The gel or the leaf of the aloe plant is commonly used topically for minor burns, skin irritation, and would healing. Aloe gel is also ingested as a gastrointestinal cleansing agent. Currently, clinical trials are under way regarding the immunostimulating activity of aloe (Blumenthal in Eskinazi, 1999).
Capsicum	Cayenne or red pepper. Used for muscle soreness, arthritic pain, and pain from shingles (Blumenthal in Eskinazi, 1999).
Chamomile	The flowers of this plant are used in teas for antiinflammatory and antispasmodic activity (Blumenthal in Eskinazi, 1999).
Dong Quai	A traditional Chinese medicine, its numerous preparations are used for analgesic, antispasmodic, and antiinflammatory effects. It is used most commonly for dysmenorrhea (Blumenthal in Eskinazi, 1999).
Echinacea	The plant's roots, leaf, flower, and seeds have been used for their antiviral and antiinflammatory actions. Clinical trials in Germany are in progress to determine effectiveness (Blumenthal in Eskinazi, 1999).
Feverfew	Historically this herb has been used as an antispasmodic and analgesic for menstrual cramps and most recently for migraine prophylaxis (Blumenthal in Eskinazi, 1999).
Flaxseed	The dried ground seeds of this plant are used for irritable bowel and diverticulitis (Decker, 1999).
Garlic	The German Commission E has established the efficacy of garlic in lowering low-density cholesterol (Blumenthal in Eskinazi, 1999). An evidence-based report from the Agency for Healthcare Research and Quality (AHRQ, 2000) found short-term cardiovascular benefits from garlic use. The full report details amounts and types of preparation, in addition to data concerning use in cancer and adverse effects.
Ginger	The root of this plant has been shown to prevent motion-sickness (Blumenthal in Eskinazi, 1999).
Ginkgo	The leaf of this plant is used for stimulating peripheral circulation and for antiplatelet-activating activity (Blumenthal in Eskinazi, 1999).
Ginseng	This herb is used for its tonic effect. It is believed to increase energy and decrease fatigue (Decker, 1999).
Kava Kava	The male plant's flowers are used to treat nervousness, anxiety, stress, and insomnia (Decker, 1999).
Licorice	Commonly used in China to treat chest and throat irritation, it is an adrenal gland stimulant or tonic. Licorice extract is used in Europe for gastric and duodenal ulcers (Blumenthal in Eskinazi, 1999).
Peppermint	The leaf of the plant is commonly used in teas for enhancing digestion. In Europe it is used for irritable bowel syndrome (Blumenthal in Eskinazi, 1999).

Continued

Table 13-1 Selected Complementary Alternative Modalities—cont'd

Type	Description
Botanicals—cont'd	
Saw Palmetto	The berries of this plant have a mild estrogenic antiandrogenic effect. It is also used for diuresis and chronic cystitis and, in Europe, for benign prostatic hypertrophy (Decker, 1999).
St. John's Wort	The yellow flowers of this plant are used to treat anxiety and depression. It has also been used to treat insomnia and gastritis (Decker, 1999).
Valerian	This aromatic root has been used as a sedative and sleep aid (Blumenthal in Eskinazi, 1999).
Diet and Nutrition	
Gonzalez plan (an offshoot of the Kelly regimen)	Recently Nicholas Gonzalez received funding from the National Cancer Institute to study the effects of diet and nutritional supplements for patients with pancreatic cancer. This modification of the Kelly regimen from the 1970s includes a patient-tailored diet and nutritional supplementation including pancreatic enzymes, hydrochloric acid, raw beef organs, and detoxification with coffee enemas (Gordon & Curtin, 2000).
Gearson therapy	A metabolic therapy that includes diet, nutritional supplementation, detoxification, and enzyme therapy to fight disease and strengthen the immune system. The Gearson Institute in California oversees a clinic in Tijuana, Mexico, that offers Gearson treatments to cancer patients. The National Cancer Institute reviewed 50 of Gearson's case studies in 1959 and found that Gearson failed to meet the criteria for evaluating clinical benefit. More recent studies reported subjective benefits, including pain relief, fewer side effects from conventional therapy, less weight loss, and a better quality of life (Gordon & Curtin, 2000).
Pritikin diet	A dietary regimen that is very low in fats (less than 10% of daily calories), low in cholesterol, and high in complex carbohydrates and fiber. The regimen includes at least 45 minutes of walking daily. This diet was shown to decrease total low-density lipoprotein cholesterol and triglyceride levels (Nurse's handbook, 1998).
Ornish program	This program consists of a low-fat vegetarian diet, regular exercise, and stress management. The diet provides about 1800 calories a day. The diet allows 2 oz of alcohol daily. The regimen requires 1 hour of walking, meditation, or yoga for stress reduction and support group attendance. Cardiac patients on the Ornish program for 1 year reported significant decreases in angina. Angiograms of those on the Ornish plan showed overall reductions of arterial blockages (Nurse's handbook, 1998).
Macrobiotic diets	Originally from Japan, macrobiotic diets became popular in the 1960s. Macrobiotic principles espouse that Western diets including dairy products, meat, and fatty processed foods cause an over-accumulation of toxins and cause imbalance. A macrobiotic diet consists of 50% whole grains, 5% to 10% beans and bean products and sea vegetables, 5% to 10% seasonal vegetables, 25% to 30% fruits (moderated as needed) and some fish. All foods must be organic, locally grown, and seasonal. Studies have shown that those who follow a macrobiotic diet have favorable cardiovascular profiles and the protective benefits of soy products (lower breast cancer rate). Currently, antidotal accounts by cancer patients have found that macrobiotics extended and enhanced their lives. Some have claimed a cure from cancer. No studies are available to verify the efficacy of macrobiotics as a treatment for cancer (Gordon & Curtin, 2000).

Biological-Based Therapies

This category has a great deal of activity in the community because of the popular use of nutritional programs, dietary supplements, herbal preparations, and therapies or products to treat special conditions or diseases. For example, glucosamine supplements for arthritis, bee pollen supplements for autoimmune diseases, diet programs such as by Drs. Pritikin and Ornish, megavitamin regimens, macrobiotic diets, antioxidant supplements, and melatonin supplements all are biological based. The range of herbal medicine choices is huge.

Aromatherapy and hydrotherapy have entered the public domain in multiple products from candles to body oils to massage kits. Aroma as therapy differs from simply selecting scents; choices for use as therapies are highly selective based on multiple factors and may be introduced complementary to other interventions. Allergies or sensitivities to aromas are not uncommon, but proper informed use can bring soothing relief and relaxation.

Many herbal products are available over the counter at local health food stores or pharmacies; others must be prepared at ethnic apothecaries. Studies have shown glucosamine and chondroitin supplements to give moderate to large relief of symptoms due to osteoarthritis (McAlindon, LaValley, Gulin, & Felson, 2000). Similarly, injectable gold has been shown to be effective for short-term treatment of swollen joints due to rheumatoid arthritis, although toxicity was a risk for some clients (Clark et al., 1999). However, the popular herb Echinacea has been found ineffective in preventing colds or reducing cold symptoms (Turner, Riker, & Gangemi, 2000).

Interactions with food, conventional medicines, and herbal products occur, but as a body of knowledge the implications of consecutive or concurrent use are relatively unknown. For example, St. John's wort, which has been used successfully for decades to treat depression and perimenopausal symptoms, was found to produce reduced blood levels of indinavir, an HIV protease inhibitor (Piscitelli, Burstein, Chaitt, Alfaro, & Falloon, 2000). Nutrition and lifestyle changes are modalities of high interest to nurses.

Manipulative and Body-Based Methods

Physiatrists and therapists in rehabilitation, chiropractors, osteopathic physicians, massage therapists, and certain alternative practitioners manipulate the musculoskeletal system during treatments. Rehabilitation practitioners are interested in myofascial release as an adjunct to pain management. The diversity of practitioners ranges from licensed chiropractors to therapists performing massage, shiatsu, reflexology, rolfing, and acupressure for soft tissues and deep muscle manipulation. Some programs, such as *Reiki* and therapeutic touch are also energy therapies. Nurses have some practice in this category, whereas physical therapists use methods such as those originated as Feldenkrais, Alexander, Trager, and others (Davis, 1997). Although chiropractors, massage therapists, and some others receive standardized training and are licensed, the methods referred to as "bodywork" are practiced by many persons who have no license or classification and under a vast array of labels. The safety and effectiveness of many techniques in this category are ready for critical research.

Energy Therapies

These therapies deal with two types of energy fields. The first is from endogenous fields within the individual's body, and the other is from exogenous fields (external energy). Bioelectromagnetic (BEM) research has identified endogenous radiation, extremely low-level light known as *biophoton emission.* It is thought that both the positive and negative results of exogenous fields may be mitigated by endogenous fields. According to Freeman and Lawless (2001, p. 463), "The energy of the biophotons and processes involving their emission, as well as other endogenous fields of the body, may prove to be involved in energetic therapies, such as healer interactions." Also reported in Freeman and Lawless (2001), the regrowth and healing capacities of animals, even lower animals, comes from the animal's brain. If the brain is malfunctioning, rehabilitation is unsuccessful. "This phenomenon may be an explanation for how a healer may empower a patient to overcome systemic disease through imagery or persuasion" (p. 461). *Qi gong, Reiki,* healing touch, and therapeutic touch are examples in which the therapist accesses a healing energy force that flows through to facilitate healing for the individual. The therapist must be able to enter into a centered state of consciousness and continually assess and evaluate the process while directing energy. Based on the research initiated by Krieger (1979) (later joined by Kunz), the principle of "undivided wholeness" is one that resonated with nurses. They have embraced therapeutic touch in research and practice, including a North American Nursing Diagnosis Association (NANDA) diagnosis of "energy field disturbance" (Gordon, 2000, p. 105).

As a nursing intervention, therapeutic touch is defined as "attuning to the universal healing field, seeking to act as an instrument for healing influence, and using the natural sensitivity of the hands to gently focus and direct the intervention process" (McCloskey & Bulechek, 2000, p. 655).

Quinn (1984) found therapeutic touch effective in reducing anxiety in patients hospitalized with cardiovascular disease. Sixty patients were divided into noncontact therapeutic touch and placebo therapeutic touch groups. Anxiety scores were significantly reduced in patients receiving therapeutic touch but not in the placebo group. Eckes-Peck (1997) studied 82 patients older than 55 years with degenerative arthritis. Subjects served as their own controls for 4 weeks and then received either therapeutic touch or progressive muscle relaxation once a week for 6 weeks. Pain intensity and distress were significantly reduced in the therapeutic touch group.

Wirth (1992) completed a double-blind study on the effects of therapeutic touch on wound healing. All participants (N=46) were given a skin punch biopsy that produced full-thickness dermal wounds of the lateral deltoid muscle. They extended the biopsied arm through a door for 5 minutes each day, unable to see whether they received intervention. Half the subjects received therapeutic touch, whereas the control subjects received no treatment. By day 16, 13 of the 23 therapeutic touch subjects had complete wound healing, whereas none of the 23 control group subjects were healed. Although many research findings support therapeutic touch, results are mixed; one critical review of the research literature raises questions about the evidence supporting the efficacy of therapeutic touch (O'Mathuna, 2000), and a clinical study questions assumptions of its unabridged safety as an intervention (Engle & Graney, 2000). The American Holistic Nursing Association (AHNA) certifies practitioners in healing touch for health care professionals. Closely aligned with Krieger's therapeutic touch and rogerian theory, it is a hand-mediated energetic healing intervention acquired by participating in a 2- to 3-year program of study, including quantum physics (Mentgen & Bulbrook, 1994).

The use of electromagnetic field energy relies on devices maneuvered by the individual or a therapist. Static and time-varying magnetic products have achieved popular use for pain relief, muscle spasms, osteoarthritis, and multiple sclerosis. Low-level laser therapy (classes I, II, and III) has been used as noninvasive treatment for reducing rheumatoid arthritis symptoms associated with morning stiffness, range of motion and function, and local swelling. Randomized controlled clinical trials (RCCTs) yielded conflicting results with some benefits for reduced pain and stiffness after a month of treatment. Overall additional research is needed, especially regarding specific details such as dose, intensity, and site (Brosseau et al., 2000).

There has long been an interest and belief in healing properties from electromagnetic fields. Many products, ranging from wrist or knee magnets to magnetic mattress pads, are available widely in the market. To date, research evidence indicates some hope for improving outcome in sleep and certain neurologic disorders and pain management; other evidence is not yet clear (Valbona & Richards, 1999).

NATIONAL CENTER FOR COMPLEMENTARY AND ALTERNATIVE MEDICINE

The NCCAM, located within the National Institutes of Health (NIH) of the U.S. Public Health Service, is part of the U.S. Department of Health and Human Services. The NCCAM was mandated by Congress in 1998 (Omnibus Appropriations Bill; public law [PL] 105-277, 11 Stat.2681]). Originating as the Office of Alternative Medicine (OAM) in 1991, it became established solidly under the NIH Revitalization Act of 1993 (PL 103-43). The complex and challenging mission of the NCCAM is to identify complementary and alternative therapies, examine patterns of use, investigate efficacy and safety, disseminate information, validate outcomes, and train practitioners to integrate tested therapies into mainstream health care practice and gain reimbursement. Today, the NCCAM has established clinical research and project centers, an information clearinghouse, a system for organizing and conducting clinical trials, advisory panels for managing specific data such as for cancer treatment, and various transgovernmental agency and advisory groups.

Clinical research, including formal clinical trials to determine the safety, clinical activity and efficacy, and potential problems of currently known and available therapies and substances, is NCCAM's highest priority. Initially five specialized research centers across the nation received funding to study the use of complementary and alternative medicine in areas of aging, arthritis, craniofacial disorders, neurological disorders, women's health, and cardiovascular disease in African-Americans. Examples of specific research topics reveal many are important to rehabilitation, such as the safety and efficacy of:

- Acupuncture in treating (separately) knee osteoarthritis, fibromyalgia, and back pain
- Melatonin for sleep disorders in Parkinson's disease
- Saw palmetto extract for benign prostatic hyperplasia
- Triple antioxidant regimen in decreasing activity of multiple sclerosis
- Self-hypnosis, acupuncture, and osteopathic manipulation for muscle tension in children with spastic cerebral palsy
- Ginkgo biloba for decreasing the incidence of dementia and Alzheimer's disease in very old persons (NCCAM, 2000).

EVIDENCE-BASED PRACTICE

By now, *evidence-based practice* has become another phrase for ensuring quality of service, therapeutic interventions, remedies, and preparations. The process examines the abilities of the practitioner, as well as the rigor of research to evaluate safety and effectiveness. At stake are reimbursement for effective products and therapies and eventual integration of proven therapies into mainstream conventional medicine and education. The field of knowledge is boggling minds with information about new findings and resources. However, a great backlog of investigation falls behind public demands and usage. Gathering evidence and disseminating findings are lengthy processes in and of themselves. The timeline is extended further by safeguards for research on human subjects and translations of studies published in foreign languages.

Clinical decisions are based on a critique of the research literature to form conclusions about what is safe, effective, and economically sound; to determine that more evidence is needed; or to declare interventions as outright unsafe or ineffective. A scheme for ranking evidence of research findings combines ranking of several medical groups.

The Cochrane Collaboration (CC) provides an international register of RCCTs in alternative research. A not-for-profit organization that prepares, maintains, and disseminates systematic, current reviews of RCCTs and/or controlled clinical trials, the CC issues reports of interest to groups across all areas of health care, such as specific treatments in rehabilitation. The CC uses a similar scheme in evaluating research findings suitable for clinical practice. Evidence must be accompanied by sufficient information about use of the therapeutic technique, instrument, or preparation, such as the dose response, strength, frequency, intensity, cautions, and adverse effects. Lack of standardization, purity of ingredients, and poor control of cause and effect are examples of quality issues (Ezzo, Berman, Vickers, & Linde, 1998).

Monitoring Claims for Cure

When cure is not forthcoming, persons with terminal, chronic, or disabling conditions may seek hope wherever promised, regardless of evidence. The Food and Drug Administration (FDA) is the government agency charged to protect consumers from danger, fraud, false expectations, and ineffective or unacceptable claims. The FDA requires pharmaceutical companies and manufacturers of dietary supplements and other health products to meet stringent standards, involving costly and lengthy procedures, whenever the label promises cure for a specific condition. However, products that are intended to improve health undergo less scrutiny, essentially just a review of their labels for false claims about cures. With more than 29,000 dietary supplements alone, the over-the-counter market is difficult to monitor and evaluate (Adams, 2000).

Composition and standards for preparation vary among companies and products. Certainly many products do help individuals, and nearly 70% of households use some type of vitamin, herbal product, or supplement. Other products do not help, and sales of ineffective products prey on the hopes of desperate clients and families. Recently a news article detailed how a young entrepreneur was helping individuals access drugs and preparations through his website. Although banned nearly 20 years ago by the FDA, laetrile was offered for sale on the site (Lagnado, 2000).

Organizational Collaboration

The NCCAM collaborated with a group of national organizations to enhance speed and improve quality of research reports from clinical investigations. The gold standard for evaluating any intervention has been recognized as the RCCT. This method sits directly in the domain of scientific approaches of conventional medicine and will be fraught with problems that are methodological, philosophical, and concerned with feasibility (Margolin, Avants, & Kleber, 1998). Critical evaluation of research conducted worldwide and databases of information gathered with organizational collaboration will assist in providing data about the validity and reliability of findings.

In fact, the FDA has announced a pilot program to encourage pharmaceutical companies to submit information from their clinical trials to a website as a contribution to a federal and private registry. Because Medicare reimbursement is tied to results of clinical trials, clients will have a vested interest in several ways. Some who have chronic conditions may choose to participate in trials with varying degrees of risk, others may seek payment for procedures or medications, and health providers may be bombarded with appropriate and inappropriate requests for services from clients (FDA on-line, 2000, www.clinicaltrials.gov/databank). Rehabilitation nurses are in positions to serve as advocates for clients on either hand: to protect them from improper participation in trials or use of products and services, or to assist them in gaining access to efficacious interventions. Becoming knowledgeable and staying current must be tempered with understanding the implications and evaluating the outcomes on individual client bases.

Once the NCCAM scientifically investigates the effectiveness of a treatment or procedure and determines the type of evidence needed, one or more of the following organizations conduct systematic reviews for evidence.

- Centers for Disease Control and Prevention (CDC) has direct access to providers and skill in survey research.
- Cancer Advisory Panel for Complementary and Alternative Medicine (CAPCAM) operates in collaboration with the National Cancer Institute (NCI) to target evaluation of cancer treatment proposals.
- Agency for Healthcare Research and Quality (AHRQ), formerly the Agency for Health Care Policy and Research (AHCPR), offers publications about best practices and guidelines for professionals and consumers.
- The CC reports can be used when deciding whether to use research findings in practice.
- Topics discussed at NIH Consensus Development Conferences sponsored by NCCAM are pertinent to practice and research.

Dissemination of Information

Not only are clients becoming active partners in their health care, in some instances they are researching and directing their care using information and resources from around the world, such as from the FDA-sponsored clinical trials database and registry mentioned earlier. Dissemination of information in reputable channels is important for providers. Alternative and complementary health care and related interventions have captured a great deal of attention in research, publications, conference proceedings, and practice settings, and dozens of schools of medicine, nursing, and allied health now include courses in these fields.

The Richard and Hinda Rosenthal Center for Complementary and Alternative Medicine at Columbia University is a resource on the World Wide Web for databases concerning alternative health care (Box 13-3). And the NCCAM has its own clearinghouse for dissemination of information about the program and research findings to providers and the public. The NCCAM maintains a citation index since 1963 available through the National Library of Medicine's MEDLINE database. The Combined Health Information Database (CHID) contains information about alternative

Box 13-3 Websites

- NCCAM website: http://nccam.nih.gov
- CAM Citation Index: http://nccam.nih.gov/nccam/resources/search.cgi
- Combined Health Information Database: http://chid,nih.gov
- Rosenthal Center: http://cpmcnet.columbia.edu/dept/rosenthal/
- Cochrane Collaboration: http://www.cochrane.dk
- Agency for Healthcare Research and Quality: http://www.ahrq.gov/
- The Office of Minority Health, Public Health Service has begun a project Assuring Cultural Competence in Health Care: Recommendations for National Standards and an Outcomes-Focused Research Agenda: http://omhrc.gov/CLAS/po.html
- A federal and privately funded on-line registry of clinical trials, both those proposed with opportunities for participation and completed trials: http://www.clinicaltrials.gov/database
- A website devoted to exposing fraudulent practices and claims or to debunking commonly held misconceptions, as a consumer protection: http://www.quackwatch.com

health consolidated with other governmental health materials and data.

REFERRAL TO A PRACTITIONER OF ALTERNATIVE MEDICINE

Increasingly, traditional or alternative practices are in the mainstream of health care. It is inevitable that rehabilitation nurses will encounter practitioners of alternative medicine or therapies, and likely they will personally use them. At times the nursing assessment and plan for care will differ from a client or family view of what is or what should be done. Lifestyle preferences, religious beliefs, family system patterns, and traditions of healing may not match a nursing or team plan of care. Traditional healers may join the team or collaborate, or the client may request a referral, use alternative therapeutics independent of the team, or rely on cultural practices in tandem with conventional rehabilitation practices.

Cultural competence includes sensitivity to clients' desires and preferences to use alternative therapies. Care is provided in ways that are acceptable, respectful, and relevant to the client's worldview. Critical thinking requires that nurses become aware of their own biases and gaps in their knowledge about a cultural group. Although no one can learn about all cultural beliefs and practices and persons differ widely in their own adherence to cultural practices, nurses can focus on those groups with whom they come into contact more regularly. Continuous learning is part of gaining competence. Clients have a right to meet their culturally based health care needs as much as possible. However, this right does not require providers to conform to situations or participate in practices that are illegal or unsafe or to violate and refute their own moral or religious beliefs. It does require that nurses be very clear about the rationale for decisions.

Collaboration with and referral to a practitioner of alternative health care without criteria for evaluating the person and the practice (Box 13-4) can be problematic. Practitioners, such as chiropractors and some therapists, may be licensed by the state, but practice laws and licensure requirements differ among states. To complicate the process, many alternative providers have no established education or training, no formal organization, and no standard name for their practice. For example, more than 30 titles fall under the category of bodyworks. Claims against alternative practitioners are minor, perhaps 5% of the medical malpractice claims. Many health insurers are providing coverage for certain alternative practices or providers, and making a referral is not usually difficult. However, when working in collaboration with an alternative provider or making a referral to an unknown practitioner, liability issues may emerge should the person suffer injury due to negligence or inappropriate care (Studdert et al., 1998; Eisenberg, 1997).

Box 13-4 Suggestions When Making a Referral to a Practitioner of Alternative Medicine

Determine whether the practitioner:
- Holds membership in specialty organizations or associations
- Is certified or accredited by specialty area
- Has liability insurance for practice
- Honors (does not violate) professional practice acts of conventional medicine professionals
- Obtains reimbursement or coverage from insurance companies
- Attends continuing education or other workshops
- Is known to other providers (conventional and alternative) in the community
- Communicates with the team members about the plan for care
- Uses safe practices and ethical behaviors, as far as can be ascertained, and avoids practices known to be unsafe or ineffective per RCTs
- Provides treatment options and indicates length of the treatment
- Does not continue process or treatments indefinitely
- Has no public, professional, or client complaints against the practice or provider for personal misconduct

NURSING PROCESS

Assessment

Conceptual frameworks that may be useful include the Health Belief Model, Leininger's transcultural model, Roger's Science of Unitary Man, and Neuman's Systems Model; all are discussed in Chapter 2.

Cultural Assessment

Recognize that the community and familial environments are part of the client's assessment. Elicit the client's explanatory model of the health condition or situation; ask for the person's own description of the condition.

- What does it mean to you or your family that you have this disease or disability?
- What do you think is the cause of the problem? Does it have a name? Why do you think it happened?
- Explain how you think this disease or disability will work. How long will it last? How sick or disabled do you think, or do others say, you are?
- What should be done to treat the condition? What have you or someone else done already? Did it work?
- Who could best treat this condition? What are problems or concerns that you have about the treatment? What support is available from your family, religious group, or community? Do you need help in contacting these groups?
- What do you plan to do? What can you expect as a result of treatment or lack of treatment?
- Are nontraditional, complementary, or alternative healers involved? What treatments are under consideration? What assistance is needed to accommodate this approach?
- Are there legal or ethical considerations? How best can these be addressed?

- What will not work or should not be done in the situation? Are there things you believe you should not talk about or say?
- What would you like the result or outcome to be?

Learning and asking about specific areas will provide better understanding of the meaning of data collected during the assessment.

Learn About

- History of the culture
- Client's perception of personal identification with the culture
- Client/family degree of acculturation with the dominant society
- Where they place themselves regarding intraethnic diversity
- Language skills (assess oral and reading/writing separately)
- Education level and socioeconomic status
- Length of time they have lived in the United States

Ask About

- Lifestyle, preferences, and prohibitions
- Dietary habits or needs
- Religious and spiritual values
- Traditional healing practices and the use of nutraceuticals, over-the-counter medications, and complementary and alternative medical practices.

Cultural assessment is complex and involves moving past ethnocentric assumptions. For example, the title of aunt or mother to a child of some cultures may not be restricted to biological or family roles. Assess the client and family perceptions of space, time, sex roles, kinship ties, and family relationships. Nonverbal communication, gestures, and facial expressions are not credible measures for understanding what is really happening and are misinterpreted often by members of differing cultures. Evaluate for specific biological or genetic conditions that are associated with certain heritages. Collection of data about cultural phenomena takes time and a trust relationship.

Giger & Davidhizar (1999) list six cultural phenomena that are evident in all cultural groups in varying degrees of application. These are communication, space, time, biological variations, environmental control, and social organization. Assessment and intervention are enriched with these kinds of data. Self-care differences among cultural groups are important for rehabilitation nurses to identify before instituting plans for care or engaging in mutual goal setting with clients and families. Table 13-2 represents religious variables of the dominant groups in North America.

Assessing the Therapeutic Relationship

Many clients or families rely on cultural, lay, or folk remedies or alternative therapies; essentially, they formulate their own plan of care apart from the rehabilitation program (Box 13-5). Learn client expectations of a rehabilitation nurse, especially for self-care and therapeutic relationships. What are the person's experiences with assistive devices or technology?

Goals

Goals for rehabilitation nurses are to become culturally competent, sensitive, and relevant and to be able to broker between the client and family culture and the culture of rehabilitation.

Interventions

Use strategies of the culture broker role to bridge or mediate between the client culture, the conventional rehabilitation system, and traditional and/or alternative medical systems.

- Clarify information, values, and expectations
- Broker concepts, such as self-care among client and team members
- Encourage building trust and therapeutic relationships
- Ensure client and family fully comprehend information and consent
- Discuss problems, misconceptions, and disagreements openly
- Facilitate using conflict resolution and negotiation skills
- Integrate family and religious and cultural values and beliefs into the person's plan for care as safely and possible
- Arrange for interventions with sensitivity to variations in perceptions, such as for time, space, lifestyle, dietary needs, and communication

Use translators cautiously. Age, sex, intraethnic animosities, class issues, and prohibitions about sharing personal information may lead to collecting inaccurate data and a client experiencing mistrust or even fear of harm. Consider how many persons are able to speak a language fluently or conversationally but remain unfamiliar with medical terminology or correct descriptions of health problems.

Many therapeutic interventions that are alternative practices are performed commonly by rehabilitation nurses. Examples of interventions known to have benefits are listed in Box 13-6.

Rehabilitation nurses may choose to pursue education and training in complementary practices for shiatsu, reflexology, biofeedback, behavioral management, herbal medicine, acupuncture, therapeutic touch, *Reiki,* and other specific healing methodologies (Rankin-Box, 1995). Other chapters in the text contain information about specific alternative interventions for particular conditions.

Outcomes

Outcomes are for cultural competence and sensitivity in rehabilitation practice and for the perceptions and expectations of client, family, and providers to be based on trust to build the therapeutic relationship.

Evaluation

Rehabilitation nurses may encounter issues with regulations and standards of practice. "Many (alternative and comple-

TABLE 13-2 Variations among Selected Religious Groups

Religion	Sacraments or Rituals	Religion and Healing	Diet and Medication	Treatment Protocols
Buddhism	Three Treasures, Buddha, Dharma, Sangha; ritual symbolizes entry into Buddhist faith	Meditation to achieve peace, truth, and enlightenment; illness may be viewed as a test of strength	Generally vegetarian diet; refrain from alcohol and tobacco; medication may be refused	Any procedure that prolongs life, such as transplant, is encouraged because longevity assists in attaining enlightenment
Christian Science	Baptism and communion	Healing is through prayer and spiritual regeneration; disease is considered a mental error	No restrictions in diet; usually refrain from alcohol and caffeine; medication is forbidden	Blood and blood products are avoided; rarely organ donors
Hinduism	*Karma,* everyone is born into a position based on a previous life, *Samaras,* reincarnation	Illness is punishment for sins, possibly from another life; some believe in faith healing	May choose not to eat meat; no medication restrictions	None
Islam	Observe Friday as the Sabbath; pray 5 times/day facing Mecca; may request confession when dying	May choose not to shorten or terminate life; ritual cleansing of the dead in preparation for burial	No pork or alcoholic beverages; no medication restrictions; fasting during Ramadan	Organ donation, creamation, and autopsy are prohibited
Judaism	Circumcision on 8th day after birth by mohel; observe the Sabbath each Saturday	Medical care must be provided by a physician; autopsy may be permitted, and burial of all body parts is required	No pork or shellfish; do not mix dairy and meat products at the same meal; food must be kosher; no medication restrictions	Generally none; in some branches, abortion on demand is not acceptable
Protestantism	Baptism, communion, confirmation, and last rights in some denominations	Prayer and anointing are common; laying on of hands in some denominations; some view illness as punishment or an act of Satan	Vary; some prohibitions on alcohol, coffee, tea, or tobacco; fasting on religious holidays for some denominations; no medication restrictions	Generally none
Catholicism	Baptism, communion, confirmation, reconciliation, matrimony, Holy Orders, anointing of sick	Sacrament of the sick administered by a priest, includes anointing, communion, and blessing; baptism for critically ill newborns; may request a visit from a priest when ill	Fasting on certain religious holidays; no medication restrictions	Abortion is forbidden; only natural birth control is accepted; sterilization is forbidden

From Kozier, B., Erb, G., Wilkinson, J.M., & Van Lewven, K. (1998). *Fundamentals of nursing concepts process and practice.* Menlo Park, CA: Addison-Wesley.

Box 13-5 Assessing Plans for Alternative Interventions

Assess whether the client and family plan for any alternative or cultural intervention is:
- Safe, legal, feasible, reasonable, or ethical
- Detrimental or harmful or has adverse effects
- Compatible with client and team goals for rehabilitation
- Related to religious beliefs or practices
- Fully understood, including consequences

mentary) strategies have long been in the purview of nursing practice. Regulatory changes in nurse practices acts and the professional practice acts of other professionals related to alternative medicine differ by state and must be carefully monitored by nurses" (Geddes & Henry, 1997).

Evidence-based practice, such as that guided by information from the CC, international studies, and findings from NCCAM-sponsored research programs, will evaluate methods, techniques, and interventions from alternative and conventional medical systems by their quality, safety, and efficacy.

Box 13-6 Nursing Practices Useful as Complementary Interventions

Relaxation response
Guided imagery
Visualization
Meditative approaches
Energy transfer
Aromatherapy
Massage
Therapeutic humor and laughter
Reframing
Cognitive redirecting
Therapeutic touch
Therapeutic exercises
Targeted therapies for music, art, or dance
Pain management
Support and self-help groups
Diet and nutrition
Prayer and intercessory groups
Sports and leisure use
Pet companionship
Self-regulatory and stress-reduction techniques
Lifestyle modifications or cessation programs for smoking
Substance abuse and related habitual conditions
Communication, education, and counseling skills

ALTERNATIVE REHABILITATION

Rehabilitation was regarded as unconventional until after World War II. Even then it was considered a last resort for clients. Now the outcomes resulting from therapeutics, processes, and principles that comprise rehabilitation are being researched as an entity. Preventive as well as restorative and maintenance benefits from rehabilitation are possible. Engstrom and Hauser (2000) found physical rehabilitation to improve motor scores on the Functional Independence Measure (FIM, see Chapter 8), with related perceptions of quality of life for clients with multiple sclerosis.

In another study persons who participated in a cardiac rehabilitation program improved their overall health, exercise capacity, and energy levels and reduced their depression. Depression has been associated with coronary artery disease. Future research can be anticipated once findings from the human genome project are released for study and practice. New issues continue to arise as alternatives within conventional medicine, such as debates about acceptance and regulations for therapeutic use of marijuana (Mitka, 1999).

SUMMARY: NURSING AND ALTERNATIVE CARE

Nurses were among the first professionals to promote alternative and complementary modes of health and healing. A holistic approach is central to nursing, nurses understand care apart from cure, and nurses encourage self-care in the therapeutic process. They recognize that at times healing arises from the person's own participation, whether from biological, psychosocial, spiritual, or other resources. Many techniques identified as alternative or complementary have been embraced by and practiced within professional nursing. Relaxation techniques, stress reduction or smoking cessation programs, lifestyle management, and therapeutic exercise are long-time nursing interventions, whereas Krieger's (1979) work on therapeutic touch remains an extension of practice for many nurses. Nurses also are comfortable working with clients from diverse backgrounds and with using proven alternative therapeutics to complement conventional practices. They understand how body, mind, and spirit interrelate so that a person may have mental and spiritual health alongside a terminal body condition.

And prevention is in vogue. The goals of *Healthy People 2010* include helping persons to maintain optimal functional abilities and promoting healthier, longer lives. However, despite funds devoted to cure of chronic, disabling conditions, minimal support targets prevention and early intervention.

Ideally, research findings supporting prevention in control of chronic conditions such as Parkinson's disease or Alzheimer's disease and arthritis may diminish focus on cure alone. Clearly safety, efficacy, and quality must be rigorously pursued in evidence-based research. Perhaps nurse advocates will direct more attention to improving the physical and social environment, potential for self-healing, and life satisfaction for persons with chronic, disabling, or developmental conditions.

The call is for an integrated health system, rather than conventional, alternative, or complementary medicine and therapeutics (Sobel, 1979; Fontanarosa & Lundberg, 1998). Many treatments, interventions, and therapeutics originating outside Western medicine have been proved safe and to have merit, especially when practiced by a trained practitioner and used properly. Similarly, more openness in global relationships has resulted in regard and acceptance of the results of rigorous and controlled research conducted by professionals in other countries.

CRITICAL THINKING

Mrs. Mehol had breast cancer, bilateral mastectomies, and reconstructive surgery approximately 5 years ago. After surgery she was treated with chemotherapy and did well for 2 years, when she began having respiratory symptoms and was diagnosed with metastasis to her liver and lung. She received a stem cell transplant and did well for 18 months, when she again had shortness of breath. At this time she had metastases to her lungs, liver, and bone. She began a regimen of chemotherapy, 2 weeks on and 1 week off. Although she had typical symptoms from the chemotherapy, nausea, and tiredness, she was able to continue her activities and generally felt well on her week off treatment. Approximately 6 weeks ago, Mrs. Mehol started to have severe back pain radiating down both legs. Magnetic resonance imaging confirmed a fracture of T4 with compression of the disk. She began a regimen of pain medications in addition to her other medications. For the first time since initial diagnosis, she is now concerned about quality of life issues. She said that the amount of pain medication necessary to control her pain made her "groggy and clouded her mind."

- What kinds of information about Mrs. Mehol are necessary before suggesting complementary interventions?
- Speculate about the relationship between Mrs. Mehol and those taking care of her.
- What complementary interventions may be helpful for Mrs. Mehol?
- How can you best intervene to help Mrs. Mehol?

Mr. Joseph, a robust 46 year-old man, is recovering from a herniated disk at L5. He is married and has two teenage children. Before his injury, in addition to working more than 40 hours a week at an office job, he ran about 5 miles a day, 5 days a week. He had been extremely active in sports and played tennis and hockey at least twice a week. Since his diagnosis, he has begun a program of physical therapy, stretching exercises, and moderate walking. He refuses pain medication other than nonsteroidal antiinflammatory drugs. He is unhappy about his inactivity and is irritable and restless.

- What additional information about Mr. Joseph is necessary before suggesting complementary interventions?
- Speculate about the relationship between Mr. Joseph and the physician and therapists working with him and about his relationship with his family.
- What complementary interventions may be helpful to Mr. Joseph?
- How can you intervene to help Mr. Joseph?

REFERENCES

Adams, C. (2000, February 22). Splitting hairs on supplemental claims. *Wall Street Journal,* Section B, p. 1.

Agency for Healthcare Research and Quality. (2000). *Garlic effects on cardiovascular risks and disease, protective effects against cancer, and clinical adverse effects summary* (Evidence Report/Technology Assessment, No. 20) [On-line]. Washington, DC: Author. Available: http://ahrq.gov/clinic/garlicsum.htm.

Austin, J.A. (1997). Why patients use alternative medicine—Results of a national study. *Journal of the American Medical Association, 279,* 1548-1553.

Benson, H. (1996). *Timeless healing, the power and biology of belief.* New York: Simon & Schuster.

Bienfield, H. & Korngold, E. (1995). Chinese traditional medicine: An overview. *Alternative Therapies, 1*(1), 42-50.

Brosseau, L., Welch, V., Wells, G., deBie, R., Gam, A., Harman, K., Morin, M., Shea, B., & Tugwell, P. (2000). Low level laser therapy (classes I, II, and III) in the treatment of rheumatoid arthritis (Cochrane review). *The Cochrane Library* (Issue 2). Oxford: Update Software.

Callahan, E.J., Bertakis, K.D., & Azari, R. (2000). The influence of patient age on primary care resident physician-patient interaction. *Journal of the American Geriatrics Society, 48,* 30-35.

Cassell, J.L. (1985). Disabled humor: Origin and impact. *Journal of Rehabilitation, October/November/December,* 59-62, 85.

Clark, P., Tugwell, P., Bennet K., Bombardier, C., Shea, B., Wells, G., & Suarez-Almazor, M.E. (1999). Injectable gold for rheumatoid arthritis (Cochrane review). *The Cochrane Library* (Issue 3). Oxford: Update Software.

Davis, C.M. (Ed.). (1997). *Complementary therapies in rehabilitation: Holistic approaches for prevention and wellness.* Thorofare, NJ: Slack.

Decker, G.M. (1999). *An introduction to complementary and alternative therapies.* Pittsburgh: Oncology Nursing Press.

Eckes-Peck, S.D. (1997). The effectiveness of therapeutic touch for decreasing pain in elders with degenerative arthritis. *Journal of Holistic Nurses, 15* (2), 176.

Eisenberg, D.M. (1997). Advising patients who seek alternative medical therapies. *Annals of Internal Medicine, 121,* 61-69.

Eisenberg, D.M., Davis, R.B., Ettner, S.L., Appel, S., Wilkey, S., Van Rompay, M., & Kessler, R.C. (1998). Trends in alternative medicine use in the United States, 1990-1997. *Journal of the American Medical Association, 280,* 1569-1575.

Eisenberg, D.M., Kessler, R.C., Foster, C., Norlock, F., Calkins, P., & Delbanco, T. (1993). Unconventional medicine in the United States. *New England Journal of Medicine, 328,* 246-252.

Eliopoulos, C. (1999). *Integrating conventional & complementary therapies: Holistic care for chronic conditions.* St. Louis: Mosby.

Engebretson, J. (1996). Comparison of nurses and alternative healers. *Image—Journal of Nursing Scholarship, 28*(2), 95-99.

Engle, V.F., & Graney, M.J. (2000). Biobehavioral effects of therapeutic touch. *Image—Journal of Nursing Scholarship, 32*(3), 287-294.

Engstrom, J.W., & Hauser, S.L. (2000). Physical rehabilitation improves disability and quality of life perception in patients with multiple sclerosis. *Harrison's online* [On-line]. New York: McGraw-Hill. Available: http://www.medscape.com/HOL/articles.

Eskinazi, D. (1999). *Botanical medicine efficacy, quality assurance, and regulation.* New York: Mary Ann Libert.

Ezzo, J., Berman, B.M., Vickers, A.J., & Linde, K. (1998). Complementary medicine and the Cochrane Collaboration. *Journal of the American Medical Association, 280*(18), 1628-1630.

Fadiman, A. (1997). *The spirit catches you and you fall down: A Hmong child, her American doctors, and the collision of two cultures.* New York: Farrar, Straus and Giroux.

Fiscela, K., Franks, P., Clancy, C.M., Doescher, M.P., & Banthin, J.S. (1999). Does skepticism towards medical care predict mortality? *Medical Care, 37*(4), 409-414.

Flexner, A. (1910). *Medical education in the United States and Canada: A report to the Carnegie Foundation for the Advancement of Teaching.* New York: Carnegie.

Fontanarosa, P.B., & Lundberg, G.D. (1998). Alternative medicine meets science. *Journal of the American Medical Association, 280*(18), 1618-1619.

Freeman, L., & Lawless, G.F. (2001). *Mosby's complementary & alternative medicine: A research-based approach.* St. Louis: Mosby.

Geddes, N., & Henry, J.K. (1997). Nursing and alternative medicine. *Journal of Holistic Nursing, 15*(3), 271-282.

Gelberg, L., Andersen, R.M., & Leake, B.D. (2000). The behavioral model for vulnerable populations: Application to medical care use and outcomes for homeless people. *Health Services Research, 34*(6), 1273-1314.

Giger, J.N., & Davidhizar, R.E. (1999). *Transcultural nursing* (3rd ed.). St. Louis: Mosby.

Gordon, J.S., & Curtin, S. (2000). *Comprehensive cancer care integrating alternative, complementary, and conventional therapies.* Cambridge, MA: Perseus Publishing.

Gordon, M. (2000). *Manual of nursing diagnosis* (9th ed.). St. Louis: Mosby.

Haddad, L.G., & Hoeman, S.P. (2000). Home healthcare and the Arab-American client. *Home Healthcare Nurse, 18*(3), 189-197.

Harwood, A. (1971). The hot-cold theory of disease: Implications for treatment of Puerto Rican patients. *Journal of the American Medical Association, 216*(7), 1153-1158.

Hoeman, S.P. (1989). Cultural assessment in rehabilitation nursing practice. *Nursing Clinics of North America, 24,* 277-289.

Hoeman, S.P. (Ed.). (1992). *Proceedings of the interdisciplinary rehabilitation delegation to the People's Republic of China, March, 1992.* Spokane, WA: People-to-People International, Citizen Ambassador Program.

Hoeman, S.P. (1996). Intraethnic diversity. *Home Healthcare Nurse, 14*(7), 32.

Hoeman, S.P. (1997). Alternative health and complementary therapies: Application to advanced practice nursing in rehabilitation. In K. Johnson (Ed.), *Advanced practice nursing in rehabilitation: A core curriculum* (pp. 64-72). Glenview, IL: Rehabilitation Nursing Foundation.

Hoeman, S.P. (1998). Dynamics of rehabilitation nursing. In G. Goldstein & S.R. Beers (Eds.). *Rehabilitation* (pp. 71-87). New York: Plenum Press.

Hoeman, S.P., & Nordin, B. (2001). *Children with complex medical situations and their families in Sweden and the United States.*

Hudson, R. (1987). *Disease and its control.* New York: Praeger.

Hufford, D.J. (1995). Cultural and social perspectives on alternative medicine: Background and assumptions. *Alternative Therapies, 1*(1), 53-61.

Hunt, L.M., Arar, N.H., & Akana, L.L. (2000). Herbs, prayer, and insulin: Use of medical and alternative treatments by a group of Mexican American diabetes patients. *Journal of Family Practice, 49*(3), 216-223.

Jacobs, J., & Moskowitz, R. (1996). Homeopathy. In Micozzi, M.S. (Ed.). *Fundamentals of complementary and alternative medicine* (pp. 67-78). New York: Churchill Livingstone.

Johnson, J.E. (1999). Older rural women and the use of complementary therapies. *Journal of Community Health Nursing 16*(4), 223-232.

Jonas, W.B. (1998). Alternative medicine—Learning from the past, examining the present, advancing to the future. *Journal of the American Medical Association, 280*(18), 1616-1617.

Keegan, L. (1994). *The nurse as healer.* Albany, NY: Delmar.

Kelly, M.L, & Fitzsimons, V.M. (2000). *Understanding cultural diversity culture, curriculum, and community in nursing.* Boston: Jones and Bartlett.

Kleinman, A., Eisenberg, L., & Good, B. (1978). Culture, illness and care: Clinical lessons from anthropologic and cross-cultural research. *Annals of Internal Medicine, 88,* 251-258.

Krieger, D. (1979). *The therapeutic touch.* Englewood Cliffs, NJ: Prentice-Hall.

Krippner, S. (1995). A cross-cultural comparison of four healing models. *Alternative Therapies, 1*(1), 21-29.

Lagnado, L. (2000, March 22). Laetril makes a comeback on the Web. *Wall Street Journal,* Section B, p. 1.

Leininger, M. (1978). Two strange health tribes: The Gnisrun and the Enicidem in the United States. In M. Leininger (Ed.), *Transcultural nursing: Concepts, theories, and practices.* New York: John Wiley & Sons.

Lumsden, D.B., Baccala, A., & Martire, J. (1998). T'ai chi for osteoarthritis: An introduction for primary care physicians. *Geriatrics, 53*(2), 84-88.

Maley, M. (1997). Nurse complementary therapists: A return to healing. *Caring Magazine, October,* 48-53.

Margolin, A., Avants, S.K., & Kleber, H.D. (1998). Investigating alternative medicine therapies in randomized controlled trials. *Journal of the American Medical Association, 280*(18), 1628-1629.

McAlindon, T.E., LaValley, M.P., Gulin, J.P., & Felson, D.T. (2000). Glucosamine and chondroitin for the treatment of osteoarthritis: A systemic quality assurance and meta-analysis. *Journal of the American Medical Association, 283,* 1469-1475, 1483-1484.

McCloskey, J.C. & Bulechek, G.M. (Eds.). (2000). *Nursing interventions classifications (NIC)* (3rd ed.). St. Louis: Mosby.

Meleis, A.I., Isenberg, M., Koerner, J.E., Lacey, B., & Stern, P. (1995). *Diversity, marginalization, and culturally competent health care: Issues in knowledge development* [Monograph]. Washington, DC: American Academy of Nursing.

Mentgen, J., & Bulbrook, M.J. (1994). *Healing touch: Notebooks.* Lakewood, CO: Healing Touch.

Micozzi, M.S. (Ed.). (1996). *Fundamentals of complementary and alternative medicine.* New York: Churchill Livingstone.

Mitka, M. (1999). Therapeutic marijuana use supported while thorough proposed study done. *Journal of the American Medical Association 281*(16), 1473-1475.

Murray-Garcia, J.L., Selby, J.V., Schmittdiel, J., Grumbach, K. & Quesenberry, C.P., Jr. (2000). Racial and ethnic differences in a patient survey: patients' values, ratings, and reports regarding physician primary care performance in a large health maintenance organization. *Medical Care 38*(3), 300-310.

National Center for Complementary and Alternative Medicine. *The NCCAM Y2K strategic plan* (draft, 11-12, 29-30). Silver Spring, MD: U.S. Government [On-line]. Available: http://nccam.nih.gov/nccam/strategic/newleft1.html.

Nurse's handbook of alternative and complementary therapies. (1998). Springhouse, PA: Springhouse Corporation.

O'Mathuna, D.P. (2000). Evidence-based practice and reviews of therapeutic touch. *Journal of Nursing Scholarship, 32*(3), 279-286.

Parsons, T. (1951). *The social system.* New York: Free Press.

Paul, B.D. (Ed.). (1955). *Health, culture, & community: Case studies of public reactions to health programs.* New York: Russell Sage Foundation.

Peck, S.D. (1998). The efficacy of therapeutic touch for improving functional ability in elders with degenerative arthritis. *Nursing Science Quarterly, 11*(3), 123-132.

Piscitelli, S.C., Burstein, A., Chaitt, D., Alfaro, R., & Falloon, J. (2000). Indinavir concentration and St. John's wort. *Lancet, 355,* 541-548.

Pizzorno, J.E., Jr. (1996). Naturopathic medicine. In Micozzi, M.S. (Ed.), *Fundamentals of complementary and alternative medicine* (pp. 163-182). New York: Churchill Livingstone.

Quinn, J.F. (1984). Therapeutic touch as energy exchange: Testing the theory. *Advanced Nursing Science, 6*(2), 42.

Rankin-Box, D. (Ed.). (1995). *The nurses' handbook of complementary therapies.* Edinburgh: Churchill Livingstone.

Reid, L.D., Wang, F., Young, H., & Awiphan, R. (1999). Patients' satisfaction and their perception of the pharmacist. *Journal of the American Pharmaceutical Association 30*(6), 835-842.

Rivera, C.R. (1999). Reiki therapy: A tool for wellness. *Imprint, February/March,* 3-1-3.

Smyth, J.M., Stone, A.A., Hurewitz, A., & Kaell, A. (1999). Effects of writing about stressful experiences on symptom reduction in patients with asthma or rheumatoid arthritis: A randomized trial. *Journal of the American Medical Association 281,* 1304-1309.

Sobel, D.S. (Ed.). (1979). *Ways of health: Holistic approaches to ancient and contemporary medicine.* New York: Harcourt Brace Jovanovich.

Spencer, J.W., & Jacobs, J.J. (1999). *Complementary/alternative medicine an evidenced-based approach.* St. Louis: Mosby.

Starr, P. (1982). *The social transformation of American medicine.* New York: Basic Books.

Studdert, D.M., Eisenberg, D.M., Miller, F.H., Curto, D.A., Kaptchuk, T.J., & Brennan, T.A. (1998). Medical malpractice implications of alternative medicine. *Journal of the American Medical Association, 280*(18), 1610-1615.

Turner, J.G., Clark, A.J., Gauthier, D.K., & Williams, M. (1998). The effect of therapeutic touch on pain and anxiety in burn patients. *Journal of Advanced Nursing, 28,* 10-12.

Turner, R.B., Riker, D.K., & Gangemi, J.D. (2000). Ineffectiveness of Echinacea for prevention of experimental rhinovirus colds. *Antimicrobial Agents Chemotherapeutics, 44,* 1708-1709.

U.S. Department of Health and Human Services. (2000). *Healthy People 2010: Conference edition* [On-line]. Available: http://web.health.gov/healthypeople/document.

Valbona, C., & Richards, T. (1999). Evolution of magnetic therapy from alternative to traditional medicine. *Physical Medicine and Rehabilitation Clinics of North America, 10*(3), 729-754.

Van den Ende, C.H.M., Vliet Vlieland, T.P.M., Munneke, M., & Hazes, J.M.W. (1999). Dynamic exercise therapy for rheumatoid arthritis (Cochrane review). *The Cochrane Library* (Issue 3). Oxford: Update Software.

Villaire, M. (1999). Healing touch therapy makes a difference in surgical unit. *Critical Care Nurse, 19*(1), 104.

Waksman, B.H. (1994). Can psychoneuroimmunology help explain disease? The example of multiple sclerosis. *Advances: The Journal of Mind-Body Health, 10*(4), 16-20.

Wellin, E. (1985). Water boiling in a Peruvian town. In B.D. Paul (Ed.). *Health, culture & community: Case studies to public reactions to health programs* (pp. 71-103). New York: Russell Sage Foundation.

Wirth, D.P. (1992).The effect of non-contact therapeutic touch on the healing rate of full thickness dermal wounds. *Subtle Energies, 1*(1), 1.

Wolf, S.L., Barnhart, H.X., Kutner, N.G., McNeeley, E., Coogler, C., & Xu, T. (1996). Reducing frailty and falls in older persons: An investigation of tai chi and computerized balance training. Atlantic FICSIT group (Frailty and Injuries: Cooperative Study of Intervention Techniques). *Journal of the American Geriatric Society 44,* 489-497.

Wong, J.Y. & Rapson, L.M. (1999). Acupuncture in the management of pain of musculoskeletal and neurologic origin. *Physical Medicine and Rehabilitation Clinics of North America 10*(3), 531-545.

Zborowski, M. (1958). Cultural components in response to pain. In E.G. Jaco (Ed.), *Patients, physicians, and illness.* Glencoe, IL: The Free Press.

Ziporyn, T. (1992). *Nameless diseases.* New Brunswick, NJ: Rutgers University Press.

Zola, I.K. (1991). Bringing our bodies and ourselves back in: Reflections on a past, present, and future "medical sociology." *Journal of Health and Social Behavior, 32*(March), 1-16.

Movement, Functional Mobility, and Activities of Daily Living

14

Shirley P. Hoeman, PhD, MPH, RN, CRRN, CS

Mr. George was quite excited. This was the afternoon his family came to watch him walk down the parallel bars in physical therapy. After many weeks of rehabilitation, he was able to walk the length of the room by using his hands on the bars for support. He walked slowly, leaning heavily on the right side, grinning into the video camera held by his wife. Therapists, family members, his primary rehabilitation nurse (Mrs. Ethros), and other clients in the room applauded. His daughter had a cake with candles, and everyone celebrated; the family gave gifts to the therapists.

Later that evening, he discussed the event with Mrs. Ethros as she assisted him with his bowel program in the privacy of his room. The two had been working extensively on bowel retraining, and outcomes had been consistently good all week. As they discussed home management, no one came to applaud, no one videotaped the session, there were no gifts for the nurse, and certainly there was no cake!

During the evening report, Mrs. Ethros told about Mr. George's great day in therapy and then, almost as an afterthought, mentioned the bowel program. Mr. Terran, the oncoming nurse for the night shift, laughed. He said, "Well Jean, I think you do not give proper credit to your nursing expertise. Just how far and how often do you think Mr. George will walk without a successful bowel program?"

A major goal of rehabilitation nursing is to assist clients in improving motor function and preventing functional loss. Although movement is critical to a person's capacity for interaction with the environment, most adults take their ability to move for granted until it becomes painful, restrained, or impaired. More than 54 million persons in the United States have some limitations in their activities due to chronic health problems; within 10 years the prevalence rate is expected to increase by 50% (Centers for Disease Control and Prevention [CDC], 2000). This chapter is concerned with movement as science and therapeutic intervention and with improving functional mobility for clients, particularly for performing activities of daily living (ADLs) and instrumental ADLs (IADLs).

Medical prescriptions for exercise versus rest have vacillated since ancient times; conventional medicine considered bed rest important to healing in the 1940s, even on maternity wards. Although ideas about the merits of activity have come down on the side of mobility, whether in obstetrics units, cardiac units, or surgical wards, immobility and functional limitations continue to represent tremendous challenges for the practice of rehabilitation nursing.

In 1967 Olson wrote the classic nursing article about "hazards of immobility," outlining the extent of damage to virtually all of the person. Every rehabilitation nurse is aware of the potential for any or all systems of the body, mind, and spirit to break down as consequences of immobility, disuse, or even poor positioning, all of which may be preventable. Problems resulting from immobility arise rapidly and are noticeable within a day even in healthy persons, possibly because some changes begin at the cellular level, and can be local, regional, or systemic. Clients in rehabilitation are at high risk for problems because of the very nature of their chronic and disabling or multiple trauma conditions, from specific impairments or complications and at times from use of the assistive devices or adaptive equipment that affords them mobility or function.

Persons who are immobile may develop depression, disorientation, irritability, lack of energy or interest, incontinence, feelings of imbalance, increased pain or aching, and general malaise. Inappropriate medication regimens, disrupted sleep, lack of sensory or cognitive stimulation, poor nutrition and low fluid balance, social isolation, and feelings of powerlessness may contribute as much to functional loss and further reduced mobility as a specific disease or impairment.

FUNCTION AND ACTIVITY

The numbers of very old persons are increasing at disproportionate rates in the population. Figure 14-1 illustrates how age and sex influence performance of physical activities, ADLs, and IADLs for persons aged 70 to 85 years and older. In general, the percentage of persons reporting difficulty with performing ADLs and IADLs doubles between those age groups; interestingly persons may be able to perform physical activities longer than ADLs or IADLs. Certain conditions are associated with limitations in ADLs. Their incidences in persons older than 70 years are as follows: arthritic conditions, 11%; heart disease, 4%; stroke and respiratory diseases, 3% each; and diabetes, 2% (CDC, 1994).

Comorbidity is an increasing concern. Rehabilitation nurses have a role in helping clients manage multiple and increasingly complex problems and to prevent additional chronicity or impairment. Rehabilitation nurses have neglected conducting, utilizing, and supporting rigorous research in areas that are important to their practice and to their clients, such as neurology (Thorn, 2000), clinical epidemiology, and prevention of chronic, disabling conditions. A review of the research literature indicates many opportunities for improving outcomes for clients. For instance, researchers conducting a large multisite study of community-dwelling women aged 65 years and older moved beyond data about disabilities that are associated with certain diseases. They examined whether particular combinations of diseases in women were related to their developing specific types of disabilities. They found that combinations of diseases paired synergistically to promote kinds of disabilities, and the problems often were more complex than the total

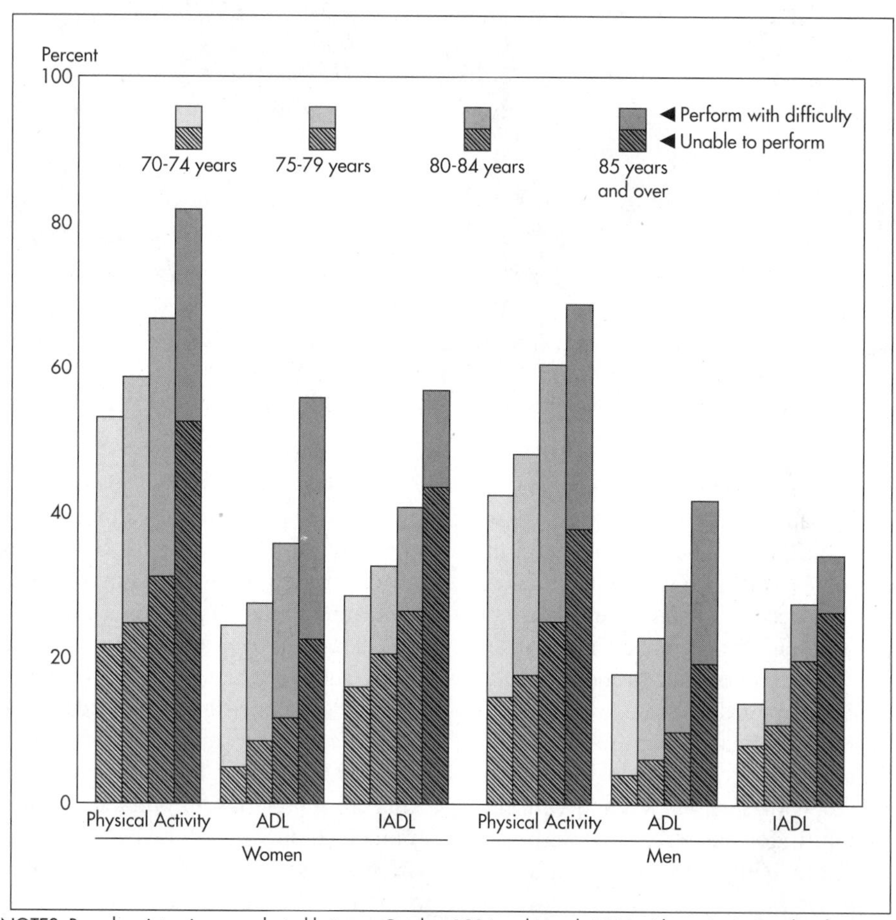

NOTES: Based on interviews conducted between October 1994 and March 1996 with noninstitutionalized persons. See Technical Notes for definitions of physical activities, activities of daily living (ADL) and instrumental activities of daily living (IADL).

SOURCE: Centers for Disease Control and Prevention, National Center for Health Statistics, 1994 National Health Interview Survey, Second Supplement on Aging.

Figure 14-1 Percentage of persons 70 years and older who have difficulty performing one or more physical activities, activities of daily living *(ADL),* and instrumental activities of daily living *(IADL)* by age and sex: United States, 1995. (Data from the Centers for Disease Control and Prevention, National Center for Health Statistics. [1994]. *National health interview survey, second supplement on aging.* Atlanta: Author.)

from the diseases measured independently. Although the prevalence of chronic diseases was high among all of the women, particular combinations of conditions or interactions among diseases yielded different functional outcomes (Fried, Bandeen-Roche, Kasper, & Guralnik, 1999).

Need for assistance with ADLs and IADLs is not limited to elderly persons; 9.4 million adults aged 18 years and older receive assistance of some type. Nearly half are younger than 65 years, and 4 of 5 (79%) live in the community, outside institutions (Spector, 2000). The most recent survey results available showed 2.5 million persons needed assistive technology they did not have, primarily because they lacked the means to pay for it (LaPlante, Hendershot, & Moss, 1992).

These figures do not take into account the number of children with needs for assistance in home and school. During the past 5 years, activity limitations for those younger than 18 years have increased by 33% for girls (4.2% to 5.6%) and by 40% for boys (5.6% to 7.9%) (CDC, 1999/2001). Furthermore, these children (31%) tended to be more sad and depressed than their peers (17%) who were without limitations (CDC, 1997). *Healthy People 2010* goals aimed at reducing disparities in access to health services target an increase in the proportion of children and adolescents who spend at least 80% of their time in regular education programs; 60% is the target (Healthy People 2010, http://web.health.gov/healthypeople/document). Environment, family resources, and access to services also influence outcomes for children with functional limitations placing them at risk for developmental difficulties (Hogan, Rogers, & Msall, 2000). With ethnicity, not only is the prevalence of chronic conditions greater, limitations preventing school attendance are found more commonly among children from African-American and Hispanic heritage (Newacheck, Stoddard, & McManus, 1993).

MOVEMENT THEORIES

Movement theories are important to rehabilitation nurses because their concepts and principles are used with clients to promote recovery and enhance compensation for altered or impaired functional abilities. Although physical and occupational therapists consider movement theories in depth, rehabilitation nurses are responsible for assessing, implementing, and evaluating movement and function in the context of each client's unique situation and environment.

According to classic movement theories, motor development occurs as a process of maturation of the central nervous system (CNS). Pioneers in the field identified specific developmental sequences and incorporated certain behaviors of early motor development into various treatment programs. Because of the belief that the process of motor development ends with neural maturation, it has become a marker for completed developmental processes, often referred to as *milestones*. In contrast, from the life-span view the processes of age-related changes in motor behaviors, such as learning, maturation, and aging, are conceptualized as lifelong phenomena. Behavioral change results from interactions between many intrinsic and extrinsic factors, such as physical growth and neural maturation, as well as supportive versus risk environments.

Models of CNS Control

Theories formulated in movement science suggest explanations for normal movement and effective interventions. Two models of CNS control of movement are the hierarchy of reflexes (Walshe, 1961; Katz & Akpom, 1976) and the various systems models; others are motor relearning programs, synergy models, constraint-induced models, and biobehavioral approaches.

Hierarchy of Reflexes

In the hierarchy of reflexes, motor development progresses in a vertically ranked order from reflexive to voluntary control with maturation. Initially, primitive reflexes regulated at the spinal cord level control movement. When the CNS matures, higher level righting and equilibrium reactions controlled by the brainstem and midbrain emerge. Thus a child does not walk until sequentially higher levels of the CNS mature sufficiently to allow independent balance and locomotion; equilibrium represents a still higher level of maturation. A number of pediatric assessments and interventions, such as sensorimotor techniques, are based on this model. It follows in this model that these higher levels deteriorate with aging, defaulting to the primitive reflex controls.

Neurodevelopmental Treatment Approaches

These ideas underlie the neurodevelopmental (NDT) treatment programs intended to influence the hierarchy of the CNS toward normal movement, such as those proposed by Rood (superficial stimulation of the skin by stroking, icing, or brushing), Brunnstrom (patterns of synergy for voluntary control of movement), Knott, the Bobaths, and Voss (Bly, 1991).

Because rehabilitation nurses have used the Bobath NDT approach (Bobath, 1978) extensively in the care of persons after stroke (Phipps, 1991; Borgman & Passarella, 1991), a review of its basic tenets follows. With the Bobath approach, clients learn the sensation of movement, not the movement itself. When brain damage occurs and sensation is altered or impaired, sensation is shunted to developing abnormal patterns of posture and movement that are incompatible with performing normal activities. Clients attempt to halt or break the abnormal patterns by regaining control over motor output, rather than by modifying sensory input. Initially nurses provide stimuli to enable clients to learn basic postural and movement patterns that elicit the righting and equilibrium responses while inhibiting abnormal patterns. Eventually these patterns can be elaborated on so the client can perform functional skills. Every skilled activity is conducted within the context of patterns for postural control, righting, equilibrium, and other protective reactions. Sensory input from the corrected motor patterns is essential for the person to develop improvement in motor control.

Systems Models

The systems or distributed control models advance the idea that movement is a product of complex interactions of multiple systems. The person is active, as well as reactive, in a continuously changing environment, but the physiological body also is a mechanistic mass subject to the forces of gravity and inertia. The CNS is one part of the multiple interwoven systems and subsystems that share in the control process, and connections are highly sensitive; movement is one outcome. As a nonlinear concept, systems are complex, dynamic, adaptive to the environment, and emerging; the popular chaos theory exemplifies nonlinear phenomena. Dynamic pattern theory (DPT) is another nonlinear example familiar to rehabilitation nurses. As the name implies, DPT focuses on movement patterns and how or why changes in the pattern occur and then how to make them retrievable or available again.

Interactions among the CNS and other (e.g., peripheral) nervous systems lead to patterns. Some patterns may be instinctive, and others may be learned, but they vary in stability and with the environment or situation. That is to say, clients can find more than one way to perform activities depending on their physical and cognitive abilities and the environment. Thus a rehabilitation nurse assists a client with medication to manage pain that prohibited transfer from a wheelchair and then installs support bars and elevates the toilet seat to facilitate transfer to the commode, resulting in improved independent function. Complex systems models have been used to explain changes in balance across the life span and as a basis for certain interventions for imbalance and postural control.

Other Approaches

Other recognized approaches include *proprioceptive neuromuscular facilitation (PNF)* based on a neurophysiological theory. A proposed program includes moving the extremities in patterned spiral and diagonal movements and a rapid stretch technique. The *Feldenkrais method,* a neuropsychomotor approach, is based on the client's perceptions and lifestyle and includes strategies for sensory, emotional, cognitive, and movement components. Sister Elizabeth Kenny used similar principles as part of her treatment for poliomyelitis. The notion is that personal habits of movement occur unconsciously. When lost or altered, they can be reconstituted through sensory and motor systems learning and adapting.

The Feldenkrais method is client centered in that it proposes a facilitative environment that minimizes pain, adjusts to the person's tempo, avoids fatigue, and relies on a trust relationship with the provider. The provider uses verbal, visual, and kinesthetic cues without touch to lead the client into and through the desired movement. Instructions are very specific: "Lift your hand off your lap. Point your index finger at your mouth reflected in the mirror. Look at the hand and finger and think about them. You can do that better by propping your elbow on the armrest. Touch the mirror where your mouth is reflected mirror; trace the outline of your mouth." As clients experience the movement, exploring and adapting to perform the action, they also gain a sense of success and awareness or discovery of the movement (Jackson-Wyatt, 1997). Although this approach is provided mainly by physical therapists, rehabilitation nurses need to have an understanding of it and may read further in specific books on the topic. Chapter 13 contains more information about other alternative and complementary modalities.

Also recognized is the Carr-Shepherd approach to motor relearning, a skill acquisition concept often associated with clients who have brain injuries but also used in other situations. The premise is that persons have memory stores of learned motor programs that can be retrieved through an organized process. The activity is analyzed to determine whether a client's inability to perform is due to impairment or environment and whether the person is conducting normal or compensatory movements. Next, the person is instructed to practice problematic or missing steps in the activity individually and then the whole activity. When the pattern of movement is accomplished, the client can try to perform the activity in another environment until, finally, it is relearned and can be transferred to other situations (Carr & Shepherd, 1987).

A number of new approaches have appeared in the past few years; they often are argued to be paradigm shifts in conceptual frameworks for movement science and therapy. The Pilates method is one program offered to therapists. It is based on synergistic principles and incorporates holistic principles, including breathing, centering, and concentrating, among others. In other approaches many complementary techniques that employ technology are used, such as biofeedback or electrical stimulation.

A concept advanced in the literature is constraint-induced movement therapy for motor recovery. The argument is that nonuse of an extremity after stroke becomes a learned behavior that is further supported or reinforced by teaching a client compensatory movement to perform activities. This occurs during the time before any spontaneous recovery has been evidenced. In one study, for 2 weeks, researchers restrained the unaffected extremity and trained the affected extremity for clients with chronic hemiparesis after stroke ($n = 5$), replicating an earlier study. They found improved quality in use of the affected extremity, speed of task performance, and functional ability (Kunkel et al., 1999). This is an approach for rehabilitation nurses to examine in research and to carefully evaluate for utilization in practice.

Behavioral Interventions

Behavioral approaches may include *kinesic* and *somatic* interventions that nurses use to assist clients with stress reduction or pain management, such as biofeedback, therapeutic massage, progressive relaxation, or therapeutic touch. Biofeedback is a method of autonomic nervous system control through self-regulation. Clients are given continuous data feedback about their biological function, such as heart rate, body temperature, or muscle activity via auditory or visual signals, such as those emitted from electromyelograms. As clients attempt to perceive the workings of their internal biologic systems, they attempt to control them by incorporating themselves into the system as part of a "feedback loop." Their efforts are complementary to exercise programs.

NORMAL MOVEMENT

Learning the basics of voluntary and normal movement is a precursor to understanding movement dysfunction. Physical and occupational therapists, as well as rehabilitation nurses, practice using the principles and techniques detailed in this chapter, making them particularly important areas for interdisciplinary collaboration. A great deal of education directed toward families and clients concerns ways to meet and maintain functional goals. Maximal mastery of functional mobility is a key component of improved outcomes, optimal independence, and continued well-being for clients.

Although rehabilitation nurses have an extraordinary investment in mobility, few studies pursue it as a theoretical concept. Nurses examine mobility as a deficit or altered state, examine mobility as the opposite of the undesirable state of immobility, or investigate interventions that improve mobility. A great deal of effort is directed at preventing the consequences of immobility, such as pressure ulcers, pneumonia, contractures, and a host of other negative outcomes. Nurses also consider the capacity of the neurological and musculoskeletal system enabling a person to move and to do so in purposeful ways. For the most part, nurses tend to regard mobility in the physical sense, that is, focusing on ability or impairment and the level of assistance a person needs.

However, movement represents a key component in a person's ability to interact with the environment and adapt. It is dynamic in that its capacities change with development, health status, and other multiple dimensions. In a holistic view, nurses consider movement from physical, cognitive, social, spatial, political, temporal, or environmental parameters (Chan & Heck, 2000). In this view functional abilities, as expressed through performing ADLs and IADLs, are measures related to mobility that incorporate the environment, mental competence, and some degree of social interaction in addition to the more obvious physical actions.

Motor Development

Human motor development proceeds in an orderly and purposeful fashion from birth. As the nervous system matures, genetically based movement patterns become more elaborate, and primitive reflexes disappear and are replaced by higher level responses. Thus an infant's Moro and tonic neck reflexes are expected to disappear before righting and equilibrium responses emerge. In normal development, skills are acquired at certain specified stages and become less random and coarse; they develop into sequences that are more purposeful and synchronized, forming the basis for stability and posture. Posture and movement are intertwined for learning motor skills and producing goal-directed activities. Once learned and perfected through practice, motor skills become nearly automatic, requiring little conscious thought to execute correctly, unless the pathways are disrupted. This principle is evident in the skills a child gains by repeatedly placing a plastic shape through a correspondingly shaped hole.

Voluntary Motor Activity

Voluntary motor activity involves the cerebral cortex, the descending pathways of the spinal cord, and the anterior horn of the spinal cord; the cerebellum, brainstem, and basal ganglia contribute as well. Simply, voluntary motor impulses from the cortex travel through the anterior corticospinal tract or cross at the medulla level and descend through the lateral corticospinal tract to the anterior horn cells and to the skeletal muscles. The effect of the nerve impulse on muscle physiology is a complex interaction that results in muscle activity. Diffuse lesions, such as with closed head injury, may damage the surface and deeper structures of the brain. Figure 15-6 illustrates the physiology.

The primary areas of the cerebral cortical regions of the CNS execute voluntary movement, but the supplementary motor area controls programming of complex sequences into rapid, discrete movements. New motor programs are assembled in the premotor area. The posterior parietal areas direct attention to objects of interest in visual space and form strategies for eye and arm movement and their coordination in space. Cognitive functions related to movement occur in the prefrontal cortex with accessory functions from the basal ganglia.

ALTERED MOVEMENT

In a complex physiology, damage to the cerebral cortical regions of the brain results in problems with planning, sequencing steps, smoothly coordinating, and timing of movements, as well as potential for disruption in predicting movement from sensory data (Guyton & Hall, 1996). Thus, with injury to the cerebellum, deficits in coordination may appear; cerebral palsy reflects problems with motor planning. Circumscribed cortical lesions, ranging from stroke to gunshot to penetrating wounds, result in dysfunctional motor planning in the related areas of function. It follows that the site and extent of motor impairment correlate with the acquired lesions of the cerebral cortex. Accompanying deficits in sensory, cognitive, and perceptual processing also influence the alteration in motor control. Table 14-1 delineates clinical signs of disrupted motor function at three levels of the nervous system.

Upper Motor Neuron Syndrome

Clinically upper motor neuron syndrome caused by lesions of the cortical, subcortical, and spinal cord areas is important in the care of clients. Nurses must anticipate and recog-

TABLE 14-1 Clinical Signs of Disrupted Motor Function at Three Levels of the Nervous System

Level	Clinical Signs	Examples of Causative Disorders
Suprasegmental	Weakness or paralysis of voluntary movement Increased muscle stretch reflexes; reflex arc intact (after "spinal shock") Some muscle atrophy secondary to disuse EMG normal	Spinal cord lesions such as trauma, infarct, tumor, and hemorrhage
Segmental	Weakness or paralysis of voluntary movement Decreased or absent muscle stretch reflexes (reflex arc disrupted) Marked muscle atrophy secondary to denervation (↓ trophic factors) EMG changes: fibrillation, giant polyphasic action potentials (denervation supersensitivity)	Brainstem lesions affecting cranial nuclei: tumors infarct, hemorrhage Cerebellopontine angle tumors compressing cranial nerves Polyneuropathies such as Guillain-Barré syndrome, alcoholic polyneuropathy, diphtheritic polyneuropathy, and toxic chemical polyneuropathy
Myoneural junction	Weakness or paralysis of voluntary movement Muscle stretch reflexes intact No muscle atrophy EMG diminished: muscle able to contract when directly stimulated; pattern of ↓ contraction varies with disorder	Chronic: myasthenia gravis (may have acute episodes of life-threatening myasthenic or cholinergic crisis); Eaton-Lambert syndrome (myasthenic symptoms associated with carcinoma); acute: botulism, curare, succinylcholine, "nerve gas," organophosphate insecticides

From Chipps, E., Clanin, N., & Campbell, V. (1992). *Neurological disorders.* St. Louis: Mosby.
EMG, Electromyelogram.

nize the potential responses, for example, autonomic dysreflexia. Resultant deficits in performance (negative symptoms) include paresis, weakness and fatigue, and reduced fine motor skills, especially manually; poor tone and loss of strength occur. The positive symptoms are important because they reflect altered motor movements that are of concern to rehabilitation nurses. These include altered exaggerated reflex responses (especially hypertonic stretch reflexes), uncertain autonomic control, increased muscle tone, and conditions that result from their dysfunction, such as spasticity or chorea (Table 14-2).

At any given time, some cells in a muscle are contracted while others are relaxed, resulting in muscle tone required to maintain normal posture. Motor control influences the power of muscle contractions through the number of motor units involved and the frequency of nerve stimulation. Abnormal muscle tone is characterized as *hypertonic,* as with spasticity, when stimuli are uninhibited and create a state of imbalance and muscles resist passive movement. The "clasped knife" phenomenon occurs in a spastic extremity when a muscle is stretched. Initially the muscle contracts and then just as suddenly it relaxes in tension release (Habel, 1997).

Interestingly spasticity may enable function for some clients, such as those with muscle weakness or partial paralysis of the lower extremities (paraparesis). For example, some clients are able to harness momentum from the increased tone in their antigravity muscles and have sufficient power to make a standing transfer (assisted for safety and as needed) from the wheelchair to the toilet.

Injury or disease affecting the upper motor neuron pathway produces continued muscle contractions with spastic tone and exaggerated reflexes. The greater than normal muscle tone produces spasticity and dysfunctional posture and positioning. Spasticity is a concern when it inhibits movement or leads to complications, especially contractures, although some have found ways to use the components of their spasticity to benefit certain movement, such as transfers. Spasms may make sitting in a wheelchair not only intolerable but also unsafe, whereas others may experience pain or poor bladder control. Dexterity and rest may be compromised when upper body and extremity spasticity occurs, making ADLs or even personal hygiene difficult.

Those with cerebral palsy find their posture, movement, or position may stimulate muscle tone leading to spasticity. Consider how spastic movements can thwart learning for a child sitting in a wheelchair and attempting to attend to classroom instructions. Scissoring steps, due to spasms from the hip and lower extremities, may impair ambulation for some. However, as a child with cerebral palsy develops and grows, it becomes difficult to control muscle tone and provide stretch to appropriate muscles to prevent fixed contractures. Children with muscular dystrophy have progressive and often rapid loss of muscle tissue, reduced strength, and a tendency to develop contractures; new muscle fibers do not develop.

TABLE 14-2 Definitions of Altered Motor Movements

Movement	Definition	Comments
Ataxia	Uncoordinated and irregular movements; may present with staggering gait and postural imbalance Altered proprioception may cause imprecise movements	Altered gait is due to congenital or acquired lesions in the spinal cord or cerebellum Friedreich's ataxia is associated with hereditary sclerosis Ataxia-type behaviors may occur in speech, aphasia, or breathing
Athetosis	Involuntary movements of the extremities and distal limbs characterized by slow, writhing activity Client cannot maintain one position, and movement is essentially continuous	Typically noted with certain cerebral palsy movements or with lesions in the basal ganglia or tabes dorsalis
Ballism (ballismus)	Violent, uncoordinated jerking or flinging of the limbs	Associated with extrapyramidal disorders; may occur as hemiballismus
Chorea	Involuntary movements, usually of the proximal limbs, that are rapid, jerky, and forceful; not purposeful and are irregular and arrhythmic	Chorea is also a suffix for specific conditions such as Huntington's or Sydenham's chorea Persons may attempt to mask movements by including them in movements for planned actions
Clonus, also clonic spasm	Clonus implies involuntary skeletal muscle actions that rapidly alternate between relaxing and contracting	Clonic reflex action occurs as a result of stretching skeletal muscles when upper motor neuron lesions are present
Apraxia	Difficulty or inability to execute complex motor planning or coordinated gait and other familiar movements Alternatively, steps in task performance may be conducted out of sequence, or familiar objects and tasks are not related	Sufficient strength and balance and sensory skills may be present, but person is unable to complete a sequence for performing ADLs or uses a known object inappropriately (motor apraxia) With sensory apraxia, the person may not perceive the purpose of an object
Flaccid	Lack of muscle tone that may result in atrophy and disuse Characterized by soft, weak, and floppy qualities; muscles lack coordination	Indicator of poorly innervated muscle tone, often after lower motor neuron damage or lesions Performance of ADLs, strength, and postural alignment may be compromised
Hyperreflexia	Exaggerated quality and response of reflexes	An example is what occurs with spinal cord injury and autonomic hyperreflexia
Reflex	Involuntary, unconscious, and immediate reaction or response to stimuli Reflexes are simple or complex and very specific; some are related to stages of development	Neuromuscular reflex responses have specific parameters; inappropriate responses may be part of diagnostic criteria
Rigidity	Increased tension in both agonist and antagonist muscles produces stiff, hard, inflexible muscles that resist movement	Extrapyramidal system lesions such as with Parkinson's disease eventually affect postural reflexes, as evidenced in poor initiation of movement and cogwheel rigidity Affects mobility and function Other examples are with upper brainstem lesions that cause the extremities to stiffen and extend, or with resistance to passive range of motion after brain damage and coma
Spasm, spastic	Involuntary, transient muscle contraction with sudden onset; often associated with a specific type of spasm May be used to describe a quality of gait, hemiplegia, or paraplegia	Spastic is an old word for certain disability conditions; also was used to describe the neurogenic (spastic) bladder in some situations Spasms vary in intensity and duration
Spasticity	Muscles that are hypertonic and have increased resistance to stretch demonstrate spasticity Prime locations are flexors of the arms and extensors of the legs; other muscles can be affected	Movements are difficult and uncoordinated Pain, weakness, and inability to move properly may impair sleep, medical procedures, and ADLs; may even cause urinary retention

Continued

TABLE 14-2 Definitions of Altered Motor Movements—cont'd

Movement	Definition	Comments
Spasticity—cont'd	Deep tendon reflexes are increased while superficial reflexes are decreased; there may be weakness	Risk is high for damage to skin and development of contractures With conditions such as multiple sclerosis formation of plaque in the brain causes spasticity accompanied by pain, fatigue, and stiffness that inhibit function (Gelber & Jozefczyk, 2000)
Tremor	Involuntary and repetitive movements described as quivering, quick movements that are rhythmic and nonpurposeful; movements may be fine or coarse Opposing muscle groups, usually the distal limb such as the hand, respond to alternating muscle contraction and relaxation	Tremor often associated with Parkinson's disease; a resting tremor, it may disappear during planned movements Intentional tremors are with diseases of the cerebellum, such as multiple sclerosis, trauma, vascular conditions, and toxin-related or tumors Cause of tremor may be familial, senile, toxic-metallic related, convulsive, psychogenic, or other (Gillespie, 1991)
Akinesia; also a root word for kinesia terms (e.g., hyperkinetic or bradykinesia)	Loss of voluntary muscle movement that may be associated with motor or psychic factors	Kinesiology is the study of movement that is important for an understanding of gait and exercise along with other facets of mobility

Compiled from Anderson, K.N., Anderson, L.E., & Glanze, W.D. (1998). *Mosby's medical, nursing, and allied health dictionary* (5th ed.). St. Louis: Mosby; and Braddom, R.L. (1996). *Physical medicine and rehabilitation.* Philadelphia: WB Saunders.
ADLs, Activities of daily living.

Alternately hypotonia is evidenced in the flaccid or floppy tone of a preterm newborn at risk. Continued flaccid tone leads to muscle atrophy and corresponding loss of muscle mass and reduced strength. This situation can arise from prolonged immobility or result from neurological or muscular disorders.

Lower Motor Neuron Pathway

Because the lower motor neuron is the final pathway actually terminating in a skeletal muscle, loss of function through disease or trauma results in flaccid paralysis or loss of both reflex and voluntary movements. It follows that persons who have stroke, brain injury, spinal cord injury (SCI), multiple sclerosis, or cerebral palsy are candidates for spasticity (St. George, 1993). The person who experiences a stroke often develops hemiplegia with paresis. The motor dysfunction may appear as breathing or swallowing deficits.

The Extrapyramidal System

The extrapyramidal system refers to the multiple different motor control areas that exist apart from the corticospinal-pyramidal pathways. A number of specific neurotransmitters operate in the basal ganglia, namely dopamine, γ-aminobutyric acid (GABA), acetylcholine, norepinephrine, serotonin, and enkephalin. Dopamine and GABA function as inhibitors, creating negative cybernetic (feedback) loops between the cerebral cortex and the basal ganglia and thus providing stability to the system. Loss of smooth, coordinated, accurately moving muscle activity results in damage to the cerebellum or basal ganglia and in turn creates imbalance in the extrapyramidal system (Guyton & Hall, 1996). Righting and equilibrium responses are threatened. Delay in carrying out or slow initiation of movement signals cerebellum problems because that is where movement parameters are specified and preprogrammed movements are initiated.

Disturbances in these areas of the nervous system result in posture and movement dysfunctions that become evident in the gait, balance, posture, and other disjointed, choppy motions. These may be affected after stroke, and Parkinson's disease is a commonly related diagnosis. Gait may be ataxic, staggering, or wide stepped, with marked muscular rigidity and bradykinesia.

Coarse tremor accompanied by other involuntary movements, such as chorea, athetosis, and facial grimacing, may appear. Tremors may be barely noticeable or so severe as to be disabling; the frequency, location, and action may vary. Postural or resting tremor is a classic movement with Parkinson's disease that may arise with abnormality in the basal ganglia of the brain (Marjama-Lyons, 2000).

Recovery Patterns

Recovery of cortical lesion damage follows a developmental sequence in that it returns from reflex to voluntary control, from mass to discrete movement, from tone before voluntary movements, and from proximal to distal control. Nonpurposeful extensor and flexor synergy patterns of the extremities may occur as a precursor to voluntary motor return, appearing as mass contractions of muscles in upper and lower extremities. For example, the elbow and knee or finger and toe both flex, or the shoulder and the hip abduct. Although a pattern of spontaneous recovery of voluntary motor control is possible after stroke, factors such as the degree or amount, particular functions, length of time, and lag time for returns are unpredictable and individual. Recovery of motor functions may cease at any point or level; recovery speed may indicate the level of function attainable. Cells in the brain that have been destroyed by the insult will not regenerate, and the specific functions are diminished or altered. Diseases of the cerebellum and basal ganglia are degenerative. To date, recovery due to neural changes is not expected, and the focus is on medication therapy and compensatory function through rehabilitation. For persons who have SCI, movement and functional abilities can be suggested from the level of the lesion or injury on the spinal cord. Table 14-3 illustrates this point.

ANATOMY AND PHYSIOLOGY RELATIVE TO MOVEMENT

In a physical sense, movement consists of an involuntary action, a reflex process, or a conscious and deliberate choice to have muscles act on bones, joints, and ligament and tendon structures. It also depends on neurological direction and stimulation and cognitive goals. The skeletal structure protects vital organs of the body and provides a frame for the skin and muscles with their underlying contents; it contributes to movement.

Musculoskeletal Structures

Bones

Bones manufacture red blood cells, store salts and minerals, and bear the weight of the body. Calcium metabolized with vitamin D is essential to bone health and repair; the parathyroid hormone acts to regulate the process. Loss of bony structure occurs with non-weight-bearing status (local stress); inadequate nutrients, especially calcium with vitamin D; chronic conditions or disuse, such as arthritis; and trauma, among other causes. As discussed in Chapter 21, osteoporosis is one consequence of non-weight-bearing exercise; trauma may induce heterotopic ossification, and poor nutrition affects bone mineralization.

Bones are joined in configurations that allow them to move in specific ways in concert with muscle actions. Different types of joints (e.g., hinge, gliding, pivot, or ball and socket) allow certain types of movements. Joint movements involving flexion, extension, rotation, abduction, and adduction movements are related to performing range of motion (ROM) exercises, positioning and alignment, and similar interventions.

Joints

Joints and movement are interrelated; joints enable movement, and movement maintains joints. The hyaline cartilage that lines joint surfaces receives nourishment from synovial fluid as it flows in and out of the joint during movement. The viscous synovial fluid cannot supply nourishment to the joint without movement; thus joint immobility leads to deterioration of the joint structures, notably cartilage. Situations that lead to restriction or immobilization of joints, such as casting, severe guarding due to pain, paralysis, non-weight-bearing status, altered or reduced muscle control, or abuse and trauma, are detrimental to joint function. Joint mobility and maintenance underlie, in part, the rationale for performing ROM exercises.

Tendons and Ligaments

Tendons are strong, fibrous bands without elasticity that attach muscles to bones. Ligaments have some elasticity enabling them to connect bones and cartilage, bridge visceral organs, and secure joints; some are part of joint synovial membranes. The longitudinal collagen fibers that make up tendons and ligaments are overlooked often, until the person experiences their presence through pain or immobilization. Recovery from damage or disuse of tendons and ligaments is a lengthy process. With contractures, tendons and ligaments become involved with immobility of muscles, joints, and surrounding tissues.

Muscles

The focus in this chapter is on skeletal or striated muscle; the other two types are viscera and cardiac. Muscles provide heat through contraction, produce motion and strength, and maintain posture. Strength is greater in larger muscles and in those with wider bulk. Muscle fibers have characteristics that enable them to contract, extend, flex, and demonstrate irritability and elasticity. As they respond to stimuli, they can shorten and thicken, stretch, and return to the original shape. Table 14-4 describes major events of muscle contraction and relaxation (Thibodeau & Patton, 1999, p. 319).

Muscle fibers can produce isotonic, isometric, or isokinetic motions. Isotonic contraction shortens the muscle as the fibers contract, but without increasing internal tension leading to movement. Isometric contraction against stable resistance maintains the length of the muscle but increases the tension or force generated by the muscle; thus no body movement occurs. These actions are illustrated in Figure 14-2. The underlying principle is building strength by lifting or moving and holding weight against the force of gravity while in various positions. Less common, isokinetic muscle movement occurs when muscle contracts maximally throughout its entire ROM and requires special equipment, such as that used in sports training and rehabilitation programs.

Every muscle movement involves a primary muscle mover, the agonist that is responsible for eliciting a particular movement; synergist muscles assist agonists in their ac-

Table 14-3 Physical Effects and Functional Outcomes of Spinal Cord Injury

Level of Injury	Motor/Sensory Effects	Functional Potential
C1 through C3	No voluntary movement or sensation below the level of the injury Remaining function in the trapezius, sternomastoid, and platysma muscles allowing head and neck movement with varying degree of control Diaphragm and intercostal muscles paralyzed Sensory losses include occipital region of head, ears, and some areas of face	Ventilator dependent Completely dependent for care Limited mobility potential with voice-, chin-, or breath-controlled wheelchair
C4	As above but neck accessory muscle function intact plus potential for partial function of diaphragm Some shoulder movement	May be able to breathe without ventilator for intervals May have limited self-feeding ability with adaptive sling
C5	Deltoid and biceps function present, which adds shoulder strength, elbow flexion, and good control of head and neck Unopposed trapezius and levator scapulae action may cause shoulders to elevate Full sensation to head, neck, upper back, and chest and lateral parts of upper arms Phrenic nerve intact to diaphragm	Independent breathing but poor lung capacity Tidal volume 300 ml Improved hand-to-mouth coordination permitting self-feeding, oral care, dressing of upper body, all with assistive aids Dependent in other areas of care Needs assistance to transfer Electric wheelchair for mobility
C6	Action of brachioradialis added, permitting wrist dorsiflexion and some grasp; some wrist extension Unopposed action of biceps and deltoids pulls the arms into abducted forearm flexed position Sensation present over lateral aspects of entire arm, thumb, and index finger	Independence in feeding and grooming with adaptive equipment Can assist with dressing, transfers, and elimination Independence with manual wheelchair Can drive a car with hand controls
C7	Diaphragm and accessories can compensate for losses of intercostal and abdominal muscles and support normal breathing Elbow flexion and extension present; wrist flexion and some finger control Sensation to middle finger and part of ring finger	Potential for independent living Can achieve independence in feeding, bathing, dressing, transfer, wheelchair mobility, and elimination care
C8	Addition of adductor and internal rotator muscles balance muscle function and eliminate abnormal arm and shoulder positions Full sensation to hand; finger flexion	Moderate to full control of shoulders, arm, wrist, and fingers Should be able to live independently
T1 through T5	No voluntary movement or sensation below the level of the injury Full control of upper extremities Some intercostal and thoracic muscle function Sensation intact to arms and midchest/midback	Pulmonary function within acceptable norms; tidal volume 500-700 ml Independent in self-care; manual wheelchair Potential for full-time employment
T6 through T10	Increasing control over abdominal and trunk muscles Sensation steadily increasing to level of umbilicus and midback	Balance improves with each segment of abdominal muscles No interference with respiratory function Full independence in care; manual wheelchair Employment reasonable expectation, can participate in sports activities
T11 through L5	Progressively adds function of hip flexors, knee extension, knee flexion, and ankle dorsiflexion Slight foot movement added at L4 Sensation intact to lower abdomen, hips, anterior surface of legs, selected sections on posterior of legs No sensation present in groin, genitals, anus, or portions of buttocks	Independent in self-care Ambulation with long leg braces possible but tires easily
S1 through S5	Progressive return of full control to legs, ankles, and feet Progressive control of bowel, bladder, and sexual function; sensory function to groin, anus, and posterior aspects of legs and feet	Independent in self-care Independent ambulation; short braces may be used for support

From Phipps, W.J., Sands, J.K., & Marek, J.F. (1999). *Medical-surgical nursing: Concepts and clinical practice* (6th ed.). St. Louis: Mosby.

TABLE 14-4 Major Events of Muscle Contraction and Relaxation

Excitation and Contraction

1. A nerve impulse reaches the end of a motor neuron, triggering the release of the neurotransmitter acetylcholine
2. Acetylcholine diffuses rapidly across the gap of the neuromuscular junction and binds to acetylcholine receptors on the motor endplate of the muscle fiber
3. Stimulation of acetylcholine receptors initiates an impulse that travels along the sarcolemma, through the T tubules, to sacs of the SR
4. Ca^{++} is released from the SR into the sarcoplasm, where it binds to troponin molecules in the thin myofilaments
5. Tropomyosin molecules in the thin myofilaments shift, exposing actin's active sites
6. Energized myosins cross bridges of the thick myofilaments, bind to actin, and use their energy to pull the thin myofilaments toward the center of each sarcomere; this cycle repeats itself many times per second, as long as adenosine triphosphate (ATP) is available
7. As the thin filaments slide past the thick myofilaments, the entire muscle fiber shortens

Relaxation

1. After the impulse is over, the SR begins actively pumping Ca^{++} back into its sacs
2. As Ca^{++} is stripped from troponin molecules in the thin myofilaments, tropomyosin returns to its position, blocking actin's active sites
3. Myosin cross bridges are prevented from binding to actin and thus can no longer sustain the contraction
4. Since the thick and thin myofilaments are no longer connected, the muscle fiber may return to its longer, resting length

From Thibodeau, G.A., & Patton, K.T. (1999). *Anatomy & physiology* (4th ed.). St. Louis: Mosby.
SR, Sarcoplasmic reticulum.

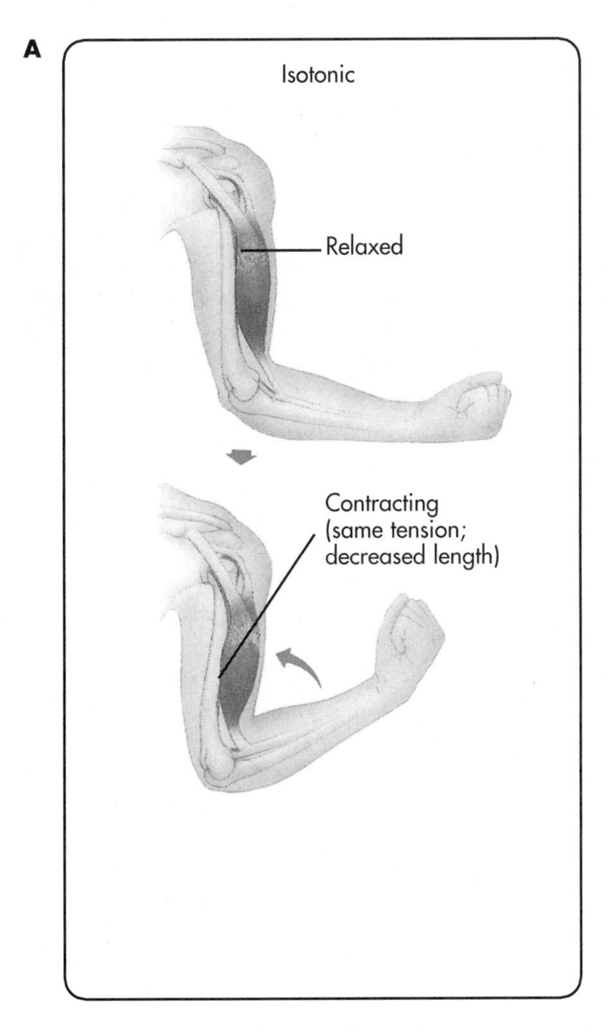

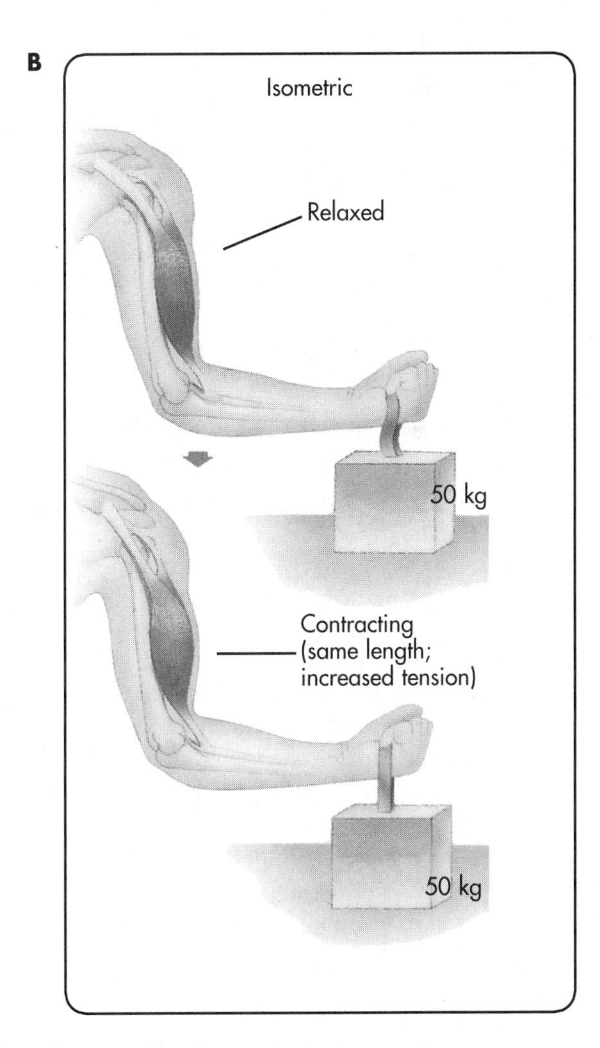

Figure 14-2 Isotonic and isometric contraction. **A,** In isotonic contraction, the muscle shortens, producing movement. **B,** In isometric contraction, the muscle pulls forcefully against a load but does not shorten. (From Thibodeau, G.A., & Patton, K.T. [1999]. *Anatomy & physiology* [4th ed.]. St. Louis: Mosby.)

tions. Antagonist muscles work to oppose agonist muscles, just as the name implies. When the biceps brachii muscle contracts (agonist) to flex the forearm, the triceps brachii muscle relaxes (antagonist). The coracoid and brachialis muscles function as synergists because they contract to allow elbow flexion. Synergist muscles can be retrained in some instances to perform the function of agonists, such as when optimizing function with paralysis after stroke or SCI, or for clients using upper extremity prostheses.

Motor control and movement depend on muscle development and function as evidenced in strength, gross and fine motor coordination, fluidity of planned movements, balance, and cognition. Muscle strength is an important factor in movement often related to factors such as postural control, functional capacity, endurance, bone mass, and overall health status, including reduced falls and mental outlook. Standard muscle strength tests may yield unreliable results for clients who experience pain or immobility at various positions, or midway through ROM. The same may be true for those who are fatigued, experience early morning stiffness, take particular medications, or have cognitive or sensory alterations.

Muscle tone can be determined in one way by the amount of resistance that occurs when performing passive ROM for a client who is cooperative and relaxed. With immobility, muscle fibers shorten and stiffen, predisposing them to reduced ROM, in some instances contributing to contractures. When tone becomes flaccid, muscles correspondingly lose their bouncing stretch capacity, and the resulting stiffness resists extension and may account for some of the hypertonic stretch response with spasticity. The negative-feedback mechanisms described earlier are essential to muscle tone; it follows that muscle tone becomes flaccid with unconsciousness or coma.

Sequelae to Congenital Conditions

Certain musculoskeletal problems occur later in life as sequelae to congenital conditions, such as cerebral palsy or spina bifida. Children with a tethered cord as a complication of myelomeningocele are at risk for loss of motor strength with mixtures of spasticity and flaccidity, asymmetrical involvement of the lower extremity, paraplegia, scoliosis or kyphosis, and other complex problems, many involving mobility. The involvement of hip, knees, feet, and spine intensifies with the developmental and aging processes. Mobility often includes bracing and orthotics, supplemented by crutches or special canes, making energy conservation important. Weight bearing and upright positioning are important to body image and self-esteem for children and adolescents. These actions may reduce contractures and help with skin integrity and bowel and bladder function; weight bearing also may reduce obesity and strengthen bones. The parapodium and its modification, the swivel walker, have proved helpful with socialization and education for children, but most will need to have a prescribed wheelchair to use for daily mobility (Hoeman, 1997).

EFFECTS OF EXERCISE

Findings from multiple studies reveal that even in older populations exercise, especially weight-bearing exercise, has benefits for improving muscle strength and related factors noted above, such as postural control. After an exercise and strengthening program, alertness and ability to pay attention were important results that led to improved postural stability and consequently reduced the risk for falls in older persons who had intact vision (Topp, Estes, Dayhoff, & Suhrheinrich, 1997).

For a number of years, rehabilitation specialists have been aware of the benefits of muscle exercise programs using weight training. During the past decade, these programs were found to increase strength and performance in persons with postpolio syndrome (Agre et al., 1996). Improvements were found for those with progressive neuromuscular disease and myasthenia gravis (Lohi, Lindberg, & Andersen, 1993). Exercises to increase endurance and aerobic exercise capacity are effective for persons with osteoarthritis, cystic fibrosis (Dunlevy, Douce, Hill, Baez, & Clutter, 1994), and muscular sclerosis, among others. Closely monitored aerobic exercise has improved fitness and prevented secondary disabilities for persons with mixed physical disabilities.

Both aerobic and strength training are known to forestall, even reverse, age-related changes in muscle function for older persons, as well as increase endurance and improve overall health status (Miller, 1995). Changes related to the aging process are detailed in Chapter 30. However, reduced bone density and muscle mass, along with reduced strength, balance, ROM, and so forth, place older persons at risk for frailty and all the accompanying problems; falls are a ready example. Gait training may be another technique to help older persons with balance (Galindo-Ciocon, Ciocon, & Galindo, 1995), certainly for those who live independently at home. Findings from studies of the effects of generalized exercise programs for older women indicate improved passive ROM for hips, knees, and ankles (Hubley-Kozey, Wall, & Hogan, 1995) and in dynamic postural stability (Lord, Ward, & Williams, 1996).

Regular exercise can be beneficial when performed in a variety of ways depending on the client's situation and functional goals. Safety is essential for any mobility or therapeutic exercise program and includes proper use of body mechanics for the provider. Before a client is medically stable, the intent is to prevent contractures or atrophy; avoid pain or joint damage; and maintain muscle tone, strength, and function. Impaired sensation and cognition present special challenges. Determination of the type, amount, and level of independence in exercise is a team function.

MOVEMENT AND SELF-CARE

The organizing framework for this book builds on self-care activities necessary for participation in everyday life (Roper, Logan, & Tierney, 1996). Ideally clients will choose to participate and accept responsibility for performing self-care, often correlated with components of ADLs, to the limits of their ability. Certainly this is the goal in rehabilitation. However, heavy reliance on goals established by the rehabilitation system may detract from those mutually set by clients and providers. Rehabilitation nurses serve as advocates to ensure that clients have maximum autonomy, independence, and participation in setting goals that are appropriate and to ensure that achievement will promote higher life quality and satisfaction.

At times, a goal is modified so that clients are able to direct others in performing self-care activities according to their preferences; indeed, some cultural norms will dictate that others perform the care for the person. Others advocate assertiveness training for clients to help them accomplish their objectives effectively. The person's motivation and ability to learn to perform self-care directly influences the outcome. Chapter 11 describes teaching and learning strategies for clients and families. Shortened lengths of stay in rehabilitation facilities and minimal services in other levels of care challenge rehabilitation teams to find ways to ensure that clients and families are prepared to continue to perform self-care skills when they return to home and community. In this chapter the focus is on understanding individual potential and improving clients' abilities to perform self-care in ADLs and IADLs with optimal independence.

Self-care, as expressed through performing ADLs and IADLs, is a functional mobility of great interest to rehabilitation nurses. Self-care includes dressing, eating, toileting, bathing, and grooming activities. IADLs are skills for independent living that include shopping, cooking, cleaning, doing laundry, managing personal finances, developing social and recreation skills, handling emergencies, and the like. Specific instruments and information for evaluation and outcome of function are found in Chapter 8. Multiple systems and factors influence functional mobility (Table 14-5).

Responsibility and Self-Care

Performing self-care is a personal matter beginning with rituals, habits, timing, and methods of carrying out these activities learned from families and cultures in childhood. Although Orem (1995) developed the theoretical foundations for self-care in nursing practice, her work again specified deficits. In rehabilitation nursing the focus is on strengths and optimal levels of function with participation by the client. Self-care requires clients to accept responsibility at the same time that they experience an intensely client-centered process involving the rehabilitation team.

Home environment, culture, education and socioeconomic status, and access to goods and services influence a person's approach to self-care. Altered or impaired mobility and their response to the situation affect clients' abilities in self-care. Inability to carry out self-care leads clients to ineffective behaviors such as fear of falling, social isolation, reduced self-esteem, depression, loss of purpose and role function, and undue reliance on caregivers or learned helplessness.

TABLE 14-5 Systems and Factors Influencing Functional Mobility

System or Factor	Influence on Functional Mobility
Central nervous system	Controls muscle tone, reflexes, paresis or paralysis, coordination, balance, motor development, and system status
Musculoskeletal system	Source for muscle strength, range of motion, joint stability, body alignment and postural control, and positioning; associated with endurance or fatigue and influenced by nutrition, sleep, stress, and general health status
Sensory system	Senses of visual-auditory-olfactory-tactile sensation are related to coordination, pain and other proprioception, and vestibular and spatial orientations; supplies visual support for balance, sensory intake, stimulation, and expression
Cognitive-perceptual factors	Related to attention, orientation, memory, comprehension and taking or following directions, judgment, and planning; perceptual deficits affect hand-eye coordination, figure-ground or depth perception, and agnosia, apraxia, or neglect with distortion of body image
Psychosocial and emotional factors	Coping behaviors and style, beliefs and practices, concerns or fears, interest and motivation affect self-care attitude and sense of responsibility
Environmental and technological factors	Architectural barriers, unsafe communities or home conditions, or lack of assistive devices and/or poorly prescribed adapted equipment deter self-care
Social, cultural, and economic factors	Beliefs and practices, including stigma about impairment; inability to pay or gain access to services; and insufficient resources may foster distrust of health system
Other	Overall health status, chronic diseases or impairments, specific problems such as hypotension-hypertension, seizures, or the like; age and developmental stage are factors influencing self-care and functional mobility

Specific Conditions and Functional Mobility Impairment

Specific conditions and impairments predictably affect performance of self-care as evidenced in ADLs and IADLs. Table 14-6 illustrates the relationship between impairments affecting self-care and certain chronic, disabling disorders. Self-care ADLs consist of multiple components requiring specific skills to complete the task.

TABLE 14-6 Examples of Conditions Affecting Self-Care

Conditions	Disorder
Paralysis or paresis of a hand	CVA, SCI, cerebral palsy, MD, TBI, arthritis
Decreased sensation of a hand or arm	SCI, TBI, CVA
Incoordination of upper extremities	Cerebral palsy, TBI
Perceptual deficits such as body image disturbances, spatial disorientation, and apraxia	Amputations, CVA, TBI
Hemianopsia	CVA
Limited range of motion; surgical procedure causing musculoskeletal limitation	Arthritis, SCI, CVA
Poor or weak hand grasp	SCI, MD, MS, arthritis
Amputation of an upper extremity	Amputation of an upper extremity
Limited endurance	Arthritis, MS, MD, SCI
Spasticity, ataxia, tremors	Parkinson's disease

CVA, Cerebrovascular accident; *SCI,* spinal cord injury; *TBI,* traumatic brain injury; *MD,* muscular dystrophy; *MS,* multiple sclerosis.

Certainly cognition and perception underlie function and bring memory, attention, orientation, and concentration or direction following, and problem-solving skills to bear in carrying out functional activities (Knight, 2000). Hand-eye coordination and sensory status affect a client's ability to carry out self-care activities in the proper manner. Apraxia is an important example because with this perceptual impairment, a client may be physically able to perform the activity but cannot produce purposeful, organized movement to do so. The particular impairment is related to the site of the lesion or injury in the brain as shown in Table 14-7.

Personal preferences and habits, cultural practices, and socioeconomic status are factors. However, persons who have problems with access to areas of their home or the community, lack of assistive devices, or concerns about safety cannot function at optimal levels of independent function regardless of their physical or cognitive functional abilities.

ASSESSMENT

Integrated neurological and musculoskeletal assessments are essential to evaluation of movement and mobility and are conducted with optimal levels of ADL and IADL performance in mind. Assessment tools for ADLs and IADLs, such as the Barthel and Katz rating scales and the Functional Independence Measure, are presented in Chapter 8. These scales have stood with modification over time; studies are examining psychometric properties of new scales, such as those designed for persons with specific conditions.

Subjective Assessment

Subjective assessment begins with data about the history of the specific problem and an overall review of past function,

TABLE 14-7 Apraxia

Type	Impairment Produced	Lesion Site
Constructional	Impairment in producing designs in two or three dimensions Involves copying, drawing, or constructing	Occipitoparietal lobe of either hemisphere
Dressing	Inability to dress oneself accurately Makes mistakes, such as putting clothes on backwards, upside-down, or inside-out, or putting both legs in the same pant leg	Occipital or parietal lobe usually in nondominant hemisphere
Motor	Loss of kinesthetic memory patterns, which results in patient's inability to perform a purposeful motor task although it is understood	Frontal lobe of either hemisphere, precentral gyrus
Idiomotor	Inability to imitate gestures or perform a purposeful motor task on command May be able to do task spontaneously	Parietal lobe of dominant hemisphere, supramarginal gyrus
Ideational	Inability to carry out activities automatically or on command because of inability to understand the concept of the act	Parietal lobe of dominant hemisphere or diffuse brain damage as in arteriosclerosis

From Phipps, W.J., Sands, J.K., & Marek, J.F. (1999). *Medical-surgical nursing: Concepts and clinical practice* (6th ed.). St. Louis: Mosby.

including ability to perform ADLs and IADLs, and activities in the household and community. Identify assistive devices and adapted equipment, along with the reason for having them and how the client uses them. Elicit clients' perceptions of their function and goals for lifestyle including vocation or education or leisure.

Describe limitations in access or ability and identify problems related to health status, impairments, or conditions. Inquire about comorbid conditions affecting mobility or self-care, such as pain; sensory, communication, or cognitive impairments; energy or endurance level; sleep hygiene; household or environmental stressors; and safety concerns, such as poor balance. Evaluate psychosocial, emotional, and cultural factors affecting mobility or performance of ADLs. Clients returning home benefit from a home and community assessment as detailed in Box 14-1.

Medical history includes surgeries; details of cardiovascular, pulmonary, rheumatologic, neurologic, or musculoskeletal conditions; and a family history. Describe the type, location, and severity of impairment or injury, along with any comorbid conditions and the potential for infection or other untoward effects.

The review of systems focuses on skin, gastrointestinal, respiration, circulation, regulatory control, elimination, eating and nutrition, sexuality, and integrated neuromuscular systems, as well as cognitive and emotional status. Review

Box 14-1 Home and Community Assessment: Access Considerations

Outdoors

Parking and distance from entrance
Location of mailbox
Storage of vehicle and access to home from the storage area
Access to home: width of doors; ability to turn key, open and close doors; need for ramps, handrails
Lighting in entrances
Community buildings used regularly; access to these buildings
Access to private or public transportation: distance from home, cost, assistance required, ability to operate own vehicle safely
Parking areas marked for handicapped; adequate space to maneuver
Width, height of incline of ramps, sidewalks

Indoors: General

Thresholds, floor obstructions, steps inside home
Arrangement of furniture and ability to use
Location of telephone
Ability to raise/lower windows
Floor coverings: slippery scatter rugs; whether wheelchair can be maneuvered
Location of all rooms; ability to maneuver a wheelchair or assistive device
Location of fuse box
Ability to control heat
Width of walkways, doorways, halls: space to maneuver
Access to outlets; ability to change light bulbs
Type of furniture and ability to use safely
Elevator: threshold, timing of door, adapted for hearing and visual impairments

Indoors: Kitchen

Access to stove, sink, cupboards, storage, work space, refrigerator, contents, other appliances
Countertop and sink height; opening under sink for wheelchair access
Ability to operate faucets, use microwave, reach knobs on stove
Convenient arrangement of appliances

Indoors: Bathroom

Height of sink and toilet, shower/tub, and location of faucets
Space for maneuvering wheelchair or assistive device
Threshold for shower
Ability to use facilities safely
Presence, location of grab bars, securely anchored

Indoors: Bedroom

Height of bed
Access to closet, ability to reach rods, storage area
Firmness of mattress
Ability to transfer in and out of bed safely; adequate space around bed
Arrangement of furniture: space to maneuver

Safety Considerations

House number clearly visible and readable for quick identification during an emergency
Locks secure; deadbolts; ability to use
Ability to see and talk to visitor at the door without being seen
Steps, porch, front door lighted and protected from the weather
Nonslip doormat
Ability to use telephone, emergency response system
Ability to control water temperature
Wiring, outlet covers for children
Smoke detectors: type, location, access
Lighting in rooms, hallways; access to control lights inside and outside home
Ability to respond to a fire emergency: fire exits/access, use of stairs instead of elevator, use of fire extinguisher, fire drills
Use of oxygen: precautions and appropriate signs in home
Access to telephone, radio, television while in bed
Use of space heaters: type, location
Location of knobs on stove, safety around stove, cleanliness of stove; ability to use good judgment when cooking
Ability to dispose of infectious materials safely
Safe play area
Ability to transport food from kitchen to table
Ventilation in all rooms
Pest-free method of trash storage

medications with attention to allergies and adverse effects, multiple medication use, and signs of misuse of medications or substances.

Objective Assessment

Following are guidelines for assessment of musculoskeletal and neurological functions related to movement. However, movement and self-care abilities are complex and involve multiple functions, such as cognition, swallowing, or communication as presented in specific chapters. Recovery occurs in varying degrees and at different rates but in predictable patterns. Baseline assessment data should be documented and clients reassessed at regular intervals or when change occurs. Specialized evaluations, such as a client's ability to return to work or to drive a car, involve expertise from the interdisciplinary team.

Physical Examination

Observe for respiratory status, skin color and turgor, and posture and alignment. Note stooped shoulders, involuntary movements, unusual gait or gestures, signs of weakness or pain during activities, and overall appearance. Inspect body for shape, symmetry, length of extremities, abnormalities, redness, edema (positional), and nodes (at joints) or protrusions. Palpate for turgor, tone, and response of tenderness, pain, or tightness.

Assess joints for ROM, stability, tightness, impingement, pain or grating on movement, edema, heat or redness, and nodules or unusual protrusions. During ROM exercises rehabilitation nurses have opportunities to assess the quality of muscle movements. Appendix 14A is a guide for assessment of a client's movement based on normal degrees of joint motion conducted before initiating a program of ROM exercises.

Assess muscle strength using a manual muscle test (MMT) to score, as in Table 14-8. Evaluate for relative strength against resistance, when grasping and squeezing, for equality on both sides of the body and in proximal and distal positions, and for ability to flex and relax. Grip the client's hand as in a handshake, both using right hands; repeat with left hands. Handgrips reveal strength and function. Observe for intact pincer grasp, uneven hand strength, contractions, spasticity, or flaccidity and note pain.

For example, poor triceps muscle strength will impair movement that involves pushing or pulling over the head. The client raises the arm straight overhead, bends at the elbow, and moves the hand behind the head. With the nurse's hand on the forearm, the client pushes against the resistance. Spasticity, reduced ROM, or weakness may render the push against resistance nonfunctional for activities without modifications.

Assess muscle tone by evaluating deep tendon reflexes (DTRs) and examining neurological responses. Assess motor stretch reflexes by striking tendons over muscle groups and observing for overresponse or underresponse of muscle contractions and involuntary muscle movements (Table 14-9). Evaluate reflexes for symmetry, hyporeflex-hyperreflex activity, abnormal or inappropriate response to stimulus (such as appearance or persistence of primitive reflexes such as reflex grasp or tonic neck), or contraction to adjoining muscles (Table 14-10).

Assess cranial nerves for function, with special attention to motor control related to vision and eye control, proprioception, speech, and swallowing.

Assess sensory status beginning with sensation on the trunk and extremities. Use side-to-side symmetrical testing beginning distal to the body. Assess superficial and deep pain, pressure, touch, and temperature. Document on a dermatome map or similar figure. See Chapter 24 for additional information. Apraxia is discussed in Table 14-7 and in Chapter 25. Sensory and motor qualities and cerebellar function are involved in a

TABLE 14-8 Muscle Function and Strength Scales

Grade	Scale	% Function	Muscle Level Assessment
5	Normal	100 or full	Full ROM against gravity with full resistance
4	Good	75	Full ROM against gravity with some resistance
3	Fair	50	Full ROM with gravity
2	Poor	25	Passive movement, full ROM
1	Trace	10	Slight contractility, no movement
0	Zero	0 or none	No contractility

Adapted from Barkauskas, V., Baumann, L.C., Stoltenberg-Allen, K., & Darling-Fisher, C. (1998). *Health & physical assessment* (2nd ed.). St. Louis: Mosby.
ROM, Range of motion.

TABLE 14-9 Motor Stretch Reflexes

Reflex	Assesses
Biceps reflex	C5-C6 functions
Patellar reflex	L2-L4 functions
Achilles reflex	S1-S2 functions
Triceps reflex	C6-C8 functions
Brachioradial reflex	C5-C6 functions
Abdominal reflex	Lower thoracic cord reflex centers; associated with multiple sclerosis
Plantar reflex (seen with Babinski's sign)	Upper motor neuron damage; normal reflex during first year of life

TABLE 14-10 Deep Tendon Reflex Response Ratings

Grade	Deep Tendon Reflex Response
0	No response
1+	Sluggish or diminished
2+	Active or expected response
3+	More brisk than expected; slightly hyperactive
4+	Brisk, hyperactive, with intermittent or transient clonus

From Seidel, H.M., Dains, J.E., Ball, J.W., & Benedict, G.W. (1995). *Mosby's guide to physical examination* (3rd ed.). St. Louis: Mosby.

client's ability to actually plan and then carry out movement, as well as the sequence of movements. Thus, include hands-on observation of a client's specific perceptual motor or sensory problems when unable to perform self-care in ADLs.

Assess proprioception and sense of position in space (kinesthesia perception) for upper and lower extremities. Ask the client to close both eyes while holding his thumb between your thumb and forefinger. As you move the thumb up and down, ask the client to identify the positions. If a position is identified incorrectly, repeat this process with other joints, such as the wrist, elbow, and shoulder. For the lower extremity, begin with the big toe and progress to the ankle, knee, and hip.

Next, strike a tuning fork and place it on the bony prominences of the extremities. Clients then report where and when they can feel the vibrations. Additionally assess the client's ability to identify familiar objects through touch, such as closing the eyes and then recognizing a coin held in the hand as a quarter.

Assess balance and coordination while sitting and during activities. Ask the person to rapidly touch the thumb to each finger or to rotate the hands from supine to prone. Or ask the client to touch his or her nose and then your finger; move your finger and repeat in several positions.

Observe for control of balance at the abdomen and trunk and strength, which are necessary for dressing and household skills, such as cooking. While the client moves forward in the seat of a chair, observe from behind; cross both arms to fold across the chest with elbows aimed to the front. Observe for compensatory balancing when pushing the upper body side-to-side and front-to-back while seated. The person seated in a chair or at the side of the bed may slump or sway to one side.

Assess the ability of a client with SCI to rotate the neck and trunk by looking behind over each shoulder while keeping the hips straight in place. Upper extremity activities can be modified, such as using over-the-head dressing techniques, when trunk rotation is limited.

Assess balance and coordination during mobility activities, such as when moving in and out of the bed, during transfers, and during ambulation. Use the Romberg test for persons able to stand with their eyes closed and feet together. However, use precautions against falls because loss of balance is possible and is a positive sign of cerebellar problems. Observe for swaying, leaning, reeling, or if standing, taking a step backward to maintain balance.

Assess gait pattern, arm swing, balance and steadiness, gait during turns, and whether the client moves to the intended destination. Observe for involuntary movements or gait patterns associated with specific conditions such as:

- **Hemiplegia:** A stiff gait with toes on the affected side scraping the floor due to reduced flexion of the knee and swing from hip. The affected arm does not swing with the unaffected footstep; the shoulder may slouch.
- **Parkinson's disease:** A festinating gait with initial hesitation, followed by small, shuffling steps. Client may appear to march in place because of difficulty in beginning to walk and then be unable to halt once in motion. The body and head appear to lean forward with the arms extended back, not swinging with gait.
- **Multiple sclerosis:** A scissor gait may appear; slow steps may be due to bilateral spasticity in the legs.
- **Other:** Persons with lower motor problems may appear to be stepping up stairs although walking on a flat surface. Those with progressive neuromuscular disease may develop a waddling gait.

Assess client's safety and performance of ADLs and IADLs. Evaluate the level and amount of physical, mental and cognitive, and emotional assistance needed, as well as types of assistive devices. Observe for actions that indicate a client is using accessory muscles or compensatory movements to aid function. Many of these movements may be effective and purposeful; others are unsafe or detrimental and indicate problems in individual situations. Box 14-2 describes actions that may represent problems or lead to further disabilities.

NURSING DIAGNOSES

Nursing diagnoses include impaired mobility, self-care deficit, and inability to perform ADLs independently.

GOALS

Client goals include optimal independence as much as possible, prevention of complications and further disability, maximal function for potential and opportunities, life satisfaction and effective coping, access to the community and quality social interaction, and safety.

NURSING INTERVENTIONS

Therapeutic interventions for mobility and self-care are core principles of rehabilitation nursing practice. Because

Box 14-2 Potential Problems in Function or Movement

Assess further when a client is observed improvising or compensating movement by:
- Holding onto a handrail to pull the body while going up stairs
- Holding onto a bed side rail or bedcovers to pull to sitting in bed
- Leaning to one side and using both hands on the handrail while going down the stairs or a ramp
- Holding onto furniture or doorways and watching the feet while walking in the house
- Lifting a leg (or arm) with the opposite leg (or arm) or holding onto clothing, such as the pants leg (or sleeve)
- Tilting the head to reach back or side of head while grooming hair
- Pushing up, rocking forward and back, and/or leaning the body over for momentum ("nose over toes") when rising to stand from a chair
- Leaning over from the waist without bending the knees and then using one hand on the thigh, as if it were a prop, to assist in getting upright
- Turning to reach for an object and then using the other arm or an object to support the reaching arm at the elbow or wrist
- Positioning a chair before sitting down by using the front or back of the knees and then using the back of the knees to guide sitting down; using the torso and hips to lean against a table or chair
- Reaching and leaning with the body rather than with an arm
- Walking with a lean to one side, a limp, or other variation of gait
- Scanning ineffectively when eating or grooming
- Rolling or scooting the body, sliding forward in a seat, or other maneuvers to move off a bed or out of a chair

of the amount of information necessary to present the interventions, mobility content is arranged in the following sections: therapeutic exercises, therapeutic positioning, activities for mobility in the bed, transfers, ambulation and gait training, wheelchairs, and environmental assistive devices. Interventions for self-care include performing personal care and hygiene, dressing, bathing, and toileting. Content on eating and swallowing is in Chapter 17, bowel and bladder elimination in Chapters 19 and 20, and cognition in Chapter 26.

INTERVENTIONS FOR MAINTAINING MOBILITY

The importance of improving or maintaining mobility to prevent deconditioning (disuse syndrome) and medical complications has been well established earlier. Mobility is foundational to performing ADLs and IADLs. To meet these goals, rehabilitation nurses are concerned with a client's functional outcomes with mobility in therapeutic exercise and positioning, bed activities, transfers, use of assistive devices or adaptive equipment such as wheelchairs, and ambulation including gait. What follows here are detailed interventions for achieving mobility goals.

Therapeutic Exercise

Regular exercise is an essential intervention for persons with or without impaired physical mobility. Before a client is considered medically stable to begin an active physical or occupational therapy program, the rehabilitation nurse implements a program of exercise based on assessment of the person's overall condition. Therapeutic exercise is used in the home and community to help clients maintain function and prevent further problems. The intent is to prevent contractures or atrophy and maintain muscle tone, strength, and function.

Safety is a consideration for any mobility or therapeutic exercise program. For instance, joint damage is possible with passive or active ROM, especially if sensation to the extremity has been impaired; spasticity and flexion contractures may be aggravated in some with upper motor neuron damage. Exercises use isotonic contractions, producing movement of joint and muscle, or isometric contractions, shortening muscle fibers without apparent movement of the limb or joint. Examples of specific concerns include autonomic dysreflexia with SCI, altered respiratory and regulatory functions, poor postural response or hypotension, dizziness or fainting, skin damage, impaired cognition, headache and visual disturbance, increased pain, and falls.

Rehabilitation nurses teach the exercise program to both client and family or other caregivers and encourage active participation, demonstrate the exercise program, lead client and family through practice, observe client and family redemonstrate the exercises, and delegate responsibility for the exercise program to client and family as an ADL.

Range-of-Motion Exercises

ROM exercises (joint ROM or ROM) is a precise set of actions taken to move the joints through their range, as possible for individual clients. ROM can be passive (performed for the person), active (performed by the person independently), or active with assistance. Appendix 14A illustrates proper ROM exercises that include instructions for the entire body.

ROM exercises are isotonic exercises used to prevent muscle contractures or atrophy; to maintain muscle tone, strength, and function; and to forestall many problems that occur with reduced mobility. The exercise program of ROM must be performed correctly to be effective and safe. Damage to the joints, pain, and other problems may result from improperly administered ROM exercises. Appendix 14A provides a visual review and written instructions for passive, active, and functional ROM. A goniometer is used to measure the angle of flexion of a joint.

Rehabilitation nurses have primary responsibility for ensuring that ROM exercises are performed properly, safely, and at regular intervals, as well as for educating others to perform them. As with all rehabilitation interventions, clients are encouraged to perform as many ROM exercises as independently as possible. A client's ADLs, especially those for personal hygiene, offer opportunities to integrate ROM exercises into daily living. A team approach is essential when developing strategies for ways to perform ROM exercises when a client has chronic disabling conditions, specific impairments, or complications such as contractures, spasticity, pain, or paralysis.

The principles of teaching and learning apply, and the caregiver demonstrates learning by giving the nurse a "return demonstration" of the exercises. Ideally two caregivers practice on each other for the demonstration. In addition to establishing correct movements, this technique affords them the experience of the exercise movements and of being passive recipients. In the community the family, home health care aides, volunteers, and other caregivers may learn to perform ROM with supervision.

Passive ROM exercises are performed for the person. A client performing active ROM may find exercises easier to learn when they are demonstrated first and supplemented with diagrams, and then return the demonstration to ensure accuracy and effectiveness. As with other forms of exercise, persons with similar disabilities may be grouped during the day for "range" exercises, or a client and family member may exercise together. A cable or on-line facility television station, a videocassette tape of ROM exercises, or programs of simple bed exercises may encourage and stimulate participation.

ROM exercise modifications for persons with specific impairments, such as hemiplegia or paraplegia, incorporate methods that aid movement of extremities using the unaffected extremities. For example, a client laces the fingers of the unaffected hand through those of the affected hand for support to exercise; raising one arm above the shoulder supports and raises the other, and flexing and extending the unaffected arm at the elbow assist reciprocal action in the other. To move the legs through their ROM, a client may combine the unaffected arm and leg, depending on strength and balance. With paraplegia a person may exercise the legs and feet while sitting in bed because the bed assists in maintaining balance and supports the legs and feet.

Isometric Exercises

Isometric exercises contract muscle fibers without movement of limbs or joints and thus require voluntary participation (see Figure 14-2). The nurse teaches a client how to perform the activity and then monitors and evaluates the results of the exercise. Energy expenditure, pain, postural stability and balance, cognition, and safety are considerations for any exercise plan.

Sometimes referred to as *muscle-setting exercises,* the most common isometric exercises are abdominal-setting, quadriceps-setting, and gluteal-setting exercises. For abdominal-setting exercises, place one hand on the client's abdomen while he or she tenses the abdominal muscle. The muscle is contracted and held for 10 seconds and then released. Remind clients, especially those who have had myocardial infarctions or brain injuries, to maintain a normal respiratory pattern during the exercise. For quadriceps-setting exercises a client contracts the long muscles in the thighs; for gluteal-setting exercises the buttocks are pinched together. Other muscle groups such as the perineal, biceps, and triceps may be contracted isometrically.

Another type of isometric exercise contracts a muscle group against an object, for example, pushing or plantar flexing the feet against a footboard for 10 seconds or less to prevent circulatory stasis. This isometric exercise is resistive because the footboard provides resistance to the activity of the muscles of the legs and feet.

Alternative and Complementary Measures

An increasing number and variety of alternative interventions are proving effective as exercises or as complementary interventions. Chapter 13 contains more information, but exercises including yoga, tai chi, and various stretching regimens are important to clients' mobility. Biofeedback and/or electrical stimulation, such as with transcutaneous electrical stimulation (TENS), may maintain or increase muscle strength and tone; biofeedback complements isometric exercise.

Prevention through Fitness

Preventive exercises are important for all clients, and examples of routines are readily available, including exercises specific to preventing low back pain and maintaining overall fitness. Exercise equipment; repetitive motion machines; a wide range of styles and sizes of balls, weights, and balance and posture aids; computer-assisted gait programs; and more are available to support therapeutic exercise to improve or maintain movement. Many adjuncts to exercise are objects common to the home or readily available in the community. For example, consider using the large, flat elastic bands designed for stretching to exercise the legs and feet as shown in Figure 14-3. Or use wooden dowels, a cane, or shortened broom handles to maintain posture and stretch during exercises from the chair. Canned goods can be used as weights, soft pliable balls squeezed in the hand, and large balls used for balance or tossing against a wall or to another person. Straight-back, steady chairs are good supports and balance while exercising, and mats and cushions help with yoga and floor exercises.

Exercises Specific to Conditions

Therapeutic exercises can be tailored to assist clients who have specific conditions with their mobility and to prevent additional problems. Exercises to prevent osteoporosis are

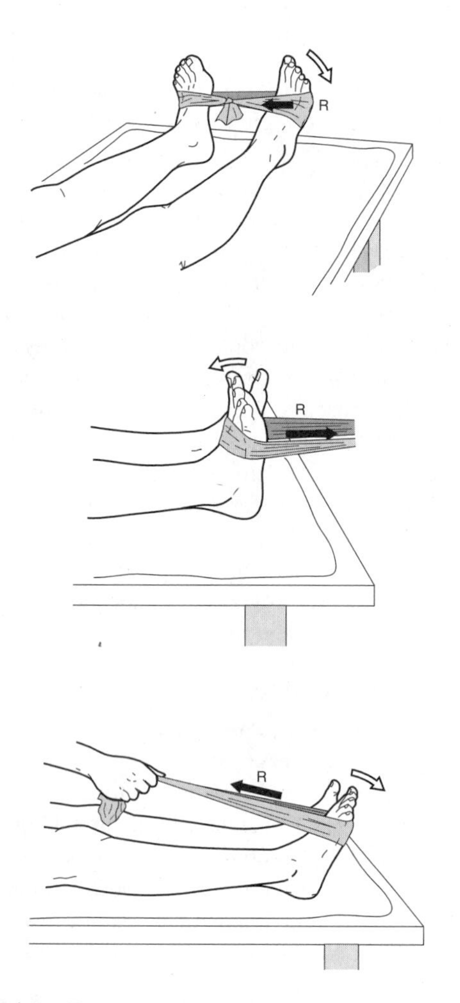

Figure 14-3 Examples of exercise using elastic bands. *R* and *dark arrow* indicate direction of resistance. *Light arrow* indicates direction of foot movement while exercising. (Redrawn from Kisner, C., & Lynn, A.C. [1990]. *Therapeutic exercise: Foundations and techniques* [2nd ed.]. Philadelphia: FA Davis.)

simple to perform provided the person has the ability and can perform them safely (Figure 14-4). Safety involves knowing contraindications as well as interventions, and Figure 14-5 illustrates exercises to be avoided with osteoporosis.

A good deal of success with exercise begins with thinking about it in terms of everyday activities. For instance, view personal hygiene and ADLs as opportunities for performing therapeutic and preventive exercises within the person's abilities and in a safe environment. Kegel exercises help with control of certain incontinence problems, relaxation and breathing exercises aid in respiration, and oral-facial movement benefits conditions such as Parkinson's disease, as detailed in Box 14-3.

Posture, balance, and strength training with improvement in muscle tone can be of benefit after stroke, with Guillain-Barré syndrome, after brain injury, or with multiple sclerosis. Clients with upper body mobility can perform stretching and flexibility exercises for the head and neck and upper extremities, including the shoulder, hand, and wrist, from the wheelchair. Those with postpolio syndrome, Lyme disease, or other fatigue-related conditions need to modify exercises to control for pain and endurance levels; conversely, proper exercise programs may yield gains in strength, tolerance, and respiratory function.

Body Mechanics

Rehabilitation nurses both practice and teach families and other caregivers the principles of proper body mechanics (Box 14-4). These are used not only for lifting and carrying but for nearly every movement in practice. In this busy, rushed health scene, nurses must take time to perform care effectively and safely for themselves as well as for clients; actually, maximum benefits occur when the two are taken together. In rehabilitation, rushing a client is not a standard of care. It takes time to explain; allow the client to do as much as possible; assess the person's readiness, capability, and understanding of the particular action; conserve energy; avoid pain or contraindicated movement; and ensure safety. Only then can action begin.

Therapeutic Positioning

Therapeutic positioning is essential for preventing the complications of immobility when a person must spend time with restricted mobility, whether prescribed or due to impairment or activity intolerance. Positioning involves not only mechanical placement of the body but also changes or repositions, mobility in place, and positions specific to the person's condition or needs. A plan for regular change in position is foundational for preventive care. Variables influencing change in a client's position include degree of independent or self-initiated movement, comfort, and fatigue; loss of sensation; symptoms such as edema; overall physical and mental status; specific disease or condition requirements; and devices or equipment such as casts, prostheses, or bracing.

General guidelines for positioning are subject to individual needs, regulatory guidelines, or facility and agency policies. Clients who experience discomfort after 30 to 60 minutes of lying prone need to be repositioned, whereas those who are able to shift their weight every 20 to 30 minutes and move independently may change total position every 2 to 4 hours. Loss of sensation, paralysis, coma, and edema are indications for position changes every 2 hours or more frequently because the client is unable to inform the nurse of discomfort or pain and because edematous, paralyzed tissue is more sensitive to pressure than normal tissue. Chapter 16 provides detailed information about maintaining skin integrity.

Time of day may influence repositioning. For instance, when a client's overall condition permits, positioning every 4 hours during the night may be desirable to promote a more restful sleep. A turning and positioning schedule posted at

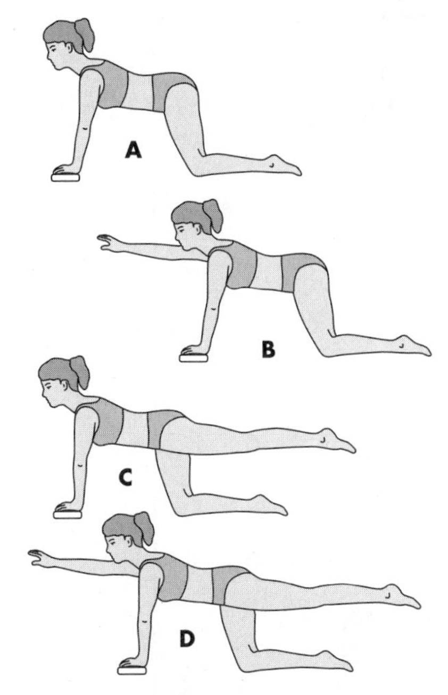

All Fours Arm/Leg Lifts
Position yourself on your hands and knees, with your hands directly under your shoulders and your knees directly under your hips (A). Your back should be flat or slightly arched. Lift one arm and hold for 3 seconds (B). Repeat with the other arm. Then lift one leg and hold for 3 seconds (C). Repeat with the other leg. If you can do these exercises comfortably, try lifting your right arm and left leg simultaneously (D), and then your left arm and right leg.

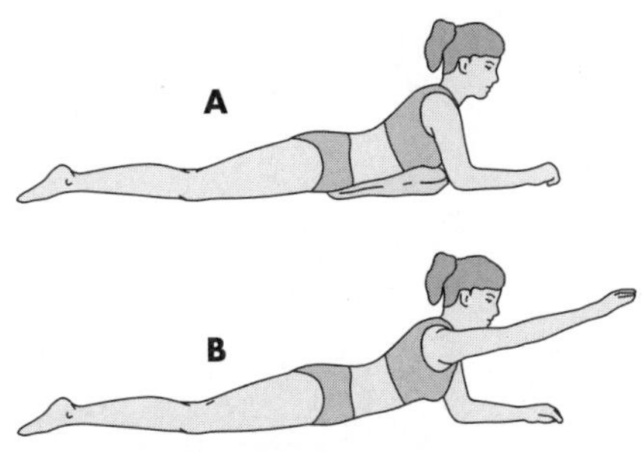

The Elbow Prop
Lie on your stomach with your elbows holding the weight of your upper body (A). Stay in this position for 5 minutes the first day; gradually increase the time to half an hour. You may be more comfortable if you put a pillow under your stomach. The elbow prop position helps reverse the effects of bad posture by passively decompressing the vertebrae and disks. To exercise the back as well, reach the right arm forward (B), then the left, and repeat.

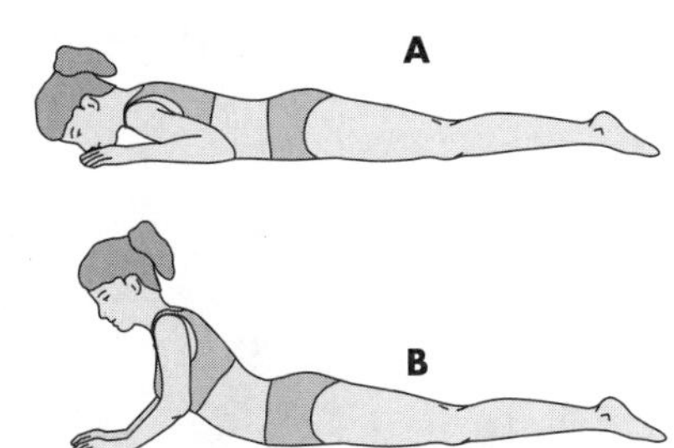

Prone Press-ups with Deep Breathing
Start out in a conventional "push-up" position (A). Arch your back, pinching your shoulder blades together (B). As you push up, inhale; as you lie down, exhale. Keep elbows partially bent to protect the back. Make sure you don't lift your pelvis.

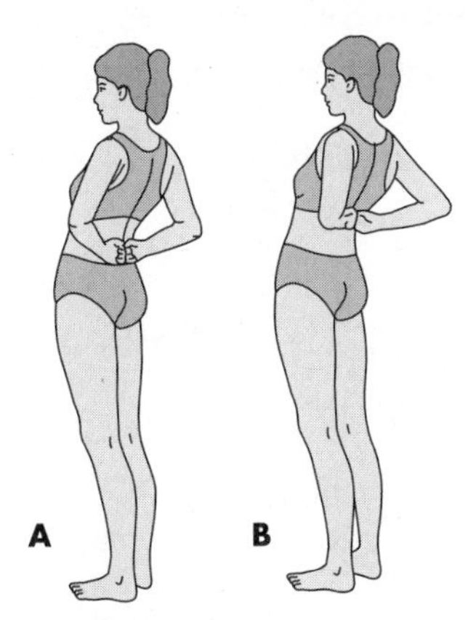

Standing Back Bend
Put your fists on your lower back. Arch backwards slowly while taking a deep breath (A). Relax and put your arms down, then repeat, this time with the fists on the middle back (B).

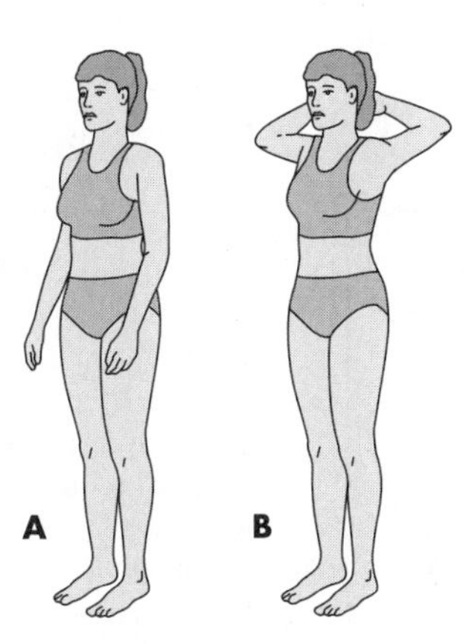

Isometric Posture Correction
Stand as tall as you can, with your chin in, not up (A). Place your palms against the back of your head. Simultaneously push your hands against your head while pinching your shoulder blades together (B). Hold for 3 seconds, then relax for 3 seconds. Maintain an erect posture throughout the exercise.

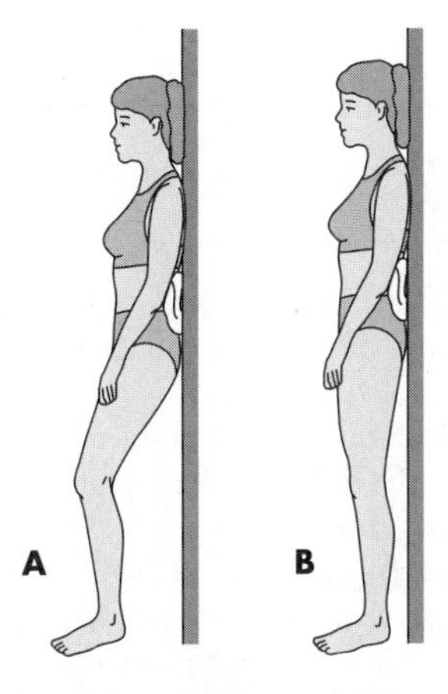

Standing and Pelvic Tilt
Stand with your feet about a foot from the wall, with your knees slightly bent and your back straight (A). Use a towel to support your lower back. Slide up and down, keeping the back straight and the stomach muscles contracted. You should be able to plant your feet closer to the wall as you improve.

Figure 14-4 Exercises for prevention of osteoporosis. (From Phipps, W.J., Sands, J.K., & Marek, J.F. [1999]. *Medical-surgical nursing: Concepts and clinical practice* [6th ed.]. St. Louis: Mosby.)

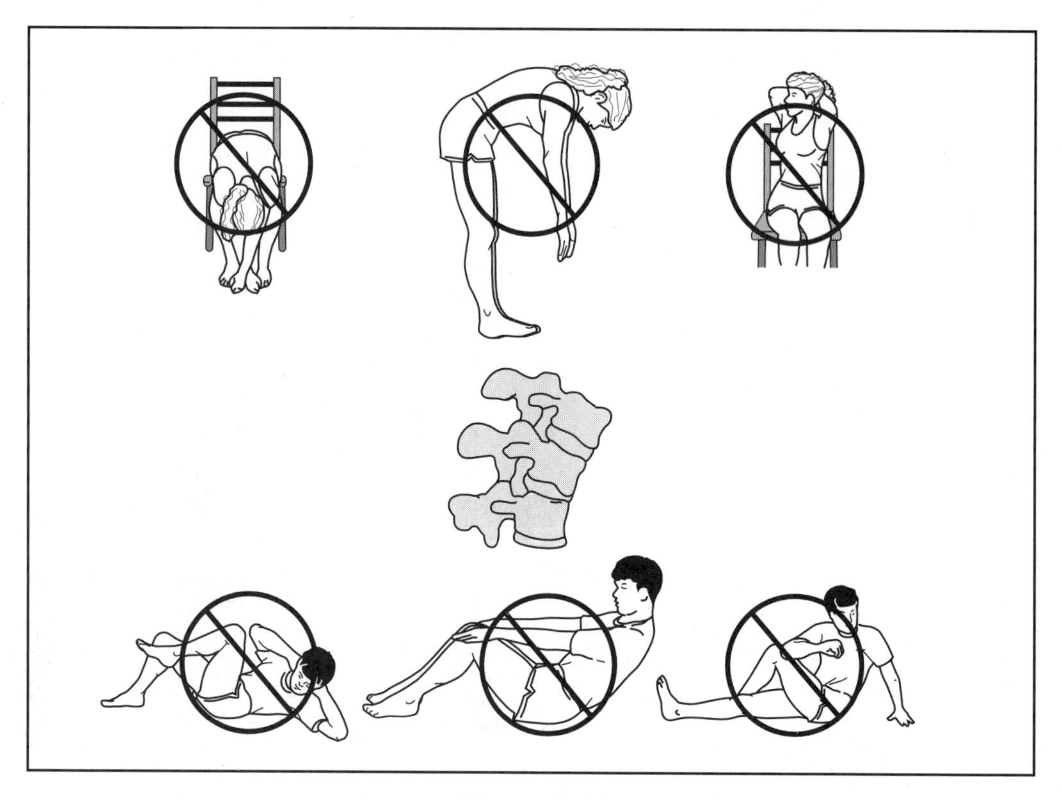

Figure 14-5 Spinal flexion exercises to be avoided with osteoporosis. (From Robinson, D., Kidd, P., & Rogers, K.M. [2000]. *Primary care across the lifespan.* St. Louis: Mosby.)

Box 14-3 Oral-Facial Exercises

Repeat each exercise three to five times:

- Slowly open and close the mouth, pressing the lips to close tightly and open widely
- Pretend to give a kiss, exaggerating puckered lips
- Smile broadly, let relax, and repeat, pushing up the facial cheeks
- Open the mouth wide, and with the lips form an "o" shape, keeping the mouth wide; then close lips tightly and repeat
- Open the mouth and stick the tongue out straight as far as possible; hold it in place without touching the mouth or lips; then pull it back and push out rapidly
- Stick out the tongue and try to touch the nose, then the chin; next lick all around the lips, touching every corner of the mouth
- Rapidly repeat sounds for MA-MA, KA-KA, LA-LA, then rest; try combining the sounds, as with KALA-KALA, MALA-MALA
- Wrinkle nose, raise the eyebrows and wrinkle the forehead, and then relax and repeat
- Open and close the mouth quickly
- Mimic exaggerated chewing motions with the mouth opening and closing with each chew

Box 14-4 Principles of Body Mechanics

- Maintain good posture with back straight, knees slightly bent, and weight over center of body
- Maintain a wide base of support using both sides of the body equally
- Bend from the hips and knees and do not use the back muscles to perform work
- Move in close to the object or person; hold them close in to the body, do not reach in front or above the head
- Push or pull instead of lifting, making smooth, fluid movements
- Do not twist the body, pivot, or shift the feet to turn
- Get help if necessary and use aids such as lifting sheets, mechanical lifts, trolleys, or carts
- Use transfer or gait belts, seat belts, transfer boards, and other safety devices
- Evaluate the environment for any potential tripping, slipping, or other hazards before moving or lifting
- Report any injury or problems and seek evaluation and treatment early

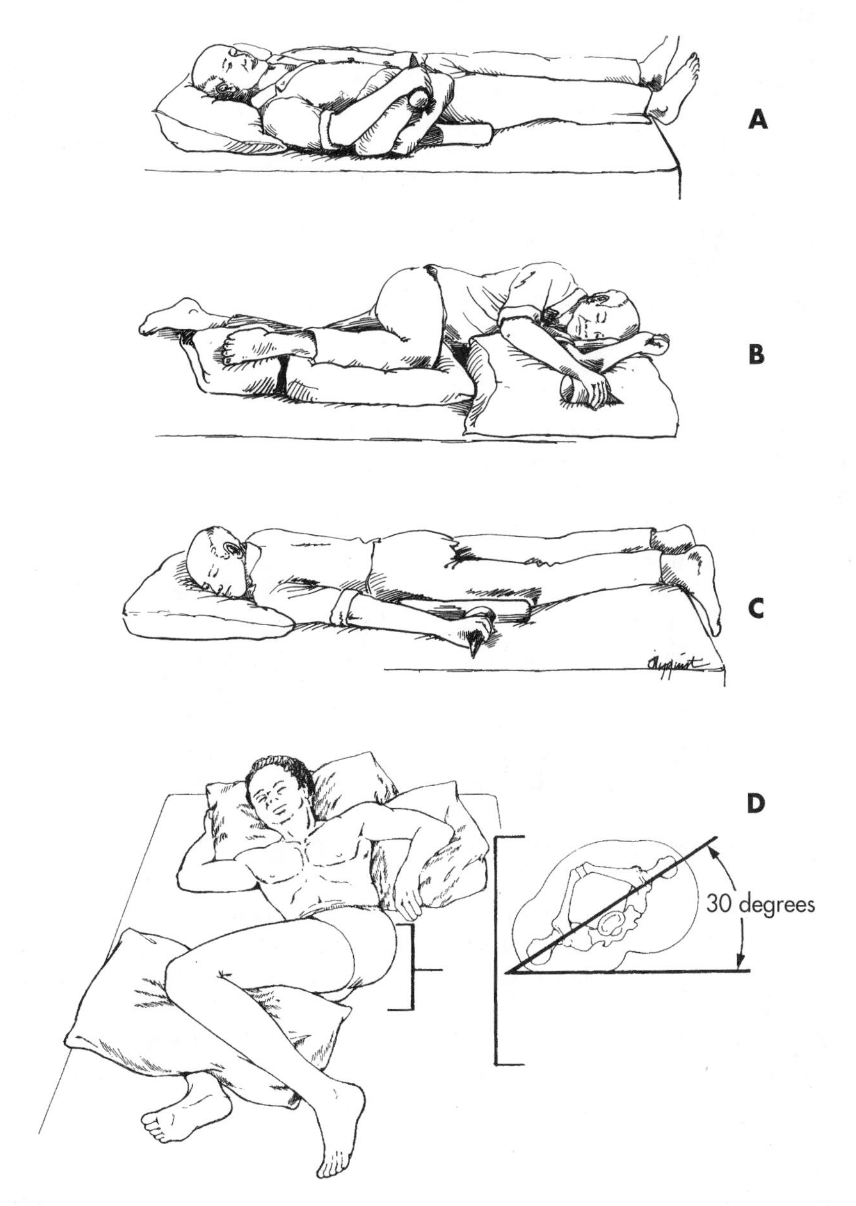

Figure 14-6 **A,** Supine position with trochanter roll to prevent external rotation of the hips. **B,** Lateral position with hand cone to prevent flexion contracture of the hand. **C,** Prone position with trochanter roll and hand cone. **D,** Thirty-degree lateral position at which pressure points are avoided. (**D** from Bryant, R.A. [2000]. Acute and chronic wounds: Nursing management [2nd ed.]. St. Louis: Mosby.)

the bedside reinforces teaching for client and family, provides initiative for position changes, encourages responsibility by client and family, and stimulates feedback from all parties. In a facility or home, use every opportunity to teach the individual and family, have them demonstrate procedures, and mutually prepare for the next phase of care.

Basic Positions

Classic basic positions are supine (back-lying), lateral (side-lying), prone (abdomen-lying), semiprone, and thirty-degree lateral (Figure 14-6). Specific positions after total hip arthroplasty and below-knee amputation are shown in Chapter 21. Because seemingly small details may affect a client's mobility outcome, positions are described and illustrated.

Supine Position. Assist the client to lie on the back (Figure 14-6, *A*), providing a small, flat pillow to support the head, neck, and upper shoulders. The arms lie along the sides of the body in a neutral position, with elbows extended and palms downward. Vary the position of the upper extremity by abducting the shoulder slightly using a small pillow or pad and then elevating the forearm and hand. Other upper extremity positions include full abduction of the shoulder with extension of the elbow and wrist or full abduction of the shoulder with a 90-degree elbow flexion and with the arm and hand positioned upward or downward.

Extend the hips and use a trochanter roll to support them in place. Avoid placing pressure on the back of the legs, which may damage blood vessels, resulting in phlebitis. The knees are extended or slightly flexed, but too great a degree of flexion at the knee may lead to flexion contracture with impairment of posture and gait. Position the feet to form a right angle with the leg. Footboards have not proven effective in preventing contractures or footdrop; however, some type of support usually maintains the desired angle of flexion, such as adjustable footboards, firmly folded blankets or pillows, resting leg splints with footplates, or high-top sneakers. Precautions in using these devices are in the Positioning Aids section.

Lateral Position. Assist the client to lie on one side (Figure 14-6, *B*) with a firm pillow to support the head and neck. Position the lower arm at the side with the uppermost arm supported by a pillow to prevent pressure on the chest. Flex the upper leg at the hip and knee and position on a pillow in front of the lower leg to minimize pressure on the lower leg. Place another pillow behind the back to maintain this side-lying position. After a stroke, the side-lying positioning incorporates the Bobath NDT approach and promotes a client's lying on the affected side as tolerated. From this position the client begins to establish weight bearing and lengthens the trunk, which later helps to counteract altered posture while sitting and standing. Positioning the person on the affected side may stimulate improved muscle tone through weight bearing in preparation for the bilateral weight bearing necessary to move up in bed, move on and off the bedpan, and stand.

Generally, in this position the bottom shoulder lies slightly ahead of the rest of the body, with the hip, knee, and shoulder in some degree of flexion. When positioning the individual who has had a stroke in the side-lying position on the affected side, the nurse should place the head in a neutral position, with the lower shoulder brought forward with the arm extended and the palm facing up and the hips and knees flexed. In this position on the unaffected side, the shoulder is placed away from the spastic pattern associated with hemiplegic posture. A towel or small pillow placed under the trunk at waist level helps elongate the affected side (Olson, 1967).

Prone Position. Before placing a client in a prone position, review the medical record and assess the person for any possible contraindications, such as increasing intracranial pressure or cardiopulmonary distress. Assist the person to lie on the abdomen (Figure 14-6, *C*). Turn the head to one side to facilitate breathing and drainage of oral secretions. Place a small pillow under the head for comfort and another between the chest and the umbilicus to relieve pressure on the chest or breasts. Extend the hips and knees and support them on pillows. The feet and toes are supported by another pillow or are positioned between the edge of the mattress and the bed frame to prevent pressure areas. In the prone position a client may feel most comfortable with arms flexed over the head or extended along the body in a neutral position. The client is in the semiprone position when resting on the side with the uppermost arm and leg placed farther forward.

Thirty-Degree Lateral Position. Place the client supine with the pelvis tilted at a 30-degree angle to the bed (Figure 14-6, *D*). All extremities are flexed at either the elbow or knee and supported on pillows. This position alleviates pressure on points, but a repositioning schedule is important because one hip supports weight. Attention to the client's lower back and overall proper alignment and support are essential; carefully assess the effects on those with shoulder problems.

Sitting Position. With so much attention placed on mobility, the act of sitting and features of seating are often undervalued. Not only does the ability to sit with balance and trunk control become preliminary to transfers, it enables the person to have an upright view of the world. All clients sit with their feet placed flat on the floor and the hips well back in the seat, with weight distributed evenly over the hips. Weight shifts are useful techniques for clients who have sufficient upper body strength and function and who are able to perform them safely from a chair or wheelchair or who have assistance available for wheelchair back tilting. They offer some exercise and help prevent pressure areas from developing.

Positioning Aids

Details of the chair and any inserts affect outcomes. Measure the depth, width, and height of the chair for sitting position and to help the client avoid leaning to one side or the other. Pillows can be used with caution if the chair seat is too wide or too deep to allow the hip and knees to be placed at right angles; however, pillows may cause the thighs to roll inward or form lumps, among other problems. Proper seat cushions and back supports make a great difference in comfort and alignment. A seat is firm and wide and does not slump or sag into a slinglike shape, unless prescribed for a specific purpose. Never use doughnut-shaped cushions; although these commonly are found as foam or rubber devices, they may impair circulation and increase potential for impaired skin integrity.

Place a small stool for the feet if the height of the chair seat does not allow the person to place both feet flat on the floor or, if in a wheelchair, use the footrests. Clients should wear shoes when seated; they offer a great deal of protection. When clients sit up in bed or in a chair, instruct them to avoid positions that encourage spastic patterns to develop, avoid bending the residual limb at the knee after amputation, and maintain proper hip angles after hip surgery. Place the affected shoulder forward using a pillow for support, if needed, and avoid a slouching posture. The affected arm rests on a table at a comfortable height or in the wheelchair on an armrest of proper height and support.

Specialty beds and devices for the skin are discussed in Chapter 16. Aids used in positioning are listed in Table 14-11 and illustrated in Figures 14-7 and 14-8.

Clients with Lower Limb Amputations

Clients who have lower limb amputations may turn prone for care or lie prone during the day for short times. Positioning cautions are listed in Box 14-5. The client uses strengthening activities for the upper body, such as lifting and turn-

TABLE 14-11 Positioning Aids

Positioning Aid	Description of Use	Comments on Use
Pillows	Use pillows to position, stabilize, support or bridge beneath a pressure area Substitute rolled or folded towels, bath blankets, or foam squares covered with washable material Maintain proper alignment of body	Check contents for any materials that may cause allergic responses Do not allow to bunch or pack into hard lumps Pillows must fully support the extremity or body part Do not use foam or rubber seat doughnuts
Trochanter rolls	Prevents outward rotation of the hip when in a supine position Place the roll beneath the hips from the top of the iliac crest to approximately 6 inches above the knee Form a roll along the outer aspect of the thigh (see Figure 14-6, *A* and *C,* for proper placement)	Commercial trochanter rolls may be replaced with a flannel sheet or bath blanket folded into thirds lengthwise and rolled under toward the client
Foot supports	These have not been found to be effective and are no longer used; they may initiate spasticity in some Clients wear shoes for protection	A footboard may keep the bedcovers off the feet if that is needed Special boots and sheepskin covers are discussed in Chapter 16
Hand rolls	Used to maintain position and prevent contractures from developing	Hard cones, not soft rolled materials, are used
Splints or orthoses Upper limb and lower limb differ; the most common lower limb orthoses are ankle-foot (short-leg braces) Knee-ankle-foot orthoses (long-leg braces) have joints at the knee Pediatric orthoses range from a standing frame to the parapodium and swivel walker to spinal orthoses for scoliosis, such as the Milwaukee brace Figure 14-8 illustrates a molded ankle-foot orthosis Special shoes often are necessary when clients have orthoses	Two types are static and dynamic (includes functional): static is rigid, providing support without movement; dynamic allows some movement and may be used to stretch a contracture If an orthosis is deemed functional, its purpose is to improve function, as with a person slowly recovering from a chronic condition Orthoses may be highly specific as for rheumatoid arthritis, spinal cord injury, burns, scoliosis, carpal tunnel syndrome, and other nerve and joint inflammations Use of slings for shoulder subluxation after stroke is no longer encouraged; slings are not used when the person is sitting or lying down	Orthoses should be as basic as possible, comfortable, and easy to maintain; ideally they will not have an undesirable appearance Client may wear an orthosis intermittently until it is tolerated but will be more likely to use it if it adds function Some splints, such as a static volar orthosis, may cover large and sensate areas of the body such as the forearm and hand and thus decrease sensory input; others may work on larger joints using the effects of gravity and weight At times, orthoses are used in conjunction with casting Volar resting splint maintains the wrist, thumb, and fingers in extension (Figure 14-7)
Casts are composed of various materials, including plaster, plastic, and fiberglass May cover small or large portions of the body	Casts are used in rehabilitation in a variety of situations: after multiple trauma, especially with fractures; to prevent pain and cardiopulmonary complications that may accompany postural problems with scoliosis; and in burn care to prevent contractures with scarring Casts may have a role in preventing contractures such as those caused by rheumatoid arthritis or with flaccid muscles	Therapists may use serial casting; rehabilitation nurses are responsible for maintaining skin integrity, circulation, and other standards of care for persons using casts After x-ray, a client receives a cast, usually to provide additional extension, and then has a new cast applied each week, which is removed daily for personal hygiene and observation

Continued

TABLE 14-11 Positioning Aids—cont'd

Positioning Aid	Description of Use	Comments on Use
Abductor wedge or pillow (illustrated in Chapter 21)	Abductor wedge is designed specifically for use after surgical total hip replacement; it maintains the legs in abduction position necessary to keep the prosthesis positioned until the muscles, soft tissues, and incisions heal Knee immobilizer may be added to control flexion of the knee to the hip on the prosthesis side Client must not exceed an angle of 90 degrees of flexion between the knee and hip, a concern with seating or toileting as recovery continues	Clients may wear antiembolism stockings after the surgery; muscle tone and strength, skin integrity, and prevention of thromboses are priorities Positioning and turning schedules take into account the person's age, comorbid conditions, risk factors such as osteoporosis or obesity, or conditions such as diabetes or rheumatoid arthritis Schedules for positioning take into account the daily schedule, socialization opportunities, and client preferences to allow the person as much control as possible while otherwise being immobilized Early ambulation is monitored closely (Chapter 21)

Box 14-5 Positioning Cautions for Clients with a Lower Limb Amputation

Clients with a lower limb amputation should **NOT:**

- Place a pillow under the hip or knee when in bed
- Lie in bed with knees bent or cross the legs
- Place a pillow under the back when lying supine in bed
- Put a pillow between the thighs
- Elevate the lower end of the bed under the knees
- Allow the residual limb to roll in or turn in toward the other leg
- Let the legs fall outwards while lying supine
- Rest the residual limb over the edge of the bed or a chair
- Sit with the residual limb bent
- Stand with the residual limb resting on the bar of a walker or grip of a crutch

ing in bed using an overhead trapeze. In a wheelchair or chair, the residual limb is supported extended straight using the leg rest or residual limb board.

Activities for Mobility in Bed

Activities for a person who is in bed consist of turning from side to side; bridging and changing positions to relieve pressure points; moving up and down or to the side of the bed; and, if possible, sitting up in the bed. For clients with total dependence, others perform the work of moving. A client who can move with some assistance or use adaptive equipment can participate if able to follow instructions; those without functional limitations may be in bed for other reasons and move independently as prescribed. Useful devices are an overhead trapeze, bed side rails, ropes or cords tied to foot rails, or other firm and secure places to grasp and pull up on as appropriate.

Caregivers use principles of body mechanics whenever working with a person who is dependent. To move this client in, out, and around the bed, raise the bed to a comfortable working height at approximately hip level, which coincides with the provider's center of gravity. When a bed cannot be raised, consider placing the bed legs or frame securely on blocks to achieve the proper height. Lock the bed if it is on casters, or brace it against a wall, so movement off the blocks is not possible. The height allows the nurse to stand with knees slightly flexed and legs positioned apart in a wide base of support. The large muscles of the legs and buttocks, rather than the small muscles of the back, are used to move the client. As the nurse moves, weight is transferred from one leg to the other in the direction of movement.

Turning

When turning a client to the side, stand on the side of the bed toward which the individual is to be turned. Position the person's arms on the abdomen and cross the far leg over the near leg at the ankle (except if contraindicated, as with total hip replacement). The nurse stands with knees slightly bent and one leg forward, the other back. One hand is positioned beneath the client's far shoulder, and the other hand is placed beneath the hips on the far side. Using a smooth, complete motion, transfer weight from the forward leg to the back leg, thereby moving the client to a side-lying position.

A client who has hemiplegia or paresis may learn to bridge or elevate the hips off the bed, a movement used to

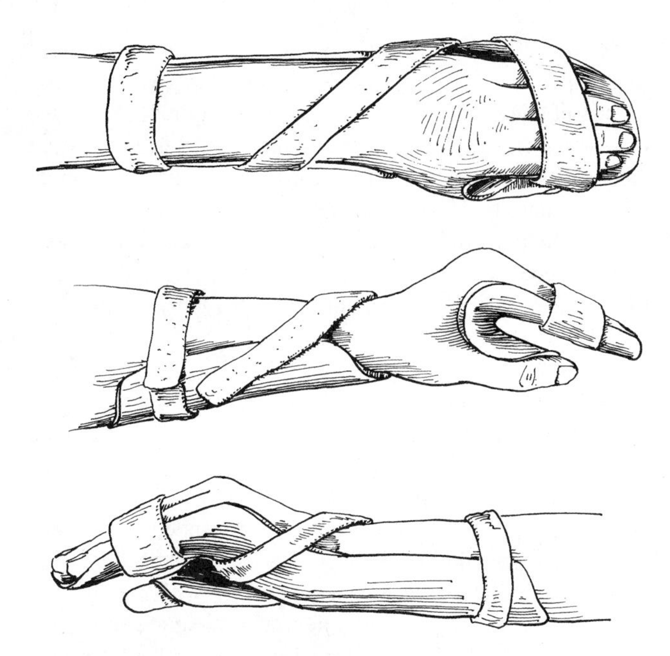

Figure 14-7 Volar resting splint provides support to the wrist, thumb, and fingers, maintaining them in position of extension.

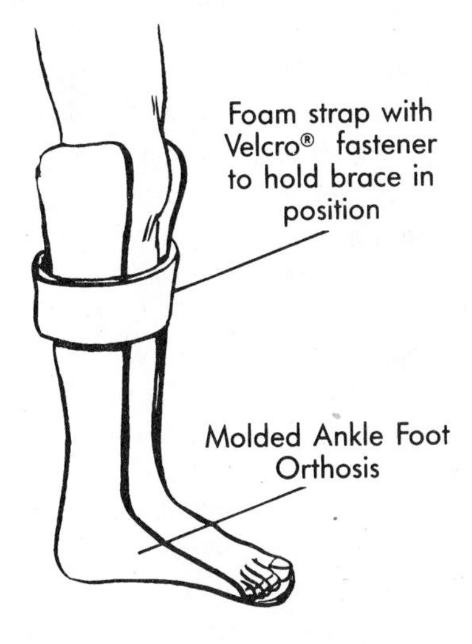

Figure 14-8 Plastic braces can be molded to the client's foot and leg and can be either long or short. (From Hoeman, S.P. [1990]. *Rehabilitation/restorative care in the community.* St. Louis: Mosby.)

get on a bedpan. The nurse bends the client's knees, instructing the client to place the unaffected foot over the affected one to stabilize it. The nurse then places a hand on top of the client's affected knee to move it down toward the feet and places the other hand under the affected hip to direct the lifting movement of the hips (Borgman & Passarella, 1991). Pressure exerted over the knee causes the hip to rise automatically. Bridging is also used with lower body dressing techniques discussed later in this chapter.

Moving in the Bed

In moving the client who is dependent toward the top or bottom of the bed, two caregivers are more energy efficient. The method of moving may depend on the client's weight and breadth. For a person within the average weight range, two persons can effect the move efficiently. Using the hands as levers, with elbows bent, one caregiver slides the arms under the client's upper back. One caregiver's arm is positioned under the shoulders, the other arm under the waist. The other caregiver supports the client's lower back, positioning one arm at the client's waist, the other below the client's hips. Both caregivers stand at the same side of the bed and mentally "divide" responsibility for moving a portion of the client's height and weight. Using their arms as levers, one caregiver supports the client under the shoulders and under the waist, while the other supports under the waist and at the hips. Each caregiver stands with knees slightly flexed and one foot forward. At a given count both caregivers transfer their weight to move the client in one smooth, continuous motion toward the top of the bed, taking care to avoid friction or shearing of the skin.

A single caregiver can move a client to the side of the bed by following the same principles of picturing the client in "thirds," a section at a time. Begin by moving the client's head and shoulders, then the waist and hips, and finally the legs and feet. Safety for client and caregiver and proper body mechanics are essential.

The client with some upper body strength and lower limb mobility can assist to move up toward the head of the bed. The client grasps the side rails, pulls up with the arms, and pushes the soles of both feet down into the mattress, which thrusts the body upward in bed. The head of the bed or a trapeze suspended on a Balkan frame or over-bed frame is useful for a client to pull up on for bedpan positioning or while the bed is being made. A physical therapist evaluates a client's ability to use a trapeze and teaches exercises that can be performed in the bed to strengthen the upper extremities. Continued dependence on side rails or a trapeze is not encouraged unless a client must have them available at home.

The client with hemiplegia or paresis after a stroke can be assisted to the side of the bed using the Bobath NDT approach. The client is instructed in sequential steps to:

1. Clasp the hands and stretch them forward
2. Bend the knees
3. Turn the head and took in the direction of the turn
4. Swing the extended arms to the side of the turn
5. Let the knees follow to complete the turn (Borgman & Passarella, 1991)

Encouraging Client Participation

When a client is able to assist in activities in bed, the nurse encourages participation and provides instruction. To turn to the side of the bed, the client is taught to pull up on the side rail with either upper extremity. When side rails are not available, a client is taught to place an immobilized arm on the abdomen so that it is not "left behind" during the turn or to position the arm carefully when turning onto the affected side. The affected leg is positioned over the other ankle to make the task of turning simpler and ensure the leg is in alignment.

If one or both legs are mobile, then a client can facilitate turning by pushing in the direction of the turn with the sole of the foot. The nurse emphasizes that the sole of the foot, rather than the heel, is used to prevent damage to the skin.

Activities Out of the Bed

Activity out of bed may be a nursing prescription for clients who are completely dependent, as well as for those who require some assistance. Generally a client is moved out of bed to a chair or wheelchair to provide a change in physical position and minimize the effects of immobility, as well as for a change in surroundings. Assess readiness to sit in a chair; monitor vital signs, balance, alertness, and level of comfort before the client moves from a high Fowler's position or dangling; supervise carefully. Assess circulation to the lower extremities with the legs dangling and apply compression or antiembolism stockings or elastic bandages before activity out of bed and to prevent venous stasis. Place the legs and feet fully supported on an elevated wheelchair footrest or on a stool to reduce edema and venous stasis.

Transfers

The client who is able to perform transfers is able to move form the bed to other locations and out of doors. Important transfers are to a chair or wheelchair, the commode or toilet, the bathtub or shower, and perhaps a vehicle and then back to the bed. The person's functional abilities and overall status determine the level of assistance necessary.

Transferring a Dependent Client

Transferring a person who is dependent from bed to a chair requires mechanical devices or trained personnel using lift transfers or pivot transfers, as described in the following section. Once a client is seated, monitor body alignment and sitting posture and time weight shifts.

Mechanical Devices. The most commonly used mechanical device is the pneumatic lift. A client is positioned on a one- or two-piece sling connected by chains to a crossbar on the lift. Pumping the hydraulic mechanism allows the lift to carry a person in a seated position off the bed. Because the lift is stable with a broad base of support and is adjustable, it may be possible to wheel the person while suspended in the lift sling from the bed to a chair or commode. As the pressure is released slowly from the hydraulic pump, the client descends into the seat. Depending on the person's size and impairment, one, two, or three caregivers may be required to transfer the client safely to a chair. The lift slings may be left in place beneath the person until he or she returns to bed or may be removed for use with others. Turn hooks on the slings away from the client to prevent injury and line the sling for hygiene.

Lift Transfer. Two caregivers can transfer clients who are of average weight from the bed to a chair. Elevate the bed surface until slightly higher than the chair. One nurse stands at the head of the bed and uses both arms to reach under the client's arms and across, using opposite hands to grasp the client's wrists. The other caregiver supports the client's legs and feet. Using proper body mechanics, the caregivers lift the client out of bed on a predetermined count and glide the client into the chair. When a client is heavier than average, four caregivers use a sturdy lift sheet, one at each of the person's shoulders and one at each of the knees. At the predetermined count, the caregivers use the lift sheet to slide the client above the surface of the bed and then into the seat.

Pivot Transfer (Assisted). When weight bearing is not contraindicated, a client who is dependent can be pivot transferred from bed to a chair. In a pivot transfer the person is brought to a sitting position on the side of the bed. The client's arms are positioned around the nurse's neck and shoulder with the nurse's arms passing under the client's arms to support the lower back. The nurse then flexes the knees and thighs and rocks back and forth with the client to gain momentum. When both client and nurse are ready, the nurse shifts weight from the forward leg to the back leg, lifting the client off the bed and turning the client toward the chair. The nurse shifts weight from the back leg to the forward leg, bending at the hip and knee as the client is lowered into the chair.

Positioning in the Chair. The nurse evaluates the seated posture of a client; ideally the client has a straight, slightly relaxed back; hips and knees flexed at 90 degrees; and feet flat on the floor. If the chair is too high, use a footstool but evaluate alignment and any pressure on the legs. Pillows placed at either side prevent a client from leaning toward one side when a chair is too wide. A pillow at the back prevents "slumping" or "slinging" should a chair be too deep. When a chair is too low, the hips and knees are flexed more acutely than is desirable, predisposing contractures. A foam pad or pillow placed under the client before transfer to the chair may alleviate the problem. Clients and family are taught to reposition each hour while sitting in a chair. When able, a client shifts weight every 15 minutes by leaning forward, to the right, or to the left.

Assisting a Client to Transfer

Clients who are independent for short periods or who require minimal assistance may find a pivot transfer useful. Figure 14-9 illustrates the steps in pivot transfer from a wheelchair to the toilet as performed by a person wearing a lower extremity prosthesis.

Clients who are partially dependent can increase their independence by using several techniques to transfer from one place to another. Techniques described in the following section are for a client with paraplegia or hemiplegia, and using a transfer board. The nurse encourages client participation, teaches sequential steps for each technique, is available for assistance, and ensures a safe environment and technique such as transfer belts or other safety devices.

Client with Paraplegia. A client who has paraplegia or limited mobility below the waist, such as with bilateral

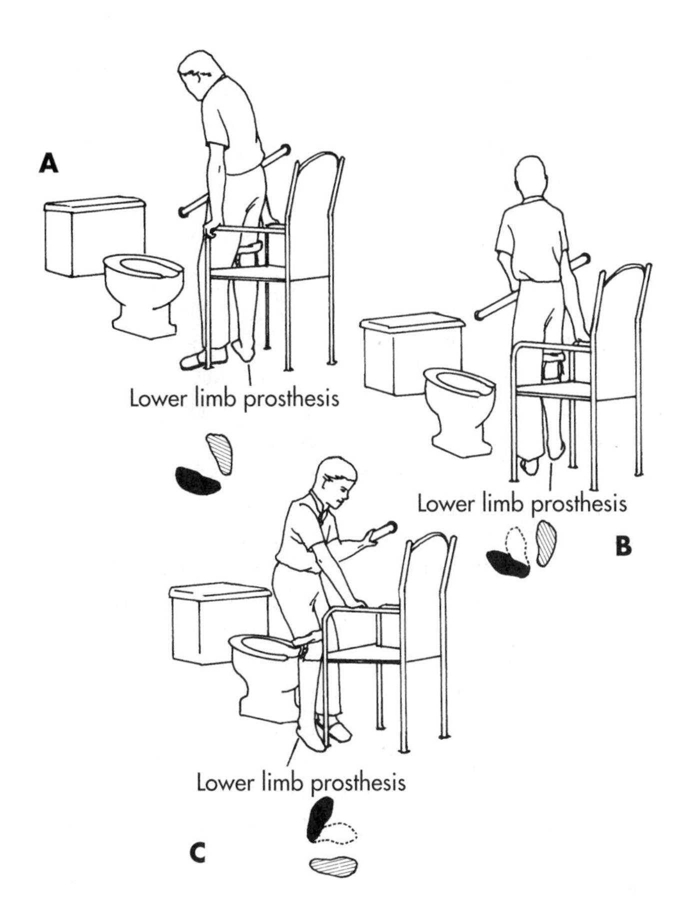

Figure 14-9 Pivot transfer for the client wearing a lower limb prosthesis. **A,** Client is shown wearing a lower limb prosthesis on the affected leg. First, lock any braces or casters; lock the knee of the prosthesis if applicable. **B,** Client will pivot with weight on the residual limb (the unaffected leg). **C,** Residual limb provides the main support and balance for the transfer. Be sure to assist the client as necessary for safety. (From Hoeman, S.P. [1990]. *Rehabilitation/resorative care in the community*. St. Louis: Mosby.)

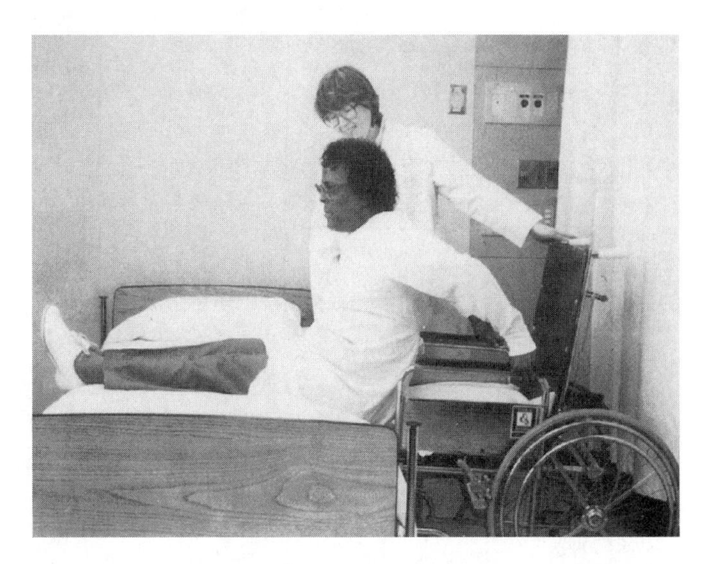

Figure 14-10 This technique enables a client with good balance and upper extremity muscle strength to transfer independently.

lower extremity amputation, can use the following transfer. The chair is placed perpendicular to the middle of the bed. Bed casters and commode or wheelchair wheels are locked, and footrests are removed. The client rises to sit and then uses upper extremity strength to turn the trunk and legs in line with the chair. With the client's back seated nearest the seat of the chair, the person reaches backward with both arms to grasp the armrests and moves the hips and legs from the bed backward into the seat of the chair. As the chair is moved away from the bed, the client lowers the legs carefully as in Figure 14-10. When proficient, a client may use a push-up and side-to-side transfer.

Client with Hemiplegia. The person with less muscle strength and/or sensation on one side of the body, such as the person with hemiplegia, can learn an independent standing transfer in many situations as described and illustrated in Figure 14-11.

When incorporating the Bobath NDT approach, the chair is placed at an angle to the bed on the client's affected side. Lock the chair and remove the armrest closest to the bed. Assist the person to the side of the bed, and position the feet flat on the floor with the heels under or slightly behind the knees. Assist the client to clasp the hands and extend the arms, leaning forward until the head and trunk are in position over the feet. The nurse then leans over the client's back and assists the client in moving the hips. The nurse rocks back, shifting the weight to the back foot, and pivots while turning the client's hips toward the chair, affected side first. The nurse shifts weight forward and the client is lowered gently to the chair or other seating (Borgman & Passarella, 1991).

Transfer Board. A transfer board assists mobility for the client who has limited function of the lower extremities. A transfer belt is used as needed for safety and for the caregiver to grasp when offering assistance. Several styles of transfer boards are available, some promoting a client's ability to "lift and bounce" across the board, but the principle is the same. Although often referred to as *sliding,* a client does not slide literally on the transfer board because this would lead to impaired skin integrity. Wheelchair or chair placement at a 45-degree angle beside the bed is essential for a smooth transfer. Lock brakes or casters and remove any armrests, as possible. Ideally the bed and chair are the same height. Place the transfer board bridging the chair and the bed; a client needs a clear path to avoid brushing against the wheel when moving to or from a wheelchair.

With assistance the client leans to position a portion of the transfer board under the buttocks and then sits and regains balance. Using the upper extremities, the client performs a series of "little push-ups" across the board. Those with a great deal of upper body strength may pull themselves toward the far armrest of the chair, but skin friction and shearing must be prevented. Either way, the hips and lower extremities are moved over the transfer board and into the chair. The client tilts the other way and removes the board.

A transfer board may be used to facilitate movement between a variety of seating areas: the chair and tub, the

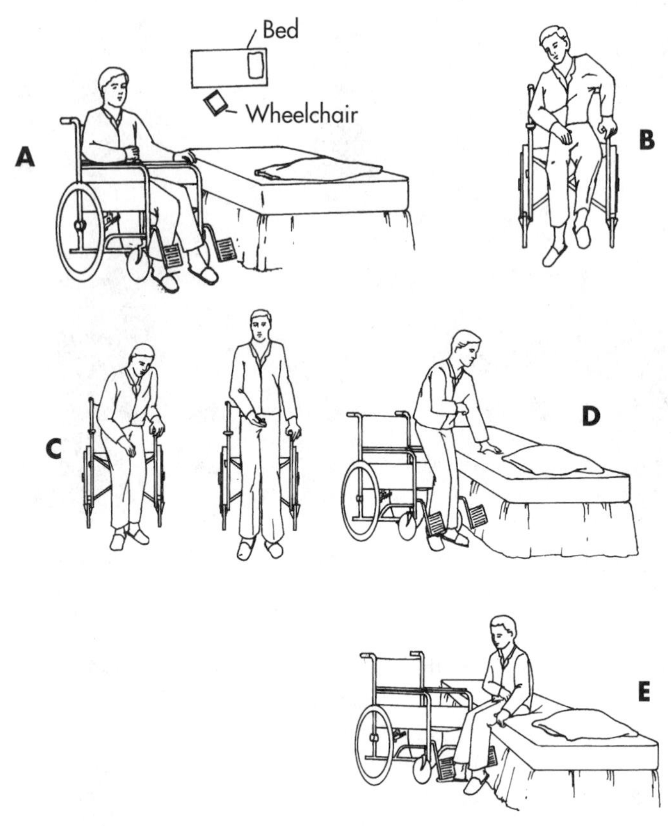

Figure 14-11 Independent standing transfer. **A,** Lock brakes and lift footrests. Angle the wheelchair close to the bed, facing the head of the bed, preferably on the client's unaffected side. Instruct the client to place both feet flat on the floor. **B,** Unaffected foot should be placed directly beneath the wheelchair seat. It will be slightly behind the affected foot. Client's unaffected hand should be on the armrest, and client should be sitting to the front of the wheelchair seat. **C,** As the client leans forward on the unaffected foot and pushes on the armrest, he or she will rise to a standing position. **D,** Client should continue to use the armrest and keep his or her feet slightly apart for safety and balance. If the client is tall, an adjustable-height armrest may be needed for the client to stand erect and safely maintain balance. **E,** Client uses his or her unaffected arm to balance and support himself or herself on the edge of the bed. The client should be instructed to take short side steps to turn toward the unaffected side. When the client's back is perpendicular to the side of the bed, he or she can sit. (From Hoeman, S.P. [1990]. *Rehabilitation/restorative care in the community.* St. Louis: Mosby.)

chair and toilet, the chair and car, and so forth. Generally the physical therapy department initiates upper extremity strengthening and the training with the client; the nurse reinforces instruction and provides encouragement for the client to integrate the transfer into daily activities.

Ambulation and Gait Training

Goal setting and attainment for functional independence in ambulation is a team effort in which the client is an active participant. A physical therapist works with the client to propose a safe ambulation plan that is reinforced in all team areas and in the community. A plan may include isometric and therapeutic exercises designed to prepare the muscles used in walking, provide practice in maintaining sitting and standing balance, gain ability for passive standing, and select adaptive equipment and assistive devices used with specific gait-training techniques.

Preambulation Activities

Preambulation activities, which involve exercises to prepare muscles for standing and walking, begin early and begin in the bed. Isometric exercises strengthen muscles of the lower extremities and trunk, including the gluteal, abdominal, and upper extremity muscles. Other therapeutic exercises preparatory to walking are modified sit-ups in the supine position and modified push-ups in the prone position. Gaining sitting balance is important. The client sits at the side of the bed with both feet resting firmly on the floor or supported by a footstool. Offering only needed assistance and monitoring for safety, the provider instructs the client to raise the arms left, right, forward, and upward. A client who is able to maintain balance can begin an ambulation program. When walking with crutches is the goal, sitting push-ups are initiated while sitting in a locked wheelchair or very sturdy armchair; both upper extremities support body weight.

Ideally a client will progress to work on standing balance. The client learns to come to a standing position and practices until performed safely. The client slides to the edge of the bed or chair, keeping the feet back and under the body. The person pushes down with the legs and arms while leaning the trunk forward to come to a standing position. Some need assistance but may be able to use assistive devices to compensate. Initially clients stand near a stable support until they can maintain an erect position and trunk balance while moving the extremities. Fall prevention is important, especially for elderly persons, who may experience imbalance due to arm movement, changes in gait patterns, or increased body sway. Activities that increase vestibular stimulation, such as passive rocking in a chair, may improve balance. Passive standing activities precede transfer and standing; they prepare the cardiovascular system to adjust to the change in circulatory demands from recumbent to erect positions.

Assistive Devices for Standing

Many assistive devices are used to support passive standing, such as a tilt table or standing frame. A client is transferred to a tilt table in physical therapy. In moving from a supine position, safety straps secure the person to the table as both feet rest on a foot support. After baseline blood pressure and pulse are recorded, the tilt table is elevated slowly to a 15-to 20-degree angle. The degree of tilt increases in 5- to 10-degree increments until the client can tolerate a standing position for 10 to 30 minutes. Blood pressure; pulse; dependent edema of the lower extremities; skin mottling; and sensations of faintness, dizziness, or headache are monitored. After prolonged bed rest or with poor cardiovascular response, a client may wear elastic wraps or stockings or an abdominal binder. Benefits of tilt table activities include relief of pressure on gluteal areas, maintenance of postural reflexes, enhanced bladder and bowel function, unimpeded chest expansion, and psychological motivation to participate in an ambulation program.

A standing frame or table is used for passive standing activities that help a client adjust to transfer from sitting to immediate upright standing without the incremental increases to erect position of the tilt table. Standing frames have stabilizers, either padded supports at the knees and abdomen or actual tabletop surfaces. Posterior stabilizers include heel cups, knee stabilizers, and pelvic or gluteal supports. With a standing frame the client can enjoy the physiological and psychological rewards of an erect position, while improving standing balance and leaving upper extremities free for activity. Children may use standing tables in school to practice being upright, to provide visualization and stimulation in learning or performing activities, and to promote inclusion with peers. Specially sized pediatric standing frames are available. When a client develops functional ability to ambulate, the physical therapist prescribes assistive devices or equipment for the specific disability and initiates client and family education. In the community, rehabilitation nurses monitor and continue work with clients through community agencies.

Assistive Devices for Ambulating

We all use assistive devices everyday: remote controls, electric can openers, automatic garage door openers, sensor lights, telephone headsets, computers, and so forth. In rehabilitation assistive devices or adapted equipment are used to improve function and access by eliminating barriers in the environment or by creating new environments. Changes in structure, ergonomic and task modification, safety measures, combined therapy approaches, and adjustments in ambiance are examples. Assistive devices can reduce or ameliorate the impact of functional impairments, add support and stability to correct balance, provide strength, improve flexibility and motor control, and increase sensory abilities. Devices can aid in healing, help in performing mobility activities, protect from damage or further injury, or enable return to activity.

Selecting Assistive Devices or Adapted Equipment

Devices and equipment require careful selection for a variety of reasons. Rehabilitation nurses in case manager roles work with the client and the team in determining the appropriate prescriptions within the economic, social, cultural, environmental, and physical parameters. Considerations include not only the initial cost but also maintenance, service, and repair costs; availability of replacement parts; reliability; and durability. Clients may demonstrate a need for a device, it must fit in the home or workplace, and they must be able to learn to operate it and be safe and comfortable while using it. Equipment must be acceptable and fit the person's lifestyle. If others are to assist with the device, they must be able to maneuver and manage it; portable equipment must fit into vehicles and not be too heavy or unwieldy. The environment is important when equipment requires access to electrical outlets; special supplies and battery chargers tips should not be worn, and all parts must be connected securely.

The particular assistive device or piece of equipment selected for a client depends on the physical limitations, disease or medical status, self-esteem and body image, lifestyle, and financial situation. Those with full use of and strength in their upper extremities but limited lower extremity function due to amputation, fracture, paraparesis, or paraplegia may use crutches. Broad-based canes or three- or four-footed canes are used for weakness or paralysis of one side of the body. A walker is prescribed when generalized weakness occurs in upper and lower extremities, such as in older persons with arthritis, hip fracture, or neuromuscular diseases. The physical therapist measures a client's height, weight, and specific needs for each device and piece of equipment; crutches, canes, and walkers are not shared.

Whether in the facility or community, rehabilitation nurses monitor the client's posture, body alignment, endurance, awareness, safety, and technique. Schedule time to evaluate walking in areas typical of daily living; many facilities have realistic virtual lifestyle units. Client education includes:

- Caring for equipment or devices
- Coming to a standing position
- Walking properly (gait training)
- Maneuvering stairs or curbs
- Returning to a sitting position
- Managing after a fall, such as by coming to a sitting or erect position

Crutches. Crutch walking begins when a physical therapist measures a client for crutches, which may be done in community settings. Measure crutch length by marking the floor 2 inches out from and 6 inches ahead of the tip of the shoe; the client holds the crutch handgrip and flexes the elbow at 30 degrees. Measure the distance from 2 inches below the client's axilla to the mark on the floor. The handgrip, never the axilla, supports body weight.

Gait Patterns with Crutches. Gait patterns depend on individual abilities. Standard patterns are a four-point alternate, a two-point, or a swing gait with the crutch. Regularly examine crutches, canes, and walkers to ensure the tips are not worn and all parts are connected securely.

The four-point alternative gait complements limited muscle strength or questionable balance; a client with a very stable and safe gait pattern may use the four-point gait to ambulate slowly. Begin from a standard crutch stance, elbows slightly flexed and crutch tips placed on the floor 6 inches out from the side of the shoe and 6 inches away from the shoe toes. The crutch axillary bar rests 2 inches below the axilla and is pressed against the chest for lateral stability. The four-point gait pattern is left crutch, right leg, and right crutch, left leg. Repeat until the destination is reached.

The two-point gait resembles a walking gait pattern. Although more rapid than a four-point gait, the two-point gait requires better balance because only two points of contact occur with the floor at any given time. Begin from a standard crutch stance to shift weight to advance the right leg and left crutch simultaneously. Follow through with the left leg and right crutch, and continue the pattern to destination.

Swing gaits are used for persons who are unable to bear weight on a lower extremity, such as after hip or leg fracture or amputation. Swing gaits vary from a slow but stable swing-to or step-to gait to a rapid but more complex swing-through gait. In the step-to swing gait, begin from a standard crutch stance, placing no weight on the affected extremity. Lift both crutches to move them forward 4 to 6 inches as one unit; whenever the client bears weight on the unaffected extremity, weight is shifted onto the crutches. The client steps up to the crutches and repeats the step-to gait process. In the step-through or swing-through gait, begin from a standard crutch stance. Again move both crutches 4 to 6 inches ahead as a single unit as the client supports weight on the unaffected extremity. This time, when the client shifts weight onto the crutches, the unaffected leg is swung through to set down in advance of the other leg, landing ahead of the crutches. Repeat the process to destination.

Canes. Canes are available in many styles with features for specific needs and lifestyles; for example, a straight cane makes a single point of contact with the floor, whereas four- or three-footed canes provide broader bases of support but are bulkier to handle. Examples of various canes are shown in Figure 14-12. Canes can be unsafe when selected incorrectly, fitted improperly, or maintained poorly. Environmental hazards (especially wet, slippery, or uneven pavement) may lead to falls.

A person's cane length is equal to the distance between the greater trochanter and the floor. To be measured properly, a client stands with elbows slightly flexed when the cane tip is set on the floor about 6 inches to the side of the foot.

To walk, the client stands with weight on both feet and on the hand holding the cane. The cane is held on the unaffected side; clients tend to place the cane on the affected side. Advance the cane 4 to 6 inches, move the affected leg up to the cane, and support weight on the affected leg and the cane. Continue by moving the unaffected leg past the cane; repeat the process to destination.

Walkers. Walkers vary in structure and purpose; they are measured as described above for canes. Persons able to maintain balance and lift the walker can use one of the lightweight, adjustable, pickup walkers. Reciprocal walkers are suitable when a client might lose balance and fall backward when lifting a regular walker. Rolling walkers, with or without a seat, may prove too unstable for some but have appeal because they help conserve a client's energy. As with other ambulation devices, check the environment for potential hazards.

With the pickup walker, the client advances the walker, steps forward in equal-sized steps using each leg in turn, ensures balance, and repeats by advancing the walker. Alternatively, advance the pickup walker and set it down; step with the right foot, advance the walker, and set it down; and step with the left foot and continue the gait pattern. Remind clients to set the walker down in turn and not to step while the walker is off the floor. When using a walker, the client attends closely to coordinating movements with placing weight on the walker or the feet, as shown in Figure 21-12.

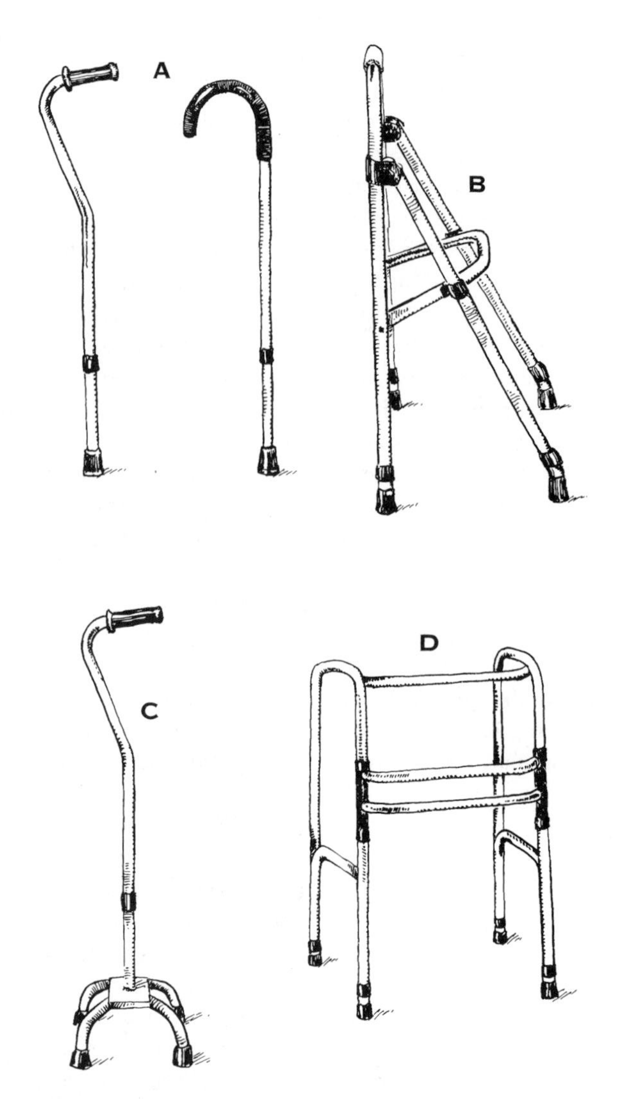

Figure 14-12 Assistive devices for ambulation. **A,** Straight canes. **B,** Pickup walker. **C,** Quad cane. **D,** Standard walker.

Orthotics and Bracing. These assistive devices are discussed in Table 14-11 and have direct involvement with ambulation. A person may use a short leg orthosis for walking and support of the affected lower extremity with hemiplegia. Because this lower limb orthosis (brace) is attached to the shoe and extends to just below the knee, it can prevent the ankle from pronating by raising the toes during walking and striking the heel back to the floor. Corrective shoes, inserts, and other devices are used routinely with orthotics.

Long leg braces, or knee-ankle-foot orthoses (KAFOs), are hinged at the knee to allow bending. KAFOs provide stability at the knee, ankle, and foot and may combine with crutches or a walker and other devices for functional ambulation, such as with paraplegia; however, the energy expenditure is enormous.

Although some controversy persists, electrical stimulation and other innovations promote functional ambulation. Research using new technologies as ambulatory aids has dealt with limited groups, such as persons with SCI. New directions in research and technological advances are changing the way the rehabilitation team and the public view potential for clients with impaired movement and function.

Prosthetic Devices. Amputation and prostheses are discussed in detail in Chapter 21. For mobility purposes, use of a prosthetic device after lower limb amputation is more stable and acceptable than a walker or crutches. Techniques for fitting and use of prostheses change with new information and products, but some basic principles apply. Early fitting after surgery may enable ambulation soon thereafter; however, permanent prosthetic devices are not fit until shrinkage subsides in the residual limb. A prosthetist-orthotist constructs highly individualized prostheses based on prescriptions from the physiatrist. Basically the lower limb prosthesis for a person with an above-the-knee amputation consists of a socket, joints at the hip and knee, a suspension system, and a foot and ankle. Specialized cushioned feet and unique knee joints, such as for athletic activities, and computer-assisted design and computer-assisted manufacture (CAD-CAM) represent only a few of the innovations in prosthetics. Because of the diversity of the components available, the prescription and construction are complicated.

The prosthesis should be functional and easy to care for while appearing as natural as possible. Prosthetic design takes the following into account:

- Length and condition of the residual limb
- Size of the client's foot
- Client's general status
- Client's age, weight, agility, and endurance
- Client's lifestyle, social goals, and vocation
- Cosmesis, including shape and skin tone
- Financial status and payment coverage
- Individual motivation and family support

Once fitted with a prosthesis a client continues gait training using a four-point or swing gait; many maneuver independently while wearing the prosthesis. A client is taught to avoid the habit of a pelvic tilt while standing and during ambulation.

Client education includes daily inspection of the surgical site and residual limb for redness, abrasions, or irritation. Instruction stresses hygiene, gentle care, edema prevention, positioning to prevent contractures, and care of prosthetic stockings and limb. Clients are cautioned to consult a prosthetist to assess or make any mechanical alterations or adjustments, as well as for regular maintenance.

Wheelchairs and Mobility

Scope of Wheelchair Use

When used 9 hours a day, the average life span of a wheelchair in the United States is about 2 years; children outgrow their wheelchairs more rapidly. Architectural barriers, village or countryside terrain, social construction of disability, and cost are a few of the factors that restrict wheelchairs for persons in many countries; they are a scarce commodity with little regard to fit or condition. As a result persons have restricted access, impaired socialization, and reduced independence and opportunity for self-support. In a few countries persons with disabling conditions have established cottage industries for constructing wheelchairs. Although significantly less sophisticated than the multiple varieties and prescriptions available from manufacturers in the United States and other industrialized countries, these locally constructed wheelchairs provide transportation and are available. In the United States and developed countries, wheelchairs have become highly developed in style, technology, function, and features.

Wheelchair Modifications

Although some clients may reject a wheelchair, the benefits of access, energy conservation, upright seated posture, and diverse activity usually outweigh issues of self-esteem or a psychological need to ambulate. Competitive sports have entered the mainstream, and wheelchair sports, dancing, and travel promote physical, emotional, and social rehabilitation. Zola (1991) makes a clear point about the differences between a person "using" and being "confined to" the wheelchair.

Wheelchairs are as diverse as the persons who use them. The prescription for a wheelchair often lists specific recommendations for modifications for a client's needs. Wheelchair height and width are based on the client's physical dimensions and requirements for seated posture. The back and seat of a wheelchair can be modified to accommodate anti-pressure devices and additional positioning supports. High backs, reclining backs, and other types provide head and neck support or options to an erect seated position. In early transfers from the bed to a wheelchair, a client may perform a simple sliding transfer into a wheelchair fitted with a back that flattens out completely. Elevating the wheelchair back helps the client into a seated position.

Folding wheelchairs, many with detachable armrests and foot or leg rests to facilitate transfers, are transported easily. Clients with upper body strength learn to load their own wheelchairs into a car. Cars may be fitted with hand controls, and persons who pass a driver's examination can operate their own vehicles. Vans equipped with hydraulic lifts and fold-down ramps allow clients to elevate into the vehicle while sitting in the wheelchair. The weight of the chair and the size and type of tires are considerations when a client is traveling within or outside the home. Generally, heavier chairs with durable tires are better suited to the outdoors; those with lightweight frames, high-quality bearings, and tubular tires may be designed specifically for sports and racing.

As a rule, modifications in wheelchair design increase costs and maintenance complexity. Manual hand controls, as well as electronic touch and breath control, can propel a wheelchair. Companies are active in developing energy-efficient components to improve manual propulsion, ergonomic designs, and technological boosters for a variety of client needs. Electric wheelchairs with microprocessors and computer technology are on the horizon; robotics will be a part of the new technology (Cooper, 1999).

Wheelchair Prescription Criteria

Traditionally, rehabilitation nurses evaluated clients and prepared wheelchair prescriptions. Today wheelchair design is a team activity, often involving the client and family, physical therapist, case manager or rehabilitation nurse, vendors, and others.

Criteria for prescription of wheelchairs as the primary mode of mobility include the following:

- Energy expenditure and conservation
- Function, access benefits, and safety
- Cost, maintenance fees, and durability
- Physiologic and specific disease factors
- Cosmetic and psychosocial factors
- Growth and development
- Client lifestyle and occupational and educational goals

Client Education

Client education includes learning to:

- Transfer to and from the wheelchair
- Change position and shift weight while seated in the wheelchair and check for signs of pressure
- Perform basic wheelchair maintenance
- Propel or operate the wheelchair safely and reliably

Wheelchair Accessibility

In the community accessibility is an issue. It is essential to know the environment where the wheelchair will be used. Doorways and room dimensions are measured, as are exits, entrances, and areas for ramp placement; building access, levels of living area, and transportation to and from living areas are considered. Also consider the feasibility of transfer from the wheelchair into a traditional motor vehicle, requirements of specialized or modified vans, amount and kind of assistance available, and emergency services on call.

Environmental Assistive Devices

Assistive devices and adapted equipment improve access and mobility. Although the Americans with Disabilities Act legislation has opened public places in many ways, a person who can ambulate on a level surface for a short distance still may be denied access to the upstairs of their home or yard. Children may attend school but have difficulty participating in field trips or social activities outside their own controlled environment. Environmental assistive devices can make an amazing difference in many situations; however, each device must be evaluated critically with consideration of the client's lifestyle and environment before cost and maintenance are incurred or storage space is used.

Examples of improvements include ramps; elevators; permanent and portable lifts; altered or expanded doorways; robotic and electronic controls; wheelchair-tread devices; and all sorts of modified home spaces, such as modified cooking areas, worktable heights, bathroom accessories, and grooming or household aids. Increasingly equipment and spaces are being modified to allow persons to participate in recreational and leisure pursuits.

Technology Aids

Advances in technology may be the hallmark of the century. Ergonomic designs are used in the home, school, and workplace, especially for work on computers. Computers are outfitted with ergonomic devices including mouse pads, keyboards with large keys, padded or shaped frames, Braille keys, special on/off switches, and height adjustment devices. Specially designed chairs and lumbar wedges are also available.

Computer software for augmentative communication, screen readers, remote controls, and voice recognition and instant message systems on the World Wide Web are only a beginning. Computer software with digital, rather than analog, control circuitry and a modem interface can be used to make changes or modifications in assistive devices and other products on-line, regardless of location or distance.

Improvements in interactive voice response systems allow clients to receive recorded messages and enable them to contact health providers and others for help or information (Piette, 2000). Rehabilitation nurses can receive clients' reports of their condition, clinical data, and other information, as well as communicate from the rehabilitation center with colleagues while they are working in the client's home. A telephone touch-tone keypad or voice recognition technology may change the quality of care and mode of delivery for clients, especially those who live at home in remote or difficult areas. The World Wide Web has many sites for information about assistive devices and technology (e.g., http://www.wapd.org/assistive and http://www.abledata.com).

INTERVENTIONS FOR SELF-CARE IN ADLs

Clients improve their self-esteem when they achieve maximum independence in personal care. A person may need to break tasks into sequential units and complete as many as possible and may require assistance with others. Repetition, practice, and demonstrations help with learning. Limiting distractions in the environment, choosing a client's best time for work on activities, and encouragement help with concentration. Findings from the assessment relate directly to the level, style, and type of self-care activity. Clients can be challenged to meet their potential, but the nurse relies on assessment to recognize when impairments interfere and plans modifications or assistance. Safety and energy conservation are ongoing concerns.

The components of self-care include performing personal care, dressing, bathing, toileting, and eating. Self-care activities may be subject to cultural and ethnic beliefs and practices about washing or bathing and personal care that may vary among individuals or families. Ask client or families about special rules, customs, or rituals they may use in self-care activities. As a rule, never remove amulets, pins, necklaces, bracelets, or hair ornaments without permission. Do not cut hair or nails without permission; do not dispose of hair, nail trimmings, or other body remnants except as directed by a client or family member.

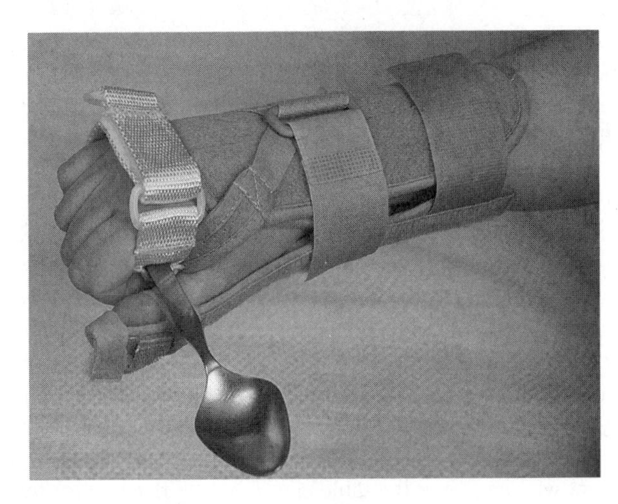

Figure 14-13 Universal cuff contains a pocket that can grip many self-care items. This one is attached to a splint to support the wrist. (From Sorrentino, S.A. (2000). *Mosby's textbook for nursing assistants* (5th ed.). St. Louis: Mosby.)

Personal Care

Personal care activities consist of personal hygiene, grooming, oral hygiene, and menstrual management. The interdisciplinary team evaluates a client's needs, but in the home setting the client, family, and rehabilitation nurse may devise and improvise ways for clients to accomplish self-care. Many assistive devices to help with personal care are available commercially or can be constructed in the home. For example, when holding an object, such as a nail clipper, cosmetic jar, or drinking cup, is a problem, suction cups keep it in place while being used. Built-up handles on toothbrushes or razors offer a better grip for those with arthritis or a weak grasp, and hair gel and toothpaste are among the products available in pump tubes. Mirrors, toilet paper holders, shoehorns, and various styles of reachers are available with long and curved handles. One of the more versatile devices is the universal cuff that can be used to grip and maneuver many items (Figure 14-13).

Hair Care

Certain activities with hair care are difficult for many persons who are older regardless of whether they have impairments. Keeping the hair washed may be difficult for those who cannot lean over, raise hands above the head, maneuver the hands, or balance the torso to wash the hair. Some may be able to sit on a shower seat and wash their hair as part of a shower. Others will need assistance, such as lying supine for a shampoo with a shower tray or clean pan placed behind the head to collect rinse water.

Left-sided hemiparesis or hemiplegia may cause neglect when combing hair at the back of the head, and clients need cues and reminders. Alternatively a client with right hemiplegia and agnosia might misconstrue a comb to be a toothbrush and put it in the mouth. Demonstrating use of the comb enables this person to use it properly. Built-up handles or a universal cuff helps those with difficulty in gripping or moving smoothly. Loops strapped to items such as brushes enable a client, including a person with C5 or C6 SCI, to slide a hand through the space and use the brush.

Nail Care

Nail care may be difficult for a person who cannot manage implements or reach the feet, who experiences pain, or who has problems bending or balancing. With aging, nails tend to become thickened or brittle, and calluses and ingrown toenails may develop, placing persons with diabetes or peripheral vascular problems at risk for complications. Hand care and nail care are challenging when a client has a fixed grasp or closed position, reduced ROM, or pain in the hand. With loss of sensation, the person may not be aware of early signs of infection; ingrown nails; or dry, cracked tissues around or in the nail beds. A magnifying glass that can be stabilized or worn about the neck may help those with impaired vision to inspect the nails.

Oral Hygiene

One of the most neglected areas of personal care for clients who cannot brush their teeth adequately is oral hygiene. Older persons have bone loss and thinner oral mucosa that is less resistant to disease. Absent teeth or ill-fitted dentures contribute to difficulty with eating and poor nutrition that is amplified with deficits, such as dysphagia or pocketing of food. Chronic illness, lowered resistance, and medication regimens may lead to poor dental health. Finding resources may be difficult for clients with badly damaged teeth or gum disease compounded by impaired mobility or involuntary movements. As advocates, rehabilitation nurses can assist dentists to understand a client's specific needs, with ways to make clients comfortable and with modifications for care.

Grooming

Grooming activities enhance self-esteem and improve hygiene. Shaving may be unwise for men and women taking anticoagulant medications or who have restricted movement or paresis. Depilatory creams or electrolysis may be solutions when an electric razor is not an option. Deodorant often is applied easier in the supine position when one extremity is flaccid or spastic. Raise the affected extremity over the head using the unaffected extremity and apply deodorant. A client who can sit at the table can move the flaccid arm forward and, reaching underneath in the space created, apply deodorant.

Cosmetics contribute to body image for women who wear them regularly. Jars can be opened with one hand when the base of the container is stabilized to a table with a suction cup. The client grasps the tube near the screw top with the unaffected hand. The thumb and index finger twist the cap or flip the top of snap caps. Alternatively the tube is held between the knees, and the sides of both hands are used to twist the top. A similar technique works with toothpaste and other tubes. Clients with neglect may ignore one side of the face and need feedback for correct application of cosmetics.

Menstrual Management

Menstrual management is one of the most difficult tasks for women with lack of sensation, impaired strength or dexterity, or mobility problems, such as spasticity. A woman must be able to remove outer clothing and underwear, position herself, remove and dispose of the soiled tampon or pad, wipe and cleanse the perineum area, get up or transfer from the toilet, and rearrange clothing (Duckworth, 1986).

Recommended adaptations for managing menstruation include adapted positions and use of mirrors, self-sticking sanitary pads, prepared or packaged wipes, and loose underwear. Adapted clothing is available; simply replacing the crotch flap in underwear may work well. One version is a flap extending over the crotch from the front to the back waistband and secured with Velcro or a Velcro-attached flap. Loops sewn several places on the sides of the underwear can help with pulling up and down.

Assess the ability of a woman to lean forward and maintain postural control to manage the task. With sufficient balance, hand dexterity, and maneuverability to slide her pants forward, she may sit on a raised toilet seat or front edge of the wheelchair seat and insert a tampon. To use sanitary pads instead, she must bridge the hips upward while leaning against the back of the wheelchair; this will enable her to slide a pad backward.

A woman able to transfer from a wheelchair to the toilet may use a long-handled mirror, a grasper similar to an assistive toilet paper holder, and a knee spreader if abduction is difficult. If strength is sufficient but balance is poor, she can lean to one side holding onto a bar or locked wheelchair. The mirror is important when sensation is impaired. Others may find managing clothing too cumbersome and choose to change lying down and bridging while in the bed.

A woman having problems with coordination, such as with cerebral palsy, may use a grab bar or find kneeling helps to support a stable position and manage clothing. Most of these adaptations are difficult to accomplish in public, where privacy, cleanliness in public rest rooms, grab bars, and paper supplies may be lacking.

Dressing

Modifications or designs in clothing, assistive or adapted devices, and dressing techniques enable clients with restricted ROM to achieve optimal independence in dressing. Wearing personal clothing signifies wellness and improves body image. Those who use a wheelchair can evaluate clothing for style while sitting and practical use during transfers. Fabrics that are durable and easy care, fit over appliances, drape free of wheels, and are in nonrestricting styles are available readily.

The Internet features sites to obtain clothing designed for persons with impairments. A good amount of personal clothing worn before the illness or injury can be modified. Features include large buttons or hooks, elastic waists, front closures, zipper pulls, stretch fabrics, loops or extension tabs, and Velcro closures. Support and prosthetic stockings are hand washed every other day and hung to dry to prolong life of the stockings; furthermore, perspiration may cause skin breakdown and odors. Stockings with elastic, knee-high stockings, and tight tube socks all impede circulation.

Persons in spica casts or traction, with urinary collection devices, or with reduced muscle strength can wear extra-large shirts that pull overhead, skirts or pants with wide tops (10 to 12 inches bigger than hip size), longer length skirts, and skirts or pants with drawstring or elastic waists. With single leg casts or antiembolism stockings, a boot is worn on the other leg (Mather, 1987).

Clothing must fit with the weather, the person's condition, any sensory impairment, and the environment. It also must not lead to complications. For example, jeans can lead to skin breakdown if the heavy center back seam cuts into the skin or can shear the skin during positioning or transfer. Also important but often overlooked are protective clothing, such as headgear and footwear. Clients wear shoes with solid toes whenever out of bed; many will have prescriptive footwear. Persons with sensory deficits will not feel heat, bumping against a chair leg, or pressure on unprotected feet. Shoes with Velcro closures or elastic inserts have replaced most laced shoes, but a one-handed shoe tie is possible. Assistive devices include a long-handled shoehorn and a sock pull.

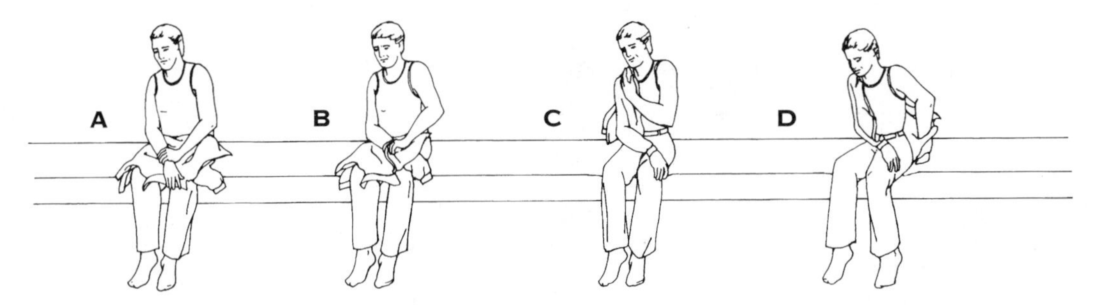

Figure 14-14 Dressing in a shirt (or button-style dress). Check your client's ability to balance before beginning. The client who has one side of the body affected should sit to put on a shirt or shirt button-styled clothing. **A,** Client lays the shirt inside-up with the collar at his knees. **B** and **C,** Client uses his unaffected hand to lift the affected hand into the armhole and pull the sleeve over his affected shoulder. **D,** Client uses a tossing movement to place the shirt and other sleeve behind him. He can reach behind him with his unaffected hand and insert it into the shirt sleeve to finish dressing. (From Hoeman, S.P. [1990]. *Rehabilitation/restorative care in the community.* St. Louis: Mosby.)

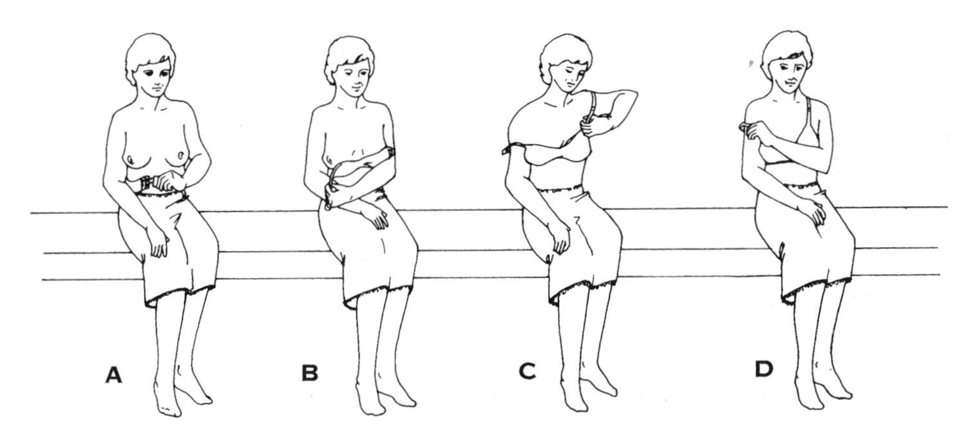

Figure 14-15 Dressing in a back-closure bra. Client must be able to sit and balance safely. **A,** Client puts the bra on backwards around her waist. Be sure cups are positioned correctly. If the client cannot fasten hooks, Velcro may work instead. Use a safety strap if needed. **B,** Client turns the bra to the front. She uses her unaffected hand to insert the affected arm into the strap. **C,** She inserts her unaffected arm into the other strap and positions the bra. **D,** Client uses her unaffected hand to position the strap on the affected side and to adjust the bra. (From Hoeman, S.P. [1990]. *Rehabilitation/restorative care in the community.* St. Louis: Mosby.)

Balance, dexterity, and ROM are key factors in a client's ability to pull on socks or to put on a front-button shirt (Figure 14-14).

Women experience difficulty with bras when using one hand or with restricted ROM. A regular back-fastened bra may be a better choice than front-fastened or over-the-head sports bras. Figure 14-15 illustrates the steps in bra dressing. If hooks are a problem, cover them with Velcro; however, Velcro may be difficult to manage with one hand, and hooks can irritate the skin. A snap clothespin holding the bra to the top of pants or underwear can mimic a stable handhold while the unaffected hand closes the hooks or the Velcro. If the client can maneuver overhead, a sports bra or Lycra stretch bra stitched closed can be pulled down into position. Persons with multiple sclerosis, amputations, hemiplegia, or spinal cord injuries may be able to manage, whereas someone with arthritis may choose to step into a bra and pull it up if stretch is sufficient. Information contained in Box 14-6 suggests dressing aids and techniques for persons who have specific conditions. Use educational principles adjusted to specific deficits and impairments when a client is learning dressing techniques. Assess a client's cognitive, emotional, and physical status with attention to mobility before beginning. If necessary, establish a means of communication, such as with eye blinks, head nods, finger movements, or communication devices. After 30 to 40 minutes of attempts, offer assistance to maintain an atmosphere of encouragement without frustration. Plan to provide cues, repetition, and reinforcement for activities and keep environmental distraction minimal. Figures 14-16 and 14-17 illustrate several movements for dressing in pants depending on the person's abilities.

Box 14-6 **Dressing Aids and Techniques for Specific Conditions**

A. Persons who have limited ROM such as with arthritic conditions
  1. Use large buttons or zippers with a loop on the pull tab
  2. Replace buttons, snaps, and hooks with Velcro or zippers
  3. Use garments made from stretchable fabrics
  4. Eliminate bending to tie shoelaces; use elastic shoelaces or other adapted shoe fasteners
  5. Use stocking aids
  6. Pick up items from the floor before donning them and after removal, and remove clothes from hangers using reaches
  7. Push stockings off heel of foot using dressing sticks

B. Persons who have neurologic disorders (when dressing while seated in a wheelchair, put on clothing in the following order: stockings, undergarments, braces [if worn], pants, shoes, and shirt or dress)
  1. To put on stockings while in bed, pull one leg into flexion, or to a cross-legged position in a chair, slip sock over foot and pull on; avoid elastic tops or garters (Pedretti & Zoltan, 1990)
  2. To put on pants and underwear in bed, pull or roll to a sitting position
     a. If balance, health status, and mobility permit, lean forward to work pant legs over feet; then pull pants up to hips
     b. While retaining the grip at the pant waist, lie back onto bed and roll from hip to hip while pulling the garment up over the buttocks (Figure 14-17)
  3. To put on pants and underwear in a wheelchair, slide to the front of the seat and then lean against the seat back
     a. Pull one leg into a flexed position and put foot into pant leg; put foot through pant leg and pull rest of pants up past knee on that side; repeat with other leg
     b. Work pants up as high as possible in this forward-seated position and gather excess pant material in front
     c. Perform a "push-up" and raise the buttocks, thighs, and pant tops from the seat while repositioning self to back portion of wheelchair seat
     d. Hold pant waist and slide or "butt-walk" down into pant tops; repeat lift/slide until pants are positioned properly
     e. To remove pants, unfasten while sitting in the forward part of the wheelchair seat, hook the waistband with the thumbs, and perform another "push-up" while backing out of the pant top; repeat as necessary
  4. Shirts, sweaters, and dresses that open down the front should be donned while in the wheelchair; some clients may need to modify traditional methods because of balance deficits
     a. Open garment on lap with collar facing toward chest and opening up
     b. Put arms into sleeves and pull over elbows
     c. Put garment on over head, pull the back down, adjust and button
  5. If putting on shoes while in bed, bend at the waist from a sitting position and put shoes on immediately after donning pants; if dressing in a wheelchair
     a. Cross legs above knee, lean over at the waist and rest torso on lap, then pull shoe on with both hands; return to upright sitting, repeat with other leg

        or

     b. Slide to front of wheelchair seat and lean back onto seat back; pull one leg into a flexed position with one hand, put shoe on foot with free hand (Pedretti & Zoltan, 1990)

C. Persons who have hemiplegia or hemiparesis (when client has balance problems, encourage dressing while seated in a sturdy armchair or a locked wheelchair, organize clothing, and arrange within easy reach or use reaching devices)
  1. Put on shirts using either techniques mentioned for persons with neurologic impairment or by inserting the affected arm first (Figure 14-14)
  2. Put on pants by crossing the affected leg over the other leg; work affected foot through pant leg, but do not pull pants past knee or it may become difficult to insert the other leg; to pull pants up several methods are possible
     a. If able to do so safely, stand to pull pants over the hips; to prevent pants from sliding down before they are fastened, place affected hand into a pocket or hook a finger/thumb into belt loop
     b. Position pants as high as possible while in seated position, elevate the hips by pushing down on floor with other leg and lean back against chair; pull pants up, then lower the hips back into chair to fasten pants
  3. Remove pants using method mentioned for persons with neurologic conditions; instruct client to sit to the front of the seat, unfasten pants, hook thumbs in waistband, and then back out of pants
  4. Another way to put on shoes is to cross the legs while in a seated posture

Box 14-6 Dressing Aids and Techniques for Specific Conditions—cont'd

As a general rule when working with individuals who have hemiplegia, insert the affected extremity into clothing first. Modified dressing techniques also may include dressing while in bed or using a wall or doorjamb for support when balance or stamina are altered.

D. Persons who have perceptual problems
   1. When teaching a client with visual agnosia, encourage client to feel parts of clothing that will assist in recognizing the object—for example, client may trace the line of buttons on the front of the shirt or practice drills to name different pieces of clothing (Zoltan et al., 1986)
   2. Clients with dressing apraxia may benefit from using the following techniques
      a. Instruct client who has difficulty positioning a garment to place it on the bed or lap with buttons or zipper facing down
      b. Use labels to distinguish front from back and right from wrong side
      c. When buttoning a shirt, begin at the bottom matching the lowest buttonhole
      d. Use touch to determine whether the button is pushed through the buttonhole (Zoltan et al., 1986)
   3. When teaching clients who have disturbances of body scheme, always touch the body part when instructing client to place clothing on that part; it may be necessary to continue this touching through the dressing activity
   4. Clients who have unilateral neglect need to have the neglected side stimulated
      a. Place clothes on client's neglected side, then teach scanning techniques to enable client to "find" clothes
      b. While dressing, client is instructed to pay attention to the neglected side
      c. Initially, frequent cueing to continue dressing that side will be necessary
      d. Use the same sequence of dressing because this will become a "built-in" cueing system, triggering client to the neglected side at a certain point in the dressing routine
      e. Finally, always speak and teach client while at the affected side
   5. Clients with figure-ground visual difficulty benefit from organizing drawers and separating types of clothing
      a. Client must be taught to slow down and carefully look for items of clothing that may be "lost"
      b. Lay clothes on a background that is unlike the color or pattern of the clothing
      c. Keep clutter from the self-care area (Zoltan et al., 1986).
   6. Clients with cognitive deficits such as memory problems, inattention, poor judgment, lack of insight, limited problem-solving ability, difficulty with abstraction, and poor mental flexibility can benefit from using an approach to dressing skills focusing on
      a. Being consistent
      b. Using verbal cueing
      c. Using self-cueing: vocalizing step-by-step sequence for dressing
      d. Scanning the environment
      e. Controlling the amount and duration of stimuli
      f. Using memory aids such as cue cards with the steps of dressing listed (Stewart, 1993); tape cue cards to a bathroom mirror or top of a wheelchair lapboard
      g. Acknowledging family and client preferences and lifestyle

E. Persons who have amputations of limbs (person with upper extremity amputations may use some of the same one-handed methods employed by clients with neurologic conditions; persons with lower extremity amputations, however, may have dynamic standing balance impairments that interfere with pulling up pants [Pedretti & Zoltan, 1990]; most other dressing procedures can be performed while seated)
   1. Pants may need to be pulled up in bed using the "hip roll" form side to side
   2. If client has sufficient body strength, "bridging" techniques may allow enough room to pull up the pants while in bed or in a chair (Figure 14-17)
   3. Remove pants by unfastening while seated and merely using supported standing to let them fall
   4. Older persons or those with diabetes who have incurred amputations may have problems donning or doffing shoes and socks and managing shoelaces; clients may need to use techniques or assistive devices such as shoehorn or sock aid (Pedretti & Zoltan, 1990)
   5. An extended shoehorn may also be used to push shoe and sock from the foot

F. Persons who have cognitive problems

   Chapter 26 details interventions for persons who have cognitive problems listed according to nursing diagnosis

---

ROM, Range of motion.

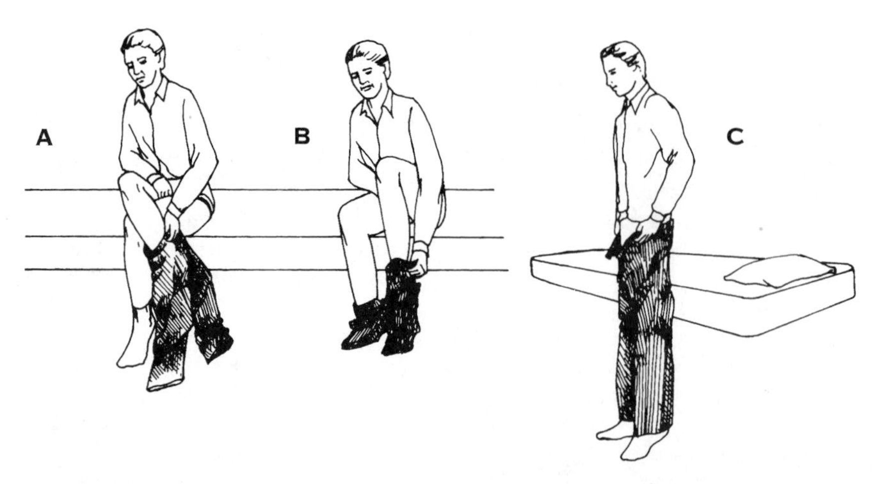

Figure 14-16 Dressing in pants while standing to balance. Check client's ability to sit or stand and balance safely. **A,** While sitting, the client uses his unaffected hand to lift his affected leg across his unaffected knee. He pulls his pants leg completely over his affected foot and ankle. If he cannot lift or cross his leg, assist him or elevate his affected leg on a box or stool so that he does not lean over. **B,** Client inserts his unaffected leg fully through the other pants leg. He uses his unaffected hand to pull the pants up on both legs as high as he is able. **C,** If the client can safely stand, he holds onto the pants and the waist with his unaffected hand. He pulls the pants on and adjusts the waist and zipper. The client never bends over to pull his pants. (From Hoeman, S.P. [1990]. *Rehabilitation/restorative care in the community.* St. Louis: Mosby.)

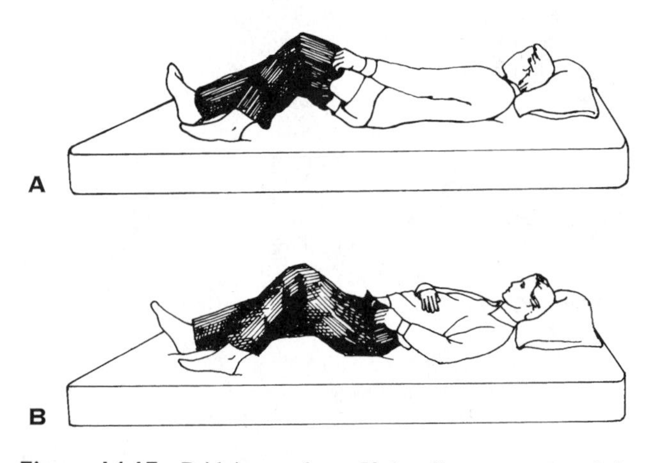

Figure 14-17 Bridging to dress. If the client cannot stand, he lies down on the bed. **A,** Client flexes his unaffected knee, keeping his foot flat on the bed. **B,** As the client pushes down on the bed, his hips elevate. Client uses his unaffected hand and arm to pull up his pants and fasten them. (From Hoeman, S.P. [1990]. *Rehabilitation/restorative care in the community.* St. Louis: Mosby.)

Bathing and Toileting

Independence in toileting is a major goal for clients, so despite potential difficulties, any who are able to use the bathroom receive encouragement and assistance to do so safely. Modesty, privacy, and dignity are important for clients in any toileting or bathing situation. Because persons who are wet, soapy, and loosely dressed are moving on or off the hard surface of the toilet or in and out of the shower or tub, it is no surprise that the bathroom is a prime location of accidents. Many safety measures are structural adaptations, such as:

- Countertops with space for grooming items
- No electrical razors or hairdryers near water
- Electrical outlets for the mirror positioned away from the sink
- Insulated or covered hot water pipes under the sink
- Nonslip surfaces and controlled hot water temperature
- Properly installed safety bars
- Elimination of clutter and loose towels, clothing, or rugs

Safety or grab bars are essential equipment in the bathroom and must be installed as shown in Figure 14-18. A client may rely on bars to lower into sitting or pull up on bars to rise from a tub or toilet seat. Nonslip materials are applied on the floor and in the tub or shower.

Access is a concern in home bathrooms, where space to turn around or complete a transfer is cramped or inaccessible by wheelchair. Narrow bathroom doors can be removed, enlarged, or converted into sliders for access. Sink tops, countertops, mirrors and electrical outlets, bathtub rims, and tub enclosures are not of a size, style, or height for transfers from a wheelchair. Lowering the sink, countertop, and mirror and opening space under the counter allows a client to sit in a wheelchair while grooming. A walk-in or roll-in shower stall, with or without a shower seat or a shower table, is an option when a tub is unmanageable and the bathroom can be reconfigured. Wheelchairs have a variety of toileting options, such as a commode seat with under-the-seat bucket.

Benches and tub seats are available in a variety of sizes, heights, styles, colors, and adjustable features. A larger seat is preferable when assisting a client to move and bathe. Bath

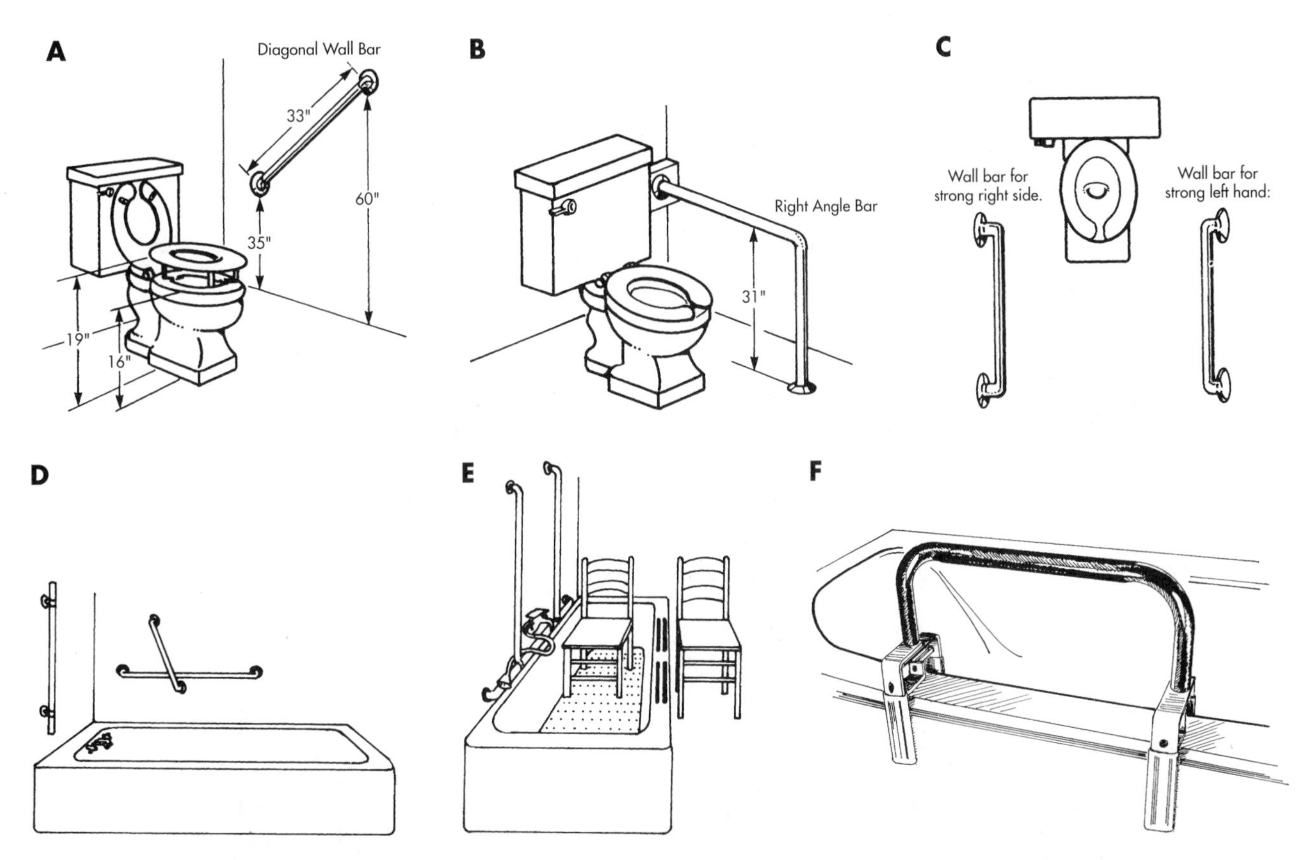

Figure 14-18 Safety grab bars. **A,** Diagonal wall bar next to commode. If commode seat is too low, making it difficult for client to get up, it may have to be raised by using a raised toilet seat. Be sure the raised seat is secure. **B,** Right-angle wall bar. **C,** Wall bars should be securely fastened to avoid a fall and should be at a 45-degree angle. Bar should be 2 to 4 inches away from the wall on the client's strong side. **D,** Grab bars are placed within reach for a seated or standing transfer into a tub. Grab bars must be firmly attached to wall studs. **E,** Homemade shower seat, nonslip bath mat, and grab bars promote shower safety. Tub chair legs are cut to reduce the height of the chair so the seat is level with the chair placed outside the tub. **F,** Bathtub bars. (From Hoeman, S.P. [1990]. *Rehabilitation/restorative care in the community.* St. Louis: Mosby.)

mats, hand-held shower hoses, bath mitts and soap bags with nonallergenic products, suction cups or wall-mounted dispensers, universal cuffs with extended holders on Velcro for holding toilet paper or razors, long-handled mirrors and back brushes, and premoistened wipes are only a few of the assistive devices available.

Clients who are able to transfer can use the pivot method (see Figure 14-9) or an independent standing transfer (see Figure 14-11) when moving from the wheelchair to the toilet. Some persons may use a transfer board to move from one seat to another, to transfer to toilet seats that are the height of the wheelchair, and to transfer to the tub (Figures 14-19 and Figure 14-20). Use a transfer belt for safety; lock wheels on the wheelchair; and assess the client's alertness, balance, and motivation.

SUMMARY

Movement science is a complex field of study of interest to all members of the interdisciplinary team. Rehabilitation nurses working with clients and their families in facilities and in community settings need to understand the theoretic basis of movement, as well as the structure and function of muscles, joints, bones, and nerves. A complete and integrated assessment of the musculoskeletal and nervous systems enables the nurse to formulate diagnoses and set realistic goals with clients that complement the interventions of other members of the rehabilitation team. Educating a client and family about reasons for and methods of optimizing mobility increases the probability of follow-through, maintenance of optimal independence, effective coping and adjustment, and prevention of further disability or complications.

CRITICAL THINKING

The Agency for Healthcare Research and Quality (AHRQ) recently awarded $45 million over the next 5 years for research to identify ways to eliminate racial and ethnic health disparities. Granted awards will fund Excellence Centers

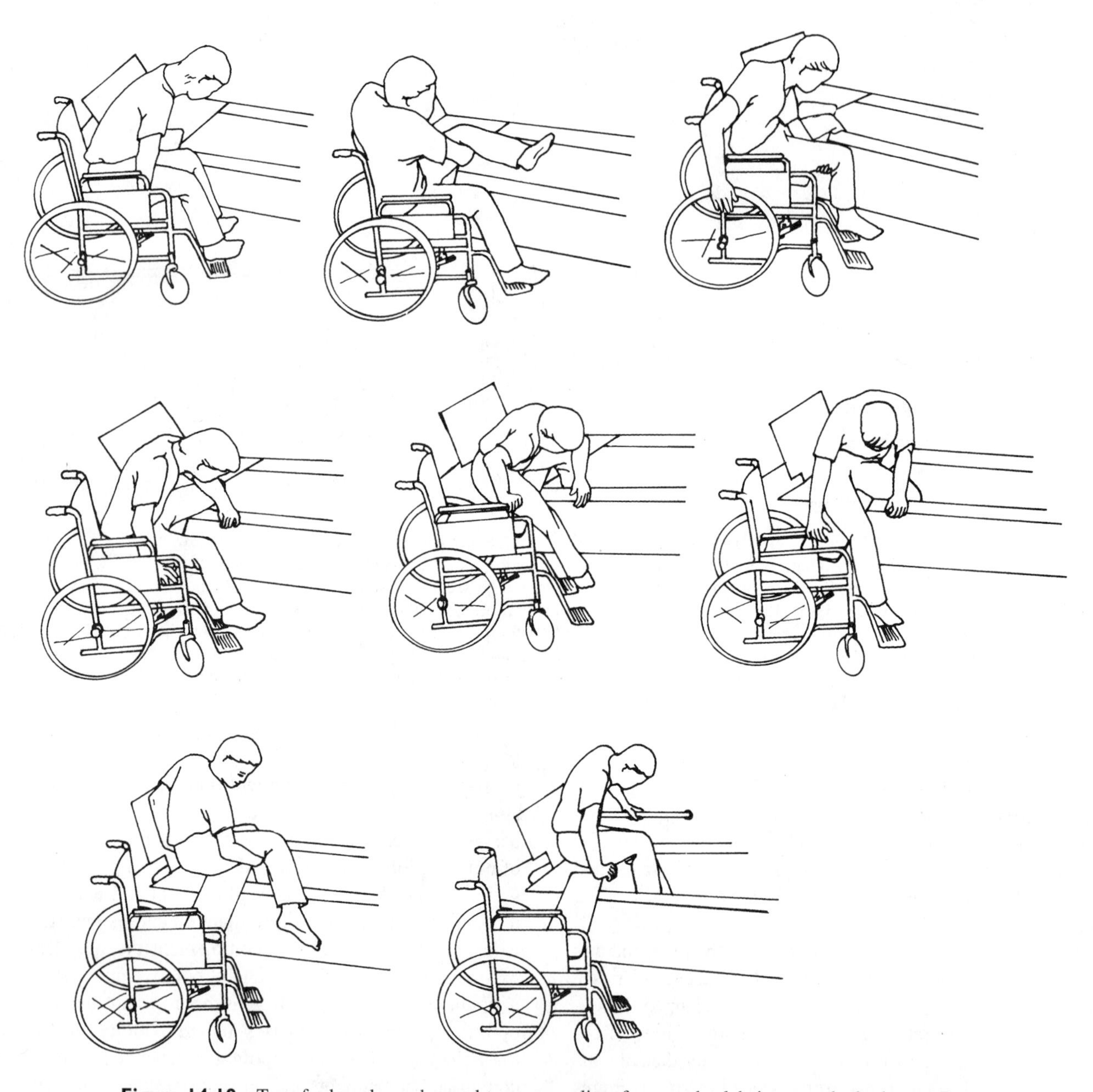

Figure 14-19 Transfer board may be used to move a client from a wheelchair onto a bathtub seat. Because the client's safety is a priority, assistance with a transfer belt may be needed. (From Hoeman, S.P. [1990]. *Rehabilitation/restorative care in the community.* St. Louis: Mosby.)

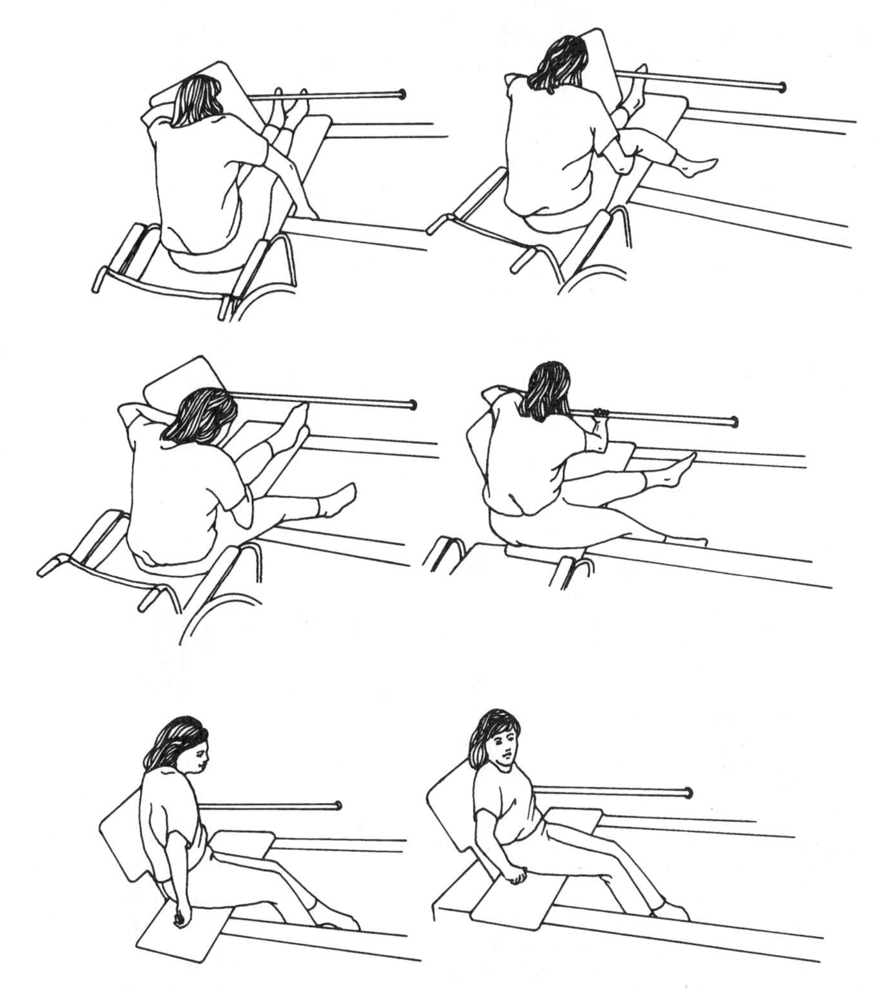

Figure 14-20 Some clients place both feet into the tub before performing a transfer from a wheelchair to a tub. (From Hoeman, S.P. [1990]. *Rehabilitation/restorative care in the community.* St. Louis: Mosby.)

to Eliminate Ethnic/Racial Disparities (EXCEED)(AHRQ, 2000). Develop a proposal for a multidimensional research project that would improve outcomes in this topic for persons with functional limitations affecting their self-care. Break the project down into four to seven studies, as the agency requests, and identify a program for research eligible for funding.

REFERENCES

Agency for Healthcare Research and Quality. (2000). *EXCEED research projects.* Available: http://www.ahrq.gov/. Washington, DC: Author.

Agre, J.C., Rodriguez, A.A., Franke, T.M., Surggum, E.R., Harmon, R., & Curt, J.T. (1996). Low-intensity, alternate day exercise improves muscle performance without apparent adverse effects in postpolio patients. *American Journal of Medicine and Rehabilitation, 75*(1), 50-58.

Bly, L. (1991). A historical and current view of the basis of NDT. *Pediatric Physical Therapy, 3,* 131-135.

Bobath, B. (1978). *Adult hemiplegia: Evaluation and treatment.* London: Heinemann.

Borgman, M.F., & Passarella, P.M. (1991). Nursing care of the stroke patient using Bobath principles: An approach to altered movement. *Nursing Clinic of North America, 20,* 1019-1035.

Carr, J.H., & Shepherd, R.B. (1987). Movement science: Foundations for physical therapy in rehabilitation. London: Heinemann.

Centers for Disease Control and Prevention, National Center for Health Statistics. (1994). *National health interview survey, second supplement on aging.* Atlanta: Author.

Centers for Disease Control and Prevention, National Center for Health Statistics. (1997). *National health interview survey.* Atlanta: Author.

Centers for Disease Control and Prevention. (1999/2001). *Trends in disability prevalence and their causes: Proceedings of the Fourth National Disability Statistics and Policy Forum.* Washington, DC, & San Francisco, CA, May 16, 1997. National Institutes on Disability and Rehabilitation Research. Disability Statistics Rehabilitation Research and Training Center, 1998.

Centers for Disease Control and Prevention. (2000). *Disability and health.* Atlanta: Division of Birth Defects, Child Development, and Disability and Health. Available: http://www.cdc.gov/nceh/cddh.

Chan, A., & Heck, C.S. (2000). Mobility in multiple sclerosis: More than just a physical problem. *International Journal of MS Care [serial online], 3,* 35-40. Available: http://mscare.com.

Cooper, R. (1999). Technology for disabilities. *British Medical Journal, 7220,* 1290-1292.

Duckworth, B. (1986). Overview of menstrual management for disabled women. *Canadian Journal of Occupational Therapy, 53,* 25-29.

Dunlevy, C.L., Douce, F.H., Hill, E., Baez, S., & Clutter, J. (1994). Physiological and psychological effects of low-impact aerobic exercise on young adults with cystic fibrosis. *Journal of Cardiopulmonary Rehabilitation, 14,* 47-51.

Fried, L.P., Bandeen-Roche, K., Kasper, J.D., & Guralnik, J.M. (1999). Association of comorbidity with disability in older women: The women's health and aging study. *Journal of Clinical Epidemiology, 52*(1), 27-37.

Galindo-Ciocon, D.J., Ciocon, J.O., & Galindo, D.J. (1995). Gait training and falls in the elderly. *Journal of Gerontological Nursing, 21*(6), 10-17.

Gelber, D.A., & Jozefczyk, P.B. (2000). The management of spasticity in multiple sclerosis. *International Journal of MS Care [serial online], 1*(1), 5-11. Available: http://mscare.com.

Gillespie, M.M. (1991). Tremor. *Journal of Neuroscience Nursing, 23*(3), 17-174.

Guyton, A.C., & Hall, J.E. (1996). *Textbook of medical physiology* (9th ed.). Philadelphia: WB Saunders.

Habel, M. (1997). Muscle tone abnormalities. *Rehabilitation Nursing, 22*(3), 118-123, 130.

Hoeman, S.P. (1997). Primary care for children with spina bifida. *Nurse Practitioner, 22,* 60-72.

Hogan, D.P., Rogers, M.L., & Msall, M.E. (2000). Functional limitations and key indicators of well-being in children with disability. *Archives of Pediatric and Adolescent Medicine, 15,* 1042-1048.

Hubley-Kozey, C.L., Wall, J.C., & Hogan D.B. (1995). Effects of a general exercise program on passive hip, knee, and angle range of motion of older women. *Topics in Geriatric Rehabilitation, 10*(3), 33-44.

Jackson-Wyatt, O. (1997). Feldenkrais method and rehabilitation. In Davis, C.M. (Ed.), *Complementary therapies in rehabilitation* (pp. 189-197). Thorofare, NJ: Slack.

Katz, S., & Akpom, A. (1976). A measure of primary sociobiological functions. *International Journal of Health Sciences, 6,* 493-506.

Knight, M.M. (2000). Cognitive ability and functional status. *Journal of Advanced Nursing, 31*(6), 1459-1468.

Kunkel, A., Kopp, B., Muller, G., Villringer, K., Villringer, A., Taub, E., & Flor, H. (1999). Constraint-induced movement therapy for motor recovery in chronic stroke patients. *Archives of Physical Medicine and Rehabilitation, 80,* 624-628.

LaPlante, M., Hendershot, G., & Moss, A. (1992). Assistive technology devices and home accessibility features: Prevalence, payment need, and trends. In *Advance data from vital and health statistics* (No. 217). Hyattsville, MD: National Center for Health Statistics.

Lohi, E.L., Lindberg, C., & Anderson, O. (1993). Physical training effects in myasthenia gravis. *Archives of Physical Medicine and Rehabilitation, 74,* 1178-1180.

Lord, S.R., Ward, J.A., & Williams, P. (1996). Exercise effect on dynamic stability in older women: A randomized controlled trial. *Archive of Physical Medicine & Rehabilitation, 77,* 232-236.

Marjama-Lyons, J. (2000). *Tremor and what to do about it.* National Parkinson's Disease Foundation on-line. XXI(1), Winter, 2000. http://www.parkinson.org/tremor.htm.

Mather, M.L.S. (1987). The secret to life in a spica. *American Journal of Nursing, 85,* 56-58.

Miller, R.G. (1995). The effects of aging upon nerve and muscle function and their importance for neurorehabilitation. *Journal of Neuro Rehabilitation, 9,* 175-181.

Newacheck, P.W., Stoddard, J.J., & McManus, M. (1993). Ethnocultural variations in the prevalence and impact of childhood chronic conditions. *Pediatrics, 91*(5), 1031-1039.

Olson, E.V. (1967). The hazards of immobility. *American Journal of Nursing, 67,* 779-797.

Orem, D. (1995). *Nursing concepts of practice* (5th ed.). St. Louis: Mosby.

Pedretti, C.W., & Zoltan, B. (1990). *Occupational therapy practice skills for physical dysfunction.* St. Louis: Mosby.

Phipps, M.A. (1991). Assessment of neurological deficits in stroke: Acute-care and rehabilitation implications. *Nursing Clinics of North America, 23,* 956-970.

Piette, J.D. (2000). Interactive voice response systems in the diagnosis and management of chronic disease. *American Journal of Managed Care 6*(7), 817-827.

Roper, N., Logan, W., & Tierney, A. (1996). *The elements of nursing: A model for nursing based on a model of living* (4th ed.). Edinburgh: Churchill-Livingstone.

Spector, W. (2000). *Characteristics of long term care users* (Publication No. 00-0049). Washington, DC: Agency for Healthcare Research and Quality.

St. George, C.L. (1993). Spasticity: Mechanisms and nursing care. *Nursing Clinics of North America, 28*(4), 819-826.

Stewart, A. (1993). *Care of traumatic brain injury. Rehabilitation Manual, CEU Program.* Boston: Kimberly Quality Care.

Thibodeau, G.A., & Patton, K.T. (1999). *Anatomy and physiology* (4th ed.). St. Louis: Mosby.

Thorn, S. (2000). Neurological rehabilitation nursing: A review of the research. *Journal of Advanced Nursing, 31*(5), 1029-1038.

Topp, R., Estes, P.K., Dayhoff, N., & Suhrheinrich, J. (1997). Postural control and strength and mood among older adults. *Applied Nursing Research, 10*(1), 11-18.

Walshe, F.M.R. (1961). Contributions of John Hughlings Jackson to neurology. *Archives of Neurology, 5,* 119-131.

Zola, I. (1991). Bringing our bodies and ourselves back in: Reflections on a past, present, and future "medical sociology." *Journal of Health and Human Behavior, 32*(March), 1-16.

Zoltan, B., Siev, E., & Freishtat, B. (1986). *The adult stroke patient: A manual for evaluation and treatment of perceptual and cognitive dysfunction* (2nd ed.). Thorofare, NJ: Slack.

APPENDIX 14A: RANGE OF MOTION: PASSIVE, ACTIVE, AND FUNCTIONAL

I. Terms: range of motion (ROM; amount of movement present in a joint)
   A. Types of ROM
      1. Flexion: bending of joint
      2. Extension: straightening of joint
      3. Abduction: motion away from midline
      4. Adduction: motion toward midline
      5. Circumduction: circular movement
      6. Internal/external rotation
      7. Pronation/supination of elbow
      8. Plantar flexion: downward motion of foot at ankle joint
      9. Dorsiflexion: upward motion of foot at ankle joint
   B. Passive ROM: nurse moves the extremity so that full motion occurs at the joint
   C. Active ROM: client uses muscles to do the moving
   D. Functional activities of ROM: many activities of daily living produce full ROM (e.g., rolling over in bed, sitting up, getting dressed); ROM can be done in conjunction with bed bathing, bed positioning, and mobilization activities
   E. Progressive resistive exercises: muscles begin to work against gravity, enhancing the strength of the muscle

II. General nursing interventions
   A. Explain all activities to client and ensure safety
   B. Reinforce all teaching to client and family
   C. Move client's arms and legs gently during ROM and move within client's tolerance and flexibility
   D. Support the extremity above and below the joint being treated
   E. Give passive ROM when client is in the supine position
   F. Perform each exercise 5 to 10 times during each treatment

G. Assess the motion of the involved side against the ROM of the uninvolved side
H. Perform ROM on all extremities if client is immobilized
I. Nurse should use proper body mechanics

III. Specific ROM exercises: upper extremity
A. Shoulder flexion/extension
1. Support the arm at the wrist and elbow; shoulder is in extended position

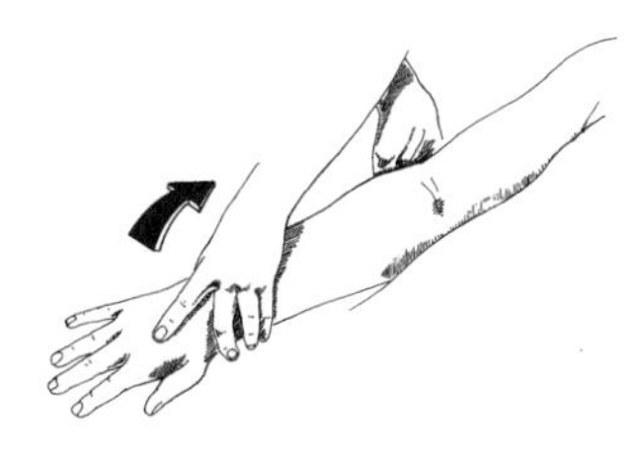

2. Lift the arm straight over client's head; flexion occurs as the arm is lifted up and back

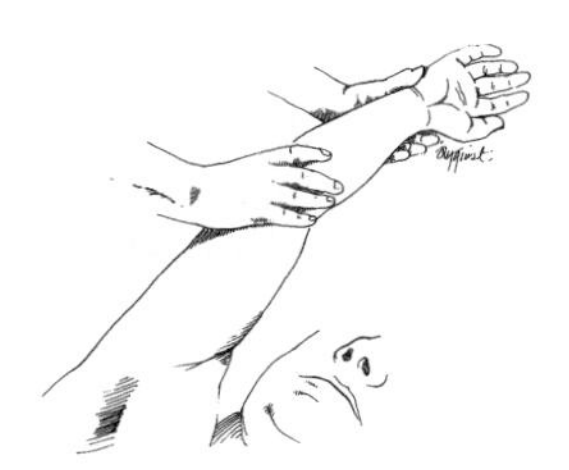

3. Rest the arm flat on the bed above the head
4. Bend client's elbow if there is not enough room for the entire motion

B. Shoulder abduction/adduction
1. Support the arm at the wrist and elbow, with client's palm facing his or her body
2. Slide the arm sideways away from the body, which produces shoulder abduction; sliding the arm toward the body produces shoulder adduction

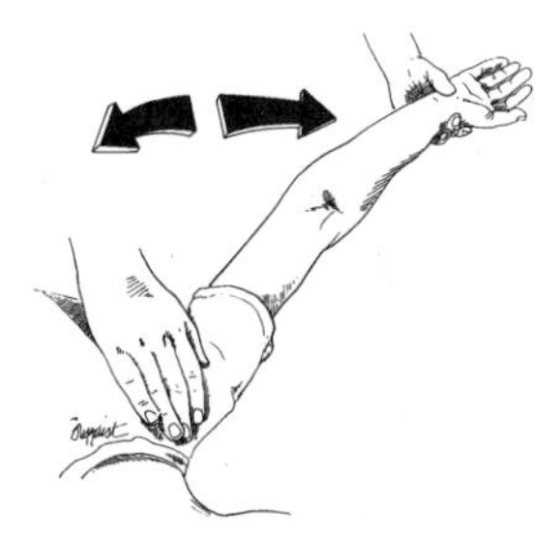

3. Allow the arm to roll or turn over when it reaches about a 90-degree angle with the shoulder
4. Bend the client's elbow if there is not enough room for the entire movement

C. Shoulder external/internal rotation
1. Support client's hand and shoulder
2. Bring the arm away from the client's side, forming a 90-degree angle with the body
3. Keep the elbow bent 90 degrees and the arm supported on the bed
4. Press down on the shoulder toward the bed
5. Move the client's hand backward until the back of the hand touches the bed; as the forearm is brought up and back, external rotation occurs at the shoulder joint

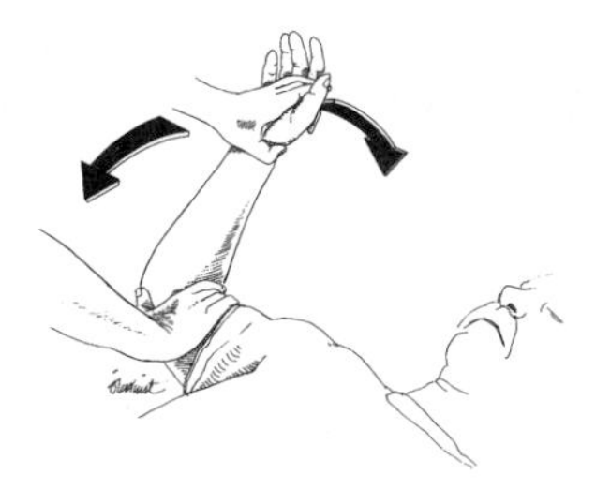

6. Move the client's hand forward until the palm touches the bed; as the forearm is brought down, internal rotation occurs at the shoulder joint

D. Elbow flexion/extension
1. Support the elbow and wrist
2. Bend the client's arm to touch the hand to the shoulder, producing elbow flexion

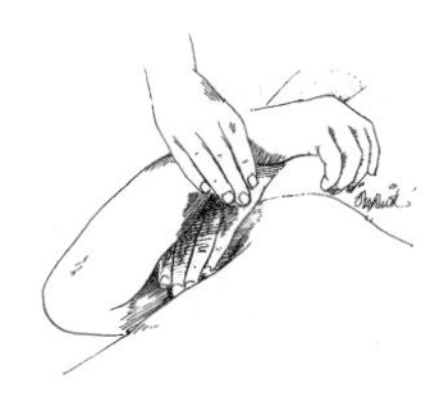

3. Straighten the arm toward the bed, producing elbow extension

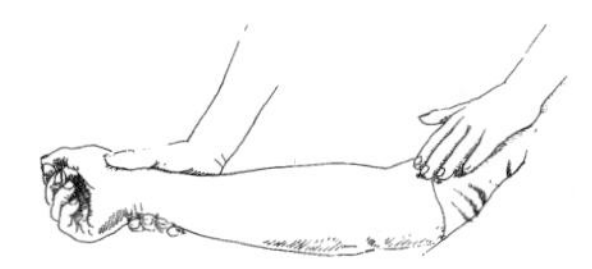

E. Forearm: pronate/supinate
1. Support the upper arm and wrist
2. Turn the palm of the client's hand toward the feet; rolling the forearm downward places it in pronation

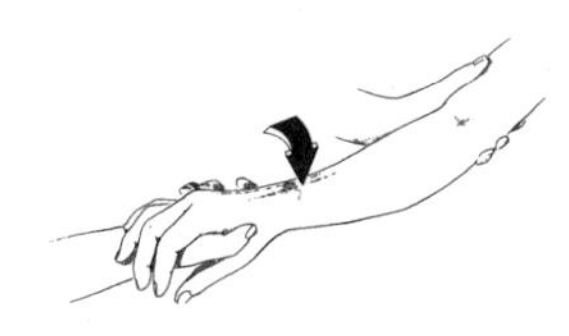

3. Turn palm of client's hand upward from the feet; this places the forearm in supination

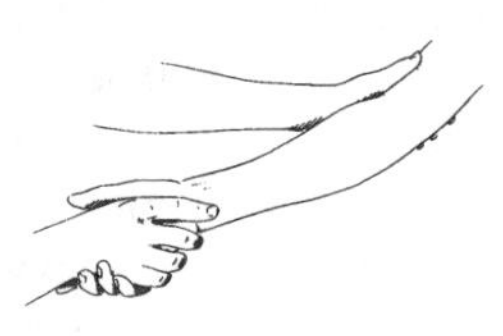

F. Wrist
1. Support the client's wrist and hand and hold client's fingers in the other hand; bend wrist forward and make a fist, producing wrist flexion

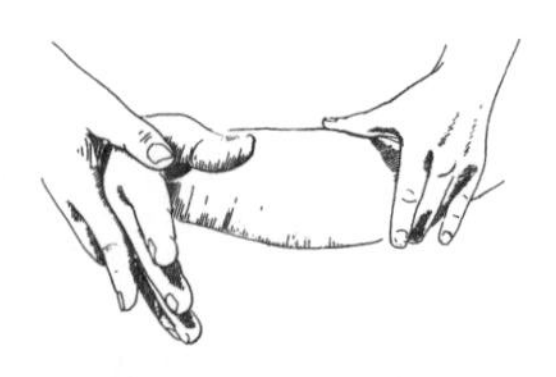

2. Bend wrist backward and extend fingers, producing wrist extension

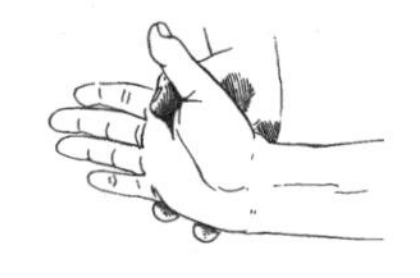

3. Move the wrist laterally, producing radial and ulnar deviation

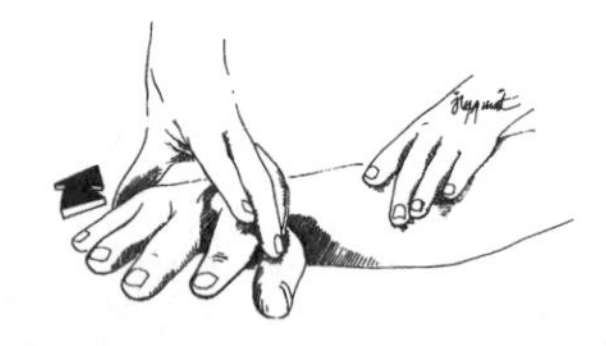

G. Fingers
1. Support client's hand by holding the palm of the hand
2. Bend all fingers at once into a closed fist, producing flexion

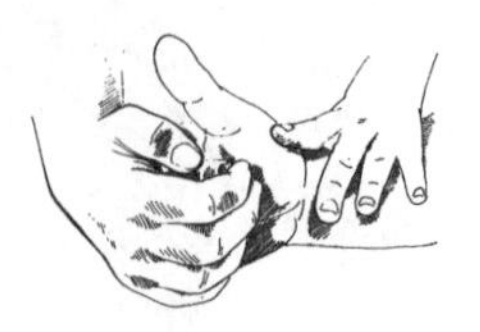

3. Straighten all fingers at once (described as an open fist), producing extension

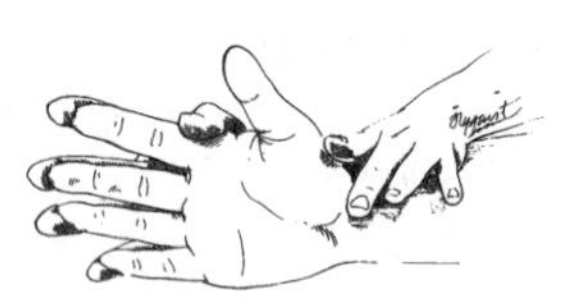

4. Each finger is separated (abducted) and brought back together (adducted)

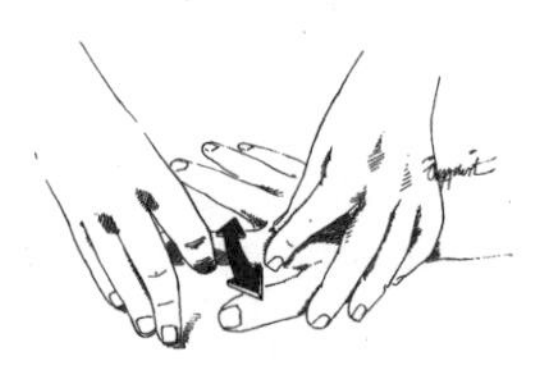

H. Thumb
1. Support the client's hand by holding the fingers straight with one hand
2. Thumb flexed toward and extended away from the fourth digit

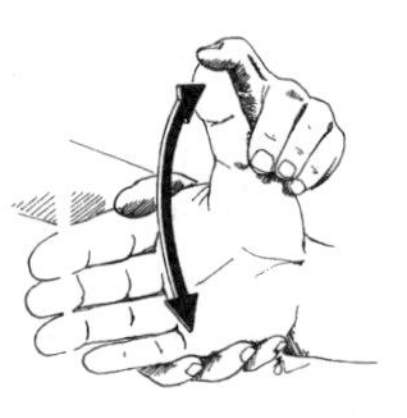

3. Pull the thumb away from the palm; thumb is abducted and adducted in relation to the other fingers

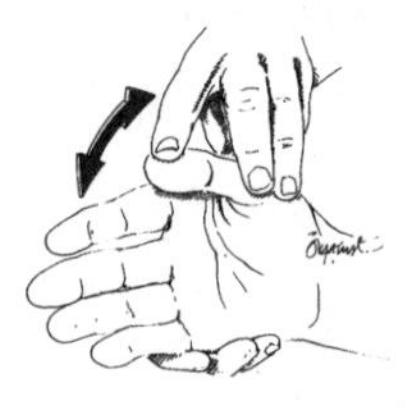

4. Stretch the web space between the thumb and index finger

I. Thumb opposition
1. Support the hand as in thumb abduction

2. Move the thumb toward the little finger in opposition to the base of each of the other four digits

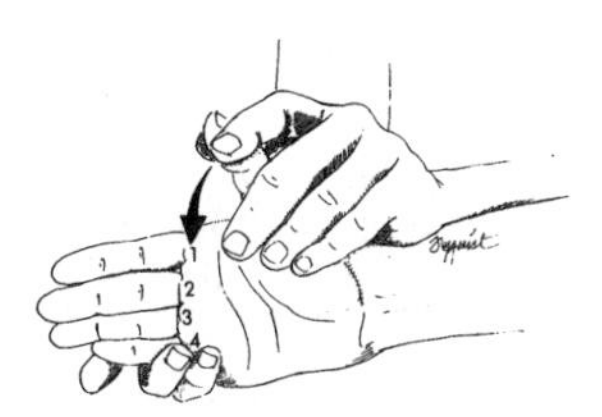

3. Move the thumb through a semicircle design

IV. Specific ROM exercises: lower extremity
   A. Hip flexion/extension
      1. Support under the client's knee and heel
      2. Raise the knee toward the chest, producing flexion

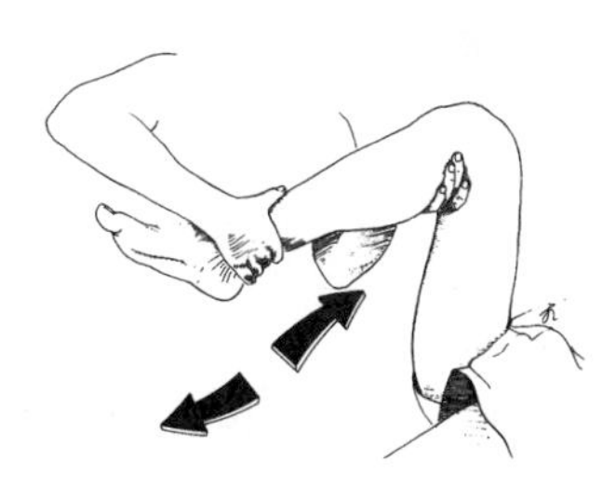

      3. Bend the hip as much as possible; allow the knee to bend slightly or within client's tolerance
      4. Sliding the leg forward produces extension
   B. Hip flexion/strength
      1. Support under client's knees and heel
      2. Lift client's leg straight and as high as possible
      3. Hold for count of 5
      4. Lower the leg gently
   C. Hip abduction/adduction
      1. Support client's knee and heel, keeping the leg in "toes up" position
      2. Move the leg away from the midline of the body, abducting the hip

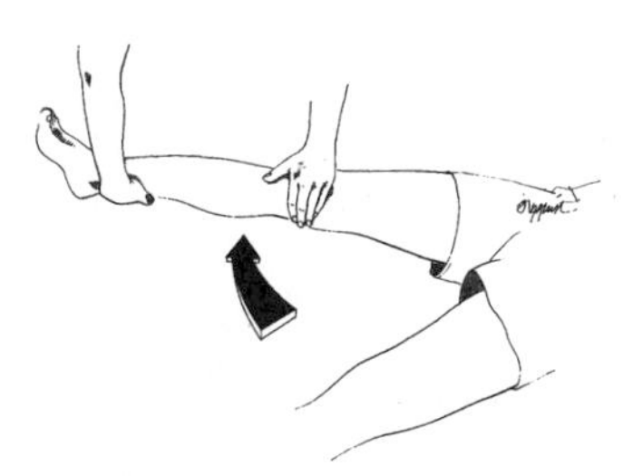

      3. Move the leg toward the midline of the body and cross over the other leg, adducting the hip

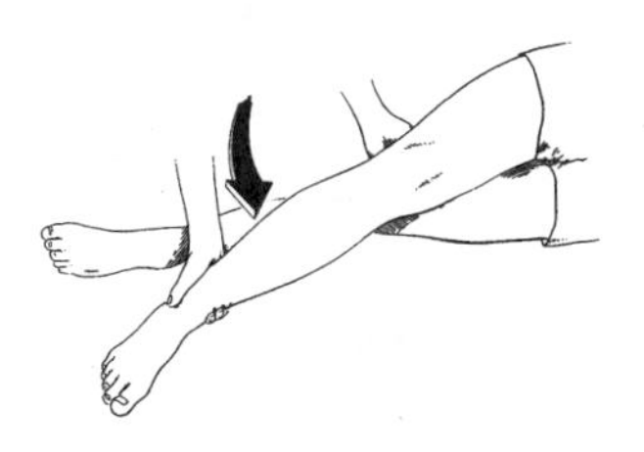

   D. Hip internal/external rotation
      1. Support under client's knee and heel
      2. Bend the hip up to 90 degrees and bend the knee up to 90 degrees
      3. Turn the lower leg toward you, keeping the hip and knee in place
      4. Turn the lower leg away from you, keeping the hip and knee in place
      5. Do not force this motion
   E. Hip internal/external rotation
      1. Support client's leg by placing hand on top of client's knee and ankle
      2. Roll the leg inward

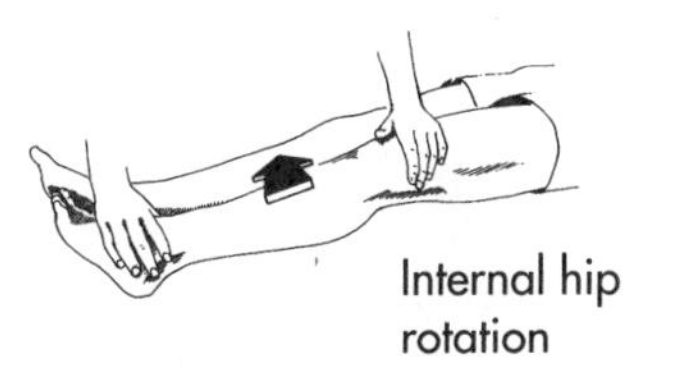

      3. Roll the leg outward

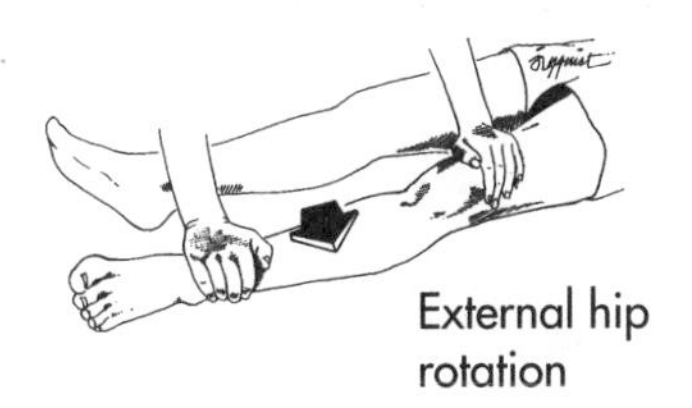

   F. Knee flexion/extension
      1. Support the leg as necessary at the heel and behind the knee
      2. Flex the hip high 90 degrees
      3. Bend the knee in a position of flexion

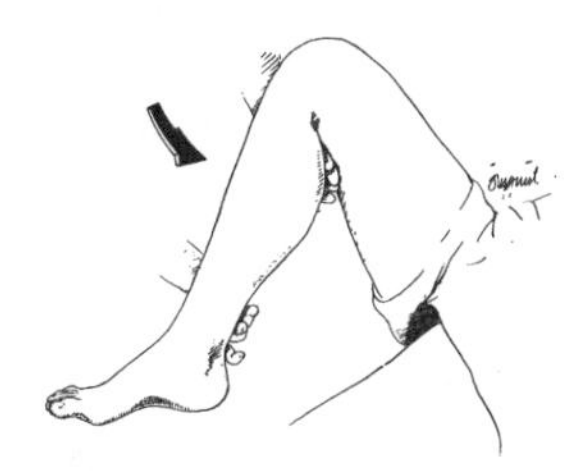

4. Movement of lower leg upward produces knee extension; hip is also in extension

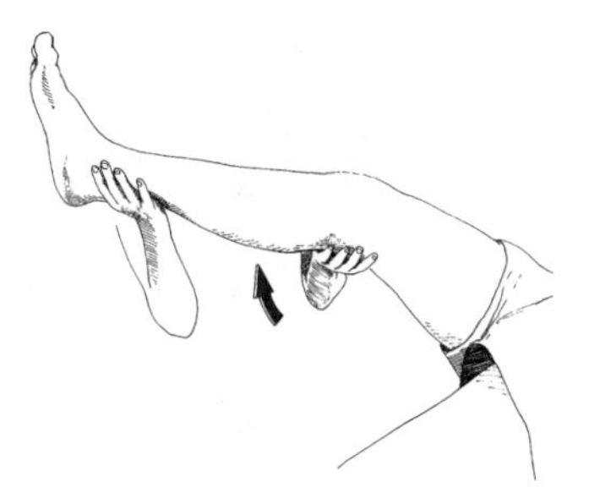

G. Heel cord stretching
   1. Support client's calf with one hand and press downward on client's leg with the other hand
   2. Pull down on the heel
   3. Press your forearm against the client's foot, pushing it toward the leg

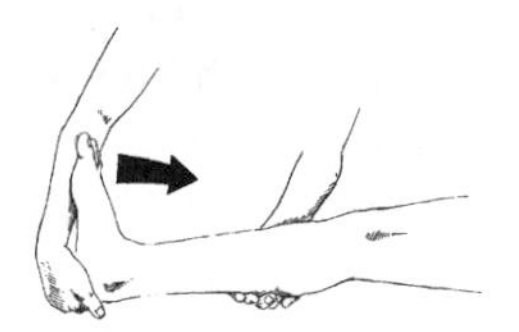

   4. Hold for count of 5 and relax

H. Toe flexion/extension
   1. Support client's foot
   2. Bend all toes downward, producing flexion
   3. Push all toes backward, producing extension

I. Ankle
   1. Support client's leg with one hand and hold the foot with the other hand
   2. Pressure with the palm of the hand against the ball of the foot produces ankle dorsiflexion

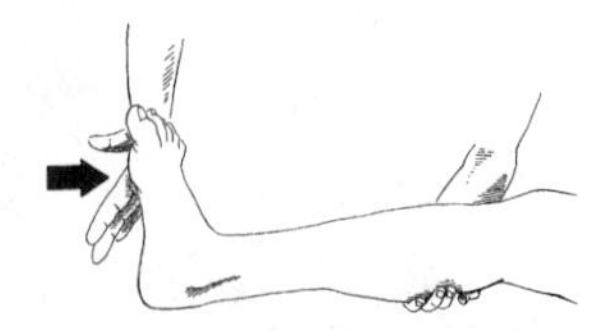

   3. Pressure against the top of the foot produces ankle plantar flexion

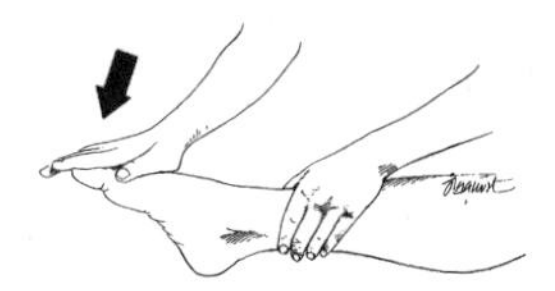

   4. Turning the foot inward produces ankle inversion

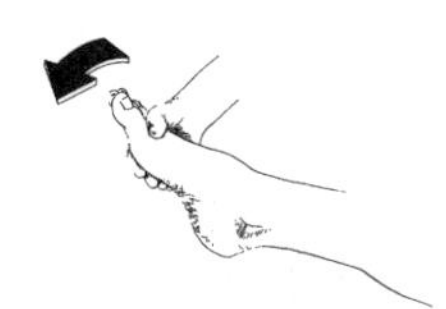

   5. Turning the foot outward produces ankle eversion

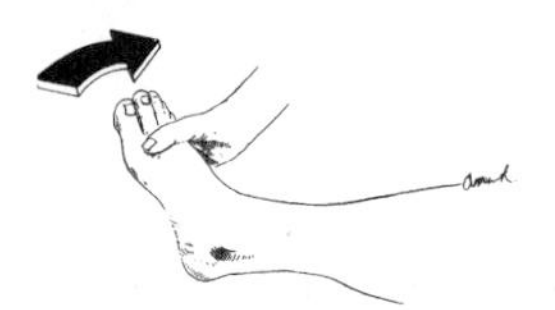

Neurophysiology 15

Joan P. Alverzo, PhD(c), MSN, CRRN

ORGANIZATION OF THE NEUROLOGICAL SYSTEM

The neurological system is composed of a network of subsystems organized to provide both the regulation of the internal environment of the body and the capacity to interact with the external environment. Whereas some functions can be localized to specific regions of the neurological system, many functions rely on the interaction of several regions working together to produce the desired effect.

Embryological Development

The embryological development of the neurological system begins early in the first trimester of pregnancy with the thickening of the ectoderm into a neural plate that quickly evolves into a neural tube, later closing and evolving to become the central neurological system. Embryological development involves a number of states including dorsal induction, ventral induction, proliferation, migration, organization, and myelination. Interruption in the rapid evolution of the neurological system can result in a number of birth defects.

Normal growth and development of the neurological system begins in the subcortical (below the cortex) region with the brainstem and spinal cord. The spinal cord mediates a number of reflexes from an early stage of prenatal development that appear and/or disappear at scheduled intervals. The cranium of the infant is composed of several bones that fuse after birth with connective tissue to allow for normal growth. The connections between bone plates are called sutures. At the juncture of the bone plates are spaces or fontanelles that remain open for a number of months after birth. Although some change in the circumference of the skull is normal through the age of 5 years, abnormal growth may signal abnormalities, including increased intracranial pressure or early suture closure.

Disorders

Defects in the neural tube closure result in anencephaly (without cerebrum), encephalocele (protrusion of the brain through a defect in the skull), meningocele (protruding sac of meninges through a defect in the spine or cranium), and myelomeningocele (protruding sac of meninges and spinal cord through the spinal cord). The incidence of these defects is 0.7 to 1.0 per 1000 births. Depending on the severity, these defects may be fatal (Figure 15-1).

Defects in the cranium include acrania (without cranium), craniosynostosis (premature closure of sutures), and a number of cranial deformities. Microcephaly (reduced brain growth) is associated with significant mental retardation. Congenital hydrocephalus (increased cerebrospinal fluid [CSF]) may be the result of obstruction, overproduction of CSF, or reduced reabsorption of CSF.

Encephalopathy is the result of embryologic malformation or environmental causes. *Cerebral palsy* is a general term used to refer to many different disabling diseases of childhood. These diseases may result from a combination of factors, from genetic to environmental.

Cellular Structure

The cells of the neurological system are highly differentiated. The neuron is the functional unit of nerve transmission and includes a cell body, nerve fiber or axon, and synapse. Neurons are specialized, each performing a specific task, and are categorized as sensory neurons, association neurons, and motor neurons. Groups of cell bodies are called *ganglia* in the peripheral nervous system and *nuclei* in the central nervous system (CNS). Nerve fibers can be myelinated to carry impulses more rapidly than unmyelinated axons. Supporting cells provide nutrition and other supports to the CNS. Astrocytes provide nutrition and facilitate transport of substances across the blood-brain barrier. Schwann cells

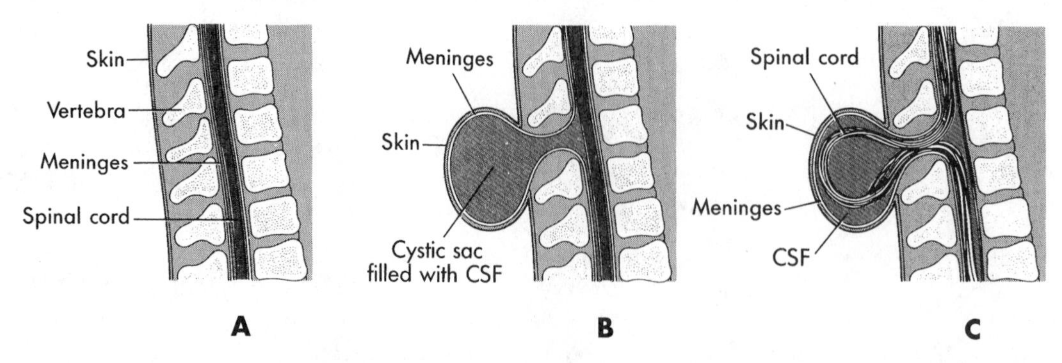

Figure 15-1 Myelodysplasia is classified according to the pathophysiology of the lesion or defect of the spinal cord and surrounding structures. **A,** Normal spine. **B,** Meningocele. **C,** Myelomeningocele. (From McCance, K.L., & Heuther, S.E. [1998]. *Pathophysiology: The biological basis for disease in adults and children.* [3rd ed.]. St. Louis: Mosby.)

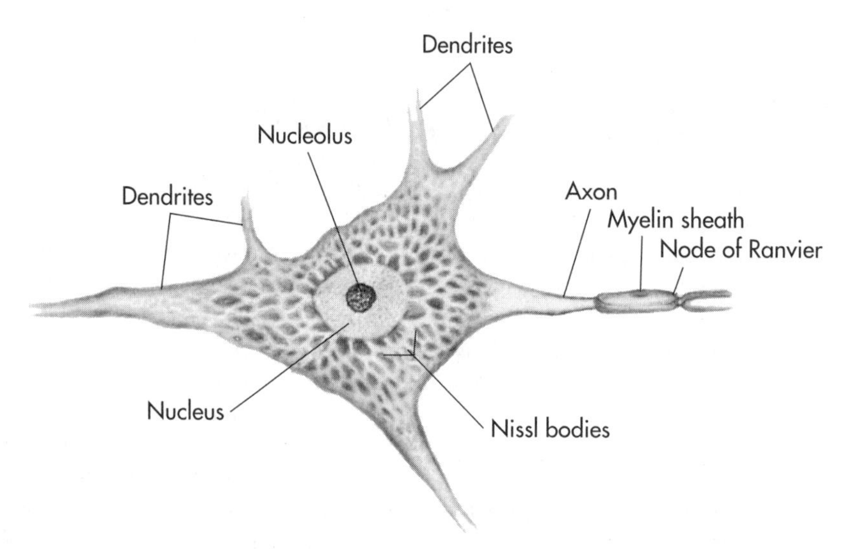

Figure 15-2 Diagram of neuron with composite parts. (From Rudy, E.B. [1984]. *Advanced neurological and neurosurgical nursing.* St. Louis: Mosby.).

produce myelin outside the CNS, and oligodendrocytes produce myelin inside the CNS. Ependymal cells are involved in the production of CSF (Figure 15-2).

Nerve impulses are generated and conducted through electrical and chemical means. Synapses are gaps between neurons that rely on neurotransmitters to conduct nerve impulses. There are more than 30 substances that act as neurotransmitters, and they can act to excite or inhibit the neurons on which they act. Many diseases of the neurological system have become associated with specific neurotransmitters, and a number of drugs to treat disease are targeted at manipulating neurotransmitters.

Disorders

Diseases associated with a decrease in the neurotransmitter acetylcholine include Alzheimer's disease and myasthenia gravis. A number of mood disorders and schizophrenia are associated with changes in serotonin levels. Parkinson's disease is the result of a defect in the dopamine-secreting neurons of the substantia nigra. Phenothiazine tranquilizers can cause tremors, bradykinesia, and rigidity, referred to as Parkinson's syndrome.

Neurotransmitters are also crucial in sleep cycles, and deficits in neurotransmitters such as serotonin can result in sleep disorders. Histamine is involved in arousal, secretion of pituitary hormones, and thermoregulation. γ-Aminobutyric acid (GABA) inhibits synaptic function, and drugs that increase GABA are used to treat seizures and pain syndromes. Substance P is a neurotransmitter in pain transmission, and morphine blocks substance P, thus reducing pain.

Multiple sclerosis is a disorder diffusely involving CNS myelin. The age of onset is between 20 and 40 years, and this disorder is a leading cause of neurological disability in early childhood. The pathogenesis is unknown, but most

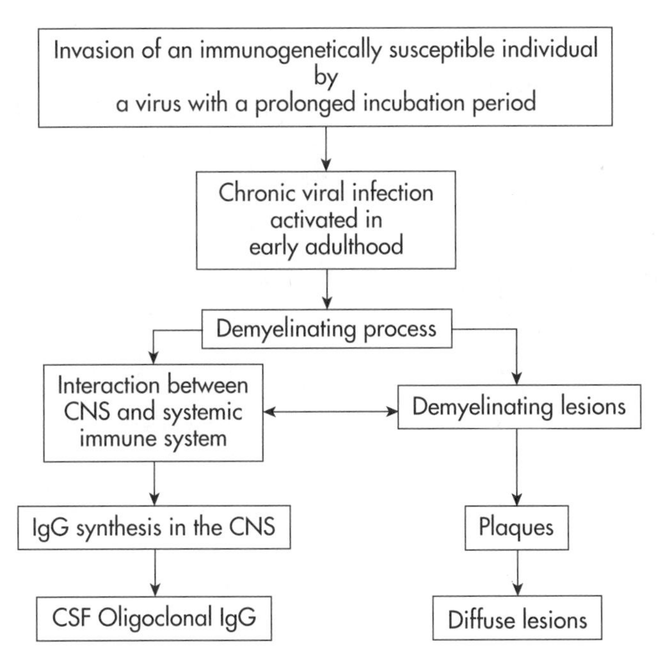

Figure 15-3 Etiopathogenic model for multiple sclerosis. The initiating or trigger event is presumed to be invasion by a virus with a prolonged incubation period, causing an altered immune response. The resulting chronic viral infection or other environmental insult becomes active in early adulthood, provoking the demyelinating process. *CNS,* Central Nervous System; *IgG,* immunoglobulin G; *CSF,* cerebrospinal fluid (From McCance, K.L., & Huether, S.E. [1998]. *Pathophysiology: The biologic basis for disease in adults and children* [3rd ed.]. St. Louis: Mosby.)

theories suggest an immunogenetic-viral cause. The progression is unpredictable and may include corticospinal syndrome, brainstem syndrome, cerebellar syndrome, or cerebral syndrome. Paroxysmal attacks, including the worsening of symptoms, may occur abruptly with short duration or may lead to progressive symptoms (Figure 15-3).

Protective Structures

The neurological system is protected by a number of structures that prevent injury by providing a physical barrier, cushioning, and skeletal support. The skull, or cranium, is a bony structure formed by eight bones that fuse during childhood to make up the cranial vault. The floor of the cranium is an irregular surface containing openings and several depressions or fossae. Because of its rough surface, the floor of the cranium can cause damage to brain tissue when trauma occurs.

The vertebral column is composed of a series of vertebrae that provide protection and support to the spinal cord. There are 31 vertebrae, and they are divided into cervical, thoracic, lumbar, and sacral vertebrae. The vertebrae provide flexibility of movement, as well as support for weight bearing, particularly in the upright position. Intervertebral disks provide cushioning between vertebrae.

Three protective membranes surround the brain and form the meninges. They are the dura mater, the arachnoid membrane, and the pia mater. The space between the skull and the dura is called the *epidural space* and is the location of several arteries. The space between the dura and arachnoid membrane contains several veins and is called the *subdural space.* The space between the arachnoid and pia mater is called the *subarachnoid space* and contains cerebral spinal fluid. A number of membranes or invaginations further define the structure of the brain. The falx cerebri separates the two hemispheres, and the tentorium cerebelli separates the brainstem from the cerebrum. Increased intracranial pressure can cause herniation of the cortex across the tentorium, referred to as *transtentorial herniation* or *supratentorial herniation,* creating pressure on the brainstem (Figure 15-4).

The cerebral spinal fluid circulates in the subarachnoid space and through the ventricles of the brain, the meninges, and around the spinal cord. This is a closed system with approximately 600 mL of fluid under 120 to 180 mm of water pressure. CSF is manufactured in the choroid plexus of the ventricles, travels through a number of foramen or openings between the ventricles, and circulates in the subarachnoid space to surround the brain and spinal cord. It is reabsorbed into venous circulation through the arachnoid villa.

Disorders

Trauma can result in a fracture of the cranium or a skull fracture that can be simple or compound. A basilar skull fracture is a break in the floor of the cranium and may result in leaking CSF from the nares or ears. Trauma to the vertebral column can result in a vertebral fracture, often with associated damage to the spinal column. In addition, trauma can result in injury to intervertebral disks with associated damage to the spinal column.

A number of pathologic processes can occur involving the meninges and CSF. Meningitis is an inflammation of the meninges that can be bacterial, viral, fungal, or simply inflammatory. Hydrocephalus, defined as excess fluid in the cranial vault and/or subarachnoid space, can have a number of causes. As a result, there are many types of hydrocephalus, including communicating, noncommunicating, and normal pressure. A number of hemorrhages can occur in and around the meninges of the brain, including subdural hematoma (slowly accumulating venous blood), epidural hemorrhage (rapidly accumulating arterial blood or venous blood), and subarachnoid hemorrhage (bleeding into the subarachnoid space).

Regions of the Brain

The brain is composed of a number of regions, each with a different function. The medulla oblongata, or myelencephalon, located most caudally in the brainstem, is the "crossroads" between the brain and the spinal cord, with all spinal cord tracks passing through this region, some cross-

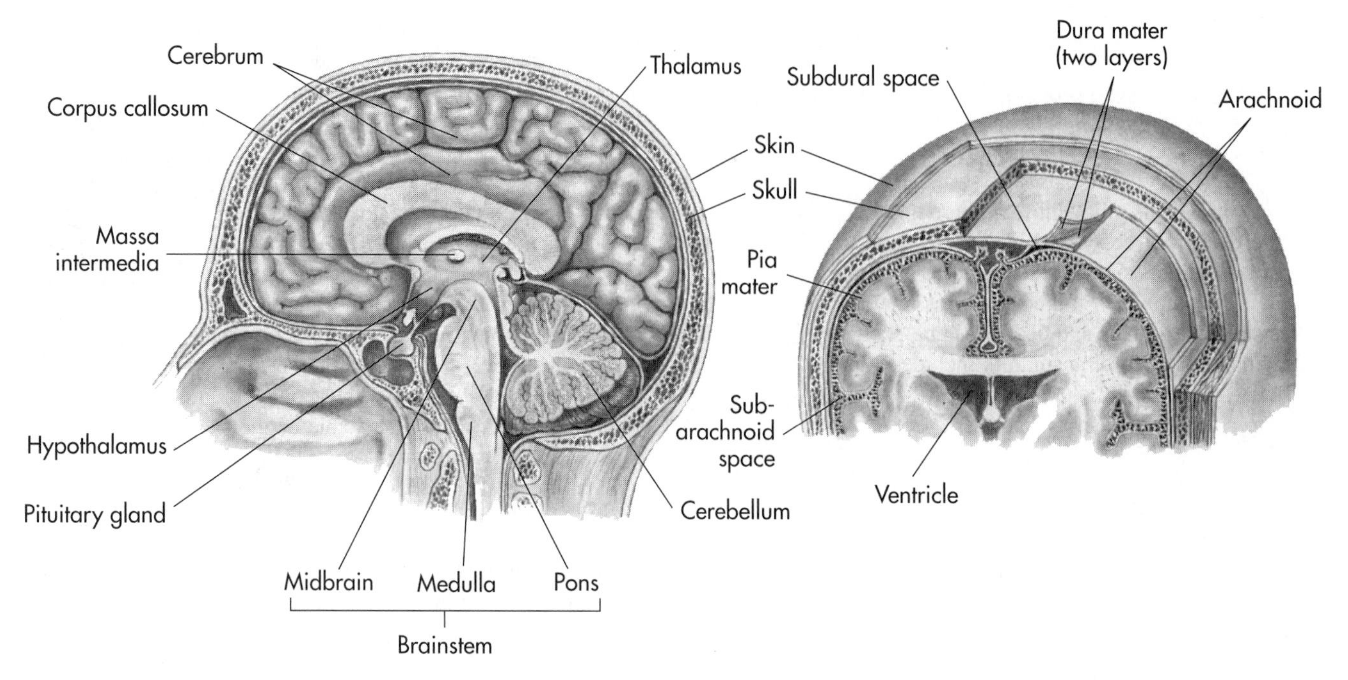

Figure 15-4 Meninges of brain. (From Thompson, J.M., McFarland, G.K., Hirsch, J.E., & Tucker, S.M. [1998]. *Mosby's clinical nursing* [4th ed.]. St. Louis: Mosby.)

ing from one side to the other. It is also a center for respiratory and cardiac function. The hindbrain, or metencephalon, is composed of the cerebellum, contributing to coordination, and the pons. The midbrain is composed of a number of structures, including the superior and inferior colliculi, red nuclei, substantia nigra, and cerebral peduncles. Combined, these structures play a critical role in a number of activities including motor coordination, hearing, and vision.

The forebrain in composed of the telencephalon, including the cerebrum and basal ganglia, and the diencephalon, including the thalamic structures. The cerebrum is composed of the frontal, parietal, occipital, and temporal lobes. Often considered the center of executive functions, the cerebral cortex participates or oversees a broad range of functions. A simplified version of functions associated with the cerebral lobes is as follows: frontal, motor/executive/affective; parietal, sensory; temporal, hearing/speech; and occipital, vision. Specific regions of the lobes of the cerebral cortex may perform specialized functions, for example, facial recognition in the parietooccipital junction. However, more often several regions may act together to perform a particular function, such as dressing, which may combine activity within the parietal lobe along with the frontal lobe premotor area and the motor strip. The right side of the cerebrum generally controls the left side of the body, and the left cerebrum controls the right side of the body. The right thalamus receives sensation from the left side of the body, and the left thalamus receives sensation from the right side of the body. Chapter 25 contains additional illustrations of the brain.

The basal ganglia are a group of nuclei that lie under the cerebral cortex and include the putamen caudate, caudate nucleus, lentiform nucleus, and globus pallidus. The basal ganglia are part of the extrapyramidal system, modulating involuntary motor activity into coordinated and complex efforts. The diencephalon is composed of thalamic structures. The largest nucleus is the thalamus, a sensory relay station and modulator between the spinal cord tracts, the brainstem, the basal ganglia, and the cerebral cortex. The hypothalamus maintains the internal environment and determines behavioral patterns. The hypothalamus exerts primary control over many body functions through the neuroendocrine pathways. The subthalamus is located beneath the thalamus and is an important component of the extrapyramidal system.

Cranial Nerves

Twelve pair of cranial nerves (CN) connect to the brain and brainstem. The CN have mixed, motor, and sensory functions as listed in Table 15-1.

Disorders

Trauma to the brain can result in a variety of deficits according to the region or regions affected. Hematomas and contusions can result from trauma, and the region of injury may be localized or diffuse. Concussions are, by definition, diffuse. Missile injuries such as gunshot wounds produce a

TABLE 15-1 Cranial Nerves and Their Functions

Cranial Nerves	Function
Olfactory (I)	Sensory: smell reception and interpretation
Optic (II)	Sensory: visual acuity and visual fields
Oculomotor (III)	Motor: eyelid raising, most extraocular movements
	Parasympathetic: pupillary constriction, lens shape change
Trochlear (IV)	Motor: downward, inward eye movement
Trigeminal (V)	Motor: jaw opening and clenching, chewing, and mastication
	Sensory: sensation to cornea, iris, lacrimal glands, conjunctiva eyelids, forehead, nose, nasal and mouth mucosa, teeth, tongue, ear, facial skin
Abducens (VI)	Motor: lateral eye movement
Facial (VII)	Motor: movement of facial expression muscles except jaw, eye closure, labial speech sounds (b, m, w, and rounded vowels)
	Sensory: taste—anterior two thirds of tongue, sensation to pharynx
	Parasympathetic: secretion of saliva and tears
Acoustic (VIII)	Sensory: hearing and equilibrium
Glossopharyngeal (IX)	Motor: voluntary muscles for swallowing and phonation
	Sensory: sensation of nasopharynx, gag reflex, taste—posterior one third of tongue
	Parasympathetic: secretion of salivary glands, carotid reflex
Vagus (X)	Motor: voluntary muscles of phonation (guttural speech sounds) and swallowing
	Sensory: sensation behind ear and part of external ear canal
	Parasympathetic: secretion of digestive enzymes; peristalsis; carotid reflex; involuntary action of heart, lungs, and digestive tract
Spinal accessory (XI)	Motor: head turning, shoulder shrugging, some actions for phonation
Hypoglossal (XII)	Motor: tongue movement for speech sound articulation (l, t, n) and swallowing

From Seidel, H.M., Dains, J.E., Ball, J.W., & Benedict, G.W. (1995). *Mosby's guide to physical examination* (3rd ed.). St. Louis: Mosby.

specific track of damage, but with enough force, may produce a contrecoup injury (damage on the side opposite the injury). Brain injury from motor vehicle accidents are often coup-contrecoup injuries (damage on the side of the injury and on the opposite side) and are generally more diffuse (Figure 15-5).

Another important type of injury results from acceleration/deceleration forces on the brain, often with a rotational component. This is called *diffuse axonal injury* and leads to loss of consciousness and disconnection between various regions as a result of stretching and/or tearing of nerve fibers. This is often not seen on examinations, such as a magnetic resonance imaging (MRI), but may account for the bulk of long-term deficits after traumatic brain injury. Tumors are another source of brain injury, and the region of damage can vary.

Among the many diseases involving regions of the brain is Parkinson's disease. Huntington's chorea is also a disease of the basal ganglia marked by choreiform and athetoid movements. Supranuclear palsy is a deterioration of basal ganglion structures of the brain and is marked by progressive loss of motor and cognitive function.

Spinal Cord

The spinal cord arises from the medulla and extends to the conus medullaris at the vertebral level L2, providing a communication pathway between the brain and peripheral nerves as well as mediating the reflex arc. The cord is made up of both gray mater (nuclei) and white mater (myelinated axons and tracts). The cell bodies are contained in the central butterfly-shaped gray mater. The posterior or dorsal horn receives sensory or afferent signals, and the anterior or ventral horn is the location for motor or efferent fibers.

The sensory tracts carry impulses to the brain and cross from one side of the cord to the other, either at the level of entry into the cord or at the medulla. The three major sensory tracts are the posterior dorsal columns, the spinothalamic tracts, and the spinocerebellar tracts. The posterior dorsal column is heavily myelinated and carries discriminating touch, vibration, pressure, and kinesthetic sensation to the parietal lobes of the cerebrum and sensory areas of the thalamus. The spinothalamic tract has a synapse in the cord at the level of entry, has a second synapse in the thalamus, and terminates in the parietal lobe mediating pain and temperature. The spinocerebellar tract is an unconscious pathway for body position and remains ipsilateral, terminating in the cerebellum and facilitating balance and posture.

The motor tracts carry impulses from the brain, cross in the medulla to the other side of the spinal cord, and carry messages down the spinal cord. The motor tract synapses with spinal nerves originating in the cord and terminating in

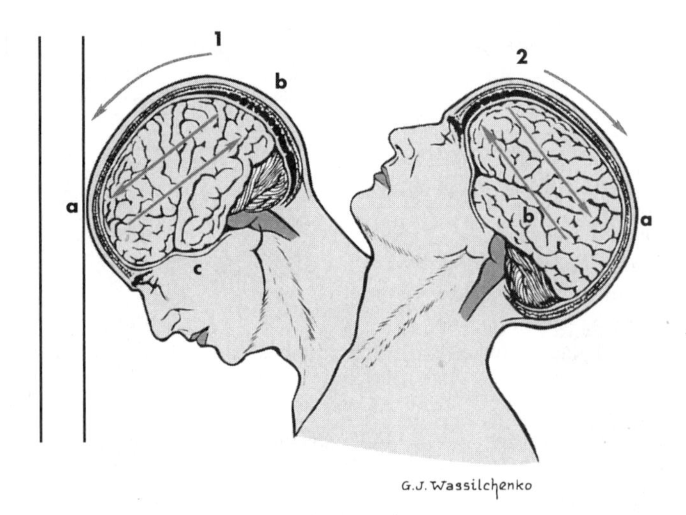

Figure 15-5 Coup and contrecoup head injury after blunt trauma. *1,* Coup injury: impact against object; *a,* site of impact and direct trauma to brain; *b,* shearing of subdural veins; and *c,* trauma to base of brain. *2,* Contrecoup injury: impact within skull; *a,* site of impact from brain hitting opposite side of skull; and *b,* shearing forces through brain. These injuries occur in one continuous motion; the head strikes the wall (coup) and then rebounds (contrecoup). (Modified from Rudy, E.B. [1984]. *Advanced neurological and neurosurgical nursing.* St. Louis: Mosby.)

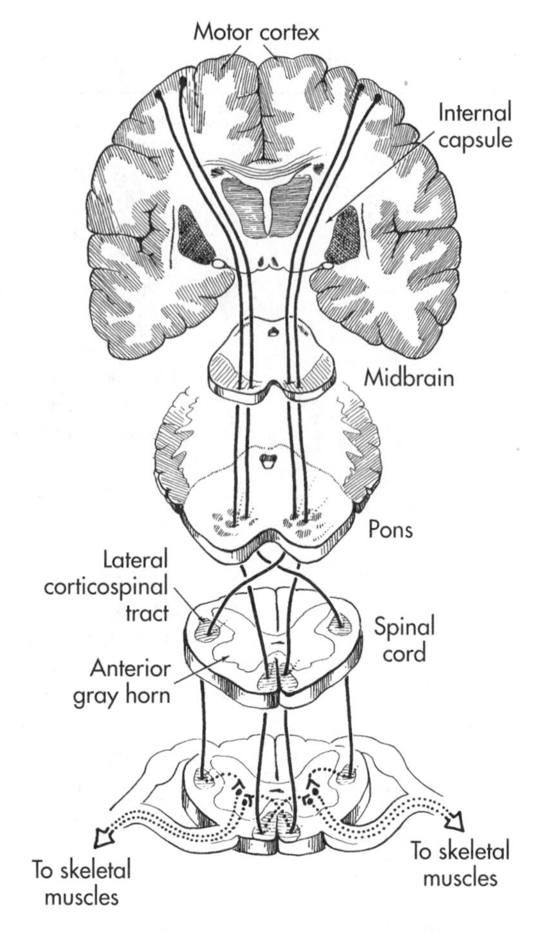

Figure 15-6 Voluntary motor impulses from the cortex to skeletal muscles. Impulses arising in the cortex descend directly through the anterior corticospinal tract or cross at the level of the medulla and descend through the lateral corticospinal tract to anterior horn cells.

the peripheral tissue. The corticospinal and reticulospinal tracts are two major motor tracts, although there are a number of other motor tracts. The corticospinal tract arises in the motor cortex of the frontal lobe, travels through the internal capsule and cerebral peduncles, and crosses in the medulla (Figure 15-6). It is called the *pyramidal tract* (passing through the pyramids of the medulla) and controls voluntary movement on the opposite side of the body. Some fibers do not cross in the medulla and control truncal motor function. The reticulospinal tract influences motor response and originates in the brainstem with lateral and medial divisions that integrate extrapyramidal function (involuntary motor movement for coordination involving nonpyramidal tracts), with the combined motor output exiting the cord as a common pathway.

The spinal nerves synapse with the peripheral regions of the body. There are 31 pairs of spinal nerves that are divided into anterior (motor) and posterior (sensory) roots. The upper spinal nerves exit the cord and travel horizontally, and the lower spinal nerves exit the cord and travel almost vertically toward the lower pelvic floor and lower extremities, forming the cauda equina or "horse tail" of nerves within the spinal canal. Groups of spinal nerves are bundled in a unit or plexus. The cervical plexus is composed of the first four cranial nerves and includes the phrenic nerve. The brachial plexus (C5-T1) divides into the radial, medial, and ulnar nerves. Thoracic nerves exit the cord individually, and the lumbar-sacral plexus branches into the obturator, femoral, and sciatic nerves (Figure 15-7).

The reflex arc is composed of an afferent/sensory neuron, an efferent/motor neuron, and an effector muscle or gland. Cell bodies are contained in gray matter of the central cord and mediate the reflex without cortical participation. Reflexes may be normal or abnormal; for example, the Babinski reflex is abnormal when present. The stimulus for a reflex may result in no response (areflexia), a normal response, an extreme response (hyperreflexia), or clonus when there is repeated hyperreflexia. Depending on the extent and nature of injury to the nerves or tracts, reflexes may be present, absent, or abnormal.

Upper motor neurons connect the brain with the anterior horn of the spinal cord and, in turn, the lower motor neuron. The corticospinal or pyramidal tracts are examples of upper motor neurons. Upper motor neuron impulses originate in the motor strip of the frontal lobe, and any interruption in the transmission of those impulses to the anterior horn of the spinal cord is considered an upper motor neuron injury. Any injury from the brain down to and including the T12/L1 ver-

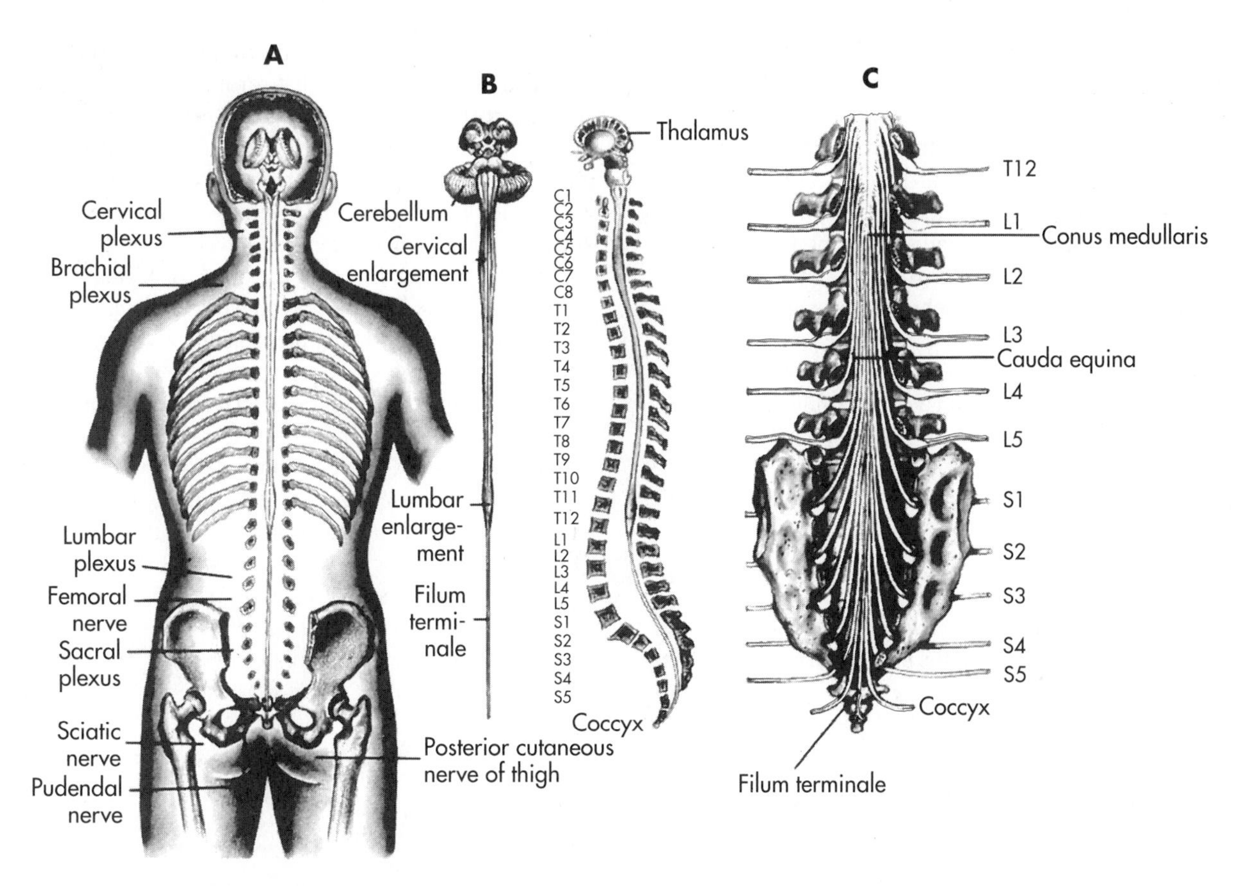

Figure 15-7 Spinal cord within vertebral canal and exiting spinal nerves. **A,** Posterior view of brainstem and spinal cord in situ with spinal nerves and plexus. **B,** Anterior view of brainstem and spinal cord. **C,** Enlargement of caudal area showing termination of spinal cord (conus medullaris) and a group of nerve fibers constituting the cauda equina. (From Rudy, E.B. [1984]. *Advanced neurological and neurosurgical nursing.* St. Louis: Mosby.)

tebral level, which is the end of the spinal cord, is defined as an upper motor lesion. This may include spinal cord injuries that transect the tracts in the cord as well as head injury, stroke, and multiple sclerosis. The upper motor neuron lesion is marked by loss of voluntary control of motor function and alteration of reflexes due to reduced inhibition or modulation. Thus the clinical presentation is often hyperreflexia, spasticity, retention of muscle mass, and loss of voluntary movement (paralysis) or weakness. Reflexes may, as a result of CNS damage, evolve from hyporeflexia to hyperrreflexia, but never the reverse.

Lower motor neurons transmit messages from the anterior horn of the spinal cord to the peripheral muscles. In order for a reflex to occur, all portions of the lower motor neuron must be functional. Damage to the lower motor neuron will result in an interruption in the reflex arc, with resultant flaccid paralysis, absent or hypoactive reflexes, and severe muscle atrophy. Damage to the spinal cord below the vertebral level of L2 is defined as a lower motor neuron lesion, with resultant problems with bowel and bladder function as well as sexual dysfunction including absence of an erection.

Spinal shock is a temporary syndrome associated with spinal cord trauma. The spinal cord as a whole shuts down within hours of the injury, and during the period of spinal shock, it may be difficult to determine the extent of injury. Spinal shock creates an exaggeration of the actual injury, and it may last days to weeks. In an upper motor neuron injury, spinal shock is considered over when there is a return of the pudendal reflexes, including the anal wink.

Disorders

Traumatic damage to the spinal cord can vary from complete transection to flexion injuries, extension injuries, partial injuries, or a mixed syndrome of motor and sensory deficits. The American Spinal Cord Injury Association (ASIA) developed a classification system for determining the location and extent of deficits after spinal trauma. Complete injuries generally indicate a complete functional transection of the spinal cord, with loss of both sensory and motor function. Partial injuries can result in motor deficits, sensory deficits, or mixed deficits, such as Brown-Sequard syndrome with the loss of motor on one side of the body and loss of sensory on the other side. Central cord syndrome, anterior cord syndrome, and Horner syndrome are other specific clinical entities.

A number of diseases affect the spinal nerves. Guillain-Barré syndrome is an ascending loss of peripheral nerve function that may extend to loss of respiratory control, which is temporary and generally reversible, although the reversal may be incomplete. Amyotrophic lateral sclerosis, commonly referred to as Lou Gehrig disease, is a loss of anterior horn cells that is progressive and eventually causes death. Poliomyelitis is a nonprogressive disease of the anterior motor horn cells of the spinal cord, resulting in a lower motor neuron syndrome. Multiple sclerosis is a deterioration of the myelin sheath surrounding neurons and is generally progressive.

Vascular Supply

The carotid arteries and vertebral arteries carry the supply of arterial blood from the heart to the brain. The carotid arteries branch into the external carotid supplying the surface of the face and skull and the internal carotid supplying the front or anterior part of the brain. Unlike the neural connection of the body to the brain, the blood supply stays on the same side; thus an impairment in the right carotid artery affects the right side of the brain. The internal carotid arteries become the anterior and middle cerebral arteries. However, the internal carotid arteries first join the circle of Willis, a circuit of arteries connected together in the very center and base of the brain that acts as a backup mechanism to ensure a collateral arterial blood supply in the event of the failure of a single artery. The anterior cerebral artery supplies the basal ganglia, corpus callosum, inner or medial surface of the cerebral hemispheres, and superior surface of the frontal and parietal lobes. The middle cerebral artery supplies the frontal, parietal, and temporal lobes, primarily on the lateral surface (Figure 15-8).

The two vertebral arteries join to form the basilar artery and later branch to form the posterior cerebral arteries. Like the carotid arteries in the front of the brain, the vertebral ar-

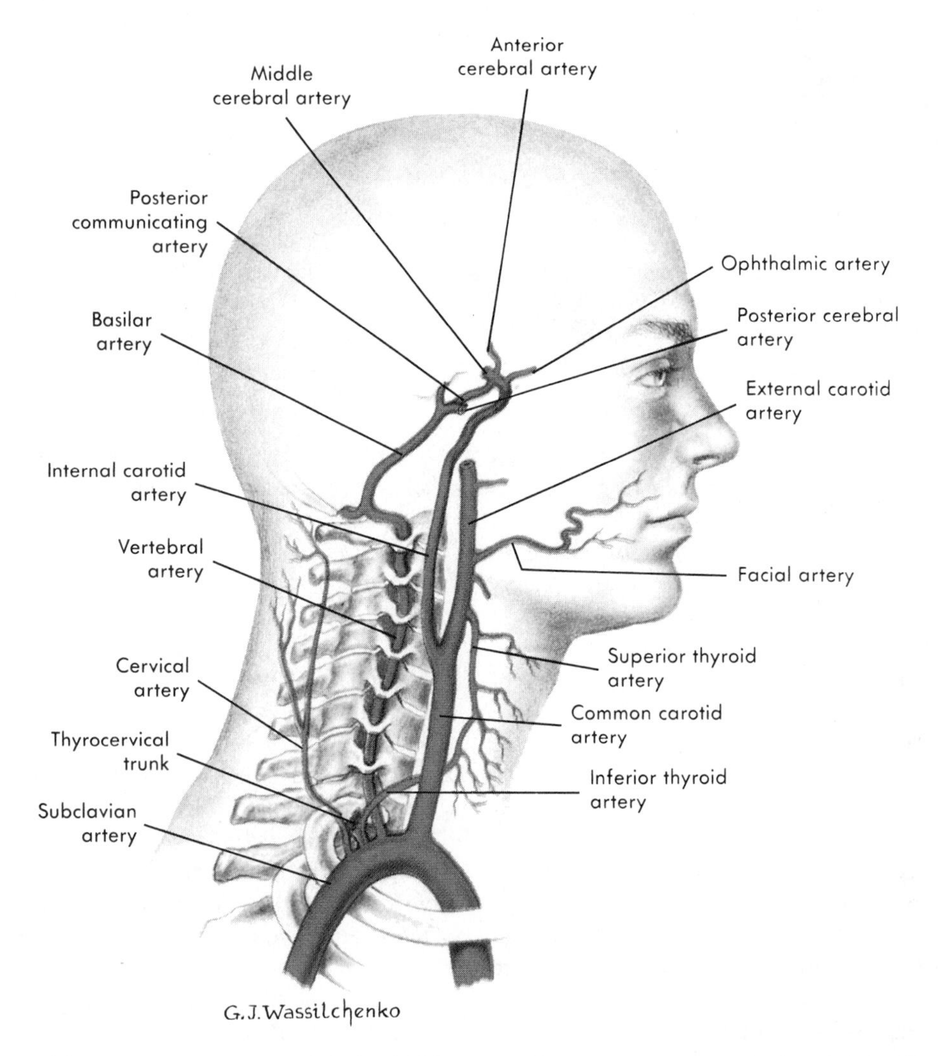

Figure 15-8 Anatomic diagram of circle of Willis. (From Chipps, E., Clanin, N., & Campbell, V. [1992]. *Neurologic disorders.* St. Louis: Mosby.)

teries first join the circle of Willis before branching out. The basilar artery divides at the level of the midbrain and becomes the posterior cerebral arteries. The posterior cerebral arteries supply the diencephalon, as well as the temporal and occipital lobes. Arteries on the surface of the brain are called *superficial* or *conducting arteries,* and those projecting into the brain are called *penetrating* or *nutrient arteries.*

Branches of arteries off the vertebral artery and branches of arteries off the aorta provide arterial flow to the spinal cord. The anterior and posterior spinal arteries originate from the vertebral arteries at the level of the brainstem and descend along the spinal cord. Arteries originating from the aorta follow the path of spinal nerves through the vertebral column and divide into the anterior and posterior radicular arteries.

Disorders

Cerebral vascular accident (CVA) refers to any deficit in the vascular supply to the brain. Abnormalities include damage to the wall of the vessel, rupture of the vessel, occlusion from a thrombus or embolus, or a change in blood flow. The resultant effect on brain tissue is ischemic or hemorrhagic, either of which may lead to infarction. Thrombotic strokes result from disease or inflammation of the vessel wall, most often from the accumulation of plaque. They may be transient, such as transient ischemic attacks, with symptoms clearing in 24 hours; or may evolve to completed strokes, resulting in permanent damage. Embolic strokes generally originate in the heart, aorta, carotid arteries, or thoracic aorta, with the embolus traveling distally until it becomes lodged in the lumen of a vessel it cannot pass through. The location of damage from a vascular infarct is determined by the artery involved and the brain tissue that is compromised.

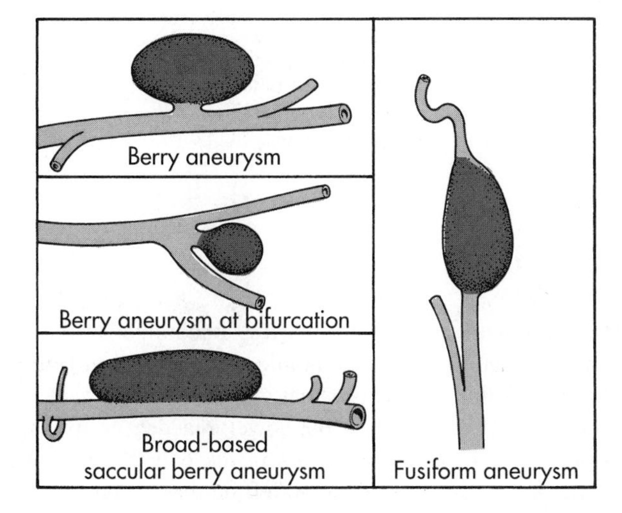

Figure 15-9 Types of aneurysms. (From McCance, K.L., & Huether, S.E. [1998]. *Pathophysiology: The biologic basis for disease in adults and children* [3rd ed.]. St. Louis: Mosby.)

Hemorrhagic strokes can result from hypertension, a ruptured aneurysm, an arteriovenous malformation, or a bleeding disorder. The location of the hemorrhage determines the type and extent of damage. In order of frequency, the locations of hemorrhagic strokes include the basal ganglia, cortex, thalamus, and cerebellum. Intracranial aneurysms may be genetic or may be caused by trauma, inflammation, or cocaine use. Most are located in or near the circle of Willis (Figure 15-9). An arteriovenous malformation is a bundle of anomalous blood vessels connecting the arterial and venous systems and may be located in any area of the brain, and symptoms due to a rupture generally occur between the ages of 10 and 20 years. Intracranial aneurysms due to arteriosclerosis, congenital anomaly, trauma, inflammation, or infection, occur most often near or on the circle of Willis. Often more than one aneurysm is present, and the peak incidence is between 35 and 60 years of age. Lacunar strokes are small infarcts generally caused by hypertension. They are most often located in the basal ganglia, internal capsule, and brainstem and may result in specific deficits of only sensory or motor deficits.

Autonomic Nervous System

The autonomic nervous system regulates the internal organs by balancing sympathetic and parasympathetic innervation to maintain equilibrium and/or respond to body demands. It is an involuntary system for the most part and includes components of the central and peripheral nervous systems. The sympathetic nervous system mobilizes energy to respond to real or perceived threats through a mechanism of "fight or flight." The cell bodies for the sympathetic system are located in the spinal cord between T1 and L2 and are collectively called the *thoracolumbar division.* Impulses leave the cord and travel to the sympathetic ganglia, a series of bead-shaped neuron groupings that run parallel to the spinal cord, and travel to the internal organs including the circulatory system (Figure 15-10).

The parasympathetic system is generally oppositional to the sympathetic system, acting to restore equilibrium and conserve energy. Innervation for the parasympathetic system begins in cranial nerves III (oculomotor), VII (facial), IX (glossopharyngeal), and X (vagus), as well as in the sacral region of the spinal cord. Internal organs are innervated, and in the pelvic region the pelvic nerve is composed of a group of preganglionic axons, innervating the viscera of the pelvic cavity (Figure 15-11).

The autonomic nervous system functions with the use of several neurotransmitters that are also used by neurons in the CNS. Acetylcholine is released by the preganglionic neurons of both the sympathetic and parasympathetic systems and initiates cholinergic transmission. Norepinephrine or adrenaline is released by postganglionic sympathetic neurons of the sympathetic division only and is considered an adrenergic transmission. Adrenergic and cholinergic effects,

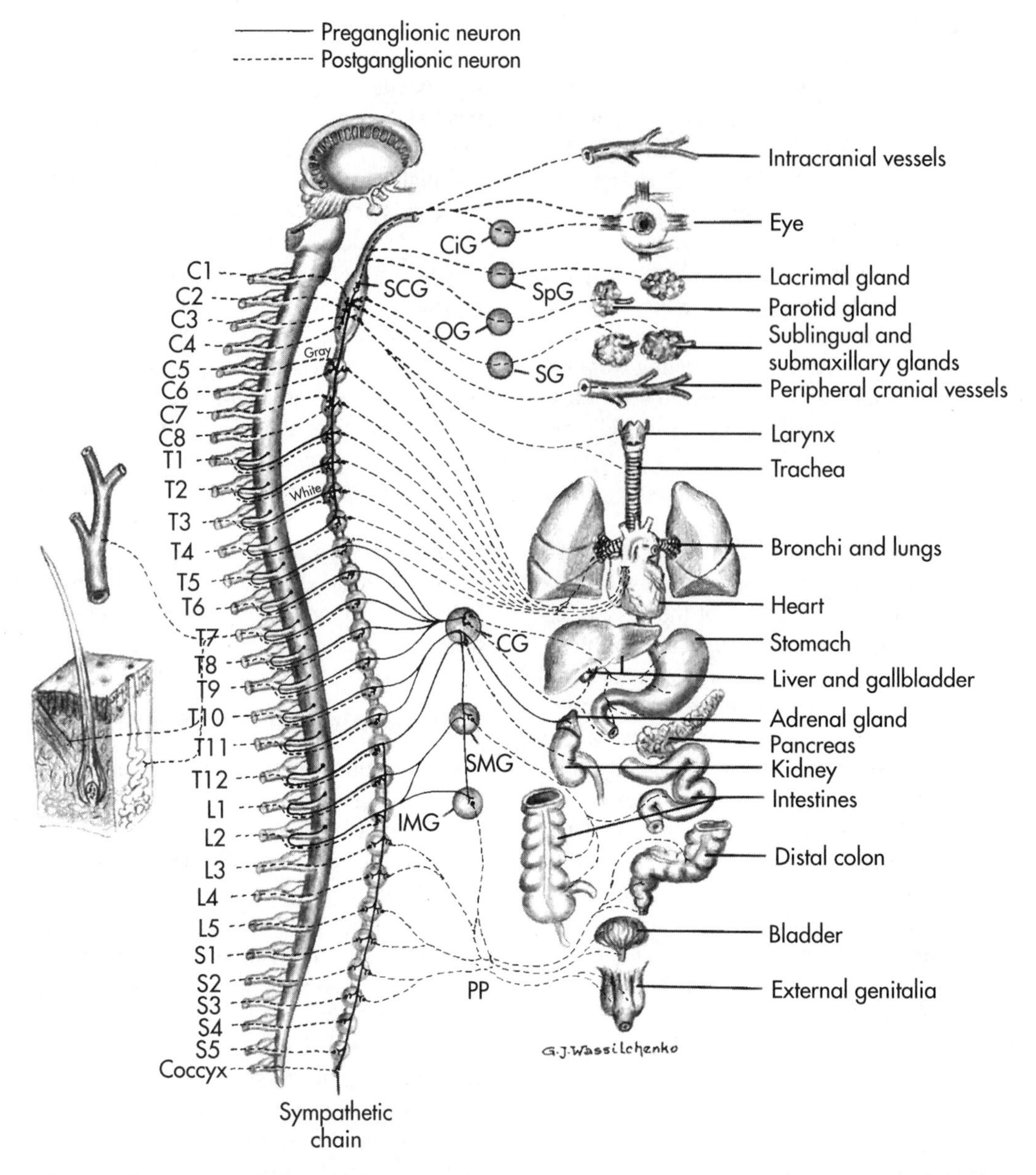

Figure 15-10 Sympathetic division of the autonomic nervous system. *CiG,* Ciliary ganglion; *SpG,* sphenopalatine ganglion; *SCG,* superior cervical ganglion; *OG,* otic ganglion; *SG,* submandibular ganglion; *CG,* celiac ganglion; *SMG,* superior mesenteric ganglion; *IMG,* inferior mesenteric ganglion; *PP,* pelvic plexus. (From Rudy, E.B. [1984]. *Advanced neurological and neurosurgical nursing.* St. Louis: Mosby.)

for the most part, produce opposite effects on each organ. The receptor sites for these adrenergic neurotransmitters are divided into alpha and beta receptors and are further subdivided into alpha 1 and 2, and beta 1 and 2 receptors. Each receptor site responds differently to adrenergic (adrenalin) and cholinergic (acetylcholine) innervation, creating complex patterns of contraction and relaxation. The sympathetic nervous system produces a more widespread response (e.g., a fight-or-flight response to a perceived threat), whereas the parasympathetic system is more localized (e.g., bladder contraction).

Disorders

In clients with spinal cord injuries, autonomic dysreflexia is a malfunction of the autonomic nervous system (Figure 15-12). The initial stimulus that triggers this reflex can be distention of the viscera of the bowel, bladder, or abdomen or stimulation of pain receptors in the pelvic region. Removal of the trigger is essential; left untreated, the situation may become fatal. Chapter 19 contains a detailed algorithm for autonomic dysreflexia.

Bladder and bowel deficits in rehabilitation clients result from defects in the central and peripheral nervous systems

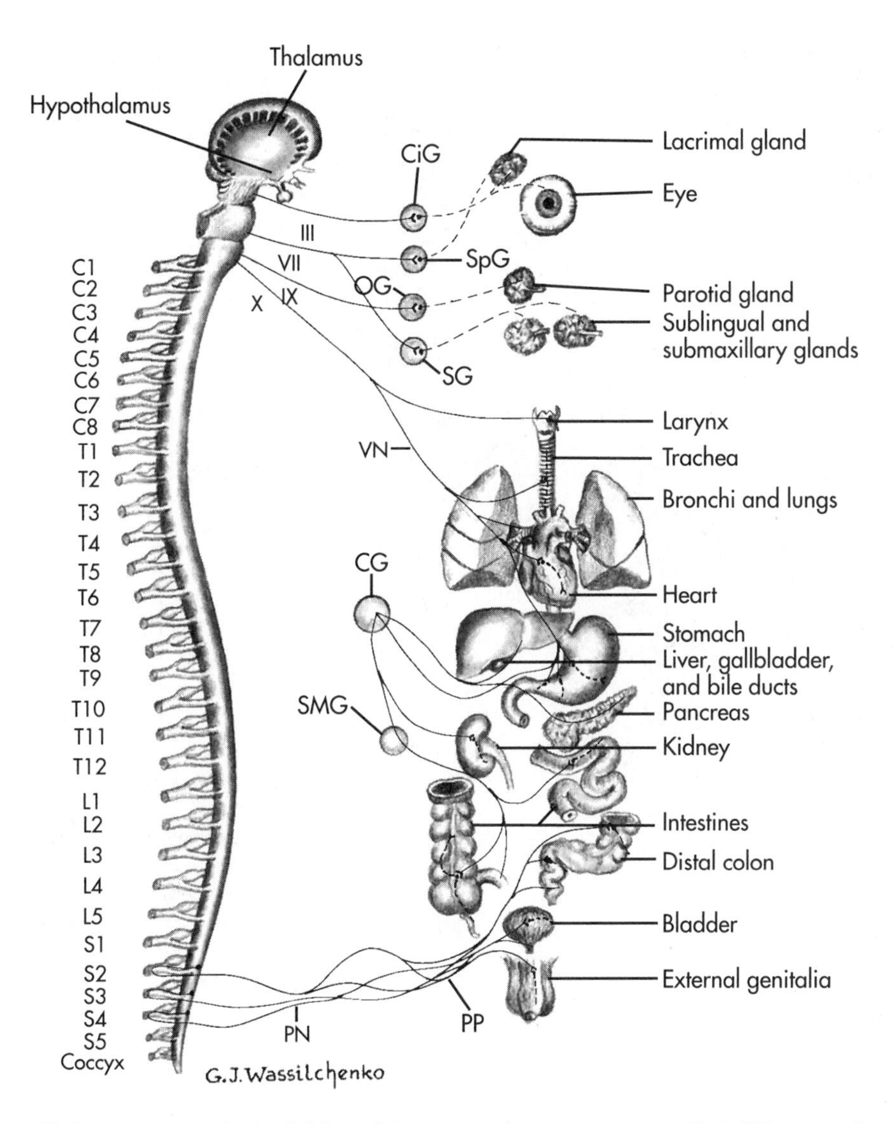

Figure 15-11 Parasympathetic division of the autonomic nervous system. *CiG,* Ciliary ganglion; *SpG,* sphenopalatine ganglion; *OG,* otic ganglion; *SG,* submandibular ganglion; *VN,* vagus nerve; *CG,* celiac ganglion; *SMG,* superior mesenteric ganglion; *PP,* pelvic plexus; *PN,* pelvic nerve. Fibers of the parasympathetic system pass through the celiac ganglion and superior mesenteric ganglion, but these ganglia are not part of the parasympathetic system. (From Rudy, E.B. [1984]. *Advanced neurological and neurosurgical nursing.* St. Louis: Mosby.)

and/or defects in the autonomic nervous system. Normal micturition relies on filling of the bladder under the regulation of the sympathetic division and emptying of the bladder innervated by the parasympathetic division. Bowel function relies on parasympathetic activity to innervate peristalsis and sympathetic activity to relax the bowel. Spinal cord injury and a number of neurological diseases can interrupt both voluntary control and regulation of the bowel and bladder, whereas brain deficits as a result of injury or disease can interrupt sensory and motor control.

Extrapyramidal System

The extrapyramidal system is composed of a number of structures that complement motor function and do not transmit within the pyramidal tract. In contrast to the pyramidal system, which is voluntary and, when injured, is marked by moderation of muscle tone, the extrapyramidal system is largely involuntary and provides for integrated and smooth movement. The structures of the extrapyramidal system are the basal ganglia and the cerebellum.

Disorders of the extrapyramidal system can be temporary or permanent, and include disorders of posture and movement that differ significantly from pyramidal disorders such as paralysis and hyperreflexia. Basal ganglia motor syndromes result in either an absence or excess of movement and have associated alterations in muscle tone and posture such as chorea, athetosis, and dystonia. Chapter 14 contains more information on involuntary movements. Cerebellar motor syndromes result in disorders of gait and balance,

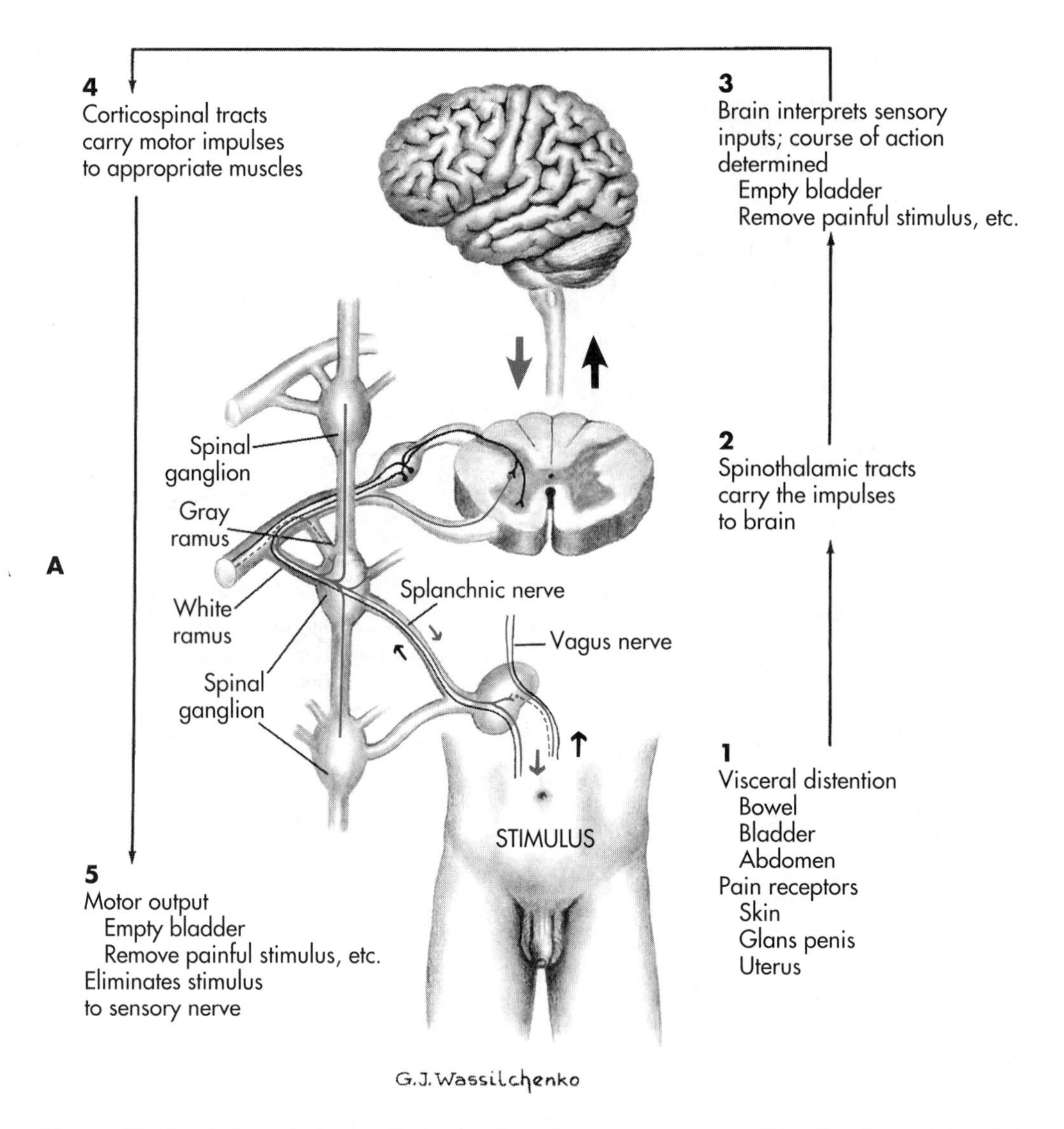

Figure 15-12 Autonomic hyperreflexia. **A,** Normal response pathway. (Modified from Rudy, E.B. [1984]. *Advanced neurological and neurosurgical nursing.* St. Louis: Mosby.)

poor coordination, and loss of control of the force and direction of movement.

Parkinsonism can be classified as either Parkinson's disease (Chapter 22) or secondary parkinsonism. Secondary parkinsonism is associated with trauma, infection, atherosclerosis, toxins, anoxia, or drug intoxication. Huntington's chorea, a hereditary disease involving diffuse damage to the basal ganglia and cerebral cortex, appears in mid-life. It is characterized by abnormal movement (choreiform or chorea) and progressive dementia along with psychiatric symptoms.

Limbic System

The limbic system, often referred to as the affective brain, is buried in the cerebrum and is responsible for emotion. The limbic system includes the hypothalamus, amygdala, hippocampus, septal nuclei, cingulate, orbital frontal lobes, and several other minor structures. Limbic activity is closely linked with temporal lobe activity. In the animal kingdom the limbic system is largely responsible for emotionality that is protective to an organism and closely linked to survival. Some of the survival emotions that originate in the limbic system are rage, hunger, thirst, and sex drive. In addition, memory is integrated with the limbic system, including the laying down of new memory and the retrieval of old memory related to emotional response.

The limbic system is highly integrated, facilitating rapid response. In human beings the limbic system continues to initiate emotionality, but the frontal cortex in conjunction with other cortical regions modulates the response. For example, the impulse to punch another person is interrupted by frontal lobe mediation based on the memory that punching another person has consequences that are undesirable, such as being arrested. Interruption in the inhibition of the limbic system by the frontal lobe results in emotional responses be-

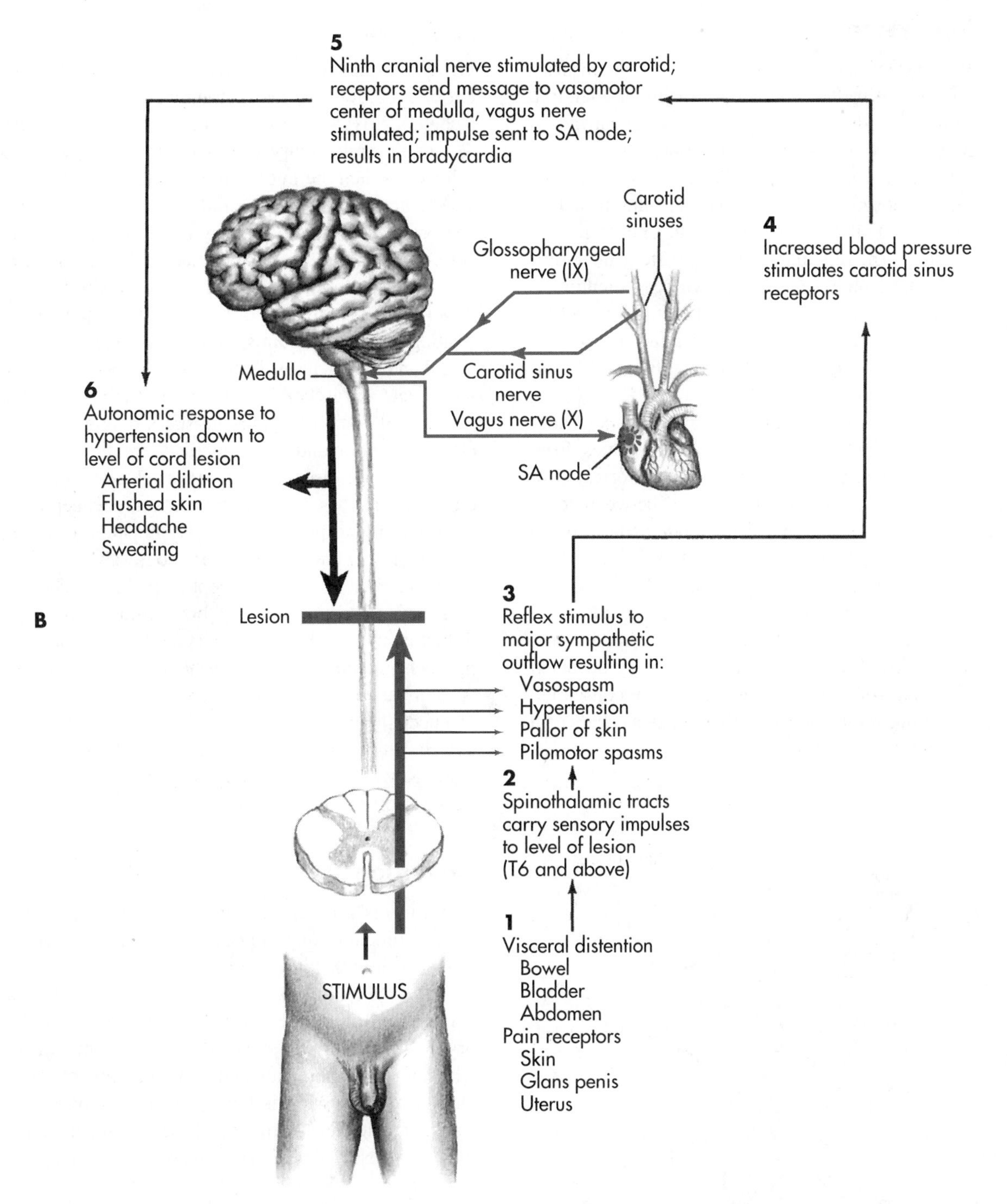

Figure 15-12, cont'd Autonomic hyperreflexia. **B,** Autonomic dysreflexia pathway.

ing displayed, largely unchecked, referred to as *lability* or *emotional incontinence.*

Disorders

Behavioral disorders, particularly after traumatic brain injury, include agitation, anger, hypersexuality, overeating, and hyperactivity. These disorders are most prominent during the initial recovery from coma, decreasing in prominence over time. However, some behavioral disorders may persist depending on the extent and nature of the injury. Memory deficits inhibit the ability to lay down new memory and to retrieve old memory. Memory deficits can occur in brain trauma, brain tumors, and a number of diseases, including dementia. Temporal lobe epilepsy includes personality changes, sexual disturbances, emotional outbursts, and exaggerated mood. The temporal lobe and the amygdala have very low seizure thresholds, increasing the risk for seizure activity.

Attention System

The attention system determines the state of consciousness, including arousal, as well as content of thought or attention. Full consciousness indicates being fully awake and aware as well as the capacity to respond appropriately to external stimuli. The attention system includes the reticular activating system, composed of the medulla, reticular formatio, substantia nigra, red nucleus, and cortex; the brainstem; and the limbic system. The reticular activating system and brainstem primarily determine wakefulness, whereas attention to the environment includes the additional function of the limbic system and cortical regions. The tentorium is the projection of dura mater that separates the cerebellum and brainstem from the cerebral hemispheres (Figure 15-13).

Level of consciousness is a critical clinical index of neurological status and includes a range of possible states, from being in a deep coma to being fully alert and oriented to time, place, and person. The range of states between coma and full consciousness are poorly defined but include confusion, disorientation, lethargy, obtunded, and stupor. Alterations in consciousness may be accompanied by changes in patterns of breathing, in pupillary response, in oculomotor response (doll's eyes), and in motor response. The Glasgow Coma Scale (GCS) (Chapter 26) is a universally accepted measure of the state of coma. Changes in level of consciousness are important indicators of a physiological change in neurological function.

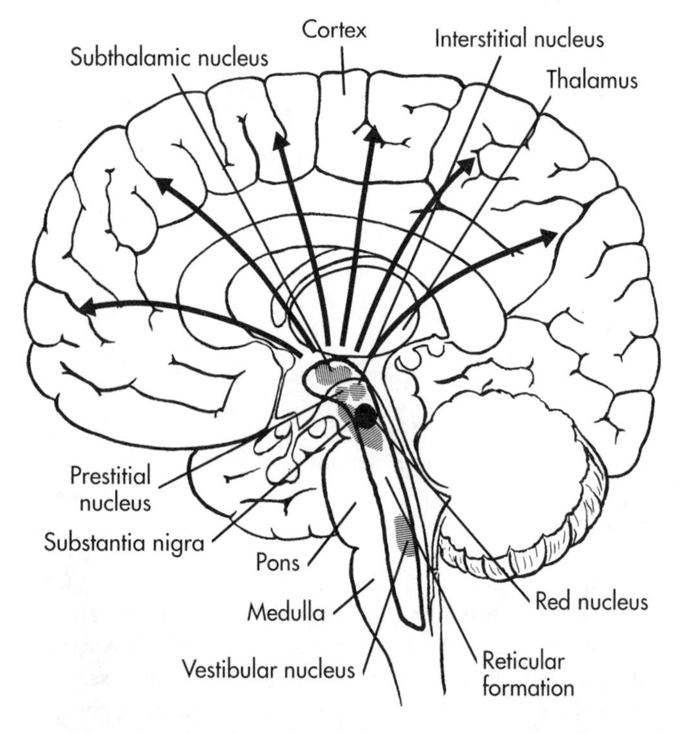

Figure 15-13 Reticular activating system. (From Thompson, J.M., McFarland, G.K., Hirsch, J.E., & Tucker, S.M. [1998]. *Mosby's clinical nursing* [4th ed.]. St. Louis: Mosby.)

Disorders

Deficits in the attention system may be the result of a number of conditions, including trauma, tumor, vascular defects, ischemia, toxicity, disease, and/or psychogenic disorders. Traumatic brain injury is a frequent cause of altered consciousness, and the initial injury to the brain in moderate to severe brain injury is generally associated with decreased cerebral perfusion followed by increasing intracranial pressure due to edema that may peak several days after the injury. Transtentorial herniation of the cerebral hemispheres down onto the brainstem directly impacts on the reticular activating system structures, and the associated coma is profound and often causes death. Brain tumors as well as vascular defects and ischemia of the brain such as by stroke may result in alterations in consciousness ranging from coma to altered attention and including disorientation.

Among the diseases that can produce metabolically induced alterations in consciousness are encephalopathies. In children, encephalopathies may be static or nonprogressive, such as cerebral palsy, or progressive, such as metabolic deficiencies. Static encephalopathies such as cerebral palsy are often the result of brain injury during gestation or birth, and the extent of injury may vary from motor impairment to cognitive impairment and seizure disorders. A number of inherited metabolic disorders may result in encephalopathy, including phenylketonuria (PKU) and Tay-Sachs disease. Acute encephalopathies in children include Reye's syndrome, drug-induced encephalopathy, and lead poisoning.

Cognition

Cognition is a composite of a number of separate mostly cortical functions that can be categorized using the computer model of input, storage, processing, and output. Reception includes the ability to attend to stimuli and select, acquire, classify, and integrate information. Storage includes memory and learning, in contrast to processing or thinking, which is the organization and reorganization of information. Output or expression is how the information is communicated or acted on. Although these are separate functions, they are closely linked with much interdependence on one another.

Input or sensory cognitive functions include the sensation and perception of stimuli and rely on the arousal process, triggering the process of cognition to begin. Sensation includes all of the sensory organs of hearing, vision, taste, smell, and touch and the transmission of the information to the brain for perception. Perception is continually processing vast numbers of sensations and includes awareness, recognition, discrimination, patterning, and orientation. Disorders of perception include a number of agnosias, which are disorders of recognition.

Storage, or memory, is essential to all learning as well as to the ability to go beyond basic impulses and provide a context to information and decision making. Disturbances in memory can cause tremendous impairment in function that may be temporary or permanent. Memory can be divided into primary memory including registration and short-term storage, and secondary memory, including the consolidation, long-term storage, and retrieval of memory. Memory defects can range from altered consciousness to amnesia and forgetting.

Processing, or thinking, includes the combination of two bits of information and the ability to make sense of them. Thinking includes a number of complex cognitive processes such as reasoning, judgment, and problem solving. The process of thinking is a function of the whole brain and is not localized to any particular region. It is important to distinguish various aspects of cognitive function from intelligence. Defects in cognitive function do not necessarily indicate lower intelligence. In understanding the effect of brain damage on cognitive function, intelligence has limited use.

Output or expression includes all aspects of observable behavior, including speech, physical gestures, facial expressions, and drawing or writing. It is important to note that disorders of expression do not indicate that other aspects of cognitive function are necessarily impaired. Disorders of expression include apraxia, constructional disorders, and aphasias. Apraxia is a defect of purposeful expression, often unconscious, that requires sequencing of motor activity. Constructional disorders, often classified as apraxias, include visual-spatial defects and an inability to recognize spatial relationships. Aphasia and dysphasia refer to deficits in language formulation. There are several classifications of aphasia, and defects may include expression, programming sequence, conduction, and comprehension.

Disorders

Deficits in cognition can be genetic or acquired and are often associated with brain damage and/or diseases that also affect other aspects of neurological function. Brain damage as a result of brain injury, neurological disease, or stroke can result in variations in cognitive function, including coma, memory disturbances, thinking disturbances including reasoning, and/or disorders of expression. Therefore cognitive deficits are often reported as additional diagnoses to be more specific. Neuropsychological testing can provide a comprehensive picture of cognitive deficits for an individual client.

Acute confusional states may result from toxicity such as alcohol or drug intoxication, diseases of the nervous system, or in association with systemic diseases such as fever or heart failure. Dementing diseases include Alzheimer's disease, Creutzfeldt-Jakob disease, Huntington's disease, Parkinson's disease, and progressive supranuclear palsy. Aging is associated with an increased risk of organic deterioration, with some cognitive changes that are considered normal aging and others that indicate underlying pathology.

16 Skin Integrity

Kelly M. M. Johnson, MSN, RN, CFNP, CRRN
Grace Nolde-Lopez, MSN, RN, CWCON, CRRN

Marta was a beautiful 11-year-old Tarahumara Indian girl from the remote Sierra Madre Mountains of Mexico. The Tarahumara Indians are an indigenous people of the Sierra Occidental of Mexico who live and work in the mountains and canyons above Chihuahua, Mexico. The area is remote and rugged, with most Tarahumara families living in caves in the mountains and canyons. When Marta was injured by gunfire and left with paraplegia, she was sent to a remote village in the mountains to live with and care for other persons with disabilities. Marta developed a pressure ulcer and was treating herself and other villager's pressure ulcers with sugar and bandages. After many months of living with a nonhealing ulcer, Marta was sent to a California facility to receive rehabilitation and management of her pressure ulcer. Marta's grade III ischial ulcer quickly healed without the need for surgical intervention. She was fitted with an appropriate wheelchair for the terrain in which she lived and was also provided with primary and backup cushions. The rehabilitation nurses, in collaboration with the interdisciplinary team, spent a great deal of time teaching Marta how to care for her skin and how to prevent further occurrences of pressure ulcers. Marta would be expected to continue in her role as a caregiver to other persons with higher level spinal cord injuries and other debilitating conditions, so her education included information on the care of pressure ulcers and prevention techniques. Marta was taught about moist wound healing, and the nurses showed her how to sterilize water, how to make saline solution, and how to fabricate dressings from available materials. All written materials were sent home with Marta in Spanish to be used for education with her community. Marta was seen for a reevaluation the next year, and she had no further occurrences of pressure ulcers.

This chapter presents nursing diagnoses, interventions, and outcomes for preservation and management of skin integrity. A research-based practice and a sound understanding of the physiological basis of skin management will enable the rehabilitation nurse to select interventions that are most effective in preventing alteration in skin integrity and restoring a wound with the least energy expenditure by clients. The appropriate use of interventions reduces emotional and monetary cost to the client, the family, and the health care system.

Alterations in skin integrity account for untold amounts of pain, suffering, and dollars expended for health care. Failure to maintain skin integrity will extend the length of stay in a health care facility, increase health care costs, increase comorbidities, increase nosocomial infections, and increase other complications (Allman, Goode, Burst, Bartolucci, & Thomas, 1999). Pressure ulcers may also interfere with an individual's ability to perform self-care tasks and resume social roles. In some instances loss of skin integrity can be life-threatening. Ultimately, pressure ulcers and related problems prevent many individuals from reaching their potential for independent function; for others they add to impairment, further disability, or prohibit employment. Pressure ulcers are any lesions produced by excessive, unrelieved pressure that results in damage of the underlying tissue (Panel for Prediction and Prevention of Pressure Ulcers in Adults [PPPPUA], 1992/1994). Descriptions of pressure sores, decubitus ulcers, or bedsores that imply the bed or recumbent position, rather than pressure, are causes are inaccurate (Maklebust & Margolis, 1995).

ECONOMIC IMPLICATIONS

The Agency for Healthcare Research and Quality (AHRQ) (formerly the Agency for Health Care Policy and Research [AHCPR]) clinical practice guideline on prevention of pressure ulcers notes that the total national cost of pressure ulcer treatment exceeded $1.3 billion (AHCPR, 1992/1994), an estimated $2000 to $30,000 per pressure ulcer (National

Pressure Ulcer Advisory Panel [NPUAP], 1989). Leg ulcers cost about $1 billion per year, or about $2000 per ulcer. They are complications adding to cost by lengthening hospital stay, extending recuperation time, delaying return to home and work, and adding risks for other complications (Bryant, Shannon, Pieper, Braden, & Morris, 1992). Economic changes in the health care arena have caused the health care system to become increasingly cost conscious and outcome oriented. Pressure ulcers must be viewed as preventable and not a de facto complication of illness and immobility (Copeland-Fields & Hoshiko, 1989). Venous ulcers affect an estimated 2.5 million persons, with a treatment cost totalling $2.5 billion to $3.5 billion, or about $2750 per ulcer (Hess, 2000; Schonfeld, Nilla, Fastenau, Mazonson, & Falanga, 2000).

INCIDENCE AND PREVALENCE

Despite increased awareness of the incidence and prevalence of pressure ulcers, improvements in assessment of risk, extensive research on prevention and management, and ongoing development of prevention and treatment products, pressure ulcers remain one of the most prevalent and costly complications in health care. Each year in the United States 60,000 persons die of pressure ulcer–related medical complications (Kynes, 1986), and more than 1 million persons in acute care and skilled nursing facilities have pressure ulcers (Tourtual et al., 1997).

Age is a definitive factor, with incidence rates for those older than 70 years at 7.7% to 23.1% (Allman, 1997), soaring to 23% to 37% in hospitalized elderly clients (Allman et al., 1986). Prevalence rates in older persons continue to be high at 11.6% to 27.5% (Schue & Langemo, 1998) and in hospitals as high as 36.4% (Baeczak, Barnett, Childs, & Bosley, 1997). Being elderly and receiving some type of institutional care is a high risk factor for developing pressure ulcers. Brandeis, Morris, Nash, and Lipsitz (1990) conducted a large-scale longitudinal multisite study of elderly persons and found a prevalence rate of 17.4%; strikingly 83.4% of persons who developed ulcers had been treated in the hospital. Brandeis et al. compared their data with Berlowitz and Wilking's (1989) finding of a 33% prevalence rate, which was attributed to older age, reduced ambulation, altered continence, and presence of chronic, debilitating conditions. Those in nursing homes fare no better, with an incidence of 10.8% to 38.5%; prevalence ranges are 1.2% to 11.2% (Berlowitz, Bezerra, Brandeis, Kader, & Anderson, 2000).

Few factors stand alone; as with many chronic and disabling conditions, many factors lead to complications, but immobility and pressure stand out. Hospitalization and health status are notable in development of pressure ulcers among all clients. Clients who were hospitalized due to trauma (n = 148) had prevalence rates of 20.3% after 2 days (Watts et al., 1998), whereas the incidence of pressure ulcers among clients in critical care was 12%, 82% of which developed in the first 72 hours after admission (Carlson, Kemp, & Shott, 1999).

Health status influences outcome; clients who were predominately postsurgical acquired stage I ulcers, whereas those with chronic conditions that affected tissue perfusion, such as respiratory diseases (50%) and diabetes mellitus (12%), developed pressure ulcers. The group who developed pressure ulcers had lower hemoglobin levels and spent more time in bed and less time in a chair than clients who did not develop problems (Olsen et al., 1996). Persons with spinal cord injury (SCI) have great risks for developing pressure ulcers; this is discussed later in the chapter.

ANATOMY AND PHYSIOLOGY OF THE SKIN

The nurse providing coordination and delivery of skin and wound care requires a thorough understanding of the normal physiologic processes and the factors that alter them (Waldrop & Doughty, 2000).

Skin Integrity

A cross-section of the skin is represented in Figure 16-1. The functions of the skin are thermoregulation of body temperature, protection from injury, sensation, metabolism, communication, and identification. The epidermis shields the underlying tissues against water loss, mechanical injury, and effects of harmful chemicals; when unbroken it prevents microorganisms from penetrating the skin. The fibrous connective tissue of the dermis supports the epidermis. Tough, elastic, and flexible, this layer contains fibroblasts that synthesize and secrete the two main proteins, collagen and elastin. Collagen gives skin its tone and tensile strength (Wysocki, 2000), and elastin provides elastic recoil (Moore & Dalley, 1999).

The blood supply to the skin serves two important functions: oxygen and nourishment for the skin and thermoregulation for the body. The avascular epidermis is nourished by the blood supply (microcirculation) in the dermal and hypodermal layers (Bates-Jensen, 1998).

Circulation and sweating account for the thermoregulatory activity of the skin. Vasodilation dissipates body heat; vasoconstriction maintains it and shunts heat to underlying body organs. Sweat glands under control of the nervous system respond to temperature changes and emotional stimulation. Evaporation of moisture on the skin through the sweat glands lowers body temperature. The skin protects the body against mechanical, chemical, viral, bacterial, and ultraviolet insults and prevents excess loss of fluids and electrolytes. Vitamin D assists with calcium and phosphate metabolism and is important to the mineralization of bone and teeth. Vitamin D is synthesized in the skin with exposure to sunlight.

Communication with the environment and interactions for safety depend on the transmission and interpretation of pain, temperature, touch, and pressure sensations. These

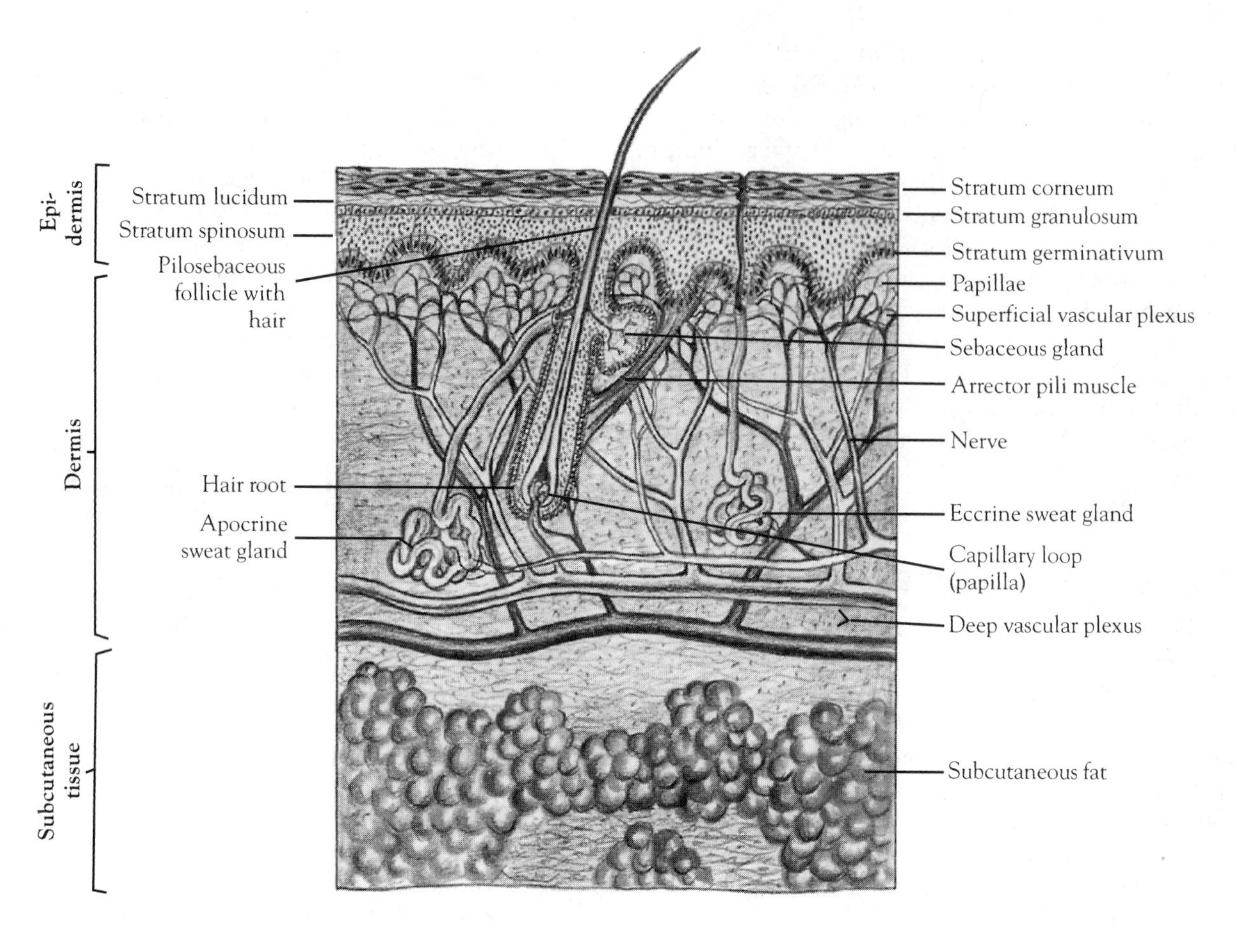

Figure 16-1 Structures of the skin. (From Thompson, J.M., McFarland, G.K., Hirsch, J.E., & Tucker, S.M. [1997]. *Mosby's clinical nursing* [4th ed.]. St. Louis: Mosby.)

stimuli are transmitted through nerve cell receptors located in the skin, and resulting messages are transmitted to the cerebral cortex through the spinal cord and autonomic nervous system. The skin also functions as an organ of communication and identification, contributing to appearance and nonverbal communication. Facial skin expresses smiling, frowning, pouting, and grimacing as a means of conveying feelings and projecting body image. Physical changes in skin can affect the person from a psychosocial as well as a physical aspect. For example, disfigurement can influence feelings about self-image, especially for adolescents who are sensitive about their appearance and very susceptible to lowered self-esteem. Changes during the aging process can influence self-perception and self-esteem.

ALTERED FUNCTION OF THE SKIN

A number of factors can alter the characteristics of the skin: aging, sun exposure, hydration, nutrition, skin-cleaning products, and medications (Boynton, Jaworski, & Paustian, 1999; PPPPUA, 1992). Many changes occur in skin throughout the life span that increase the susceptibility to injury and extend time for wound healing. Decreases in epidermal turnover (rate is doubled by 35 years of age), slower epithelialization, and reduced vitamin D production and inflammatory response occur with aging. Diminished sensory receptors decrease awareness of when the skin is being damaged, and reduced numbers of sweat glands, diminished vascularity, and reduction of subcutaneous fat result in less thermoregulation. Reduced immunocompetence makes skin more prone to cancer and infection, and capillary fragility and dermal-epidermal junction changes allow more bruising and tearing (Kudravi & Reed, 2000). The changes of aging skin impair the ability to distribute pressure effectively and vascularize compromised tissue, especially when elderly clients are confronted with several stressors at one time. Elderly skin simply is more susceptible to forces of pressure, shear, and friction.

Ultraviolet rays accelerate aging of the skin, increase the risk of cancer, and reduce the immunocompetence of the skin. A number of factors affect skin hydration, including the amount of sebum in the skin and the relative environmental humidity. Reduced hydration will lead to dryness with itching and scaling and may contribute to decreased resistance to skin breakdown. Many nutrients, including protein, carbohydrates, fats, vitamins, and minerals, are required to maintain healthy skin and prevent injury. Balanced dietary intake should be sufficient in most cases to maintain

TABLE 16-1 Role of Selected Nutrients in Wound Healing

Nutrient	Function
Protein	Cell multiplication, antibody production, wound remodeling; promotes angiogenesis and collagen synthesis
Carbohydrates	Provide energy to leukocytes and fibroblasts; cofactor for synthesis of fatty acids and some amino acids
Vitamin A	Promotes epithelialization and collagen synthesis; factor in inflammatory response
Vitamin B complex	Promotes protein synthesis; enhances antibody formation to promote immunity; cofactors in enzyme systems and cellular development; amino acid metabolism
Vitamin C	Hydroxylation of amino acids; immune reaction; promotes collagen synthesis for scar formation, capillary formation, and capillary permeability
Vitamin D	Absorption and metabolism of calcium from small intestine necessary for collagen maturation
Vitamin E	Antiinflammatory action; role in wound healing poorly understood
Vitamin K	Protein synthesis; prothrombin synthesis; synthesis of blood clotting factors VII, IX, X
Amino acids	Protein synthesis
Albumin	Maintenance of capillary colloid osmotic pressure
Essential fatty acids	Provide energy to leukocytes and fibroblasts; building blocks for prostaglandins; provide cellular membrane integrity
Copper	Component of enzyme systems in collagen maturation strength; hemoglobin synthesis
Iron	Hydroxylation of amino acids for collagen synthesis; supports oxygen transport via red blood cell formation
Magnesium	Activates enzymes for protein synthesis
Zinc	Role in vitamin A transport and plasma vitamin A concentration; promotes collagen and noncollagen protein activity in granulation tissue; stabilizes cellular membranes; cofactor in enzyme systems

From Andrychuk, M.A. (1998). Pressure ulcers: causes, risk factors, assessment and intervention. *Orthopaedic Nursing, 17*(4), 65-82.

healthy skin and prevent injury; inadequate nutrition will influence the health of the skin and wound healing. Many experts consider nutrition to be an extremely critical factor—second only to immobility—in the causation of pressure ulcers (Ayello, Thomas, & Litchford, 1999).

Vitamins C, A, and E; zinc; protein; and individual amino acids all have been identified as necessary for prevention of pressure ulcers and for adequate wound healing (Thomas, 1997). Malnutrition has been reported in 52% to 85% of institutionalized elderly persons (Zulkowski, 1999). Hypoproteinemia leads to interstitial edema, which impairs the cellular transport of oxygen and nutrients. Vitamin C deficiencies can lead to capillary fragility and an impaired immune system (Ayello, Thomas, & Litchford, 1999; Stotts, 2000). Low serum albumin levels have been highly associated with pressure ulcer development (Bates-Jensen, 1998).

Two prospective studies show evidence that poor diet—especially inadequate intake of calories, protein, and iron—is a causative factor in pressure ulcer development (Bergstrom & Braden, 1992; PPPPUA, 1992). However, obese persons have many nutritional deficits and may have malnutrition despite their adequate calorie intake (Gallagher, 1997). Those with long-term tetraplegia are often in a hypometabolic state and frequently restrict their intake to control their weight, but they also have a significant increase in resting energy expenditure when a pressure ulcer is present (Lui, Spungen, Fink, Losada, & Bauman, 1996). Table 16-1 displays the role of select nutrients in wound healing, and Figure 16-2 contains the AHCPR algorithm of recommendations for nutritional assessment and support for a client who has an existing pressure ulcer.

Skin-cleaning products influence health of the skin. Alkaline soaps reduce the thickness and number of cell layers in the stratum corneum. Excessive use of skin-cleaning products removes the sebum coating and its antibacterial and antidehydration properties, leading to dryness and increased opportunity for infection. Many classifications of medications can affect the skin; corticosteroids interfere with epidermal proliferation, and others have photosensitizing effects. A thorough review of the medication profile of every client is essential to assess for possible medication effects on the skin.

Alteration in Skin Integrity: Contributing Factors

Alterations in skin integrity have a number of causes and contributing factors. Many are preventable; some are not. Even with diligent nursing care, some clients may develop alterations in skin integrity because of compromised medical status. Rehabilitation nurses must teach appropriate strategies to prevent skin problems at all levels of care, as well as how to best manage skin problems when they do occur.

Mechanical forces are frequent contributors to skin compromise and ultimately to skin breakdown. *Friction* is a mechanical force that occurs when the skin moves against a support surface, such as when extremities are brushed across a mattress. These movements can be inadvertent, as in spasticity, or due to carelessness. In its mildest form, friction produces skin tears—abrasions limited to the epidermal and dermal layers (Pieper, 2000). Friction decreases the amount of external pressure required to produce a pressure ulcer,

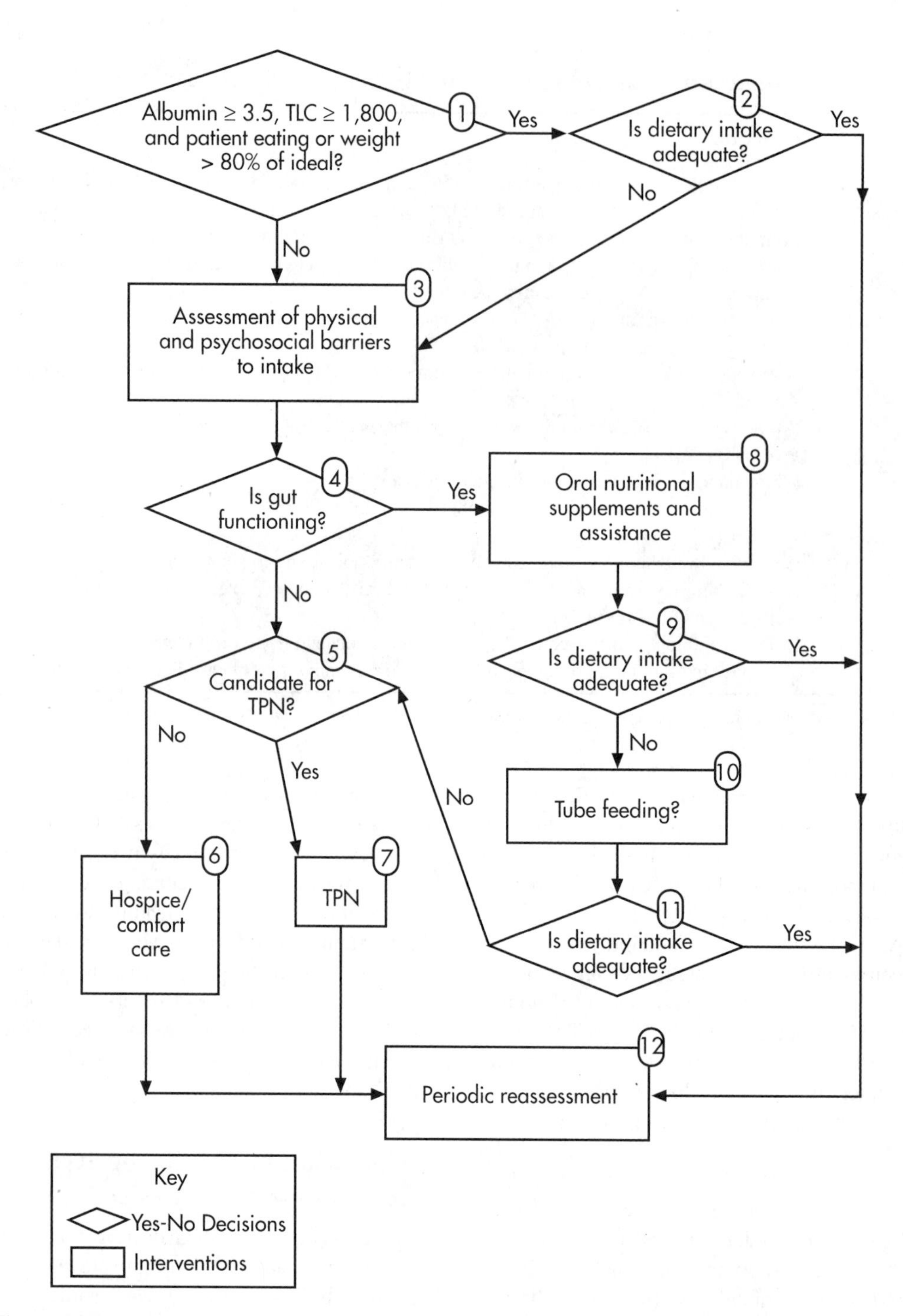

Figure 16-2 The AHCPR algorithm details recommendations for nutritional assessment and support for the client who has an existing pressure ulcer. *TLC,* Total lymphocyte count; *TPN,* total parenteral nutrition. (From Bergstrom, N., Bennett, M.A., Carlson, C.E., et al. [1994]. *Treatment of pressure ulcers: Clinical practice guidelines* [No. 15, AHCPR Publication No. 95-0652]. Rockville, MD: U.S. Department of Health and Human Services, Agency for Health Care Policy and Research.)

and when pressure combines with shear, friction contributes to extensive injury (PPPPUA, 1992).

Shear likewise contributes to pressure areas and other skin injuries. Shear injury occurs when the skin remains stationary and the underlying tissue shifts (PPPPUA, 1992). Shearing forces (Figure 16-3) are produced when adjacent surfaces slide over one another (Bryant, 2000). Early on Reichel (1958) found that shearing forces caused blood vessels to become angulated, disrupting the arteries of the skin from the blood supply of the muscle. The typical shear injury presents as a wound with a large amount of undermining. Common causes of shearing are spasticity, poor sitting posture, poor bed positioning, and sliding rather than lifting. When the head of the bed is elevated between 30 and 90 degrees,

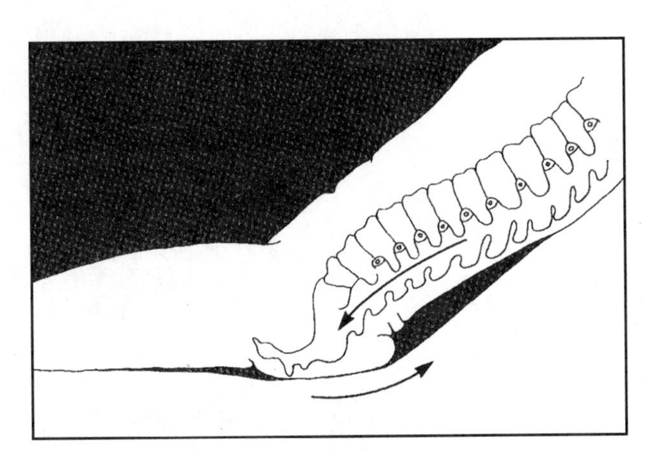

Figure 16-3 Shearing force. (From Bryant, R.A. [Ed.]. [2000]. *Acute and chronic wounds* [2nd ed]. St. Louis: Mosby.)

the client may slide down, producing shearing forces. The sacrum, with the attached muscle and fascia, slides down while the skin stays in place; this causes shearing (Pieper, 2000). Shearing is frequently responsible for the triangular lesions found over the sacrum and coccyx.

Skin tears occur when forces of minor friction or shearing cause the epidermis to separate from the dermis at the dermal-epidermal junction. The resulting injury is generally referred to as a *skin tear;* these most commonly occur on the extremities of older adults (Payne & Martin, 1993a, 1993b). Skin tears can result from such varied activities as grasping an extremity, dressing, bathing, performing a transfer, and scraping against objects such as tables and chairs (Bryant, 2000). Epidemiological studies suggest that at least 1.5 million skin tears occur each year in adults who are in institutions (Thomas, Goode, LaMaster, Tennyson, & Parnell, 1999).

Evidence supports that *moisture* alone can make the skin more susceptible to injury (PPPPUA, 1992). Moisture causes weakening of the connective tissue of the skin, making it five times as likely to become ulcerated as dry skin (Maklebust & Sieggreen, 1996). When exposed to prolonged moisture from sweating, urinary and fecal incontinence, and wound drainage, the skin can become macerated and develop a rash or become infected, predisposing it to pressure ulcer formation. Several researchers found incontinence to be a major risk factor for development of pressure ulcers. *Incontinence* is a major risk factor and the most reliable predictor for pressure ulcer formation, especially fecal incontinence (Allman, 1989) or urinary incontinence occurring with both friction and neurological disorders (Haalboom, den Boer, & Buskens, 1999).

External pressure applied to the skin for prolonged or unrelieved periods and in amounts in excess of capillary closing pressure will produce ischemia in underlying tissue. The blood vessels dilate in response to anoxia, leakage of fluid from the blood vessels causes interstitial edema, and forward flow of blood is impeded. The cells continue to produce metabolic byproducts that accumulate because they cannot be transported out as a result of vessel compromise. The amount of damage depends on pressure exerted and tissue involved. Cellular death can result (Alterescu & Alterescu, 1998).

Many chronic wounds can develop on the lower legs and feet due to *vascular damage.* Skin ulcers result from venous insufficiency, arterial insufficiency, and neuropathies. Although each produces wounds with unique characteristics (Table 16-2), accurate diagnostic studies to identify causes and comprehensive management using defined protocols are necessary to improve outcomes in hospital and community settings (Ghauri et al., 2000).

Immobility, a high risk factor for pressure ulceration, is discussed further in Chapter 14; closely related is inactivity. The less physically active the person, the greater the susceptibility to pressure ulcers. Those confined to bed and those using wheelchairs are more likely to develop pressure ulcers. There is a positive relationship between overall health and well-being and increased activity (PPPPUA, 1992).

Altered sensory perception, especially the inability to detect sensations that would indicate the need to change position, is rated as a highly critical factor for pressure ulcer development. Rehabilitation nurses placed sensory perception third behind immobility and inactivity as a risk very characteristic of clients with pressure ulcers (Copeland-Fields & Hoshiko, 1989).

Chemical damage to the skin may result from fecal and urinary incontinence, harsh products used in cleansing the skin and wounds (e.g., alcohol, povidone-iodine, and antacids), poorly contained drainage from acute and chronic wounds, and drainage from percutaneous tubes. Skin irritation also occurs when skin care products are used improperly. Choose skin cleansers carefully and use them appropriately to avoid disrupting the normal acid pH of the skin (Fiers, 1996). *Epidermal stripping* is the inadvertent removal of the epidermis by mechanical means such as tape removal (Bryant, 2000).

Radiation can damage the epidermis, presenting with dry skin due to destruction of sweat and sebaceous glands. Radiation reduces fibroblasts and destroys the cell nucleus, which can result in wide, shallow, irregularly bordered wounds. Radiation-induced ulcers appeared after being latent for 7 months to 8 years (Goldberg & McGinn-Byer, 2000). Irradiated skin requires continual assessment for changes and care to protect against mechanical and chemical assault.

Studies examining the role of smoking in the development of pressure areas for individuals with SCI found a positive correlation; the more persons smoked, the greater their incidence of pressure ulcers (Niazi, Salzberg, Byrne, & Viehbeck, 1997).

Researchers correlated increased body temperature with increased risk of pressure ulceration. Elevated temperature may put increased demands for oxygenation on already compromised tissue (Pieper, 2000). Diaphoresis can cause skin to become macerated, increasing risk. Heat can injure the skin due to excess thermal energy or accelerated meta-

Table 16-2 Wound Characteristics by Types

	Arterial Ulcer	Venous Ulcer	Diabetic Ulcer	Pressure Ulcer	Vasculitic Ulcer
Predisposing factors/cause	PVD, diabetes mellitus, advanced age	Valve incompetence in perforating veins, history of deep vein thrombophlebitis and thrombosis, failed calf pump, history of venous ulcers or family history of ulcers, obesity, age, pregnancy (in women with a family history of venous ulcers)	Diabetic client with peripheral neuropathy and/or peripheral vascular disease	Multiple medical diagnoses, age, impaired mobility, decreased mental status, poor nutritional status, incontinence, impaired circulation	Often accompanied by history of recurrence; almost always accompanied by connective tissue disease and systemic inflammatory conditions
Location and depth	Usually distal to impaired arterial supply, between toes or tips of toes, over phalangeal heads, around lateral malleolus, at sites subjected to trauma or rubbing of footwear; usually relatively shallow, but may be deep	May occur anywhere between the knee and ankle, with medial and lateral malleolus most common sites; usually shallow	Any sites on the foot and lower limb subjected to repetitive pressure, friction, shear, or trauma: plantar aspect, metatarsal heads (especially first and fifth), big toe, heel; shallow to deep, may have tracking and/or undermining	On heels, sacrum, coccyx, occiput, any bony prominences subjected to pressure, friction, or shear; depth ranges from persistent red, blue, or purple area of intact skin (depending on skin color) to deep destruction and loss of tissue	Below malleolus-foot dorsum; shallow
Wound bed and wound appearance	Pale, gray, or yellow, with no evidence of new tissue growth; necrosis or cellulitis may be present; almost always accompanied by desiccated eschar in wound bed; often accompanied by exposed tendons	Variable appearance, frequently ruddy, "beefy" red, granular tissue; calcification in wound base common; superficial fibrinous, gelatinous necrosis may occur suddenly with healthy-appearing granulation tissue underneath	Granular tissue unless PVD is present; often has deep necrotic area; may be dry; cellulitis or osteomyelitis may be present; neuropathic ulcers almost always accompanied by eschar and often accompanied by exposed tendons	Extensive necrotic tissue may be present; extensive undermining, sinus tracts, or tunneling may be present (tissue necrosis is usually greater than suggested by the external appearance of the epidermal defect)	Typically arise from small reddened areas that continue to increase in size; necrotic with marked vascularity; wound bed contains mixed necrotic and red granulation tissue
Exudate/drainage	Minimal exudate	Frequently moderate to heavy exudate	Low to moderate exudate; infected ulcer may have purulent drainage	Exudate amount varies	Exudate amount varies

Wound shape and margins	Smooth, even, regular; shape will conform to injury if caused by trauma; "punched out" appearance	Tend to be large with irregular margins	Smooth, even; may be small at surface with large subcutaneous abscess, characterized by callus around the ulcer and undermined edges	Usually well-defined; shape frequently is round but will conform to cause of ulcer and may be irregular if large	Irregular, blistering edge; purple-red, hemorrhagic, "angry looking" intense surrounding erythema
Surrounding skin	Pale, blanched, gray, cool, thin; no hair on legs/toes; little or no edema; often accompanied by livedo reticularis	Pigmented, edematous, macerated; characterized by hyperpigmentation, dermatitis, and lipodermatosclerosis; often accompanied by livedo reticularis; atrophie blanche may be present	Dry, thin, frequently callused; periwound hyperkeratosis common and indicates continued pressure	Should be dry; clinical infection indicated by redness, warmth, induration or hardness, and/or swelling	Hyperemic; characterized by atrophie blanche, livedo reticularis, and purpura; often accompanied by hyperpigmentation
Pain	Often accompanied by severe pain at rest and numbness, paresthesias; pain often increases with leg elevation; pain may also increase with ambulation (time of onset depends on severity of disease)	Varies unpredictably; small but deep ulcers around malleoli are typically the most painful; pain often improves with leg elevation	No sensation, or constant or intermittent numbness or burning; neuropathic ulcers almost always accompanied by numbness and paresthesias	Varies	Often accompanied by severe pain at rest, numbness, paresthesias
Healing	Must have increased/adequate blood supply to heal	Epithelialization often fails despite good granulation; average time to healing (based on combined literature) is 53 weeks, depending on degree of venous insufficiency, extent of lipodermatosclerosis, and presence of cardiovascular disease	Client must comply with diet, glucose regulation, exercise, and foot care/wear; aggressive revascularization and appropriate antibiotics may be needed for healing; custom or specialized shoes will reduce pressure and help prevent a recurrence	Must eliminate/reduce pressure, shear, and friction and implement appropriate skin care for healing	Must control the inflammatory process and establish adequate circulation to heal

From *Advances in skin and wound care.* (2000). *13*(1), 41. Springhouse, PA: Springhouse.
PVD, Peripheral vascular disease.

bolic activity induced by elevated temperature. Avoid hot water for daily cleansing and hygiene and minimize force and friction applied to the skin, especially tissue massage over bony prominences. There is no evidence to support the efficacy of this intervention, and there is evidence that indicates massage can lead to deep tissue trauma (Buss, Halfens, & Abu-Saad, 1997; PPPPUA, 1992). On the other hand, decreased circulation from extremely cold temperatures may make the skin more susceptible to breakdown. Hypothermia blankets or ice bags may cause a thermal burn.

Psychosocial factors influence pressure ulcer formation. Anderson and Andberg (1979) found life satisfaction, self-esteem, and practice of responsibility to be significant. In two studies of stress resulting from the transfer of elderly persons to a nursing home, Braden (1988, 1998) found that elevated cortisol levels placed the person at risk for pressure ulcer development. Cortisol directly affects immune function and will cause delayed wound healing (Waldrop & Doughty, 2000; Padgett, Marucha, & Sheridan, 1998). In persons with disabilities, a number of psychosocial factors may apply, including adjustment to disability, family environmental support, vocational opportunity, and financial constraints. Krause (1998) correlated the number of pressure areas found in a population of individuals with SCI with poorer adjustment in nearly every area of life studied. Harding-Okimoto's (1997) evidence suggests that persons with SCI who develop pressure ulcers have lower measures of self-concept and body image.

Children have different psychosocial problems with regard to skin integrity: the presence of a supportive parent or caregiver and good past experiences with the health care system can positively influence a child's cooperation level. Children fear loss of control, pain, and change in body image. Adolescents have increased stress with perceived alterations in body image, which causes them to question their value as human beings (Garvin, 1990).

WOUND HEALING

Wound healing is a complex series of events. To manage wounds properly, the rehabilitation nurse must understand the process to intervene appropriately at the right time. The approach to nonhealed wounds remains a clinical problem. Better understanding of the wound healing cascade is an interdisciplinary challenge (Witte & Barbul, 1997). Wounds heal by the process of regeneration or scar formation. The type of closure depends on the type of tissue damage. Regeneration is the restoration of normal tissue structure by the production of undamaged "like" cells (PPPPUA, 1992). Only certain body tissues can regenerate: epithelial, endothelial, and connective tissue. Epidermal, dermal, bone, and muscle tissue can be healed by regeneration. Healing in the muscle and bone by regeneration is impaired by infection, lack of vascularization, or innervation. When these complications are present, the wounds close by scar formation. Scar formation is a process of repair by connective tissue (Waldrop & Doughty, 2000).

Classification

Wound healing has three levels, or intentions. Wounds with no tissue loss are closed by primary intention. Examples are wounds in which the edges are approximated and closed surgically or with tape or glue. These wounds heal quickly with minimal scar formation provided there is no infection or secondary breakdown (Kenney, 1998).

Wounds with tissue loss that require connective tissue to fill the defect may close by secondary intention. Because the wound edges are difficult or impossible to approximate, the wounds are left open to heal by scar formation. Healing time depends on the extent of tissue loss and whether healing is prolonged by infection. Examples of these wounds are burns, wound dehiscence, and pressure ulcers (Waldrop & Doughty, 2000; Kravitz, 1996).

Tertiary intention refers to wounds in which primary closure is delayed or wounds that are deliberately left open for drainage and then closed. The wounds form more scar tissue than a wound with primary closure but less than a wound with secondary closure (Carlson et al., 1992; Disa, Carlton, & Goldberg, 1992).

Phases

Wound repair is a cascade of physiologic responses initiated by tissue trauma that can be divided into phases: defensive, proliferative, epithelization, and maturation. The extent of the wound will determine the extent of activation of each phase of wound healing. This process happens interactively, with overlap between the stages (Waldrop & Doughty, 2000).

The defensive phase is the body's first response to injury with hemostasis and inflammation. The primary outcomes of this phase are control of bleeding and a clean wound base. Hemostasis results from trauma to tissue disrupting the vascular supply. Released blood contacts collagen to activate coagulation factors, causing an aggregate of platelets. Fibrin clots then form, acting as the initial wound closure, and serve as scaffolding for invading cells, such as neutrophils, monocytes, fibroblasts, and endothelial cells (Witte & Barbul, 1997). Key to wound healing is the subsequent breakdown of platelets releasing potent growth factors that attract the cells and products needed to begin healing. Hemostasis seems to be the critical factor in initiating the wound-healing process. This may be important to understanding the stagnant nature of chronic nonhealing wounds. Poorly vascularized and often resulting from compromised vascularization, these wounds may lack the necessary stimulus to promote wound healing (Waldrop & Doughty, 1992).

In the inflammation stage vasodilation ensues as a result of histamine release. There is increased blood vessel permeability, vasocongestion, and leakage of serous fluid into the surrounding tissue. Initially leukocytes protect the wound from bacterial invasion, and within several days macrophages arrive. Macrophages play an important role throughout the wound-healing process by assisting with wound debridement, producing growth factors, and stimulating collagen synthesis (Waldrop & Doughty, 2000). This defensive phase last 3 to 4 days. Nurses understand and support the need for the inflammatory process to occur and monitor progress because suppression of inflammation in the first days of a wound's existence will affect the wound's overall quality of healing (Anstead, 1998). Nurses also are aware of factors that might alter the process, such as steroid therapy or decreased oxygenation. The clinical picture of the wound during this phase is red, hot, and edematous.

The desired outcome of the proliferative phase is to fill the wound defect with connective tissue and cover it with epithelium. There are three major stages to this phase: granulation, contraction, and epithelialization (PPPPUA, 1992). In the process of granulation, neoangiogenesis and collagen synthesis combine to provide a new capillary network and to nourish the collagen tissue filling in the wound bed. These two processes are simultaneous and codependent. Neoangiogenesis (the production of new blood vessels) is stimulated by hypoxia. Vessels are formed from the wound edges and advance inward, joining at the center of the wound. Collagen synthesis occurs simultaneously in a number of complex events. The fibroblast is the key cell during this phase of healing, rapidly synthesizing collagen and other connective tissue. The collagen fibers gradually thicken and assume parallel orientation, which provides the increased tensile strength of the wound (Witte & Barbul, 1997). The tissue formed by this process is called *granulation tissue.* Tiny round projections of connective tissue are noted on the surface of the wound, which appears translucent and red. It is vascular, is fragile, and bleeds easily. As the wound heals, the new vessels will recede.

Contraction is the reduction of the size of the tissue defect by the inward movement of the tissue and the surrounding skin. This is a desirable response because it decreases the size of the wound, and with that the healing time (Calvin, 1998). In wounds where there is good mobility of surrounding tissue (e.g., sacral wounds), this occurs easily; however, it is more difficult where tissue is not movable (e.g., bony prominence, trochanteric area) (Waldrop & Doughty, 2000; PPPPUA, 1992). The exact mechanism of wound contraction is not known; some suggest the myofibroblast is responsible (Witte & Barbul, 1997).

In the epithelialization stage, cells of the intact epidermis reproduce and migrate over the defect. In epidermal and dermal wounds, epithelial cells proliferate and cross the wound bed in the first 24 hours. Epidermal tissue is formed at the wound edges. The wound quickly regenerates. In wounds healing by secondary intention, the wounds cannot repair until the wound bed is established. Epithelial cells do not migrate across a dry wound bed. In a dry wound the epidermal cells must tunnel down to a moist level to begin migration. In wounds limited to the epidermis and dermis where scabs have been allowed to develop, the epithelial cells first must secrete collagenase to remove the scab before epithelial migration. In healing large wounds, epithelialization is limited to about 3 cm from the edges of the wound. Chronic wounds with "rolled" edges will not be able to migrate epithelial cells from the nonproliferative edges. The rolled edges, or *epiboly,* can be treated with a silver nitrate stick applied to the edges. The silver nitrate will burn off the nonproliferative edges and leave clean epithelial edges stimulated to migrate and close the wound. If this does not work, surgical intervention may be indicated (PPPPUA, 1992). The proliferative phase lasts from day 3 to day 21, during which rehabilitation nurses ensure clients have adequate nutrition, hydration, and oxygenation.

Maturation is the phase of remodeling that begins when the wound is closed with connective and epithelial tissue. Collagen production stabilizes; fibers organize and increase the tensile strength of tissue. Activities during this last phase determine the strength and mobility of scar tissue. If there is an alteration in the remodeling of collagen fibers, contractions or adhesions can occur. The healed tissue will achieve only 80% of previous tissue strength, and scars will be less elastic than intact skin. Support for healing during this phase recognizes the decreased strength of tissue; the healing process continues for up to 2 years.

Influential Factors

Many factors influence wound healing, including tissue perfusion, nutritional status, infection, hematopoietic abnormalities, aging, diabetes, smoking, steroid and immunosuppressive therapy, radiation therapy, sensorimotor dysfunction, and obesity (Stotts, 2000; Motta, 1993). Children have better capacity for wound repair but have fewer reserves to combat systemic attack. Factors that are detrimental to wound healing in children include their easily upset electrolyte balance, sudden changes in body temperature, and rapid spread of infection (Garvin, 1990). Table 16-3 summarizes the major factors and their impact on wound healing. To aid wound healing, each factor must be evaluated and incorporated into the client's plan of care.

WOUNDS COMMONLY MANAGED BY REHABILITATION NURSES

Nurses in rehabilitation settings most often encounter three categories of wounds: pressure ulcers, diabetic ulcers, and dermal ulcers caused by arterial and venous problems. Pressure ulcers have been discussed under a variety of names: decubitus ulcer, bedsores, and pressure sores. Pressure ulcers can develop anywhere there is unrelieved pressure; therefore names that describe pressure ulcers as having been

TABLE 16-3 Influencing Factors for Wound Healing

Factor	Effect
Decreased tissue perfusion and oxygenation (hypotension, hypovolemia, hypoxia)	Impairs collagen synthesis, leading to inadequate tensile strength of connective tissue Decreases epithelial proliferation and migration Reduces tissue resistance to infection
Decreased nutritional status	Impairs inflammatory response/delays healing Impairs collagen synthesis Impairs immune system
Infection	Prolongs inflammatory phase Induces additional tissue destruction Delays collagen synthesis Prevents epithelialization
Hematopoietic abnormalities	
Red blood cells ↓	Decrease oxygenation of the wound
Platelets ↓	Delay of hemostasis and the cascade of healing events
Aging	Delays inflammatory response Produces capillary fragility Reduces collagen synthesis Slows neoangiogenesis Slows epithelialization
Diabetes	Decreases collagen synthesis Induces leukocyte dysfunction (secondary to hyperglycemia)
Smoking	Decreases oxygen to the wound secondary to coagulation in small blood vessels and vasoconstriction
Steroids	Inhibit epithelial proliferation Impair inflammatory response Decrease growth factor available for wound healing Increase wound vulnerability to infection Inhibit epithelial proliferation Impair inflammatory response Decrease macrophage activity Increase wound vulnerability to infection
Immunosuppressives	Impair inflammatory process Increase susceptibility to infection Prolong healing process
Radiation	Reduces fibroblast proliferation Inhibits inflammatory response
Sensorimotor dysfunction in affected part	Decreases inflammatory response secondary to decreased vasomotor response
Obesity	Decreases vascularity of adipose tissue Increases tension on wound

Data from Doughty, D., & Waldrop, J. (2000). Wound-healing physiology. In Bryant, R.A. (Ed.), *Acute and chronic wounds: Nursing management* (2nd ed.). St. Louis: Mosby.

caused by the bed or a recumbent position are inaccurate. The term *pressure ulcer* is more accurate and descriptive. It reflects the cause—excessive pressure resulting in ischemia and ulceration (Bryant et al., 1992). The PPPPUA (1992) defines a pressure ulcer as any lesion caused by unrelieved pressure resulting in the damage of underlying tissue.

Pathogenesis of Pressure Ulcers

Byrne and Salzberg's (1996) review of the literature revealed more than 200 factors that contribute to the development of pressure ulcers. Primary contributing factors include pressure, friction, shear, and moisture, the most important being pressure (Wywialowski, 1999). Secondary factors include mobility status, sensorimotor function, nutrition, age, hemopoietic changes, diabetes, circulatory dysfunction, fecal incontinence, medications, and psychosocial issues. Braden and Bergstrom's (1987) classic conceptual schema (Figure 16-4) divides factors into intrinsic and extrinsic forces and provides a model displaying the interactive nature of pressure ulcer development. Pieper (2000) and Russell (1998) divide risk factors into three categories: extrinsic (e.g., pressure and shear), intrinsic (e.g., general health, nutrition, and mobility), and external (e.g., long times without movement, such as waiting on a stretcher in an emergency department).

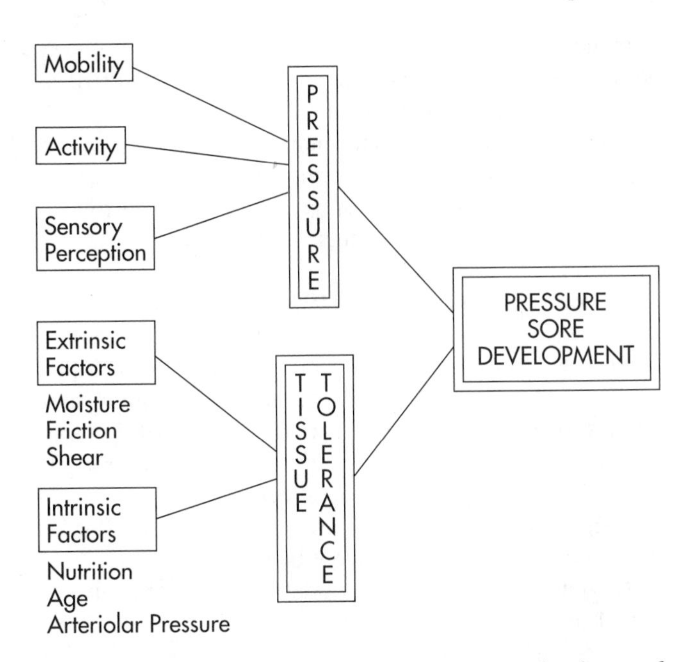

Figure 16-4 Braden and Bergstrom's conceptual schema of pressure sore risk factors. (From Braden, B., & Bergstrom, M. [1989]. A conceptual schema for the study of the etiology of pressure sores. *Rehabilitation Nursing, 14*[5], 258.)

Pressure

Of the three aspects—intensity, duration, and tissue tolerance to pressure—pressure is most important and the cause of pressure ulcers is prolonged, uninterrupted mechanical loading of tissue (Pieper, 2000; PPPPUA, 1992). The critical issue of pressure and its effects on tissue were defined by early researchers. Husain (1953) developed the concept of tissue tolerance and demonstrated the relationship between time and pressure. By exerting a force for 2 hours, microscopic ischemic changes in tissue were produced, and when the same force was applied for 6 hours, total muscle destruction occurred (International Association for Enterostomal Therapy [IAET], 1991). Experiments with dogs and cats defined time-pressure relationships; 70 ml of pressure applied continuously for 2 hours produced pathological changes. An important inverse relationship of pressure and time was evident when intense pressure applied for a short duration was as damaging as lower intensity pressures exerted for extended periods (Kosiak et al., 1958; Kosiak, 1959).

Tissues can tolerate much higher cyclic pressures than constant pressures. If pressure is relieved intermittently every 3 to 5 minutes, higher pressures can be tolerated (Kosiak, 1959). Pressure needs to be relieved frequently over time and reduced over the surface-skin interface. This translates to the clinical practice of weight shifting every few minutes to extend safe sitting times and the use of 2-hour minimum turning times in bed or frequent small position changes in bed to provide pressure relief (Norton, McLaren, & Exton-Smith, 1975/1962; PPPPUA, 1992; Staas & Cioschi, 1991).

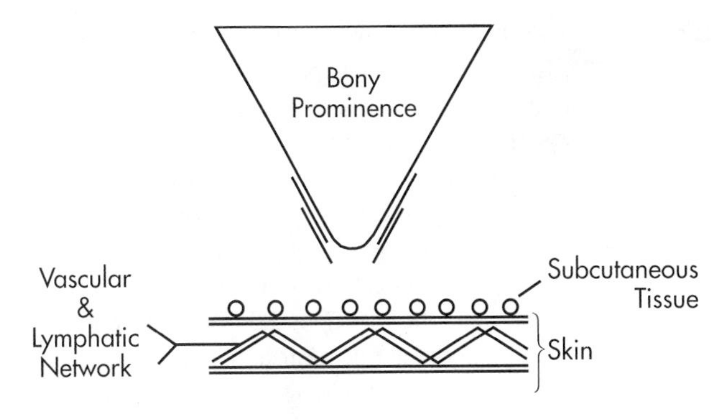

Figure 16-5 Pressure cone. (Adapted from Slater, H. [1985]. *Pressure sores in the elderly.* Pittsburgh: Synapse.)

Muscle is more sensitive than skin to pressure. When muscle is damaged without skin breakdown, a second application of less pressure and less time can result in an ulcer. This is clinically important in the need to relieve pressure at the first sign of skin impairment, blanchable hyperemia, and allow time for tissue recovery.

Pressure is transmitted from the body surface to the underlying bone. Greatest pressure is over the bone, distributed in a conelike fashion, with the base of the cone on the underlying body surface (Figure 16-5). This explains why the greatest damage occurs at the muscle layer and not at the skin surface. Thus, although only a small skin defect or reddened area presents, a large area of undermining has developed below the surface of intact skin. The damage begins at the bone—soft tissue interface, not at the skin surface, and extends downward, generating a cone-shaped pressure gradient, with the point of the cone at the skin surface. The damage evident on the skin then becomes the "tip of the iceberg," making a larger deep area of necrosis and ischemia.

Kosiak (1959) and Lindan (1961) determined the amount of pressure human skin is subjected to in supine and sitting positions. In the supine position pressures greatly exceeded 32 mm Hg in the areas under the occiput, spine, sacrum, and heels. Pressure under the buttocks was greater than 70 mm Hg. In the sitting position the ischial tuberosity had pressures exceeding 300 mm Hg. Earlier research by Landis (1930) demonstrated 32 mm Hg to be arteriolar closing pressure and 15 mm Hg to be venous closing pressure. Capillary closing pressure is the minimum pressure needed to collapse the capillary. Lindan (1961) demonstrated that pressure causes tissue damage by closure of blood vessels, resulting in tissue necrosis.

These early capillary blood-flow studies were done in the fingertips of young, healthy men. More recent capillary closure studies have shown much lower pressures needed to collapse capillaries in elderly and debilitated subjects and that these pressures can vary over different sites on the body. There is some difficulty extrapolating these data to the skin to support surface-interface pressure. The pressures found by indirect measurements at the skin to support the surface interface may not accurately reflect the picture of blood flow through the capillaries (Bryant, 2000; Pieper, 2000). Clinically this led to searching for support surfaces that reduce the skin to support surface pressure below 32 mm Hg.

Clinical Aspects. Clinically the facets of pressure (intensity, duration, and tissue tolerance) produce concern for clients with the inability to relieve pressure over a skin surface. The progression of tissue changes occurs in response to obstruction of capillary blood flow. With reactive hyperemia (blanching hyperemia) the blood vessels dilate to compensate for periods of anoxia. The skin appears flushed. This may be difficult to note in dark-skinned individuals because the discoloration appears as a deepening of normal ethnic color or as a purple hue to the skin. When compressed with a fingertip, the area will blanch and return to color immediately as the finger is lifted. The area may exhibit slight edema, feel warm to touch, and clients with intact sensation may report pain. At this stage relief of pressure can reverse tissue damage. With nonreactive hyperemia (nonblanching hyperemia), vasodilation continues as a response to the anoxia. Dark-skinned persons exhibit deepened skin color, a purple to gray skin hue, and changes in skin texture. The skin damage now appears bright red to dark purple. When compressed, the area does not blanch. The area is cool to touch and may feel hard (indurated) or soft and boggy. The tissue damage is not reversible at this stage (Pieper, 2000; Bates-Jensen, 1998).

Special Populations at Risk. Risk factors for development of pressure ulcers may be specific to different populations and higher in some groups. All risks are not equal, and incidence rates are not distributed evenly across populations. Variations need more study before predictions can be made. For instance, persons with fractures are at greater risk than those admitted to hospitals for elective orthopedic procedures. However, hospital nurses were found not to recognize the high risk because they did not document preventive measures or begin treatment until after pressure ulcers began in clients with hip fractures (Gunningberg, Lindholm, Carlsson, & Sjoden, 2000).

Clients with SCI are at extremely high risk for pressure ulcers. The first studies of prevalence of pressure ulcers with SCI were conducted with soldiers after World War II and reported rates of 57% to 85% (Kosiak et al., 1958). A prevalence rate of 25% to 40%, with greater improvement evident in rehabilitation and SCI units (prevalence 15% to 30%) (Allman, 1997), is attributable to better understanding of prevention and overall interventions during initial management of persons with SCI. Preventing recurrence remains a challenge because 35.2% of initial pressure ulcers recur in this population and 42.2% recur in those who also smoke (Niazi et al., 1997).

Pressure ulcers are the most common complication of SCI for persons living in the community, a 33% prevalence rate (Eastwood, Hagglund, Ragnarsson, Gordon, & Marino, 1999), compared with an 8.7% prevalence rate in home care settings (Allman, 1997). Compounding the obvious factors of reduced mobility, activity, and sensory perception, clients with SCI have unique factors that may increase their risk, as discussed in the following section.

Some relationships are not confirmed clearly. Lower education level related positively with increased risk and severity of ulcers (Schryvers, Stanc, & Nance, 2000) at follow-up; it was not a factor during acute rehabilitation (Carlson, et al., 1992).

Although Lloyd and Baker (1986) found no relationship between severity of pressure ulcer and level of injury, a higher incidence of pressure ulcer in persons with quadriplegia than in those with paraplegia occurred during initial hospitalization but not at follow-up. Carlson et al. (1992) found that the higher the level of injury during acute care, the greater the incidence of pressure ulcer; however, no associated significance was found between increased level of injury and rehabilitation and follow-up phases.

Completeness of injury did relate significantly between complete lesions and increased incidence of pressure ulcers at follow-up. According to the Frankel scale (indication for presence or absence of sensation and motor activity below injury level), those with more complete lesions had greater incidence of pressure ulcers during rehabilitation and follow-up. All who developed pressure ulcers in rehabilitation recorded the highest factor of complete injury on the Frankel scale (Frankel et al., 1969). Of major interest is that no one who had any preserved function below the level of injury developed a pressure ulcer during rehabilitation and follow-up. It appears that even nonfunctional preserved motor activity reduces the risk of pressure ulcers.

It would follow from the discussion and the prevalence rates discussed above that a history of pressure ulcers correlated highly with having pressure ulcers at follow-up (Carlson et al., 1992; Niazi et al., 1997). Not surprising, newly injured persons with SCI had extended hospital stays when pressure ulcers were present (Burnett, Kolakowsky-Hayner, Gourley, & Cifu, 2000).

Common Sites of Pressure Ulcers. Pressure ulcers occur most frequently over bony prominences, the sacrum, ischial tuberosity, trochanter, and calcaneus (Figure 16-6). In acute care hospitals the most common sites for clients to develop pressure ulcers are the sacrum and heels (Baeczak et al., 1997; Tourtual et al., 1997), but they will occur anywhere on the body where soft tissues are compressed. The most common cause was positional pressure (47.4%), and the second and third leading causes were cervical collars (23.7%) and tracheostomy/endotracheal tubes (10.5%) (Watts et al., 1998). Cervical collars cause skin breakdown at the chin and the occiput (Black, Fenn-Buderer, Blaylock, & Hogan, 1998). The rehabilitation nurse carefully monitors clients with splints, orthoses, and orthopedic immobilizers, such as halo jackets. The sacrum is the most common site for severe pressure ulcers for clients with SCI (Carlson et al., 1992), due in part to time spent on a spine board or the operating table. Early medical manage-

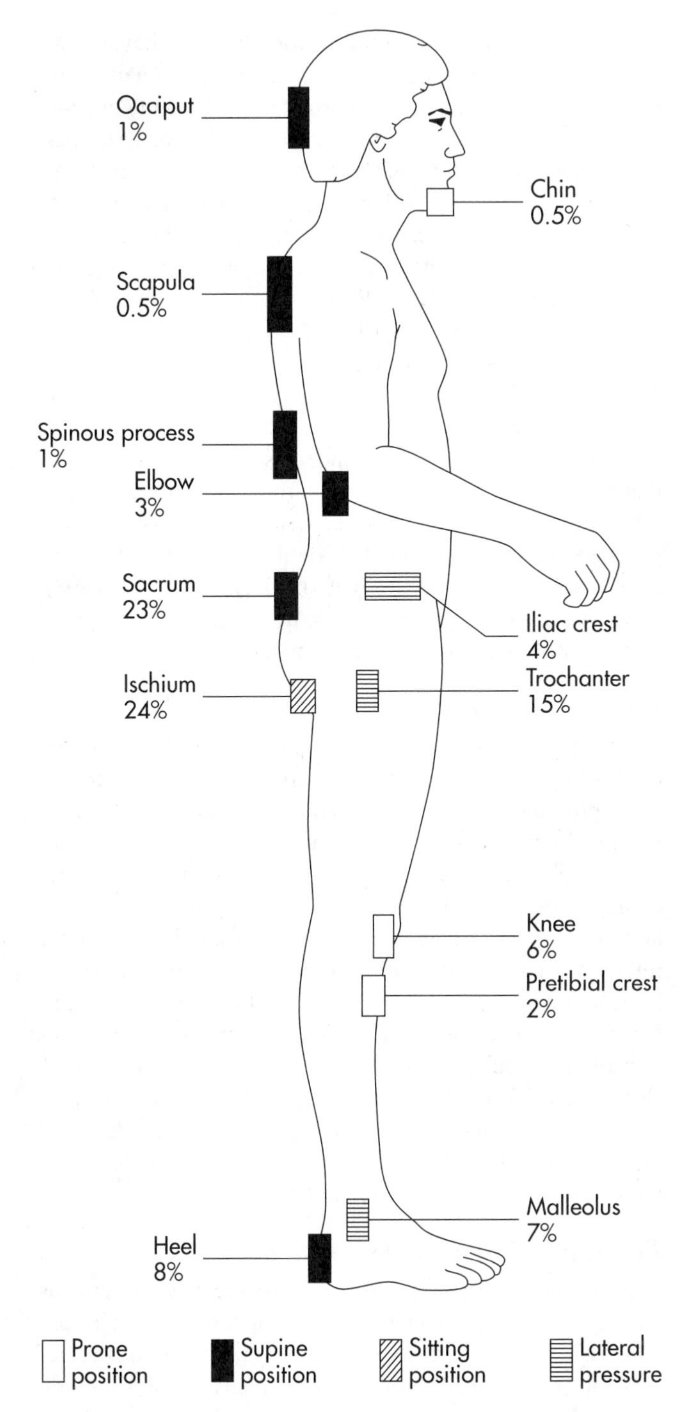

Figure 16-6 Common sites for pressure ulcers and frequency of ulceration per site.

ment on bed rest without adequate pressure relief and more time in a wheelchair contribute to increased incidence at the ischial tuberosities and the feet. Nearly half (47%) of all ulcers discovered during follow-up were on the foot, toes, plantar surfaces at the metatarsal heads, outer edges of the foot, heels, and malleolus of the ankle (Calson et al., 1992). In a study of children aged 10 weeks to 13 years, the occiput was the site of greatest pressures, changing to the sacrum as the child aged. This is not surprising considering the percentage of body weight the child's head represents. A child's positioning needs must be considered separately from the adult's.

Diabetic Ulcers

Diabetic ulcers are a second category. Clients with diabetic peripheral neuropathy experience varying degrees of symptoms from sensory, motor, or autonomic origins or a combination. Loss of sensation is most problematic because it predisposes the foot to trauma and skin breakdown. Motor neuropathies result in muscular atrophies of the foot, leading to bony deformity and gait changes; putting undue stress on the foot; and leading to pressure, shear, and friction problems (Armstrong, Lavery, & Harkless, 1996).

Autonomic neuropathies often lead to absence of sweating, which leads to increased heat and drying of skin. The foot is the most common location of diabetic ulcers. As much as 20% of persons with diabetes will experience foot complications during their lifetime. Of the 125,000 lower extremity amputations performed each year, it has been estimated that between 56% and 83% are directly attributable to diabetes mellitus (Mulder, 2000).

Venous and Arterial Wounds

The third category has two situations, arterial insufficiency and venous insufficiency. It is important to note that some clients have both arterial and venous ulcers and that treatment for one type of ulcer may exacerbate the symptoms or alter the healing of the other type.

Insufficient arterial perfusion to an extremity causes arterial ulcers (Scully, 1999). Less common than venous ulcers, they are more difficult to manage with the complexity of disease processes and complications. The lack of perfusion to the lower extremity creates great difficulty for wound healing. Peripheral vascular disease is the associated disease entity with arterial insufficiency. It involves the arteries, veins, and lymphatics. Assessment includes pedal pulses and measurement of the ankle-brachial index. Symptoms can be treated, but there is no cure for peripheral vascular disease. Surgical intervention is the most likely outcome (Sieggreen, Cohen, Kloth, Harding, & Stotts, 1996).

Venous insufficiency leads to venous ulcers that result from disorders of the deep venous system. Most commonly the origin is damage to incompetent valves from thrombosis in the deep or superficial veins (Scully, 1999). Damage occurs to the veins or calf muscle pump, resulting in high venous pressure in the deep veins (venous hypertension). Precursors include clinical conditions that trigger a sequence of events promoting edema and perhaps dermal ulceration (Hess, 2000). When a disease process alters the flow of blood forward, dysfunction ensues, resulting in increased hydrostatic pressure and venous hypotension, leading to dermal ulceration. The diseases contributing to venous insufficiency are listed in Table 16-2. Venous pressure promotes extravasation of erythrocytes and fibrinogen, leading to a cascade of events that eventually ends in tissue death and dermal ulcers. Assessment for venous ulcers includes pedal pulses and measurement of the ankle-brachial index (Sieggreen et al., 1996). Venous ulcers generally require only noninvasive intervention. Compression and elevation along with topical wound care are the interventions most commonly required (Harris, 1996). Successful wound healing is multivariant and requires a cohesive team approach using guidelines for care (Hess, 2000; Ghauri, et al., 2000). Important to note is that a person can have both arterial and venous ulcers, and the treatment for one type may exacerbate symptoms or alter healing of the other.

NURSING MANAGEMENT OF SKIN

Maintaining skin integrity and management of acute and chronic wounds is a major component of rehabilitation nursing. The rehabilitation nurse is the team member primarily responsible for assessing skin, implementing prevention strategies, treating wounds, and teaching the client and family prevention techniques for the home setting and treatment modalities for home management if alteration in skin integrity occurs. A systematic approach to management of the skin and assessment are vital components of overall health assessment for every client. Regular and ongoing assessment of the skin is of particular importance to clients in need of rehabilitation nursing services because of the nature of their illness, injury, and disability.

Assessment

The skin assessment is used to establish a baseline of skin status that can be monitored for changes over time. A health history is critical and includes data about acute and chronic medical problems and surgeries or hospitalizations. Of particular importance to document are alterations in motor or sensory function, neuropathies, diabetes, anemias, nutritional compromise, autoimmune diseases, immune suppression, cardiovascular problems, respiratory disease, or other systemic disease.

An overview of skin health includes the usual skin condition, skin care habits, previously diagnosed and treated skin problems, color changes, dryness, ecchymosis, lesions, masses, pruritus, sensory changes, temperature changes, and texture changes. Note medications, particularly steroids and antibiotics, and allergies. Assessment of activity levels specifies ambulation and bed mobility status, extremity movement, pain, contractures, and paralysis. Evaluate bowel and bladder continence and any ostomies. Nutrition and fluid assessment with intake and laboratory values may be appropriate (Aranovitch, 1993).

The health history includes assessment of functional health patterns that relate to the client's situation, and interwoven throughout are cultural factors that may have implications for skin management. A safety assessment commonly is overlooked but is important in establishing whether a client has deficits or lives in an unsafe environment for performing activities of daily living. Damaged skin, even burns, is a concern for many children and older persons and those with impairments. Psychosocial assessment includes current and past mental status with inquiry into depression and substance use or abuse (Barkauskas, Stoltenberg-Allen, Baumann, Darling-Fisher, 1998).

Inspect the skin for variations in color or pigmentation, wrinkling, lesions, masses, hygiene, and changes. Palpation augments inspection to determine skin temperature, moisture, texture, and turgor. Evidence-based practice prescribes that the skin must be inspected thoroughly and regularly in rehabilitation and in all areas, especially high-risk places or pressure points. Additionally examine the extremities for edema and pulses and the feet (Barkauskas et al., 1998). Other assessments pertinent to skin integrity are range of motion, motor and sensory function, and mobility.

Ethnic Considerations

Darkly pigmented intact skin requires careful assessment because it does not blanch when pressure is applied over a bony prominence and bruises show differently. Natural or halogen light is preferable to fluorescent light because it imparts blue tones to dark skin. Skin photographs give better definition because the light helps to visualize the skin area and provides documentation for monitoring changes or for reference. Palpate the skin tone, temperature, especially heat, and edema; ". . . assess for erythema and/or inflammation with localized changes in skin temperature in comparison to the surrounding tissue, edema, and/or induration" (Bennett, 1995, p. 35). Many acceptable variations occur in all skin colors; in absence of a baseline, ask the client and family to describe what they may perceive as changes or alterations in skin or to clarify questions.

Pressure Ulcer Risk Assessment

The purpose of risk assessment is to identify individuals at risk for development of pressure ulcers, to target specific risk factors, and to define early intervention strategies for prevention. Identifying individuals at risk is central to prevention because interventions are targeted to them (PPPPUA, 1992; Stotts, Deosaransingh, Roll, Newman, 1998) to avoid adverse outcomes and minimize cost (Xakellis, Frantz, Lewis, & Harvey, 1998). Risk factors were discussed earlier with emphasis on populations that are elderly, have reduced mobility, and have compromised health status.

Risk assessment scales are tools to identify populations at highest risk for developing altered skin integrity and to concentrate efforts and allocate resources toward appropriate situations (Pieper & Weiland, 1997; Pieper, Sugrue, Weiland, Sprague, & Heimann, 1997). Although current risk assessment scales offer standardized measures of risk, their predictive value in rehabilitation populations, such as those with

SCI, requires continued investigation (Baggerly & DiBlasi, 1996; Bergstrom, Braden, Kemp, Champagne, & Ruby, 1998; Schue & Langemo, 1998; Stordeur, Laurent, & D'Hoore, 1998), as well as instrument development and subsequent psychometric testing (Salzberg et al., 1998). Pediatric skin assessment tools are being developed (Waterlow, 1997).

Risk assessment scales measure items for immobility, incontinence, nutritional factors such as inadequate dietary intake and impaired nutritional status, and altered level of consciousness. Clients are assessed on admission to rehabilitation and assigned scores; assessment is repeated at periodic intervals during hospitalization and again at follow-up. The scores are used to determine an individual's risk and are correlated with an appropriate level and type of preventive intervention. The Norton scale and the Braden scale are two valid assessment tools that are used commonly in a variety of settings.

The Norton scale (Table 16-4) assesses five factors related to development of pressure ulcers: physical condition, mental condition, activity, mobility, and incontinence. The nurse rates a client for each factor on a scale from 1 to 4. The lower the score on the scale, the greater the risk to the individual. Combined scores range from 5 to 20. Norton determined that a combined score of 14 indicated onset of risk, and a score of 12 and below indicated a high risk of pressure ulcer formation. The scale does not have rater guidelines that may lead to lower interrater reliability; however, when tested with other scales, development of pressure ulcers was predictable (Pieper, 2000).

The Braden scale (Table 16-5) is used to assess six client factors: mobility, activity, moisture, sensory perception, nutrition, and friction and shear. Each subscale has a range from 1 to 4, except the factors of friction and shear, which are rated from 1 to 3. A combined score may range from 4 to 23; an individual with a combined score of 16 or below is considered at risk.

Wound Assessment

Rehabilitation clients may present with alterations in skin integrity for a variety of reasons. For instance, a postsurgical wound may heal poorly, or an unsuccessful attempt to prevent breakdown in a person with paralysis may lead to a pressure ulcer. A client with diabetes may present with a foot ulcer, or a person with arteriovenous insufficiency may present with a venous-stasis ulcer. Assessment sets the rationale for deciding when and how to treat any wound, to evaluate the efficacy of treatment, and for communication of needs or consultations with other caregivers (PPPPUA, 1994). Team members must use a standard assessment system to ensure that multiple providers can make ongoing comparisons of the wound to identify problems and determine effectiveness of interventions. It is paramount that all members of the team responsible for assessing wounds use assessment tools and processes consistently and accurately.

Wounds are monitored following a regular schedule at least weekly (PPPPUA, 1994) to provide consistent assessment of wound healing and timely evaluation if changes are required in the treatment plan. An initial assessment of a wound determines the cause or source of the wound. Distinction is made between wounds that are surgical and those that are nonsurgical and between acute and chronic to help in choosing specific interventions. The rehabilitation nurse may improve outcomes by initially determining both causative and contributing factors to a wound's development.

An in-depth assessment of the wound bed reveals the characteristics; tissue type including presence of granulation tissue, tissue color, drainage, and odor are examined and documented. Similarly, surrounding tissues are examined, and erythema, maceration, induration, and other indicators of tissue health are documented in the assessment. The location and size of the wound are two essential elements. Accurate notation of the location is as complete as possible and described in anatomical terms; the wound is located on the ischium, not the lower buttock (Baranoski, 1995). Wound measurement requires accuracy and consistency that are imperative to document the effectiveness of interventions on wound healing (Langemo, Melland, Hanson, Olson, & Hunter, 1998). A variety of tools are used: tape measures, rulers, concentric tracing circles, wound photography, planimetry, three-dimensional wound gauges, and wound

TABLE 16-4 Norton Scale

		Physical Condition		Mental Condition		Activity		Mobility		Incontinent		
		Good	4	Alert	4	Ambulant	4	Full	4	Not	4	
		Fair	3	Apathetic	3	Walk/help	3	Slightly limited	3	Occasionally	3	
		Poor	2	Confused	2	Chair-bound	2	Very limited	2	Usually/urine	2	Total
Name	Date	Very bad	1	Stupor	1	Bed-bound	1	Immobile	1	Doubly	1	Score

From Norton, D., McLaren, R., & Exton Smith, A.N. (1975/1962). *An investigation of geriatric nursing problems in hospitals.* London: Churchill Livingstone.

TABLE 16-5 Braden Scale for Predicting Pressure Sore Risk

				Date of Assessment	
Sensory perception Ability to respond meaningfully to pressure-related discomfort	**1. Completely limited:** Unresponsive (does not moan, flinch, or grasp) to painful stimuli, due to diminished level of consciousness or sedation, *or* Has limited ability to feel pain over most of body surface.	**2. Very limited:** Responds only to painful stimuli. Cannot communicate discomfort except by moaning or restlessness, *or* Has a sensory impairment that limits the ability to feel pain or discomfort over half of body.	**3. Slightly limited:** Responds to verbal commands but cannot always communicate discomfort or need to be turned, *or* Has some sensory impairment that limits ability to feel pain or discomfort in 1 or 2 extremities.	**4. No impairment:** Responds to verbal commands. Has no sensory deficit that would limit ability to feel or voice pain or discomfort.	
Moisture Degree to which skin is exposed to moisture	**1. Constantly moist:** Skin is kept moist almost constantly by perspiration, urine, etc. Dampness is detected every time client is moved or turned.	**2. Moist:** Skin is often but not always moist. Linen must be changed at least once a shift.	**3. Occasionally moist:** Skin is occasionally moist, requiring an extra linen change approximately once a day.	**4. Rarely moist:** Skin is usually dry; linen requires changing only at routine intervals.	
Activity Degree of physical activity	**1. Bedfast:** Confined to bed.	**2. Chairfast:** Ability to walk severely limited or nonexistent. Cannot bear own weight and/or must be assisted into chair or wheelchair.	**3. Walks occasionally:** Walks occasionally during day but for very short distances, with or without assistance. Spends majority of each shift in bed or chair.	**4. Walks frequently:** Walks outside the room at least twice a day and inside room at least once every 2 hours during waking hours.	
Mobility Ability to change and control body position	**1. Completely immobile:** Does not make even slight changes in body or extremity position without assistance.	**2. Very limited:** Makes occasional slight changes in body or extremity position but unable to make frequent or significant changes independently.	**3. Slightly limited:** Makes frequent though slight changes in body or extremity position independently.	**4. No limitations:** Makes major and frequent changes in position without assistance.	

Nutrition Usual food intake pattern	**1. Very poor:** Never eats a complete meal. Rarely eats more than ⅓ of any food offered. Eats 2 servings or less of protein (meat or dairy products) per day. Takes fluids poorly. Does not take a liquid dietary supplement, *or* Is NPO and/or maintained on clear liquids or IV for more than 5 days.	**2. Probably inadequate:** Rarely eats a complete meal and generally eats only about half of any food offered. Protein intake includes only 3 servings of meat or dairy products per day. Occasionally will take a dietary supplement, *or* Receives less than optimum amount of liquid diet or tube feeding.	**3. Adequate:** Eats over half of most meals. Eats a total of 4 servings of protein (meat, dairy products) each day. Occasionally will refuse a meal but will usually take a supplement if offered, *or* Is on a tube feeding or TPN regimen, which probably meets most of nutritional needs.	**4. Excellent:** Eats most of every meal. Never refuses a meal. Usually eats a total of 4 or more servings of meat and dairy products. Occasionally eats between meals. Does not require supplementation.	
Friction and Shear	**1. Problem:** Requires moderate to maximum assistance in moving. Complete lifting without sliding against sheets is impossible. Frequently slides down in bed or chair, requiring frequent repositioning with maximum assistance. Spasticity, contractures, or agitation leads to almost constant friction.	**2. Potential problem:** Moves feebly or requires minimum assistance. During a move skin probably slides to some extent against sheets, chair, restraints, or other devices. Maintains relatively good position in chair or bed most of the time but occasionally slides down.	**3. No apparent problem:** Moves in bed and in chair independently and has sufficient muscle strength to lift up completely during move. Maintains good position in bed or chair at all times.		
				TOTAL SCORE	

 A conceptual schema for the study of the etiology of pressures sores. *Rehabilitation Nursing, 12,* 8-16.
NPO, Nothing by mouth; *IV,* intravenously; *TPN,* total parenteral nutrition.

molds. Rulers, tracing, and photography are used commonly. Other methods have proved to be too costly, inconsistent in measurement, and complicated or time consuming for clinical use (Cooper, 2000).

Rulers. Linear measurement is a relatively simple and accurate method of measuring wounds. It is advisable for clinicians to determine a consistent method of measuring and documenting wound measurements in their setting. One recommended method is to envision the face of a clock and then measure wounds from the 12 to 6 o'clock positions and the from the 9 to 3 o'clock positions. Although this may not always reflect the widest dimension of a wound, it provides for a consistent measure that will detect changes (Bates-Jensen, 1998).

Wounds with depth and sinuses need further measurement to picture the wound accurately. Because it may be difficult to detect changes in this type of wound, consistently repeated measurements will, over time, depict a "trend" to the wound repair process (Cooper, 2000). Use the end of an applicator without the cotton to measure the depth as the applicator shaft enters the wound. The cotton tipped end is not used because the cotton can dislodge in the wound. Use the clock face method described above to document the wound, but include descriptions of any tunneling and undermining. For example, 20 mm tunneling at the 5 o'clock position or 10 mm undermining from the 11 to 3 o'clock positions.

Tracing. Sterile plastic rulers and concentric circles are a way to make one-time-use tracings of the wound or ulcer surface. Wounds can be difficult to trace depending on their location, and a client's position can change the shape of a wound opening. Tracings can be useful to describe a pattern of progress (Cooper, 2000; Motta, 1993).

Photography. Wound photography with instant and delayed-exposure cameras can be used to assess and document wound progress. When available, a digital camera transfers wound photographs and series of photographs directly to a computerized medical record. Serial photographs of the wound document progress over time. The camera records rough size of the wound (this improves if a ruler is placed alongside of the wound), color of the wound, presence of exudate, and appearance of the surrounding skin. Photographs do not accurately capture depth or color of tissue (Cooper, 2000) but are helpful when a number of clinicians evaluate a wound. With improved technology, the enhanced digital photography system's quantitative evaluation enables evaluation and measurement of wound volume; "a picture of a wound is worth thousands of dollars" (Salcido, 2000).

Ultrasonic Measurement Tools. Ultrasound scanners have potential for wound management including pressure ulcers and burns. They can capture and reproduce images of soft tissue at high resolution via laptop computers and then store the images or send them via e-mail to another clinician for interpretation. Scans can be viewed six at a time for comparison (Salcido, 2000).

Documentation. Proper documentation of wounds and ulcers is essential and includes the following:

- Determine the cause and type of the wound
- Describe the anatomic location of the wound
- Measure the wound size and depth in millimeters/centimeters
- Stage the wound, using standard tools
- Describe the wound edges (well defined to indistinct)
- Perform linear measurement of undermining and tunneling (sinus tracts)
- Describe the wound bed including notation of the presence or absence of necrotic or granulation tissue, presence or absence of exudate and odor, and description of the surrounding tissue (e.g., indurated, edematous, red) (Bates-Jensen, 1998; Cooper, 2000)

Staging of Pressure Ulcers

Standardized measurement of pressure ulcers involves the nurse grading or staging wounds to classify the degree of tissue damage observed. The most frequently used staging system is that recommended by the NPUAP and the AHCPR in their document *Pressure Ulcers in Adults: Prediction and Prevention* (1992) (Table 16-6).

TABLE 16-6 Staging of Pressure Ulcers

Stage	Description
I	Nonblanchable erythema of intact skin; the heralding lesion of skin ulceration. Reactive hyperemia can normally be expected to be present for one half to three fourths as long as the pressure-occluded blood flow to the area; it should not be confused with a stage I pressure ulcer.
II	Partial-thickness skin loss involving epidermis and/or dermis. Ulcer is superficial and presents clinically as an abrasion, blister, or shallow crater.
III	Full-thickness skin loss involving damage or necrosis of subcutaneous tissue that may extend down to, but not through, underlying fascia. Ulcer presents clinically as a deep crater with or without undermining of adjacent tissue.
IV	Full-thickness skin loss with extensive destruction; tissue necrosis; or damage to muscle, bone, or supporting structures (e.g., tendon or joint capsule). Undermining and sinus tracts may also be associated with stage IV pressure ulcers.

From Panel for Prediction and Prevention of Pressure Ulcers in Adults. (1992). Pressure ulcers in adults: prediction and prevention (Clinical Practice Guideline No. 3, AHCPR Publication No. 92-0047). Rockville, MD: Agency for Health Care Policy and Research, Public Health Service, U.S. Department of Health and Human Services.

Staging systems, although extremely valuable, have a number of inherent limitations. Staging can be used only when the wound bed can be visualized; if covered by necrotic tissue, the wound is labeled *unable to stage.* Staging depends on a gross description of the tissue involved (epidermis versus muscle) and requires the evaluator to have clinical knowledge to recognize and differentiate between tissue layers. Healing wounds have tissue that can be difficult to classify, and granulation tissue does not fit into the classification schema. Thus healing of pressure ulcers cannot be staged with these descriptors (Cooper, 2000).

When a wound is healing, it does not become a lower stage wound. A stage III wound would be noted as a healing stage III wound and would not progress to a stage II wound. Accurate staging of wounds is of particular importance to many clients receiving home health care because their continued care and reimbursement for support products are based on the stage of their wound. Adopting a universal classification system will provide uniformity to the language of pressure ulcers. Researchers will be able to compare results of studies on factors contributing to prevalence and incidence and on the effectiveness of preventive interventions and wound care modalities (NPUAP, 1989).

Data concerning the skin and skin care activities are gathered from the client's health history and physical assessment. Analysis of the data and conclusions about nursing intervention are influenced by current nursing knowledge and past nursing experience. The nursing diagnoses reflect identification of the client's strengths and limitations to assist nurses in determining interventions.

Nursing Diagnosis

As with any area of nursing practice, nursing diagnoses are useful to the rehabilitation nurse in describing their clinical judgments about health-related conditions, projecting outcomes, and planning interventions. Nursing diagnoses applicable to skin management with clients in rehabilitation are listed in Table 16-7. The primary diagnoses are impaired skin integrity and risk for impaired skin integrity. The associated or contributing diagnoses might include altered health maintenance, altered nutrition (less than body requirements), impaired physical mobility, impaired bed mobility, impaired transfer ability, impaired wheelchair mobility, self-care deficit, uncompensated sensory loss, and knowledge deficit (Gordon, 2000).

Rehabilitation Nursing Outcomes

Outcomes define a client's state that follows and can be expected to be influenced by an intervention (Johnson, Maas, & Moorhead, 2000). Rehabilitation nurses are accountable for instituting means to improve client outcomes. Reimbursement and health care payment structures are dependent on nursing assessment, diagnoses, outcomes, and interventions. Table 16-7 displays relevant outcomes for several identified diagnoses related to skin integrity.

Rehabilitation Nursing Interventions

Nursing interventions include any treatment, based on clinical judgment and knowledge, that a nurse performs to enhance client outcomes (McCloskey & Bulechek, 2000). Nursing interventions relevant to selected skin management diagnoses and outcomes are listed in Table 16-7. Details of specific interventions are in the following section.

Prevention

Nursing intervention for skin management is targeted primarily at prevention. As with most health issues, prevention is the most cost-effective management when compared with the costs of treating a pressure ulcer or other alteration in skin integrity (Xakellis et al., 1998). As previously mentioned, risk for alteration in skin integrity is an integral part of health assessment and will guide the prevention efforts of the rehabilitation nurse. The plan of care would include items to address identified risk factors.

The AHCPR recommends four target goals: (1) identify at-risk individuals who need prevention and the specific factors placing them at risk; (2) maintain and improve tissue tolerance to pressure in order to prevent injury; (3) protect against the adverse effects of pressure, friction, and shear; and (4) reduce the incidence of pressure ulcers through educational programs (PPPPUA, 1992). Further clarification of the recommendations for skin care and early treatment from the AHCPR guideline include (American Hospital Association, 1997):

- Inspect the skin of all at-risk individuals at least once a day; pay particular attention to bony prominences
- Document results of skin inspection
- Cleanse the skin at the time of soiling and at routine intervals; individualize the frequency of skin cleansing according to need and/or client preference
- Avoid hot water and use a mild cleansing agent that minimizes irritation and dryness of the skin
- During cleansing, take care to minimize the force and friction applied to the skin
- Minimize environmental factors leading to skin drying, such as low humidity (less than 40%) and exposure to cold; treat dry skin with moisturizers
- Avoid massage over bony prominences
- Minimize skin exposure to moisture due to incontinence, perspiration, or wound drainage
- Minimize skin injury due to friction and shear forces through proper positioning, transferring, and turning techniques; friction injuries may be reduced by the use of lubricants, protective films, protective dressings, and protective padding
- When apparently well-nourished clients develop an inadequate dietary intake of protein or calories, first attempt to discover the factors compromising intake and offer

TABLE 16-7 Nursing Diagnoses Applicable to Skin Management

Nursing Diagnosis	Nursing Outcomes Classification (NOC)	Nursing Interventions Classification (NIC)
Risk for impaired skin integrity	Risk reduction Risk control Tissue integrity Tissue perfusion	Pressure management Pressure ulcer prevention Risk identification Self-care assistance Foot care intervention Health education
Impaired skin integrity/pressure ulcer	Tissue integrity Wound healing Tissue perfusion Nutrition Self-care Fluid balance Immobility consequences Treatment behavior	Health education Pressure ulcer care Skin care: Topical treatment Describe characteristics of the ulcer at regular intervals, including size, stage, location, exudate, granulation or necrotic tissue, and epithelialization Monitor color, temperature, edema, moisture, and appearance of surrounding skin Keep ulcer moist to aid in healing Cleanse skin around the ulcer with mild soap and water Debride ulcer as needed Cleanse ulcer with the appropriate nontoxic solution, working in a circular motion from the center Note characteristics of any drainage Apply dressings as appropriate Monitor for signs and symptoms of infection in the wound Position every 1-2 hours to avoid prolonged pressure Use specialty beds and mattresses as appropriate Use devices on the bed that protect the client's skin Ensure adequate dietary intake Initiate consultation of an enterostomal therapy nurse as needed
Deficient knowledge: skin management	Knowledge: skin care and treatment regime Knowledge: prevention of pressure ulcers	Health education Learning facilitation Learning readiness enhancement Teaching: pressure ulcer prevention, development, treatment Teaching: prescribed diet and nutrition management
Impaired nutrition: less than body requirements	Nutritional status: nutrient intake	Fluid/electrolyte management Fluid monitoring Nutritional counseling Nutrition therapy Nutritional monitoring Weight management/weight gain assistance Teaching: prescribed diet
Impaired mobility	Body positioning: self-initiated	Exercise promotion Exercise therapy Positioning Self-care assistance

Data from Johnson, M., Maas, M.L., & Moorhead, S. (2000). *Nursing outcomes classification (NOC)* (2nd ed.). St. Louis: Mosby; McCloskey, J.C., & Bulechek, G.M. (2000). *Nursing interventions classification (NIC)* (3rd ed.). St. Louis: Mosby; and North American Nursing Diagnosis Association. (2001). *Nursing diagnosis: definitions and classification 2001-2002* (4th ed.). Philadelphia: Author.

support, including nutritional supplements, as needed; for nutritionally compromised individuals, implement a plan of nutritional support and/or supplementation.

Additional recommendations for mechanical loading and support surfaces from the AHCPR guideline include (American Hospital Association, 1997):

- Reposition any individual in bed who is assessed to be at risk for developing pressure ulcers at least every 2 hours if consistent with overall client goals; teach clients using wheelchairs to shift their weight every 20 minutes
- For individuals in bed, use positioning devices such as pillows or foam wedges to keep bony prominences from direct contact with one another
- Maintain the head of the bed at the lowest degree of elevation consistent with medical conditions and other restrictions; limit the amount of time the head of the bed is elevated

- Use lifting devices such as a trapeze or bed linen to move (rather than drag) individuals in bed who cannot assist during transfers and position changes
- Place any individual at risk for developing pressure ulcers on a pressure-reducing device, such as a foam, static air, alternating air, gel, or water mattress, when he or she is lying in bed
- For chair-bound individuals, use a pressure-reducing device; do not use doughnut-shaped devices

According to the AHCPR guideline, educational programs for the prevention of pressure ulcers should (American Hospital Association, 1997):

- Be structured, organized, comprehensive, and directed at all levels of health care providers, clients, and family caregivers
- Include information on cause of and risk factors for pressure ulcers, risk assessment tools and their application, skin assessment, selection and/or use of support surfaces, development and implementation of an individualized program of skin care, demonstration of positioning to decrease risk of tissue breakdown, and instruction on accurate documentation of pertinent information
- Identify persons responsible for pressure ulcer prevention, describe each person's role, and be appropriate to the audience in terms of level of information presented and expected participation

Bed Support Surfaces

The AHCPR guidelines recommend the use of bed support surfaces for pressure relief in high-risk individuals. With numerous products on the market, careful assessment of the client's specific need for a bed support surface is essential to selecting the appropriate product. The products are costly, and improper choices actually may interfere with physical independence of some clients. Numerous investigators have measured the characteristics, properties, and effectiveness of bed support surfaces. Most findings indicate that bed support surfaces reduce the incidence of pressure ulcers, but the product type does not necessarily make a difference (Aranovitch, Wilber, Slezak, Martin, & Utter, 1999; NPUAP, 1997; Whittemore, 1998).

When pressure-reducing devices were compared with standard hospital beds, clients cared for on a standard hospital mattress had much greater incidence of pressure ulcers. However, comparisons of two types of pressure-reducing devices found no significant differences in incidence and severity of pressure ulcers (PPPPUA, 1992). Table 16-8 outlines a variety of bed support surfaces and advantages and disadvantages for each.

Because one bed support surface is not necessarily superior to another for reducing pressure ulcers, other considerations are reviewed when making a selection. Conine, Choi, and Lim (1989) suggest "user friendliness" as a guide. Qualities for consideration include:

- Costs: initial, maintenance, and replacement
- Regulations (hospital safety codes)
- Client pleasing: comfort, stability, temperature, noise, and suitability of weight (bed and chair)
- Caregiver pleasing: difficulty in moving and transferring, frequent need to calibrate and monitor equipment, and service and repair availability

The high-technology end of replacement beds usually is retained for the most difficult skin problems. Two studies examined reduced cost and rapidity of healing as factors for choosing beds. Strauss, Gong, Gary, Kalsbeek, and Spear (1991) found home air-fluidized therapy for pressure ulcers was no more costly than alternative therapy, and it reduced hospitalizations. Ferrell, Osterweil, and Christenson (1993) showed low-airflow beds provided substantial improvement over foam mattresses for healing pressure ulcers and did so more rapidly.

Support surfaces are categorized by their mechanical features; they are pressure-relieving or pressure-reducing surfaces. Pressure-relief systems consistently keep surface tissue pressure below capillary closing pressure. Use of pressure-reducing surfaces results in lower pressures when compared with a standard hospital mattress (Pieper, 2000; IAET, 1991). Support surfaces are available as overlays (support surface placed over the hospital mattress), replacement mattresses, and specialty beds. Figure 16-7 illustrates current AHCPR guidelines for management of tissue loads. Support surfaces are reviewed for their ability to distribute pressure, avoid humidity buildup, and insulate (Conine et al., 1989).

Overlays and replacement mattresses are the most common types of support surfaces. Once again, multiple options are available, and products change often. Mattress overlays help with pressure reduction but do not provide complete pressure relief. The higher the density of the product, the more pressure is distributed and air is circulated. Clients need to be monitored for their own responses to pressure relief.

The physical environment and a client's abilities are considerations when choosing an overlay system. For example, if the height of the bed or seat is increased with the overlay, assisted or independent transfers may become difficult for both client and caregiver. Or an overlay may create a safety problem, such as a client rolling over the side rails and off the bed. A person can become wedged between the overlay and the side rails. Caregivers may need a step stool to provide care and cautions about the use of proper body mechanics to avoid back injury. Replacement mattresses have surface characteristics similar to those of overlays but have the advantage of providing the depth needed to increase density or flotation without the additional height problem of an overlay (Pieper, 2000).

Water systems come as overlays and replacement systems. Water systems must be checked for proper inflation so that the person floats; they should not be underfilled or overfilled. Water motion may be a problem for some persons. Baffle systems on some models control water activity. Turning individuals on water surfaces can be more difficult. Additional concerns are weight of the mattresses (they are not supported by flooring in some homes), punctures, and

Table 16-8 Support Surfaces for the Bed

Product/Goal	Description	Client Selection	Advantages	Disadvantages	Nursing Interventions
Mattress replacement/pressure reduction	Replaces standard hospital mattress and fits on bed frame Most are constructed of bonded layers of different foam densities Covered with conformable, cleanable, bacteriostatic cover	No skin breakdown, but client at risk Stage I, II, or III ulcer and client can be positioned off area Only 1 ulcer Cooperative with repositioning	Multiple client use Reduces use of overlay devices Does not add height to mattress Easy to clean Low maintenance	May be too hot for some clients, particularly spinal cord injured Initial expense may be higher than standard mattress Foam will deform over time and will lose effectiveness	Use with turning schedule Mattress must be oriented properly on bed frame (i.e., "head" or "feet") Massive body fluid spills should be cleaned immediately Multiple layers of pads and linens on top of surface decrease effectiveness
Static overlay/pressure reduction	Lies on top of mattress Constructed of foam or air-filled polyvinyl	As above, plus: For clients up to 200 lb; assess heavier clients on a case-by- case basis	Inexpensive Air-filled, easy to clean	If punctured, air-filled overlay will leak Adds height to mattress Air-filled overlays often require "hand checks" to determine whether client is "bottoming-out" Foam may be infection-control concern	Use with a turning schedule Do not overinflate air-filled overlay Position properly over mattress Multiple layers of pads and linens on top of surface decrease effectiveness
Alternating air-filled overlay/pressure reduction	Overlay consists of different configurations of chambers through which air is pumped at regular intervals to provide inflation and deflation of the chambers Interface pressures may be lower than capillary closing pressure when chambers are deflated but are then higher than capillary closing pressure when chambers are inflated (trochanter pressures commonly higher in both phases)	Client at low to moderate risk Only one ulcer present; stage I or II Able to reposition and stay repositioned with individualized turning Not recommended for clients over 175 lb	Easy to clean Pump reusable	Motion may feel uncomfortable to client Assembly required Motor may be noisy Pressure under trochanters is commonly higher than capillary closing pressure	Use with a turning schedule Position properly over mattress Multiple layers of pads and linens on top of surface decrease effectiveness

Gel-filled overlay/pressure reduction	Pads constructed of silicon or polyvinyl chloride available in a variety of shapes and sizes	Skin intact and client at low risk Client able to be repositioned and stay repositioned Avoid use with clients over 175 pounds	Low maintenance Easy to clean Multiple client use possible	Expensive Limited research on effectiveness Heavy	Use with a turning schedule Monitor for friction/shear Multiple layers of pads and linens on top of surface decrease effectiveness
Low-air-loss overlay or bed/pressure reduction	Available as a specialty bed or as a mattress overlay Air-filled pillows deflate for emergency or transfer Instant seat deflates when getting client out of bed Able to raise head and foot of bed with controls	Deep stage III or IV ulcers Severe intractable pain Anticipate immobility for several days Flap rotation, grafts Preferred device for pressure relief because has all benefits of regular hospital bed (i.e., raised head or foot of bed) As client's status changes, a step-down device may be indicated	Transfers in/out of bed possible Portable motor with overlay makes bed transfer possible	Expensive; client should be stepped down to less expensive product when possible Bed surface material is slippery, and clients may slip or slide Transfers in or out of bed may be difficult	Client should be repositioned as able Know how to operate bed/overlay Do not use Chux beneath client; use incontinence pads provided with bed overlay, which allow airflow
Oscillation therapy (with low air loss)/pressure reduction and pulmonary support	Same as above, plus: Can be set to rotate client from side to side	Use when client has acute respiratory distress; may help prevent pulmonary complications Contraindicated for clients in cervical or skeletal traction As client's status changes, so may need for pressure relief or pressure reduction Reevaluate at least every 5 days	May have significant positive effect on multiple body systems	Expensive	Know how to operate bed Assess client for shear if bed rotating
Fluid mattress overlay/pressure reduction and shear/friction relief	Available as specialty bed or mattress overlay Fluid-filled mattress that conforms to client's body to decrease pressure Slippery mattress cover to reduce shear/friction Static; requires no motor or external power source	Deep stage III or IV ulcers Intractable pain Immobility Flap rotation/grafts Continent or controlled incontinence	Transfers in or out of bed easy Requires no external energy source	Heavy	Client should be repositioned as able Do not try to eliminate wrinkles in mattress cover; wrinkles are supposed to be there

Continued

Table 16-8 Support Surfaces for the Bed—cont'd

Product/Goal	Description	Client Selection	Advantages	Disadvantages	Nursing Interventions
High air loss (fluidized bed)/pressure relief	Bed frame containing silicone-coated beads; provides pressure relief when air is blown through beads, making them behave as if they were a liquid Some able to raise head of bed only by placing foam wedges; newer generation beds include mechanical control to elevate head Replaces regular bed	Deep stage III or IV ulcers Intractable pain Immobility Flap rotation/grafts Client bedridden or transfers with limited frequency	May assist in management of copious wound drainage or incontinence Procedures facilitated by turning bed off Traction can be used on bed frame Less frequent turning schedule may be possible	Warm, dry air from bed may dehydrate client/wounds Room may be warm from bed motor Width and height of bed can make client access difficult Difficult to transfer client in or out of bed Clients may feel/become disoriented or report feeling weightless Size/weight of bed too large for most home use	Clients should be on a turning schedule with special attention to heels Apply moisturizer to skin at least twice a day Know how to operate bed Assess client for dehydration Report leakage of beads from bed (safety and health issue) If client too warm, notify manufacturer Difficult to transfer client in or out of bed

From Andrychuk, M. A. (1998). Pressure ulcers, risk factors, assessment and intervention. *Orthopaedic Nurse, 17*(4), 65-81.

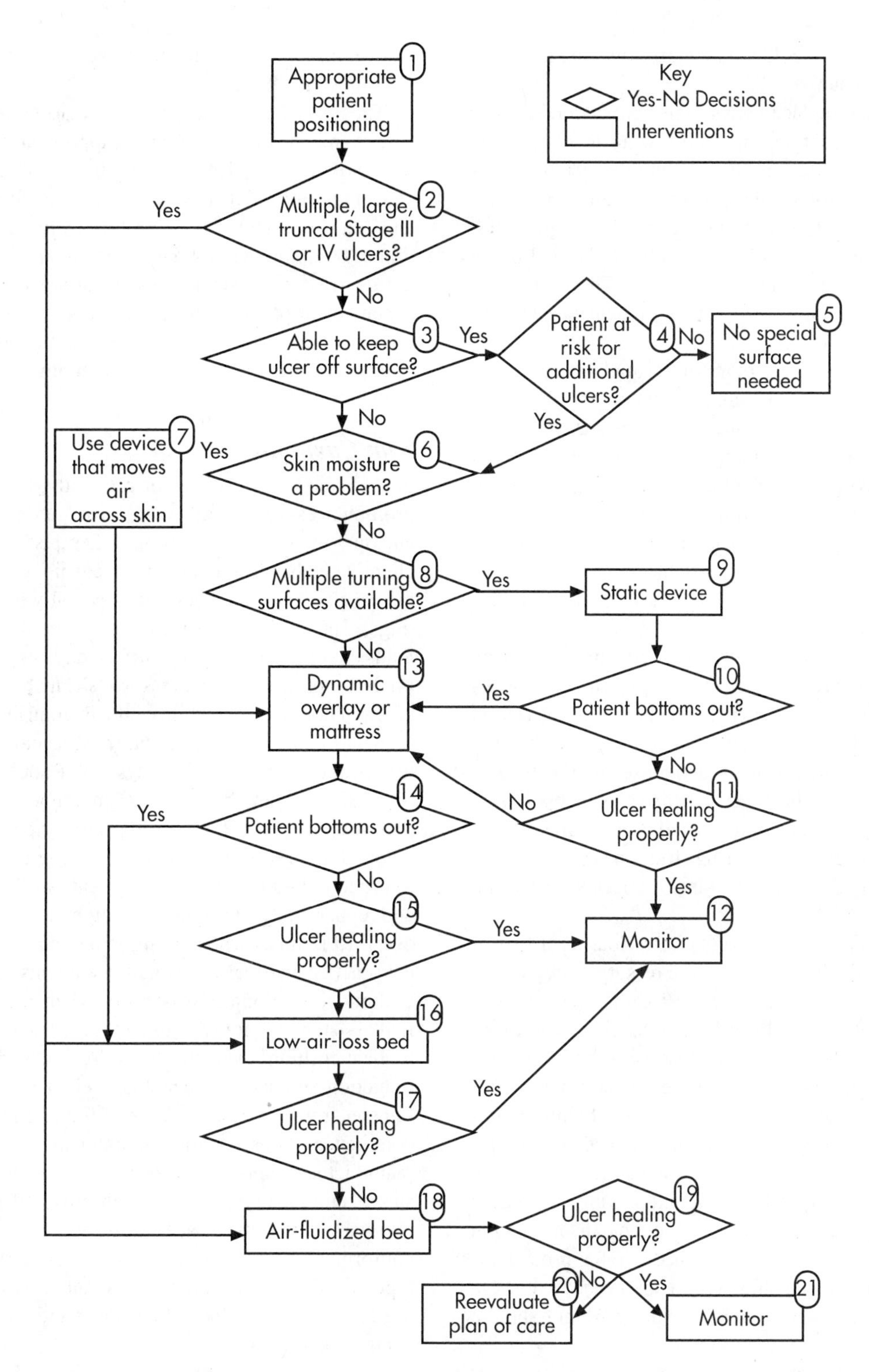

Figure 16-7 The AHCPR algorithm for management of tissue loads assists the nurse to choose support surfaces that help distribute pressure and reduce friction and shear on the tissue. (From Bergstrom, N., Bennett, M.A., Carlson, C.E., et al. [1994]. *Treatment of pressure ulcers: Clinical practice guidelines* [No. 15, AHCPR Publication No. 95-0652]. Rockville, MD: U.S. Department of Health and Human Services, Agency for Health Care Policy and Research.)

temperature (some need heat controls). The manufacturer may recommend not raising the head of the bed, although some water mattresses have compartments to allow this.

Gel overlay and replacement systems usually are combined with foam. These are easy-to-clean, low-maintenance, puncture-resistant systems without the disadvantages of moving water or difficulty with turning clients. Disadvantages include weight, which creates problems for both the caregiver and the client, and expense. Temperature guidelines provided by the manufacturer need to be checked.

Some gels get harder in cold temperatures, making them unusable in cold climates.

Air overlays and replacement systems are divided further into static-air, alternating-air, and low-air-loss systems. Static air mattresses force air through interconnected tunnels (bulbous cells) to provide the proper pressure and subsequently require skilled monitoring to check for proper inflation. Some models allows for cells (bulbs) to be tied off to give pressure relief over designated areas. These are low-maintenance systems designed for multiclient use but are easily punctured and expensive.

Alternating air mattresses pump air through interconnecting tunnels, alternating intervals of inflation and deflation. They are promoted as devices to reduce pressure and stimulate circulation. Their advantages are similar to those of static-air systems, with the added client concerns about noise and inflation and deflation. With both static-air and alternating-air systems, there is the added concern for safe transfers. They do not provide a stable base and may be problematic for clients with poor hand and trunk control (Conine et al., 1989).

Low-air-loss mattresses fill channels with air and provide for air movement around the skin. This feature reduces moisture perspiration problems and helps to reduce friction and shear. As with the alternating-air overlay and replacement systems, puncture problems and noise are drawbacks.

Specialty beds are the most expensive of support surfaces. They replace the hospital bed and provide pressure relief, as well as decreased shearing, friction, and moisture. High-air-loss, low-air-loss, and kinetic specialty beds are available.

High-air-loss beds allow the client to float on a bed of silicone-coated, air-fluidized beads. Pressure relief is not absolute on these beds; studies have found pressures over capillary closure in heels (PPPPUA, 1992); however, existing pressure ulcers heal faster on these beds, and fewer ulcers develop. High-air-loss beds are extremely helpful for clients after skin flap surgery because the flotation provides minimal pressure to tissue at the surgical site and reduces the problems of friction and shear. Concerns with this bed include dehydration, wound drying, increased client and room temperature, and client disorientation (Pieper, 2000). The bed can be turned off for procedures and transfers. The height and weight of the bed can be a problem, although newer models are lighter weight and are height adjustable.

Low-air-loss beds provide a series of interconnected air-filled bladder pillows around the bed. Each pillow is filled and calibrated for proper inflation and to provide airflow. The head of bed can be elevated, and transfers are easier; however, the surface is very slippery. There is decreased shearing and friction, but transfers may pose a safety concern.

Kinetic beds provide continuous motion and may be combined with an air-loss feature. These primarily are used as management for multiple problems of immobility, usually from trauma. The ability to relive pressure is one feature (Bryant et al., 1992).

The heels are known to be particularly vulnerable to pressure even on pressure-reducing support surfaces (Blaszczyk, Majewok, & Sato, 1998). A number of commercially available pressure-relief devices, such as sheepskin booties and foam boots, can help protect from shearing and friction or bumping the foot during transfers. Heel protectors do not decrease or dissipate pressure appreciably. Devices that elevate the foot totally from the support surface are most effective when pressure relief is needed (Yetzer & Sullivan, 1992) and are the only ones recommended for pressure relief.

Seat Cushions

Seat cushions are critical for protecting the skin over bony prominences for clients who have motor-sensory deficits and are in a sitting position. Therapists may evaluate a client's needs and recommend a cushion, but rehabilitation nurses also make the decision, especially in community settings. The purpose of a cushion is to distribute pressure loads over the entire sitting surface and keep excess pressure off bony prominences. Pressure, shear, heat, moisture and postural control and stability all can contribute to the development of a pressure ulcer and must be considered in selection of a cushion or seating system (Rappl, 1998). Recommendations from the AHCPR guideline on prevention of pressure ulcers (PPPPUA, 1994) are for persons to be repositioned at least every hour when sitting up in a chair or be returned to bed (Figure 16-8). Clients with cognitive ability and upper body strength are taught to shift their weight every 15 minutes when sitting in a chair. However, in clinical practice and real-life situations, clients may spend hours without repositioning, especially when they require maximal assistance to transfer in and out of bed. When selecting a chair cushion, evaluate the following variables: pressure reduction and stability benefits, weight if it is necessary to transfer from the cushion, ease of transfer from the cushion, continence status, cushion maintenance requirements and manufacturer support, reimbursement by the individual's insurer, durability, type of cushion cover (the cover needs a two-way stretch material to prevent shear and to allow for conformability without increasing pressure), and design or type of cushion (an air-filled donut-shaped device is not used because it acts like a tourniquet and reduces blood flow centrally).

Wound Care

First and foremost in wound care is identifying the cause of the wound. Failure to address the cause of the wound will result in a nonhealing wound despite appropriate local and systemic treatment (Waldrop & Doughty, 2000). It cannot be stressed enough that topical care supports the wound; the healing comes from removing the cause and addressing systemic concerns. Local wound care is critical to provide an ideal healing environment.

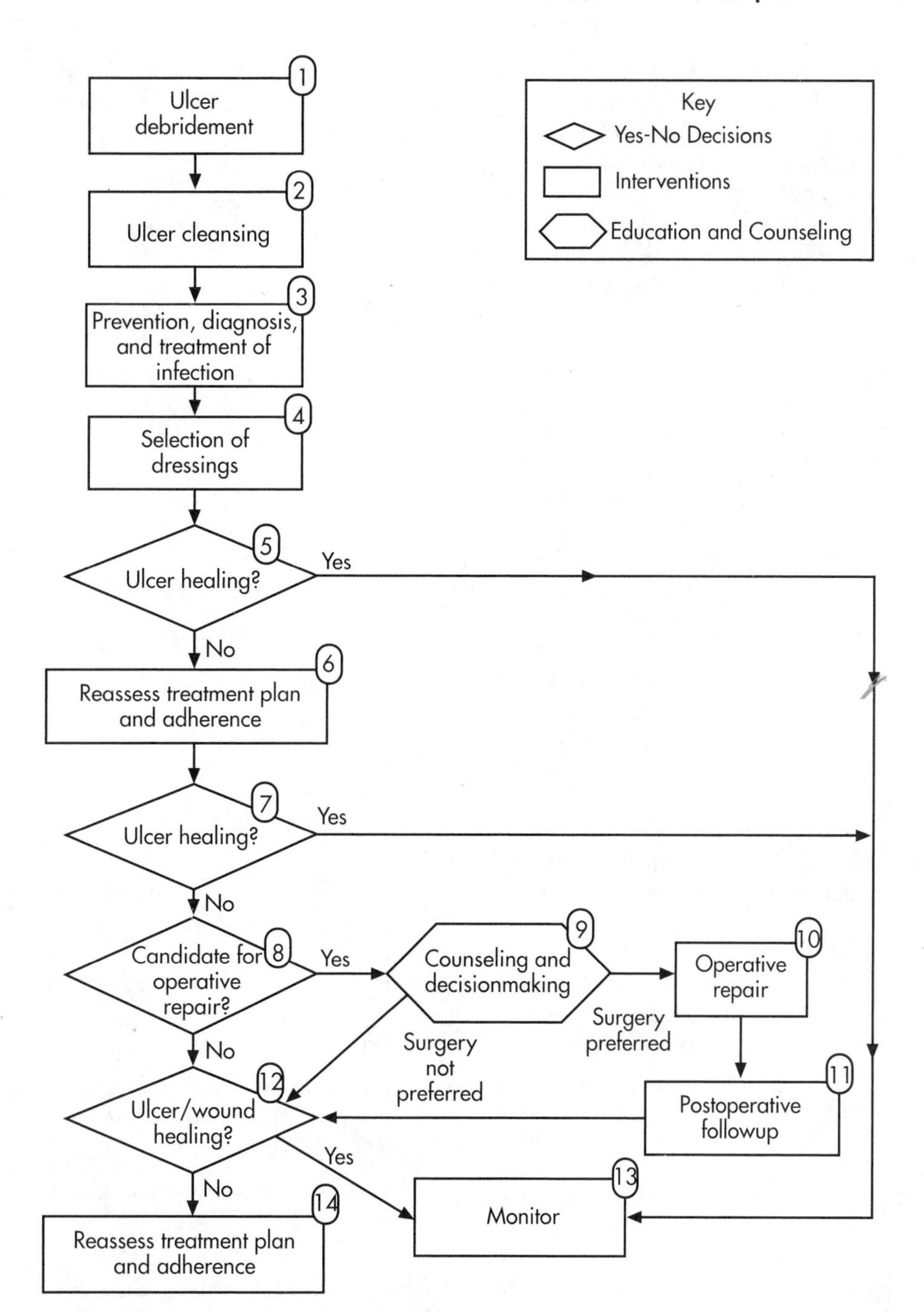

Figure 16-8 The AHCPR algorithm for treatment of pressure ulcers. (From Bergstrom, N., Bennett, M.A., Carlson, C.E., et al. [1994]. *Treatment of pressure ulcers: Clinical practice guidelines* [No. 15, AHCPR Publication No. 95-0652]. Rockville, MD: U.S. Department of Health and Human Services, Agency for Health Care Policy and Research.)

Key Principles for Local Wound Care. Local wound care involves cleansing and debriding the wound, treating and controlling infection, absorbing excess exudate, eliminating dead space, maintaining moisture, and covering the wound. Cleansing the wound makes it easier to assess and promotes growth of healthy tissue. Cleansing removes bacteria and surface contaminants and protects a healing wound.

Debridement of necrotic tissue that prolongs the inflammatory process and promotes bacterial growth can be accomplished with selective methods, which remove only nonviable tissue, or by nonselective methods. Selective methods include surgical or sharp, autolytic, enzymatic, and osmotic debridement. Nonselective methods include wet-to-dry dressings, pressurized irrigation, and whirlpool. Surgical or sharp debridement uses a scalpel, scissors, and forceps.

Autolytic debridement is facilitated by covering the wound with a moisture-retentive dressing such as a hydrocolloid or transparent film. Usually within 72 to 96 hours of occlusion, the necrotic tissue begins to liquefy as the polymorphonuclear leukocytes, macrophages, and bacteria in the wound fluid provide endogenous enzymes to continue autodigestion. Enzymatic debridement involves topical application of an exogenous enzyme that digests necrotic tissue. Collagenase (Santyl) and Travase are examples. They break up the collagen fibers that hold the necrotic tissue within the wound base. Eschar is removed or cross-hatched for the enzyme to be effective.

Osmotic debridement is accomplished through the absorption of exudate, bacteria, and wound debris using osmotic agents such as calcium alginates, dextranomer beads, and hydrocolloid beads and pastes. Surgical laser debridement is being used by surgeons on an outpatient basis. It has superior qualities because of its instant hemostasis and sterilization of the wound (Ramundo & Wells, 2000).

Nonselective methods such as wet-to-dry dressings remove necrotic tissue when removed but also remove fragile epithelial cells and newly formed granulation tissue and increase client discomfort. Pressurized irrigation and whirlpool are also nonselective and are used to remove necrotic tissue but are discontinued once the wounds are clean and granulation tissue is present (Baharestani, 1999).

Infection prevents wound healing by prolonging the inflammatory phase, delaying collagen synthesis, inhibiting epidermal migration, and competing for oxygen for tissue repair. Diagnosis is by culture, and treatment follows with culture-specific antibiotic therapy.

Absorb excess exudate to prevent maceration of surrounding tissue or any inhibiting of wound repair. Because moisture is a contributing factor in wound development, use one of the many materials available for keeping skin surfaces dry while drawing away moisture. Creative use of the products can assist with moisture control in a variety of situations. Other acceptable moisture barriers include ointments, sealants, or solid wafers. Absorption of excess exudate differs from the principle of maintaining a moist surface. A moist wound environment promotes tissue growth because it prevents cell death and promotes migration of epidermal tissue. Thus a moist wound environment enhances all phases of wound healing.

Obliterate dead space formed by tissue destruction beneath the wound, such as sinus tracts. Dead spaces provide a medium for bacterial growth and can contribute to abscess formation and inhibit the healing process. Covering the wound adds a protective coat to resist bacterial invasion and prevent trauma to the wound bed, as well as helping support a moist wound environment (Motta, 1993; Rolstad, Ovington, & Harris, 2000).

Figure 16-9 displays the AHCPR algorithm for treatment of pressure ulcers (PPPPUA, 1994).

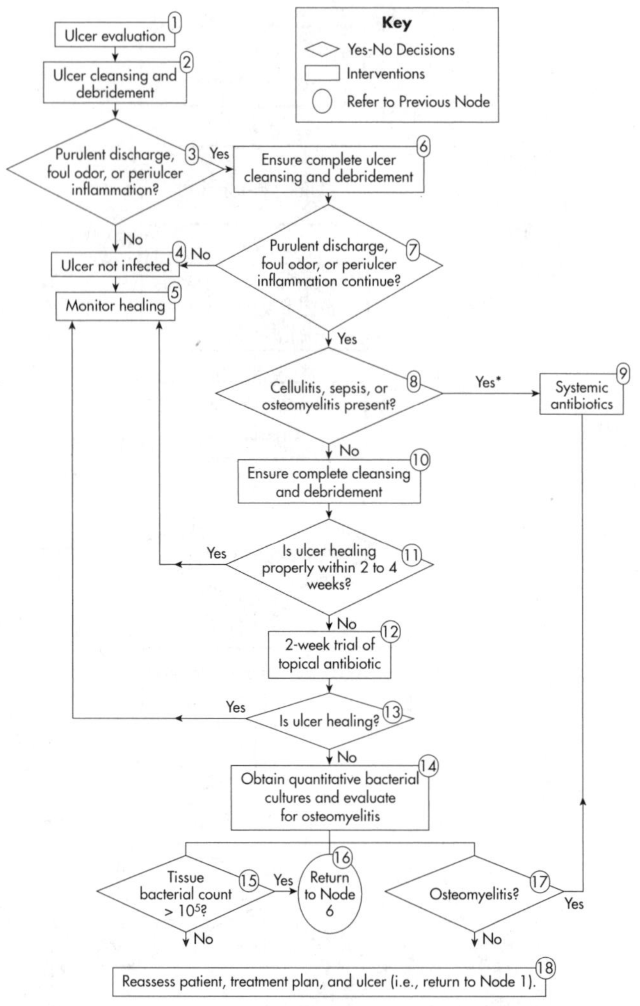

Figure 16-9 Managing bacterial colonization and infection. (From Bergstrom, N., Bennett, M.A., Carlson, C.E., et al. [1994]. *Treatment of pressure ulcers: Clinical practice guidelines* [No. 15, AHCPR Publication No. 95-0652]. Rockville, MD: U.S. Department of Health and Human Services, Agency for Health Care Policy and Research.)

Wound Cleansing. Controversy continues about what constitutes proper wound cleansing. Nurses need to be knowledgeable about the action of cleansing solutions on tissues, specifically during each phase of wound healing. In a clean proliferating wound, the goal is to promote the health of cells. The AHCPR recommends using normal saline solution with enough irrigation pressure to enhance wound cleansing without causing trauma to the wound bed (PPPPUA, 1994). However, commercially available mild wound cleansers vary from safe to toxic (Table 16-9). Trauma inflicted by the cleansing process must be justified by the effectiveness of the procedure. Extremely dirty wounds require more mechanical force and stronger cleansing solutions, but as the wound becomes cleaner, the mechanical force and cleanser strength can be decreased proportionally.

Some support leaving the wound surface of clean wounds alone and allowing the supportive exudate to heal the wound. Antiseptic cleansers such as povidone-iodine, acetic

TABLE 16-9 Toxicity Index for Wound and Skin Cleansers

Test Agent	Toxicity Index*
Shur Clens	1:10
Biolex	1:100
Saf Clens	1:100
Cara Klenz	1:100
Ultra Klenz	1:1,000
Clinical Care	1:1,000
Uni Wash	1:1,000
Ivory Soap (0.5%)	1:1,000
Constant Clens	1:10,000
Dermal Wound Cleanser	1:10,000
Puri-Clens	1:10,000
Hibiclens	1:10,000
Betadine Surgical Scrub	1:10,000
Techni-Care Scrub	1:100,000
Bard Skin Cleanser	1:100,000
Hollister	1:100,000

*The dilution required to maintain white blood cell viability and phagocytic efficiency.

From Bergstrom, N., Bennett, M.A., Carlson, C.E., et al. (1994). *Treatment of pressure ulcers: clinical practice guidelines* (No. 15. AHCPR Publication No. 95-0652). Rockville, MD: U.S. Department of Health and Human Services, Agency for Health Care Policy and Research.

acid, Dakin's solution, and hydrogen peroxide should not be used for routine wound cleansing because of their harmful effects on healing tissue (Rolstad et al., 2000). Povidone-iodine damages granulation tissue and may cause iodine toxicity (Eaglstein, 1986). Acetic acid is effective against *Pseudomonas aeruginosa* but also damages proliferating tissue. Dakin's solution is irritating to granulation tissue as well as surrounding tissue. Although hydrogen peroxide provides mechanical cleansing, it is harmful to new tissue, and the air bubbles formed can cause air emboli if introduced into sinus tracts.

Culturing of wounds is also controversial. All chronic wounds are considered contaminated because multiple organisms are present. Cultures (swabs) of the surface of the wound will uncover multiple organisms, but these represent contaminants within the wound bed rather than a pathogenic agent producing a clinically relevant wound infection. When an organism is cultured from the tissue of a wound in a non-immunocompromised client, a colony forming unit (CFU) count of more than 10 CFU/ml indicates an invasive wound infection. This culture must be obtained from the depth of the lesion or from a wound biopsy specimen. Proper technique is essential to confirm the diagnosis of infection. Always first cleanse the wound well with saline solution or water, removing the excess necrotic debris. Do not swab exudate, pus, eschar, or heavily fibrous tissue (Fowler, 1998).

A wound infection is managed by systemic sensitivity-guided antibiotic therapy. Topical agents will not adequately treat an infection (Rubano & Kerstein, 1998). Metronidazole will reduce odor in pressure ulcers, however it must be used in combination with another dressing and will not substitute for systemic antibiotics (Motta, 1993). In general, wounds are cultured when there are signs of infection: fever, edema, induration of the surrounding wound bed, and erythema. Drainage may be copious and foul smelling or minimal. Figure 16-9 reflects the AHCPR recommendations for management of bacterial colonization and infection (Figure 16-8 PPPPUA, 1994).

Wound Dressings. A variety of available wound dressings are available to enhance the natural physiological wound environment, provide thermal insulation, and protect the wound from bacteria and trauma (Rolstad et al., 2000). The moist environment permitted by dressings heals pressure ulcers more quickly and effectively. More investigation is needed to compare dressing choices and wound outcome. Although dressings are selected on the basis of clinical assessment of the wound characteristics matched with the qualities of a particular dressing. When wounds do not progress, review the cause and systemic effects because failure to improve may signal infection or systemic problems or simply a need for an alternate dressing product.

Appendix 16A summarizes dressing options in management of pressure ulcers (PPPPUA, 1994).

Growth factors have gained popularity in treatment of chronic ulcers. Most studies of growth factors have been conducted in clients with foot ulcers, primarily diabetic ulcers, but other chronic wounds including pressure ulcers and venous ulcers are under investigation. Growth factors affect the wound-healing process, including cell metabolism, differentiation, and growth (Mulder, Haberer & Jeter, 1999). Becaplermin (Regranex) is the most well known and studied growth factor, and it is approved by the Food and Drug Administration.

Anabolic Steroids. Systemic use of anabolic steroids is also gaining acceptance in wound management. Oxandrolone and human growth hormone (HGH) have been shown to increase lean body mass and protein stores and improve the healing rate of wounds. Use of these anabolic steroids has not presented serious side effects (Demling & De Santi, 1998, 1999).

Electrical Stimulation. Electrical stimulation also is gaining acceptance as a modality in wound management. The theory is that when an electrical current is applied, energy transfers to the wound and facilitates healing because it enhances the body's own bioelectrical system to attract the cells of repair, change the cell membrane permeability, enhance cellular secretion through the cell membranes, and orient cell structures. Electrical stimulation has shown positive effects on increasing blood flow, reducing edema, wound debridement, control of infection, improved wound oxygenation, and improved scar formation (Sussman & Byl, 1998).

Negative Pressure Wound Therapy (Vacuum-Assisted Closure). Controlled negative pressure can be used to evacuate wound fluid, stimulate granulation tissue, and decrease bacterial colonization (Mendez-Eastman,

1998). It also improves nutrient delivery to the wound by increasing blood perfusion. Proven cost-effective in home care, it is useful in treating chronic wounds and in closing contoured wounds by assisting the rate of "graft take" (Hartnett, 1998; Philbeck et al., 1999; Blackburn et al., 1998).

Surgical Management. When wounds reach stage III to IV, surgical closure becomes an option. Early closure of the wound will decrease loss of fluid and nutrients, improve the client's general health status, and lead to earlier mobilization and reentry into society. Unfortunately rates of recurrence and surgical failures are high (Goodman, Cohen, Armenta, Thornby, & Netscher, 1999; Yamamoto, Tsutsumida, Murazumi, & Sugihara, 1996), so clients must be at optimal nutritional and health status. Those with a serum albumin levels less than 3 benefit from nutritional intervention before surgery and may not be good candidates for healing. Disa et al. (1992) caution that additional prospective study is needed to conclude who will benefit most from surgical closure. An open-cell foam sponge is placed into the wound bed, sealed with adhesive tape, and subjected to subatmospheric pressure via an evacuation tube controlled by a computerized pump. The pump is programmed to deliver negative pressure according to the wound assessment (Broussard, Mendez-Eastham, & Frantz, 2000). Surgical closure of chronic pressure ulcers allows clients to mobilize quickly and return to work, family, or school without bed rest and potential complications from immobility.

Education. Preventing pressure ulcers is an integral component of rehabilitation practice. A comprehensive program includes prevention as a key means of improving outcomes. The AHCPR clinical practice guideline on prevention of pressure ulcers has an overall goal to reduce the incidence of pressure ulcers through educational programs that are structured, organized, comprehensive, and directed to all levels of providers, clients, families, and caregivers (PPPPUA, 1992, 1994). Rehabilitation nurses have long recognized the importance of coordinated and comprehensive education and value an interdisciplinary approach. More outcome studies are needed to support early correlations of clients' involvement in care with increased awareness of pressure ulcer risk factors, assessment, and early treatment for SCI (Andberg, Rudolph, & Anderson, 1983; Krouskop, Noble, Garber, & Spencer, 1983).

A comprehensive program for clients and families must encompass the behavioral component of wound prevention and management including individual responsibility. Dai and Catanzaro (1987) developed a paradigm for relating interreactions among individual health beliefs, modifying factors, and cues to action with skin care compliance. Individuals who believed they were susceptible to pressure ulcers were more likely to comply with skin care interventions than those who perceived the severity of pressure ulcers. Chapter 11 details client education, including plans for specific populations. Clients learn all elements of skin care: nutrition, causes of pressure ulcers and preventive techniques, safety precautions, management of equipment and supplies, and treatment of any existing sores, emphasizing prevention and early detection.

SUMMARY

Pressure ulcer prediction, prevention, and treatment is a national concern, as evidenced by the attention it has received from such groups as the NPUAP and the PPPPUA. The costs in morbidity, mortality, and dollars are high. Nurses play pivotal roles in maintaining skin integrity and in predicting, preventing, and treating pressure ulcers. Evidence-based practice is becoming a norm for professional nursing. As information about risk factors is disseminated and incorporated into practice, nurses can influence prevention and outcomes (Gerrish et al., 1999).

CRITICAL THINKING

Rehabilitation nurses are well aware that too many clients arrive in rehabilitation settings with existing pressure ulcers developed during their acute care or long-term care experiences. These persons lose opportunities for restoration and functional abilities; some losses, such as with contractures, are not recoverable. Because prevention and management of skin integrity are nursing responsibilities, some rehabilitation nurses consider part of their role to be educating their colleagues in other settings about ways to improve outcomes. Discuss how nurse-to-nurse education and consultation would best be accomplished and what information and rehabilitation principles would apply in specific areas of nursing practice.

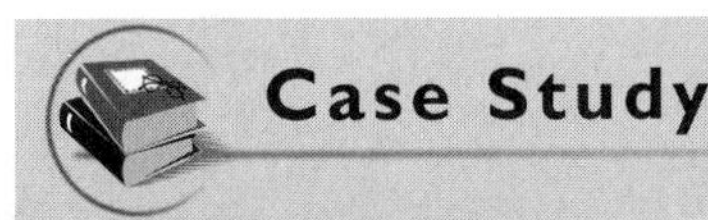

Case Study

John is a 72-year-old man who had a cerebrovascular accident (CVA) 3 months ago. He lives at home with his wife of 50 years, who provides his personal care assistance. John is able to perform a standing pivot transfer and turn and position himself in bed with moderate assistance, but occasionally he drags his sacrum across the bed.

A tall, thin man with little interest in food, John has been admitted to the hospital for treatment of pneumonia. During the admission assessment, the rehabilitation nurse notes a stage II pressure ulcer on his sacrum. The ulcer measures 30 by 34 mm, with no measurable depth. The wound bed is desiccated and has a dark pink appearance with minimal serous drainage and no odor. The surrounding tissue is dry and intact with no erythema. John's wife states that she has been applying a triple antibiotic ointment and a dry dressing during the day and leaving the wound open at night, so that it can "breathe."

Several nursing diagnoses are appropriate for John. He presents with a pressure ulcer supported by the history, physical examination, and evaluation of the cause. Being thin and having a pressure ulcer will increase his nutritional needs. It can be deduced that a contributing cause of the pressure ulcer is the dragging of the sacrum or impaired bed mobility. There are also data that would lead the rehabilitation nurse to suspect several areas of knowledge deficit regarding prevention and management of pressure ulcers.

Nursing Diagnoses (Gordon, 2000)

- Impaired skin integrity: stage II sacral pressure ulcer
- Altered nutrition: less than body requirements
- Impaired bed mobility
- Knowledge deficit: skin care

The nursing outcomes identified for this client relate to treating the current pressure ulcer and preventing others. A stage II pressure ulcer will heal best by secondary intention because the wound does not possess the characteristics to close by primary intention or the severity to heal by tertiary intention. John will require supplemental nutrients to heal the pressure ulcer and his respiratory illness. Interventions to establish adequate nutritional intake will assist in preventing new pressure ulcers. John needs to learn to turn and position in bed more effectively and safely; his wife needs to learn how to avoid skin shearing when assisting him with bed mobility. Ensuring adequate knowledge for home care and for prevention of further skin breakdown is a major nursing intervention to improve outcomes for this couple.

Nursing Outcomes (Johnson, Maas, Moorhead, 2000)

- Wound healing: secondary intention
- Nutritional status: nutrient intake
- Body positioning: self-initiated
- Knowledge: skin care and treatment regimen, prevention of pressure ulcers

Nursing Interventions (McCloskey & Bulechek, 2000)

All of the principles of pressure ulcer prevention and treatment discussed up to this point apply as interventions in this case. The ulcer requires baseline and ongoing assessment, including treatment of the ulcer and the surrounding skin with a moist healing environment, an appropriate dressing, and infection control. Selection of a support surface and proper turning and positioning are used. An enterostomal therapy consultant may be consulted when John's needs extend beyond the rehabilitation nurse's expertise or when his problems become complex and require more in-depth intervention.

Pressure Ulcer Care: Facilitation of Healing in Pressure Ulcers

- Describe characteristics of the ulcer at regular intervals, including size, stage, location, exudate, granulation or necrotic tissue, and epithelialization
- Monitor color, temperature, edema, moisture, and appearance of surrounding skin
- Keep the ulcer moist to aid in healing
- Cleanse the skin around the ulcer with mild soap and water
- Debride the ulcer as needed
- Cleanse the ulcer with the appropriate nontoxic solution, working in a circular motion from the center
- Note characteristics of any drainage
- Apply dressings as appropriate
- Monitor for signs and symptoms of infection in the wound
- Position every 1 to 2 hours to avoid prolonged pressure
- Use specialty beds and mattresses and seating systems as appropriate
- Use devices on the bed that protect the client's skin
- Ensure adequate dietary intake
- Initiate consultation services of the enterostomal therapy nurse or other skin care resources available in your setting

Nutrition intervention is critical to promote a positive wound-healing environment as well as to account for the additional protein and other nutrients required for healing. Fluid management is an important part of nutritional status in wound healing. Thus John may require increased caloric and/or fluid intake or increases in various components of his diet, such as protein. Therapeutic diet changes may be required with appropriate diet counseling and monitoring. John needs more caloric intake than he receives at home, particularly in light of wound healing and respiratory illness. It will be important for the nurse to work with the dietitian, dietary staff, client, and his wife to select appropriate foods and quantities with supplements. His wife needs supportive, nonthreatening education about ways to help meet John's ongoing nutritional needs.

Nutrition: Less Than Body Requirements

- Fluid/electrolyte management
- Fluid monitoring
- Nutritional counseling
- Nutrition therapy
- Nutritional monitoring
- Weight management/weight gain assistance
- Teaching: prescribed diet

Problems with bed mobility, including dragging the sacrum across the bed, no doubt contributed to the development of a sacral pressure ulcer for John. Bed rest care and mobility in bed may require physical therapy evaluation and intervention, in ad-

Continued

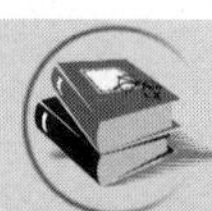

Case Study—cont'd

dition to rehabilitation nursing measures. Positioning and moving off the pressure ulcer will contribute to healing and prevent further breakdown. He may need assistance with self-care while in bed for his respiratory illness and the pressure ulcer.

Mobility: Impaired Bed Mobility
- Bed rest care
- Exercise promotion: stretching
- Exercise therapy: muscle control
- Positioning and turning
- Self-care assistance (general)

Both John and his wife a need education all areas of skin management, including health, exercise and nutrition, and specifically for the following interventions

Knowledge Deficit/Skin Care
- Health education
- Learning facilitation
- Learning readiness enhancement
- Teaching: pressure ulcer prevention, development, and treatment
- Teaching: prescribed diet and nutrition management
- Teaching: skin and wound care
- Teaching: bed mobility and turning and positioning
- Instruct family members/caregivers about signs of skin breakdown, as appropriate
- Teach client/family members wound care procedures
- Teaching: prescribed activity/exercise

REFERENCES

Allman, R.M. (1997). Pressure ulcer prevalence, incidence, risk factors, and impact. *Clinics in Geriatric Medicine, 13*(3), 421-436.

Allman, R.M., Goode, P.S., Burst, N., Bartolucci, A.A., & Thomas, D.R. (1999). Pressure ulcers, hospital complications, and disease severity: Impact on hospital costs and length of stay. *Advances in Wound Care, 12,* 22-30.

Allman, R.M., Laprade, C.A., Noel, L.B., Walter, J.M., Moorer, C.A., Dear, M.R., & Smith, C.R. (1986). Pressure sores among hospitalized patients. *Annals of Internal Medicine, 105,* 337-342.

Alterescu, V., & Alterescu, K. (1998). Etiology and treatment of pressure ulcers. *Decubitus, 1*(1), 28-35.

American Hospital Association. (1997). Here are highlights of pressure ulcer guideline. *Healthcare Benchmarks, November,* 162-163.

Andberg, M., Rudolph, A., & Anderson, T. (1983). Improving skin care through patient and family training. *Topics in Clinical Nursing, 5,* 45-54.

Anderson, T., & Andberg, M. (1979). Psychological factors associated with pressure sores. *Archives of Physical Medicine and Rehabilitation, 60,* 341-346.

Andrychuk, M.A. (1998). Pressure ulcers, risk factors, assessment and intervention. *Orthopaedic Nurse, 17*(4), 65-81.

Anstead, G. (1998). Steroids, retinoids, and wound healing. *Advances in Wound Care 11,* 277.

Armstrong, D., Lavery, J., & Harkless, L. (1996). Treatment based classification system for assessment and care of diabetic feet. *Ostomy/Wound Management, 13*(1), 33-36.

Aranovitch, S.A. (1993). The use of an assessment tool in managing placement on pressure relief surfaces. *Ostomy/Wound Management, 39*(4), 18-32.

Aranovitch, S.A., Wilber, M., Slezak, S., Martin, T., & Utter, D. (1999). A comparative study of an alternating air mattress for the prevention of pressure ulcers in surgical patients. *Ostomy/Wound Management, 45*(3), 34-44.

Ayello, E.A., Thomas, D.R., & Litchford, M.A. (1999). Nutritional aspects of wound healing. *Home Healthcare Nurse, 17*(11), 719-729.

Baeczak, C.A., Barnett, R.I., Childs, E.J., & Bosley, L.M. (1997). Fourth national pressure ulcer prevalence survey. *Advances in Wound Care, 10*(4), 18-26.

Baggerly, J., & DiBlasi, M. (1996). Pressure sores and pressure sore prevention in a rehabilitation setting: Building information for improving outcomes and allocating resources. *Rehabilitation Nursing, 21*(6), 321-325.

Baharestani, M. (1999). Pressure ulcers in an age of managed care: A nursing perspective. *Ostomy/Wound Management, 45*(5), 18-26, 28-32, 34.

Baranoski, S. (1995). Wound assessment and dressing selection. *Ostomy/Wound Management, 41*(S7A), 7S-12S.

Barkauskas, V.H., Stoltenberg-Allen, K., Baumann, L.C., & Darling-Fisher, C. (1998). *Health and physical assessment.* St. Louis: Mosby.

Bates-Jensen, B. (1998). *Wound care: A collaborative manual for physical therapists and nurses.* Gaithersburg, MD: Aspen.

Bennett, M.A. (1995). Report of the task force on the implications for darkly pigmented intact skin in the prediction and prevention of pressure ulcers. *Advances in Wound Care, 8*(6), 34-35.

Bergstrom, N., & Braden, B. (1992). A prospective study of pressure sore risk among the institutionalized elderly. *Journal of the American Geriatric Society, 40*(8), 747-758.

Bergstrom, N., Braden, B., Kemp, M., Champagne, M., & Ruby, E. (1998). Predicting pressure ulcer risk: A multisite study of the predictive validity of the Braden scale. *Nursing Research, 47*(5), 261-269.

Bergstrom, N., Braden, B.J., Laguzza, A., & Holman, V. (1987). The Braden scale for predicting pressure sore risk. *Nursing Research, 36,* 205-210.

Berlowitz, D.R., Bezerra, H.Q., Brandeis, G.H., Kader, B., & Anderson, J.J. (2000). Are we improving the quality of nursing home care: The case of pressure ulcers. *Journal of the American Geriatric Society, 48,* 59-62.

Berlowitz, D.R., & Wilking, S.V.B. (1989). Risk factors for pressure sores. *Journal of the American Geriatric Society, 37,* 1043-1050.

Black, C.A., Fenn-Buderer, N.N., Blaylock, B., & Hogan, B.J. (1998). Comparative study of risk factors for skin breakdown with cervical orthotic devices. *Journal of Trauma Nursing, 5*(3), 62-66.

Blackburn, J.H., Boemil, L., Hall, W.W., Jeffords, K., Hauck, R.M., Banducci, D.R., & Graham, W.P. (1998). Negative-pressure dressings as a bolster for skin graft. *Annals of Plastic Surgery 4*(5), 453-457.

Blaszczyk, J., Majewski, M., & Sato, F. (1998). Make a difference: Standardize your heel care practice. *Ostomy/Wound Management 44*(5), 32-40.

Boynton, P.R., Jaworski, D., & Paustian, C. (1999). Meeting the challenges of healing chronic wounds in older adults. *Nursing Clinics of North America, 34*(4), 921-932.

Braden, B., & Bergstrom, N. (1987). A conceptual schema for the study of the etiology of pressure sores. *Rehabilitation Nursing, 12,* 8-16.

Braden, B.J. (1988). The relationship between serum cortisol and pressure sore formation among the elderly recently relocated to a nursing home. *Reflections, 14,* 182-186.

Braden, B.J. (1998). The relationship between stress and pressure sore formation. *Ostomy/Wound Management, 44*(3A), 26S-37S.

Brandeis, G.H., Berlowitz, D.R., Hossain, M., & Morris, J.N. (1995). Pressure ulcers: The minimum data set and the resident assessment protocol. *Advances in Wound Care, 8*(6), 18-25.

Brandeis, G.H., Morris, J.N., Nash, D.J., & Lipsitz, L.A. (1990). The epidemiology and natural history of pressure ulcers in elderly nursing home residents. *Journal of the American Medical Association, 264,* 2905-2909.

Broussard, C.L., Mendez-Eastman, S., & Frantz, R. (2000). Adjuvant wound therapies. In R. Bryant (Ed.), *Acute and chronic wounds: Nursing management* (2nd ed.). St. Louis: Mosby.

Bryant (2000). Skin pathology and types of damage. In R. Bryant (Ed.), *Acute and chronic wounds: Nursing management* (2nd ed.). St. Louis: Mosby.

Bryant, R., Shannon, M.L., Pieper, B., Braden, B., & Morris, D.J. (1992). Pressure ulcers. In R. Bryant (Ed.), *Acute and Chronic Wounds: Nursing Management.* St. Louis: Mosby.

Burnett, D.M., Kolakowsky-Hayner, S.A., Gourley, E.V., & Cifu, D.X. (2000). Spinal cord injury "outliers": An analysis of etiology, outcomes and length of stay. *Journal of Neurotrauma, 17*(9), 765-772.

Buss, I.C., Halfens, R.J., & Abu-Saad, H.H. (1997). The effectiveness of massage in preventing pressure sores: A literature review. *Rehabilitation Nursing, 22*(5), 229-234, 242.

Byrne, D.W., & Salzberg, C.A. (1996). Major risk factors for pressure ulcers in the spinal cord disabled: A literature review. *Spinal Cord, 34,* 255-263.

Calvin, M. (1998). Cutaneous wound repair. *Wounds, 10*(1), 12.

Carlson, C.E., King, R.B., Kirk, P.M., Temple, R., & Heinemann, A. (1992). Incidence and correlates of pressure ulcer development after spinal cord injury. *Rehabilitation Nursing Research, 1,* 34-40.

Carlson, E.V., Kemp, M.G., & Shott, S. (1999). Predicting the risk of pressure ulcers in critically ill patients. *American Journal of Critical Care, 8*(4), 262-269.

Conine, T.A., Choi, A.K., & Lim, R. (1989). The user friendliness of protective support surfaces in prevention of pressure sores. *Rehabilitation Nursing, 14,* 261-263.

Cooper, D.M. (2000). Assessment, measurement and evaluation: Their pivotal roles in wound healing. In R. Bryant (Ed.), *Acute and chronic wounds: Nursing management* (2nd ed.). St. Louis: Mosby.

Copeland-Fields, L.D., & Hoshiko, B.R. (1989). Clinical validation of Braden and Bergstrom's conceptual schema of pressure sore risk factors. *Rehabilitation Nursing, 14,* 257-260.

Dai, Y.T., & Catanzaro, M. (1987). Health beliefs and compliance with a skin care regimen. *Rehabilitation Nursing, 12,* 13-16.

Demling, R., & DeSanti, L. (1998). Closure of the "non-healing wound" corresponds with correction of weight loss using the anabolic agent oxandrolone. *Ostomy/Wound Management, 44*(10), 58-62.

Demling, R., & DeSanti, L. (1999). Involuntary weight loss and the non-healing wound: The role of anabolic agents. *Advances in Wound Care, 12*(1 Suppl.), 1-14.

Disa, J.J., Carlton, J.M., & Goldberg, N.H. (1992). Efficacy of operative cure in pressure sore patients. *Plastic and Reconstructive Surgery, 89,* 272-278.

Eaglstein, W.H. (1986). Wound healing and aging. *Dermatology Clinics, 4,* 481-484.

Eastwood, E.A., Hagglund, K.J., Ragnarsson, K.J., Gordon, W.A., & Marino, R.J. (1999). Medical rehabilitation length of stay and outcomes for persons with traumatic spinal cord injury, 1990-1997. *Archives of Physical Medicine and Rehabilitation, 80,* 1457-63.

Ferrell, B.A., Osterweil, D., & Christenson, P. (1993). A randomized trial of low-air-loss beds for treatment of pressure ulcers. *Journal of the American Medical Association, 269,* 494-497.

Fiers, S.A. (1996). Breaking the cycle: The etiology of incontinence dermatitis and evaluating and using skin care products. *Ostomy and Wound Management, 42*(3), 32-34, 36, 38-40.

Fowler, E. (1998). Wound infection: A nurse's perspective. *Ostomy/Wound Management, 44*(8), 44-52.

Gallagher, S. (1997). Morbid obesity: A chronic disease with an impact on wounds and related problems. *Ostomy/Wound Management, 43*(5), 18-27.

Garvin, G. (1990). Wound healing in pediatrics. *Nursing Clinics of North America, 25,* 181-192.

Gerrish, K., Clayton, J., Nolan, M., Parker, K., & Morgan, L. (1999). Promoting evidence-based practice: Managing change in the assessment of pressure damage risk. *Journal of Nursing Management, 7*(6), 355-362.

Ghauri, A.S., Taylor, M.C., Deacon, J.E., Whyman, M.R., Earnshaw, J.J., Heather, B.P., & Poskkitt, K.R. (2000). Influence of a specialized leg ulcer service on management and outcome. *British Journal of Surgery, 87*(8), 1048-1056.

Goldberg, M.T., & McGinn-Byer, P. (2000). Oncology-related skin changes. In R. Bryant (Ed.), *Acute and chronic wounds: Nursing management* (2nd ed.). St. Louis: Mosby.

Goodman, C.M., Cohen, V., Armenta, A., Thornby, J., & Netscher, D.T. (1999). Evaluation of results and treatment variables for pressure ulcers in 48 veteran spinal cord injured patients. *Annals of Plastic Surgery, 42*(6), 665-672.

Gordon, M. (2000). *Manual of nursing diagnosis* (9th ed.). St. Louis: Mosby.

Gunningberg, L., Lindholm, C., Carlsson, M., & Sjoden, P.O. (2000). The development of pressure ulcers in patients with hip fractures: Inadequate nursing documentation is still a problem. *Journal of Advanced Nursing, 31*(5), 1155-1164.

Haalboom, J.R., den Boer, J., & Buskens, E. (1999). Risk-assessment tools in the prevention of pressure ulcers. *Ostomy/Wound Management, 45*(2), 20-26, 28, 30-34.

Harding-Okimoto, M. (1997). Pressure ulcers, self-concept and body image in spinal cord injury patients. *SCI Nursing, 14*(4), 111-116.

Harris, A.H. (1996). Managing vascular leg ulcers. Part 2: Treatment. *American Journal of Nursing, 96*(2), 40-47.

Hartnett, J.M. (1998). Use of vacuum-assisted wound closure in three chronic wounds. *Journal of Wound Ostomy and Continence Nursing 25*(6), 281-290.

Hess, C.T. (2000). Management of the patient with a venous ulcer. *Advances in Wound Care, 13*(2), 79-83.

Husain, T. (1953). An experimental study of some pressure effects on tissues with reference to the bedsore problems. *Journal of Pathologic Bacteriology, 66,* 347-382.

International Association for Enterostomal Therapy (IAET). (1991). *Standards of care for dermal wounds: Pressure ulcers* (Revised ed.). Irvine, CA: Author.

Johnson, M., Maas, M., & Moorhead, S. (2000). *Nursing outcomes classification* (2nd ed.). St. Louis: Mosby.

Kenney, I.J. (1998). Early phase wound healing by primary intention as shown by ultrasonography. *Journal of Wound Care, 7*(5), 222-224.

Kerstein, M. (1995). Moist wound healing: The clinical perspective. *Ostomy/Wound Management, 41*(7A), 37S-44S.

Kosiak, M. (1959). Etiology and pathology of ischemic ulcers. *Archives of Physical Medicine and Rehabilitation, 40,* 62-69.

Kosiak, M., & Kubicek, W.G., Olson, M., Danz, J.N., & Kottke, F.J. (1958). Evaluation of pressure as a factor in the production of ischial ulcers. *Archives of Physical Medicine and Rehabilitation, 39,* 623-629.

Krause, J.S. (1998). Skin sores after spinal cord injury: Relationship to life adjustment. *Spinal Cord, 36,* 51-56.

Kravitz, M. (1996). Outpatient wound care. *Critical Care Nursing Clinics of North America, 8*(2), 217-233.

Krouskop, T.A., Noble, P.C., Garber, S.L., & Spencer, W.A. (1983). The effectiveness of preventive management in reducing the occurrence of pressure sores. *Journal of Rehabilitation Research and Development, 20,* 74-83.

Kudravi, S.A., & Reed, M.J. (2000). Aging: Cancer and wound healing. *In Vivo, 14*(1), 83-92.

Kynes, P.M. (1986). A new perspective on pressure sore prevention. *Journal of Enterostomal Therapy, 13,* 42-43.

Landis, E.M. (1930). Micro-injection: Studies of capillary blood pressure in human skin. *Heart, 15,* 209-228.

Lindan, O. (1961). Etiology of decubitus ulcers: An experimental study. Archives of Physical Medicine and *Rehabilitation, 42,* 774-783.

Lloyd, E.E., & Baker, F. (1986). An examination of variables in spinal cord injury patients with pressure sores. *SCI Nursing, 3,* 219-222.

Lui, M., Spungen, A., Fink, L., Losada, M., & Bauman, W. (1996). Increased energy needs in patients with quadriplegia and pressure sores. *Advances in Wound Care, 9*(3), 41-45.

Maklebust, J., & Margolis, D. (1995). Pressure Ulcer: Definition and assessment parameters. *Advances in Wound Care, 8*(4, Suppl.), 6-7.

Maklebust, J., & Sieggreen, M. (1996). *Pressure ulcers: Guidelines for prevention, and nursing management* (2nd ed.). Springhouse, PA: Springhouse.

McCloskey, J.C., & Bulechek, G.M. (2000). *Nursing interventions classification* (3rd ed.). Mosby: St. Louis.

Mendez-Eastman, S. (1998). Negative pressure wound therapy. *Plastic Surgery Nursing, 18*(1), 27-29, 33-37.

Moore, K.L., & Dalley, A.F. (1999). *Clinically oriented anatomy* (4th ed.). Philadelphia: JB Lippincott.

Motta, G. (1993, April). Skin and wound care: Dressing for success. Providence, RI: Workshop American Healthcare Institute.

Mulder, G. (2000). Evaluation and managing the diabetic foot. *Advances in Skin and Wound Care, 13*(1), 33-36.

Mulder, G.D., Haberer, P.A., & Jeter, K.F (Eds.). (1999). *Clinician's pocket guide to wound repair* (4th ed.). Springhouse, PA: Springhouse.

National Pressure Ulcer Advisory Panel. (1989). Pressure ulcers prevalence, cost and risk assessment: Consensus development conference statement. *Decubitus, 2,* 24-28.

National Pressure Ulcer Advisory Panel. (1997). Management of tissue load: An excerpt from the third NPUAP slide set. *Advances in Wound Care, 10*(6), 35-38.

Niazi, Z.B.M., Salzberg, C.A., Byrne, D.W., & Viehbeck, M. (1997). Recurrence of initial pressure ulcer in persons with spinal cord injuries. *Advances in Wound Care, 10*(3), 38-42.

Norton, D., McLaren, R., & Exton Smith, A.N. (1975/1962). *An investigation of geriatric nursing problems in hospitals.* London: Churchill Livingstone.

Olsen, B., Langemo, D., Burd, C., Hanson, D., Hunter, S., & Cathcart-Silberberg, T. (1996). Pressure ulcer incidence in an acute care setting. *Journal of Wound Ostomy Continence Nursing, 23,* 15-22.

Padgett, D., Marucha, P., & Sheridan, J. (1998). Restraint stress slows cutaneous wound healing in mice. *Brain, Behavior, and Immunity,* 12, 64.

Panel for Prediction and Prevention of Pressure Ulcers in Adults. (1992). Pressure ulcers in adults: Prediction and prevention (Clinical Practice Guideline No. 3, AHCPR Publication No. 92-0047). Rockville, MD: Agency for Health Care Policy and Research, Public Health Service, U.S. Department of Health and Human Services.

Panel for Prediction and Prevention of Pressure Ulcers in Adults. (1994). Pressure ulcers in adults: Prediction and prevention (Clinical Practice Guideline No. 3, AHCPR Publication No. 92-0047). Rockville, MD: Agency for Health Care Policy and Research, Public Health Service, U.S. Department of Health and Human Services.

Payne, R.L., & Martin, M.L. (1993a). Defining and classifying skin tears: Need for common language. *Ostomy/Wound Management, 39*(5), 16.

Payne, R.L., & Martin, M.L. (1993b). The epidemiology and management of skin tears in older adults. *Ostomy/Wound Management, 26,* 26-37.

Philbeck, T.E., Whittington, K.T., Millsaph, M.H., Briones, R.B., Wight, D.C., & Schroeder, W.J. (1999). The clinical and cost effectiveness of externally applied negative pressure wound therapy in the treatment of wounds in home healthcare Medicare patients. *Ostomy/Wound Management, 45*(11), 41-50.

Pieper, B. (2000). Mechanical forces: Pressure, shear and friction. In R. Bryant (Ed.), *Acute and chronic wounds: Nursing management* (2nd ed.). St. Louis: Mosby.

Pieper, B., Sugrue, M., Weiland, M., Sprague, K., & Heimann, C. (1997). Presence of pressure ulcer prevention methods used among patients considered at risk versus those considered not at risk. *Journal of Wound, Ostomy and Continence Nursing, 24*(4), 191-199.

Pieper, B., & Weiland, M. (1997). Pressure ulcer prevention within 72 hours of admission in a rehabilitation setting. *Ostomy/Wound Management, 43*(8), 14-22.

Ramundo, J., & Wells, J. (2000). Wound debridement. In R. Bryant (Ed.), *Acute and chronic wounds: Nursing management* (2nd ed.). St. Louis: Mosby.

Rappl, L.M. (1998). Management of pressure by therapeutic positioning. In C. Sussman, & B.M. Bates-Jensen (Eds.). *Wound care: A collaborative practice manual for physical therapists and nurses.* Gaithersburg, MD: Aspen.

Reichel, S.M. (1958). Shearing forces as a factor in decubitus ulcers in paraplegics. *Journal of the American Medical Association, 166,* 762-763.

Rolstad, B.S., Ovington, L.G., & Harris, A. (2000). Principles of wound management. In R. Bryant (Ed.), *Acute and chronic wounds: Nursing management* (2nd ed.). St. Louis: Mosby.

Rubano, J.J., & Kerstein, M.D. (1998). Arterial insufficiency and vasculitides. *Journal Wound Ostomy Continence Nursing, 25*(3), 147-157.

Russell, L. (1998). Physiology of the skin and prevention of pressure sores. *British Journal of Nursing, 7*(18), 1084, 1088-1092, 1096.

Salcido, R. (2000). The future of wound measurements. *Advances in Wound Care, 13*(2), 54-55.

Salzberg, C.A., Byrne, D.W., Cayten, C.G., Kabir, R., van Niewerburgh, P., Viehbeck, M., Long, H., & Jones, E.C. (1998). Predicting and preventing pressure ulcers in adults with paralysis. *Advances in Wound Care, 11*(5), 237-246.

Schonfeld, W.H., Villa, K.F., Fastenau, J.M., Mazonson, P.D., & Falanga, V. (2000). An economic assessment of Apligraft (graftskin) for the treatment of hard-to-heal venous leg vices. *Wound Repair and Regeneration, 8*(4), 251-257.

Schryvers, O.I., Stranc, M.F., & Nance, P.W. (2000). Surgical treatment of pressure ulcers: 20 year experience. *Archives of Physical Medicine and Rehabilitation, 81*(12), 1556-1562.

Schue, R.M., & Langemo, D.K. (1998). Pressure ulcer prevalence and incidence and a modification of the Braden scale for a rehabilitation unit. *Journal of Wound, Ostomy and Continence Nursing, 25*(1), 36-43.

Scully, C. (1999). In on a limb. *Nursing Times, 95*(27), 59-65.

Sieggreen, M.Y., Cohen, I.K., Kloth, L.C., Harding, K.G., & Stotts, N.A. (1996). Commentaries on venous leg ulcers diagnostic and treatment draft guidelines. *Advances in Wound Care, 9*(4), 18-26.

Staas, W.E., Jr., & Cioschi, H.M. (1991). Pressure sores: A multifaceted approach to prevention and treatment. *Western Journal of Medicine, 154,* 539-544.

Stordeur, S., Laurent, S., D'Hoore, W. (1998). The importance of repeated risk assessment for pressure sores in cardiovascular surgery. *Journal of Cardiovascular Surgery, 39*(3), 343-349.

Stotts, N.A. (2000). Nutritional assessment and support. In R. Bryant (Ed.), *Acute and chronic wounds: Nursing management* (2nd ed.). St. Louis: Mosby.

Stotts, N.A., Deosaransingh, K., Roll, F.J., & Newman, J. (1998). Underutilization of pressure ulcer risk assessment in hip fracture patients. *Advances in Wound Care, 11*(1), 32-38.

Strauss, M., Gong, J., Gary, B., Kalsbeek, W.D., & Spear, S. (1991). The cost of home air fluidized therapy for pressure sores: A randomized controlled trial. *Journal of Family Practice, 33,* 52-59.

Sussman, C., & Byl, N. (1998). Electrical stimulation for wound healing. In C. Sussman, & B.M. Bates-Jensen (Eds.). *Wound care: A collaborative practice manual for physical therapists and nurses.* Aspen: Gaithersburg, MD.

Thomas, D. (1997). Specific nutritional factors in wound healing. *Advances in Wound Care, 10*(4), 40-43.

Tourtual, D.M., Riesenberg, L.A., Korutz, C.J., Semo, A.H., Asef, A., & Gill, R.D.F. (1997). Predictors of hospital acquired heel pressure ulcers. *Ostomy/Wound Management, 43*(9), 24-34.

Waldrop, J., & Doughty, D. (2000). Wound-healing physiology. In R. Bryant (Ed.), *Acute and chronic wounds: Nursing management* (2nd ed.). St. Louis: Mosby.

Waterlow, J.A. (1997). Pressure sore risk assessment in children. *Paediatric Nursing, 9*(6), 21-24.

Watts, D., Abrahams, E., MacMillan, C., Sanat, J., Silver, R., VanGorder, S., Waller, M., & York, D. (1998). Insult after injury: Pressure ulcers in trauma patients. *Orthopedic Nursing, July/August,* 84-91.

Whittemore, R. (1998). Pressure-reduction support surfaces. A review of the literature. *Journal of Wound, Ostomy and Continence Nurses, 25*(1), 6-25.

Witte, M., & Barbul, A. (1997). General principles of wound healing. *Surgery Clinics of North America, 77*(3), 509-528.

Wysocki, A. (2000). Anatomy and physiology of skin and soft tissue. In R. Bryant (Ed.), *Acute and chronic wounds: Nursing management* (2nd ed.). St. Louis: Mosby.

Wywialowski, E.F. (1999). Tissue perfusion as a key underlying concept of pressure ulcer development and treatment. *Journal of Vascular Nursing, 17*(1), 12-16.

Xakellis, G.C., Frantz, R.A., Lewis, A., & Harvey, P. (1998). Cost-effectiveness of an intensive pressure ulcer prevention protocol in long-term care. *Advances in Wound Care, 11*(1), 22-29.

Yamamoto, Y., Tsutsumida, A., Murazumi, M., & Sugihara, T. (1996). Long-term outcomes of pressure sores treated with flap coverage. *Plastic and Reconstructive Surgery, 100*(5), 1212-1217.

Yetzer, E.A., & Sullivan, R.L. (1992). The foot at risk: Identification and prevention of skin breakdown. *Rehabilitation Nursing, 17,* 247-251.

Zulkowski, K. (1999). A conceptual model of pressure prevalence: MDS+ items and nutrition. *Ostomy/Wound Management, 45*(2), 36-44.

BIBLIOGRAPHY

Frankel, H.L., Hancock, D.O., Hyslop, G., Melzak, J., Michaelis, L.S., Ungar, G.H., Vernon, J.D., & Walsh, J.J. (1969). The value of postural reduction in the initial management of closed injuries of the spine with paraplegia and tetraplegia. *Paraplegia, 7,* 179-192.

Harkness, G., & Dincher, J. (1996). *Medical-surgical nursing. Total patient care.* St. Louis: Mosby.

Langemo, D.K., Melland, H., Hanson, D., Olson, B., & Hunter, S. (1998). Two-dimensional wound measurement: Comparison of 4 techniques. *Advances in Wound Care, 11*(7), 337-343.

Thomas, D.R., Goode, P.S., LaMaster, K., Tennyson, T., & Parnell, L.K. (1999). A comparison of an opaque foam dressing versus a transparent film dressing in the management of skin tears in institutionalized subjects. *Ostomy/Wound Management, 45*(6), 22-24, 27-28.

APPENDIX 16A: DRESSINGS OPTIONS GUIDE*

Product	Description	Indications for Use	Contraindications
Absorption/Wound Fillers			
Used to absorb exudate and fill dead space Maintain a moist wound bed, absorb large amounts of exudate, and can provide a minimum of debridement	Exudate absorbers are usually composed of dextranomer polysaccharides starch, natural polymers, and colloidal particles Available in gel, powder, paste, bead, and granule forms	Wounds with depth requiring packing to fill dead space Exudate (minimum to moderate) Stage II or III wounds Used in combination with other wound care products Infected and noninfected wounds	Stage I wounds Dry wounds Deep tunneling or undermining wounds Wounds with dry eschar and wounds without exudate
Alginates			
Occur naturally in seaweed. Although available in the United Kingdom since the late 1940s, they have been slow to be used in the United States; absorb exudate, maintain a moist wound surface, and can be used in a variety of wounds from shallow exudative wounds to deep wounds; very absorptive and require a top dressing	Calcium, sodium, or alginic acid Naturally occurring polymer or brown seaweed derivative Gel formed by fibers interacts with exudate and exchanging sodium Insoluble in aqueous solutions Available in ropes, pads, or freeze-dried pads	Moderately to heavily exudating wounds Autolysis Moist wound healing Stage II, III, or IV wounds	Stage I wounds Dry or minimally exudative wounds Third-degree burns and black wounds
Collagens			
Manufactured in sheets, pads, particles, and gels Composed of collagen 90% and alginate 10%; combine structural support of collagen and gel-forming properties of alginate		Partial and full-thickness wounds Primary dressing Infected and noninfected wounds Tunneling wounds Minimal to heavy exudating wounds Skin grafts and donor sites	Third-degree wounds or black wounds

From Andrychuk, M.A. (1998). Pressure ulcers, risk factors, assessment and intervention. *Orthopaedic Nurse, 17*(4), 65-81.

*This product list is not exhaustive. In each category there are other products available and new products not available during development of this chapter.

Advantages	Disadvantages	Tips	Brands (Manufacturers)
No reinjury at removal Nonadherent Moist environment Absorb exudate Autolysis Conform/flexible Nonocclusive May decrease odor Inert	Not a bacterial barrier May require mixing Secondary dressings required May be expensive May desiccate wound	Can use gauze or hydrocolloid as secondary dressing Dressing change frequency varies with amount of exudate Protect surrounding skin to prevent maceration	AcryDerm Strands (AcryMed Inc.) Bard Absorption Dressing (Bard, CR Bard Inc.) Comfeel Paste (Coloplast, Sween Corp.) Comfeel Ulcer Powder (Coloplast) Cutinova Cavity (Beiersdorf AG) Debrisan Wound Cleaning Beads and Paste (J&J Medical Inc.) DermaSORB Spiral Dressing (ConvaTec) HydraGram Absorbant (Allegiance Healthcare Corp.) IODOSORB (Healthpoint Medical)† MULTIDEX (DeRoyal Wound Care) Osmocyte Pillow (Procyte Corp.) PolyWic Wound Filler (Ferris Mfg. Corp.) Stericare Absorbent Dressing (Horizon Medical Inc.) Stericare Copolymer Absorbent Dressing (Horizon Medical Inc.)
Absorb up to 20 times own weight Autolysis Conformable Fill in dead space Hemostatic properties Reduce pain Provide moist wound environment (forms a gel within the wound) Nonadherent (in presence of sufficient wound fluid) No trauma to granulating tissue on removal, if moist	Require secondary dressing May desiccate wound May have odor Labor intensive Possible systemic absorption of sodium or calcium	Some forms must be cut to wound size; others may overlap onto skin (refer to manufacturer's instructions) Dressing change varies from every 8 hours to every 3-4 days, depending on product and amount of exudate	AlgiDERM (Bard Medical Division, CR Bard Inc.) Algisite (Smith & Nephew Inc.) Algisorb (ConvaTec) CarraSorb (Carrington Laboratories Inc.) CURASORB Zinc (Kendall Healthcare Products Co.) Dermacea Alginate (Sherwood-Davis & Geck) FyBron (B. Braun Medical) Gentell Calcium Alginate (Gentell) KALGINATE (DeRoyal Wound Care) KALTOSTAT (ConvaTec) Poly Mem Alginate (Ferris Mfg. Corp.) Restore Calcicare (Hollister Inc.) SeaSorb (Coloplast-Sween Corp.) SORBSAN (Dow Hickam Pharmaceuticals) Tegagen (3M Health Care)
Conformable Absorbent Provide moist wound environment May be used in combination with topical agents Nonadherent	Require a secondary dressing		Fibracal Collagen-alginate (J&J Medical Inc.) Medifil (Biocare Medical Technologies Inc.) Skin Temp (Biocare Medical Technologies Inc.)

†Contains cadexomer iodine.

Continued

Product	Description	Indications for Use	Contraindications
Gauze			
Purpose to absorb exudate Supports moist wound healing if kept moist Most often used to fill large dead spaces or, as ribbons, to pack sinuses Should be packed lightly to prevent impairment of circulation	Fabric, woven or nonwoven Constructed from 100% cotton (natural); rayon, polyester blend (synthetic); cotton and synthetic blend Woven (preferred for wicking, packing, debridement), non-resilient Nonwoven (more absorbent, less limiting, removes easily from wound) Resilient Available in rolls, sponges or pads, ribbons of various sizes	Primary dressing Secondary dressing Minimal to heavy exudate Stage II, III, or IV wounds Fluffing Debridement Packing to fill dead space Cleansing	Stage I wounds Dry wounds Gauze should not be used over healing proliferative wounds or dry eschar

From Andrychuk, M.A. (1998). Pressure ulcers, risk factors, assessment and intervention. *Orthopaedic Nurse, 17*(4), 65-81.

Advantages	Disadvantages	Tips	Brands (Manufacturers)
Insulation Packing deep wounds, sinuses, undermining Absorption Readily available in most settings Debridement Ease of use	Not a bacterial barrier Nonselective debridement May dehydrate wound May be painful if dry at removal Bulky Expensive/labor intensive Usually requires use of a solution	When used as packing, pack loosely into wound to prevent compromise of blood flow Dressing change frequency varies with amount of exudate Protect surrounding skin from maceration with moisture-barrier ointment or skin barrier Film wipe	**All Purpose** CURITY (Kendall Healthcare Products Co.) EXCILON (Kendall Healthcare Products Co.) Gentell Bordered Gauze (Gentell) Fluftex Nonwoven (DeRoyal Wound Care) Intersorb (Sherwood-Davis & Geck) J&J Bulk Gauze (J&J Medical Inc.) LISCO (Kendall Healthcare Products Co.) Mirasorb Sponges (J&J Medical Inc.) NuGauze (Johnson & Johnson Medical Inc.) Sof-wick Sponges (J&J Medical Inc.) Steripad Gauze (J&J Medical Inc.) Topper Sponge (J&J Medical Inc.) VERSALON (Kendall Healthcare Products Co.) **Impregnated (Other Than Hydrogel)** Aquaphor (Beiersdorf-Jobst Inc.) CURASALT Sodium Chloride Dressing (Kendall Healthcare Products Co.) CURITY Non-Adhering Dressing (Kendall Healthcare Products Co.) CURITY Wet Saline Dressing (Kendall Healthcare Products Co.) DermAssist Oil Immulsion (AssisTec Medical Inc.) DermaGran Wet Dressing (Derma Sciences Inc.) Kendall Petrolatum Gauze U.S.P. (Kendall Healthcare Products Co.) Kendall Xeroform Dressing (Kendall Healthcare Products Co.) KERLIX Wet Saline Dressing (Kendall Healthcare Products Co.) KERLIX Zinc Saline Dressing (Kendall Healthcare Products Co.) Mesalt (SCA MOLYNLYCKE) Scarlet Red Ointment Dressing (Sherwood, Davis & Geck) Stericare Wet Saline Gauze Dressing (Horizon Medical Inc.) Vaseline Oil Emulsion Dressing (Sherwood, Davis & Geck) Vaseline Petrolatum Gauze (Sherwood, Davis & Geck) Xeroflo Gauze Dressing (Sherwood, Davis & Geck) Xeroform Petrolatum Gauze Dressing (Sherwood, Davis & Geck)

Continued

Product	Description	Indications for Use	Contraindications
Hydrocolloid			
Hydrocolloid wafer dressings insulate and protect the moist wound surface and absorb exudate Occlusive dressings that do not permit oxygen to diffuse into the wound, which creates low oxygen tension at the wound site that can stimulate capillary growth (Kerstein, 1995) Early in their use clinicians worried about collecting exudate; now it is understood that occlusion promotes wound healing, with growth factors allowed to proliferate beneath the dressing (Kerstein, 1995)	Hydrophilic particles formulated with hydrophobic matrices Covered by water-resistant film or foam Occlusive Opaque Varying absorption levels Available in various sizes of wafers or wraps; thin or standard thickness	Granular or partially necrotic wounds Autolysis Minimal to moderate exudating wounds Burns Donor sites Venous ulcers Stage I, II, and occasional shallow stage III wounds Used in conjunction with absorptive products or hydrogels Noncompromised arterial ulcers	Use with caution and vigilance in diabetic foot/leg wounds Infected wounds without systemic treatment with culture-specific antibiotics Muscle, tendon, or bone exposed Wounds with tracts Stage III wounds with deep tissue loss Stage IV wounds with dead space Heavily exudating wounds May be used under compression garments or devices

From Andrychuk, M.A. (1998). Pressure ulcers, risk factors, assessment and intervention. *Orthopaedic Nurse, 17*(4), 65-81.

Advantages	Disadvantages	Tips	Brands (Manufacturers)
			Roll/Wrapping Coban (3M Health Care) Confrom (Kendall Healthcare Products) DYNA-FLEX Elastic Bandage (Johnson & Johnson) FLEX-WRAP (Kendall Healthcare Products) Intersorb (Sherwood, Davis & Geck) KERLIX (Kendall Healthcare Products) Kling (Johnson & Johnson) Sof-Band (Johnson & Johnson) Sof-Kling (Johnson & Johnson) Softexe (Acme United Corp.) Sta-tite (Sherwood, Davis & Geck) **Packing/Debriding** CarraGauze (Carrington Laboratories Inc.) CURITY Packing Strips, iodoform (Kendall Healthcare Products) CURITY Packing Strips, plain (Kendall Healthcare Products) Intersorb Roll Stretch (Sherwood, Davis & Geck) Johnson & Johnson Gauze Sponges (Johnson & Johnson) KERLIX Packing Sponge (Kendall Healthcare Products) Kling Fluff Sponge (J&J Medical Inc.) MIRASORB Sponges (Johnson & Johnson) NU-BREDGE Packing & Debridement Sponge (Johnson & Johnson) Xeroflo Dressing with BTP (Sherwood, Davis & Geck)
Protection (bacterial, reinjury, insulation) Absorption Moist environment Autolysis Some protection of periwound skin Conforms/flexible	Potential for anaerobic bacterial growth Odor when removed Adhesive residue on skin or in wound Inability to visualize wound	"Defat" skin with barrier film (skin sealant); wipe before application to promote adhesion Allow 1-1.5 inch margin of intact skin around wound edges to be covered with dressing Taping edges of dressing helps prevent meltdown of edges Hold in place several seconds after application to allow body heat to help seal dressing in place Change every 3-7 days and as needed with leakage or dislodging Gel from dressing combined with wound fluid creates puslike exudate; rinse wound with saline solution or noncytotoxic wound cleanser before assessing	Comfeel (Coloplast Sween Corp.) CURADERM (Kendall Healthcare Products Co.) Cutinova (Beiersdorf-Jobst Inc.) Dermatell (Gentell) DuoDERM (ConvaTec) Hydrocol (Dow Hickman Pharmaceuticals Inc.) RepliCare (Smith & Nephew Inc.) Restore (Hollister Inc.) Signa Dress (Convatec) Tegasorb (3M Health Care)

Continued

Product	Description	Indications for Use	Contraindications
Hydrogel			
Available in impregnated sheets, gels, and granules to pour onto the wound Hydrogel dressings provide a moist wound environment and mild absorption and can be used to fill dead space; they are painless and easy to apply and remove Care should be taken to keep the dressing from the surrounding skin; the dressing must be covered with a secondary dressing	Interlacing network of polymers cross-linked to produce a matrix that traps water 80%-99% water; remainder is gel-forming material Nonadhesive Nonocclusive Transparent to translucent Hydrophilic Available in gel, sheets/wafers, impregnated gauze	Granular or necrotic shallow wounds Stage II, III, or IV wounds Provide moist environment Limited absorption required Autolysis via moisture action	Stage I wounds Wounds with copious exudate

From Andrychuk, M.A. (1998). Pressure ulcers, risk factors, assessment and intervention. *Orthopaedic Nurse, 17*(4), 65-81.

Advantages	Disadvantages	Tips	Brands (Manufacturers)
Easily removed Nonocclusive Nonadhesive Moisture at wound-dressing interface Varied amounts of absorption Promotes autolysis Conforms/flexible Soothing and may reduce pain Can be used when infection present Fills dead space	Does not provide bacterial barrier May dehydrate Potential to macerate periwound skin May be difficult to apply Usually requires secondary dressing Minimally absorptive	Use skin barrier film wipe (skin sealant) on surrounding intact skin to prevent periwound maceration Sheet/wafer forms work better on superficial wounds Dressing change schedule varies from every 8 hours to every 72 hours depending on product and amount of exudate	**Hydrogel Amorphous** Biolex (Bard Medical Division, CR Bard Inc.) Carrasyn (Carrington Laboratories Inc.) Curofil Gel (Kendall Health Care Products) Dermagram Zinc-Saline (Derma Sciences Inc.) CURASOL (Healthpoint Medical)‡ DuoDERM HYDROACTIVE (ConvaTec) Gentell (Gentell) HyFIL (B. Braun Medical Inc.) IntraSite (Smith & Nephew United Inc.) Normligel (SCA MOLYNLYCKE) Restore (Hollister Inc.) Royl-Derm (Acme United Corp.) SAF-GEL (ConvaTec) SoloSite (Smith & Nephew United Inc.)
			Hydrogel Sheet AcriDerm Advanced Wound Dressing (AcryMed Inc.) AQUASORB (DeRoyal Wound Care) CarraDress (Carrington Labs Inc.) CarraSorb M Freeze Dried Gel (Carrington Labs Inc.) ClearSite (Con Med Corp.) CURAGEL (Kendall Healthcare Products) Elasto-Gel (Southwest Technologies Inc.) FLEXDERM (Dow Hickam Pharmaceuticals Inc.) NU-GEL (Johnson & Johnson Medical Inc.) THINSite (B. Braun Medical Inc.) Transorbent (B. Braun Medical Inc.) Vigilon (Bard Medical Division, CR Bard Inc.)
			Hydrogel Dressings: Impregnated Gauze Biolex (Bard Medical Division) CarraGauze (Carrington Laboratories Inc.) ClearSite (Con Med Patient Care Systems) CURASOL (Healthpoint Medical) HydroGauze (Con Med Patient Care Systems) Restore (Hollister Inc.) Stericare (Horizon Medical Inc.)

‡Glycerin based.

Continued

Product	Description	Indications for Use	Contraindications
Nonadherent Dressings/Contact Layers			
	Impregnated gauze or nonimpregnated gauze with antishear layer Manufactured as a single layer of a woven (polyamide) net that acts as a low-adherence material when placed in contact with the base of the wound Materials allow the exudate to pass to a secondary dressing	Primary dressing for partial and full-thickness wounds Secondary (cover) dressing for infected wounds or wounds that require packing Skin donor sites and split-thickness skin grafts	Tunneling wounds Cleaning or debriding wounds Third-degree wounds
Polyurethane Foam			
Dressings have nonadherent wafers that are used to promote moist wound healing and provide absorption Highly absorptive, remove easily, and their hydrophobic surfaces repel contaminants Not self-adherent and require an additional taping or dressing to adhere to skin (Motta, 1993)	Modified polyurethane foam Inert material Semiocclusive Hydrophilic Nonadherent Varied thickness Some have carbon-impregnated layer (for odor-proofing) Available in pad form Nonlinting	Minimal to moderately draining wounds Stage II or III wounds Autolysis (minimal) Diabetic wounds Tracheostomy sites	Dry wounds without exudate Stage I wounds Deep wounds
Specialty Absorptives			
	United Multilayer product Semiadherent or nonadherent layer or highly absorptive layers of fibers, such as cellulose, cotton, or rayon May or may not have adhesive border	Primary or secondary dressing Light to heavy drainage Partial and full-thickness wounds Infected and noninfected wounds	Third-degree-burns Tunneling wounds Known sensitivity to dressing or its compounds

From Andrychuk, M.A. (1998). Pressure ulcers, risk factors, assessment and intervention. *Orthopaedic Nurse, 17*(4), 65-81.

Advantages	Disadvantages	Tips	Brands (Manufacturers)
Nontraumatic Can be used with topical agents (creams, ointments) Occlusive	May stick to wound if dries out Require secondary dressing (tape or gauze) to secure to site	Dressing change schedule varies from every 8 hours to every 24 hours	ADAPTIC (Johnson & Johnson) Aquaphor (Beiersdorf-Jobst Inc.) Conformant 2 Wound Veil (Exu-Dry Wound Care Products Inc.) Coverlet (Beiersdorf-Jobst Inc.) Cutiplast (Beiersdorf-Jobst Inc.) DERMANET Wound Contact Layer (DeRoyal Wound Care) Mepitel (SCA Molnlycke) N-Terface Interpositional Surfacing Material (Winfield Laboratories Inc.) Owens Nonadherent Surgical Dressing (Sherwood-Davis & Geck) Profore Wound Contact Layer (Smith & Nephew Inc.) 3M Tegapore Wound Contact Material (3M HealthCare) RELEASE (Johnson & Johnson) TELFA (Kendall Healthcare Products Co.)
Protection (insulation) May be used with infected wounds Conforms/flexible Nonadherent May be used with wound fillers May be used under compression garments or devices	Not a bacterial barrier May desiccate wound Requires taping or other securing method Some require specific surface applied to wound Not effective for wounds with dry eschar	Use skin barrier film (skin sealant) wipe on surrounding intact skin to prevent periwound maceration Dressing change schedule every 1-5 days depending on product and amount of exudate	Allevyn (Smith & Nephew Inc.) Carrasmart (Carrington Labs Inc.) CURAFOAM (Kendall Healthcare Products Co.) Cutinova (Beiersdorf-Jobst Inc.) FLEXZAN (Dow Hickam Pharmaceuticals) HYDRASORB (ConvaTec) LoProfile (Gentell) Lyofoam (Convatec) Odor Absorbent Dressing (Hollister Inc.) POLYDERM (DeRoyal Wound Care) PolyMem (Ferris Mfg. Corp.) TIELLE (Johnson & Johnson)
Secondary dressing over most primary dressings Nonadherent Highly absorptive Easy to apply and remove	Some may not be appropriate as a primary dressing for undermining wounds		CombiDerm ACD (Convatec) CovaDerm Adhesive (DeRoyal Wound Care) Curity Abdominal Pads (Kendall Healthcare Products Co.) Exu-Dry (Exu-Dry Wound Care Products Inc.) Multipad Nonadherent (DeRoyal Wound Care) Surgi-Pad Combine (Johnson & Johnson Medical Inc.) TenderSorb Wet Pruf Abdominal Pads (Kendall Healthcare Products Co.)

Continued

Product	Description	Indications for Use	Contraindications
Thin Films (Transparent Adhesives)			
The first occlusive dressings devised to insulate, protect, and maintain the moist wound surface Exudate can build up under the film, contraindicating its use in wounds of clients with aging, friable skin Films are good choice for dry, necrotic wounds requiring debridement	Translucent Gas permeable Polyurethane or polyethylene film Moisture vapor permeable Partial or continuous adhesive Occlusive to liquids and bacteria	Granular or necrotic shallow wounds Autolysis As secondary (cover) dressing over absorption products Stage I, II, or shallow III ulcers	Infected wounds with tracts, undermining, or heavy exudate Stage III wounds with deep tissue loss Stage IV wounds Fragile surrounding skin (long-term steroid use, etc.)
Vacuum-Assisted Wound Closure Dressing			
	Use of a negative-pressure sponge dressing into the wound to increase blood flow, increase granulation tissue and nutrients to the wound, and decrease bacterial load	Chronic wounds healing by secondary intention Avulsions Open amputations Evacuated hematomas, gunshot wounds Wound dehiscence	Osteomyelitis and wound infection

From Andrychuk, M.A. (1998). Pressure ulcers, risk factors, assessment and intervention. *Orthopaedic Nurse, 17*(4), 65-81.

Advantages	Disadvantages	Tips	Brands (Manufacturers)
Protection (from bacteria, other contaminants, and reinjury) Moist environment Autolysis Conforms/flexible Allows visual assessment of wound	Premature dressing removal may occur Minimal insulation of wounds May require drainage with puncture aspiration or frequent removal and reapplication to prevent periwound maceration Not absorptive May be difficult to apply	Cut the surrounding hair closely to promote adhesion and prevent irritation during removal "Defat" skin with barrier film wipe (skin sealant) before application Allow 1-2 inch margin of intact skin to be covered with dressing to promote adhesion Frequency of dressing change dependent on wound site and characteristics Change at least every 7 days	ACU-derm (Acme United Corp.) BIOCLUSIVE (Johnson & Johnson Medical Inc.) Blisterfilm (Sherwood-Davis & Geck) CarraFilm (Carrington Laboratories Inc.) DermAssist Transparent Site Dressing (Assistec Medical Inc.) FLEXFILM (Dow Hickam) OpSite (Smith & Nephew Inc.) POLYSKIN II (Kendall Healthcare Products Co.) PRO-CLUDE (ConvaTec) Tegaderm (3M Health Care) TRANSEAL (DeRoyal Wound Care) Uniflex (Smith & Nephew Inc.)
Increases the vascularity and oxygenation of the wound bed Maintains moist environment Removes exudate through negative pressure	Dressing removal may be painful Time-consuming Staff education is intensive		

17 Nourishment and Swallowing

Nancy H. Glenn-Molali, MSN, RN, CRRN

Mr. L was a 60-year-old man in the rehabilitation setting where I was working as a new nurse. He was always polite but very reserved. His dysphagia was a result of a cerebrovascular accident. He had a nasogastric tube and could not receive anything by mouth. One day he was particularly anxious to get to his speech therapy session. When he returned to the nursing unit, he communicated how happy he was that he had just had a few small bites of custard. His first food by mouth in more than a month! That was the first time I really thought about what it must be like to have dysphagia.

The process of swallowing (deglutition) begins in utero during the second trimester. When all swallowing mechanisms are functioning properly, we are generally unaware of swallowing once a minute when awake, or nearly 1000 times a day. An adult independently obtains and ingests proper nutrients to maintain health and function. Eating meals occurs during family or social gatherings, celebrations, or events for many cultural groups and has become associated with feelings of sharing, belonging, and friendship. When an person can no longer secure or ingest nutrients in an efficient manner, a biological, social, or psychological crisis may occur. Clients who are no longer able to swallow in a normal manner are said to have dysphagia. Dysphagia may cause clients to aspirate food or fluids resulting in aspiration pneumonia, or they may have frequent choking resulting in frustration, disappointment, and fear, which may lead to reduced nutritional intake and malnutrition. Clients may also become dehydrated. This chapter includes information on nourishment, statistics on dysphagia, anatomy and physiology of swallowing, factors associated with altered deglutition, diagnostic tests, and nursing process with outcome criteria for persons with impairments of eating or swallowing.

NOURISHMENT

The primary purpose of eating and swallowing is to provide the body with necessary nutrients and hydration. All persons need a balanced diet from the major food groups, as recommended in the U.S. Department of Agriculture (USDA) Food Guide Pyramid, and adequate hydration (at least eight 8-oz glasses of water a day), unless contraindicated due to a physiological condition.

We are what we eat is an old but true saying. Research findings support the contribution of adequate and appropriate nutrition to improved outcomes in healing, strength, tissue regeneration, and cognitive awareness. Metabolic responses to chronic illnesses, such as pulmonary diseases, and to stresses after trauma are increasingly important areas of concern for rehabilitation nurses. Severe deficiencies in several B vitamins affect brain function and behavior, including abnormal electroencephalograms, impaired memory, anxiety, confusion, irritability, and depression. Pyridoxine (vitamin B_6) deficiencies cause abnormal brain electrical activity (Harris, 1996). Cognitive impairment may be caused by a disease process, but it can also be caused by dehydration, potassium imbalance, iron-deficiency anemia, and deficiency of water-soluble vitamins. Zinc deficiency is associated with impaired immune function, anorexia, poor wound healing, and development of pressure ulcers (Shuman, 1996).

Nutrition, Medication, and Herbs

The nutritional status and medications taken by an client can have direct effects on each other. Medications include prescription medications, over-the-counter medicines, vitamins, minerals, herbs, and dietary supplements. Tables 17-1 and 17-2 give examples of some medications that affect nutritional status and some foods that affect medications. Medications can affect nutritional status by increasing or decreasing appetite, decreasing the senses of smell and taste, affecting absorption of nutrients, or altering metabolism and excretion of nutrients. Food can affect medications by altering absorption, metabolism, and excretion. Any person who takes medication is at risk for a drug-nutrient interaction. Persons at highest risk include those who take multiple medications; consume alcohol; have poor nutrition; take a vitamin, mineral, or herbal supplement; or take medications at mealtimes.

When taking a nutritional assessment, it is important to obtain information regarding intake of vitamins, herbs, and nutritional supplements. Some vitamins, when taken in excess of body requirements, can have negative effects. For example, excess vitamin A has been associated with liver injury, elevated intracranial pressure, and birth defects after maternal consumption during pregnancy. Vitamin B_6 in excess may lead to ataxia or sensory neuropathy; too much selenium may concentrate and cause damage to tissues. Excess niacin may produce liver damage, gastrointestinal distress, myopathy, cytopenia, and maculopathy of the eyes (Harris, 1996).

Many persons who use certain herbs to treat various ailments may not consider them medications. It is important to question clients on the possible use of herbs because some can cause serious illness. Some herbal preparations used for weight reduction, for example, germander, stephania, magnolia, or ma huang, have caused a range of problems including stroke, hypertension, severe kidney disease, and others.

When working with clients, care should be based on the individual's physiological, pathological, and psychosocial condition. All clients, whether at home, in a hospital, in a nursing home, or in a residential center, should have a nutritional assessment on admission as part of the nursing assessment, then every 6 months, and as their condition changes, such as with weight gain or loss and disease progression. This is particularly helpful in improving outcomes for clients with infections, impaired skin integrity, loss of

TABLE 17-1 Examples of Medications Affecting Nutritional Status

Medication	Effect on Nutritional Status
Phenobarbital, phenytoin, primidone	Interfere with intestinal absorption of calcium
Phenytoin	Metabolism requires folic acid and is accelerated by supplementation, which may cause subtherapeutic levels of the medication
Levodopa	Binds with pyridoxine and is excreted; supplemental pyridoxine may decrease effectiveness
Corticosteroids	Deplete body of ascorbic acid
Cholestyramine	Increases excretion of fat-soluble vitamins A, D, E, and K; folic acid; vitamin B_{12}; calcium; and iron
Long-term antacid or potassium chloride use	Neutralizes gastric acidity and decreases absorption of folic acid, vitamin B_{12}, and iron
Furosemide	Increases excretion of sodium, potassium, and calcium

Data from Lutz, C.A., Przytulski, K.R. (1997). *Nutrition and diet therapy* (2nd ed.). Philadelphia: FA Davis; and Burns, R.D., Carr-Davis, E.M. (1996). Nutritional care in diseases of the nervous system. In L.K. Mahan & S. Escott-Stump (Eds.), *Krause's food, nutrition and diet therapy* (9th ed., pp. 863-889). Philadelphia: WB Saunders.

TABLE 17-2 Examples of Foods Affecting Medications

Food	Effect on Medication
Amino acids in protein	Inhibit absorption of levodopa and theophylline; delay action of phenytoin
High fiber meal	Decreases absorption of digoxin
Milk, alcohol, and hot beverages	Cause premature erosion of enteric coatings
Pectin in jelly and apples	Decreases absorption of acetaminophen
Carbohydrates	Increase absorption of levodopa, phenytoin, and theophylline
Tyramine-containing foods	Cause hypertension crisis when combined with MAO inhibitors
Vitamin K (in food or supplement)	Reverses effects of warfarin

Data from Lutz, C.A., Przytulski, K.R. (1997). *Nutrition and Diet Therapy* (2nd ed.). Philadelphia: FA Davis. and Burns, R.D., Carr-Davis, E.M. (1996). Nutritional Care in Diseases of The Nervous System. In L.K. Mahan & S. Escott-Stump (Eds.), *Krause's food, nutrition and diet therapy* (9th ed.) (pp. 863-889). Philadelphia: WB Saunders.*MAO,* Monoamine oxidase.

muscle tissue, healing bones or wounds (D'Eramo, Sedlak, Doheny, & Jenkins, 1994), and potential malnutrition due to poor absorption or compromised immunity.

Psychological and Sociocultural Factors

Nutritional status is influenced not only by the physical ability to consume food but also by psychological and sociocultural factors. In the United States there are many ethnic groups, each with various food preferences, and each attaches different emotional significance to food. It is important in the assessment to identify these characteristics and to realize that cultural patterns may affect the client's nutritional choices. Additionally food is commonly associated with social events and therefore has significant psychological meaning. Traditional foods for holidays are a good example. As one ages or becomes ill, the lack of interaction at meals or lack of other meaningful social interactions can reduce nutritional intake significantly. It is difficult to change lifelong eating habits, and these can hinder the client's rehabilitation. However, highly motivated clients can often overcome these habits.

When dietary plans and menus are offered to clients from differing culture groups, the nutritional composition of ethnic or religious food selections may be calculated so that these foods are included in the plan. For example, Asian diets tend to have rice as a staple and very few dairy products. Pork and chicken are used more than beef. Mediterranean diets are high in olive oil, fruits, vegetables, cheeses, milk, legumes, and wine. Vegetarian diets vary from consuming no animal products to consuming fowl, fish, and dairy products but no red meat. Jewish dietary laws specify which animals may be eaten and how the animals are to be killed and prepared and state that meat and milk may not be combined in the same meal. Seventh Day Adventist do not consume pork, certain seafood, or fermented beverages.

Malnutrition

Many clients will be at risk for malnutrition. Risk factors for malnutrition include any of the following: cognitive impairment, social isolation, being homebound, frailty, depression, advanced age, low income, chronic disability, functional disability, poor dentition, polypharmacy, regular alcohol intake, dysphagia, or inadequate food intake. Older clients will be at a risk for dehydration because the sense of thirst diminishes with age and there is a decrease in water conservation by the kidneys. Many older clients also take diuretics and laxatives, which further deplete fluid volume. Some clients with incontinence limit fluid intake to decrease the risk of an accident, which may also contribute to dehydration.

Clients may also have inadequate nutritional intake due to a knowledge deficit. They may be unaware of what foods and nutrients compose an adequate diet, what adaptive equipment is available, or what community resources are available. Some community resources include the Women, Infants, and Children (WIC) program; food stamps; local community food programs; food banks; cooperatives; church- or religion-sponsored meal programs; social services; Meals on Wheels; and adult day care programs. Some services also provide shopping and meal preparation for elderly persons.

Diseases and Injuries

Swallowing impairments are common with many neurological diseases and can cause nutritional deficits. Other diseases and injuries, such as Alzheimer's disease, rheumatoid arthritis, and burns can put a client at risk for a nutritional deficit.

Barrett-Connor, Edelstein, Corey-Bloom, and Wiederholt (1996) found that weight loss in the elderly may be an early warning sign of Alzheimer's disease. As the disease progresses clients either have an insatiable appetite with weight gain, possibly because they forget that they have eaten or, more commonly, refuse food or forget to eat. These clients should have frequent offerings of finger foods. In the late stage the client may be unable to chew, and a diet with modified consistencies or a feeding tube may be needed.

Clients with rheumatic diseases may have anorexia due to medications, fatigue, and pain; have decreased dietary intake; and taste alterations due to xerostomia. If metabolic bone disease is present, calcium and vitamin D supplements are indicated (Touger-Decker, 1996).

Clients with any type of metabolic stress, such as sepsis, multiple trauma, burns, or surgery, require additional calories.

The energy requirements for clients who have had burns can increase as much as 100% or more, and protein requirements may triple, depending on the size and depth of the injury. This is due to stress, fluid and protein loss through the burn wound exudate, fever, infection, immobility, and hypercatabolism. A major concern is also fluid and electrolyte balance. Vitamin and mineral requirements may increase to two times the recommended daily allowance, particularly vitamins C and A because they promote wound healing (Moy, 1996; Winkler & Manchester, 1996).

Clients who have acute brain injury are generally well nourished before injury. However, because of the hypermetabolic and hypercatabolic state after injury, nutritional support is needed to prevent rapid loss of lean body mass and immunosuppression. Clients with severe brain injury have been shown to require up to twice the normal number of calories, and protein requirements can increase from approximately 0.8 g/kg to 1.5 to 2.5 g/kg. Clients also benefit from B vitamins, vitamin C, and zinc (Stanley, 1998; Walleck & Mooney, 1994).

Elderly Clients

Traditionally the term *elderly* refers to persons 65 years and older. Factors to consider when working with the elderly include:

- Glucose tolerance decreases with age, leading to an increase in plasma glucose; thus the glucose tolerance curve developed for young adults is now recognized as inappropriate for elderly persons

- Basal metabolic rate decreases by 20% between the ages of 30 and 90 years because of a decrease in lean body mass
- Kidney function can decrease by 50% between the ages of 30 and 80 years; acid-base response to metabolic challenges is slowed
- Lean body mass is replaced with fat and connective tissue
- Body protein in healthy elderly persons is 30% to 40% less than that of young adults
- Bone density is diminished

Excess Weight

It is estimated that at least 26% of adults and 25% to 30% of children in the United States are overweight or obese (Pamuk, Makuc, Heck, Reuben, & Lochner, 1998). A person is considered to be obese if he or she is 20% over ideal body weight. Persons at risk include the elderly and clients with chronic, disabling conditions; children with spina bifida or Down syndrome also have a tendency toward weight gain.

A client's nutritional status affects nearly all aspects of daily life, and it is important to consider the effect that extra weight has on a person's life. Excess weight can lead to physical and psychological problems and is often the result of a sedentary lifestyle. Eating may be a means to relieve anxiety, stress, depression, and loneliness and to pass the time. Excess weight stresses many of the body's systems in both adults and children. It increases a person's risk for joint disease, hypertension, diabetes, gall bladder disease, sleep disorders, some cancers, and menstrual irregularities. (Barlow & Dietz, 1998). It can decrease mobility and the level of functioning in all activities of daily living.

Healthy People 2000, the prevention agenda for the nation, identified being overweight as "the most significant preventable threat to health" and identified physical activity and fitness and nutrition as the top two priority areas. (Healthy People 2000). New research is finding that losing 5 to 10 lb of excess weight can positively affect a person's quality of life.

DYSPHAGIA STATISTICS

The nature of dysphagia makes it difficult to accurately identify all persons who are affected by it. Specific statistics on the nature and prevalence of dysphagia are rare, and the statistics that are available for the United States generally pertain to persons older than 60 years.

It is estimated that approximately 15 million Americans have dysphagia (Hansell & Heinemann, 1996), and about 338,393 to 624,757 persons are affected by dysphagia each year as a result of a neurological disorder. The largest group of clients with neurological disorders who have dysphagia is composed of those who have had a stroke. Approximately 213,000 persons with Parkinson's disease will be diagnosed with dysphagia each year, and approximately 240,781 persons are affected by dysphagia each year as a result of other neurological diseases (Agency for Health Care Policy and Research [AHCPR], 1999). Studies of residents in nursing homes report the prevalence of dysphagia to be between 53% and 74% (O'Laughlin & Shanley, 1998).

These statistics do not address persons younger than 60 years, including the pediatric population; thus it is difficult to truly appreciate the magnitude of the numbers of persons who are affected each year.

MECHANICS OF EATING

The ability to eat and swallow food and liquids is dependent on position and function of the oropharyngeal cavity, esophagus, cranial nerves, brain, muscles, and limbs. The mechanics of eating and swallowing comprise the anatomic structures, physiological processes of eating and swallowing, and phases of swallowing discussed in the following material.

Anatomic Structures

Swallowing is a complex neuromuscular process that requires complex communication between the central and peripheral nervous systems and coordinated actions between the oral cavity, pharynx, esophagus, larynx, muscles, cranial nerves, and brain. Ingestion of food begins in the oral cavity, which is composed of the lips, cheeks, tongue, teeth, gums, mandible, hard and soft palate, uvula, anterior and posterior faucial arches, palatine tonsils, and salivary glands (Figure 17-1).

The oral cavity is lined with different types of sensory cells that have a role in swallowing. The mechanoreceptive cells cover the largest area. These cells are concentrated most heavily at the tip of the tongue and along the midline of

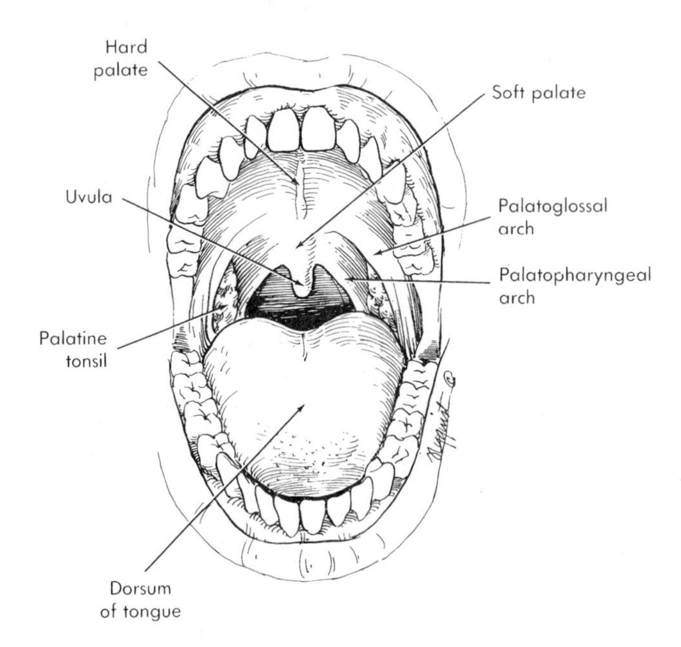

Figure 17-1 Anatomy of the oral cavity.

the palate. When the sensory cells on the palate are stimulated with pressure, peristaltic movements of the tongue are produced. Studies have shown that the amplitude of the oral peristaltic wave is greater for thickened foods, implying feedback modulation from sensory fibers in the oral cavity (Plant, 1998).

The oral cavity is also innervated by thermoreceptive and chemoreceptive cells. The spatial distribution of the thermoreceptive cells is highest along areas of the palate and tongue that come in contact with each other during swallowing. Chemoreceptive cells are distributed most densely along the tongue. The specific role of these receptors in swallowing is not known (Plant, 1998).

Pharynx

The oral cavity communicates with the pharynx via the oropharyngeal isthmus. The pharynx is a 12- to 14-cm musculomembranous tube extending from the soft palate to the cricoid cartilage, where it connects to the esophagus. It is formed by 26 pairs of striated muscles and is densely innervated with motor fibers. Three striated constrictor muscles, the superior, medial, and inferior, propel food along the pharynx during swallowing. Fibers of the inferior constrictor muscle attach to the sides of the thyroid cartilage, forming the spaces of the pyriform sinuses and ending at the cricopharyngeal muscle (Logemann, 1983), the most inferior structure of the pharynx (Figure 17-2). At rest, tonic contractions of the cricopharyngeal muscle prevent air from entering the esophagus during respiration and food from refluxing into the esophagus and up to the pharynx. The cricopharyngeal muscle relaxes to allow a bolus of food to enter the esophagus (Figure 17-3).

The pharynx is divided into three portions. The nasopharynx lies above the soft palate, and the oropharynx lies posterior to the mouth. The portion of the pharynx extending below the esophagus is the hypopharynx (Groher, 1997).

Esophagus and Larynx

The esophagus is a hollow, muscular tube approximately 23 to 25 cm long, with a sphincter at each end. The muscles of the upper third of the esophagus are striated; the muscles of the middle third are a mix of both striated and smooth. The lower third, including the lower esophageal sphincter, is smooth muscle. The bolus of food enters the esophagus from the pharynx and is transported to the stomach by the muscular peristaltic action of the esophagus.

The upper esophageal sphincter (UES) separates the hypopharynx from the esophagus. It is a high-pressure region, 3 to 4 cm in length, that prevents air from entering the stomach during swallowing and limits reflux of gastric contents into the pharynx. There are two muscles running from the cricoid cartilage to the pharynx, the pars obliqua and the pars fundiformis. The pars obliqua runs in an oblique direction superiorly and posteriorly from the lateral cricoid and blends with the inferior constrictor fibers. The pars fundiformis runs in a horizontal direction around the posterior pharynx and reinserts on the opposite side of the cricoid. The triangular gap between the pars obliqua and the pars fundiformis is Killian's triangle. Generally the pars fundiformis is referred to as the *cricopharyngeus muscle* (Wisdom & Blitzer, 1998). There are five levels of UES activity: relaxation, opening, distention, collapse, and contraction. The forces propelling the food bolus through the UES are generated by the movement of the tongue in the pharynx. The sphincter opening and closing occur during the time of maximum laryngeal elevation (Wisdom & Blitzer, 1998).

The larynx begins at the base of the tongue with the epiglottis. It is anterior to the hypopharynx at the upper end of the trachea. The spaces formed between the base of the tongue and the sides of the epiglottis are the valleculae,

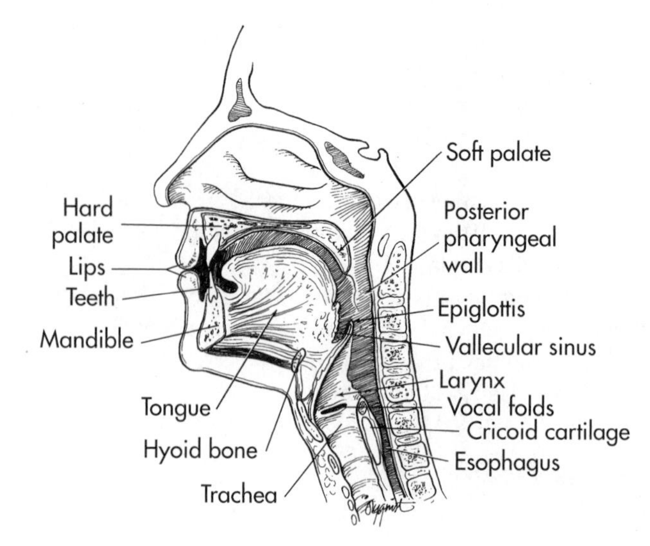

Figure 17-2 Structures associated with deglutition.

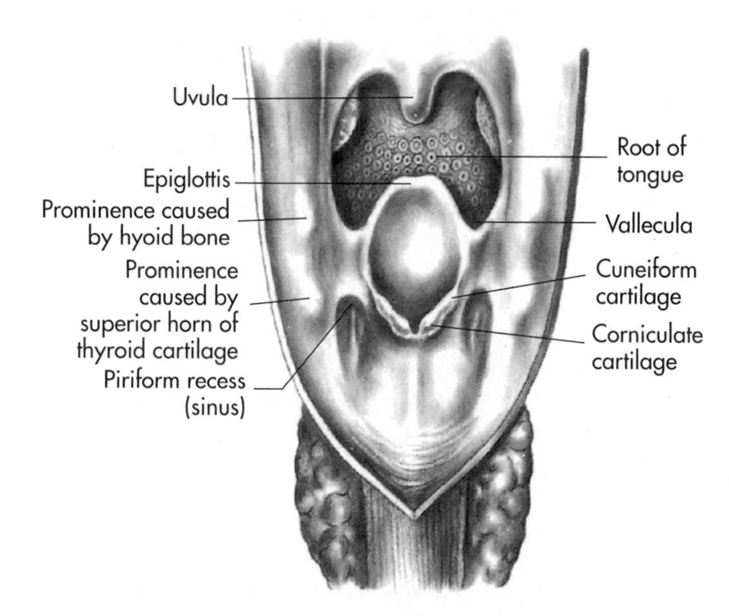

Figure 17-3 Posterior view of hypopharynx. (From Thompson, J.M., McFarland, G.K., Hirsh, J.E., Tucker, S.M. [1997]. *Mosby's clinical nursing* [4th ed.]. St. Louis: Mosby.)

TABLE 17-3 Cranial Nerves Used for Deglutition

Cranial Nerve	Function
Trigeminal (V)	
Motor	Mandibular muscles
Sensory	Maxillary, mandibular
Facial (VII)	
Motor	Submandibular and sublingual salivary glands; facial expression
Sensory	Taste: anterior two thirds of tongue
Glossopharyngeal (IX)	
Motor	Stylopharyngeus muscle
Sensory	Taste: posterior third of tongue; sensation of soft palate and uvula
Vagus (X)	
Sensory	Membrane of larynx and pharynx
Spinal Accessory (XI)	
Motor	Sternocleidomastoid Muscle
Hypoglossal (XII)	
Motor	Intrinsic tongue

where food may collect either before or after the swallow reflex is triggered. Unlike the oral cavity, the larynx has few mechanoreceptive cells; however, there are more cells with free nerve endings in the epithelium, which respond more to liquid stimulation (Plant, 1998). Other structures of the larynx include the aryepiglottic folds and the true and false vocal cords. During deglutition the larynx is elevated, the epiglottis is displaced downward, and the aryepiglottic folds and true and false vocal cords are adducted to protect the trachea (Groher, 1997; Logemann, 1998).

The brain interprets, integrates, and coordinates sensory, motor, and reflex information and activity. Six cranial nerves (V, VII, IX, X, XI, and XII) and the first three cervical nerves of the spinal cord are involved in eating and swallowing (Table 17-3).

Stimulation studies show regions in the pons and medulla that will evoke a swallowing reflex when stimulated. The motor nuclei for many of the muscles involved in swallowing are located in the brainstem. The cerebral cortex assists in the initiation of the oral and pharyngeal phases of swallowing. Muscle contraction during the involuntary phase of swallowing was previously thought to be influenced by the lower brainstem; however, recent studies indicate that the cortex may play a more significant role in facilitating swallowing (Plant, 1998).

Secondary Structures

Secondary structures involved in eating are the eyes, nose, arms, hands, and legs, which are necessary for a person to remain functionally independent; able to locate, secure, and prepare food; and deliver it to the oral cavity. Visualizing food may stimulate appetite, and movements such as the arm bringing food to the mouth, presenting food on a spoon or other utensil, and stimulating texture for oral preparation and taste are important in alerting the system to prepare for swallowing and in triggering the swallow itself (Poertner & Coleman, 1998).

PHYSIOLOGICAL BASIS

The physiological process of eating and swallowing requires the following four stages:

- Selecting and securing food
- Preparing food
- Experiencing the anticipatory stage when food is brought to and placed in the mouth
- Swallowing

A caregiver may select and secure food for a client without serious physiological consequences. However, social and psychological consequences may result when a person becomes unable to prepare food and self-feed.

The final stage of eating is the act of swallowing, which begins once food enters the oral cavity. Swallowing is a complex function accomplished only when activities within the oral cavity, pharynx, larynx, and esophagus are coordinated with interruption of respirations. Afferent, efferent, and central nervous system actions—some volitional and some reflexive—govern the entire swallowing process, which lasts 5 to 10 seconds (Logemann, 1998). Swallowing is divided into four phases:

- Oral preparatory phase: food is manipulated within the mouth, formed into a bolus
- Oral phase: food bolus is centrally located and pushed posteriorly toward the oropharynx
- Pharyngeal phase: bolus is carried by the swallowing reflex through the pharynx
- Esophageal phase: peristalsis carries the bolus to the stomach

Oral Preparatory Phase

The oral preparatory phase is a voluntary phase during which the airway remains open and nasal breathing continues. After food is placed in the mouth, the labial seal holds it in the oral cavity while it is manipulated. The type and amount of manipulation vary with the consistency of the food. Mastication uses rotary and lateral movements of the tongue and mandible to control and manipulate food while the upper and lower teeth crush food.

Mixed with saliva to form a bolus, the food is collected medially on the tongue before the swallow. Soft food may be held on the tongue or between the tongue and hard palate. Liquids are pooled and cupped between the tongue and anterior hard palate until the oral stage begins. Peripheral nerves give feedback about the position of the bolus to prevent injury to the tongue.

Oral Phase

The oral phase, also voluntary, begins as the tongue moves the bolus posterior toward the oropharynx. The bolus sits in a groove created along the center of the tongue until the tongue squeezes the bolus posteriorly against the hard palate toward the oropharynx (Figure 17-4). Within a second the bolus passes the anterior faucial arches, completing the oral phase. Cranial nerves V, VII, and XII control this phase (Table 17-3).

Pharyngeal Phase

The most complex part of swallowing is the pharyngeal phase. The person must maintain airway integrity while the bolus moves along the pharynx to the esophagus. Respirations are inhibited during this phase (Wisdom & Blitzer, 1998). Although this phase is reflexive, it must be initiated voluntarily; once initiated, it cannot be stopped. The swallowing reflex in most persons activates when the food bolus comes into contact with the anterior faucial arches. However, sensory receptors that can elicit the swallowing reflex are present in the tongue, epiglottis, and larynx (Logemann, 1983).

Once the swallowing reflex has been initiated, the following events occur: the tongue moves up and back to force the bolus into the upper pharynx; the soft palate elevates to assist in closure of the pharyngeal port to prevent entry of food into the nasal cavity; the pharyngeal constrictors initiate pharyngeal peristalsis to carry the bolus past the pharynx; the lateral walls of the pharynx are drawn up; the larynx is elevated and pulled forward to assist in closure of the larynx; the epiglottis angles down to help protect the airway (Figure 17-5); the liquid bolus generally flows to either side of the epiglottis and down the pyriform sinuses; the epiglottis checks the descent of the bolus; and the cricopharyngeal sphincter relaxes to permit the bolus to enter the esophagus (Groher, 1997) (Figure 17-6). Impulses travel to the swallowing center in the brainstem via the glossopharyngeal nerve. The fifth, seventh, tenth, and twelfth cranial nerves carry the motor impulses that produce the swallowing reflex (Table 17-3 lists cranial nerves involved in swallowing). The pharyngeal phase lasts approximately 1 second.

Laryngeal Actions

The larynx is protected in part by the downward movement of the epiglottis at an angle of approximately 135 degrees. This moves the laryngeal opening up and forward under the base of the tongue and epiglottis. Laryngeal movement with contraction of the intrinsic laryngeal muscles temporarily decreases the circumference of the laryngeal vestibule. The true and false vocal cords also adduct and the aryepiglottic folds close to provide airway protection. The larynx may close at any stage during swallowing but is already closed when the last bolus leaves the pharynx. This

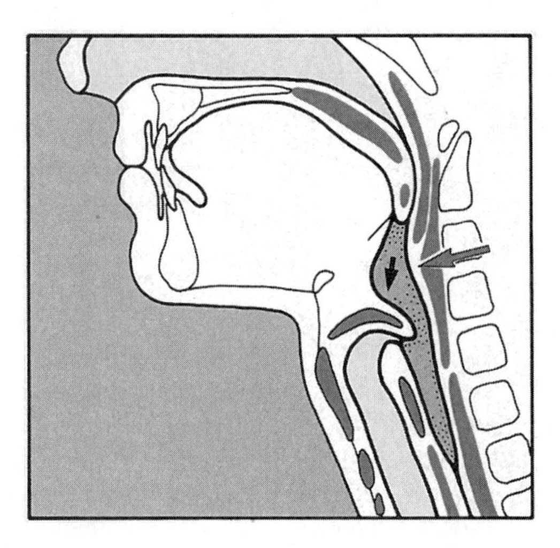

Figure 17-5 Middle pharyngeal phase. (Illustration by Barbara Cousins.)

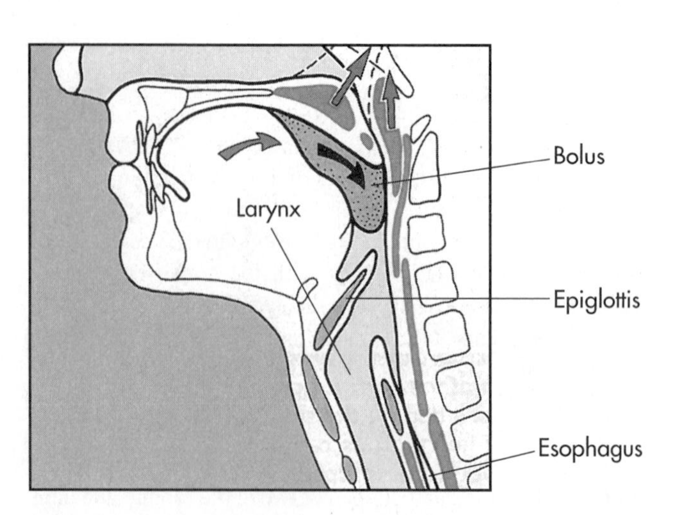

Figure 17-4 Late oral phase (bolus in swallow preparatory position). (Illustration by Barbara Cousins.)

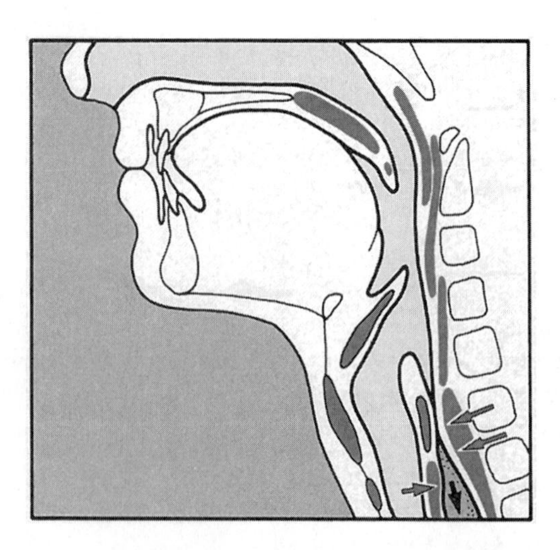

Figure 17-6 Late pharyngeal phase.

causes any food entering the larynx to be squeezed out. The downward movement of the epiglottis helps protect the laryngeal opening from bolus residue. The negative pharyngeal pressure associated with reinflation of the airway propels any residue up and traps it in the valleculae (Groher, 1997).

Esophageal Phase

Swallowing is completed with the esophageal phase, which lasts 8 to 20 seconds. As the bolus enters the esophagus at the cricopharyngeal junction, peristaltic waves respond to the swallow reflex by propelling the bolus down the esophagus. The bolus passes through the gastroesophageal juncture and into the stomach. The cricopharyngeus normally exerts a pharyngeal pressure of 15 to 23 mm Hg and must be overcome by the hypopharynx to induce the opening of the UES (Wisdom & Blitzer, 1998).

Maintaining and Protecting Airway Integrity

Both food and air share the pathways of the pharynx. Consequently, to avoid aspiration while eating, respirations (airflow) must cease for approximately a half second during movement of the food bolus through the pharyngeal phase of the swallow. Food is not permitted into the larynx and trachea. The mechanisms for airway protection are sensory cues and reflex arcs and motor activity. Respiration and swallowing are coordinated functions. The following events maintain and protect the airway during swallowing: the tongue moves posteriorly to push the bolus into the pharynx; the soft palate elevates to help block the nasopharyngeal opening; and the larynx is elevated and pulled forward, causing the epiglottis to tilt down and help protect the airway. The liquid bolus flows around each side of the epiglottis, and the vocal cords adduct to close off the trachea (Plant, 1998; Groher, 1997). The vocal folds normally close before initiation of the pharyngeal swallow and simultaneous with elevation of the larynx. Closure of the airway starts at the vocal folds and progresses in a superior direction (Groher, 1997).

The gag reflex is a protective mechanism that prevents unwanted material from entering the pharynx, larynx, or trachea. It does not occur during the normal act of swallowing. Sensory mechanisms that trigger the gag reflex differ from those involved in swallowing, and motor control of the gag reflex is opposite the motor coordination activated in swallowing, as it forces food up and out of the pharynx. It has been demonstrated that absence of a gag reflex is not a clinical sign of dysphagia. Approximately one third of persons without dysphagia either do not have a gag reflex or have a diminished one. The presence of a gag reflex does not protect against aspiration. Clients with dysphagia can have a normal gag reflex (Leder, 1996).

SWALLOWING CHANGES ACROSS THE LIFE SPAN

Swallowing is a complex neuromuscular process, and many factors can impair its efficiency. Age, neuromuscular impairments, and certain structural deficiencies that may alter swallowing are discussed.

Infants

The fetus begins swallowing in the womb during the twelfth week of gestation. The current concept of swallowing development in infants is that sensory inputs from the mouth and pharynx during feeding stimulate development of the regions in the brain that are responsible for various feeding movements, which then generate more refined movements. The system reciprocates in both its peripheral and central aspects (Groher, 1997).

For term infants the sucking reflex, present at birth and throughout the first 7 months, begins the swallow. Anatomy and swallowing patterns of infants differ from those of adults. An infant's oral cavity is smaller, causing the tongue to fill a greater part of the mouth and to rest more anteriorly. The larynx is suspended higher in the pharynx and acts as a sphincter; the jaw, tongue, cheeks, and lips move as a single unit. The tongue elevates during sucking and then thrusts the liquid to the posterior oral cavity. These actions are coordinated with the pharyngeal swallow. The anterior to posterior sucking movements of the tongue make the intake of even soft solids difficult before the third to fourth month (Groher, 1997). Infants do not distinguish between liquids and solids until the fourth month (Derkay & Schechter, 1998).

As the infant grows, the lower jaw extends downward and forward, and the sucking pads are reabsorbed, thereby increasing the intraoral space. The infant begins to learn new voluntary suck patterns and to suppress the reflexive suckle patterns. There is an increased closing action of the lips, and the tongue motion becomes a raising and lowering of the body of the tongue. This up-and-down motion helps to pull soft food and liquid into the oral cavity. Most infants complete this transition by 9 months of age (Darrow & Harley, 1998).

Respirations in the sucking pattern follow in a sequence of inhalation, swallow, and exhalation. In some term infants, preterm infants, and neurologically compromised infants, feeding apnea may lead to hypoxia or bradycardia.

Children

Children develop patterns and behaviors associated with eating as part of development. A child with impaired swallowing still needs to be able to experience eating- and food-related events appropriate for the culture and age, such as finger foods for toddlers. The same child can be expected to develop food preferences and may use eating as a manipulative tool if too much attention is focused on eating.

Clinicians who work with children are becoming increasingly aware of the influence that early abnormal feeding performance has on the patterns of feeding in the neurologically impaired child. Abnormalities of breathing and positioning in the infant have a cumulative effect in the developing child. Abnormalities in feeding, respiration, and posture affect the development of the muscles and skeleton in the mouth, pharynx, and larynx, causing further abnormalities and difficulties in feeding and swallowing (Bosma, 1997).

The child with poor head and trunk control, altered or dependent sitting balance, and impaired swallowing, as occurs with cerebral palsy, requires special attention to posture, head position, lip and mouth control, eating and swallowing techniques, and feeding environment. This child may retain oral and swallowing reflexes that are expected to disappear in infancy, making risk of aspiration while eating extremely high (Helfrich-Miller, Rector, & Straka, 1986).

Adults

Changes in mastication and deglutition generally do not occur in normal healthy adults until the eighth decade. The anatomy and function of the oral cavity may change with decreased sensation in the oral cavity, increased connective tissue in the tongue, loss of dentition, and decreased masticatory strength. Poorly fitting dentures can interfere with the oral preparatory phase by causing poorly formed boluses (Plant, 1998). Other changes may include reduced pharyngeal peristalsis, with some of the bolus often remaining in the pharynx, increased pharyngeal transit times and total duration of motor response, decreased size of the opening of the cricopharyngeal sphincter, decreased esophageal peristalsis, and increased esophageal transit time (Logemann, 1998; Rademaker, Pauloski, Colangelo, & Logemann, 1998). In one study the respiratory cycle was interrupted more often in the inspiratory phase in elderly persons as compared with the expiratory phase in younger persons (Ozer, 1994). Robbins, Levine, Wood, Roecker, and Luschei (1994) found a decrease in lingual pressures in two separate studies.

NEUROMUSCULAR DISEASES

Neuromuscular diseases often affect multiple body systems and functions, including swallowing. The complex innervation of the eating and swallowing process allows multiple variations of impairment to occur, involving minute steps during any one or more stages or phases (Willig, Paulus, Lacau Saint Guily, Beon, & Naavarro, 1994). Major neuromuscular impairments that can affect swallowing are summarized in Table 17-4, along with the phase of deglutition affected and the impairment that results.

Impairments in the oral preparatory phase commonly result from poor sensation and perception about the quantity and location of the food in the mouth. Impaired motor control of muscles and tongue movement during mastication may leave food improperly chewed or pocketed to the side of the mouth, where the anterior and posterior faucial arches form cavities.

Impaired pharyngeal motility results in a poorly coordinated swallowing reflex. Food then becomes lodged within

TABLE 17-4 Neuromuscular Diseases Associated with Poor Deglutition and the Resulting Impairment

Phase of Deglutition/Disease	Impairment
Oral Preparatory	
Cerebral palsy	Poor suck reflex, inappropriate reflexive behaviors
Parkinson's disease; myasthenia gravis; ALS; left, right, bilateral, and brainstem cerebrovascular accidents; multiple sclerosis (when cranial nerve XII is involved)	Poor mastication, foods inadequately chewed
ALS; left, right, bilateral, and brainstem cerebrovascular accidents; Huntington's chorea; myasthenia gravis; Parkinson's disease; head trauma	Poor tongue control and mobility
Oral	
Bilateral and brainstem cerebrovascular accident	Delay in swallow reflex
Huntington's chorea, head trauma, cerebral palsy, Parkinson's disease, multiple sclerosis (when cranial nerve IX is involved)	Choking or coughing
Left, right cerebrovascular accident	Lingual hemiparesis
Pharyngeal	
Parkinson's disease; ALS; multiple sclerosis; left, right, bilateral, and brainstem cerebrovascular accident; poliomyelitis	Impaired pharyngeal motility and peristalsis
Cerebrovascular accident, myasthenia gravis	Residue remains in valleculae and pyriform sinuses
Myotonic dystrophy, head trauma, ALS, Huntington's chorea	Aspiration

ALS, Amyotrophic lateral sclerosis

the valleculae or pyriform sinuses and drains into the trachea, causing aspiration. Aspiration occurs most commonly during the oral phase when the swallowing reflex is delayed and the bolus of food or liquid is allowed to invade the larynx. The most experienced bedside observers do not identify 40% of the clients who aspirate (Logemann, 1983). Clients who have had a cerebrovascular accident may exhibit lingual hemiparesis, which interferes with tongue control and preparation for swallowing.

Clients with the same neurological disease will exhibit different symptoms, and the onset of dysphagia will occur at different stages of the disease. Clients must always be treated as individuals, and the interventions should be based on the client's specific symptoms and situation.

Specific Neurological Impairments

Clients with amyotrophic lateral sclerosis (ALS) often have difficulty with oral transit and initiating swallowing; thus mealtimes become prolonged. They may also have palatal and pharyngeal weakness and isolated choking with liquids. Interventions may include dietary changes to a modified consistency with soft, cohesive foods such as macaroni casseroles and custards. The use of calorie-dense foods and liquids with increased taste, temperature, and texture sensation may combat weight loss and food boredom. Clients should also have regular swallowing evaluations to monitor disease progression.

Clients who are no longer able to meet their caloric needs because of food spillage, slow eating with inadequate time for meals, and respiratory fatigue may require a percutaneous endoscopic gastrostomy (PEG) tube (Wisdom & Blitzer, 1998; Groher, 1997).

Clients with Parkinson's disease may have difficulty during the oral, pharyngeal, and esophageal phases of swallowing. The severity of the disease does not correspond to the severity of dysphagia. Interventions may include feeding and dietary modifications, coordinating medications with mealtimes to maximize their positive effects, and offering small, frequent meals with increased sensory input. Small, frequent meals offer psychological benefits by allowing clients to feel that they do not need to finish a large meal in a short time, thus allowing them to enjoy the meal, and it reassures clients that they will not go hungry if they do not finish a meal (Wisdom & Blitzer, 1998; Groher, 1997).

It is not unusual for clients with multiple sclerosis to deny difficulty with swallowing. This can be due to cognitive deficits or because they are not aware of the swallowing difficulty. In the early stages the clients may have occasional choking, especially when fatigued. In the later stages of the disease, the swallowing difficulties are in the oral cavity and pharynx, with delayed swallowing reflex and reduced pharyngeal peristalsis. Some clients have also reported abnormal taste. Interventions include necessary feeding modifications, decreased distractions at mealtime, and increased awareness of sensory cues (Wisdom & Blitzer, 1998).

The client with myasthenia gravis may have slow and weak tongue movements, fatigue during deglutition, and bolus residue in the oropharynx. Chewing and swallowing abilities may deteriorate during meals. Interventions include coordinating medications with meals and limiting physical activity, including talking, before eating to maintain strength (Groher, 1997).

Strokes occurring in both hemispheres were previously believed to cause dysphagia; however, new findings demonstrate that strokes occurring in one hemisphere can cause dysphagia. Clients with damage to the left hemisphere are more likely to have impairments in the oral phase, whereas damage to the right hemisphere causes deficits in the pharyngeal phase. Systematic tongue-to-palate interaction is fundamental to successful oral food transport. Chi-Fishman, Stone, and McCall (1998) and Daniels, Brailey, and Foundas (1999) found lingual incoordination in clients with subcortical lesions in the periventricular white matter, as well as in clients with unilateral left hemisphere damage and clients with unilateral right hemisphere damage.

Commonly, neuromuscular impairments involve more than one stage of swallowing (Glenn, Araya, Jones, & Liljefors, 1993). Robbins, Logemann, and Kirshner (1986) found all participants of their study who had Parkinson's disease "exhibited abnormal oropharyngeal movement patterns and timing during the volitional oral and pharyngeal phases of swallowing." Clients with chronic, progressive diseases such as cerebral palsy, Parkinson's disease, multiple sclerosis, and amyotrophic lateral sclerosis often have progressive difficulty with swallowing.

ANATOMIC IMPAIRMENTS

Cleft lips and cleft palates, anatomic impairments found in children, require surgical correction. A cleft in the lip may be only a small notch, or it may extend to the floor of the nose; cleft palates occur alone or in conjunction with cleft lips. These anatomic impairments may involve only the uvula or may extend through the hard and soft palates, exposing one or both nasal cavities. Until surgical repair is completed, nasal regurgitation complicates the tasks of sucking and swallowing liquids, nutritional intake is compromised during an infant's stage of rapid growth and development, and health status may be affected. All of these are serious consequences to be prevented and avoided.

Pharyngoesophageal diverticulum, or Zenker's diverticulum, in the cervical esophagus is an abnormal muscular pouch that forms either above the cricopharyngeal muscle through Killian's triangle or below the cricopharyngeal muscle. The exact cause has not been established; however, in some clients it is associated with esophageal disease. It is more common in men between 60 and 80 years of age. The symptoms include regurgitation of undigested food, foul breath, fullness in the neck, weight loss, and nighttime cough with aspiration. Surgery is usually required to correct this dysfunction (Groher, 1997)

Persons who have had radical head and neck surgery often experience impaired swallowing. The severity of the impairment varies with the location, cause of the surgery, and swallowing mechanisms that have been affected. Esophageal cancers tend to develop in such a way that by the time symptoms are present the cancer is advanced and incurable. Curative treatment is surgery; however, the 5-year survival rate is only about 5% (Groher, 1997).

Other less common causes of dysphagia include prolonged mechanical ventilation (Tolep, Getch, & Criner, 1996); tracheostomy tubes, which can reduce elevation and anterior movement of the larynx; improperly fitting hard cervical collars, which can restrict laryngeal elevation (Houghton & Curley, 1996); neck overextension in clients with halo fixators; excessive neck flexion with Philadelphia collars; and inadequate head support in high-back wheelchairs. Other causes are cervical spine surgery with an anterior approach (Kirshblum, Johnston, Brown, O'Connor, & Jarosz, 1999), cervical osteophytosis (McGarrah & Teller, 1997), and acquired immunodeficiency syndrome (AIDS) (Martinez & Nord, 1995).

FEEDING TUBES

A goal for all clients is to avoid the prolonged use of feeding tubes. However, in the early stages of treatment one may be necessary to provide the nutrients needed to maintain or achieve metabolic balance. The person with dysphagia who is unable to swallow safely uses alternative means for nutrition. For short-term nutritional intervention, the rehabilitation nurse tests the person for an active gag reflex and assesses the risk for aspiration.

The nasogastric method is commonly used by clients who have some gag reflex, provided they are awake and alert. Huggins, Tuomi, and Young (1999) found that fine-bore (French 8 × 85 cm) and wide-bore (16 × 122 cm) nasogastric tubes slowed swallowing in healthy persons; however, the small-bore nasogastric tubes slowed swallowing less. The smaller tubes are also less irritating with less nasopharyngeal erosion and less compromise of the gastroesophageal sphincter. A nasogastric tube in a client with dysphagia can cause increased difficulty with swallowing of saliva, regurgitation of gastric contents, and suppression of the cough reflex. A nasointestinal method is used for a client without a gag reflex and with a history of aspiration.

A surgically placed feeding tube is the method of choice for most long-term assisted nutritional programs, including clients who receive nutritional care at home. The most commonly used tubes are gastrostomy, jejunostomy, and esophagostomy; children may have a gastrostomy button. A commonly used third alternative nutritional method is via PEG. Percutaneous gastrostomies can be performed with local anesthesia and result in fewer complications than surgical procedures (Sands, 1999).

Clients and families are taught to recognize and report signs of complications such as postoperative edema, bleeding, tube dislodgment, peritonitis, aspiration, skin irritations, or diarrhea. The most serious complication associated with any method is aspiration. The potential for aspiration is lessened when the client is sitting up in a chair or is in bed with the head of the bed elevated at least 45 degrees while being fed and for the hour that follows.

Clients receiving any type of tube feeding should be monitored daily for edema, dehydration, fluid intake and output, and stool output and consistency (including caloric composition and density). A weight should be taken at the same time, in the same amount of clothing (as little as possible), at least three times a week. Serum electrolytes, blood urea nitrogen (BUN), creatinine, and blood count should be checked 2 to 3 times a week, and a chemistry profile should be done weekly (Bradford, 1996; Sands, 1999).

Not all medications can be crushed and given via the tube, and some may not be available in a liquid form; thus substitutions may be needed. Some medications that cannot be crushed are benzonatate, diclofenac, diltiazem, isotretinoin, omeprazole, orphenadrine, pentoxifylline, and piroxicam (Miller & Miller, 1995). Other medications that should not be crushed include those that have SR (sustained release), SA (sustained action), XL (extended release), -bid, -dur, -ten, or –slow in the name. Capsules containing a liquid, capsules that are sealed, and enteric-coated tablets also should not be crushed (Glenn-Molali, 2001). Medications also may affect swallowing processes, as described in Box 17-1.

When a client is able to take adequate oral nutrition, the tube is removed. Accurate calorie and nutritional data are indicators as to whether a person can maintain adequate oral intake; however, these must be carefully assessed before the

Box 17-1 Examples of Medications That Can Affect Swallowing

An important part of the nursing assessment is evaluating all of the client's medications. This includes prescriptions, over-the-counter medicines, vitamins, minerals, and herbs. Many different types of medications can have a negative effect on swallowing

- Medications with sedative effects can cause confusion or disorientation, which may decrease the client's swallowing abilities
- Antispasticity medications may affect swallowing ability by decreasing the strength of the involved muscles
- Neuroleptics can cause extrapyramidal reactions
- Anticholinergics may cause altered salivation
- Any medication with xerostomic side effects, such as anticonvulsants, antihistamines, antihypertensives, cold medications, and diuretics, can adversely affect swallowing by drying the oral and pharyngeal mucosae and decreasing the saliva necessary to help illicit the swallowing reflex
- Other medications that do not directly affect swallowing may affect eating by decreasing appetite

Data from Harris (1996) and Groher (1997).

tube is removed. Premature removal and subsequent reinsertion of a feeding tube may add to discomfort for a client, be viewed as regression, or lead to depression for the client or family.

A tracheal glucose assay test can be used for clients who have a tracheostomy or translaryngeal intubation and are receiving tube feedings to detect aspirated feeding formula.

NURSING ASSESSMENT

The nursing assessment involves both collection and interpretation of data. It is central to understanding a client's nourishment patterns and eating process and identifying specific deficits. A complete assessment includes a history of difficulties in eating, a measurable review of food and fluid intake, evaluation of laboratory data, interpretation of findings from diagnostic studies, and a physical assessment.

Nursing History

The purpose of the nursing history as it relates to eating and swallowing is to establish the present eating patterns of the client and the patterns before the illness or injury, to describe any present difficulties, to determine areas of evaluation for the physical assessment, and to evaluate the client's need for education. The history should focus on the following four broad areas:

- Ability of the client to obtain and prepare food
- Adequacy of the diet and nutritional habits and preferences
- Ability of the client to bring food to the mouth
- Ability of the client to chew and swallow food

The assessment questions are divided into the four areas listed above. Different questions may be more important depending on where the care is being provided: community, clinic, acute care, rehabilitation, or long-term care setting.

Obtaining and Preparing Food

Caregivers who obtain and prepare food should be present, if possible, to offer information when taking the history regarding nutritional adequacy of the diet, how food is prepared, personal or ethnic rules about food or eating, when foods are served, and similar data that might affect a client's intake. When a client shops for and prepares food, ask the following questions in the history:

- How do you get to the store? How often do you shop?
- What storage and preparation facilities are available to you at home?
- Do you have any difficulty preparing food?
- Are cooking areas accessible and safe? For example, is there a fire extinguisher and a place for sharp knives?
- Are meals prepared from a standing or a sitting position? Are any adaptive devices used?
- Is there any difficulty with mobility?
- Is there sufficient strength and dexterity in the arms and hands to manipulate, open, and prepare foods?

Adequacy of the Diet, Nutritional Habits, and Preferences

- Has a special diet ever been recommended by your physician? If yes, what is the diet? How closely do you follow the special diet?
- Has there been a recent change in weight? If yes, what is the reason?
- Do you eat alone?
- Are meals eaten out or is take-out ordered? If yes, how often, what are the usual restaurants, and what foods are ordered?
- Are any meals provided and brought to the home by someone else?
- How many meals/snacks are eaten each day?
- What fluids (water, juice, soda) and how much do you drink each day?
- Do you drink any alcohol? How often and how much?
- What is the typical intake of foods and fluids over 3 days?
- Which medications, both prescription and over the counter, do you take? Which vitamins, herbs, or supplements do you take?
- Do you take medications with meals?
- Are there any cultural or religious preferences?
- Are there any foods you will not or cannot eat (due to allergy or intolerance)? If yes, what are they?
- Is there a particular type of food used (canned, frozen, vegetarian)?
- How much money is available for food on a weekly basis?

Economics and access to affordable fresh foods can play an important role in the types of food available to the client. Convenience or prepared foods may be easier but commonly are more expensive and many contain unwanted fat and salt. Fresh foods may have more nutrient value but are more difficult to prepare and store, and they be may be more expensive out of season. The social aspect of eating may also affect nutritional status; persons who eat alone are at greater risk for poor nutrition.

Ability of the Client to Bring Food to the Mouth

- Do you feed yourself? If yes, do you have any difficulties?
- Is any adaptive feeding equipment used?
- Are you able to open individual food containers/packages?
- Do you tire easily or become short of breath while eating?
- Do you sit in any particular position while eating or soon after? Can you sit upright during meals without difficulty?

Ability of the Client to Chew and Swallow Food

The next phase of the history elicits the client's ability to swallow food effectively. If the client answers yes to any of the following questions, question how long the symptom has been present. Factors to be considered include the following:

- Is there a history of aspiration pneumonia?
- Is there pain with swallowing?
- Do foods get stuck in the throat?
- Are solids washed down with liquids?
- Is there difficulty with swallowing solid or soft foods?
- Is there difficulty with swallowing liquids?
- Do foods need to be cut into very small pieces?

- Do foods or liquids regurgitate nasally?
- Is there choking or coughing when eating or drinking?
- Are foods/fluids modified to help with eating or drinking?
- Do you need to be in a particular position when eating or drinking?
- Do you use any special techniques/movements to help you swallow?

Psychosocial Factors

By the end of the history the nurse should be able to assess the following through conversations with the client:

- The degree to which loneliness or depression is contributing to a poor nutritional intake
- The amount of fear the person has regarding eating
- The degree to which lifelong eating habits are contributing to a poor nutritional intake
- The degree of willingness and motivation the client has to work in a rehabilitation program

Physical Assessment

As part of the nursing assessment it is important to determine the client's ability to understand and follow directions. Poor subjective data form an unreliable basis for the physical assessment of the client's ability to obtain and prepare food, place food in the oral cavity, and swallow food. The physical assessment begins with examination of the head and neck and should include the following:

- Assess the client's head control while the client is in a seated position.
- Assess facial symmetry.
- Inspect the lips for color, symmetry, and moisture. Malignant lesions of the oral cavity may occur on the lips (and under the tongue).
- Assess whether the client is drooling, indicating poor control of oral fluids.
- Ask the client to close the lips tightly.
- Ask the client to open the mouth. Assess internal symmetry.
- Inspect the mucosa of the oral cavity and the tongue (with dehydration they will appear dry). Check for lacerations, indicating biting while chewing
- Inspect the teeth for number and condition.
- If there are dentures, inspect for proper fit. Ask the client to remove them (or remove dentures if client is unable to remove them) and inspect the underlying gums.
- Test cranial nerve XII (hypoglossal) by inspecting the tongue for irregular movement or asymmetry, both while the tongue is in the mouth and when protruded. Ask the client to move the tongue side to side and in and out rapidly.
- Test cranial nerves IX (glossopharyngeal) and X (vagus) by asking the client to say "ah." The uvula and soft palate should rise. Deviation of the uvula is found with paralysis. When the uvula is touched with a tongue depressor, a gag reflex occurs, indicating intact motor function of the vagus nerve. Although the gag reflex is closely associated with the swallowing reflex, it does not have to be present for the normal swallow to occur. Evaluate the voice for hoarseness or nasal quality.
- Inspect the pharynx for color, edema, and ulcerations. This observation includes the anterior and posterior faucial arches and palatine tonsils.
- Test cranial nerve V (trigeminal) for strength and symmetry by asking the client to clench the teeth, chew, and move the lower jaw side to side against the resistance of the examiner's hand. The examiner palpates the temporomandibular area to determine muscle strength during contraction. The sensory component of the nerve is tested by asking the client to identify sharp and dull sensations on the sides of the face, forehead, and cheeks. The two sides should be compared to each other.
- Test cranial nerve VII (facial) by observing throughout the examination for the presence of tics and unusual movements or asymmetry of the face. Test motor function by observing the client's ability to clench the teeth, smile, raise the eyebrows, wrinkle the forehead, purse the lips, whistle, and blow. Dentures should be in place if worn by the client. The sensory component of this cranial nerve is used to identify sweet and salty tastes. Sugar or salt may be placed on the anterior two thirds of the tongue.
- Test cranial nerve XI (spinal accessory) by asking the client to raise the shoulders against resistance of the examiner's hands and by asking the client to turn the head against resistance. Inability to raise the shoulders indicates damage on the ipsilateral side, and inability to turn the head is indicative of damage on the contralateral side from the head turn (Voss, 1994).
- If indicated, test the client for the presence of primitive reflex behaviors usually seen only in infants and which, when present in later life, indicate a disturbance of the upper motor neuron system (e.g., after a brain injury). These reflexes include the rooting reflex, stimulated by stroking the lips or corners of the mouth and having the client's head reflexively turn toward the stimulus. The tonic neck reflex, sometimes called the fencing position. The tonic neck reflex is a total body pattern that occurs by turning the head to one side, resulting in extension of the extremities on the face side and flexion of the extremities on the skull side.
- Throughout the examination, evaluate the client's voice. Oral and palatal dysfunction are highlighted by dysarthria or hypernasality.
- Ask the client to cough. Is it forceful? If not, ask the client to cough forcefully.
- Ask the client to swallow water. Can the client form a seal with the lips? How long does it take to complete the swallow? Does the client have difficulty initiating the swallow? Does the client use any compensatory techniques?

- Does the client have a moist, wet voice after swallowing water? Does the client frequently clear the throat?
- Check the client's temperature. Is it elevated? An elevated temperature 30 minutes after eating food can be indicative of aspiration.

The remainder of the physical examination should focus on the client's ability to eat independently. If the client has difficulty with arm or hand range of motion or coordination, dietary staff may prepare foods that can be eaten more easily. A description of the difficulty the client has with feeding is helpful when performing the physical assessment. The following areas should be assessed:

- Does the client have sufficient mobility, muscle strength, and control to lift utensils from the plate to the mouth?
- Are grip and strength sufficient to hold eating utensils?
- Does a tremor or involuntary movement interfere with coordination?
- Can the client cut food?
- Is the client limited to the use of one hand?
- Is there sufficient muscle strength and head control to remain sitting upright for meals?
- What is the client's visual acuity? Is vision limited (e.g., hemianopsia)?

The nursing history and physical assessment should provide data to describe the client's disability and to form the basis for the nursing diagnoses.

Diagnostic Tests

The most commonly used diagnostic tests for identifying dysphagia include the bedside swallow examination (BSE), modified barium swallow with videofluoroscopy, and videoendoscopy.

The purpose of the BSE is to identify clients who may be at risk for aspiration. The BSE may be an informal clinical examination or a structured assessment. The informal examination may consist of the clinician asking the client a few questions and then placing two fingers on the thyroid notch between the hyoid bone and larynx. As the client swallows, the clinician should feel the larynx move up and forward. There should be equal movement on both sides of the larynx. If elevation of the larynx is not felt, it may indicate that the cricopharyngeus did not open properly and that the epiglottis did not tilt downward adequately to protect the trachea.

A structured BSE consists of taking a detailed history regarding the medical condition, surgeries, and medications that may cause dysphagia; performing a physical examination of the client's face, mouth, and throat (see Physical Assessment section and previous paragraph); and observing the client swallow different amounts and consistencies of food and fluid. (AHCPR, 1999)

Videofluoroscopic swallow study (VFSS), or modified barium swallow, allows viewing of the oral cavity, laryngopharynx, and cervical esophagus. During the test the client swallows small amounts of a liquid, puree, or solid mixed with barium. As the client manipulates the bolus in the oral cavity and swallows, the fluoroscopic study is recorded on videotape. Videotaping of the swallowing study allows clinicians to have repeated viewing and slow-motion analysis.

Compensatory techniques, head positions, and a client's tolerance for swallowing foods and liquids of different consistencies can be evaluated, and all four phases of swallowing can be assessed. With repeated testing, clinicians must inform clients about their exposure to some amounts of radiation (Ozer, 1994). However, the dosage used is not considered a major concern (Wright, Boyd, & Workman, 1998).

Video endoscopic swallow study (VEES)/fiberoptic endoscopic swallow study (FEES) is a procedure that uses a fiberoptic nasopharyngoscope to enable a clinician to visually examine a client's palate, pharynx, and larynx. The clinician is also able to observe a swallow and any secretions that are pooling and assess the sensation of the upper aerodigestive tract. The client is then given fluids and foods of different consistencies to swallow. Dye may be added to the food to increase its visibility, and the study is recorded on videotape for client teaching and biofeedback. The equipment is portable, and no radiation is used for this test. The test can also be conducted throughout a meal to identify fatigue factors (Bastian, 1998).

Fiberoptic endoscopic evaluation of swallowing with sensory testing (FEESST) combines the endoscopic evaluation of swallowing with a technique that determines laryngopharyngeal sensory discrimination thresholds. An air-pulse stimulus is delivered through the endoscope to the mucosa innervated by the superior laryngeal nerve. The stimulus elicits a brainstem-mediated airway protection reflex (Aviv et al., 2000)

Manometry is used to obtain information on the strength, timing, and sequencing of pressure events in the esophagus during deglutition. A catheter with pressure transducers is positioned within the esophagus; once in place, the transducers measure pressures as the client swallows. Usually the transducers are positioned to measure pressures in the UES, the esophagus, and the lower esophageal sphincter. Manometry is used to identify disruptions in the peristaltic waves through the pharynx and esophagus and to diagnose impairments of the upper or lower esophagus.

Manofluorography combines monometry with videofluoroscopy (Bastian, 1998).

Pulse oximetry is used to identify the occurrence of aspiration of food or fluids by detecting hypoxia (Farrell & O'Neill, 1999) while the client is eating or drinking. Clients who exhibit aspiration or laryngeal penetration without clearing have a significant decline in Spo_2 (Sherman, Nisenboum, Jesberger, Morrow, & Jesberger, 1999). Collins and Bakheit (1997) found that pulse oximetry was a reliable method of diagnosis of aspiration in most clients with dysphagia. It is easy to use, is noninvasive, and provides immediate information.

The nurse uses a stethoscope placed at the client's throat to listen for cervical breath sounds as the client swallows.

The purpose of cervical auscultation is to evaluate a client for the risks of tracheal aspiration. Auscultation with an accelerometer transduces surface body movements to an acoustic signal. Auscultation with a laryngeal microphone provides a broader spectrum sound of tissue and fluid movement and breath exchange. A stethoscope will detect low-frequency breath sounds (Zenner, Losinski, & Mills, 1995). Takahashi, Groher, and Michi (1994) suggest using the site over the lateral border of the trachea immediately inferior to the cricoid cartilage and evaluating the swallowing sounds from repeated swallows. Their research supports using either side of the trachea. Hamlet, Penney, and Formolo (1994) found that two stethoscopes had superior overall acoustical performance: the Littman Cardiology II and the Hewlett-Packard Rappaport-Sprague with a medium bell and small diaphragm.

Auscultation does not currently have a common nomenclature, and there are no data to support the correlation of acoustic sounds with specific swallowing events. Additionally clinicians require extensive training. However, Zenner et al. (1995), with two extensively trained and experienced clinicians, reported favorable results using this technique to diagnose dysphagia in a long-term care setting.

The Exeter dysphagia assessment technique (EDAT) is noninvasive and records the respiratory patterns, contact of the lips or tongue with a spoon, and associated swallow sounds that occur during eating and drinking. Bidirectional airflow is recorded through a plastic catheter supported under the nose. Spoon contact is recorded by completion of a circuit between an indifferent electrode and an electrode forming part of the spoon handle. Swallow sounds are recorded by a microphone positioned next to the throat. The signals obtained by the three sources are recorded and reproduced in a chart. The chart is then analyzed by a clinician. This technique may be used to assist in the diagnosis of dysphagia, and Pinnington, Muhiddin, Lobeck, and Pearce (2000) found it to be a reliable and effective tool.

The simple two-step swallowing provocation test (STS-SPT) was reported by Teramoto, Matsuse, Fukuchi, and Ouchi (1999) to be helpful in differentiating clients predisposed to aspiration from those with normal swallowing function. A bolus injection of 0.4 or 2.0 ml of distilled water was given through a small nasal catheter at the suprapharynx while the client was in a supine position. The STS-SPT was estimated by the swallowing response and latent time for swallowing after the bolus injection. The latent time was assessed with a stopwatch from bolus injection to the onset of swallowing. Swallowing was identified by visual observation of laryngeal movement.

NURSING DIAGNOSIS

The priority nursing diagnosis that may be used for eating and swallowing deficits from the nutritional-metabolic pattern are listed in Table 17-5, along with the suggested nursing interventions (NIC) and nursing outcomes (NOC).

Other nursing diagnoses that may be applicable to the client with eating and swallowing impairments are from health perception–health management pattern and the cognitive-perceptual pattern.

1. Self-feeding deficit
2. Self-bathing hygiene deficit (specify level)
3. Health-seeking behaviors (specify)
4. Altered health-seeking maintenance (specify)
5. Ineffective management of therapeutic regimen (specify area)
6. Risk for ineffective management of therapeutic regimen (specify area)
7. Effective management of therapeutic regimen

TABLE 17-5 Suggested Priority Nursing Diagnoses, Nursing Interventions, and Nursing Outcomes for a Client with Dysphagia

Nursing Diagnosis	Nursing Intervention	Nursing Outcome
Imbalanced nutrition: less than body requirements or nutritional deficit	Nutrition management Nutrition therapy Nutritional monitoring Swallowing therapy	Nutritional status Nutritional status: nutrient intake Nutritional status: food and fluid intake
Impaired swallowing (uncompensated)	Swallowing therapy Aspiration precautions	Swallowing status Swallowing status: oral phase Swallowing status: pharyngeal phase Swallowing status: esophageal phase
Risk for aspiration	Aspiration precautions	Aspiration control
Risk for deficient fluid volume	Fluid monitoring Fluid management	Fluid balance Hydration

Data from Johnson, M., Maas, M.L., & Moorhead, S. (2000). *Nursing outcomes classification (NOC)* (2nd ed.). St. Louis: Mosby; McCloskey, J.C., & Bulechek, G.M. (2000). *Nursing interventions classification (NIC)* (3rd ed.). St. Louis: Mosby; and North American Nursing Diagnosis Association. (2001). *Nursing diagnosis: definitions and classification 2001-2002* (4th ed.). Philadelphia: Author.

8. Ineffective family management of therapeutic regimen
9. Health-management deficit (specify area)
10. Risk for health-management deficit (specify area)
11. Noncompliance (specify area)
12. Risk for noncompliance (specify area)
13. Knowledge deficit in proper nutrition, adaptive equipment, or availability of community resources

Goals

The goals for the client having difficulty with eating and swallowing or the family may include all or some of the following:

1. Maintains adequate nutrition
2. Maintains adequate body weight
3. Demonstrates and uses compensatory postures
4. Demonstrates and uses compensatory swallowing techniques
5. Demonstrates ability to swallow modified foods and fluids
6. Verbalizes understanding of the importance of modifications in consistency of foods and fluids
7. Shows no evidence of aspiration
8. Improves or maintains fluid volume
9. Demonstrates improved ability to feed self
10. Demonstrates ability to use adaptive equipment
11. Demonstrates improved ability to participate in oral hygiene
12. Verbalizes understanding of measures to prevent and alleviate choking
13. Verbalizes understanding of proper nutrition
14. Verbalizes understanding of importance of following prescribed dietary restrictions
15. Verbalizes understanding of available community resources to assist in providing adequate nutrition

Goals established by the nurse and client relate to the nursing diagnoses and are based on information obtained from the client during the nursing assessment, from family members, and from home assessment data. Impaired swallowing may result because of a poor swallowing reflex. The nurse may decrease the episodes of aspiration and choking by reinforcing compensatory swallowing techniques, making the swallowing process safer. Fluid-volume deficit, or risk for fluid-volume deficit, means increasing liquid intake either through alternate forms or by more frequent feedings. For someone with an inadequate swallowing process, liquids are often more difficult than foods to swallow. As a result the client may have a great deal of fear when taking liquids. It is important to maximize the safety of the swallowing process and to provide encouragement when the client is taking liquids.

Inadequate caloric intake, particularly of solid foods, necessitates alternate and more frequent feedings. If poor intake is a result of depression, the underlying problem must be addressed. A complete diet history that includes food preferences and the significance of food to the client should be completed to find foods the client might eat. If the client is consuming too many calories, the goal is to reduce caloric intake by substituting reduced-calorie foods. Often it is necessary to look for meaningful activities that the client can use to substitute for time previously spent eating.

NURSING INTERVENTIONS

Once an assessment is completed, nursing diagnoses are formulated, and goals are established, specific nursing interventions must be considered. All clients are individuals, and the interventions must be tailored for the specific impairment. The priority NIC that may be used for eating and swallowing deficits from the nutritional-metabolic pattern are listed in Table 17-5 with the nursing diagnosis and NOC. Other NIC (McCloskey & Bulechek, 2000) that may be applicable to a client with dysphagia include:

1. Diet staging
2. Airway suctioning
3. Intravenous therapy
4. Oral health maintenance
5. Self-care assistance: feeding
6. Teaching: prescribed diet
7. Health education

Interventions

All clients need proper body posture and alignment during mealtimes with any necessary modifications for their situation. Proper body alignment helps to stimulate the central nervous system and minimize food entering the trachea by narrowing the airway.

See Box 17-2 for general mealtime recommendations for a client who is dysphagic and taking a diet with modified food consistencies. These suggestions should be altered as necessary for each client. Feeding recommendations for these clients include:

- If the client has poor head control and the head falls forward, hold the head up by placing the palm of your hand on the client's forehead for support
- Initially use teaspoon-sized bites of soft food that are easy to swallow (custards, purees); observe laryngeal elevation before offering the next bite
- Place a half teaspoonful on the middle to back part of the tongue; however, if the client has tongue or facial paralysis or has had a partial laryngectomy, the correct placement is on the unaffected intact side, not midline, to provide maximum sensory stimulation
- Place the spoon firmly on the tongue to stimulate removal of food from the spoon
- If swallowing does not occur, remove the spoon from the client's mouth
- Instruct the client to move the food toward the rear of the mouth

Box 17-2 Recommendations for Dysphagic Clients on a Diet with Modified Consistencies

- Place the client in an upright sitting position with the head in the midline and both arms supported on the table; use positioning aids if needed; the upright sitting position is the most efficient for eating and drinking and allows a more adequate swallow to be performed
- For many clients the head-down/chin-tuck position (so the neck is flexed and the chin is approximately three fourths of the way down toward chest) will provide better airway protection and decrease the risk of aspiration.
- Keep the client upright for 30 minutes after the meal to decrease esophageal reflux
- Throughout the meal observe the client for signs and symptoms of aspiration and change in respiration rate, color, voice quality, and coughing (Miller & Chang, 1999; Groher 1997)
- Be sure room is well lighted with minimal distractions, the television off and the environment quiet, conversations kept to a minimum to discourage the client from eating and talking, although brief conversation allows assessment of the client's voice quality
- Encourage the client to participate in feeding as much as possible
- Sit down when assisting the client to eat; this communicates time and willingness to help
- Allow at least 30 to 45 minutes for feeding a client with dysphagia
- Let the client see and smell the food

- Check that the client's lips are sealed, or the swallowing reflex will not begin; manually seal the lips together or use a jaw control maneuver to pull the jaws together
- Medications may need to be given in custard, jelly, or blended flavored gelatin instead of applesauce because it tends to fall apart during swallowing.
- If fatigue is a factor, offer nutritious snacks between meals or small, frequent meals.

Additional interventions for all clients with dysphagia include monitoring weight, hydration, and caloric intake (Box 17-3). Adequate fiber should be offered to prevent constipation, and the client and family should be taught compensatory swallowing techniques and educated about the specific swallowing difficulty and care.

Dietary Modifications

It is often suggested that thick liquids and pureed foods be offered to the client with dysphagia; however, these are not always the safest options. The diet modifications must be specific to the physiology of the swallowing disorder.

Clients who have difficulty managing liquids eat a modified diet without liquids or a diet using liquids of a specified consistency. The texture or consistency of the foods the client eats may also need to be modified. Most institutions have dysphagia diets that categorize liquids by consistency (Box 17-4) and foods by texture or consistency.

Hot and cold liquids may be thickened by adding a commercial thickening agent or a household food product, such as instant potato flakes and instant baby rice cereal. For commercial thickening agents refer to the product information for obtaining the proper consistency. Some thickening agents will hold the thickness or consistency as mixed, whereas others will continue to thicken the liquid over time. It is important for the persons using the thickening agent (nurses, nursing assistants, dietitians, dietary aides, etc.) to be familiar with the product characteristics and to be notified when an institution changes products. During digestion

Box 17-3 Additional Interventions for Clients with Dysphagia

- Weight is a key indicator of the degree of difficulty the client may have with eating and should be monitored closely. Whether in the hospital or at home, clients should be weighed at least weekly in the same amount of clothing to monitor weight changes.
- Dehydration is a major concern for clients with dysphagia, particularly for those unable to safely tolerate thin liquids. Dehydration can lead to electrolyte imbalance and confusion. Clients should have liquids of modified consistency offered throughout the day and supplemental intravenous lines if necessary to maintain adequate hydration.
- Intake and output (I&O) and calorie counts assist in monitoring the nutritional intake of the client. It is important that these records be filled out correctly because this information is often used to determine whether a client is able to have a feeding tube removed. Most facilities have specific forms for this purpose.

Box 17-4 Classification of Liquid Consistency

- **Thin:** Water, broth, milk, fruit juices (except prune), nutritional supplements, coffee, and tea
- **Medium thick:** Prune juice, nectars, tomato and vegetable juices, and thick milkshakes
- **Medium thick plus:** Honey consistency to which a thickening agent has been added
- **Spoon thick:** Too thick for a straw and require a spoon; these substances "plop" at room temperature, like frozen shakes, custard, pudding, yogurt, and liquids thickened with a commercial thickening agent.

Curran (1997).

Box 17-5 Classification of Food Consistency

Stage 1: Food does not fall apart or require chewing; similar to mashed potatoes (e.g., plain yogurt, pureed meat with gravy, ice cream, pudding)
Stage 2: Soft, moist foods that cling together without small food particles; similar to pudding; no chewing is required (e.g., pureed meats and vegetables, mousse, souffle)
Stage 3: Food is mashed and easy to chew (e.g., soft casseroles, ground meats with gravy)
Stage 4: Diced, finely chopped, or bite-size whole foods; foods that fall apart easily should be avoided

starch-based thickeners, as opposed to vegetable gum thickeners, release 98% of the fluid back into the digestive tract (Vartan, 1989).

Modifications in food consistency are divided into four stages or levels (Box 17-5). As a client progresses to a new level, the foods from the previous level may still be consumed (Gilbride & Spector, 1996). Most diets of modified consistencies are low in fiber. To prevent constipation, bran may be added to many dishes and prune juice thickened to the necessary consistency.

Choking (a protective maneuver for the airway) is frightening for a client but unfortunately may be expected to occur at times in persons with swallowing difficulties. If coughing and choking can be minimized, fear and anxiety associated with feeding will be decreased. When coughing or choking begins, the nurse instructs the client to flex at the waist or neck if possible. Waist or neck flexion assists in more efficient airway clearance. If food becomes lodged in the larynx and compromises breathing and the client is unable to speak, the Heimlich maneuver should be used.

Milk and milk products should be avoided because these tend to form tenacious secretions that are poorly handled. If the client can chew, a textured food may be more desirable. Above all, the nurse should encourage the client and family to keep the diet flexible and reevaluate it often to avoid monotony.

Compensatory Postures and Swallowing Techniques

Interventions are individualized for each client based on the findings from diagnostic tests so that the client, family, and nurse are able to work effectively with the speech/swallowing therapist. Tables 17-6 and 17-7 list compensatory postures and swallowing techniques and their benefits and the physiological disorders for which they are used. Box 17-6 describes how to do the swallowing techniques.

Sensory Stimulation

Sensory stimulation heightens sensitivity of sensory receptors involved in facilitation, initiation, efficiency, and safety of swallowing. Techniques include placement of food in specific locations within the oral cavity and modification in bolus volume, consistency, temperature, and taste. Because swallowing impairments usually occur in conjunction with impairments of the oral cavity, pharynx, larynx, and esophagus, the sensory stimulation techniques should be tested during radiographic evaluation. Clients with partial or complete sensory loss within the oral cavity or with impaired facial and lingual muscle strength may not be able to safely manage and control the bolus. The bolus may spread throughout the oral cavity and spill out of the lips or fall prematurely over the back of the tongue into the pharynx. The client with lingual hemiparesis may need the bolus placed on the unaffected side of the tongue. The client with difficulties propelling the bolus to the back of the oral cavity may require placement of the bolus on the back of the tongue (Martin-Harris & Cherney, 1996).

Modifying the consistency of a bolus can affect the onset and duration of swallowing events. The consistency of the bolus affects the transit time through the oral cavity and pharynx. Thick liquids move more slowly than thin liquids; thus thick liquids are recommended to clients with delayed pharyngeal swallow. Thick liquids may also be suggested for clients with incomplete laryngeal elevation and closure because a thick liquid is less likely to penetrate the unprotected larynx. Thin liquids may be recommended for clients with cricopharyngeal dysfunction or decreased pharyngeal clearance (Martin-Harris & Cherney, 1996).

Modifying the bolus size to a small volume may assist the client prone to aspiration due to a pharyngeal swallow delay because a small bolus will not enter the pharynx as quickly as a large bolus. A larger bolus may be needed by other clients to initiate oral bolus transit. Additionally, larger bolus volumes increase the extent and duration of laryngeal elevation, laryngeal closure, and pharyngoesophageal segment opening (Martin-Harris & Cherney, 1996).

For clients with decreased oral sensation or poor initiation of oral transport, cold stimulus facilitates more rapid posterior tongue movements and pharyngeal swallow. Other clients swallow efficiently with a warm bolus. Logemann and Pauloski (1995) demonstrated that clients with pharyngeal swallow delay showed a significant improvement in oral onset of swallow using a sour bolus.

Adaptive Equipment

For the client who has a self-feeding deficit, the nurse can work closely with occupational and physical therapists in muscle strengthening, coordination, and use of adaptive equipment. The nurse's role is to assess intake and imple-

TABLE 17-6 Compensatory Postures: Postural Changes Affect How Gravity Moves Food through the Pharynx

Position	Benefit	Physiological Disorder
Head-down/chin-tuck position: lowering head so neck is flexed and chin is approximately three fourths of way down toward chest	Widens valleculae; epiglottis covers more of airway, resulting in increased protection and decreased risk of aspiration; decreases pressures at cricopharyngeal muscle	Delayed reflex and reduced laryngeal closure
Head back: gently and slowly tossing head back	Moves food more rapidly through the oral cavity	Reduced tongue movement
Head turned toward affected or less functional side	Increases vocal fold adduction; closes pharynx on side to which head is turned, causing bolus to travel down opposite side of pharynx; reduces resting tone of cricopharyngeal muscle	Unilateral pharyngeal dysfunction, reduced laryngeal closures or unilateral laryngeal dysfunction, cricopharyngeal problems
Head tilted to more functional side	Gravity directs food down more functional side of pharynx	Unilateral damage to tongue and pharynx
Head turned and chin down	Affects direction of bolus and increases airway protection	Reduced laryngeal closure
Head back and turned	Moves bolus quickly through oral cavity; sets direction of bolus	Decreased tongue function, decreased laryngeal closure, unilateral pharyngeal weakness
Lying on one side with head supported	Removes effects of gravity	Reduced peristalsis, reduced laryngeal elevation

Adapted from Logemann, J.A. (1991). Approaches to management of disordered swallowing. *Bailliere's Clinical Gastroenterology, 5,* 269-280; and Miller, R.M., & Chang, M.W. (1999). Advances in the management of dysphagia caused by stroke. *Physical Medicine and Rehabilitation Clinics of North America, 10*(4), 925-941.

TABLE 17-7 Swallowing Techniques

Technique	Benefit	Physiological Disorder
Thermal stimulation	Increases sensitivity of swallow reflex; results short lived	Decreased oral awareness, delayed pharyngeal swallow
Superglottic swallow	Increases voluntary airway protection, voluntary closure of glottis before and during swallow; ensures pulmonary air volume for throat clearing	Delayed pharyngeal swallow, impaired vocal cord closure
Mendelson maneuver	Allows voluntary increase in laryngeal elevation time and opening of cricopharyngeal sphincter, prolongs airway closure	Decreased laryngeal elevation or opening of cricopharyngeal sphincter
Effortful swallow	Improves weakness of tongue base	Reduced posterior movements of tongue

Adapted from Logemann, J.A. (1991). Approaches to management of disordered swallowing. *Bailliere's Clinical Gastroenterology, 5,* 269-280; and Miller, R.M., & Chang, M.W. (1999). Advances in the management of dysphagia caused by stroke. *Physical Medicine and Rehabilitation Clinics of North America, 10*(4), 925-941.

ment and reinforce the compensatory techniques and use of adaptive equipment. Examples of adaptive equipment include scoop dishes, plate guards, and silverware modified for easy grasp and effective cutting and eating (Figures 17-7 and 17-8). Nonskid pads or a wet cloth may be used under dishes to prevent slipping.

Use of a straw requires complex functioning of the oral musculature and is often not recommended for clients with dysphagia. If the client can drink from a cup, remember that when the glass is less than half full, it becomes necessary to tilt the head back to drink. This position increases the risk of aspiration and should be avoided. Specially designed cups are available, or a cutaway cup can be made easily by cutting a semicircular portion out of a paper cup. This allows the client to tilt the cup further without tilting the head (Figure 17-8).

Box 17-6 How to Implement Swallowing Techniques

Thermal Stimulation

- Chill laryngeal mirror in ice for 1 minute
- With back of mirror lightly touch both sides of mouth 5 times on each side; use short light strokes
- Have client swallow
- Repeat a total of 5 times, rechilling mirror between
- Repeat 3 to 4 times per day

Superglottic Swallow (May Be Done With or Without Food in the Oral Cavity)

- If using food, place food in mouth
- Have client inhale and hold breath
- Ask client to swallow while holding breath (cover tracheostomy tube if applicable)
- Have client cough or clear throat after swallowing without inhaling again
- Repeat 10 times, 3 to 4 times per day

Mendelson Maneuver (May Be Done With or Without Food in the Oral Cavity)

- Ask client to place hand on larynx
- Have client swallow and feel larynx left at its highest position
- If using food, ask client to place food in mouth
- Have client swallow and again hold larynx in highest position during the swallow; client then releases hold
- Repeat 3 to 5 times, 3 to 4 times per day

From Logemann J.A. (1991). Approaches to management of disordered swallowing. *Bailliere's Clinical Gastroenterology, 5*, 269-280.

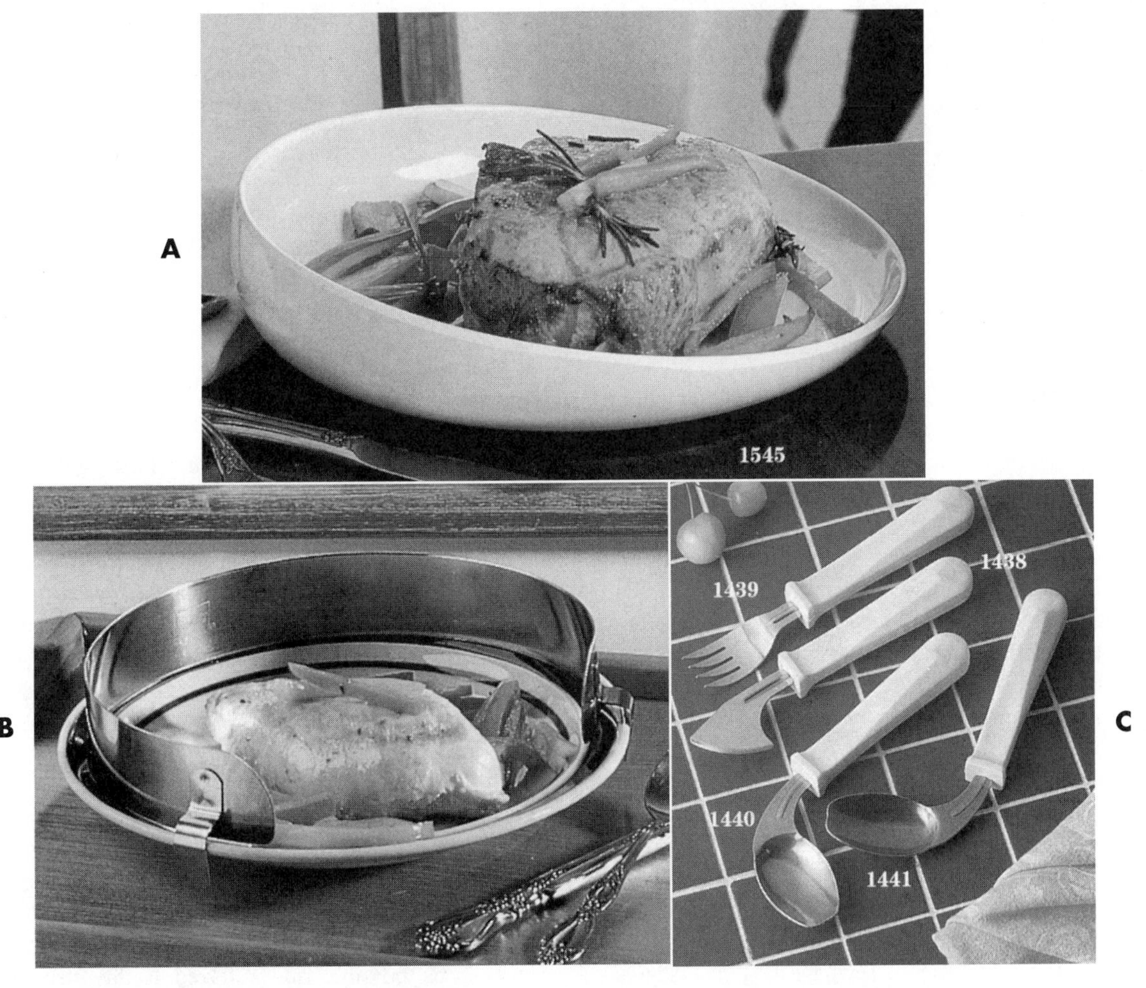

Figure 17-7 A, Scoop dish. B, Food guard. C, Easy-hold utensils. Knife blade will cut in both slicing and rocking motions. (Courtesy Sammons Preston, a Bissell Healthcare Company, Bolingbrook, IL.)

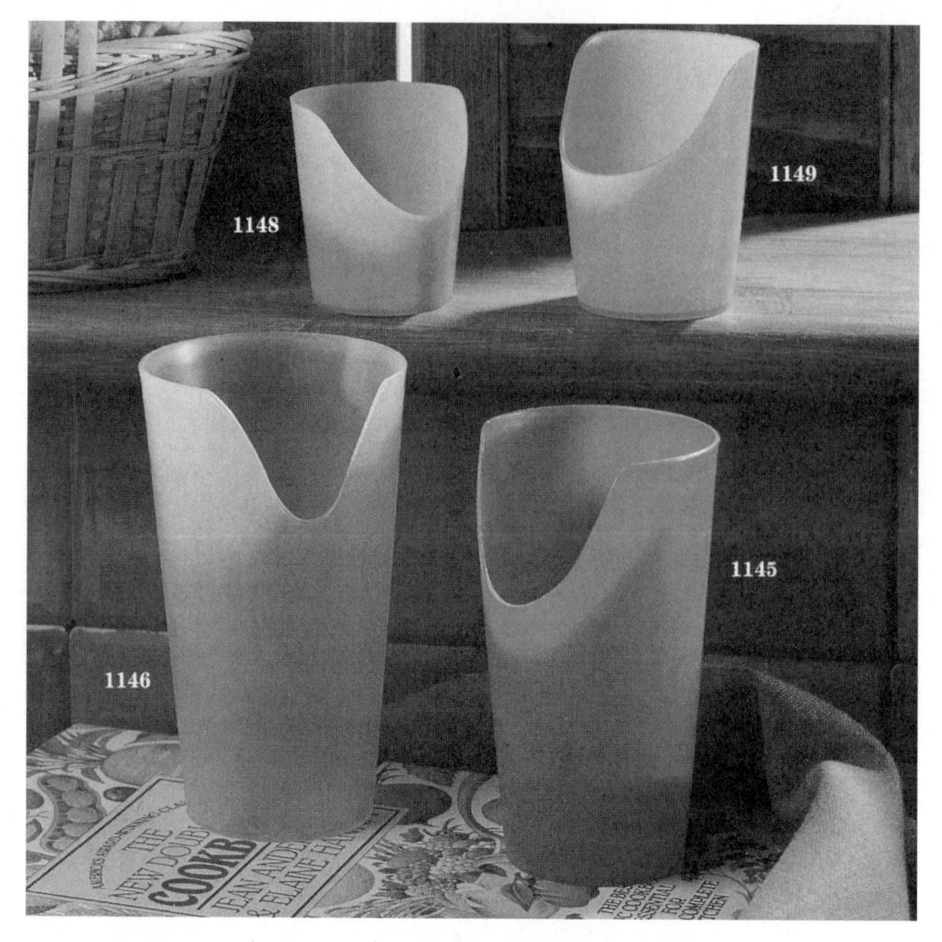

Figure 17-8 Tumbler with a special cutout for the nose allows the client to drink without tipping the head back. (Courtesy Sammons Preston, a Bissell Healthcare Company, Bolingbrook, IL.)

Oral Hygiene

It is important to remind or assist the client with maintaining good oral hygiene. Dentures and partial plates should be worn to help support oral structures, give contour to the mouth, and promote normal movements (Miller & Chang, 1999). The oral cavity should be cleaned after each meal, and all food particles and pocketed food removed. Artificial saliva and humidified air may be beneficial to some clients because mouth breathing can cause drying of oral structures and promote bacterial growth.

Client and Family Education

In addition to understanding the exact nature of the eating deficit, the client and family need to be involved in establishing goals and planning care. Without client and family cooperation, the rehabilitation process will be less effective. The role of the rehabilitation nurse includes promoting good communication with the family. Throughout the system, between care-plan meetings, and elsewhere the nurse is an advocate for the family, explains new treatment approaches, and reports progress. The client and family should demonstrate knowledge of dietary modifications, the hazards of offering "unsafe" food even when requested by the client, use of adaptive equipment if needed, the process for feeding, and performance of emergency measures in the event of choking.

When the client has excessive caloric intake, it is necessary to work with the family and client. For this client food commonly is substituted for other activities or used as a reward. Family members may bring food to the client because it brings pleasure. The nurse can work with the client and family to develop other positive forms of reinforcement and long-term goals for rehabilitation and to help the client to see the consequences of overeating.

Rehabilitation Team Interventions

Eating and swallowing deficits are complex, multifaceted disorders that require the nurse to collaborate with other rehabilitation team professionals. All clients presenting with neuromuscular or neurological disorders should be evaluated for a swallowing impairment as early in the assessment process as possible and referred to the necessary team members (Hoeman & Glenn-Molali, 1999). Many facilities now have dysphagia teams or programs that are usually led by a speech-language pathologist, nurse, or occupational therapist (Glenn, Araya, Jones, & Liljefors, 1993). The members of the team and their roles vary by institution, but the key members are the physician, nurse, speech-language pathologist, occupational therapist, dietitian, and physical therapist.

The physician is responsible for coordination of the client's medical management and must order the initial referral to the dysphagia team. The physician must also write orders for any dietary modifications.

As noted earlier, physical therapy helps improve muscle tone, strength, and coordination. Treatment is directed at improving muscle tone for the primary eating muscles as well as secondary muscles of the arms, legs, head, and neck.

The occupational therapist performs self-feeding evaluations, recommends and teaches the use of adaptive equipment and exercises to improve hand control and coordination, and offers assistance in food preparation techniques. The therapist also may recommend meaningful activities for the client to engage in during the day as a substitute for eating.

The speech-language pathologist may perform a bedside swallow evaluation and determine the need for diagnostic tests. On the basis of results of the screening or testing, the speech pathologist may design a program of exercises for the oropharyngeal musculature and identify what compensatory swallowing techniques and postures are to be used. They also work with clients on speech deficits.

The dietitian helps develop a menu plan that meets the nutritional, socioeconomic, and cultural requirements of the client and teaches the proper diet to the client and family. The dietitian also monitors nutritional status.

The nurse conducts a complete history and physical assessment and in-depth self-feeding and swallowing assessments. The nurse also monitors the client's weight, caloric and fluid intake, and laboratory studies for hydration and nutritional status. A primary nursing responsibility is working with the client and family to reinforce feeding and swallowing skills and to communicate progress to other team members. Demonstrated abilities on the unit or in a feeding group may differ from abilities in a private session with a therapist.

NURSING OUTCOMES

The priority NOC that may be used for eating and swallowing deficits from the nutritional-metabolic pattern are listed in Table 17-5 with the nursing diagnosis and NIC.

Other nursing outcomes (Johnson, Maas, & Moorhead, 2000) that may be applicable for the client experiencing difficulty with eating and swallowing include:

1. Nutritional status: energy
2. Nutritional status: body mass
3. Respiratory status: airway patency
4. Respiratory status: gas exchange
5. Oral health
6. Self-care instrumental activities of daily living
7. Self-care: hygiene
8. Self-care eating
9. Knowledge: treatment regimen
10. Knowledge: treatment procedures
11. Knowledge: diet

For the client with a progressive neuromuscular disorder, maintaining the maximum level of independence in eating and attaining adequate nutritional intake are realistic goals. Clients with neurological insults (e.g., cerebrovascular accident, head trauma) may anticipate a return to near-normal function after an active rehabilitative period, but this depends on the extent of the injury. Three months appears to be the critical period in which maximum return of function can be anticipated (Logemann, 1983).

RESEARCH

Treatments that are currently being researched include use of medication and use of nerve grafts. Perez, Smithard, Davies, and Kalra (1998) gave clients who had dysphagia 2 weeks after a stroke slow-release nifedipine for 4 weeks and reported improvement in pharyngeal transit times and swallow delay. Arai et al. (1998) gave an angiotensin-converting enzyme (ACE) inhibitor to clients with a history of stroke and symptomless dysphagia. They reported improvement in symptomless dysphagia in 10 of the 16 clients. The specific improvements were not discussed. Other researchers are investigating the use of nerve grafts to restore sensory and motor function in the larynx by implanting a local nerve or a neuromuscular pedicle into the intrinsic laryngeal muscles (Aviv, Mohr, & Blitzer 1997).

SUMMARY

Physiologically eating and swallowing are essential to person's survival. Psychologically food and the ability to eat are important to feelings of self-worth. Socially many activites revolve around food. When one can no longer eat without difficulty, fear is commonly an overriding emotion. It includes not only fear for one's survival and ability to function but also fear of or actual loss of significant social interactions.

The nurse is crucial in identifying clients who may be at risk for or who have an eating or swallowing deficit. The nurse is the primary advocate in assisting these clients and their families in receiving the necessary interventions in all types of settings. The nurse has the knowledge and ability to draw in other rehabilitation team members as needed. Patience, understanding, and the ability to teach the client and family about this aspect of rehabilitation have many positive rewards and outcomes for the client, family, and nurse.

CRITICAL THINKING

Mr. W, recently widowed and living alone, is a 78-year-old man referred to community health nursing services on discharge from a 1-night stay at an acute care hospital. He was referred for wound care to his head after a fall during a "minor" right cerebrovascular accident. During the nursing assessment, as the client is drinking juice, the nurse observes that he is coughing frequently.

1. What questions would be important to ask Mr. W?
2. Which areas of the nursing physical assessment would be key?
3. Which nursing diagnosis would be applicable?
4. Which NIC would be applicable?
5. Which NOC would be applicable?
6. Which rehabilitation team members would be brought in?
7. Which diagnostic tests are anticipated?
8. What would be important areas for client education?

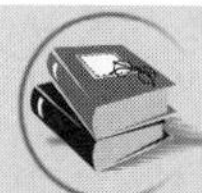

Case Study

Mrs. G is a widow who moved to the Mid-Atlantic area from Puerto Rico after the death of her husband 6 years previously to live near her two married daughters. She speaks only Spanish and lives alone in a small city apartment located in a culturally diverse community. In addition to having diabetes, she had a stroke 2 months previously and was referred to a rehabilitation center in the next city. She was discharged with only mild residual muscle weakness but persistent dysphagia. Unable to return to her former neighborhood apartment, she lived near the rehabilitation center and was treated by a speech-language therapist, a physical therapist, a home health aide, and the rehabilitation nursing consultant from the visiting nurse association. Two immediate goals are to work with Mrs. G to stabilize her nutritional status and to continue the gains she made with swallowing while in the rehabilitation center.

Mrs. G has been refusing to eat her meals and appears to be anxious about eating and swallowing. On several occasions, she began shouting and waving her hands when lunch was served, refusing to eat the food or to work with the speech therapist. The physical therapist was a young man who spoke some Spanish in his own home, but Mrs. G would not communicate with him about her concerns other than to tell him, "I had this illness because I am being punished for bad things in my life, and now God has allowed someone, a spirit I think, to place a spell on me."

The home health aide told the nurse that Mrs. G's daughter was present the next day and translated for Mrs. G; Mrs. G claimed that she was being given food to make her sick, not better. The aide was concerned that Mrs. G was taking medicines she obtained from a relative and using over-the-counter purgatives. The nurse arranged to meet with the daughter and Mrs. G at lunch and to check the medications in the house. After a discussion with the daughter, the nurse met with the interdisciplinary team. A dietitian and an *espiritisa,* a traditional Puerto Rican healer, were invited as consultants. The spiritual healer met privately with Mrs. G and agreed to return the following week. With improved trust and rapport, Mrs. G and the team were able to concentrate on the therapeutic regimen. With proper evaluation and client/family education about common symptoms, swallowing problems can be managed effectively for clients in their home. Presently Mrs. G is on a waiting list for housing in a senior complex in her old neighborhood.

The rehabilitation nurse consultant prepared a staff in-service program based on the discussions with Mrs. G's daughter and the *espiritisa,* and this led to mutually agreeable goals and interventions. The staff improved the outcome for Mrs. G by providing culturally sensitive and relevant care. One therapist remarked, "Learning about things that influenced Mrs. G's care was a bit like unraveling a mystery . . . about why she wouldn't do things. We thought she was being stubborn, or worse, we thought she had undetected residual damage from the stroke, and of course, her diabetes was a concern. I learned a lot about making assumptions and about the importance of cultural values."

For example, Mrs. G would not speak to the young male physical therapist because she was uncomfortable discussing personal information with a man, especially because his family background was Cuban, not Puerto Rican. The importance of finding a translator who is acceptable to the client involves more than a common language. In fact, there is a great deal of diversity among the Spanish language dialects within the many Hispanic/Latino groups in the United States. Furthermore, modesty, privacy, age, and gender issues were extremely sensitive for Mrs. G.

Beliefs about spiritual causes of illness, or illness as punishment, are held by some Hispanic/Latino persons. Self-medication, especially laxatives or purgatives, may be used to rid the body of disease, and various herbs are added to teas or foods to replace strength. Mrs. G was at risk for imbalance in the dietary management of her diabetes. Some persons, like Mrs. G, believe that there are diseases incurred only by a Puerto Rican and that these can be cured only by an *espiritisa.* Having the traditional healer involved in planning culturally relevant and sensitive care reduced Mrs. G's stress, improved her perception of her health, and provided essential information to the team.

Dietary differences, including mealtime and food preferences, had not been incorporated into Mrs. G's nutritional plan. The team discovered that Mrs. G preferred to have four meals a day, consisting of a light breakfast, a main meal at lunch, a small supper, and another supper after 8 PM. Mrs. G's daughter assisted the dietitian in preparing the diabetic menus in Spanish and in using foods from Puerto Rican markets in her old neighborhood.

Mrs. G had accused the team of trying to harm her because they had offered her "hot foods for a hot condition." Like many persons from Hispanic cultures (or from Asian cultures, as in the case of those who believe in yin and yang), she believed that a balance among the humoral areas is essential for maintaining health. According to this belief, an illness or disease may have hot or cold properties; foods are similarly categorized based on their having hot or cold properties, apart from their temperature or nutritional attributes. Thus offering a hot food for a hot condition contributes to imbalance and may be perceived as harmful or hazardous to health, such as was the case with Mrs. G. An exact list of foods considered hot or cold is best assembled by each client or family because there are variations among cultural groups. In addition, many persons will respond affirmatively to a health professional's questions regarding their use of medications, adherence to treatments or procedures, and dietary practices. *Yes* may be a polite response, an elusive one, or simply the easiest answer for some persons. Therefore a cross-cultural dietary assessment and evaluation may prevent misunderstandings and build trust.

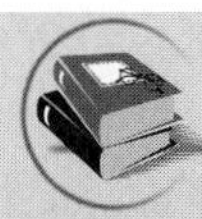

Case Study—cont'd

Cross-Cultural Dietary Assessment and Intervention

- Assess individual food preferences, snack or meal patterns, and the symbolic use or meaning of foods, and determine what foods are taboo or inedible for the client and his or her family. Consider the budget available for food.
- Assess the client and his or her family for cultural food habits and preferences, available foods or substitutes, and means of food preparation. Consider the time and place of meals and whether eating is accomplished alone or as a social or group event.
- Assess lifestyle, socioeconomic, and religious patterns that influence food habits. Evaluate whether the client believes in the hot or cold properties of foods; whether foods should be kosher, vegetarian, or related to other specific diets; and whether there are restricted stimulants, including coffee or tea, or other dietary requirements. Determine whether beliefs or practices can be used to treat a client's condition from a traditional or cultural perspective (e.g., medicinal foods or beverages). Learn whether ceremonial or religious observations are important to the client and his or her family, such as observing Ramadan, which may influence responses to medication, treatment outcomes, or dietary needs. Enlist traditional healers to participate when possible.
- Evaluate how the client's health or specific medical condition is affected by food patterns or habits. Consider ways to incorporate foods and habits that are neutral or not detrimental to health into the therapeutic regimen. Use traditional preferred foods whenever possible (case study courtesy of S. Hoeman).

The USDA has many free publications to assist with food selection for healthy nutrition. The USDA Food Guide Pyramid has been adapted for various ethnic and cultural diets, including Mediterranean, vegetarian, Asian, and Latin-American. A listing of websites begins at http://www.nal.usda.gov/fnic/etext/000023.htm. Ethnic sites are at http://www.oldwayspt.org/html/p (at the end of this website address, leave a space after the last *p* and then add the desired special diet [e.g., med.htm, veg.htm, asian.htm, or latin.htm]).

REFERENCES

Agency for Health Care Policy and Research. (1999, July). *Diagnosis and treatment of swallowing disorders (dysphagia) in acute-care stroke patients* (Evidence Report/Technology Assessment No. 8.; prepared by ECRI Evidence-Based Practice Center under contract No. 290-97-0020.; AHCPR Publication No. 99-E024). Rockville, MD: Author.

Arai, T., Yashuda, Y., Takaya, T., Toshima, S., Kashiki, Y., Yoshimi, N., & Fujiwara, H. (1998). ACE inhibitors and symptomless dysphagia. *Lancet, 352,* 115-116.

Aviv, J.E., Kaplan, S.T., Thomson, J.E., Spitzer, J., Diamond, B., & Close, L.G. (2000). The safety of flexible endoscopic evaluation of swallowing with sensory testing (FEESST): An analysis of 500 consecutive evaluations. *Dysphagia, 15,* 39-44.

Aviv, J.E., Mohr, J.P., & Blitzer, A. (1997). Restoration of laryngeal sensation by neural anastomosis. *Archives of Otolaryngology Head and Neck Surgery, 123,* 154-160.

Barlow, S., & Dietz, W. (1998). Obesity evaluations and treatment: Expert committee recommendations. *Pediatrics, 102*(3), e29.

Barrett-Conner, E., Edelstein, S. I., Corey-Bloom, J., & Wiederholt, W. C. (1996). Weight loss precedes dementia in community dwelling older adults. *Journal of the American Geriatric Society. 44, 1147-1152.*

Bastian, R. (1998). Contemporary diagnosis of the dysphagic *Otolaryngologic Clinics of North America 31*(3), 489-506.

Bosma, J.F. (1997). Development and impairments of feeding in infancy and childhood. In M. Groher (Ed.) *Dysphagia diagnosis and management* (pp. 289-312). Boston: Butterworth-Heinemann.

Bradford, S. (1996). Methods of nutritional support. In L.K. Mahan, & S. Escott-Stump (Eds.) *Krause's food, nutrition and diet therapy* (9th ed., pp. 425-448). Philadelphia: WB Saunders.

Chi-Fishman, G., Stone, M., & McCall, G.N. (1998). Lingual action in normal sequential swallowing. *Journal of Speech, Language & Hearing Research, 41*(4), 771-786.

Collins, M., & Bakheit, A. (1997). Does pulse oximetry reliably detect aspiration in dysphagic stroke patients? *Stroke, 28*(9), 1773-1775.

Curran, J.E. (1997). Nutritional considerations for dysphagia. In M. Groher (Ed.), *Dysphagia: Diagnosis and management* (pp. 289-312). Boston: Butterworth-Heinemann.

Daniels, S.K., Brailey, K., & Foundas, A.L. (1999). Lingual discoordination and dysphagia following acute stroke: Analyses of lesion localization. *Dysphagia, 14,* 85-92.

Darrow, D.H., & Harley, C.M. (1998). Evaluation of swallowing disorders in children. *Otolaryngologic Clinics of North America, 31*(3), 405-418.

Derkay, C.S., & Schechter, G.L. (1998). Anatomy and physiology in pediatric swallowing disorders. *Otolaryngologic Clinics of North America, 31*(3), 397-404.

D'Eramo, A.L., Sedlak, C., Doheny, M.O., & Jenkins, M. (1994). Nutritional aspects of the orthopaedic trauma patient. *Orthopedic Nursing, 13,* 13-20.

Farrell, Z., & O'Neill, D. (1999). Towards better screening and assessment of oropharyngeal swallow disorders in the general hospital. *Lancet, 354*(9176), 355-356.

Gilbride, J.A., & Spector, S. (1996). Nutritional considerations for the stroke patient with dysphagia. In L.R. Cherney, & A.S. Halper (Eds.). *Topics in stroke rehabilitation* (pp. 51-68). Frederick, MD: Aspen.

Glenn, N., Araya, T., Jones, K., & Liljefors, J. (1993). A therapeutic feeding team in the rehabilitation setting. *Holistic Nursing Practice, 7,* 78-81.

Glenn-Molali, N. (2001). Personal communication with pharmacists. Havre de Grace, MD.

Groher, M. (1997). *Dysphagia: Diagnosis and management* (3rd ed.). Boston: Butterworth-Heinemann.

Hamlet, S., Penney, D.G., & Formolo, J. (1994). Stethoscope acoustics and cervical auscultation of swallowing. *Dysphagia, 9,* 63-68.

Hansell, D., & Heinemann, D. (1996). Improving nursing practice with staff education: The challenges of dysphagia. *Gastroenterology Nursing 6,* 201-206.

Harris, D.R. (1996). *Diet and nutrition sourcebook.* Detroit: Omnigraphics.

Healthy People 2000. (2000). www.health.gov/healthypeople.

Helfrich-Miller, K.R., Rector, K.L., & Straka, J.A. (1986). Dysphagia: Its treatment in the profoundly retarded patient with cerebral palsy. *Archives of Physical Medicine and Rehabilitation, 67*(8), 520-525.

Hoeman, S.P., & Glenn-Molali, N. (1999). Community approaches for evidence-based practice in dysphagia. *Nutrition in Clinical Practice, 14*(5), S31-S34.

Houghton, D.J., & Curley, J.W. (1996). Dysphagia caused by a hard cervical collar. *British Journal of Neurosurgery, 10*(5), 501-502.

Huggins, P.S., Tuomi, S.K., & Young, C. (1999). Effects of nasogastric tubes on the young, normal swallowing mechanism. *Dysphagia 14,* 157-161.

Johnson, M., Maas, M., & Moorhead, S. (2000). *Nursing outcomes classification (NOC)* (2nd ed.). St. Louis: Mosby.

Kirshblum, S., Johnston, M.V., Brown, J., O'Connor, K.C., & Jarosz, P. (1999). Predictors of dysphagia after spinal cord injury. *Archives Physical Medicine and Rehabilitation, 80,* 1101-1105.

Leder, S. (1996). Gag reflex and dysphagia. *Head and Neck, March/April,* 138-141.

Logemann, J.A. (1983). *Evaluation and treatment of swallowing disorders.* San Diego: College Hill Press.

Logemann, J.A. (1998). *Evaluation and treatment of swallowing disorders* (2nd ed.) Austin, TX: PRO-ED.

Logemann, J.A., & Pauloski, B.R. (1995). Effects of a sour bolus on oropharyngeal swallowing measures in patients with neurogenic dysphagia. *Journal of Speech & Hearing Disorders, 38*(3), 556-564.

Martin-Harris, B., & Cherney, L.R. (1996). Treating swallowing disorders following stroke. In L.R. Cherney & A.S. Halper (Eds.), Topics in stroke rehabilitation (3rd ed., pp. 27-40). Frederick, MD: Aspen.

Martinez, E.J., & Nord, H.J. (1995). Significance of solitary and multiple esophageal ulcers in patients with AIDS. *Southern Medical Journal, 88*(6), 626-629.

McCloskey, J., & Bulechek, G. (2000). *Nursing interventions classification (NIC).* St. Louis: Mosby.

McGarrah, P.D., & Teller, D. (1997). Posttraumatic cervical osteophytosis causing progressive dysphagia. *Southern Medical Journal, 90*(8), 858-860.

Miller, D., & Miller, H. (1995). Giving medication through the tube. *RN, 58*(1), 44-46.

Miller, R.M., & Chang, M.W. (1999). Advances in the management of dysphagia caused by stroke. *Physical Medicine and Rehabilitation Clinics of North America, 10*(4), 925-941.

Moy, A. (1996). Restorative rehabilitation with burn injuries. In S.P. Hoeman (Ed.), *Rehabilitation nursing: Process and application* (p. 650). St. Louis: Mosby.

O'Laughlin, G., & Shanley, C. (1998). Swallowing problems in the nursing home: A novel training response. *Dysphagia, 13,* 172-183.

Ozer, M. (1994). *Management of persons with stroke.* St. Louis: Mosby.

Pamuk, E., Makuc, D., Heck, K., Reuben, C., & Lochner, K. (1998). *Socioeconomic status and health chartbook. Health, United States.* Hyattsville, MD: National Center for Health Statistics.

Perez, I., Smithard, D.G., Davies, H., & Kalra, L. (1998). Pharmacological treatment of dysphagia in stroke. *Dysphagia, 13,* 12-16.

Pinnington, L., Muhiddin, K., Lobeck, M., & Pearce, V. (2000). Interrater and intrarater reliability of the Exeter dysphagia assessment technique applied to healthy elderly adults. *Dysphagia, 15,* 6-9.

Poertner, L., & Coleman, R. (1998). Swallowing therapy in adults. *Otolaryngologic Clinics of North America, 31*(3), 561-579.

Plant, R. (1998). Anatomy and physiology of swallowing in adults and geriatrics. *Otolaryngologic Clinics of North America 31*(3), 477-489.

Rademaker, A.W., Pauloski, B.R., Colangelo, L.A., & Logemann, J.A. (1998). Age and volume effects on liquid swallowing function in normal women. *Journal of Speech, Language, & Hearing Research, 41*(2), 275-285.

Robbins, J.A., Logemann, J.A., & Kirshner, H.S. (1986). Swallowing and speech production in Parkinson's disease. *Annals of Neurology, 19,* 283-287.

Robbins, J., Levine, R., Wood, J., Roecker, E., & Luschei, E. (1994). Geriatrics. Swallowing physiology related to normal aging. *Rehabilitation R&D Progress Reports, December*(30-01), 108-9.

Sands, J. K. (1999). Management of persons with problems of the intestines. In W.J. Phipps, J.K. Sands, & J.F. Marek, *Medical-surgical nursing* (6th ed., pp. 1313-1372). St. Louis: Mosby.

Sherman, B., Nisenboum, J.M., Jesberger, B.L., Morrow, C.A., & Jesberger, J.A. (1999). Assessment of dysphagia with the use of pulse oximetry. *Dysphagia, 14,* 152-156.

Shuman, J.M. (1996). Nutrition in aging. In L.K. Mahan & S. Escott-Stump (Eds.), *Krause's food, nutrition and diet therapy* (9th ed., pp. 287-308). Philadelphia: WB Saunders.

Stanley, K. (1998). Assessing the nutritional needs of the geriatric patient with diabetes. *Diabetes Educator, 24*(1), 29-36.

Takahashi, K., Groher, M.E., & Michi, K. (1994). Symmetry and reproducibility of swallowing sounds. *Dysphagia, 9,* 168-173.

Teramoto, S., Matsuse, T., Fukuchi, Y., & Ouchi, Y. (1999). Simple two step swallowing provocation test for elderly patients with aspiration pneumonia. *Lancet, 353*(9160), 1243.

Tolep, K., Getch, C.L., & Criner, G.J. (1996). Swallowing dysfunction in patients receiving prolonged mechanical ventilation. *Chest, 109*(1), 167-172.

Touger-Decker, R. (1996). Nutritional care in rheumatic diseases. In L.K. Mahan & S. Escott-Stump (Eds.), *Krause's food, nutrition and diet therapy* (9th ed., pp. 889-898). Philadelphia: WB Saunders.

Vartan, K.S. (1989). Perspectives on practice: Understanding instant food thickeners. The role of starches and gums in hydration. Lancaster, PA: American Institutional Products.

Voss, H. (1994). The neurologic assessment. In E. Barker (Ed.), *Neuroscience nursing* (pp. 49-92). St. Louis: Mosby.

Walleck, C., & Mooney, K. (1994). Neurotrauma: Head injury. In E. Barker (Ed.), *Neuroscience nursing* (pp. 324-351). St. Louis: Mosby.

Willig, T.N., Paulus, J., Lacau Saint Guily, J., Beon, C., & Naavarro, J. (1994). Swallowing problems in neuromuscular disorders. *Archives of Physical Medicine and Rehabilitation, 75,* 1175-1181.

Winkler, M.F., & Manchester, S. (1996). Nutritional care in metabolic stress: Sepsis, trauma, burns, and surgery. In L.K. Mahan & S. Escott-Stump (Eds.), *Krause's food, nutrition and diet therapy* (9th ed., pp. 663-680). Philadelphia: WB Saunders.

Wisdom, G., & Blitzer, A. (1998). Surgical therapy for swallowing disorders. *Otolaryngologic Clinics of North America, 31*(3), 537-538.

Wright, R., Boyd, C., & Workman, A. (1998). Radiation doses to patients during pharyngeal videofluoroscopy. *Dysphagia, 13*(2), 113-115.

Zenner, P.M., Losinski, D.S., & Mills, R.H. (1995). Using cervical auscultation in the clinical dysphagia examination in long term care. *Dysphagia, 10,* 27-31.

BIBLIOGRAPHY

Hamdy, S., Aziz, Q., Rothwell, J.C., Crone, R., Hughes, D., Tallis, R.C., & Thompson, D.G. (1997). Explaining oropharyngeal dysphagia after unilateral hemisphere stroke. *Lancet, 350*(9079), 686-692.

Logemann, J.A. (1991a). *Swallowing disorders II workshop.* Evanston: Northwestern University.

Logemann, J.A. (1991b). Approaches to management of disordered swallowing. *Bailliere's Clinical Gastroenterology, 5,* 269-280.

Mahan, L.K., & Escott-Stump S. (Eds.). (2000). *Krause's food, nutrition and diet therapy* (10th ed.). Philadelphia: WB Saunders.

Respiration and Pulmonary Rehabilitation

18

Jean K. Berry, PhD, RN
Joyce H. Johnson, PhD, RN
Kim Vander Ploeg, MS, RN

It was my first home visit with Mr. B, although I had met him previously during his screening for our 12-week rehabilitation program. He had already passed his screening exercise tests, and his chronic obstructive pulmonary disease (COPD) was still in the moderate category. He experienced quite a bit of shortness of breath with activity, but he was eager to begin his exercise training program. Both he and his wife were excited about the possibility of improvement in his symptoms.

As I brought the exercise bike into his house, I asked him where I should place it, since he would be spending quite a bit of time with it during the next 12 weeks. Most clients put bicycles in a room away from the living area, out of the way of others, but near a TV or other form of entertainment as a distractor while they exercise. I was surprised when Mr. B said, "put the bike in front of my living room picture window. I want to see and be seen by everybody while I'm working out." His wife had already cleared the area. Needless to say, I knew Mr. B was going to be a pleasure to work with.

Rehabilitation nurses deal with clients who have multiple, complex respiratory conditions. Assessment of pulmonary function has been identified as a long-term predictor for overall survival rates in a 29-year follow-up prospective study of men (n = 554) and women (n = 641) between the ages of 20 and 89 years old. This makes it a valuable assessment and evaluation tool at all levels of care (Schunemann et al., 2000).

Respiratory disability has a considerable physical, psychosocial, and financial impact on the client, family, and society. The multidimensional nature of impaired breathing presents a complex and difficult problem for the rehabilitation team to develop an adequate plan of care. From the client's perspective, problems are breathlessness, a productive cough, fatigue, and poor tolerance of physical exercise and activities of daily living (ADLs). Clients may experience shortness of breath at meals or difficulty with swallowing; inability to cough effectively makes removing secretions a problem; and fatigue is significant with chronic lung disease.

From a pathophysiological perspective the primary problems are ineffective airway clearance, altered breathing patterns, and/or ineffective gas exchange. The most common respiratory problems in rehabilitation are seen in clients with chronic obstructive pulmonary disease (COPD), cystic fibrosis (CF), bronchopulmonary dysplasia (BPD), and neuromuscular disease involving the respiratory muscles. Consistent early intervention can often alleviate respiratory symptoms and prevent further deterioration. In rehabilitation the team collaborates and assumes responsibility for early diagnosis and treatment of potential and actual respiratory problems, reducing morbidity and mortality. In the home, clients learn to recognize and treat both potential and actual respiratory problems in the earliest stages before they become life-threatening. A partnership relationship between clients and the rehabilitation team plays a vital role in clients learning how to manage their respiratory problems.

This chapter reviews the concepts for pulmonary rehabilitation and broad goals for both clients and programs. Specific physiological processes necessary for ventilation and gas exchange are discussed. Alterations in ventilation and gas exchange characterize respiratory problems experienced by clients in rehabilitation, specifically those with COPD, CF, BPD, and neuromuscular diseases involving the respiratory muscles. Respiratory physiology and the nursing process are frameworks used to manage common respiratory problems related to airway clearance, breathing patterns, and gas exchange. Essential components of a pulmonary rehabilitation program are outlined for inpatient and outpatient settings.

CONCEPTS FOR PULMONARY REHABILITATION

The concepts for pulmonary rehabilitation resulted from experiences of physicians who contracted tuberculosis in the late 1800s. Dr. Charles Denison, a pulmonologist suffering from pulmonary hemorrhages due to tuberculosis, left his home in Connecticut for the climate in Colorado. Exercise during his recuperation produced a feeling of well-being. In 1895, he published a monograph of the first program of exercise, which included breathing exercises, for "pulmonary invalids" suffering from the residual effects of tuberculosis. Another pioneer of pulmonary rehabilitation, Dr. Albert Haas, contracted tuberculosis in 1932 during his medical school training in Budapest. Convalescence at that time included months or years of prolonged inactivity and bed rest. Bored, the young student asked for his medical books so that he could continue to study. He observed that maneuvering his heaviest books did not tire him; instead the physical activity produced well-being, improved appetite, and weight gain (Casaburi & Petty, 1993). Subsequently, pilot projects and scientific conferences stimulated others' interest in this approach and hope for improved quality of life for clients with chronic lung disease. Since then, rigorous scientific trials have produced evidence that pulmonary rehabilitation reduces symptoms, increases functional ability, and improves quality of life in individuals with chronic respiratory disease. From being regarded as a last-ditch effort to manage clients with severe respiratory impairment, pulmonary rehabilitation has evolved as an integral part of the clinical management and health maintenance of clients with chronic respiratory disease. Pulmonary rehabilitation includes the following client goals: reduction of symptoms, decreased disability, increased participation in physical and social activities, and an overall improvement in the quality of life of individuals with chronic respiratory disease (American Thoracic Society [ATS], 1999).

Methods for achieving these goals are diverse, but all pulmonary rehabilitation programs contain four components: exercise training, education, psychosocial/behavioral intervention, and outcome assessment (ATS, 1999). Programs may be instituted in hospital, outpatient, or home settings according to individual monitoring, cost, or access needs.

RESPIRATORY PHYSIOLOGY

Structure and Function

Airways are either conducting airways or respiratory units. Conducting airways extend from the nose through the terminal bronchioles and function as conduits, distributing but not exchanging gases throughout the lungs (Figure 18-1). Respiratory units extend from the respiratory bronchioles to the alveoli and are the areas for oxygen and carbon dioxide exchange. The circumference of individual airways decreases with each branching, whereas the aggregate circumference increases. In larger airways, inspired air moves by bulk flow, but the velocity of airflow decreases as the aggregate circumference of the airways increases. The velocity of airflow is very slow in the smaller airways, and in the alveoli, air moves by diffusion of gases.

Conducting Airway

The mucosa of the nasopharyngeal region is well-vascularized, enabling inspired air to be heated to body temperature and humidified by the time it reaches the trachea. Because the airway is lined with ciliated columnar epithelium and mucus-secreting cells and glands, any large airborne particle gets trapped in the mucous layer before it reaches the trachea. The entire tracheobronchial region is lined with ciliated epithelial cells, mucus-secreting cells, and mucous glands (see Figure 18-1). Smaller airborne particles are trapped in the mucous layer in this region, and only the tiniest particles reach terminal respiratory units. The mucus and cilia lining the conducting airways protect the respiratory system and serve as a major defense mechanism, the mucociliary escalator. The normal volume of secretions is approximately 100 ml/day (Copstead, 2000). Closure of the epiglottis, located at the entrance to the larynx, protects the airway from aspiration during swallowing and allows intrathoracic pressure to develop during coughing or the Valsalva maneuver. Sensory fibers in the larynx and tracheobronchial tree are sensitive to chemical and mechanical irritants that stimulate a cough. The cough reflex can be depressed by neurological dysfunction, unconsciousness, or anesthesia. It may become less sensitive with age, increasing the risk of infection in the upper respiratory tract.

Gas Exchange Units

The terminal respiratory unit, or acinus, consists of respiratory bronchioles, alveolar ducts, and alveoli. As alveoli begin to appear as outgrowths of the airways in the smaller bronchioles, increasing in number with each generation, they provide a surface area for gas exchange about the size and surface of a tennis court.

Ventilation

Ventilation is the movement of air into and out of the lungs and can be likened to a "pump" for the lungs. The process of ventilation involves the central nervous system, peripheral nervous system, rib cage, and respiratory muscles. When respiratory centers in the brain send messages via the central and peripheral pathways to the respiratory muscles, they contract and generate the pressure differences required for airflow.

Alveolar ventilation is the amount of air that actually reaches the alveoli and participates in gas exchange. Alveolar ventilation is less than the volume of inspired air because the conducting airways, including the trachea and large bronchi, are anatomical dead space not directly communicating with alveoli. Alveolar ventilation is unevenly distributed, with a greater fraction of ventilation flowing to the

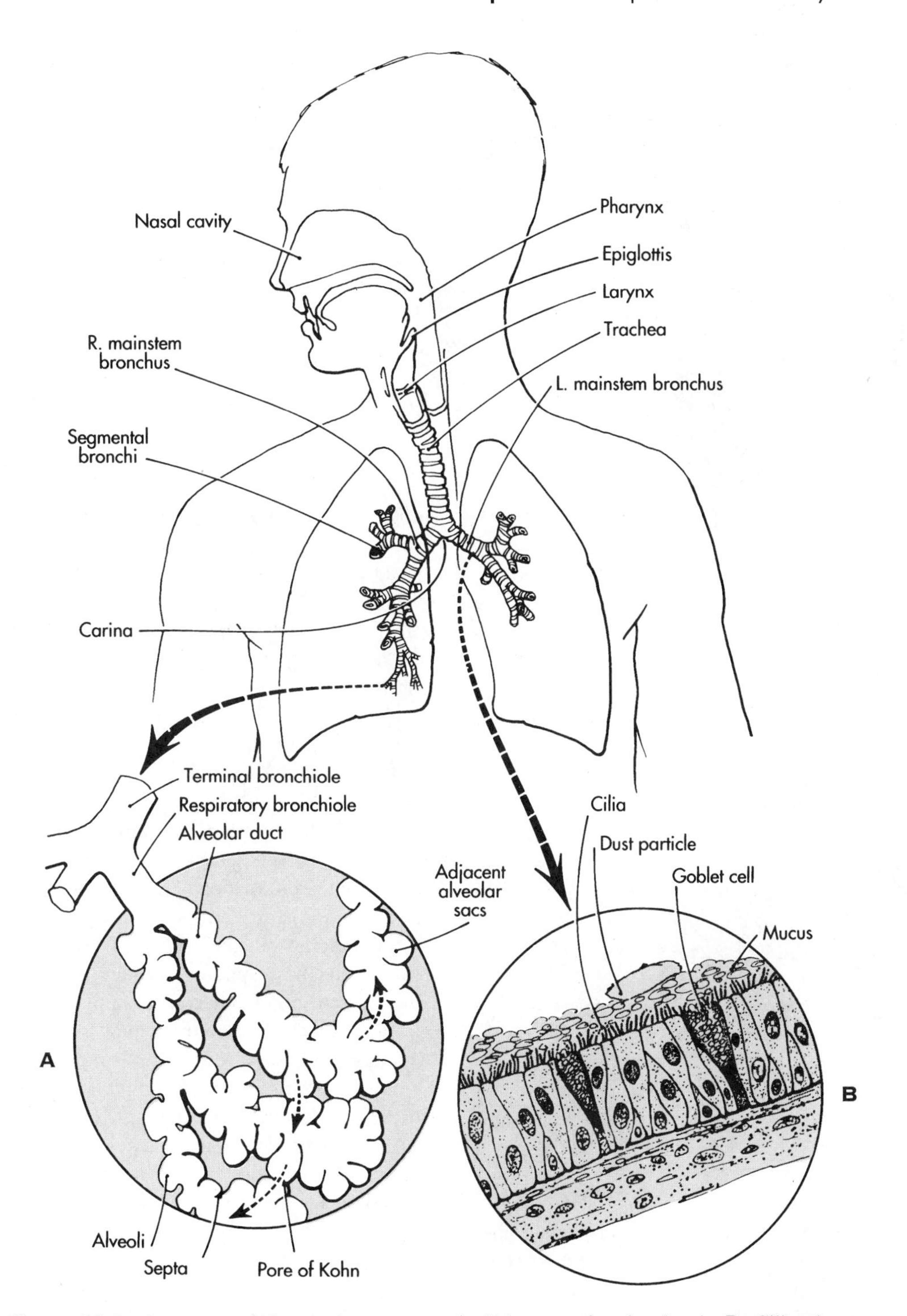

Figure 18-1 Structures of the respiratory tract. **A,** Pulmonary functional unit. **B,** Ciliated mucous membrane. (From Price, S., & Wilson, L. [1997]. *Pathophysiology: Clinical concepts of disease.* [5th ed.]. St. Louis: Mosby.)

bases of the lungs in the upright body position (Copstead, 2000).

Mechanics of Breathing

Strength of both inspiratory and expiratory muscles of respiration functions in the same manner as other skeletal muscles. Strength declines with aging, in malnutrition, and with a sedentary lifestyle; in women with less muscle mass than men, there is less muscle strength. The diaphragm is the primary muscle of *inspiration* (Figure 18-2). Innervated by the phrenic nerve at C3, C4, and C5, its dome shape is attached peripherally to the lower rib cage. When the diaphragm contracts, it pulls downward on the lungs, decreasing intrapleural, intrathoracic, and airway pressures, creating the pressure gradient for inspiratory airflow. Diaphragm contraction

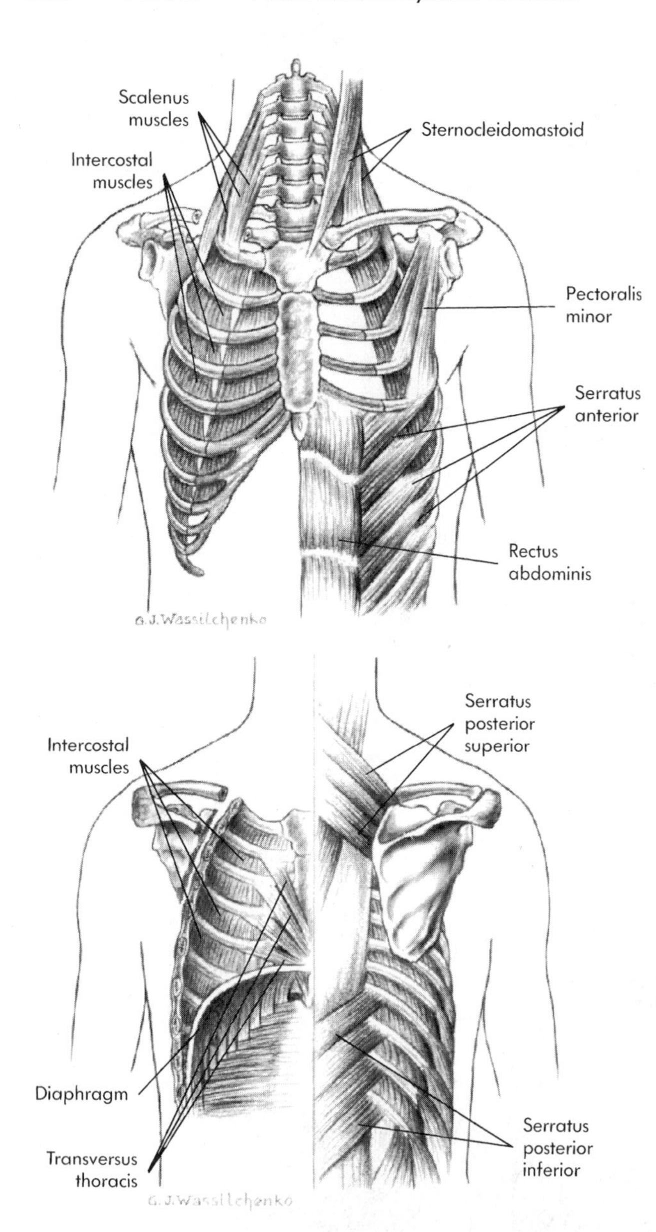

Figure 18-2 Inspiratory muscles of the chest aid in inspiration and expiration. (From Wilson, S.F., & Thompson, J.F. [1990]. *Respiratory disorders.* St. Louis: Mosby.).

pushes downward on the abdominal cavity increasing abdominal pressure. Normal *expiration* is passive with elastic recoil of the lungs. Expiratory muscles are recruited to maintain high levels of ventilation during exercise and forced expiratory maneuvers, such as a cough (Frownfelter & Dean, 1996).

Lung Compliance

Compliance refers to the elasticity of the lungs. Static compliance is the change in pressure necessary to inflate the lungs to a given volume. Normally, lung pressure-volume characteristics are influenced by surfactant that reduces the surface tension of alveoli, increasing their compliance and stabilizing them. Without the stabilizing effect, the smaller alveoli tend to collapse at low lung volumes during expiration. For example, with pulmonary fibrosis, the stiff lungs have decreased compliance and resist inflation, therefore alveolar ventilation is harder (Copstead, 2000). *Airway resistance* determines the pressure required to generate a given airflow. Resistance to flow is inversely related to the diameter of the airways. Inflammation or obstruction of the airways and increased tone of airway smooth muscle can decrease airway diameter. Increased airway resistance increases the work of breathing, as with COPD, CF, and asthma.

Control of Breathing

Breathing can be modified by involuntary and voluntary control (Figure 18-3). Involuntary control occurs through activity of respiratory centers in the brainstem, peripheral chemoreceptors, central chemoreceptors, and respiratory motor neurons. Voluntary control arises from the cerebral cortex. The basic spontaneous rhythm of breathing is established in the *respiratory centers.* Chemoreceptors, proprioceptors, and the vagus nerve send afferent input to the respiratory centers where the sensory information is coordinated and neural output is initiated via the spinal motor neurons and efferent nerves.

Central chemoreceptors are aggregates of cells in bilateral areas of the medulla that are distinct from respiratory center neurons. They are sensitive to elevations in carbon dioxide (CO_2) and the hydrogen ion concentration (H^+) in the surrounding extracellular fluid and respond by increasing the minute ventilation (V_E). *Peripheral chemoreceptors,* located at the bifurcation of the common carotid arteries and along the aortic arch, respond to a decrease in partial pressure of arterial oxygen (PaO_2) of less than 60 mm Hg by stimulating the respiratory centers to increase ventilation. They also respond to decreases in pH and increases in CO_2 by signaling the respiratory center for increased breathing. Voluntary control of respiration is regulated by the *cerebral cortex.* Breathing patterns are modified by conscious control for talking, laughing, crying, and swallowing, and activity depends on the state of wakefulness. The voluntary conducting pathways in the spinal cord are distinct from those involved in involuntary regulation. Fibers from involuntary pathways can be injured even though the voluntary pathways remain intact, and vice versa.

Gas Transport

Oxygen Transport. Most oxygen is transported to the peripheral tissues bound to hemoglobin (Hb); minimal oxygenation is in the form of dissolved O_2 (Copstead, 2000). The difference in alveolar and pulmonary capillary PO_2 establishes the gradient for the diffusion of O_2 across the alveolar-capillary membrane. The arterial PO_2 in turn drives the binding of oxygen with Hb. Box 18-1 illustrates the normal range of values for arterial blood gases. Delivery of O_2 to the tissues requires adequate cardiac output and tissue perfusion. As arterialized blood perfuses the tissues, O_2 is unloaded because of the lower PO_2 at the tissue level.

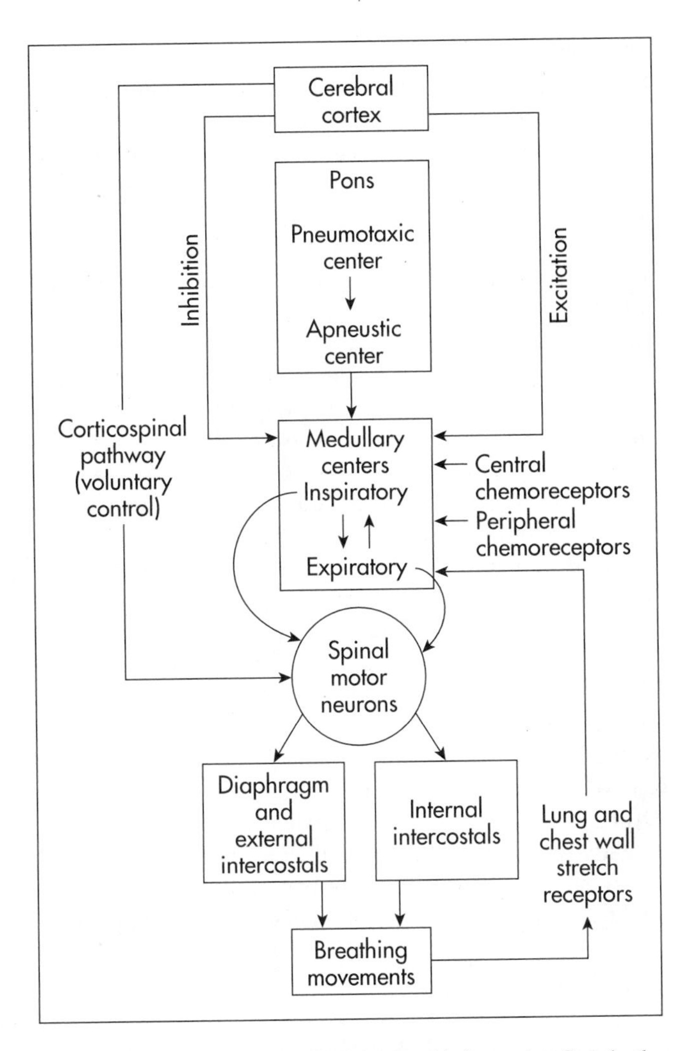

Figure 18-3 A hypothetical diagram of information flow in the respiratory control system, including some of the inputs that establish respiratory drive. The feedback loops based on the effect of ventilation on blood gas composition are not shown. (From Moffett, D.F., Moffett, S.B., & Schauf, C.L. [1993]. *Human physiology* [2nd ed.]. St. Louis: Mosby).

Carbon Dioxide Transport. Carbon dioxide transport deals with the amount of CO_2 produced as an end-product of metabolism and depends on metabolic activity and dietary intake. CO_2 is transported from the peripheral tissues as carbonic acid (an insignificant amount), dissolved in plasma (5% to 10% of total), as carbamino compounds (20% to 30% of total), or as bicarbonate (60% to 70% of total). Elimination of CO_2 via the lungs depends on an adequate level of alveolar ventilation (V_A).

Gas Exchange

Pulmonary Circulation

The pulmonary vascular bed is a low-resistance system. Normal distribution of pulmonary blood flow is influenced passively by posture and exercise. When a person is at rest, perfusion of the pulmonary capillary bed is greatest in the dependent portions of the lungs; when a person is upright, perfusion is greatest at lung bases; and when a person is in the side-lying position, perfusion is greatest in the inferior portion of the dependent lung. This uneven distribution of pulmonary blood flow is caused by hydrostatic pressure differences within the pulmonary vascular system. Due to gravity, hydrostatic pressures are greater in the dependent regions, distending the vessels and increasing the rate of flow. Mild exercise increases both cardiac output and pulmonary blood flow, leveling hydrostatic pressures and blood flow distribution in the pulmonary vascular bed (Copstead, 2000).

Box 18-1 Normal Range for Arterial Blood Gases

PO_2: 80-100 mm Hg
PCO_2: 35-45 mm Hg
pH: 7.35-7.45
HCO_3^-: 22-26 mEq/L

From Pagana, K.D., & Pagana, T.J. (1998). *Mosby's manual of diagnostic and laboratory tests.* St. Louis: Mosby.

Diffusion

Oxygen diffuses down its concentration gradient from the alveolar gases, across the alveolar-capillary membranes, through the plasma, across the red blood cell membrane, and within the red blood cell to combine with Hb. The rate of diffusion is directly proportional to the alveolar-capillary gradient of PO_2 (the difference in gas partial pressures between the two sides of the alveoli) and the cross-sectional area of the alveolar-capillary membrane. In addition, the rate of diffusion is inversely proportional to the length of the diffusion path. Theoretically the diffusion capacity can be reduced by destruction of alveolar-capillary surface area, as occurs in COPD, or by a lengthening of the diffusion path, as occurs in interstitial fibrosis. However, multiple factors must be present to impair gas exchange on the basis of a true diffusion defect.

Ventilation-Perfusion Relationships

Efficient gas exchange depends on ventilation of the alveoli, perfusion of the pulmonary capillary bed, and matching ventilation and perfusion. Uniform distribution of ventilation and perfusion throughout the lungs is ideal for gas exchange, but even distribution of ventilation and perfusion is not a normal situation. When an individual is positioned upright, a greater portion of ventilation and perfusion is distributed to the base of the lungs, but the difference is greater for perfusion. Consequently the ventilation-perfusion ratio increases from the base to the apex of the lungs, with an average ratio of 0.8, an alveolar PO_2 of 104 mm Hg, and an arterial PO_2 of 100 mm Hg.

FACTORS ASSOCIATED WITH ALTERED PHYSIOLOGICAL FUNCTIONING

Major changes in physiological functioning are categorized as alterations in gas exchange or alterations in ventilation. Many chronic lung diseases are characterized by a combination of these alterations, especially in severe or advanced stages. Clinically, clients with chronic lung disease experience a slow, progressive worsening of their condition with episodic acute exacerbations secondary to upper and lower respiratory tract infections (RTIs). When impairment of lung function is mild, clinical evidence of altered functioning may be apparent only during acute exacerbations; when severe, the clinical evidence will be readily visible on a daily basis, even without exacerbations.

Aging may accentuate pulmonary problems, resulting in decreased compliance as tissues stiffen, changes in reduce tidal volumes and vital capacity, and the aggravation of underlying lung disease. Increased calcification of rib articulations may interfere with chest expansion: the chest wall stiffens and accessory muscles are recruited for resting breathing (Seidel, Ball, Dains, & Benedict, 1999).

Biological variation in the prevalence, morbidity, and mortality of COPD reveals that the incidences of chronic bronchitis and emphysema are higher in men; however, they cause increased mortality in middle-age women when associated with increased smoking exposure. International variability may be explained by differences in smoking habits, types of cigarettes, and methods of diagnosis and death reports. However, genetic susceptibility and other environmental influences on respiratory health are implicated. Frequent childhood respiratory infections are common in developing countries where environmental factors, such as poor indoor ventilation and wood burning stoves, produce toxic, irritating gases that damage respiratory membranes. Similarly, air pollution can add to existing atmospheric conditions to aggravate chronic respiratory conditions. Fuel burning, except nuclear, produces carbon monoxide and nitric oxide, which converts to nitrogen dioxide and irritates the airways. When small hydrocarbons from burning fossil fuels and strong sunlight combine into ozone and other photochemical products, this photochemical smog remains until winds disperse it. Changes in weather, especially humidity and rapid temperature drops, are difficult for clients with COPD to tolerate.

Subjective Assessment

Subjective manifestations of disease may prompt individuals to seek medical attention. Constitutional symptoms such as fever, weight loss, fatigue, and sleep disturbance may be present, justifying a review of body systems. A detailed subjective assessment of the three most common respiratory-related complaints—dyspnea, cough, and activity intolerance—and a history of symptoms and smoking behavior are essential to planning care.

Dyspnea

Dyspnea, the sensation of difficulty with breathing associated with increased effort to breathe (Gift, 1998; McCarley, 1999), manifests in many ways. Clients use different terms to describe dyspnea—shortness of breath, difficulty breathing, suffocating, and chest tightness. Dyspnea, the primary symptom for many patients with cardiopulmonary diseases including COPD, pulmonary fibrosis, asthma, pulmonary hypertension, and congestive heart disease, may occur with obesity, pregnancy, and neuromuscular diseases. Intensity may not correlate with the extent of impairment; some clients with severe lung disease report minimal dyspnea, whereas others with mild lung disease report intense dyspnea. Clinical assessment describes frequency, intensity, history of symptom onset (acute or chronic), precipitating events, duration, associated symptoms, relieving factors, and identifiable patterns.

The Borg CR10 Scale for rating of perceived exertion rates the intensity of dyspnea at rest or during physical activity (Box 18-2). Clients point to the number on the scale that best describes the intensity of their breathlessness. Clients use the scale differently—some appear in acute distress while rating their dyspnea as minimal, whereas others use the full range, reporting maximal dyspnea when they appear to be extremely dyspneic. Consequently the intensity of dyspnea is not comparable. Clients tend to use the scale consistently when rating changes in their dyspnea over time. To assess the general intensity of dyspnea, rehabilitation nurses might use one of the scales designed for large population studies of lung disease, such as the breathlessness scale

Box 18-2 Borg CR10 Scale*

0	Nothing at all	"No I"
0.3		
0.5	Extremely weak	Just noticeable
0.7		
1	Very weak	
1.5		
2	Weak	Light
2.5		
3	Moderate	
4		
5	Strong	Heavy
6		
7	Very strong	
8		
9		
10	Extremely strong	"Strongest I"
11		
•	Absolute maximum	Highest possible

*For correct usage of the scale, see Borg, G. (1998). *Borg's perceived exertion and pain scales*. Champaign (IL): Human Kinetics. CR10 Scale ©Gunnar Borg, 1982, 1998. Used with permission.

from the Recommended Respiratory Disease Questionnaire (ATS, DLD, 1978) (Box 18-3).

Chronic dyspnea contributes to functional disability when activities that produce symptoms or decrease energy are eliminated despite their importance to life satisfaction. Lifestyles and interests may change accordingly at great cost to personal, physical, social, and emotional well-being.

Cough

Coughing occurs to clear the airways of secretions and to protect them from aspiration and/or inhalation of noxious substances. A cough can be acute or chronic, associated with other symptoms (e.g., pain, wheezing, dyspnea, syncope), productive or dry, or effective or ineffective (unable to clear secretions). It is abnormal if it is persistent, irritating, painful, or productive. Thus all data about how the cough developed are pertinent. For example, the cough may follow a recent illness or RTI, be exacerbated by seasonal or environmental conditions, or occur only at a certain time of day. Chronic cough tends to worsen when a client is lying down or arising after lying down for an extended period. A cough during or shortly after eating may indicate aspiration of food or fluid into the tracheobronchial tree. Characteristics of the cough—quality, frequency, and alleviating factors or a change in usual characteristics of a chronic cough—are investigated. The presence of a cough alone is nonspecific but along with other signs and symptoms may suggest a particular diagnosis.

Assess sputum production, quantity, and character. Normally, individuals do not produce noticeable amounts of sputum, but persons with chronic bronchitis expectorate small to moderate amounts of mucoid material each day, often in the morning. The volume is greatly increased with bronchiectasis and CF. Suspect lower RTI with a change to thick yellow or green sputum. Individuals with COPD, bronchiectasis, CF, and spinal cord injury at the midcervical level are predisposed to RTIs. In CF, thick, green, and purulent sputum suggests *Pseudomonas aeruginosa* infection; foul odors in sputum signal anaerobic bacterial infections such as those caused by the *Pseudomonas.*

Hemoptysis generally originates from a problem in the airways, parenchyma, or pulmonary vasculature. Severity varies from blood-streaked sputum, as sometimes seen in chronic bronchitis, to frank bleeding, which may accompany pulmonary infarction. Commonly occurring without a diagnosis, the symptom is worrisome and requires investigation. A small amount of blood streaking in the sputum is not uncommon and usually self-limiting with CF, especially in older clients, and does not require intervention.

Box 18-3 Breathlessness Scales from the ATS-DLD Questionnaire

1. Are you troubled by shortness of breath when hurrying on the level or walking up a slight hill?
2. (If yes) Do you have to walk slower than others your age on the level because of breathlessness?
3. (If yes) Do you ever have to stop for breath when walking at your own pace on the level?
4. (If yes) Do you ever have to stop for breath after walking about 100 yards (or after a few minutes) on the level?
5. (If yes) Are you too breathless to leave the house or breathless on dressing or undressing?

Adapted from Ferris, B.G. (1978). Recommended respiratory disease questionnaires for use with adults and children in epidemiological research (part 2). *American Review of Respiratory Disease, 118,* 7-53.

Activity Intolerance

Typically, clients with respiratory disease complain of shortness of breath and easy fatigue with exercise that may relate to the severity of disease. Activity produces an abnormal heart rate, and the time needed to return to the post-activity rate is prolonged. Muscle pain or weakness in peripheral muscles may occur while an individual is engaging in physical activity, but severe dyspnea prevents clients from continuing activity.

History of Symptoms and Smoking Behavior

A chronology of health data focusing on presenting respiratory symptoms helps the health care provider to establish nursing diagnoses and develop a plan of care. Data collected include information about past or concurrent medical problems, treatment regimens, compliance behaviors, incidence of respiratory infections, and smoking habits. Questions about smoking include the age smoking began, the type and amount of tobacco used (cigarettes, cigar, pipe, snuff, chewing tobacco), current smoking habits, successful and unsuccessful attempts to quit, and reasons for continuing to smoke or for quitting. The nurse can ascertain the client's readiness to participate in a pulmonary rehabilitation program. Information about the psychosocial environment is essential assessment data for developing an appropriate plan of care.

Objective Assessment

A complete physical examination is indicated since respiratory dysfunction often results from other system impairments (Seidel et al., 1999). The following section details clinical evaluation specific to the respiratory system. When examining the chest, envision the underlying anatomy of the lungs and thorax and compare for bilateral symmetry.

Inspection

Inspection begins during the interview in a well-lighted room. Observe the client's general appearance, skin color, presence and degree of respiratory distress, character and rate of respirations, quality of voice, pattern of speech, interruptions by coughing or breathlessness, flaring nostrils, use of pursed-lip breathing (PLB), and assumed posture. For the inspiratory to expiratory ratio of breathing (I:E), the inspiratory phase is longer than the expiratory phase over most lung fields. With obstruction, as in COPD, the expiratory phase is prolonged and the I:E ratio may exceed 1:6. With the client supine and chest exposed, look for asymmetrical movement and expansion of the rib cage with breathing, use of accessory muscles of respiration, splinting secondary to pain, obstructed airflow, or paralysis of the respiratory muscles. Paradoxical motion of the abdomen during quiet breathing may indicate abnormal or absent diaphragm use, as seen with high cervical lesions of the spinal cord.

The client sits for inspection of chest shape and configuration. The anteroposterior diameter increases slightly with aging but significantly with COPD. The thoracic spine and rib cage are evaluated for deformities or abnormalities that interfere with chest expansion, causing decreased compliance and reduced lung volume. Common deformities contributing to a restrictive defect include kyphosis, scoliosis, and kyphoscoliosis. Ankylosing spondylitis causes a forward angling of the spine and an immobile spinal column that limits expansion of the chest. Trauma can cause a flail chest that appears as a paradoxical movement of a portion of the chest wall.

Cyanosis is best detected in daylight at the nail beds and buccal mucosa. Cyanosis reflects severe hypoxemia of arterial blood to a sufficient degree to desaturate Hb. Approximately 5 g/100 ml of reduced Hb must be present to change the usual color of skin to a pale tone, ranging to blue in a light toned individual. For this reason, cyanosis is not identified with anemia until hypoxemia is severe, whereas clients with polycythemia may appear cyanotic with less hypoxemia present. The most common cause for cyanosis is generalized hypoxemia (central cyanosis), but cyanosis also may occur secondary to peripheral vasoconstriction.

Palpation

Palpation is used to evaluate the underlying structure and function of the chest, detect areas of tenderness or crepitation, and assess respiratory excursion. Tenderness noted on palpation often is musculoskeletal, but the intercostal spaces are palpated for tumor, swelling, or crepitation that needs evaluation.

A variety of chest conditions alter transmission of sounds. Decreased transmission can be secondary to weakness of the voice; obstruction of the airway; or the collection of air, fluid, or tissue in the pleural space. Increased air retained in the lung, as in emphysema, decreases tactile fremitus, whereas consolidated lung tissue, as with pneumonia or tumor mass, causes increased fremitus if the airway remains patent.

Percussion

Healthy, air-filled lungs produce a different sound with percussion than do fluid-filled lungs or solid tissue. Quality ranges from dull to resonant. With increased density, resonance fades to dullness, as when percussing over solid organs, areas of consolidation, or fluid-filled spaces. Hyperresonance accompanies an increased accumulation of air, such as with hyperinflation or pneumothorax.

Diaphragm location and excursion are evaluated by percussing the lower posterior lung fields until the sound changes. The distances between levels of dullness at deep inspiration and deep expiration are compared to evaluate movement of the diaphragm. Normal excursion ranges from 4 to 6 cm. A low-lying diaphragm with limited excursion often accompanies hyperinflation. Diaphragm paralysis, atelectasis, or pleural effusion may accompany an elevated diaphragm and impaired movement.

Auscultation

Auscultation of the chest is used to evaluate the quality and intensity of breath sounds in all lung fields and adventitious lung sounds that may indicate a respiratory disorder. When possible, the client is seated, but if the client is weak or debilitated, having him or her turn from side to side enables complete examination. Prevent clients from rapid breathing that may cause dizziness. Breath sounds will be decreased or absent when the rate of airflow is decreased, as seen in persons with increased airway resistance and excessive secretions. Shallow breathing from weakness, obesity, or neuromuscular disorders will also produce diminished breath sounds, as will excess subcutaneous fat or pleural effusion.

Crackles (rales) are commonly heard with pulmonary edema, atelectasis, pneumonia, and interstitial lung disease. *Wheezes* (rhonchi) are caused by airflow through obstructed airways caused by bronchospasm, secretions, compression, mucosal swelling, and/or a foreign body.When pleural surfaces become inflamed or roughened a *pleural friction rub,* a grating sound or vibration associated with breathing, can be heard over the site of discomfort. Many conditions are associated with a pleural friction rub, including pleurisy, tuberculosis, pulmonary infarction, pneumonia, and primary and metastatic carcinoma. *Stridor,* a high-pitched sound on inspiration, is caused by an obstruction high in the respiratory tree and is characterized by a prolonged inspiratory phase with an I:E ratio of 3:1 or greater. In infants and children, stridor indicates a serious problem in the trachea or larynx that warrants immediate attention (Seidel et al., 1999).

Diagnostic Studies

Accurate medical diagnosis of a pulmonary problem includes pulmonary function tests, arterial blood gas studies, radiological studies, and laboratory data. Nurses play a major role in client and family education throughout the assessment and ongoing evaluation and collaborate with the rehabilitation team to establish a complete profile of information for informed decision making.

Pulmonary Function Testing

Pulmonary function testing that is conducted in a specialized laboratory by trained technicians provides an objective, noninvasive means of documenting pulmonary impairment. Lung volumes determined by body plethysmography or helium dilution establish the extent of hyperinflation with large lung volumes or of restrictive lung disease with small lung volumes. *Spirometry* establishes the extent of airflow obstruction and may be tested in outpatient settings to monitor effectiveness of treatment. All spirometers are calibrated regularly to meet ATS standards. The nurse coaches clients to use proper technique to attain the best flow-volume measurements; at least three acceptable efforts are recorded at each testing. The personal effort that meets ATS criteria with the highest sum of forced vital capacity (VC) and forced expiratory volume in 1 second (FEV_1) recorded is the client's reading for that day. The most useful parameters are listed in Box 18-4.

Arterial Blood Gases

Arterial blood gas values are used to evaluate oxygenation, ventilation, and acid-base balance. Arterial blood gases are routinely evaluated for PO_2, PCO_2, bicarbonate, and pH values. Many persons with pulmonary disease have a complex, mixed picture of abnormalities that can be better understood through periodic monitoring of arterial blood gas values. Blood gas measurements are objective data that determine the need for supplemental O_2. Box 18-1 contains descriptions of normal arterial blood gas values.

Pulse Oximetry

Pulse oximetry rates reflect oxygenation of the tissues in a noninvasive manner. A decrease of more than 3%, or an oxygen saturation of less than 89%, indicates desaturation. However, accuracy can vary (±5%), and alterations in oxygen saturation can be masked in smokers by elevated carboxyhemoglobin levels (Noble, 1996). Peripheral circulatory problems in areas of the probe may lead to erroneously low readings. Changes in oxygenation are verified with blood gas values or other clinical evidence of activity intolerance, such as severe dyspnea, pallor and sweating, apprehension, lack of coordination, increased labored respirations, or increased heart rate and blood pressure (Beare & Myers, 1998). Initiate oxygen administration if desaturation is confirmed. Pulse oximetry gives no information about ventilation or level of carbon dioxide in the blood, but it is a useful measure for observing trends and estimating oxygenation in clients with stable conditions in the home or rehabilitation facility. It is not a definitive method to evaluate oxygenation.

Box 18-4 Pulmonary Function Test Parameters

Vital capacity (VC): Maximum amount of air exhaled from the point of maximum inspiration
Forced expiratory volume in 1 second (FEV_1): Volume of air exhaled during the first second of the forced vital capacity maneuver
Functional residual capacity (FRC): Volume of air in the lungs at the end-expiratory position after a normal breath
Residual volume (RV): Volume of air in the lungs after maximum exhalation
Total lung capacity (TLC): Volume of air in the lungs after maximum inspiration

Radiographical Examination

A chest x-ray is a baseline evaluation and helps rule out other causes for symptoms, such as heart failure with cardiac enlargement or lung lesions from cancers. Computed axial tomography (CAT) scans are used to depict areas of emphysematous tissue and to evaluate clients for surgical therapies.

Laboratory Data

These data include standard measurements of blood count, serum electrolytes, urea, creatinine, and blood glucose. Results assist in ruling out anemias and other abnormalities that may mimic a chronic respiratory disorder.

INEFFECTIVE AIRWAY CLEARANCE

Ineffective airway clearance is defined as the "inability to effectively clear secretions or obstructions from [the] respiratory tract" (Gordon, 2000). Normal, small amounts of secretions cleared by the mucociliary system differ from the excessive secretions produced by clients with a respiratory condition, such as chronic bronchitis, CF, bronchiectasis, or lower respiratory tract infection. Problems arise when the volume of secretions is too large to be cleared by deep breathing and coughing because respiratory muscles are too weak to be effective and/or when secretions are too thick to mobilize. A study by Carlson-Catalano et al. (1998) found the following defining characteristics of ineffective breathing, listed in order of importance: difficulty with sputum, abnormal breath sounds, chest congestion, fatigue, cough, and anxiety.

To generate an effective cough, clients must have sufficient muscle strength on inspiration to take a deep breath before the cough and on expiration to generate the sudden rise in intra-thoracic pressure during the cough. Respiratory muscle strength is influenced by nutritional status and lean body muscle mass. Some clients with obstructive pulmonary disorders experience daily problems with ineffective airway clearance, whereas others have episodes during exacerbation. Individuals with a significant amount of chronic bronchitis or CF produce excessive secretions, evidenced by a productive cough every morning on arising. Unless they mobilize secretions and clear their airways daily, these clients are at risk for stagnated secretions and bacterial growth. Clients with neuromuscular disease, COPD, and CF who contract a viral or bacterial respiratory infection have further reductions in muscle strength and are at risk for ineffective airway clearance (Seemungal, Donaldson, Bhowmik, Jeffries, & Wedzicha, 2000). Viral infections cause increased secretions and promote a secondary bacterial infection of the lungs, further increasing the work of breathing. Consequently, in clients with severe respiratory muscle weakness, the increased work of breathing and reduction in respiratory muscle strength may be sufficient to trigger ventilatory failure.

Episodic problems with airway clearance occur with respiratory muscle weakness secondary to neuromuscular disease and in midcervical or higher level injury of the spinal cord. The respiratory muscles are too weak to produce effective coughing and deep breathing during a respiratory tract infection, and the virus can cause further impairment of respiratory muscle strength. Immobility, with shallow breathing and pooled stagnant secretions, compounds problems.

Subjective Assessment

Clients with ineffective airway clearance typically complain of an inability to cough up secretions and chest congestion. They also complain of dyspnea, fatigue, and anxiety.

Objective Assessment

Typically, adventitious breath sounds will include low- or high-pitched wheezes and coarse crackles that occur on inspiration or on both inspiration and expiration. Low-pitched wheezes indicate secretions in the airway that generally clear with coughing. A persistent cough and hypoxemia may signal ineffective airway clearance, and sputum suggests pulmonary disease. Sputum characteristics are documented as to amount, color, odor, and consistency and described as being tenacious, viscous, frothy, mucoid, mucopurulent, blood tinged, or having a foul odor.

Goals

The primary nursing goals for the individual with ineffective airway clearance are to establish and maintain a patent airway and adequate ventilation. Client goals include the following:

1. Maintain a patent airway.
2. Master techniques that can assist in producing an effective cough.
3. Readily mobilize secretions for expectoration.
4. Maintain adequate hydration and humidification.
5. Correct nutritional deficiencies.

Interventions for Clients with Actual or Potential Airway Clearance Problems

Nursing interventions to achieve goals augment the client's natural defense mechanisms. Specific interventions are nebulization, cough techniques, deep breathing exercises, incentive spirometry, postural drainage, percussion, vibration, hydration, and appropriate pharmacotherapy. Table 18-1 lists interventions and outcomes based on the nursing diagnosis of ineffective airway clearance.

Care Settings

Whereas ineffective airway clearance problems of many clients can be managed without invasive measures, some patients may necessitate artificial airway placement, and in severe cases, endotracheal intubation. In the latter cases, tracheostomies and care in subacute and long-term settings, as well as at home, may be necessary. Ultimately, client goals are to breathe apart from a mechanical ventilator and to function independently at home. All caregivers learn all aspects of care and suctioning when a permanent tracheostomy is required, as when a client cannot be weaned from a ventilator or effectively cough up secretions.

Hydration

Amounts of fluid that are adequate to replace fluid losses, maintain hydration, and keep mucous membranes moist facilitate the mobilization of secretions. It is not necessary to force fluids because excess fluid is excreted and does not affect the composition of respiratory secretions, and excess fluids aggravate comorbid conditions, such as heart failure. Caffeinated coffee and tea act as diuretics and are avoided or not included in daily fluid intake. However, some clients may find drinking warm fluids facilitates the coughing up of secretions and promotes hydration of mucous membranes. Monitoring fluid status includes assessing mucous membranes, skin turgor, and thirst and evaluating the urine.

All *environmental humidifiers* used during cold weather must be cleaned regularly to prevent growth of bacteria and fungi. For clients with a tracheostomy, the heat and moisture exchanger (HME) connects directly to the tracheostomy tube. It warms and humidifies inspired gases by recovering humidity from expired gases. Adult and pediatric sizes are

TABLE 18-1 Nursing Interventions and Outcomes for Ineffective Airway Clearance

Nursing Diagnosis	Suggested Nursing Interventions Classification	Suggested Nursing Outcomes Classification
Ineffective Airway Clearance	Cough enhancement Airway management Airway insertion and stabilization Artificial airway management Airway suctioning	Respiratory status: Airway patency

Data from Johnson, M., Maas, M.L., & Moorhead, S. (2000). *Nursing outcomes classification (NOC)* (2nd ed.). St. Louis: Mosby; McCloskey, J.C., & Bulechek, G.M. (2000). *Nursing interventions classification (NIC)* (3rd ed.). St. Louis: Mosby; and North American Nursing Diagnosis Association. (2001). *Nursing diagnosis: definitions and classification 2001-2002* (4th ed.). Philadelphia: Author.

available for inpatient and home use with or without mechanical ventilation. The HME is not used continuously for more than 24 hours. When a client coughs up secretions or needs suctioning, the HME is disconnected from the tracheostomy tube. If secretions or mucus adhere to the mesh inside the unit, it is replaced immediately; therefore, only clients who can independently remove the humidifier when the mesh becomes obstructed with secretions can use the HME at home.

Nebulization

Nebulization delivers water vapor or medication in fine mist droplets that travel through the respiratory system and penetrate deep within the lungs. Various methods produce droplets of varying sizes; generally the smaller the particle, the deeper the penetration into the respiratory tract. Particles of 1 to 5 mm penetrate to the periphery, particles of 5 to 10 mm are deposited in the bronchi, and particles larger than 10 mm are deposited in the upper airway passages. Aerosols are bland or medicated. A bland aerosol contains water or saline solution from a reservoir container and is delivered either at room temperature or heated. Medicated aerosols can be administered through metered-dose inhalers or nebulizers. Scientific evidence does not support the use of inhalation of bland aerosolized water or saline via mask or mouthpiece (ATS, 1995). The small amount of aerosolized water droplets that reaches the lower airways does not aid in liquefying secretions, except in the case of clients with a tracheostomy, since bland aerosols are necessary to prevent thickening of airway secretions. Hazards associated with nebulization include overhydration, airway irritation, and risk of pneumonia. Special precautions in the administration of aerosol mists include educating clients on the proper cleansing of nebulizers to prevent infection. One method of disinfecting nebulizers is to soak immersible parts in a weak vinegar solution two to three times a week and then run the nebulizer for 20 minutes before use to eliminate vinegar fumes.

Cough Techniques

Coughing is an important physiological mechanism for the removal of secretions from the respiratory tract. Maximal effect from coughing can be achieved through controlled coughing or a forced-expiratory technique called huff coughing (Frownfelter & Dean, 1996). This technique can help control coughing and remove mucus more easily. Using timing to control coughing on exhalation and while simultaneously using the arms to push on the abdomen will be less tiring for the client and more productive. Although these techniques are beneficial in clients with COPD and CF, they are difficult with clients who have dyspnea. Individuals with COPD or neuromuscular disorders may not be able to perform these techniques effectively because of collapsed airways. The cough technique is selected according to clients' needs (Frownfelter & Dean, 1996). A discussion of cough techniques follows.

Controlled Cough. A *controlled cough* consists of a slow maximal inspiration followed by holding one's breath for several seconds and then by two or three coughs.

Huff Cough. *Huff coughing* ("open glottis coughing") is a form of controlled cough designed to clear the airways while conserving energy. Clients cross their arms just below the rib cage, take a deep breath while leaning forward with arms crossed over a pillow, and exhale sharply while whispering the word "huff" several times. Whispering the word "huff" prevents closure of the glottis and reduces airway compression during the cough. Continued relaxation takes place with slow diaphragmatic breathing between coughs (Frownfelter & Dean, 1996).

Pump Cough. *Pump coughing* is a variation of the huff technique that extends the huff and improves efficiency of the effort. The client makes three short huffs and follows these with three short, easy coughs at lower lung volumes.

Quad Cough. The *quad cough* is used for persons with expiratory muscle weakness secondary to a neuromuscular dysfunction. The technique is also referred to as the *manual cough* or *diaphragmatic push* (Frownfelter & Dean, 1996). The person assisting the client positions his or her hand below the client's xiphoid process and pushes quickly on the epigastric area, diagonally inward toward the head, while the client attempts to cough. Quad-assist coughing is similar to the Heimlich maneuver. This motion should be coordinated with the client's attempt to exhale forcefully. Some clients can assist themselves by quickly compressing the abdomen. With the feet positioned on the floor or stool, the client takes a slow, deep breath through the nose and exhales, simultaneously bending forward and pressing a pillow against the abdomen. After several deep breaths and exhalations, the client coughs several times while exhaling and bending forward. Most clients will appreciate privacy during the coughing procedure because they regard sputum production as socially unattractive.

Glossopharyngeal Breathing. Clients with neuromuscular disorders with little or no respiratory muscle function can use *glossopharyngeal breathing (GPB)* to increase VC and improve cough force. To perform GPB, also known as "frog" breathing, the client traps air in the mouth and then pushes it back into the trachea with the tongue. The vocal cords remain closed until the air enters the trachea. Mastery of GPB takes time, but it is useful to assist minimal voluntary ventilation and to provide a ventilator-free time. Since GPB can be fatiguing, clients must be carefully monitored with the checking of oxygen levels with pulse oximetry (Frownfelter & Dean, 1996).

Deep Breathing Exercises

Deep breathing exercises mobilize secretions to facilitate airway clearance. Difficulty with deep breathing can be caused by weak muscles of inspiration, as with neuromuscular disorders and by pain after surgery or trauma. Maximal deep breathing is obtained in the upright position because gravity helps pull the diaphragm and abdomen downward. In the supine position the abdomen pushes upward on the diaphragm, and functional residue capacity (FRC) and decreased VC reduce the client's ability to take a deep breath. The client, sitting in upright position, takes a prolonged deep inspiration through the nose, holds the breath for at least 3 seconds, and then exhales slowly in a relaxed manner while simulating a normal sigh. Clients with COPD exhale through pursed lips for most benefit.

Incentive Spirometry

An *incentive spirometer* may facilitate efforts for lung inflation by providing visual feedback of performance based on inspiratory flow or on volume, depending on the type of spirometer used. Clients are taught to seal their lips around the mouthpiece and attempt maximum inhalation; then they hold their breath for several seconds before exhaling slowly. Generally, incentive spirometers are inexpensive, disposable, and safe, and clients do not require assistance. Deep breathing or incentive spirometry is performed three to four times a day, according to the clinical condition. Beneficial effects from incentive spirometry in persons with obstructive diseases have not been validated, but inhaling forcibly may intensify the hyperinflated condition of chronic obstructive airways.

Chest Physiotherapy

Chest physiotherapy is a general term for assistance to move airway secretions from peripheral airways to more central airways for expectoration and/or suctioning (McCloskey & Bulechek, 2000). The maneuvers include (a) chest percussion, (b) chest vibration, and (c) postural drainage techniques, used independently or in combination to assist in mobilizing secretions. Using humidifiers and bronchodilators before chest physiotherapy may facilitate airway clearance. In clients with CF, the benefits are limited to those who produce at least 25 ml of sputum per day since this modality is effective only for clients with copious sputum production (Celli, 1998), and it does not improve pulmonary function.

Chest Percussion. *Chest percussion* is performed by the health care provider who cups the hands and rhythmically strikes the targeted area of the client's chest. The cupping creates an air pocket between the hand and chest and produces a hollow, not slapping, sound on percussion. To avoid fatigue, the provider's wrists are kept loose with the elbows slightly flexed. Clients are more comfortable when percussion is performed over a thin layer of clothing. This technique requires only 2 to 3 minutes and should cause no discomfort. Chest percussion often is used in conjunction with postural drainage, chest vibration, and coughing techniques. Percussion is not performed over the sternum, vertebrae, kidneys, or tender areas and is contraindicated for clients with cardiac conditions, osteoporosis, and pleural effusion (Frownfelter & Dean, 1996).

Chest Vibration. *Chest vibration* follows percussion and is also performed by the health care provider. Chest vibrations transmit through the chest wall while the client takes a deep breath, then exhales slowly. The provider's arms and shoulders are straight with the hand placed flat over the area of the chest to be drained. An alternate tensing and contracting of the arm and shoulder muscles create vibration that continues for the duration of the client's expiration so that fine vibratory movements are transmitted to the client's chest wall. If the client does not cough spontaneously, encourage a cough after vibration or assisted coughing. Chest vibration can be repeated several times.

Postural Drainage

Postural drainage uses the principles of gravity to drain pulmonary secretions from the various segments of each lung. It is effective for clients who produce copious amounts of sputum daily (25 ml or more), such as in CF and bronchiectasis (Frownfelter & Dean, 1996). Postural drainage with percussion and vibration is the most effective combination of techniques to manage the significant secretions associated with CF in children. However, the use of postural drainage in clients with chronic bronchitis remains controversial, is contraindicated in conditions that predispose the client to increased intracranial pressure and hypertension, and has been associated with bronchoconstriction and decreases in arterial oxygenation (Frownfelter & Dean, 1996).

Twelve positions are necessary to drain various lobes and bronchopulmonary segments. The nurse examines radiographical reports to determine which lobe(s) require drainage since few require drainage in each position. Several of the positions require the client's head to be below the trunk and must be modified for clients who cannot tolerate the head-down position. The head-down position is used only when the uppermost lung segment requires drainage and is never used when increased intracranial pressure is suspected. It is used cautiously when clients are being monitored for hypoxemia, cardiovascular or hemodynamic instability, and marked bronchospasm. Oxygen may be administered or increased, unless contraindicated, in clients with compromised respiratory status.

Postural drainage should not be performed immediately before or after a meal. Before beginning, the nurse explains the procedure and provides the client with tissues and a sputum cup. Bronchodilating medications given by nebulization, if ordered, are administered approximately 15 minutes before beginning the technique to facilitate drainage through dilated airways. The client is then assisted into proper position, using extra pillows for support. Loosely fitted clothes facilitate coughing, deep breathing, and position changes. Postural drainage in clients who have spinal cord injury is performed only within the limitations of orthopedic alignment and stabilization, type of immobilization bed in use, and client tolerance and with continuous monitoring of respiratory status. If the client complains of respiratory difficulty or demonstrates unstable vital signs, immediately assist the client to a more upright position and be prepared to provide supplemental oxygen or ventilator support. Auscultation before and after postural drainage determines effectiveness of the procedure.

Percussion and vibration in conjunction with postural drainage may help secretions move into the upper airways for expectoration and suctioning. These measures fatigue clients, especially when many lung segments require therapy. A client remains in a position for 5 to 10 minutes to drain one segment of the lung. In the home, postural drainage is most effective with another person assisting. Mechanical vibrators are available to help clients who must perform this procedure alone. A recent systematic review of the literature on bronchopulmonary hygiene physical therapy in clients with COPD and bronchiectasis whose conditions are stable revealed that the effect of these techniques on lung function is not clear. No statistically significant effects on pulmonary function measurements or arterial oxygen tension were reported in seven randomized controlled studies (Jones & Rowe, 2000). However, anecdotal reports indicate that secretion mobilization and increased client comfort after therapy continue to provide a rationale for these therapies.

A schedule for performing chest physiotherapy is based on the client's needs. The procedure commonly is performed in the morning on arising to remove secretions that have pooled during the night and in the evening before going to bed to allow for optimum ventilation during sleep. A respiratory infection may increase secretions and necessitate therapy more frequently.

Pharmacotherapy

Pharmacotherapy using expectorants, such as guaifenesin, along with fluid intake are thought to stimulate respiratory tract secretions toward expectoration. Monitor effectiveness of pharmacotherapy by assessing lung sounds and cough frequency. For clients with COPD and asthma, the goal of drug therapy is to reduce the work of breathing by decreasing airflow obstruction and inflammation of the airways. Pharmacological therapy operates in a stepwise approach, adding one medication at a time. Clinical response to pharmacological therapy varies; hence the response to each drug is evaluated before another drug is added to the regimen. If clinical improvements are observed with a drug, it is continued and additional drugs are added only if the clinical response is suboptimal.

Initially, ipratropium is prescribed for its bronchodilating effects. If optimal treatment is not achieved with ipratropium, one of the inhaled β_2 agonists or inhaled corticosteroids is added to the regimen. Inhaled corticosteroids are initial routine prescriptions for clients with asthma; however, routine use in clients with COPD has not demonstrated decreased obstruction, as measured by increased FEV_1 (Postma & Kerstjens, 1999). Data from studies examining regular use of inhaled steroids for 3 to 6 months suggest improvements in health status and reduction of exacerbations. The findings need to be confirmed with further studies (Postma & Kerstjens, 1999). Oral corticosteroids are prescribed during the acute phase of an exacerbation in clients with COPD. The dose is tapered and discontinued as soon as possible because of the multiple side effects associated with their prolonged use (Katzung, 1998).

Pneumococcal vaccine with revaccination every 6 years and annual influenza vaccine are recommended for clients with COPD. Viral infections often trigger exacerbations, but broad-spectrum antibiotics are administered to prevent secondary bacterial infections, as described later in the chapter.

Inhaled medication is preferable since the same benefits can be obtained with smaller doses than when medication is given systemically, thus maximizing therapeutic effects and minimizing potential side effects. Inhaled medications are best administered with a metered dose inhaler (MDI) and spacer device to promote deposition of drugs deep into the airways. When only the MDI is used, approximately 11% to 42% (depending on particle size) of the drug is deposited in the lungs because the spray hits the back of the throat, depositing much of the drug in the oropharyngeal region (Busse & Wenzel, 2000). The percent deposited in the lung can be increased by timing of inhalation and activation of the MDI, followed by breath holding.

Timing and coordination are difficult for many clients. Spacer devices simplify the required procedure and improve deposition of the drug. With a spacer device the droplets are suspended in the device long enough for the carrier molecule to evaporate, leaving the smaller molecule of drug to be carried deep into the airways. Newer modes of medication delivery do not contain chemical hazards to the environment. Dry powder inhalers, for instance, minimize the chance for client technical error and require a simple inhalation technique. Nebulizers are used to administer inhaled medications in small children because they are very simple, whereas spacer devices are too difficult for small children to use.

For clients with CF, respiratory medications include antibiotics, bronchodilators, and cromolyn sodium. Broad-spectrum antibiotics are used during exacerbations to treat bacterial infections of the lower respiratory tract. Parenteral and oral antibiotics are used for acute exacerbations, and bronchodilators and cromolyn sodium are used for reactive airway disease. Inhaled antibiotics are used episodically or more continuously to treat chronic infection and improve respiratory status. If upper airway problems are present, nasal cromolyn sodium or nasal corticosteroids are used to treat chronic inflammation and nasal polyps. A newer mucolytic agent, rhDNase (combinant human deoxyribonuclease), is under investigation for treatment of CF.

For children with BPD, pharmacological therapy to enhance respiratory status depends on clinical manifestations. Theophylline is used in premature infants to control apneic episodes and may be continued for apnea and/or reactive airway disease. Corticosteroids are used in infants to improve respiratory status related to BPD and to facilitate weaning from mechanical ventilation. Corticosteroids also are used intermittently for exacerbations of reactive airway disease. The majority of children with BPD will have some reactive airway disease at some point in the course of their illness, and for many children this reactivity will persist into adolescence and adulthood. Bronchodilators are prescribed when there is evidence of reactive airway disease, and antibiotics are used during exacerbations with infections (Kenner, 1998).

Suctioning the Intubated Client

Tracheobronchial Suctioning. *Tracheobronchial suctioning* removes secretions when the client cannot clear the airway by coughing or by other noninvasive techniques. In rehabilitation, suctioning is avoided unless clinical indications show absolute necessity, such as in the cases of audible secretions and low-pitched wheezes (Beare & Myers, 1998). Clinical assessment of the chest to determine the need, rather than a routine schedule, prevents unnecessary suctioning. Suctioning is most effective when performed after administering bronchodilators and after mobilizing tracheobronchial secretions with the therapies previously described for airway clearance.

Tracheobronchial suctioning, although a common nursing procedure, has potentially serious complications, such as hypoxia, atelectasis, bronchoconstriction, hypotension, cardiac arrhythmias, infection, irritation of the mucous membranes, and laryngospasm (Simmons, 1997).

Nurse researchers have generated a large body of research examining techniques to minimize the potential complications of suctioning. Most studies focused on the effects of hyperoxygenation, hyperinflation, and hyperventilation before and after suctioning to minimize suction-induced hypoxemia (Wainwright & Gould, 1996; Carrol, 1998). Although the combination of hyperoxygenation and hyperinflation are effective in preventing complications for many clients, its efficacy depends on the underlying clinical condition. To date, there are no definitive evidence-based guidelines for safe and effective tracheobronchial suctioning; general guidelines, however, are listed in Table 18-2. Suctioning protocols must be modified according to the client's need for and response to suctioning. Lung sounds are assessed before and after the procedure. The client's tolerance and response to the procedure and the color, consistency, and quantity of secretions obtained are documented.

If suctioning will be required after the client leaves the facility, the caregivers should be instructed in the procedure and potential complications early in the rehabilitation process. A mirror may help the client to visualize the procedure. Clean technique can be used in the home. Catheters are not discarded but washed in a mild soap solution after each use, rinsed thoroughly, and then boiled for 5 minutes. Wrapped in a clean towel, they are ready for use. A new supply of sterile water or saline is made daily to prevent bacterial contamination. The sterile water or saline is made by adding 1 teaspoon of salt per quart of water; the solution is then stored in a sealed container. Once the receptacle has been opened, it also is boiled. Referral to a home health care agency for follow-up care allows the nurse to evaluate how the client and family are coping and to make any modifications in care. Agency social services can facilitate purchase or rental of a portable suction machine and other equipment.

Nasotracheal Suctioning. *Nasotracheal suctioning* seldom is indicated in nonintubated clients. It is traumatic and frightening to the client because of the discomfort of advancing the catheter through the nasal passages to the trachea. The procedure can exhaust clients and can further impair ventilation function in persons with borderline reserve. If necessary, its use is limited to clients who may yet be able to avoid endotracheal intubation (ATS, 1995). During nasotracheal suctioning, inform the client about the progress, move gently from one stage to the next, and prepare the client for unpleasant sensations. After suctioning, report outcomes to reassure the client.

Nasotracheal suctioning is an aseptic procedure. The principles for nasotracheal and orotracheal suctioning are listed in Table 18-3. The placement of a nasopharyngeal airway can facilitate suctioning and decrease the amount of trauma to the mucous membranes when frequently repeated suctioning is necessary, but the airway can be left in place for no more than 8 hours. Oral suctioning should not be performed until deep nasotracheal suctioning is completed. A metal or plastic (Yankauer) catheter can be used to suction the oral cavity. The client's tolerance of the procedure as well as the color, consistency, and amount of secretions obtained are documented.

Interventions for Clients with Tracheostomies

Tracheostomy Tubes

For individuals with ineffective airway clearance, a tracheostomy tube (Figure 18-4) may be inserted to (1) relieve airway obstruction, (2) protect the airway from aspiration because of impaired gag reflexes, (3) facilitate the removal of respiratory tract secretions, and (4) provide for mechanical ventilation. Clients often are admitted to rehabilitation facilities with temporary or permanent tracheostomies in place. Clients who cannot be weaned from a respirator or cannot effectively cough up secretions have permanent tracheostomies.

Commonly used tracheostomy tubes are described in Table 18-4 and are made of silicone, pliable plastic, or metal. They may have an inner and outer cannula or only one lumen and come with or without a cuff. The cuff is inflated with air when a sealed airway is desired for mechanical ventilation (Figure 18-4). In long-term care, plastic tubes are common, but metal tubes are more durable. The tracheostomy tube best suited to the client's needs is chosen. Anatomical changes such as growth, development of granulation tissue, or changes in ventilation require ongoing evaluation.

The soft-cuffed tracheostomy tube is deflated when problems arise or once every 2 to 3 days to check for overinflation. Inflation pressures are kept between 20 to 25 cm H_2O to prevent high-pressure damage to the lateral wall of the trachea. The cuff pressure is monitored three times a day with a manometer without deflating the cuff. The oropharynx is suctioned before deflation to prevent aspiration of pooled secretions above the inflated cuff. Hard cuffs are not recommended because they do not conform to the shape of trachea and therefore require higher pressures to prevent excessive leaking around the cuff. With higher pressures the

TABLE 18-2 Tracheal Suctioning of a Client with an Artificial Airway

Procedure	Rationale
Wash hands	
Explain procedure to patient	
Adjust suction regulator to 80 to 120 mm Hg (adults)	
Set oxygen flowmeter connected to manual resuscitation bag at 15 L/min	Studies show most manual resuscitation bags deliver close to 100% oxygen at 15 L/min
Apply goggles and unsterile gloves	In accordance with infection control policy
Open suction catheter package and sterile gloves	Catheter should remain protected by package
Connect catheter to suction tubing and occlude the suction finger port to test system	
Disconnect ventilator to oxygen source and attach manual resuscitator bag	
Hyperoxygenate for at least 30 seconds with manual resuscitator bag connected to 100% oxygen source	Adequate PEEP levels are maintained for patients requiring >5 cm H_2O
Put sterile gloves onto dominant hand over examination glove	One hand and catheter must remain sterile; coiling catheter around sterile hand protects catheter; two-glove technique is used to avoid contact contamination and protect second hand from organisms in secretions
Remove wrapping from catheter, maintaining sterility of one hand	
Gently insert catheter through tube as far as it will go	Advance without suction to prevent mucosal damage
Slowly withdraw catheter while applying intermittent suction: total suctioning time not to exceed 10 to 15 seconds	Remember, patient is not being adequately oxygenated at this time
Hyperinflate the patient with at least 5 breaths using the manual resuscitator bag	Application of intermittent suction prevents catheter adherence to mucosal wall; continuous suction may cause mucosal damage; catheter should be withdrawn within 10 seconds; if bradycardia or signs of hypoxia are noted, immediately withdraw catheter and oxygenate manually
Flush catheter and connective tubing with water	
Suction mouth and pharynx	Do not reenter trachea after suctioning mouth and pharynx; catheter is contaminated
Reconnect the patient to the ventilator or oxygen source	
Dispose of suction catheter	Coil catheter around gloved hand; remove glove over coiled catheter
Secure suction connection tubing over wall suction so that tip does not contact floor	Dust and particulate matter may contaminate system; do not leave tubing on bed; organisms in tubing can further colonize patient environment
Administer mouth care, if indicated; this can be performed wearing unsterile gloves	
Auscultate chest; evaluate breath sounds	
Wash hands	
Document date, time frequency of treatments, and patient's response to treatments; note nature and amount of secretions and record pertinent observations or changes in nursing progress notes; secretions should be described with regard to consistency/ease of clearing, amount, color, and odor	
NOTE: Some of these steps will be unnecessary with closed tracheal suction catheter systems	

From Beare, P.G., & Myers, J.L. (1998) *Adult health nursing* (3rd ed.). St. Louis: Mosby.
PEEP, Peak end-expiratory pressure.

cuffs press against the lateral wall of the trachea, causing necrosis of the tracheal tissue (Hooper, 1996).

Communication is a problem for clients with a tracheostomy. The fenestrated tube can be used to facilitate verbal communication; alternatively, a tracheostomy tube with no cuff or deflated cuff can be used for clients receiving mechanical ventilation. If the client is receiving positive pressure ventilation (PPV), the ventilator settings can be adjusted to provide higher airflow, allowing air to flow around the tube toward the vocal cords for speaking. The ability to tolerate this procedure will depend on the client's ventilatory stability, strength, and secretion volume. A number of additional communication aids are available, such as the Passy-Muir tracheostomy speaking valve (Frownfelter & Dean, 1996). This device fits into the tracheostomy tube opening and is a one-way valve, allowing inspiration only and forc-

TABLE 18-3 Guidelines for Nasotracheal or Orotracheal Suctioning

Procedure	Rationale
Wash hands	
Explain procedure to patient	
Adjust suction regulator to 80 to 120 mm Hg and occlude tubing with finger to test suction	Excessive vacuum pressures can cause mucosal trauma, tissue grabbing, and bleeding
Place patient in semi-Fowler position	
Apply mask, goggles, and unsterile gloves	In accordance with infection control policy
Open sterile glove, suction catheter package, and bottled water	One hand and catheter must remain sterile; 2-glove technique is used to avoid contact contamination and to protect second hand from organisms in secretions
Squeeze water-soluble lubricant onto sterile wrapper	
Encourage the patient to take 5 deep breaths (with supplemental oxygen if possible)	
Connect the catheter to suction tubing and occlude the suction finger port to test the system	
Put the sterile glove on your dominant hand over the examination glove	
With the sterile-gloved hand, remove the catheter from its paper wrapping so that it does not touch a potentially contaminated object or surface	
Dip catheter tip into lubricant and gently advance catheter through nares during inspiration 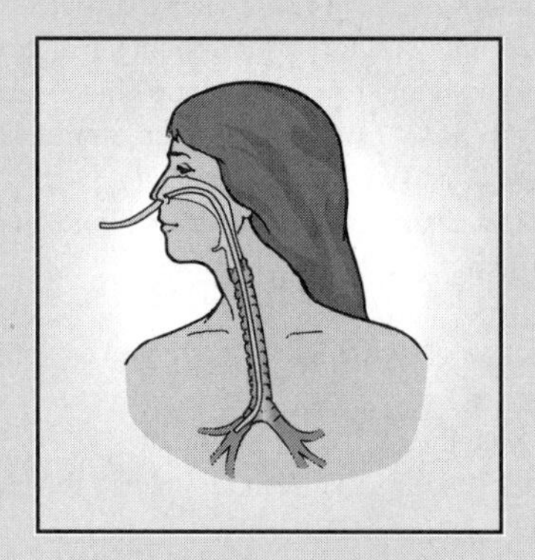	Unless contraindicated, catheter should be directed inferiorly and medially along floor of nasal passageway; when resistance is met at posterior nasopharynx, gently rotate catheter downward; if use of oral passage is necessary, inserting an oral airway facilitates control of tongue; *do not* force catheter if obstruction is met; insertion of catheter may stimulate gag reflex; be prepared to turn patient to side if vomiting occurs
Instruct the patient to cough	
Withdraw catheter 2 to 3 cm while applying intermittent suction, and rotate catheter between thumb and index finger	Continuous suction may cause mucosal damage; 10 seconds is maximum for each aspiration; if catheter "grabs" mucosa, release suction; if any complications occur, discontinue procedure, and instruct patient to breathe deeply
Repeat suction process as tolerated by the patient, allowing adequate recovery between attempts	Do not tire patient; observe for signs of cardiac or respiratory distress
Allow the patient to take several deep breaths	Hypoxemia and atelectasis can result from suctioning; both conditions may respond to oxygen administration and deep breathing
Thoroughly clear catheter and suction tubing by flushing with bottled water	
Discard catheter and gloves	Coil catheter around gloved hand; remove glove over coiled catheter
Administer mouth care frequently	
Auscultate chest; evaluate breath sounds	
Wash hands	
Document date, time, frequency of suctioning, and patient's responses to suctioning; note nature and amount of secretions, and record pertinent observations or changes in progress notes; secretions should be described with regard to consistency/ease of clearing, amount, color, and odor	

From Beare P.G. & Myers J.L. (1998). *Adult health nursing* (ed. 3). St. Louis: Mosby.

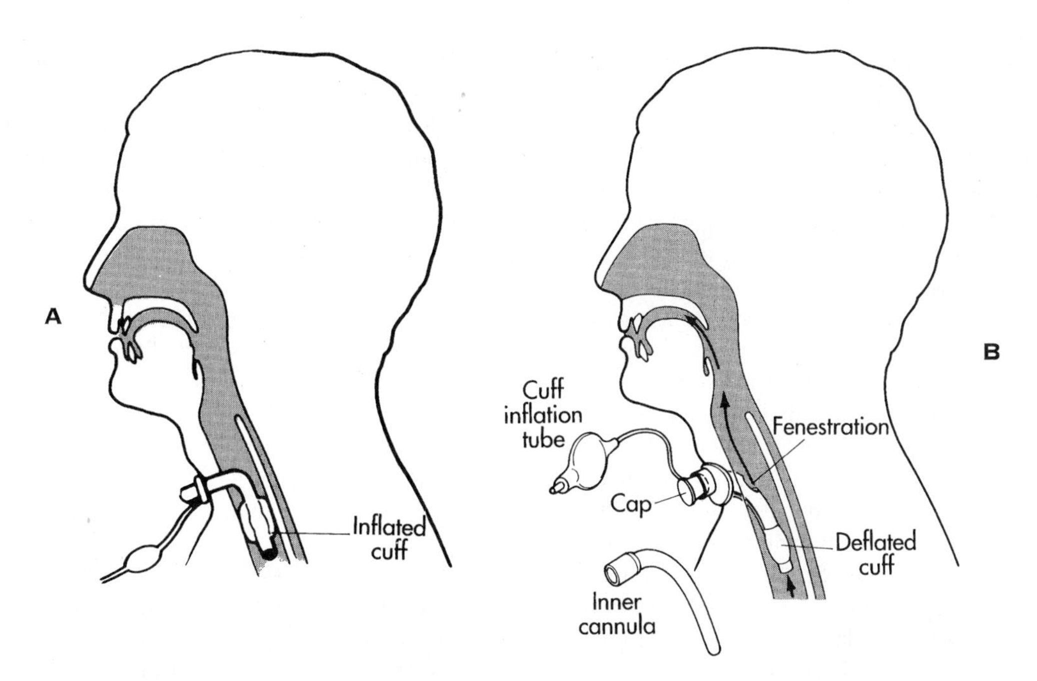

Figure 18-4 **A,** Placement of tracheostomy tube with inflated cuff. **B,** Fenestrated tracheostomy tube with cuff deflated, inner cannula removed, and tracheostomy tube capped to allow air to pass over the vocal cords. (From Lewis, S.M., Collier, I.C., Heitkemper, M.M., & Dirksen, S.R. [2000]. *Medical-surgical nursing: Assessment and management of clinical problems* [5th ed.]. St. Louis: Mosby.)

TABLE 18-4 Tracheostomy Tubes

Types	Indications
Cuffed tube with soft flexible cuff	A soft-cuffed tube is used in mechanically ventilated clients to prevent the leak of air and aspiration of secretions around the tube. Soft cuffs are less likely to cause problems with high pressures on the tracheal wall.
Fenestrated tube	Fenestrated tubes are used during weaning. They have opening(s) or fenestration(s) in the outer cannula so air can flow through the fenestrations to the larynx for speaking (see Figure 18-4). The fenestrations also allow the client to cough and expel secretions through the mouth. The cuff should be deflated before inserting the inner cannula.
Uncuffed plastic and metal tubes	Uncuffed tubes frequently are used for long-term care when the client has a functioning glottis. Metal tubes are rigid and can cause localized tissue irritation and excessive production of mucus.

ing exhalation through the upper airway. Refer to a speech pathologist to evaluate the client's need for additional communication devices. A system must be established in the home for outside communication and contact with designated persons in an emergency.

Tracheal buttons can be used for ventilatory support for only part of the day. The button is used to occlude the tracheostomy and establish normal airflow through the larynx, oral cavity, and nasal passages, allowing the client to speak and to cough. The Olympic tracheostomy button can be used as a transition before occlusion of the tracheostomy. This button maintains the stoma should a tracheostomy be needed again.

Tracheostomy Care

Rehabilitation clients with tracheostomies have special care requirements to prevent complications and maintain adequate ventilatory function. Some differences apply to the suctioning principles previously described and must be noted. With tracheostomy suctioning, the suction pressure should be reduced to only 60 to 80 mm Hg. The distal tip of the suction catheter is inserted into the tracheostomy until slight resistance is met, with care being taken not to traumatize the airway by pushing forcefully (see Table 18-2).

With a tracheostomy in place, the humidifying and warming mechanisms of the nose are bypassed. Cold, dry air causes drying of the tracheobronchial mucosa and thickening of secretions and promotes encrustation within the tube. The risk for problems of this nature can be reduced by providing humidity via a tracheostomy collar with a heated jet nebulizer (ATS, 1995).

Cannula and stoma care is performed every 8 hours using a sterile disposable cleaning kit. The inner cannula is soaked in hydrogen peroxide, cleansed with a test tube brush and pipe cleaners, and rinsed with saline solution. Be sure the inner cannula is locked securely in place on reinsertion. Cleanse the stoma site or area around the tracheostomy tube with a hydrogen peroxide solution to remove secretions. With one hand, hold the tracheostomy tube to lessen its movement and decrease the cough stimulus. Carefully cleanse the area around the stoma site, rinse with saline solution, and replace the tracheostomy dressing. Tracheostomy ties should be changed only with another person assisting to hold the tracheostomy firmly in place. If another person is not available, never remove the soiled ties until the clean ones are tied firmly in place. An extra sterile tracheostomy tube of the same size with its obturator must be immediately available at all times along with a sterile hemostat to hold the stoma open. Generally reinsertion of a tracheostomy tube is not difficult if the tracheostomy is more than 72 hours old. The physician is notified immediately.

A tracheostomy tube remains in place only as long as necessary. Complications of delayed removal include tracheal stenosis, tracheoesophageal fistula, and infection. Initiate decannulation procedures as soon as the client can maintain adequate ventilation and is able to cough and expel secretions. First, the cuff (if present) is deflated; if tolerated, the tracheostomy tube then can gradually be reduced in size. With the cuff deflated, the tube can be intermittently plugged with a tracheal button. As previously noted, the buttons allow ready access for suctioning or ventilation. Monitor the client closely at this time for respiratory distress. Initially, until "plugging" is well tolerated, the nurse should stay with the client to encourage proper breathing technique and provide reassurance. This procedure is very stressful for the client. If tracheostomy tube occlusion is tolerated and the client is able to cough and expel secretions, the tube can be removed after 24 to 72 hours. The tracheal button may remain in place if there is concern that the client may require suctioning. Once the tube is removed, place a sterile gauze piece over the stoma, and it will close spontaneously in a few days. Observe the client closely for any evidence of respiratory distress.

Education for Home Care

Clients discharged to home may participate in specialized day care during the week; ultimately, family members are responsible for some or all of the care necessary to maintain the airway. When family participate in care while the client is in a health facility, they are more apt to learn in a relaxed and unhurried manner. Inner cannula care, especially, is easier and less anxiety producing for them to learn in the structured, safe setting with the team available.

Equipment for cleaning the inner cannula and stoma includes hydrogen peroxide, dressings, and pipe cleaners or a brush to remove secretions from inside the tracheostomy tube. The primary caregiver must demonstrate competence and comfort with all aspects of care, including accidental decannulation and insertion of a new tracheostomy tube. The client should be capable of directing someone in proper tracheostomy care, and emergency telephone numbers should be readily available and visible in the home. Proper humidification of the client's air supply via a mechanical room humidifier or a portable source of humidified air or oxygen is essential; a dressing dampened with sterile water placed over the tracheostomy tube may be sufficient. However, the client is cautioned to protect the tracheostomy opening from water, inhalation of foreign substances (e.g., powder, aerosol sprays), and dry air. Adequate amounts of fluid help liquefy secretions.

Nutritional Therapies

Nutritional assessment is essential in rehabilitation of any client with chronic lung disease. Undernutrition or overnutrition is detrimental for gas exchange and respiratory health. About half of the clients with moderate to severe COPD lose lean body mass and muscle used for respiratory function. Underweight clients with COPD have higher mortality rates than those with normal weight in part because malnourishment impairs the immune system. Nutritional evaluation begins with a thorough history of food intake; height and weight measures; routine laboratory values, including albumin and serum ferritin; and total lymphocyte count. Serum albumin reflects visceral protein stores and signs of chronic malnourishment, and the lymphocyte count is an indicator of cellular immune status. Important clinical indicators for malnutrition are recent weight loss of 10% of body weight, body weight of less than 90% or greater than 120% of ideal body weight, visible muscle wasting, dietary intake changes, gastrointestinal symptoms persisting for more than 2 weeks, decreased functional capacity, and edema or ascites. In-depth nutritional assessments trigger referral to a dietitian (Berry & Braunschweig, 1998).

For clients who are hypercapnic, reduced carbohydrate intake relative to fat intake may improve the metabolic workload and decrease the amount of carbon (removed as CO_2) released through respiration. Interventions include increased consumption of calorie-rich foods, dietary supplements, and vitamins and minerals to meet the daily recommended daily allowances; problems, such as anemia, require specific interventions.

Overweight clients also are referred to a dietitian for the planning of healthy diets that include macronutrients and vitamins and minerals for good lung health but fewer calories for weight reduction. Ongoing monitoring for adherence and encouragement is necessary for either nutrition regimen.

Outcome Criteria

Health Promotion and Prevention of Illness

Smoking is detrimental to health. It irritates the mucous membranes lining the airways; stimulates mucus production; impairs ciliary function; increases vulnerability to respiratory tract infections; and is implicated in other diseases, such as pancreatic cancer. Clients and family need assistance and referral for smoking cessation. Clients must avoid environmental air pollution, remaining inside on ozone alert days, and if possible staying in central air conditioning. Air purification filters minimize the effects of indoor air pollution; however, occupational exposure to dust and irritants contribute to COPD. Clients should avoid individuals with respiratory tract infections since these clients are particularly vulnerable.

Often overlooked, oral hygiene and dental care are emphasized. The oropharyngeal area contains many organisms, including anaerobes, that can be aspirated into the lower respiratory tract. Oral hygiene and dental maintenance decrease the number of these organisms and reduce the risk of infection.

IMPAIRED GAS EXCHANGE

Impaired gas exchange is a "disturbance in oxygen or carbon dioxide exchange in the lungs or at the cellular level" (Gordon, 2000). Impaired gas exchange is seen in many clients with chronic lung disease, including COPD, interstitial lung disease, BPD, and acute infections. In pulmonary rehabilitation, clients with impaired gas exchange most commonly have COPD; whereas in general rehabilitation, clients have severe restrictive lung disease with or without concomitant lower respiratory tract infection, such as in quadriplegia secondary to spinal cord injury, Guillain-Barré syndrome, and scoliosis. All clients with impaired gas exchange also experience ineffective breathing pattern and ineffective airway clearance.

Alterations in Gas Exchange

Alterations in gas exchange are primarily reflected by hypoxemia (decreased PaO_2). Alveolar hypoventilation and abnormalities of diffusion can cause hypoxemia, but the most common cause of hypoxemia is a mismatch of ventilation and perfusion. Chronic problems with gas exchange are described in the following sections using three clinical examples of chronic lung disease: COPD, interstitial lung disease, and BPD. Acute problems with gas exchange occur with respiratory tract infections.

COPD

Clients with severe COPD demonstrate problems with gas exchange. Hypoxemia develops primarily from a mismatch of ventilation and perfusion, though diffusion limitations may contribute. Clients with chronic bronchitis develop hyperplasia of the mucous glands within the large and central airways, producing excessive secretions. When emphysema is a component, the airspaces enlarge secondary to destruction of alveoli and loss of segments of the pulmonary capillary bed. These pathological changes result in uneven distribution of ventilation to the alveoli and of perfusion to the pulmonary capillaries. Hypoxemia results when the pulmonary capillaries perfuse unventilated alveoli, dumping unoxygenated blood into the arterial side of the circulation. Similarly, ventilation is wasted by ventilating unperfused alveoli, thereby decreasing the effective V_A and increasing dead space ventilation (V_{DS}). Clients with hypoxemia develop pulmonary vascular hypertension secondary to hypoxic vasoconstriction of the pulmonary vascular bed and when prolonged, right-sided failure of the heart or cor pulmonale.

It is well-established that smoking is the major cause of COPD, though the precise mechanism is not understood. The risk of COPD is proportional to the overall lifetime exposure to cigarette smoke. Possible associations between free radical–induced oxidative damage and the development of lung cancer, emphysema, and other smoking-related disorders are under investigation (Cosio & Guerassimov, 1999). Smoke-induced lung inflammation has a pathogenic role in the development of COPD and is thought to involve many inflammatory cell types, including neutrophils, eosinophils, alveolar macrophages, and lymphocytes (Cosio & Guerassimov, 1999).

Cigarette smoking is responsible for 420,000 deaths annually in the United States and additional millions worldwide. Moreover, both active smoking and the environmental exposure to second-hand smoke cause lung cancer, heart disease, emphysema, and other diseases (Andrews, 1998). Unfortunately, studies indicate that smoking rates are rising more dramatically among adolescents than any other age group (Dappen, Schwartz, & O'Donnel, 1996). Early addiction to nicotine, the most addictive of psychoactive chemical compounds, in this vulnerable age group is more likely to lead to life-long tobacco use and increased risk of related disease (Andrews, 1998). Recently, smoking cessation interventions have been identified as a critical preventative strategy to address this growing problem.

Interstitial Lung Disease

Clients with interstitial lung disease experience problems with gas exchange, as is seen in idiopathic interstitial pulmonary fibrosis. Alveolar-capillary membranes are destroyed by progressive interstitial and intra-alveolar fibrosis. These architectural changes cause an uneven distribution of ventilation and perfusion, resulting in a mismatch of ventilation and perfusion and hypoxemia.

The etiology of interstitial lung disease includes organic and inorganic dusts, gases, drugs, poisons, radiation, allergic response, and trauma. For example, silica dust and antineoplastic drugs commonly cause interstitial lung disease. However, the etiology is unknown for many forms of interstitial lung disease, including sarcoidosis, interstitial diseases associated with the collagen-vascular disorders, and idiopathic pulmonary fibrosis (Copstead, 2000).

Bronchopulmonary Dysplasia

Characteristic features of BPD include pulmonary edema, airway obstruction, fibrosis, and areas of emphysema alternating with areas of atelectasis. Clinically these changes result in ventilation-perfusion mismatch and lead to hypoxemia (Casey, 1999). The factors most commonly identified in the development of BPD include premature birth and its inherent lung immaturity, surfactant deficiency, and lung injury caused by mechanical ventilation (barotrauma) and oxygen toxicity. Prematurity, and more specifically, low birth weight are recognized as the most important predictors of BPD; it is less commonly observed in term infants with conditions such as pneumonia, meconium aspiration, cyanotic congenital heart disease, and apnea (Hazinski, 1999). When children with BPD have respiratory tract infections that cause consolidation in portions of the lung, they experience acute alterations in gas exchange. Hypoxemia results when the pulmonary capillaries perfuse consolidated and atelectatic alveoli. The extent of consolidation and atelectasis determines the severity of hypoxemia (Kenner, 1998).

Assessment

The NANDA (North American Nursing Diagnosis Association) defining characteristics for impaired gas exchange include confusion, somnolence, restlessness, irritability, hypercapnia, hypoxemia, respiratory rate and depth change, inability to move secretions, shortness of breath, and dyspnea on exertion or at rest (Gordon, 2000). Defining characteristics reported by Carlson-Catalano et al. (1998) are abnormal blood gas levels and expressed fatigue.

Subjective Assessment

Subjective assessment includes data collection with a history of smoking behaviors; environmental risks; frequency, duration, and productivity of cough; wheezing; and recent acute respiratory or chest illnesses. Clients may report feelings of anxiousness, irritability and/or restlessness, and shortness of breath. Subjective symptoms distinguish COPD from asthma (Brewin, 1997). Breathlessness in COPD has a gradual onset with little variation and occurs primarily with activity, whereas in asthma a sudden onset with considerable variation in severity occurs at rest. In COPD, the client reports a chronic productive cough that is more severe in the morning; with asthma, the cough and sputum are acute and more severe at night.

Objective Assessment

Objective assessment of the chest of the client with COPD initially may reveal slowed respirations and wheezing on forced expiration only. As the disease progresses, hyperinflation and increased diameter of the anteroposterior diameter are evident. Impaired gas exchange is reflected in the arterial blood gas values, which are measured while the client breathes room air. The PaO_2 and oxyhemoglobin saturation will be decreased, and the $PaCO_2$ may be increased. Although arterial blood gases remain the standard for determining arterial oxygenation, changes in oxyhemoglobin saturation over time can be detected with noninvasive pulse oximetry. Arterial blood gas values are part of the baseline assessment and determine acid-base status (ATS, 1995).

Goals

The primary nursing goal is for the client to maintain adequate oxygenation without developing complications of oxygen toxicity. Client goals include the following:

1. Demonstrate improved ventilation and adequate oxygenation of tissues
2. Demonstrate normal mental status for client
3. Use effective measures to promote sleep
4. Increase efficiency of energy utilization
5. Improve activities of daily living abilities
6. Demonstrate breathing comfort without dyspnea for activities of daily living (see Table 18-5)

Interventions for Clients with Impaired Gas Exchange

The underlying causes of impaired gas exchange may be related to ineffective airway clearance and ineffective breathing pattern, as described earlier. In most cases, clients will have more than one of the related respiratory problems. Combined approaches will be warranted. If secretions are excessive and tenacious, nursing interventions related to ineffective airway clearance are appropriate; when the underlying problem is an ineffective breathing pattern, then interventions are directed at increasing breathing effectiveness.

TABLE 18-5 Nursing Interventions and Outcomes for Impaired Gas Exchange

Nursing Diagnosis	Suggested Nursing Interventions Classification	Suggested Nursing Outcomes Classification
Impaired gas exchange	Positioning Oxygen therapy Respiratory monitoring	Respiratory status: ventilation Respiratory status: gas exchange Vital signs status: cognitive ability

Data from Johnson, M., Maas, M.L., & Moorhead, S. (2000). *Nursing outcomes classification (NOC)* (2nd ed.). St. Louis: Mosby; McCloskey, J.C., & Bulechek, G.M. (2000). *Nursing interventions classification (NIC)* (3rd ed.). St. Louis: Mosby; and North American Nursing Diagnosis Association. (2001). *Nursing diagnosis: definitions and classification 2001-2002* (4th ed.). Philadelphia: Author.

Positioning

Assisting the client to lean forward at a 30- to 40-degree angle with the arms resting on the thighs or an overhead table may relieve breathlessness (ATS, 1995). Since the client is unable to use the accessory muscles of respiration, leaning forward allows more air to be removed from the lungs on exhalation and improves the upward action of the diaphragm. Position influences pulmonary function and is critical for maximum respiratory function in clients with spinal cord injury. In clients with quadriplegia or paraplegia, significant decreases in forced vital capacity (FVC) can occur with changes in posture. Assess the client's tolerance during moves from supine to upright positions, and alter therapies based on tolerance to the postural changes (Frownfelter & Dean, 1996).

Clients with unilateral lung disease are positioned from side to side routinely because gravity offers dependent portions of the lung a greater proportion of ventilation and perfusion. When the client is upright the bases receive a greater proportion of ventilation and perfusion than the apex; when the client is side-lying, the dependent lung receives the greater proportion. Clients with unilateral lung involvement have the highest arterial oxygen levels when they alternate between the semi-Fowler's position and side-lying with the uninvolved lung down every 60 to 90 minutes (Frownfelter & Dean, 1996). The heart and blood vessels may compress the lung more when the client lying on the left side; consequently, clinical guidelines call for positioning clients with unilateral lung involvement with the uninvolved side down. The client with bilateral lung involvement rests with the head elevated and on the right side (Frownfelter & Dean, 1996).

Oxygen Therapy

Oxygen is considered part of the pharmaceutical management of the client. Oxygen therapy does not treat the underlying cause of hypoxemia but does decrease the cardiopulmonary workload, allows the client to breathe easier, and reduces the effects of hypoxemia. Intermittent use of oxygen therapy can reduce breathlessness associated with exertion in COPD or restrictive lung conditions. Many clients resist the use of oxygen therapy because it symbolizes a worsening of their condition, and they may consider it inconvenient and limiting to their activities. Allow the client early on to adjust to the idea of oxygen use and its future benefits and to actively participate in selecting the type of oxygen delivery system. Educate clients that oxygen is as important as other medications and is the only therapy shown to be associated with decreased mortality in COPD (Rochester & Ferranti, 1998).

Long-term oxygen therapy (LTOT) is often prescribed for clients with severe hypoxemic COPD and to treat children who have varying degrees of respiratory insufficiency from multiple causes (Voter & Chalanick, 1996). Oxygen therapy may allow a client to return home, prolong life, and improve quality of life, but it does have potential toxicity and complications if used improperly. Although high oxygen concentrations are uncommon in rehabilitation, concentrations of oxygen for more than 24 hours may be toxic.

Clients with severe COPD are likely to require LTOT to accomplish several goals: prevention of pulmonary hypertension and cor pulmonale, reduction of secondary polycythemia, and improvement of mental functioning and exercise tolerance (Rees & Dudley, 1998; ATS, 1995). Findings over 5 years of research indicate that long-term oxygen therapy improves the quality of life and neuropsychological function and increases exercise tolerance (Rochester & Ferranti, 1998). However, a review of four randomized clinical trials concluded that LTOT improved the survival rate only in COPD clients with severe hypoxemia but not in those with moderate hypoxia or those who have arterial oxygen desaturation only at night (Crockett, Moss, Cranston, & Alpers, 1999).

Carbon dioxide retention must be evaluated when a client is breathing with an increased fraction of oxygen. It is known that carbon dioxide may rise due to a blunted hypercapnic respiratory drive that results from chronic carbon dioxide retention. Hypoxic drive becomes more critical so that an increase in inspired oxygen may actually improve the oxygen level while also reducing ventilation and increasing CO_2 pressure.

Another consideration for oxygen therapy is that higher levels of inspired oxygen may also increase the amount of wasted perfusion of poorly ventilated lung, causing greater mismatch of ventilation and perfusion. Thus, when LTOT is prescribed, the arterial blood gases are measured both when the client is on and off the planned oxygen regimen (Rees & Dudley, 1998).

Controlled low-flow oxygen (1 or 2 L) is recommended for part or all 24 hours of the day for clients with a PaO_2 level less than or equal to 55 mm Hg or a SaO_2 level less than or equal to 88%. An additional 1 L may be provided during exercise or sleep if oxygen desaturation occurs (ATS, 1995). Since the respiratory drive of the client with COPD is stimulated by a need for oxygen, oxygen delivery should not be increased beyond the level necessary to maintain adequate blood gas values. Low-flow oxygen should raise the PaO_2 value to 60 or 65 mm Hg or the O_2 saturation to 90% to 94%, as measured by oximetry.

Home Oxygen Therapy

A physician or nurse practitioner prescribes oxygen based on medical necessity and specific guidelines adopted by medicare for reimbursement. Recent changes in reimbursement (Health Care Financing Administration [HCFA]) to durable medical equipment vendors for oxygen delivery systems resulted in decreases in reimbursement levels of 25% in 1998 and an additional 5% in 1999 (Consensus Conference Report, 1999). Medicare reimbursement, most private insurance carriers, and the Department of Veterans Affairs authorize home oxygen use for conditions in which the PaO_2 level is less than 55 mm Hg or the SaO_2 level is less than 88% (ATS, 1995).

Clients also are eligible for home oxygen coverage if they have cor pulmonale with a PaO_2 level of 55 to 59 mm Hg or an SaO_2 level greater than or equal to 89% and one of the following secondary diagnoses:

1. Dependent edema, which suggests congestive heart failure; cor pulmonale on ECG; or erythrocytosis with a hematocrit value greater than 55%
2. During sleep the PaO_2 level drops to or less than 55 mm Hg or drops more than 10 mm Hg or the SaO_2 level drops to or less than 85% or drops more than 5%
3. During exercise the PaO_2 level drops to or less than 55 mm Hg or the SaO_2 level drops to or less than 85%

A certificate of medical necessity (HCFA form 484) must be completed when prescribing home oxygen. The prescription must clearly specify the number of liters per minute, minimal number of hours per day for nocturnal use, oxygen source, the method of delivery (e.g., nasal prongs), and the need for portable oxygen with conditions for use. For medicare reimbursement the prescription for oxygen must additionally include the specific respiratory diagnosis and duration, (e.g., 3 months). Arterial blood gas values are the criteria used to document the need for LTOT (Rochester & Ferranti, 1998).

Oxygen Delivery Systems. There are three methods for delivery of O_2 in the home: compressed gas in tanks or cylinders, liquid oxygen in reservoirs, and oxygen concentrators and enrichers (ATS, 1995). Refer to Table 18-6 for a more detailed description of these methods. A variety of systems are available to administer oxygen depending on the client's clinical condition, concentration of oxygen needed, degree of ventilatory support required, and his or her ability and/or desire to adhere to the therapy.

The dual-prong nasal cannula is a simple, effective way to administer low to moderate oxygen concentrations for the client with hypoxemia whose condition is stable. Each liter per minute of oxygen flow adds about 3% to 4% to the concentration of oxygen in inspired air (FiO_2) (ATS, 1995), and humidification is not required when oxygen flow rates are less than 5 L/minute. Advantages are ease of administration and the client does not have to interrupt oxygen flow to eat, cough, and perform other activities. Cannulas can cause nasal irritation, even when the oxygen is humidified. Small amounts of a water-soluble lubricant applied to the nares can reduce or prevent discomfort. Clients who are mouth breathers benefit despite receiving less oxygen since COPD improves with only low levels of flow (Dunn & Chisholm, 1998).

A basic oxygen mask is used to deliver high concentrations of oxygen in acute situations, for clients who breathe through the mouth, or for clients with advanced disease and/or severe hypoxemia. Disadvantages are that oxygen concentrations can vary depending on how tightly the mask fits the face, the level of respiratory effort, and removal of the mask to eat or speak. Oxygen masks can be combined with humidity and/or medication for aerosol therapy. When oxygen concentrations of less than 35% are required, the aerosol can be delivered by compressed air.

Although not commonly used in rehabilitation or in the home, several high-flow oxygen masks are available. The partial rebreathing mask consists of a tightly fitting mask connected to a reservoir bag and can deliver oxygen concentrations of approximately 90% to 100%. The oxygen flow rate is set between 5 and 10 L/minute to prevent the reservoir bag from completely collapsing during inspiration and to provide the system with a continuous oxygen supply. A portion of the client's exhaled gas re-enters the reservoir bag—hence the name—as it fills between breaths. The portion of exhaled gas that enters the bag is the first exhale from the respiratory tract and therefore has low CO_2 levels. The partial rebreathing mask is used primarily to deliver high concentrations of oxygen for short periods. Clients with COPD who retain carbon dioxide must receive oxygen through a controlled oxygen therapy system. The Venturi mask provides fixed concentrations of oxygen in ranges from 24% to 40% (Dunn & Chisholm, 1998).

T-pieces are used to deliver continuous oxygen through a tracheostomy tube. Humidification of inspired oxygen is necessary even at low flow rates of 1 L/minute since the upper airway passages are bypassed by the tracheostomy. The T-piece is a hard plastic tube in the shape of a T. The bottom

TABLE 18-6 Types of Oxygen Systems

Type	Advantages	Disadvantages	Important Information
Compressed gas	Ability to deliver 100% oxygen with accuracy over a wide range of liter-per-minute flow	Large, heavy unit with limited capacity	Back pressure-compensated flowmeter called for when long tubing is used with smaller E tank
Liquid oxygen	Small, light, and portable system (<10 lb)	Expensive; loses small amount of oxygen if not used	Ideal for the active patient: check insurance coverage
Oxygen concentrators	Most economical and efficient system	Not suitable for patients requiring high flow rates; somewhat noisy, and backup gas system is required in case of power outage	Does increase electric bill; most suitable for homebound patients

of the T is attached directly to the tracheostomy tube, and one of the other two ends is attached to the humidified oxygen source; the third end remains open. A tracheostomy mask also may be used to deliver humidified oxygen or medicated aerosol through a tracheostomy tube.

Alternative Delivery Systems. A number of alternative delivery systems are available to conserve oxygen and conceal the nasal prongs and tubing. Examples of these are oxygen pendants and eyeglasses with concealed oxygen tubing leading to nasal prongs. The pendant conserves oxygen, which is important because the portable oxygen tanks last longer, enabling clients to be away from home longer. The eyeglasses conceal the nasal prongs and add cosmetic improvements.

Transtracheal oxygen systems deliver supplemental oxygen directly into the trachea via a small plastic cannula that is inserted into the trachea at the base of the neck. These systems are less conspicuous than nasal prongs. A lower flow rate is required because oxygen is delivered continuously and directly into the trachea throughout inspiration and expiration, bypassing part of the anatomical dead space. Humidification of oxygen is necessary. Advantages of the system are increased portability, mobility, and comfort. Complications of transtracheal oxygen delivery are infrequent and mild, including catheter displacement, subcutaneous emphysema, and infection. The best candidates for transtracheal oxygen delivery are clients who have a strong desire to remain active, are willing to follow the care protocol, have few exacerbations, and identify a caregiver willing to actively participate in the care (ATS, 1995) (Figure 18-5).

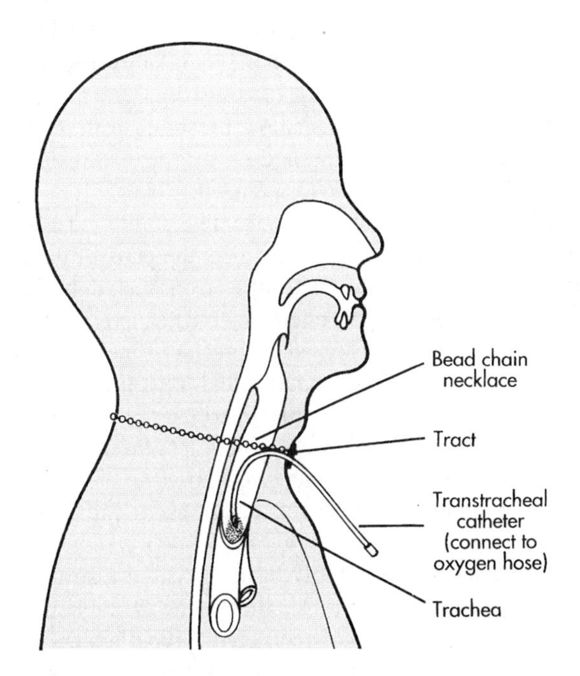

Figure 18-5 Transtracheal oxygen catheter. (From Lewis, S.M., Collier, I.C., Heitkemper, M.M., & Dirksen, S.R. [2000]. *Medical-surgical nursing: Assessment and management of clinical problems* [5th ed.]. St. Louis: Mosby.)

Once the respiratory tract has matured, catheter care begins with daily removal for washing with tap water and antibacterial soap. While in place, the catheter is irrigated twice daily with normal saline solution to prevent mucous balls from accumulating on the distal end, occluding the catheter and causing a buildup of pressure in the tubing. A "pop" when disconnecting the catheter indicates obstruction of oxygen flow.

The reservoir nasal cannula and pulse-dose demand valve device are noninvasive systems that conserve oxygen by restricting flow to the inspiratory phase of ventilation. With the reservoir system, oxygen flows continuously into the reservoir and is inhaled from the reservoir during inspiration. This system is designed with two styles: a pendant device, with standard nasal prongs and the reservoir located in a pendant at the neck, and a mustache device (which resembles a mustache), with the reservoir attached directly to the nasal prongs. The pulse-dose demand valve device conserves oxygen by sensing the beginning of inhalation and immediately delivering a bolus of oxygen (ATS, 1995). Both systems require some nasal breathing on inspiration and expiration to trigger the devices. Clients who are mouth breathers have to use a traditional system at night or the system may not be triggered, resulting in a drop in the SaO_2 level.

Education and Monitoring

Clients with COPD reduce the hours of oxygen use because they tend to sleep fewer hours and often dislike the appearance of the oxygen delivery system. Some clients associate the need for oxygen therapy with deterioration of their condition rather than as prolonging life and improving quality of life. Reframing the perception of oxygen as a drug to increase functional level and using a less conspicuous delivery system may help. The nurse must reinforce that the benefits of oxygen therapy will not be fully realized unless the client adheres to the prescribed regimen.

Since clinical signs of hypoxemia may not always be present, the nurse monitors the PaO_2 and SaO_2 levels to determine the need for and evaluation of oxygen therapy. For continuous monitoring, pulse oximetry is preferred to repeating measures of arterial blood gas values under most conditions. Pulse oximetry is *not* considered an adequate substitute for the measurement of arterial blood gases in an initial assessment or for determining blood gas values. Appropriate oxygen therapy is based on knowledge of the client's arterial blood gas values and pH. Oxygen therapy usually is titrated to maintain a PaO_2 level of 60 to 100 mm Hg, as measured by arterial blood gases, or a SaO_2 level greater than 90%, as measured by pulse oximetry. If the oxygen delivery formula is determined while the client is awake and seated upright, it may be necessary to increase the flow rate 1 L/minute during sleep.

Pulse oximetry measures total Hb saturation and does not distinguish between Hb saturation with oxygen and carbon monoxide. This is a problem with heavy smokers, because heavy smoking increases carbon monoxide levels in the blood. A heavy smoker may have a carboxyhemoglobin saturation of 8% and an oxyhemoglobin saturation of 90%, but the pulse oximeter will register 98% Hb saturation. Consequently the pulse oximeter is most useful in monitoring changes in Hb saturation in clients who are not smoking; significant changes should be verified with arterial blood gas values. Small portable pulse oximetry devices are well suited for monitoring clients continuously at rest or during exercise and for use at home to document for medicare reimbursement.

Air Travel and Oxygen Therapy

Air travel by individuals using supplemental oxygen is more commonplace today despite poor standardization of in-flight oxygen by the Federal Aviation Administration or individual airlines. The oxygen delivery system and flow rates vary considerably by airline, but all carriers offer nasal cannula delivery. Generally, airlines require 48 to 72 hour advanced notification of oxygen need by the individual's physician. Actual charges for in-flight oxygen vary from free to a fee that may be as high as $1500. It is important that potential travelers be counseled to consider charges for in-flight oxygen when selecting an airline (Stoller, Hoisington, & Auger, 1999).

Outcome Criteria

For the client with impaired gas exchange, the following outcome criteria are identified. The client will demonstrate adequate gas exchange as evidenced by the following:

1. Normal rate, rhythm, and depth of respirations for client; PaO_2 levels at 65 to 80 mm Hg and a SaO_2 level to 85% or within normal ranges for client.
2. Mental status within expected range.
3. Usual color of skin and mucous membranes.
4. Client states that sleep is adequate and uninterrupted.
5. Client states that energy level is adequate.
6. Client states breathing is comfortable and without dyspnea during activities of daily living.

INEFFECTIVE BREATHING PATTERN

Ineffective breathing pattern is defined as respiration inadequate to maintain sufficient oxygen supply for cellular requirements (Gordon, 2000). Effective breathing requires normal lung and airway structures; a feedback mechanism involving the nervous system structures that control respiration (peripheral chemoreceptors, central chemoreceptors, and respiratory neurons of the pons and medulla); intact nerve pathways to the muscles of respiration; and an intact structure of the chest wall. Damage in these components results in ventilatory failure when alveolar ventilation is insufficient to accomplish adequate gas exchange.

Dyspnea and fatigue were found to be the defining characteristics of ineffective breathing pattern (Carlson-Catalano et al., 1998). In rehabilitation, nurses most commonly address chronic problems related to ineffective breathing patterns, such as those seen in clients with obstructive lung disease and with restrictive lung disease.

Alterations in Ventilation

Alveolar hyperventilation and hypoventilation are clinically defined by the $PaCO_2$ value. Hyperventilation causes the $PaCO_2$ to fall to less than 35 mm Hg (Longenecker, 1998), usually in clients who are breathing rapidly for an extended period. Hyperventilation is a normal response to a high altitude environment, but it also appears in clients who have greatly increased anxiety levels. In contrast, alveolar hypoventilation causes the $PaCO_2$ level to rise above 45 mm Hg. Hypoventilation occurs in individuals with severe lung disease and neuromuscular disease. Ventilatory failure is the extreme form of alveolar hypoventilation, characterized by a $PaCO_2$ level greater than 45 mm Hg and a PaO_2 level less than 60 mm Hg (Frownfelter & Dean, 1996).

Alveolar hypoventilation results from either an inadequate V_E and/or an excessive V_{DS}. Inadequate V_E can be caused by alterations in respiratory mechanics, inadequate ventilatory drive, and respiratory muscle weakness. Excessive V_{DS} can be caused by either the mismatch of ventilation and perfusion or by shallow breathing.

Obstructive Defects

Clients with very severe COPD are more likely to experience chronic alveolar hypoventilation, as evidenced by chronic hypercapnia. Hypercapnia is seen most commonly in clients with COPD with a FEV_1 of less than 1 L. The precise mechanisms for the development of alveolar hypoventilation are not well understood in clients with COPD, but evidence points to blunting of the ventilatory response to chemical stimuli, such as hypoxia and hypercapnia, and/or the development of rapid shallow breathing patterns to reduce the work of breathing and protect against respiratory muscle fatigue (Montes de Oca & Celli, 2000).

In infancy, significant areas of vulnerability exist within the respiratory system. Box 18-5 lists the parts of the pediatric respiratory anatomy that differ from the adult respiratory anatomy. In pediatric clients with BPD, hypoventilation and hypercapnia are observed as a result of ineffective ventilation due to airway damage and obstruction (Casey, 1999). Characteristic interstitial markings or strand densities are evidenced on the chest radiograph. Pulmonary function is compromised by increased airway resistance, decreased compliance, increased dead space, and increased airway reactivity.

Adult clients with COPD have increased airway resistance, and respiratory muscles must generate higher forces to maintain a given level of ventilation. Hyperinflation of the chest wall places the inspiratory muscles at a mechanical disadvantage to generate the higher forces, and nutritional deficits impede muscle strength and mass. These clients are predisposed to respiratory muscle fatigue and rapid shallow

Box 18-5 Pediatric Anatomy and Physiology of the Respiratory System: Special Considerations in Children

There are many anatomical and physiological differences in children that predispose them to respiratory compromise. In a child with a respiratory disease process or condition, the differences only increase the risk of respiratory compromise.

1. Central nervous system control of breathing is immature in infants.
2. Airways in infants and children are much smaller compared with an adult.
3. In children, distal airways develop more slowly than proximal airways, providing increased resistance to airflow.
4. Supportive airway cartilage is not fully developed until school age, making it more prone to collapse.
5. The pediatric larynx is anterior and cephalad.
6. Neonates and infants are obligate nose breathers, so any obstruction of the nasal passages can become a critical threat.
7. The tongue is larger in proportion to the mouth, increasing the likelihood of airway obstruction.
8. There are decreased numbers of alveoli available for gas exchange, which contributes to a decreased respiratory reserve.
9. The chest wall is compliant due to cartilaginous ribs. Furthermore, the chest wall retracts during respiratory distress, reducing the young child's ability to maintain functional residual capacity.
10. The intercostal muscles are not fully developed until school age and may lack power, tone, and coordination, especially during times of respiratory distress.
11. The diaphragm is the primary muscle of respiration; therefore, anything that interferes with diaphragmatic movement can compromise ventilation.
12. Oxygen consumption is higher in infants and children (6-8 ml/kg/min) compared with that of an adult (3-4 ml/kg/min). Therefore, when apnea or inadequate ventilation develops in a child, hypoxia can occur more rapidly.
13. Children suffer an increased number of respiratory infections compared with the adult population.
14. Respiratory compromise accounts for the majority of pediatric arrests, *not* cardiac compromise.

breathing, which increases the V_{DS}. With severe COPD, the mismatch of ventilation and perfusion contributes to alveolar hypoventilation.

Restrictive Defects

Clients with neuromuscular disease develop alveolar hypoventilation secondary to respiratory muscle weakness and decreased compliance of the lungs and chest wall. Weakened inspiratory muscles make them unable to take a deep breath, leading to a decline in V_E. Secondly, the reduced VC leads to microatelectasis and increased stiffness of the chest wall, thereby increasing the work of breathing and further contributing to the decline in V_E.

In the early stages of neuromuscular disease, mild respiratory muscle weakness can exist without clinical consequences if the respiratory muscles are capable of meeting ventilatory demands and generating an effective cough. Respiratory muscle fatigue and ventilatory failure occur when the ventilatory demands exceed the ability of the respiratory muscles.

The extent of respiratory muscle involvement depends on the nature of the pathophysiology and its pattern of progression. In Duchenne's muscular dystrophy, respiratory muscle weakness appears early in the course of the disease and progresses slowly until death (Lyager, Steffensen, & Juhl, 1995). In amyotrophic lateral sclerosis (ALS), respiratory muscle weakness is secondary to denervation atrophy, beginning with the expiratory abdominal muscles and eventually progressing to the inspiratory muscles. In ALS the progression of respiratory muscle weakness is faster than in other neuromuscular diseases. In persons with spinal cord injury, the extent of respiratory muscle involvement depends on the level and nature of the injury. Persons with high cervical lesions (above C4) typically require mechanical ventilation; with midcervical lesions (C4 to C8) they experience severe expiratory muscle weakness and/or paralysis and mild inspiratory muscle weakness. Many spinal cord injury lesions are oblique, interrupting innervation to one side of the diaphragm and producing severe diaphragmatic weakness on only one side.

Combined Obstructive and Restrictive Defects

Clients with CF have two abnormal copies of a defective CF gene, that in turn, codes for a defective or mutant cystic fibrosis transmembrane regulator (CFTR) protein. With a mutant CFTR protein, chloride movement is inhibited, and the balance of sodium, chloride, and water is disrupted in affected cells. This imbalance results in classic findings in CF: dehydrated secretions and mucous obstruction in the ducts of exocrine glands (Hudson & Guill, 1998).

CF affects multiple organ systems to varying degrees in different individuals, but lung disease is the major cause of morbidity and mortality. Generally, clients with normal pancreatic function have milder lung disease, possibly related to improved nutritional status. The lung disease in CF results from an ongoing cycle of obstruction, infection, inflammation, and injury, with resultant restrictive elements. Dehydrated secretions block airway passages. These secretions also contain large amounts of uninhibited proteolytic enzymes, which contribute to tissue injury and impaired mucociliary transport (Hudson et al., 1998). Obstruction leads to endobronchial infection. Two bacteria primarily responsible for infections in the CF lung—*Staphylococcus aureus* and *Pseudomonas aeruginosa*—will continue to colonize the CF lung. Antimicrobial therapies that reduce bacterial colony counts offer clinical improvement.

Chronic obstruction and infection cause progressive deterioration of lung structure and function. Early changes, more prominent in the upper lobes, include air trapping; airway inflammation; and peribronchial thickening, which contribute to restrictive symptoms. As lung injury continues, changes become more diffuse with evidence of bronchiectasis, fibrosis, and cyst formation. When fibrosis develops in some tissues, restrictive lung disease compounds what began as obstructive lung disease. Box 18-6 contains a summary of mechanisms.

Subjective Assessment

Clients have a subjective feeling that ventilation requirements are not being met, and dyspnea is the chief complaint with ineffective breathing patterns. Clinical assessment includes the client's perception of the frequency, intensity, and contributing factors. Various scales (previously discussed) can be used to quantify the client's perception of dyspnea. Research suggests that worsening dyspnea is not directly related to changes in lung impairment (Lareau, Meek, Press, Anholm, & Roos, 1999). Perceptions of fatigue, another subjective complaint, are explored as to severity, time of day, and possible underlying causes. Reports of snoring, apneic episodes during sleep, and excessive daytime sleepiness indicate sleep pattern disturbance.

Objective Assessment

On physical examination, pay particular attention to changes in mental status, use of accessory muscles of respiration, pursed-lip breathing, and paradoxical abdominal breathing—findings that suggest ineffective breathing patterns and ventilatory failure (Madison & Irwin, 1998). Investigate signs of airflow obstruction, wheezing during auscultation, a prolonged forced expiratory time, obesity, and the need to assume unusual positions to relieve dyspnea.

Pulmonary function testing differentiates between restrictive and obstructive lung disease, but results are more difficult to interpret with mixed restrictive and obstructive disease. In obstructive lung disease, the time needed to forcefully exhale after full inspiration is increased; the FEV_1/FVC ratio will be low. In restrictive lung disease, air can be expelled rapidly; the FEV/FVC ratio will be high. Spirometry can measure the volume of air expelled from fully inflated lungs (Petty, 1998).

Goals

The primary nursing goals for the client with ineffective breathing pattern are to maximize ventilation and improve airflow. Client goals include the following:

1. Ventilation parameters in expected range
2. Adequate breathing pattern noted during sleep
3. No or minimal complaints of dyspnea or breathlessness at rest
4. Decreased complaints of dyspnea or breathlessness with activity
5. Decreased anxiety levels
6. Increased activity levels (Table 18-7)

Interventions for Clients with Ineffective Breathing Patterns

Nursing management is aimed at maintaining adequate ventilation through assistance, exercise training, mechanical ventilation, electrical phrenic stimulation, and anxiety reduction.

Ventilation Assistance. Persons with ineffective breathing pattern may benefit from breathing retraining techniques such as pursed-lip breathing (PLB), abdominal-diaphragmatic breathing, segmental breathing, and glossopharyngeal breathing (GPB). Breathing retraining is designed to (1) assist the client in controlling breathing patterns, (2) promote ventilation through effective breathing patterns, and (3) relieve symptoms of dyspnea.

Box 18-6 Mechanisms for Altered Ventilatory Patterns

Restrictive Lung Disease: Decreased Expansion of the Lungs

Disease states: Degenerative neuromuscular diseases, spinal cord injury, scoliosis, bony deformities of the chest wall, interstitial pulmonary fibrosis

Clinical presentation: With increasing weakness and fatigue of the respiratory muscles, clients may develop uncoordinated breathing and alternate between use of the muscles of the chest wall and the diaphragm to breathe. Paradoxical breathing (inward displacement of the abdomen with inspiration) is seen as the diaphragm weakens. Respiratory impairment can be either unilateral or bilateral, temporary or permanent. Paradoxical movement of the abdomen on inspiration becomes especially pronounced in the supine position because the diaphragm cannot fall passively.

Obstructive Lung Disease: Increased Resistance to Airflow

Disease states: Emphysema, chronic bronchitis, asthma, BPD, some cystic fibrosis

Clinical presentation: During quiet breathing, clients with moderate to severe COPD commonly demonstrate an increased respiratory rate with a normal tidal volume and V_E, even when their lung condition is stable and they are in their best state of health. During an exacerbation and/or during an episode of respiratory failure, the respiratory rate will further increase and the V_E will decrease, producing rapid, shallow breathing. The precise mechanisms for altered breathing patterns in individuals with COPD may include respiratory muscle fatigue with declines in maximum inspiratory force, and injury to the airways with subsequent stimulation of irritant receptors.

Pursed-Lip Breathing. *PLB* is a technique of exhaling slowly through partially closed, or "pursed," lips. By controlling expiration and maximum emptying of the alveoli, PLB reduces respiratory rate, minute ventilation, and carbon dioxide levels and increases tidal volume, arterial oxygen pressure, and oxygen saturation (ATS, 1999). Clients with COPD may gain some control over breathing patterns but are cautioned about increased breathlessness at rest and during exercise (Breslin et al., 1996). When teaching a client, the nurse may explain that exhaling with pursed lips increases the resistance to both the outflow and the airway pressure. The small airways remain open longer to allow more air to be exhaled. Exhalation lasts two or three times longer than inhalation to effectively empty the lungs of trapped air.

To perform PLB, instruct the client to inhale slowly through the nose (with mouth closed) and to pause slightly at the end of inspiration, then exhale slowly while relaxed through pursed lips. Folding the arms across the abdomen while sitting and bending forward while exhaling further aids complete emptying of the lungs. Counting during the technique helps pace exhalation at two or three times as long as inspiration.

Diaphragmatic Breathing. *Diaphragmatic breathing* exercises traditionally have been used in pulmonary rehabilitation to increase efficiency of the respiratory muscles while reducing the ineffective movements of the rib cage. Several studies, however, have found that diaphragmatic breathing actually reduces the mechanical efficiency of the chest wall and increases the work of breathing (Vitacca, Clini, Bianchi, & Ambrosino, 1998; Gosselink, Wagenaar, Sargeant, Rijswijk, & Decramer, 1995). One study demonstrated increased, rather than decreased, intensity of dyspnea with diaphragmatic breathing (Gosselink et al., 1995). The American Thoracic Society does not recommend routine use of diaphragmatic breathing as a training protocol for persons with COPD in pulmonary rehabilitation (ATS, 1999); however, diaphragmatic breathing been shown to strengthen a partially paralyzed diaphragm in persons with spinal cord injury. When a client is partially paralyzed, placing your hand on the diaphragm helps focus attention on it, even though the client may not be able to feel your hand (Frownfelter & Dean, 1996).

Clients who may benefit from GPB (previously described) include those who are dependent on mechanical ventilation due to respiratory muscle paralysis but who can tolerate short periods without ventilatory support and clients who have intact mental status and bulbar musculature without any obstructive lung disease. GPB also can increase voice volume for clients not dependent on a ventilator.

Exercise. *Exercise training* is foundational for pulmonary rehabilitation and may be integrated into a home or facility based program. Exercise has positive effects on dyspnea and minimizes the effects of deconditioning (Berry, Rejeski, Adair, & Zaccaro, 1999; ATS, 1999; San Pedro, 1999). Research findings indicate that specific muscle groups can be strengthened with regular training for 20 to 30 minutes, two to five times per week. Either interval or continuous training at up to 60% of maximal workload may be possible. Clients with respiratory disease usually find interval training easier to tolerate and more enjoyable than continuous bouts of training. Interval training alternates periods of work with periods of rest and elicits training effects similar to continuous training regimens. The following section describes exercises performed at home or in rehabilitation with supervision.

Upper Extremity Exercise. Clients with severe COPD report a marked increase in the perception of dyspnea with routine tasks that require arm use, especially activities associated with unsupported arm elevation (LaCasse, Guyatt, & Goldstein, 1997). Merely raising the arm increases the metabolic demand and ventilatory effort for clients with severe COPD, thus making unsupported arm exercise training a way of enhancing endurance (LaCasse et al., 1997). A simple and inexpensive unsupported arm training exercise for COPD clients is performing lifts with a lightweight dowel rod from waist to shoulder level. Adding weights to the rod will increase resistance as tolerance increases. Providing arm support, such as bracing them on a table, may increase the client's ability to perform common arm tasks.

TABLE 18-7 Nursing Interventions and Outcomes for Ineffective Breathing Pattern

Nursing Diagnosis	Suggested Nursing Interventions Classification	Suggested Nursing Outcomes Classification
Ineffective breathing pattern	Ventilation assistance	Respiratory status: ventilation
	Mechanical ventilation	
	Anxiety reduction	Anxiety control
	Exercise management	Muscle function
	Energy management	Energy conservation

Data from Johnson, M., Maas, M.L., & Moorhead, S. (2000). *Nursing outcomes classification (NOC)* (2nd ed.). St. Louis: Mosby; McCloskey, J.C., & Bulechek, G.M. (2000). *Nursing interventions classification (NIC)* (3rd ed.). St. Louis: Mosby; and North American Nursing Diagnosis Association. (2001). *Nursing diagnosis: definitions and classification 2001-2002* (4th ed.). Philadelphia: Author.

Lower Extremity Exercise. Many methods have been used to accomplish conditioning of the lower extremities, including treadmill walking (Ries, Kaplan, Limberg, & Prewitt, 1995), bicycling (Maltais et al., 1996; Vallet et al., 1997), stair climbing, walking, and swimming. Some experts believe that individuals can improve their condition by walking in corridors and on stairs instead of on treadmills or riding on bicycles because walking has been found to be more enjoyable and more representative of day-to-day activity.

Respiratory Muscle Training. Research findings support the notion that inspiratory muscle training (IMT) can be used to improve strength and endurance of the respiratory muscles, primarily in clients with COPD (Breslin, 1997). The training requires either an alinear resistive breathing device or a linear resistive breathing device. With either device the client performs IMT by breathing in and out through the device, generating high airway pressures during inspiration and normal airway pressures during expiration. The client must work hard during inspiration, whereas expiration is normal and relaxed.

There is some evidence that improvement in inspiratory muscle strength results in decreased breathlessness and increased respiratory muscle endurance (Hamilton, Killian, & Jones, 1995). Benefits of respiratory muscle training are not well-established, and it is unclear whether results signify improvements in symptoms or disability. Further research is required to establish the role for respiratory muscle training and the target specific groups it may benefit.

Outcome Assessment of Exercise Training. A group of standard outcome assessment tools are available to evaluate the effectiveness of techniques and programs. An individual's progress can be measured by incremental and submaximal exercise tests and walking tests. General health status can be evaluated with questionnaires such as St. George's Respiratory Disease Questionnaire, Pulmonary Functional Status Scale (PFSS), the Functional Performance Inventory (FPI), and other functional instruments. Exertional dyspnea can be quantified with the use of a visual analog scale (VAS) rating and the category rating (Borg) during exercise testing. Overall dyspnea may be evaluated with the Medical Research Council Scale (MRC), the Baseline Dyspnea Index (BDI), and the Transitional Dyspnea Index (TDI) (ATS, 1999).

Energy Conservation Techniques. Clients who use energy conservation techniques will enhance functional ability by performing activities when they work slowly, use proper muscle groups and body mechanics, and alternate work with rest periods. By coordinating breathing techniques with specific activities, a client can take full mechanical advantage of muscle movement to assist breathing during self-care activities. Techniques that reduce dyspnea include the following:

1. Inhaling before bending, then exhaling slowly through pursed lips while bending, and then inhaling again while returning to the upright position.
2. Moving the arms forward away from the side, or above the head, which elevates the chest and assists with inspiration.
3. Putting the hands on the hips at frequent intervals or moving the arms away from the body on inspiration while performing ADLs, such as bathing or dressing.

In addition, specific energy saving strategies will assist the client to maximize his or her energy use. Suggestions are to wear a terry cloth bathrobe after bathing to reduce the need to towel dry, sit on a stool while showering, use arm rests and hand bars for support, place items at waist height in the home, and consume foods that can be cooked in a microwave or prepared by other less time-consuming methods.

Altered Sleep Patterns. Respiratory abnormalities may cause alterations in sleep patterns, including sleep fragmentation, nocturnal oxygenation and heart rate disturbances, and resulting daytime sleepiness. Clients with COPD who snore may have obstructive sleep apnea. A recent study demonstrated that clients with COPD who snore have poor sleep quality with nocturnal hypoxemia and heart rate disorders similar to those observed in COPD clients with severe obstructive sleep apnea (Kosmas, Toukmatzi, Polychroniaki, & Damianos, 1998). Positive airway pressure treatment including bi-level (BIPAP) or continuous positive airway pressure (CPAP) support by mask can provide relief for clients with these altered sleep patterns (Loube et al, 1999; McArdle et al., 1999). These noninvasive therapies have been shown to be beneficial for clients with a wide range of both restrictive and obstructive pulmonary and neuromuscular disorders (Consensus Conference Report, 1999). Diagnostic strategies, including sleep studies, determine the best treatment strategy for individuals.

Ventilatory Support Devices. Noninvasive ventilatory support devices are mechanical means to move the chest wall by manually pushing on the stomach, chest, or back. They do not require an artificial airway, but the chest wall must be capable of effective movement. Noninvasive support devices have proven useful in respiratory muscle paralysis associated with neurological disease or injury but are inappropriate for clients with COPD. The most commonly used ventilatory support devices are rocking beds and pneumobelts.

Rocking Beds. *Rocking beds* assist ventilation by using gravity and the pressure of the abdominal contents to alternately apply and remove pressure on the diaphragm. When the client's body is tilted with the head up, the abdominal contents fall, and the diaphragm is pulled downward to assist with inhalation. Exhalation is assisted when the body is tilted head-down and the abdominal contents push against the diaphragm for expiration. Rocking beds are simple to operate and maintain and are noninvasive. Unfortunately, many clients cannot tolerate the rocking motion, nor does it control tidal volumes. The bed is best for clients who are bedridden or when used as a nighttime alternative to a ventilator.

Pneumobelts. *Pneumobelts* consist of an inflatable rubber bladder inside a corset worn around the abdomen and are most effective when a person sits upright, as in a wheelchair. As the bladder inflates, it pushes the abdominal contents up against the diaphragm, assisting with expiration. When the bladder deflates, abdominal contents and the diaphragm drop, assisting with inhalation. The pneumobelt connects to a positive pressure generator with 15 to 50 cm H_2O pressure. Some clients find the belt uncomfortable, and it does not control tidal volumes. Clients with a progressive condition may necessitate more extensive assistance; mechanical ventilation is the next step.

Mechanical Ventilation. Although care of clients who receive mechanical ventilation is primarily an acute aspect of respiratory care, some individuals require long-term mechanical ventilation. They have chronic, underlying lung disease, such as emphysema, or a neurological impairment resulting from cervical spinal cord injuries. Two commonly used ventilation devices are negative-pressure ventilators (NPVs) and positive-pressure ventilators (PPVs) (Marino, 1999).

Negative-Pressure Ventilators. NPVs that were used during the 1950s and 1960s to provide mechanical ventilation to victims of poliomyelitis have been less popular since PPVs were introduced (see Figure 1-1). Cuirass respirators replaced the "iron lung" as an alternative to the PPVs. Individuals with neuromuscular diseases are candidates for this type of ventilator. The use of a NPV in clients with COPD is not recommended (ATS, 1995). NPVs apply negative pressure around the thorax, creating a pressure gradient inside the thoracic cavity and allowing air to flow into the lungs. Unfortunately, the client is sealed off in the cumbersome device with markedly restricted mobility; however, tracheal intubation is not required.

Positive-Pressure Ventilators. PPV applies positive pressure to the airways to promote inspiration while expiration is passive. An artificial airway usually is necessary to connect the ventilator to the client, although mouthpieces can be used if only intermittent ventilation is required. The two types of PPV devices are pressure-cycled ventilators and volume-cycled ventilators. *Pressure-cycled ventilators* inflate the lungs until a predetermined pressure is reached, at which point inspiration ends and expiration begins. The volume of air delivered to the client can vary with each inspiration, depending on the compliance of the airways. For example, an individual experiencing bronchospasm quickly reaches the pressure set on the ventilator so that only a small volume of air is delivered into the lungs. In contrast, *volume-cycled ventilators* deliver a fixed predetermined tidal volume of air into the lungs; the pressure to deliver this volume of air varies depending on compliance of the lungs and chest wall. A safety valve or pressure-limit device stops the ventilator from continuing the inspiratory cycle at a preset volume, therefore preventing trauma from air being forced into the lungs at too high a pressure. Volume-cycled ventilators are preferable for hospital and home use because of the consistent volume of air delivered to the lungs. The advantages of PPVs over NPVs are better accessibility to the client and increased mobility of the client. Most clients with COPD chose assist-control ventilation, intermittent mandatory ventilation, or pressure support ventilation (ATS, 1995). Some evidence suggests that adding pressure support ventilation increases comfort, promotes client synchrony with the ventilator, and may facilitate weaning for clients with stable COPD and acute respiratory failure who maintain adequate ventilatory drive (Kirton, 1997).

Mechanical Ventilation in the Home. As a rule, ventilators developed for home use are more compact than those used in hospitals. Some self-contained and self-powered ventilators are mounted on motorized wheelchairs. A sufficient oxygen supply and suction equipment allow for mobility for up to 3 hours. Ventilators used in the home can be powered by electricity, batteries, or gas, but backup systems must be available in case of a power outage. In choosing home ventilator equipment, consideration should be given to the home environment, long-term home care commitment by the individual and family, financial considerations, and home support services. Every effort should be made to choose and modify ventilatory support devices according to client and family needs and preferences.

Usually the home physical environment is rearranged to allow room for safe, effective, and efficient operation of the equipment with maximum freedom for the client. Consider the amount of time a client spends in an area of the house or outdoors. Evaluate electrical requirements, ability to maneuver the equipment, safety, temperature, and air control. Establish schedules and equipment checks with vendors of supplies and services, as well as with the local pharmacy. A self-inflating resuscitation bag should also be accessible in case the ventilator has a mechanical failure. An emergency call system and telephone numbers will allow the client to summon help when needed. Service agencies, such as emergency medical services, electrical and telephone companies, and fire or rescue departments, are notified when a client dependent on mechanical ventilation is living in the community.

Home support services may include home health care nurses, home health aides, and respiratory therapists. Respiratory equipment is almost always maintained by the company that supplies the ventilator. Individuals discharged from the hospital with volume-cycled ventilators must understand how to operate the equipment and possible mechanical problems. Although third-party payment is available for home ventilator care, the financial arrangements are changing rapidly and can be confusing and frustrating. Referral to a case manager or social worker to assist with arrangements, planning, and reimbursement will help with the complex needs since programs and regulations vary.

Rehabilitation of persons who are dependent on mechanical ventilation necessitates a team approach. Mechanical ventilation in the home provides certain individuals with an improved quality of life within familiar surroundings and is more cost-effective than institutional care (Frownfelter & Dean, 1996). However, clients with ventilators in the home and their families necessitate frequent evaluation of their physical and psychological management.

Clients requiring long-term mechanical ventilation pose a special nutritional problem. Abdominal distention can occur because of aspiration of air into the stomach, or food may be aspirated into the lungs when a client is intubated. Cuffed tracheostomy tubes are kept inflated during meals and for 1 to 2 hours after meals to prevent aspiration. Adequate nutritional intake is important. Studies show that semistarvation in clients receiving ventilation therapy can lead to a diminished hypoxic drive, especially in clients with COPD, and a diminished hypoxic drive can precipitate respiratory failure (Berry & Braunschweig, 1998).

Differences in upper airway mechanics during sleep and wakefulness may affect air leaks around uncuffed tracheostomies. Monitor the status of any client showing signs of hypoxia and hypercapnia (increased restlessness, confusion, seizures) with oximetry. At night, some clients may require increased levels of ventilation for management.

Weaning. Weaning from mechanical ventilation is the ultimate goal for all clients who require it as a life-prolonging therapy (Manthous, Schmidt, & Hall, 1998). While it is not practical to strive for this goal in all cases, periods of freedom from mechanical ventilation may be possible for many clients. Various weaning parameters provide objective criteria to predict client readiness to sustain spontaneous ventilation with adequate oxygenation. Weaning parameters may include measurements such as inspiratory muscle strength (PImax), airway occlusion pressure, vital capacity, respiratory system compliance, and airway resistance. Although some of these measures are not available in rehabilitation, several integrative indexes have been examined for predictive ability.

One simple index is the Rapid Shallow Breathing Index that measures the respiratory rate: tidal volume ratio (breaths/min/L) during a 1-minute T-piece trial (Manthous et al., 1998). The threshold for weaning is 105 breaths/min/L. Clients who have more rapid and shallow breaths are less successful. Traditional weaning predictors have included a fraction of inspired oxygen of less than 0.5, vital capacity of 10 ml/kg or more, and PImax (or negative inspiratory force [NIF]) of at least -20 cm H_2O (Burns et al., 1995). Generally, the weaning process may be initiated with a vital capacity of at least 800 ml, provided the client is free of infection in secretions and other pulmonary or medical complications.

Several modes of ventilation have proven to be helpful during the weaning process. Pressure support (5 to 8 cm H_2O), CPAP, and T-piece trials are the most common methods used for testing readiness to wean (Manthous et al., 1998). Pressure support, a spontaneous mode of ventilation that delivers a high flow of gas early in inspiration until a predetermined pressure level is reached, has been shown to decrease the work of breathing and decrease oxygen consumption (Burns et al., 1995). CPAP is also a continuous level of positive pressure in the airways used during spontaneous breathing that assists the alveoli to remain open. The T-piece trial is used to provide humidification and oxygen but no ventilatory assistance or positive airway pressure for the client and is recommended by some as the most useful method to test readiness to wean (Manthous et al., 1998). In several studies, CPAP and pressure support were shown to significantly reduce the work of breathing in comparison with the T-piece trial. However, there is inconclusive evidence regarding the superiority of CPAP, T-piece or intermittent mandatory ventilation (IMV); thus, the consensus of research studies indicates that all of these methods are equally effective in supporting the weaning process.

Some clients who receive ventilator assistance require gradual withdrawal or weaning. Surveys have shown that IMV is the most commonly used mode of both ventilatory support and weaning (Burns et al., 1995) and allows clients to breathe spontaneously at their own tidal volume and rate. Spontaneous inspiration allows for cardiac output and venous return that are more physiologically normal than with assisted ventilation. The client receives periodic intermittent breaths from the ventilator, and then less frequently during the weaning process. Theoretically, IMV allows a smooth transition from controlled to spontaneous ventilation by gradually decreasing the mandatory ventilation rate as clients assume an increasing percentage of the total work of breathing. The diaphragm has to work constantly to maintain adequate ventilation. Since IMV is not conducive to strengthening the diaphragmatic muscle, its use is more appropriate in the client with COPD in whom strengthening of the diaphragmatic muscle is not the primary concern. This gradual process theoretically may allow time to strengthen existing respiratory muscles in preparation for withdrawal of ventilatory support.

Most importantly, with all methods, the client's status must be monitored closely for signs of respiratory distress throughout the weaning process. The use of accessory muscles, tachycardia, decrease or increase in blood pressure, tachypnea or bradypnea, and somnolence must be regarded as signs of intolerance to the weaning trial. Continuous oximetry to monitor arterial and venous oxygen saturation is helpful. The client should be encouraged in the use of proper breathing techniques, relaxation techniques to decrease anxiety, and assistive coughing techniques. The weaning process predictably is a time of high anxiety for the client. Psychological support, biofeedback with oximetry, and the use of relaxation techniques have been found to decrease anxiety. The goal of the weaning process is complete withdrawal of ventilatory support. However, each client must be evaluated on an individual basis. Some clients may tolerate breathing without the ventilator only during waking hours, whereas others may tolerate independent breathing indefinitely.

Diaphragmatic Electrophrenic Nerve Pacing Diaphragmatic electrophrenic nerve pacing provides an alternative for some clients (ventilator dependent) with respiratory paralysis who have normal phrenic nerves, diaphragms, and lungs but require ventilatory assistance during the day (Chervin & Guilleminault, 1997; Elefteriades & Quin, 1998). Most often, clients treated with diaphragmatic pacing have had high cervical quadriplegia or central alveolar hypoventilation. Diaphragmatic pacing is accomplished through high-frequency stimulation of the phrenic nerve by radio frequency transmissions from an electrode surgically attached to the phrenic nerve. A receiver implanted subcutaneously and attached to the electrode receives transmission through a battery-operated transmitter.

The major physiological limitation is diaphragmatic muscle fatigue (Chervin & Guilleminault, 1997) that can be minimized with gradual conditioning using low-frequency pacing over 3 to 6 months for adults and a longer period for children as prescribed. However, a four-pole stimulation system may shorten the conditioning time, increasing tolerance for diaphragmatic pacing. Initially, a client's regimen is 1 hour on and 1 hour off; gradually, tolerance may reach 8 to 12 hours.

Family members must be fully informed about potential mishaps and educated to adhere to a regular medical schedule and follow-up visits for the client (Chervin & Guilleminault, 1997). Pulse oximetry with an alarm and memory capacity is necessary for home monitoring. A readily available alternative method of ventilation must be available in the event of pacer failure due to external or internal components. The batteries in the transmitter are replaced each day. An emergency call system should be available to the client in the home. Diaphragmatic pacing can offer long-term advantages to a carefully selected population.

Anxiety Reduction Techniques. Dyspnea is commonly associated with high levels of anxiety, especially in clients with COPD. Taped relaxation messages and muscle relaxation exercises are effective in reducing anxiety associated with dyspnea. Music therapy has been found to be effective in reducing anxiety and promoting relaxation in clients receiving ventilatory assistance (Chlan, 1998). However, most people will not relax unless provided with a specific technique that they believe is effective.

Progressive muscle relaxation is a technique commonly used for pulmonary clients. One system of this technique alternately tenses and relaxes muscle groups. By doing so, the client becomes more aware of the differences between tension and relaxation and better able to achieve a relaxed state (DeMarco-Sinatra, 2000).

Outcome Criteria

For the client with ineffective breathing pattern, the following outcome criteria are identified. The client will demonstrate an effective breathing pattern as evidenced by:

1. Rate, rhythm, depth, and pattern of respiration and blood gas values normal for client.
2. Absence of sleep-disordered breathing.
3. Control of anxiety response.
4. Feelings of effortless breathing with activity.
5. Increased ability to tolerate increased activity levels.

CLIENT AND FAMILY EDUCATION

Education is essential to any pulmonary rehabilitation program. Separate components of a program may be difficult to evaluate, but the education process can promote changes in behaviors and increase clients' participation in learning self-management. Whether in small groups, as part of a formal program, or in a home, initial evaluation of the learning level helps identify content. Areas of teaching cover anatomy and physiology; pathophysiology of lung disease; airway management; breathing training strategies; energy conservation and work simplification; medications; self-management skills; benefits of exercise and safety guidelines; oxygen therapy; environmental irritant avoidance; respiratory and chest therapy techniques; symptom management; psychological factors such as coping, panic, control, and stress management; end of life planning; smoking cessation; travel/leisure; sexuality; and nutrition (ATS statement, 1999).

Addressing Unmet Client Needs

Smoking Cessation

Many clients with lung disease continue to smoke or be exposed to passive smoke that worsens their lung status. The smoking cessation process has five stages of behavioral change: precontemplation, contemplation, preparation, action, and maintenance. Rehabilitation team members must understand and support the smoker's stage of behavior and readiness to change, thus providing more effective assistance for successful cessation (Andrews, 1998). Because of the physical dependence on nicotine and the physiological dependence on the smoking habit, cessation interventions are tailored to each client. With any approach, include basic information about the hazards of smoking and benefits of cessation. Set a quit date as a first step when the client is willing, usually within 1 to 2 weeks of the counseling session. Behavior modification strategies may include a smoking diary with notation of social cues, cravings, and triggers associated with each cigarette smoked.

Pharmacotherapy with nicotine replacement is an option available in the form of gum, transdermal patches, sprays, and inhalers. The costs are roughly equivalent or slightly higher than the cost of smoking one to two packs of cigarettes over the same period (Andrews, 1998). Antidepressants as adjunctive therapy have shown promise. Bupropion (Wellbutrin SR, Zyban) is a weak inhibitor of neuronal uptake of norepinephrine, serotonin, and dopamine and does not inhibit monoamine oxidase. The mechanism of action of bupropion in assisting smokers to quit is unknown but seems to be unrelated to its antidepressant properties. Possible adverse reactions include rash, nausea, agitation, and migraine (Andrews, 1998). This medication is not prescribed for clients who have a history of a seizure disorder.

Follow-up is essential in supporting clients during smoking cessation programs. Contact within the first 1 to 2 weeks is recommended because relapses occur within 2 weeks. Additional follow-up 1 to 3 months after the quit date assists clients to cope with longer-term maintenance issues. If relapse occurs, the client renews the commitment to cessation and sets a new quit date. Assure the client that many persons achieve stable abstinence after five or six attempts (Andrews, 1998). Smoking cessation education should be provided for family members who smoke, as well as for clients.

Sexuality

Sexuality is often not addressed openly between clients and providers. COPD can contribute to sexual problems and precipitate feelings of apprehension, fear, and humiliation. Sexual activity may become a negative experience because of the dyspnea that accompanies the physical activity. These issues need to be addressed openly by discussing feelings and attitudes between clients and partners.

Pharmacological interventions, such as bronchodilators used shortly before sexual activity, may permit more comfortable breathing and enjoyment. Clients taking medications that depress sexual drive can discuss alternatives with the physician or nurse practitioner; alternative medications may be available. Energy-conserving positions for sexual activity are recommended for this population. If one partner can avoid placing weight on the chest of the client, this will eliminate aggravating any problems with breathing. Ultimately, energy and breathing conservation must guide all activities (Haas & Haas, 2000).

End of Life Planning

No predictions for length of life are available, with or without lung disease. Two factors are important in the longevity of a client with COPD: the age at diagnosis and the FEV_1 in relation to the age. Being relatively young at diagnosis and having a smaller FEV_1 usually mean that the disease progresses faster (Haas & Haas, 2000). Preparation and decision making for death and dying must be done for everyone, regardless of health status. Advanced directives outlining wishes with regard to mechanical ventilation are especially relevant for those with chronic lung disease. Home care with respiratory equipment is possible and may be the first choice for many with hospice care as they approach the end of their life. Death without medical intervention may appeal to some, whereas others desire medical intervention to postpone death. The process of deciding a client's wishes for managing the last phase of life are also discussed with the family, if the client agrees, so that everyone is informed, clear, and comfortable in respecting the client's decisions and wishes. Refer to Chapters 4, 28, and 35 for additional discussions on ethics, problem resolution, and advance directives.

Support Groups

Support groups can be very helpful in providing information and networking for clients with chronic pulmonary disease. Sponsored rehabilitation facilities or lung associations typically offer clients a place to meet, help with planning programs and finding guest speakers, and a forum to discuss topics of interest or to exchange tips about managing lung disease. Friendships can develop from a link with others who share similar problems and experiences. Groups may be led by rehabilitation nurses with team members, such as respiratory therapists, or by clients themselves. Other support groups are for family and friends of clients with lung disease.

NEW DIRECTIONS

Surgical therapies are available for certain clients with severe COPD. Lung volume reduction and lung transplantation offer hope for some clients with incapacitating dyspnea. Lung volume reduction has been revived and modified from earlier techniques used in the late 1950s. The benefits of *lung volume reduction* surgery occur when the diseased and functionless lung tissue is removed, giving improved function in the remaining lung tissue. Early reports indicated improvements in FEV_1 and FVC with reductions in total lung capacity (TLC) and residual volume (RV) after lung volume reduction surgery. Oxygenation also improved postoperatively; long-term effects have not been evaluated extensively. Currently, this therapy is palliative, bringing symptomatic relief and improvement in quality of life (Newsome & Ott, 1997). Further research to measure outcomes beyond 5 years as well as randomized controlled trials with examination of the various techniques are necessary to evaluate the effects (Hensley, Coughlan, & Gibson, 1999; Sciurba et al., 1996).

Lung transplant surgery has been performed successfully for at least two decades. This type of surgery has been recognized as a therapeutic option for a variety of end-stage lung diseases. For clients with COPD, cystic fibrosis, and idiopathic pulmonary fibrosis, it offers improved quality of life and longer survival. However, frequent complications result in constraints on long-term preservation of graft function and affect client survival. The availability of suitable donor lungs has been a limitation in meeting the increasing need for transplantation.

Criteria for transplantation are strict, including upper age limitations of 55 years for heart-lung, 60 years for bilateral lung, and 65 years for single-lung transplantation. Persons with chronic medical conditions and end organ damage are not considered for transplantation due to evidence of poor outcomes in these clients.

Peak effect is usually noted 3 to 6 months after the surgery. Normal pulmonary function usually is achieved after bilateral lung transplantation; in contrast, lung function improves but does not completely normalize after single-lung transplantation. At best, 1-, 3-, and 5-year actuarial survival after lung transplantation is 70.7, 54.8, and 42.6 percent, respectively, with a median survival of 3.7 years (Arcasoy & Kotloff, 1999).

Information on quality-of-life changes after transplantation is limited. Primarily, clients without complications have reported dramatic global improvement in all quality-of-life measures within several months after transplantation. Beyond that time, quality-of-life measures appear to remain stable for clients without complications but decline substantially in those with complicated courses. Common complications include graft failure, airway complications, infection, and rejection—both acute and chronic. Future areas for research include investigation of xenotransplantation, the use of animal organs for transplantation in humans and related ethical issues, and strategies to promote immune tolerance to avoid the use of life-long immunosuppressive agents. Chapter 34 discusses renal transplants.

Comprehensive pulmonary rehabilitation addresses all aspects of client and family needs. Incorporating pulmonary rehabilitation as a strategy for clients enhances outcomes and moves beyond standard medical and nursing management to far-reaching benefits with decreases in dyspnea and improvements in health status. As newer therapies are developed and validated for efficacy, they will be incorporated into rehabilitation programs across all settings.

CRITICAL THINKING

1. Robert, a 68-year-old retired schoolteacher, has been discharged from the hospital after an exacerbation of emphysema that developed into pneumonia. He was also diagnosed with congestive heart failure 2 years ago. He is to participate in pulmonary rehabilitation, and you are evaluating him for entry into the program. He has expiratory wheezing and crackles throughout the lung fields bilaterally and states that he is experiencing a "fair" amount of shortness of breath today. You note ankle swelling bilaterally and increased jugular venous distention.
   What is your evaluation of the cause of his increase in shortness of breath today?
   How should Robert be treated for his increase in shortness of breath?
2. You are taking care of a 65-year-old man with COPD who is receiving 2 L of oxygen/minute per nasal cannula. His wife suggests increasing his oxygen flow to improve his breathing. His oxygen saturation is 90% at rest.
   What can you tell his wife about increasing his oxygen flow?
   What strategies can suggest to improve his breathing?
3. You are caring for a 79-year-old woman who had a cerebral vascular accident 2 weeks ago. She has been discharged from a long-term–care setting where she was given physical therapy to assist her in rehabilitation. She is receiving 2 L of oxygen/minute per nasal cannula due to resolving pneumonia after prolonged bed rest at this facility. This morning she complains of a sharp pain in her chest and difficulty with breathing.
   What actions would you take in this situation?
   What is the most likely complication that she is experiencing?

Pediatric Case Study ⌒ *Spinal Muscular Atrophy*

Spinal muscular atrophies (SMA) are a group of inherited degenerative neuromuscular diseases of the motor neurons. Characteristics are progressive muscle weakness, severe hypotonia, muscle atrophy, and loss of reflexes; intelligence typically is normal. The three major types primarily differ with time of onset and rate of progression. Overwhelmingly, prognosis is poor, with life expectancy not exceeding young childhood.

Clinical management focuses on supportive care and preventing complications. Many children require an artificial airway and often need mechanical ventilation. The most common problems associated with these disorders are respiratory compromise and immobility. To ensure child and family transition to home successfully, the needs and abilities of all persons and the necessary services must be part of early discharge planning. One critical consideration for a child with SMA is the potential for ineffective airway clearance due to the lack of sufficient strength of respiratory muscles to generate an effective cough. The immobility that accompanies the disorder compounds problems with the difficulty of mobilizing secretions. The following case will be used to illustrate how one rehabilitation nurse prepared for the discharge of an infant with SMA with a focus on the child's respiratory status.

T.E. is a 2-year-old girl with SMA. At 6 months of age, her parents noticed she was delayed in meeting her developmental milestones and had regressed from earlier accomplished goals. She became progressively weaker until she was unable to hold her head upright. At 7 months of age, she was diagnosed with SMA. T.E. had a sister who died of respiratory failure secondary to SMA at 15 months old.

T.E. was 1 year old when admitted to the Pediatric Intensive Care Unit for a respiratory infection and respiratory failure. Due to the need for prolonged mechanical ventilation along with her inability to protect her airway, she received a tracheostomy tube. She continued to need mechanical ventilation, and home ventilation was arranged.

Today, T.E. only uses supplemental oxygen during an acute respiratory illness but continues to require mechanical ventilation. Due to the risk for aspiration, T.E. is fed via her gastrostomy tube. She has a wheelchair and leg braces.

T.E. lives with her parents in a three-bedroom home. They do not have extended family in the area to assist them. As discharge approaches, both parents are looking forward to her return home but express concerns about their ability to care for her adequately. Although nurses will assist them, the family must learn and

Continued

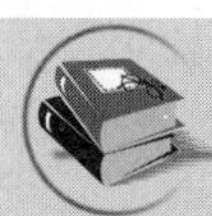

Pediatric Case Study 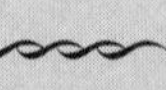 *Spinal Muscular Atrophy—cont'd*

demonstrate competency in all aspects of her care. T.E. will go home with a tracheostomy tube; a ventilator; humidification; an oxygen saturation monitor; supplemental oxygen, if needed; and a wheelchair.

Goals

The primary respiratory goals for SMA are to ensure a patent airway, foster airway clearance, and prevent respiratory infection. Since she is a child, goals include helping T.E. meet optimal levels of development to her potential.

Plan of Care: T.E.'s Potential for Ineffective Airway Clearance

1. Maintain a patent tracheostomy tube
2. Stimulate and encourage cough
3. Suction as needed
4. Monitor respiratory status
   a. Respiratory rate and synchrony with ventilator
   b. Auscultation
   c. Signs of respiratory distress
   d. Ventilator settings as ordered
   e. Mucus production
5. Assess for a change in amount and consistency of secretions
6. Provide humidification through tracheostomy tube
7. Perform postural drainage with chest physiotherapy (CPT) regularly to assist with airway secretion clearance.
8. Provide supplemental oxygen as needed
9. Teach parents aspects of T.E.'s care and have them demonstrate competency in the following areas:
   a. Tracheostomy care
   b. CPT
   c. Ventilator management
   d. Humidification
   e. Suctioning
   f. Respiratory assessment
   g. Signs of infection
   h. Monitoring equipment
10. Require that parents learn CPR before discharge
11. Provide the parents with a written plan that specifies the steps to take when T.E. shows signs of respiratory distress or deterioration
12. Arrange for home nursing

Parental Anxiety Related to Diagnosis and Impending Discharge from Hospital

1. Explore the individual concerns of each parent
2. Provide parents with information and support
3. Introduce parents to other families of children with SMA and/or tracheostomies and home ventilation
4. Provide information to parents about support groups
5. Teach parents how to care for T.E.'s discharge needs
6. Familiarize parents with T.E.'s baseline status, and teach them to recognize deviations from normal

Respiratory Teaching Areas: SMA

1. Baseline of child (respiratory status, behavior)
2. Signs/symptoms of respiratory infection, distress, and deterioration
3. Nutritional/feeding needs and strategies
4. Equipment needs: use, care, and rationale
   a. Oxygen delivery
   b. Tracheostomy care
   c. Ventilator
   d. Oxygen saturation monitor
   e. Suction devices
   f. Thermometer
   g. Humidification devices
5. Emergency care
   a. CPR training
   b. Troubleshooting tracheostomies
   c. Written emergency plan
   d. Emergency service contact
6. Infection control measures
7. Follow-up care
   a. Primary care physician
   b. Subspecialists
   c. Therapists
   d. Early intervention or infant stimulation programs

REFERENCES

American Thoracic Society, DLD (1978). *American Review of Respiratory Disease, 1(8),* 7-53.

American Thoracic Society (ATS). (1995). Standards for the diagnosis and care of patients with chronic obstructive pulmonary disease. *American Journal Respiratory and Critical Care Medicine, 152,* S77-S120.

American Thoracic Society (ATS). (1999). Pulmonary rehabilitation—1999. *American Journal of Respiratory and Critical Care Medicine, 159,* 1666-1682.

Andrews, J. (1998). Optimizing smoking cessation strategies. *The Nurse Practitioner, 23,* 47-64.

Arcasoy, S.M., & Kotloff, R.M. (1999). Medical progress: Lung transplantation. *New England Journal of Medicine, 340,* 1081-1091.

Beare, P.G., & Myers, J.L. (1998). *Adult health nursing.* St. Louis: Mosby.

Berry, J.K., & Braunschweig, C.A. (1998). Nutritional assessment of the critically ill patient. *Critical Care Nursing Quarterly, 21,* 33-46.

Berry, M.J., Rejeski, W.J., Adair, N.E., & Zaccaro, D. (1999). Exercise rehabilitation and chronic obstructive pulmonary disease stage. *American Journal of Respiratory and Critical Care Medicine, 160,* 1248-1253.

Breslin, E.H. (1997). Respiratory muscle training in the treatment of respiratory muscle dysfunction: the state of science. *Rehabilitation Nursing, 5,* 134-142.

Breslin, E.H., Ugalde, V., Bonekat, W., Walsh, S., Cronan, M., & Horasek, S. (1996). Abdominal muscle recruitment during pursed lip breathing in COPD. *American Journal of Respiratory and Critical Care Medicine, 153,* A128.

Brewin, A. (1997). Comparing asthma and chronic obstructive pulmonary disease (COPD). *Nursing Standard, 12,* 49-55.

Burns, S.M., Clockesy, J.M., Hannemann, S.K.G., Ingersoll, G.E., Knebel, A.R., & Shekleton, M.E. (1995). Weaning from long-term mechanical ventilation. *American Journal of Critical Care, 4,* 4-21.

Busse, W.W. & Wenzel, S.E. (2000). *Large and small airway dysfunction in asthma rationale for treating the entire airway. Asthma and the small airways, continuing medical education monograph.* New York: ATS Society.

Carlson-Catalano, J., Lunney, M., Paradiso, C., Bruno, J., Kraynyak Luise, B., Martin, T., Massoni, M., & Pachter, S. (1998). Clinical validation of ineffective breathing pattern, ineffective airway clearance, and impaired gas exchange. *Image—The Journal of Nursing Scholarship, 30,* 243-248.

Carrol, P. (1998). Closing in on safer suctioning. *RN, 61,* 22-27.

Casaburi, R. & Petty, T.L. (1993). *Principles and practice of pulmonary rehabilitation.* Philadelphia: WB Saunders.

Casey, P. (1999). Respiratory distress. In J. Deaco, & P. O'Neill (Eds.), *Core curriculum for neonatal intensive care nursing.* Philadelphia: WB Saunders.

Celli, B.R. (1998). Pulmonary rehabilitation for COPD: A practical approach for improving ventilatory conditioning. *Postgraduate Medicine, 102,* 159-160, 167-168, 173-176.

Chervin, R.D., & Guilleminault, C. (1997). Diaphragm pacing for respiratory insufficiency. *Journal of Clinical Neurophysiology, 14,* 369-377.

Chlan, L. (1998). Effectiveness of a music therapy intervention on relaxation and anxiety for patients receiving ventilatory assistance. *Heart and Lung, 27,* 169-176.

Consensus Conference Report. (1999). Clinical indications for noninvasive positive pressure ventilation in chronic respiratory failure due to restrictive lung disease, COPD, and nocturnal hypoventilation—A consensus conference report. *Chest, 116,* 521-534.

Copstead, L.C. (Ed.). (2000). *Perspectives on pathophysiology* (2nd ed.). Philadelphia: WB Saunders.

Cosio, M.G., & Guerassimov, A. (1999). Chronic obstructive pulmonary disease. *American Journal of Respiratory and Critical Care Medicine, 160,* 521-525.

Crockett, A.J., Moss, J.R., Cranston, J.M., & Alpers, J.H. (1999). Domiciliary oxygen in chronic obstructive pulmonary disease. In *The Cochrane Library.* Oxford: Update Software.

Dappen, A., Schwartz, R.H., & O'Donnel, R. (1996). A survey of adolescent smoking patterns. *Journal of the American Board of Family Practice, 9,* 7-13.

DeMarco-Sinatra, J. (2000). Relaxation training as a holistic nursing intervention. *Holistic Nursing Practice, 14,* 30-39.

Dunn, L., Chisholm, H. (1998). Oxygen therapy. *Nursing Standard, 13,* 57-60, 63-64.

Elefteriades, J.A., & Quin, J.A. (1998). Diaphragm pacing. *Chest Surgery Clinics of North America, 8,* 331-357.

Frownfelter, D., & Dean, E. (Eds.). (1996). *Principals and practice of cardiopulmonary physical therapy* (3rd ed.). St. Louis: Mosby.

Gift, A., (1998). Validity of the numeric rating scale as a measure of dyspnea. *American Journal of Critical Care, 7,* 200-204.

Gordon, M. (2000). *Manual of nursing diagnosis* (9th ed.). St. Louis: Mosby.

Gosselink, R.A., Wagenaar, R.C., Sargeant, A.J., Rijswijk, H., & Decramer, M. (1995). Diaphragmatic breathing reduces efficiency of breathing in chronic obstructive pulmonary disease. *American Journal of Respiratory and Critical Care Medicine, 151,* 1136-1142.

Haas, F., & Haas, S.S. (2000). *The chronic bronchitis and emphysema handbook* (2nd ed.). New York: John Wiley & Sons.

Hamilton, N., Killian, K.J., & Jones, N.L. (1995). Muscle strength, symptom intensity, and exercise capacity in patients with cardiorespiratory disorders. *American Journal of Respiratory and Critical Care Medicine, 152,* 2021-2031.

Hazinski, M.F. (1999). *Manual of pediatric critical care.* St. Louis: Mosby.

Hensley, M., Coughlan, J., & Gibson, P. (1999). Lung volume reduction surgery for chronic obstructive pulmonary disease (Cochrane Review). In *The Cochrane Library,* 3. Oxford: Update Software.

Hooper, M. (1996). Nursing care of the patient with a tracheostomy. *Nursing Standard, 10,* 40-43.

Hudson, V., & Guill, M. (1998). New developments in cystic fibrosis. *Pediatric Annals, 27,* 515-520.

Jones, A., & Rowe, B.H. (2000). Bronchopulmonary hygiene physical therapy in bronchiectasis and chronic obstructive pulmonary disease: A systematic review. *Heart and Lung, 29,* 125-135.

Katzung, B.G. (1998). *Basic & clinical pharmacology.* Norwalk, CT: Appleton & Lange.

Kenner, C. (1998). Complications of respiratory management. In C. Kenner, J. Wright Lott, & F. Applewhite (Eds.), *Comprehensive neonatal nursing: a physiologic approach.* Philadelphia: WB Saunders.

Kirton, O.C. (1997). Ventilatory support modes. In J.M. Civetta (Ed.), *Critical care* (3rd ed.). Philadelphia: Lippincott-Raven.

Kosmas, E.N., Toukmatzi S., Polychronaki, A., & Damianos, A. (1998). Consequences of severe snoring in patients with chronic obstructive pulmonary disease (COPD). *Chest, 114,* 321S-322S.

LaCasse, Y., Guyatt, G., & Goldstein, R. (1997). The components of a respiratory rehabilitation program: A systematic overview. *Chest, 111,* 1077-1088.

Lareau, S.C., Meek, P.M., Press, D., Anholm, J.D., & Roos, P.J. (1999). Dyspnea in patients with chronic obstructive pulmonary disease: Does dyspnea worsen longitudinally in the presence of declining lung function? *Heart and Lung: Journal of Acute and Critical Care, 28,* 65-73.

Longenecker, J.C. (1998). *High-yield acid-base.* Baltimore: Williams & Wilkins.

Loube, D.I., Gay, Z.P.C., Strohl, K.P., Pack, A.I., White, D.P., & Collop, N.A. (1999). Indications for positive airway pressure treatment of adult obstructive sleep apnea patients. *Chest, 115,* 863-866.

Lyager, S., Steffensen, B., & Juhl, B. (1995). Indicators of need for mechanical ventilation in Duchenne muscular dystrophy and spinal muscular atrophy. *Chest, 108,* 779-785.

Madison, J.M., & Irwin, R.S. (1998). Chronic obstructive pulmonary disease. *Lancet, 362,* 467-473.

Maltais, F., Leblanc, P., Simard, C., Jobin, J., Berube, C., Bruneau, J., Carrier L., & Belleau, R. (1996). Skeletal muscle adaptation to endurance training in patients with chronic obstructive pulmonary disease. *American Journal of Respiratory and Critical Care Medicine, 154,* 442-447.

Manthous, C., Schmidt, G.A., & Hall, J.B. (1998). Liberation from mechanical ventilation: A decade of progress. *Chest, 114,* 886-901.

Marino, P.L. (1999). *The ICU book.* Philadelphia: Lea & Febiger

McArdle, N., Devereux, G., Heidarnejad, H., Engleman, H., Mackay, T., & Douglas, N. (1999). *American Journal of Respiratory and Critical Care Medicine, 159,* 1108-1114.

McCarley, C. (1999). A model of chronic dyspnea. *Image—The Journal of Nursing Scholarship, 31,* 231-236.

McCloskey, J., & Bulechek, G. (2000). *Nursing interventions classification (NIC)* (3rd ed.). St. Louis: Mosby.

Montes de Oca, M., & Celli, B. (2000). Respiratory muscle recruitment an exercise performance in eucapnic and hypercapnic severe chronic obstructive lung disease. *American Journal of Respiratory and Critical Care Medicine, 161,* 880-885.

Newsome, E.A., & Ott, B.B. (1997). Lung volume reduction: Surgical treatment for emphysema. *American Journal of Critical Care, 6,* 423-427.

Noble, J. (1996). *Textbook of primary care medicine* (2nd ed.). St. Louis: Mosby.

Petty, T.L. (1998). Strategies in preserving lung health and preventing COPD and associated diseases: The National Lung Health Education Program. *Chest, 113*(2S), 123S-163S.

Postma, D.S., Kerstjens, H.A.M. (1999). Are inhaled glucocorticosteroids effective in chronic obstructive pulmonary disease? *American Journal of Respiratory and Critical Care Medicine, 160,* 566-571.

Rees, P.J., & Dudley, F. (1998). ABC of oxygen: Oxygen therapy in chronic lung disease. *British Medical Journal, 317,* 871-874.

Ries, A.L., Kaplan, R.M., Limberg, T.M., & Prewitt, L.M. (1995). Effects of pulmonary rehabilitation on physiologic and psychosocial outcomes in patients with chronic obstructive pulmonary disease. *Annals of Internal Medicine, 122,* 823-832.

Rochester, C.L., & Ferranti, R. (1998). Long-term oxygen therapy: What benefits for your patients? *Journal of Respiratory Disease, 19,* 133-134.

San Pedro, G.S. (1999). Pulmonary rehabilitation for the patient with severe chronic obstructive pulmonary disease. *American Journal of Medical Science, 318,* 99-102.

Schunemann, H.J., Dorn, J., Grant, B.J.B., Winkelstein, W., & Trevisan, M. (2000). Pulmonary function is a long-term predictor of mortality in the general population. A 29-year follow-up of the Buffalo Health Study. *Chest, 118,* 656-664.

Sciurba, F.C., Rogers, R.M., Keenan, R.J., Slivka, W., Gorcsan, J., Ferson, P.F., Holbert, J.M., Brown, M.L., & Landreneau, R.J. (1996). Improvement in pulmonary function and elastic recoil after lung-reduction surgery for diffuse emphysema. *New England Journal of Medicine, 334,* 1095-1099.

Seemungal, T.A.R., Donaldson, G.C., Bhowmik, A., Jeffries, D.J., & Wedzicha, J.A. (2000). Time course and recovery of exacerbations in patients with chronic obstructive pulmonary disease. *American Journal of Respiratory and Critical Care Medicine, 161,* 1608-1613.

Seidel, H.M., Ball, J.W., Dains, J.E., & Benedict, G.W. (1999). *Mosby's guide to physical examination* (4th ed.). St. Louis: Mosby.

Simmons, C.L. (1997). How frequently should endotracheal suctioning be undertaken? *American Journal of Critical Care, 6,* 4-6.

Stoller, J.K., Hoisington, E., & Auger, G. (1999). A comparative analysis of arranging in-flight oxygen aboard commercial air carriers. *Chest, 115,* 991-995.

Vallet, G., Hmaidai, S., Serres, I., Fabre, C., Bourgouin, D., Desplan, J., Varray, A., & Prefaut, C. (1997). Comparison of two training programmes in chronic airway limitation patients: Standard versus individualized protocols. *European Respiratory Journal, 10,* 114-122.

Vitacca, M., Clini, E., Bianchi, L., & Ambrosino (1998). Acute effects of deep diaphragmatic breathing in COPD patients with chronic respiratory insufficiency. *European Respiratory Journal, 11,* 408-415.

Voter, K.Z., & Chalanick, K. (1996). Home oxygen and ventilation therapies in pediatric patients. *Current Opinion in Pediatrics, 8,* 221-225.

Wainwright, S.P., & Gould, D. (1996). Endotracheal suctioning: An example of the problems of relevance and rigor in clinical research. *Journal of Clinical Nursing, 5,* 389-398.

Bladder Elimination and Continence

19

Marilyn Pires, MS, RN, CRRN-A

A parish nurse is doing grief counseling with the oldest daughter of an elderly couple. The father has just died and the daughter is worried about her mother. "With Dad gone, I am not sure what will happen with my mother. I would love to have her home with me. We have plenty of room now that the kids have all moved out. My husband is very supportive and loves my mother, but I know he just couldn't deal with her urinary incontinence. I wish there were something I could do. She gets so embarrassed and feels so bad." The parish nurse asks, "Has your mother ever been evaluated for her incontinence?" The daughter replies, "No, I don't think so; we all thought it was just something that happens when a woman gets older." The parish nurse answers, "Actually, there is a lot that can be done to treat urinary incontinence. A friend of mine is a rehabilitation nurse who has her own continence practice. If you would like, I can give you her number and you can make an appointment for your mother." The daughter responds, "Oh, that would be great! It would be such a blessing if Mom could get help for this problem. It would make the difference between having to think about a nursing home and living with us."

Care of persons with urinary incontinence has long been a priority of rehabilitation nursing practice. The majority of clients who enter a rehabilitation setting are admitted with urinary incontinence. Conversely, the majority of those leaving a rehabilitation setting are continent. The intervening variable has been specific rehabilitation nursing interventions that primarily address the management of incontinence because of neurogenic etiology and functional incontinence.

Urinary incontinence resulting from neurogenic causes represents a very small percentage of the prevalence of incontinence in the United States. Recent national recognition of the scope of the problem of incontinence represents an opportunity for rehabilitation nurses to expand their practice by developing and participating in continence programs. To do this, rehabilitation nurses must bolster their knowledge base to include an understanding of the nonneurogenic etiology of urinary incontinence and the appropriate interventions for these types of incontinence.

SCOPE OF THE PROBLEM OF URINARY INCONTINENCE

The American Urological Association (2000) defines urinary incontinence as the involuntary loss of urine. The Urinary Incontinence Guideline Panel, convened by the Agency for Health Care Policy and Research (AHCPR), defined urinary incontinence as "the involuntary loss of urine which is sufficient to be a problem" (Urinary Incontinence Guideline Panel, 1992a, 1992b). The 1996 AHCPR Clinical Practice Guideline update did not change that definition (Fantl et al., 1996). However, at the 1998 Conference on Incontinence in Monte Carlo, Monaco, specialists proposed that the World Health Organization change the classification of urinary incontinence from an ill-defined condition to a disease (Voelker, 1998). The rationale for the change is to promote diagnosis of, treatment for, and attention to the disease of urinary incontinence.

More than 13 million Americans in both community and institutional settings experience urinary incontinence (National Kidney and Urologic Diseases Advisory Board, 1994). The prevalence of urinary incontinence in persons younger than 30 years ranges from 6% to 10% in men and 5% to 16% in women (Doughty & Waldrop, 2000). Nygaard, Thompson, Svengalis, and Albright (1994) conducted a study of elite female athletes averaging about 20 years of age and found 28% of the women experienced incontinence while participating in their sport. In the 30- to 60-year age group, the average prevalence rate for women is 29% and for men ranges from 2% to 12% (Hampel et al., 1997). For community-dwelling persons older than 65 years, the prevalence of urinary incontinence ranges from 10% to 33% (Teasdale et al., 1988). The prevalence for elderly women ranges between 12% and 49% (Yarnell, Richards, & Stephenson, 1981) and between 7% and 22% for elderly men (Teasdale et al., 1988). Thus elderly women are twice as likely to be incontinent as men (Steeman & Defever, 1998). At least half of the 1.5 million residents of nursing homes are incontinent of urine at least once a day (Hampel et al., 1997). It is estimated that the annual direct cost of caring for incontinent persons of all ages in the community and in nursing homes is more than $24 billion (Wagner & Hu, 1998).

Although urinary incontinence is highly prevalent and among the four most distress-causing disorders next to anginal pain and locomotor and mental disorders (Grimby & Svanborg, 1997), many individuals do not seek treatment (Shaw, Tansey, Jackson, Hyde, & Allan, 2001). Children older than 6 years, as well as adults, are expected to maintain control of their urinary elimination. When persons become incontinent, they are often embarrassed and ashamed. Many persons believe that incontinence is an inevitable consequence of aging with which they must learn to deal (Skelly & Boblin-Cummings, 1999). Nearly a third of the women aged 45 years and older (N = 1 in every 6 women) never discuss incontinence with anyone (Maloney & Cafiero, 1999). Until recently this was also the perception of many health care professionals, including nurses. Although changes associated with aging contribute to older persons' susceptibility to incontinence, it is not a normal part of aging. It is now known that incontinence is a symptom and with proper diagnosis and appropriate interventions, most incontinence can be reversed or managed effectively (Tannenbaum, Perrin, Dubeau, & Kuckel, 2001). Research findings indicate that 80% or more of individuals with urinary incontinence may experience significant improvement in symptoms through diagnosis and treatment (Burkhart, 2000).

Rehabilitation nurses practice in many settings and work with clients across the life span. Because of this and the intimacy of interactions with clients, rehabilitation nurses are in a unique position to detect unreported bladder dysfunction and to initiate the assessment and intervention needed to offer treatment to persons with urinary incontinence. Treating urinary incontinence can significantly improve the quality of life of those with incontinence, their families, and their caregivers. Urinary incontinence results in a loss of self-esteem in children and adults and a decrease in the ability to achieve or maintain independence. In children with congenital disabilities or who have experienced trauma, incontinence may delay or prevent social interaction with other children of their own age and significantly delay or obstruct their social development and other developmental milestones. Fear of incontinence causes the person to curtail excursions outside the home, including social interaction with friends and family. Frequency of sexual activity may be severely diminished or avoided entirely (Grimby, Milsom, Molander, Wiklund, & Ekelund, 1993). Urinary incontinence is generally recognized as one of the major causes of institutionalization of elderly persons (Fantl et al., 1996).

ANATOMY AND PHYSIOLOGY

Normal Bladder Function

The urinary tract is composed of the kidneys, ureters, bladder, and urethra. The kidneys filter waste products from the blood and continuously produce urine. The ureters are bilateral muscular tubes that drain urine from the kidneys to the bladder. The ureters enter the posterior surface of the bladder at an oblique angle and function as a valve to prevent backflow of urine. The bladder is a reservoir for urine. It is a hollow muscular organ with two parts. The bladder's body is made up of the detrusor muscle, which consists of layers of intertwining smooth muscle. The other part, the trigone, is a small triangular area at the base of the bladder through which the ureters and urethra pass and is contiguous with the bladder neck. The bladder neck is 2 to 3 cm long and is part of the posterior urethra. The muscles in this area form the internal sphincter. The urethra is a tube that carries urine from the bladder out of the body. Beyond the posterior urethra, the tube continues through an extension of the deep perineal muscles. This striated muscle is called the rhabdosphincter, which in conjunction with the urogenital diaphragm, makes up the external sphincter mechanism (Gray, 2000). Figure 19-1 is a diagram of the lower urinary tract's anatomy. The external sphincter mechanism is a voluntary skeletal muscle, in contrast to the smooth autonomic muscle of the bladder body and bladder neck. The external sphincter mechanism is under voluntary control and allows a person to prevent urination even when involuntary mechanisms are attempting to empty the bladder (Guyton & Hall, 1996).

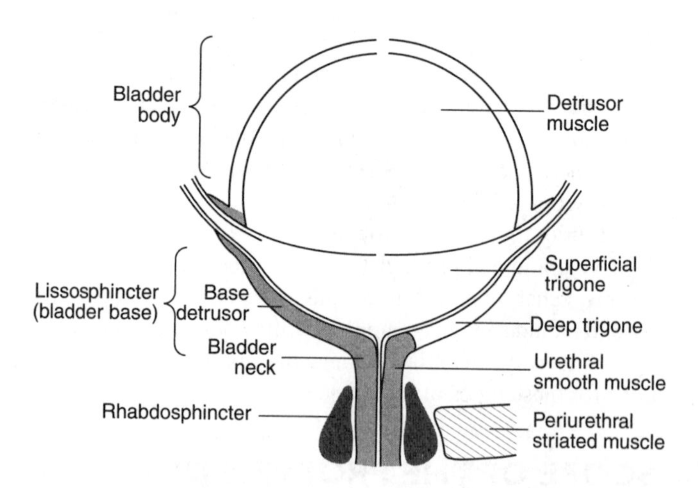

Figure 19-1 The bladder can be divided into two regions: fixed base, sometimes called the lissosphincter, and flexible bladder body containing detrusor muscle. (From Doughty, D.B. [2000]. *Urinary and fecal incontinence: Nursing management* [2nd ed.]. St. Louis: Mosby.)

Other structures that contribute to continence are the pelvic floor muscles and, in males, the prostate gland. The muscles of the pelvic floor support the bladder. They include the levator ani, pubococcygeus, internal obturator, pyriform, and the superficial and deep perineal muscles that make up the urogenital diaphragm. Voluntary contraction of these pelvic muscles results in compressing, lengthening, and elevating the urethra. For example, the voiding stream can be interrupted by voluntarily contracting the pubococcygeal muscle. In men the prostate gland is important in maintaining continence. The urethra, which passes through the prostate gland, contains both smooth and striated muscle (Rathe & Klioze, 2000).

Innervation of the Lower Urinary Tract

The nerve supply of the lower urinary tract includes parasympathetic and sympathetic fibers as well as somatic nerve fibers.

The parasympathetic nerves provide motor stimulation to the bladder, causing bladder contraction through the pelvic nerve. The pelvic nerve exits the spinal cord at S2-S4 level. The preganglionic nerves originate in the sacral cord and synapse with the short postganglionic nerves within the bladder wall (Rathe & Klioze, 2000). Parasympathetic nerves work by releasing the neurotransmitter acetylcholine. Stimulation of parasympathetic fibers causes the ureters to speed up transport of urine from the kidneys to the bladder, causes the detrusor muscle to contract, thus causing the bladder to empty, and may cause the internal sphincter to open slightly.

The sympathetic nerves mediate the storage of urine in the bladder by stimulating contractions of the bladder neck and proximal urethra. The sympathetic fibers exit the thoracic lumbar cord at the T12-L2 level via the hypogastric nerve. The preganglionic nerves originate in the thoracolumbar cord and synapse with the postganglionic fibers at the inferior mesenteric and hypogastric plexuses. The postganglionic fibers travel from these plexuses to the bladder neck and proximal urethra (Gray, 2000). Sympathetic nerves work by releasing the neurotransmitter norepinephrine. Stimulation of sympathetic fibers causes the ureters to slow the transport of urine from the kidneys to the bladder and to relax the detrusor muscle (thus facilitating storage of urine) and to constrict the internal sphincter.

Somatic innervation consists of both efferent (motor) and afferent (sensory) fibers. The efferent fibers of the somatic nervous system originate in the anterior horn of the S2-S4 segments and travel through the pudendal nerve to the external striated sphincter and the muscles of the pelvic floor. Somatic nerves work by releasing the neurotransmitter acetylcholine. The external sphincter mechanism normally is contracted, supporting bladder storage by preventing leakage of urine. This mechanism, however, can be relaxed at will, allowing urination.

Afferent fibers originate in the bladder and proceed through the pelvic and hypogastric nerves to the posterior horn of the spinal cord. Sensory fibers of the pelvic nerve are stimulated during bladder filling by mechanoreceptors in the detrusor muscle. Messages travel from the bladder to the sacral micturition center and stimulate the voiding reflex, whereas other messages are transmitted to the brain through the spinothalamic tract. Sensation permits voluntary control of the bladder. Table 19-1 lists neurotransmitters that mediate micturition.

Neural Coordination of Micturition

The micturition reflex is mediated by a complex reflex arc (Figure 19-2). During the micturition reflex, sensory messages pass from the bladder into and through the sacral cord and are coordinated by the pons. The pons coordinates the relaxation of the urethral sphincter with detrusor contraction. The pons is controlled voluntarily by the frontal cortex. If a person does not want to urinate, the frontal micturition center sends inhibitory messages from the frontal cortex through the pons, down the reticulospinal tract to the sacral micturition center and inhibits the motor messages for detrusor contraction and sphincter relaxation (Figure 19-3). Continence involves active inhibition of the complex reflex arc. There is also direct cortical control of the external sphincter mechanism. Direct corticospinal connections travel from the frontal cortex to the S2-S4 segments, then through the pudendal nerve to provide voluntary contraction and relaxation of the external sphincter mechanism (Gray, 2000) (Figure 19-4).

TABLE 19-1 Neurotransmitters That Mediate Micturition

Neurotransmitter	Innervation	Neuroreceptor	Location of Neuroreceptor	Physiological Effect
Acetylcholine	Somatic	Cholinergic	External sphincter	Bladder storage
Acetylcholine	Parasympathetic	Cholinergic	Bladder base and body	Bladder contraction
Norepinephrine	Sympathetic	Adrenergic	Alpha: bladder base, neck, and proximal urethra	Bladder storage
			Beta: bladder body	Bladder storage

Data from Doughty, D.B.. (2000). *Urinary and fecal incontinence nursing management.* (2nd ed.) St. Louis: Mosby.

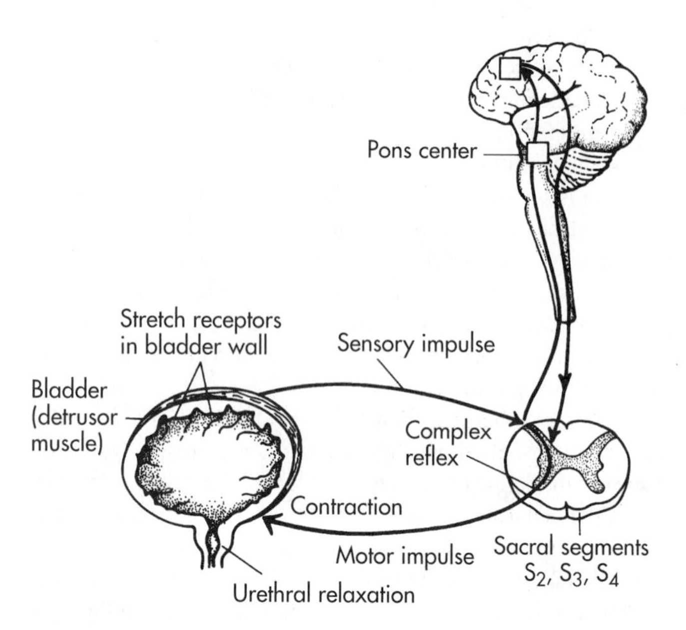

Figure 19-2 Complex reflex arc. (From Jeter, K.F., Fallen, N., & Norton, C. [1990]. *Nursing for continence.* Philadelphia: WB Saunders.)

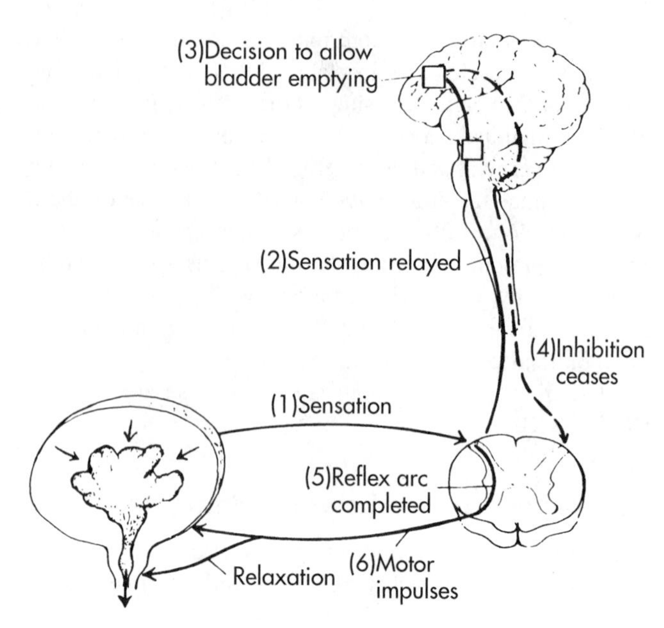

Figure 19-4 Micturition. (From Jeter, K.F., Fallen, N., & Norton, C. [1990]. *Nursing for continence.* Philadelphia: WB Saunders.)

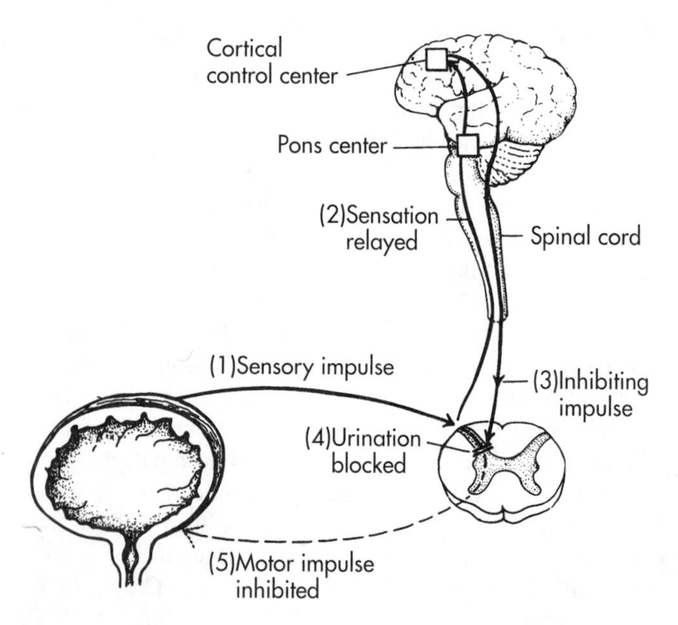

Figure 19-3 Inhibition of the reflex arc. (From Jeter, K.F., Fallen, N., & Norton, C. [1990]. *Nursing for continence.* Philadelphia: WB Saunders.)

Normal Micturition

Normal micturition consists of a filling and storage phase and a contraction and emptying phase. During the filling phase, bladder pressure rises slowly and the normal tone of the urethral sphincters and the pelvic floor muscles maintain continence. When the bladder volume reaches the micturition threshold, usually 200 to 300 ml, the person feels the urge to void and the pressure increases. To remain continent, sympathetic stimulation increases, resulting in contraction of the internal sphincter through α-adrenergic reception, which increases urethral resistance. At the same time, the sympathetic stimulation suppresses detrusor activity through β-adrenergic reception. This inhibits bladder contractility (Rathe & Klioze, 2000). Voluntary contraction of the external sphincter mechanism increases by stimulating the pudendal nerve. This reaction is known as the guarding reflex; it further increases urethral resistance (Siroky & Krane, 1982).

Eventually bladder distention increases sensory afferent stimulation, leading to voluntary coordinated micturition. During the emptying phase, voluntary inhibition of somatic stimulation to the striated external sphincter decreases resistance at the urinary outlet. There is a decrease in sympathetic nerve activity, causing unopposed parasympathetic stimulation. This parasympathetic stimulation opens the bladder neck and facilitates bladder contraction. As the detrusor contracts, bladder pressure increases as the bladder neck relaxes, urethral resistance decreases, and normal voiding occurs (Gray, 2000) (Figure 19-5).

In summary, to hold urine during the filling phase, the intraurethral pressure must exceed the intravesical (bladder) pressure. During the emptying phase, the intravesical pressure exceeds intraurethral pressure. Continence is maintained as long as the intraurethral pressure remains higher than the intravesical pressure (Guerrero & Sinert, 2001).

This normal voiding pattern can be demonstrated by a simultaneous cystometrogram (CMG), which measures bladder volume and pressure, and electromyogram (EMG), which records electrical activity of the pelvic floor muscles and sphincter (Rathe & Klioze, 2000). Figure 19-6 provides

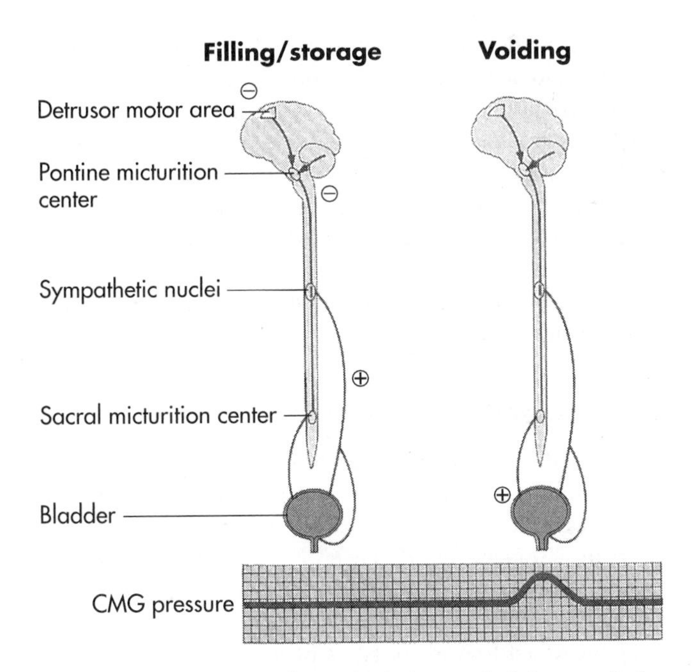

Figure 19-5 Schema of neurological control of detrusor during bladder filling and storage and during micturition. (From Gray, M. [1992]. *Genitourinary disorders.* St. Louis: Mosby.)

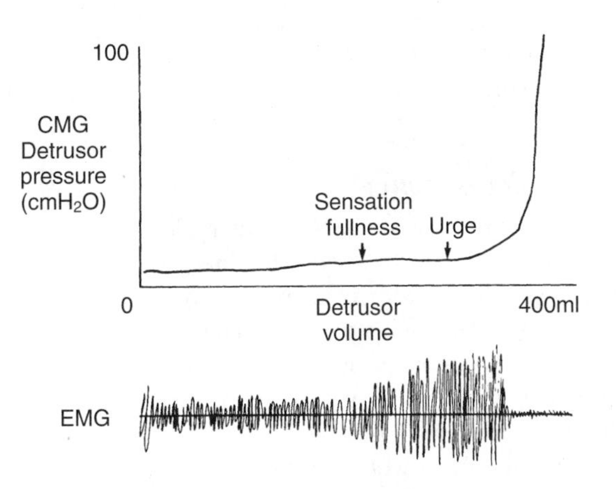

Figure 19-6 Normal results of CMG and EMG. (From Wheeler, J.S., Niecestro, R.M., & Goggin, C. [1988]. *Journal of Enterostomal Therapy,* 15[6], 244.)

normal results of a CMG and EMG. The CMG shows low bladder pressure at low bladder volumes. As the bladder fills, the person feels the sensation of fullness and the urge to void. The EMG shows increased muscle activity in the pelvic floor and sphincter muscles as the person feels the urge to void. This is the guarding reflex. As the micturition threshold is reached, the EMG activity diminishes, and the CMG shows a rapid rise in bladder pressure. These changes are consistent with the contraction of the bladder and appropriate sphincter relaxation associated with normal coordinated voluntary voiding.

Age-Related Factors in Voiding

A newborn baby voids by virtue of the complex reflex arc. As the bladder fills, stretch receptors in the detrusor send sensory messages through the S2-S4 segments to the pontine micturition center. When the impulses are strong enough, the reflex arc is completed, motor impulses cause bladder contraction coordinated with urethral sphincter relaxation, and the bladder empties. This filling and emptying cycle is repeated throughout the 24-hour period. At this stage the baby's immature central nervous system cannot consciously appreciate or voluntarily control this cycle. The child is thus incontinent. Between the ages of 2 and 3 years, a child acquires continence from the combination of two processes: societal expectation and maturation of the central nervous system. By the age of 3 years, most children have the mental and neuromuscular capacity to inhibit the reflex arc to prevent voiding and initiate voluntary voiding appropriately during the day. However, it is common for children up to 5 years old to have both periodic incontinence accidents during the day and nocturnal enuresis (Rathe & Klioze, 2000).

At puberty the pelvic genitalia become functional in both boys and girls. In boys the prostate gland grows large enough to assist with ejaculation. The growth of the prostate gland provides support for the pelvic floor and increases urethral resistance. In girls the structures of the pelvic floor mature. The tone of muscles of the pelvic floor and the urethra in women is maintained by stimulating estrogen receptors in those structures. At puberty the release of estrogen increases muscle tone of the pelvic floor and increases urethral resistance. The normal pelvic floor is illustrated in Figure 19-7, *A*.

In the adult male the prostate grows slowly until approximately age 45 years, when growth accelerates. With prostate enlargement, there is increased urethral resistance. Depending on the severity of urethral obstruction, the increased contractility needed to overcome the urethral resistance can cause the bladder to hypertrophy or decompensate, leading to urinary retention.

Women may experience temporary or permanent distortion or trauma to the pelvic floor and urethral anatomy as a result of childbirth. With normal pregnancy and delivery, postpartum exercises and return of normal estrogen levels, the tone of the pelvic floor and the integrity of the lower urinary tract usually will be restored. After menopause women experience a decrease in estrogen levels, causing atrophy of the pelvic floor structures. The urethral mucosa also becomes thin and friable, reducing coaptation, thus decreasing urethral resistance and predisposing to infection. Decreased tone of the pelvic floor may allow herniation of the urinary tract through the supporting structures, decreasing urethral resistance. Postmenopausal women may experience incontinence when bladder pressure surpasses urethral resistance such as during coughing, sneezing, laughing, or exercising.

There are other, less clearly understood, effects of aging on bladder function. For one, a decrease in bladder capacity makes the urge to void occur more frequently. Older persons experience a delayed onset of the desire to void, making it more difficult to further delay voiding. As a result an increase in the residual urine volume raises potential for urinary tract infections. Older persons experience an increase in the number of involuntary detrusor contractions, contributing to the symptoms of urgency, frequency, and incontinence. The decrease in urethral and bladder compliance is coupled with lowered maximal urethral closure pressure (Resnick & Yalla, 1985). Elderly clients also may experience functional changes in vision, mobility, and dexterity, making it difficult to locate and reach the toilet, as well as managing clothing in time to void without being incontinent (Guerrero & Sinert, 2001). All of these problems may be exaggerated by medications such as diuretics, which may increase urgency. Although urinary incontinence should not be accepted as a normal part of aging, these age-related changes predispose older persons to incontinence and are discussed in Chapter 30.

In summary, normal function of the urinary tract and continence are dependent on anatomic integrity of the bladder and urethra, an intact neurological system that provides voluntary control of micturition, the pattern of urine production, and the physical and mental ability and the psychological willingness of the person to perform tasks associated with toileting (Tanagho, 1990).

Incontinence, then, is a symptom of another problem. A symptomatic approach to the assessment and treatment of incontinence provides opportunities for rehabilitation nursing interventions to improve the quality of life of individuals experiencing incontinence.

TYPES OF INCONTINENCE

For the purpose of this chapter, incontinence is categorized into three basic types: transient, established, and neurogenic. These are somewhat artificial and overlapping classifications; however, these distinctions help to facilitate the discussion of incontinence. Transient or acute incontinence has a precipitous onset. It usually is associated with an acute medical or surgical condition and often resolves when the precipitating condition is addressed. Established, persistent, or chronic incontinence may have a sudden onset precipitated by an acute condition or it may have a gradual onset without a known precipitating cause (Ouslander, 1981; Guerrero & Sinert, 2001). Neurogenic incontinence may have a sudden or progressive onset, depending on the disease or trauma that causes the lesion within the nervous system.

Transient Incontinence

In today's complicated health care delivery system, patients are exposed to multiple and interacting factors that can contribute to urinary incontinence. This is called transient incontinence because many of these factors are reversible. The most common of these factors are included in the mnemonic DIAPPERS (**d**elirium, **i**nfection or **i**nflammation, **a**trophic vaginitis and urethritis, **p**harmaceuticals, **p**sychological conditions, conditions resulting in **e**xcess urine production, **r**estricted mobility, and **s**tool impaction) (Resnick, 1996). Clients subject to these factors need comprehensive diagnostic evaluation that focuses not only on the lower urinary tract but also on the person's general medical condition and functional status (Fantl et al., 1996). Table 19-2 lists reversible conditions that may cause or contribute to transient urinary incontinence.

Established Incontinence

Established incontinence cannot be easily reversed; it is usually caused by a pathological condition within the urinary tract or neurological system or by irreversible cognitive impairment (Brandeis et al., 1997). In 1975 the International Continence Society (ICS) established a vocabulary and classification system for the types of incontinence They originally identified four major types of incontinence: stress incontinence, urge incontinence, overflow incontinence, and reflex incontinence (Bates et al., 1979). In 1988 an updated report was issued with revised definitions of the types of incontinence (Abrams, Blaivas, Stanton, Andersen, 1988). With the addition of functional incontinence to these classifications, both the North American Nursing Diagnosis Association and the 1996 AHCPR Guidelines Panel have based their classification systems on the ICS system (Fantl et al., 1996; Gordon, 2000).

Stress Incontinence

Stress incontinence is the involuntary loss of urine when intravesical pressure exceeds the maximum intraurethral pressure in the absence of detrusor contraction (Abrams et al., 1988). Stress incontinence is characterized by sudden loss of small amounts of urine with an increase in intra-abdominal pressure during coughing, sneezing, laughing, lifting, or bending (Figure 19-7). Stress incontinence is seen more commonly in women but also may occur in men after prostatectomy.

Urge Incontinence. Urge incontinence is the involuntary loss of urine associated with a strong urge to void. Urge incontinence is divided into motor and sensory urgency. Motor urgency is ascribed to overactive detrusor function—either unstable detrusor contractions or detrusor hyperreflexia. Sensory urgency is ascribed to hypersensitivity (Abrams et al., 1988). Urine is lost in moderate to large amounts, and clients cannot reach the toilet before leakage occurs. They also report symptoms of urinary frequency and nocturia (Guerrero & Sinert, 2001). Urge incontinence is associated with supratentorial central nervous system lesions. When this is the case, it is referred to as uninhibited bladder (see the neurogenic bladder section). When there is no overt neuropathy, the cause usually is referred to as detrusor instability (Figure 19-8). The causes may be local irritation of the bladder or simply idiopathic (Gray, 2000).

TABLE 19-2 Identification and Management of Reversible Conditions That Cause or Contribute to Urinary Incontinence

Condition	Management
Conditions Affecting the Lower Urinary Tract	
Urinary tract infection (symptomatic with frequency, urgency, dysuria, etc.)	Antimicrobial therapy
Atrophic vaginitis/urethritis	Oral or topical estrogen
Pregnancy/vaginal delivery/episiotomy	Behavioral intervention; avoid surgical therapy postpartum, as condition may be self-limiting
Postprostatectomy	Behavioral intervention; avoid surgical therapy until clear condition will not resolve
Stool impaction	Disimpaction; appropriate use of stool softeners, bulk-forming agents, and laxatives if necessary; implement high fiber intake, adequate mobility and fluid intake
Increased Urine Production	
Metabolic (hyperglycemia, hypercalcemia)	Better control of diabetes mellitus. Therapy for hypercalcemia depends on underlying cause.
Excess fluid intake	Reduction in intake of diuretic fluids (e.g., caffeinated beverages)
Volume Overload	
Venous insufficiency with edema	Support stockings; leg elevation; sodium restriction; diuretic therapy
Congestive heart failure	Medical therapy
Impaired ability or willingness to reach a toilet	
Delirium	Diagnosis and treatment of underlying cause(s) of acute confusional state
Chronic illness, injury, or restraint that interferes with mobility	Regular toileting; use of toilet substitutes; environmental alterations (e.g., bedside commode/urinal)
Psychological	Remove restraints if possible. Appropriate pharmacological and/or nonpharmacological treatment
Drug Side Effects*	
Diuretics (polyuria, frequency, and urgency)	With all medications, discontinue or change therapy, as clinically possible. Dosage reduction or modification (e.g., flexible scheduling of rapid-acting diuretics) may also help.
Caffeine (aggravation or precipitation of UI)	
Anticholinergic agents (urinary retention; overflow incontinence; impaction)	
Antidepressants (anticholinergic actions; sedation)	
Antipsychotics (anticholinergic actions, sedation, rigidity, immobility	
Sedatives/hypnotics/CNS depressants (sedation, delirium, immobility, muscle relaxation)	
Narcotic analgesics (causing urinary retention, fecal impaction, sedation, delirium)	
Alpha-adrenergic blockers (urethral relaxation)	
Alpha-adrenergic agonists (urinary retention—present in many cold and OTC preparations)	
Beta-adrenergic agonists (urinary retention)	
Calcium channel blockers (urinary retention)	
Alcohol (polyuria, frequency, urgency, sedation, delirium, immobility)	

*From Fantl, J.A., Newman, D.K., Colling, J., DeLancey, J., Keeys, C., Loughery, R., McDowell, B., Norton, P., Ouslander, J., Schnelle, J., Staskin, D., Tries, J., Urich, V., Vitousek, S., Weiss, B., & Whitmore, K. (1996, March). *Urinary incontinence in adults: Acute and chronic management* (AHCPR Publication No. 96-0682, Clinical Practice Guideline No. 2, 1996 Update). Rockville, MD: U.S. Department of Health and Human Services, Public Health Service, Agency for Health Care Policy and Research.

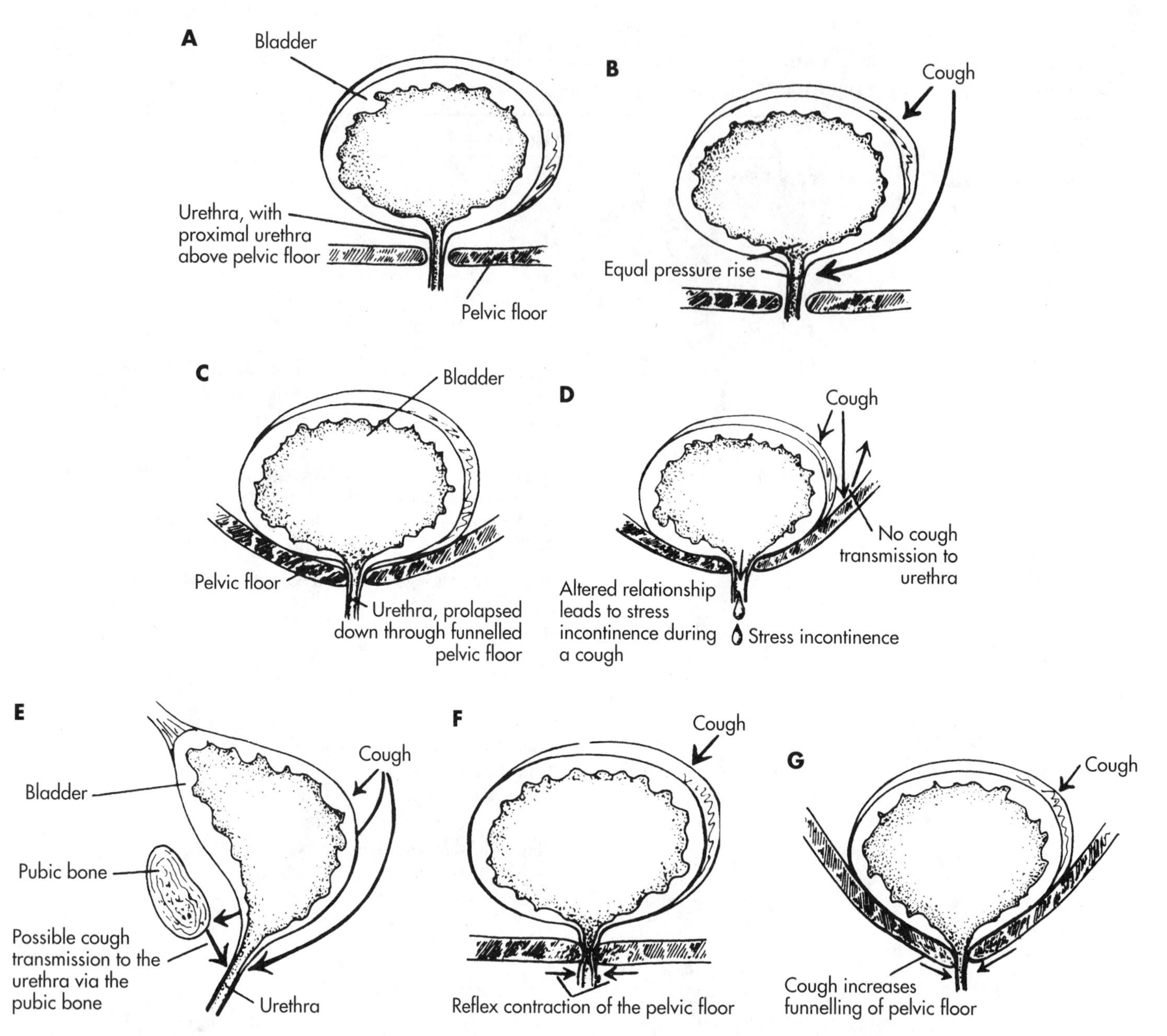

Figure 19-7 **A,** Normal anatomic relationship of bladder, urethra, and pelvic floor at rest; **B,** During a cough. **C,** In a woman with stress incontinence: at rest; **D,** During a cough. **E,** Possible cough transmission to the urethra by way of the pubic bone. **F,** Normal contraction of the pelvic floor with raised abdominal pressure. **G,** Contraction of the pelvic floor with stress incontinence. (From Jeter, K.F., Fallen, N., & Norton, C. [1990]. *Nursing for continence.* Philadelphia: WB Saunders.)

Overflow Incontinence. Overflow incontinence is occurs when any urine is lost involuntarily when associated with an overdistended bladder (Abrams et al., 1988). Overflow incontinence is characterized by continuous dribbling of small amounts of urine and frequent voiding of small amounts of urine as a result of an overdistended bladder, either because of outlet obstruction (Figure 19-9) or impaired bladder contractility (Guerrero & Sinert, 2001) (Figure 19-10). The most common nonneurogenic cause of overflow incontinence in men is prostatic hypertrophy because it causes an outlet obstruction. Although outlet obstruction is rare in women, it can occur as a complication of an anti-incontinence surgical procedure or because of severe pelvic organ prolapse (Fantl et al., 1996).

Reflex Incontinence. Reflex incontinence is defined as a "loss of urine due to detrusor hyperreflexia and/or involuntary urethral relaxation in the absence of the sensation usually associated with desire to micturate. This condition is only seen in clients with neuropathic bladder/urethral disorders" (Abrams et al., 1988, p. 9). Rarely, reflex incontinence may be seen as a result of radiation cystitis, inflammatory bladder conditions such as chemical cystitis, or interstitial

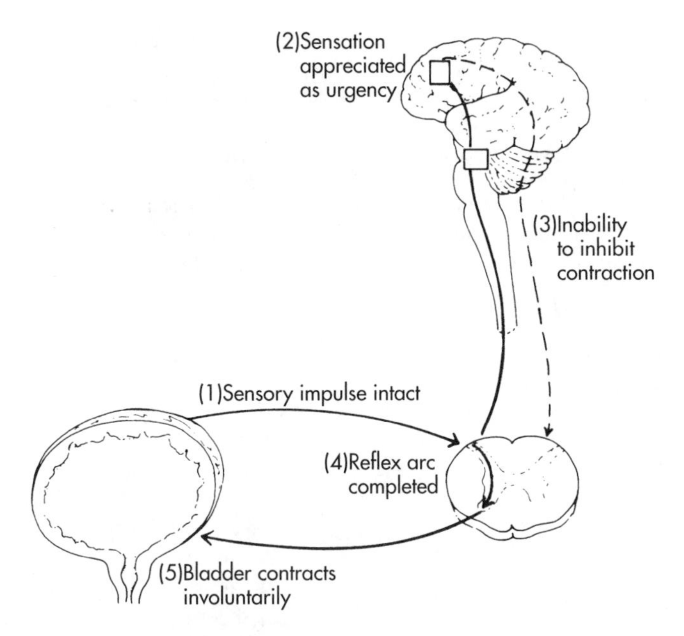

Figure 19-8 Detrusor instability. (From Jeter, K.F., Fallen, N., & Norton, C. [1990]. *Nursing for continence.* Philadelphia: WB Saunders.)

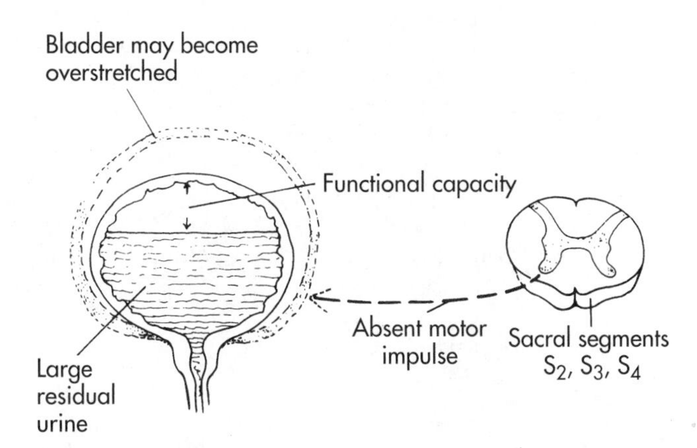

Figure 19-10 Atonic bladder. (From Jeter, K.F., Fallen, N., & Norton, C. [1990]. *Nursing for continence.* Philadelphia: WB Saunders.)

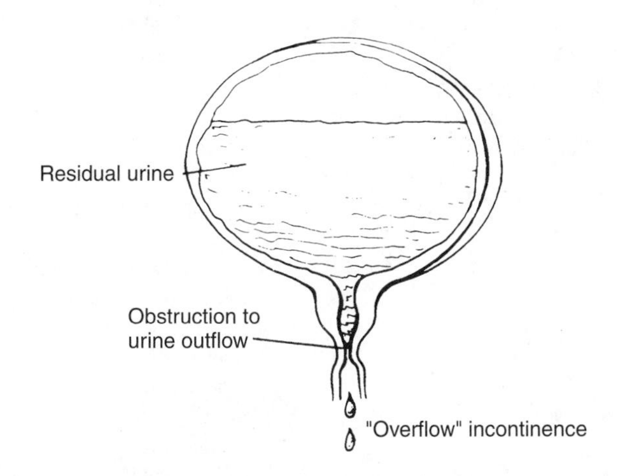

Figure 19-9 Outflow obstruction. (From Jeter, K.F., Fallen, N., & Norton, C. [1990]. *Nursing for continence.* Philadelphia: WB Saunders.)

cystitis (Fantl et al., 1996). Reflex incontinence will be covered in the neurogenic incontinence section.

Functional Incontinence. Although not identified by the ICS, functional incontinence is another major classification used by clinicians. Functional incontinence is defined as urine loss caused by problems outside the urinary tract. The lower urinary tract functions correctly, but problems in other areas effect bladder control. Functional incontinence is most often related to cognitive impairment or loss of mobility (Jirovec, 2000). Functional incontinence may also result from psychological unwillingness or environmental barriers to toilets (Bates et al., 1979). In true functional incontinence, there is normal functioning of the lower urinary tract although cognitive and physical impairment can exacerbate incontinence from other causes. Table 19-3 lists types and causes of established urinary incontinence.

Neurogenic Incontinence

Neurogenic bladder dysfunction is the most common form of bladder impairment seen in rehabilitation settings. In the community, rehabilitation nurses are the primary case managers for clients regarding incontinence; in many instances they may advocate for continence issues to be addressed in a client's care plan.

CLASSIFICATION OF NEUROGENIC BLADDER DYSFUNCTION

Neurogenic bladders are classified into five types and are labeled according to the underlying pathological process: (1) uninhibited, (2) reflex, (3) autonomous, (4) sensory paralytic, and (5) motor paralytic neurogenic bladders. Most neurogenic bladders represent a combined motor and sensory impairment. For ease of description, the types of neurogenic bladder are described here according to the schema proposed by Lapides and Diokno (1976).

Uninhibited Neurogenic Bladder

The uninhibited neurogenic bladder results from a disruption of the corticoregulatory tract or a malfunction of the supraspinal center that regulates voiding. Figure 19-11

Table 19-3 Types and Causes of Established Urinary Incontinence

Functional Type	Description	Associated Characteristics	Pathophysiology	Common Causes
Stress	Urine leakage associated with a sudden increase in intraabdominal pressure (e.g., as a result of a cough, sneeze, laugh, or exercise); amount of urine loss usually minimal to moderate	Occurs usually in the daytime only; infrequently, nocturnal incontinence may occur	Sphincter incompetence; urethral instability	Pelvic prolapse in women; sphincter weakness or damage (e.g., as a result of a prostatectomy)
Urge	Urine leakage preceded by a strong desire to void; urine loss varies from moderate to large amount	Urinary frequency, nocturia; possible suprapubic discomfort	Detrusor instability	Central nervous system damage secondary to stroke, Alzheimer's disease, brain tumor, or Parkinson's disease; interference with spinal inhibitory pathways secondary to spondylosis or metastasis; local bladder disorders such as bladder cancer, radiation effects, interstitial cystitis, or outlet obstruction
Overflow	Periodic or continuous dribbling of urine resulting from obstruction or over-distention of the bladder	Hesitancy, straining to void, weak or interrupted urinary stream; occurs day or night	Outlet obstruction or underactive detrusor	Obstruction, as from prostatic hypertrophy, bladder neck obstruction, or urethral stricture; underactive detrusor, as from myogenic or neurogenic factors (e.g., herniated disk or peripheral neuropathy secondary to diabetes mellitus); anticholinergic/antispasmodic drugs
Functional	Urine leakage associated with an inability or unwillingness to toilet appropriately because of cognitive or physical impairments, psychological factors, or environmental barriers	May be complicated by other medical problems, iatrogenic illness, or adverse stimuli	Normal bladder and urethral function	Impaired mobility or cognitive status; inaccessible toilets; depression, anger, hostility, or schizophrenia

From Wyman, J.F. (1988). Nursing assessment of the incontinent geriatric outpatient population. *Nursing Clinics of North America, 23,* 181.

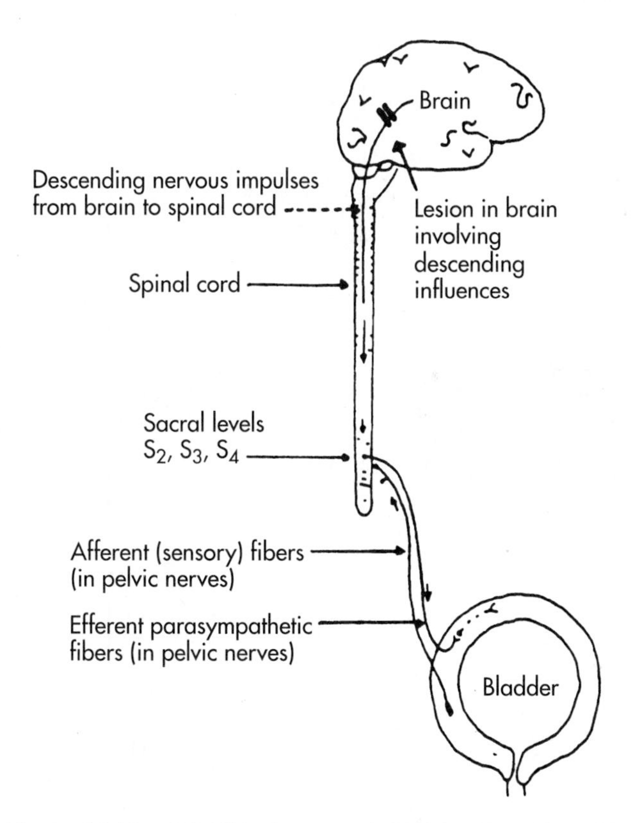

Figure 19-11 Uninhibited neurogenic bladder. (From Pires, M., & Lockhart-Pretti, P. [1992]. *Nursing management of neurogenic incontinence.* Skokie, IL: Rehabilitation Nursing Foundation.)

shows areas of the nervous system where damage may occur, and Table 19-4 lists the possible causes.

Frequent uninhibited contractions occur, but the bladder usually empties completely, resulting in no residual urine. The micturition reflex remains intact. Sensation is present because is the bulbocavernosus reflex. A CMG will demonstrate strong, uninhibited contractions as the bladder is filled. The capacity of the bladder is decreased, and involuntary voiding will take place almost as soon as the urge is perceived.

Persons with uninhibited neurogenic bladder frequently complain about the urgency and frequency of urination and nocturia. After the urge is perceived, they cannot inhibit flow. When the external sphincter is voluntarily contracted, partial control of urination, even with strong voiding contractions, is possible. The intravesical pressure, however, remains high because of the force of detrusor contractions. Anticholinergic medication may be recommended to decrease bladder contractility and increase bladder capacity (Giroux, 1988). These clients may be able to avoid incontinence by voiding before the bladder is full enough to trigger the micturition reflex. Therefore an important part of nursing intervention is scheduled voiding and attention to fluid intake, to anticipate the need to void before the urge becomes too strong. For those clients who can follow three step commands and volitionally start and stop their urinary stream, bladder training is a nursing intervention that may lead to continence. See Figure 19-12 for a treatment algorithm for uninhibited neurogenic bladder.

A Special Concern: Spinal Shock

Immediately after spinal injury, the person experiences some degree of spinal shock, a temporary condition of flaccid paralysis and loss of all reflex activity below the level of the lesion. Complete anesthesia and flaccid paralysis are present below the level of the lesion, regardless of the site of damage. The signs of spinal shock related to the urinary tract mirror the signs of autonomous neurogenic bladder–that is, reflexes are absent; perception of fullness is absent; and the bladder becomes overdistended. Findings from the CMG show a very large bladder capacity, absence of detrusor contractions, and low intravesical pressure. Spinal shock may last from a few weeks to a few months. Signs of resolution vary according to the cord level of the lesion and the type of neurogenic bladder that results, either reflex or autonomous.

Reflex Neurogenic Bladder

The reflex neurogenic bladder also is referred to as an upper motor neuron, suprasacral, spastic, or central neurogenic bladder. This type of bladder dysfunction occurs when both the sensory and motor tracts of the spinal cord, which send messages between the bladder and the supraspinal center, are disrupted. Figure 19-13 demonstrates where damage may occur, and Table 19-4 contains lists of the possible causes.

The reflex arc remains intact, and voiding is involuntary because of the lack of cerebral control and may be incomplete because of uncoordinated bladder contractions. The bulbocavernosus reflex is present and hyperactive. A CMG shows uninhibited contractions with decreased bladder capacity. The detrusor muscle frequently hypertrophies, which can lead to vesicoureteral reflux, hydronephrosis, and permanent renal damage.

The person with reflex neurogenic bladder is unable to sense fullness and is unable to void volitionally; therefore, micturition cannot be started or stopped in the normal manner. If the detrusor contraction and external urinary sphincter are coordinated, spontaneous voiding will occur when the micturition reflex arc is stimulated. If the two events are uncoordinated, however, pressure within the bladder wall will increase as the detrusor attempts to contract against the contracted external urinary sphincter. The resulting dysfunction is termed detrusor sphincter dyssynergia (DSD). Combined cystometry and EMG of the external sphincter demonstrates that during detrusor contraction, the periurethral muscle also contracts. This pattern causes increased resistance to outflow with high intravesical pressure, high residual urine volumes, and poor bladder emptying (Erickson, 1980).

TABLE 19-4 Neurogenic Bladder Dysfunction and Management

Dysfunction	Level in Neuraxis	Possible Etiology	Voluntary Control	Saddle Sensation	Bulbocavernous Reflex	Signs and Symptoms	Management
Uninhibited neurogenic	Cortical and subcortical	Newborn child, CVA, MS, cerebral arteriosclerosis, brain tumor, pernicious anemia, trauma	Initiation or inhibition diminished	Normal	Normal	Frequency, urgency, urge incontinence, nocturia, decreased bladder capacity	Scheduled voiding, anticholinergic drugs Male: external collection device (condom type) Female: "padding"
Reflex neurogenic	Spinal cord above conus medullaris	Trauma, tumor, vascular disease, MS, syringomyelia, pernicious anemia	Absent	Absent or impaired	Hyperactive	Unpredictable voiding: stream starts and stops (may initially appear as areflexic during spinal shock)	Reflex voiding with alpha blocker or IC with anticholinergic drugs, or surgery
Autonomous (areflex) neurogenic	At conus medullaris or cauda equine	Spina bifida, myelomeningocele, tumor, postoperative radical pelvic surgery, herniated intervertebral disk	Absent	Absent	Absent	Increased bladder capacity, high residual, dribbling incontinence, no bladder contractions, overflow (stress) incontinence with straining or compression	IC, Valsalva maneuver (strain), Credé's methods (if permitted)
Motor paralytic	Anterior horn cells or S2, S3, or S4 ventral roots	Poliomyelitis, herniated intervertebral disk, trauma, tumor	Absent	Normal	Absent	Voiding similar to clients with symptoms of "prostatism" strain to void, incontinence rare	IC, Valsalva maneuver (strain), Credé's methods (if permitted)
Sensory paralytic	S2, S3, or S4 dorsal roots or cells of origin or dorsal horns of spinal cord	Diabetes mellitus, tabes dorsalis	Normal initially becomes impaired with chronic overdistention	Absent	Absent	Voids only 1-3 times daily; overflow incontinence rare	Timed voiding, IC

Courtesy Rancho Los Amigos Medical Center, Downey, CA.
CVA, Cerebrovascular accident; *MS,* multiple sclerosis; *IC,* intermittent catheterization.

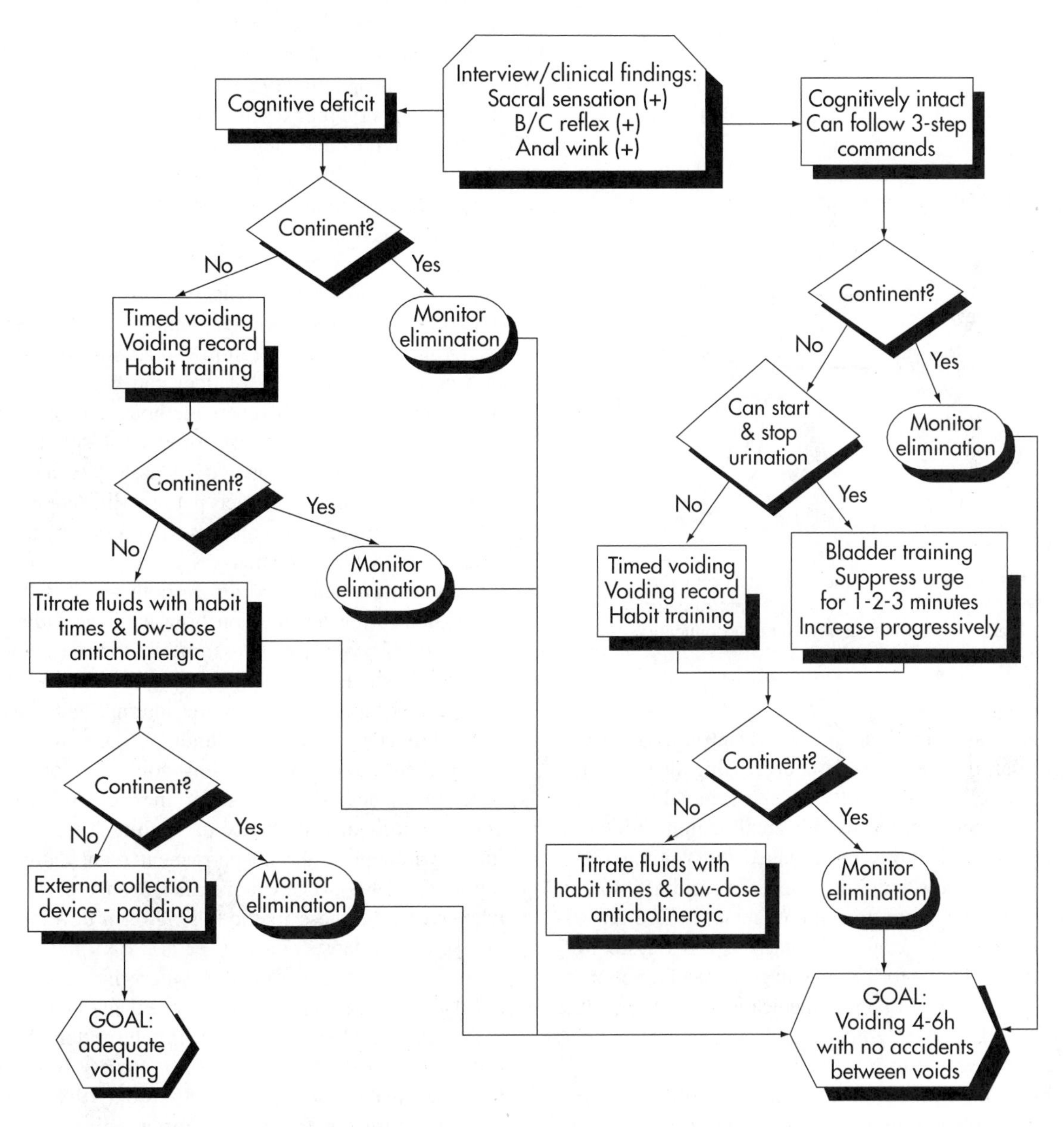

Figure 19-12 Algorithm for uninhibited neurogenic bladder. (Copyright 2000, Rancho Los Amigos National Rehabilitation Center, Downey, CA.)

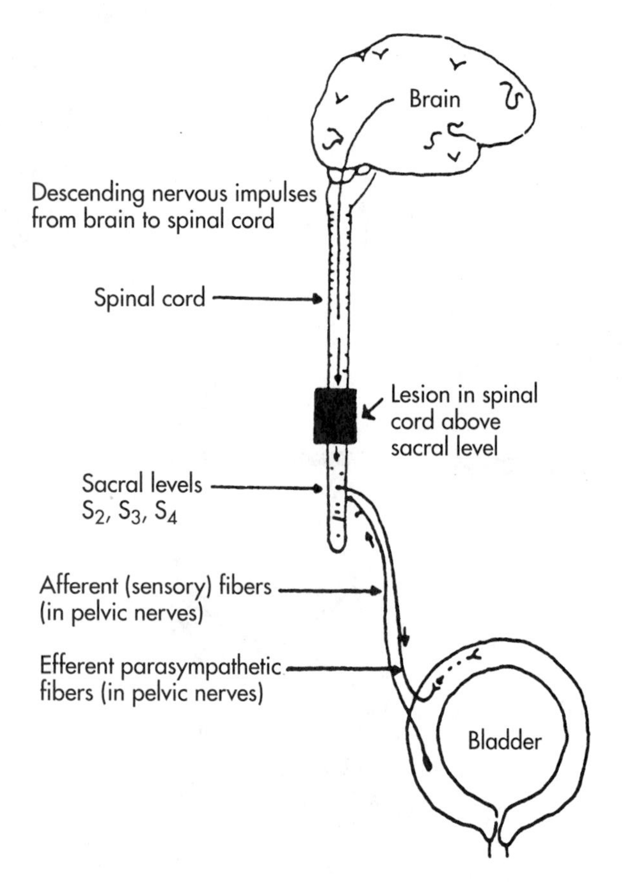

Figure 19-13 Reflex neurogenic bladder. (From Pires, M., & Lockhart-Pretti, P. [1992]. Nursing management of neurogenic incontinence. Skokie, IL: Rehabilitation Nursing Foundation.)

Drugs such as dantrolene sodium (Dantrium) and baclofen (Lioresal) may be valuable in decreasing the spasticity of skeletal muscle, including that of the external sphincter. Anticholinergic medications used in combination with these antispasmodic medications may reduce the voiding pressures enough to allow low-pressure reflex voiding (40 cm H_2O). This bladder program requires males to use an external condom and leg bag and women to use a system of padding. An alternative for those with good hand function is to increase the anticholinergic medications, allowing the person to stay dry and to empty the bladder by intermittent catheterization every 4 to 6 hours (Giroux, 1988). See Figures 19-14 through 19-16 for a treatment algorithm for reflex neurogenic bladder highlighting the options of continuous intermittent catheterization or voiding by reflex.

Autonomous Neurogenic Bladder

The autonomous neurogenic bladder also is referred to as a lower motor neuron, flaccid, atonic, areflexic, nonreflex, sacral, or peripheral bladder. It is difficult to determine when spinal shock subsides for a client who has an autonomous neurogenic bladder, because the characteristics are similar. Damage occurs to the conus medullaris or cauda equina (lesions involving the reflex arc), disrupting pathways that carry sensory impulses from the bladder to the spinal cord, motor impulses from the spinal cord to the detrusor muscle, and motor impulses from the spinal cord to the external sphincter. Figure 19-17 illustrates areas where damage may occur, and Table 19-4 lists possible causes. Autonomous neurogenic bladder is the most common neurogenic bladder dysfunction seen in children with the congenital disabilities of spina bifida and myelomeningocele.

Voiding is involuntary and occurs when the bladder overflows. Peripheral reflexes and the bulbocavernosus reflex are absent or hypoactive. Sensation and motor control also are absent. Findings from a CMG demonstrate the absence of uninhibited contractions, a bladder capacity above normal (600 to 1000 ml), decreased intravesical pressure, and residual urine.

As with reflex neurogenic bladder, the client with autonomous neurogenic bladder cannot sense fullness, cannot void volitionally, and therefore cannot start or stop voiding in a normal manner. The bladder can be partially emptied with manual pressure (Credé's methods) and straining (Valsalva maneuver). Two patterns of external sphincter activity may occur: (1) no motor activity or (2) some uncontrollable activity. In the former pattern, the client can void while maintaining low intravesical pressure; in the latter pattern, the voiding maneuvers discussed previously may increase intravesical pressure. In both patterns the amount of residual urine depends on how well the individual can expel urine by applying pressure, the tone of smooth muscle and elasticity of the bladder wall, and the amount of muscle resistance offered by the internal and external urinary sphincters (Peschers, Jundt, & Dimpfl, 2000). Recently there has been increasing concern about the safety of Credé's methods because of the potential risk of the complications of high pressure voiding, vesicoureteral reflux, hydronephrosis, and permanent renal damage (Vickrey et al., 1999). There have also been reports of clients who have used these methods long term developing rectal or vaginal prolapse (Vickrey et al., 1999). If the bladder cannot be emptied completely when the person performs a Valsalva maneuver or does Credé's methods (if permitted), or if the client preference is intermittent catheterization, then intermittent catheterization every 6 to 8 hours is the usual management program (Giroux, 1988). See Figure 19-18 for a treatment algorithm for autonomous neurogenic bladder.

Sensory Paralytic Bladder

The sensory paralytic bladder occurs when the afferent or sensory side of the micturition reflex arc is damaged. This condition is most often seen in persons with diabetes who have sensory neuropathy. Figure 19-19 shows where damage occurs, and Table 19-4 lists the possible causes.

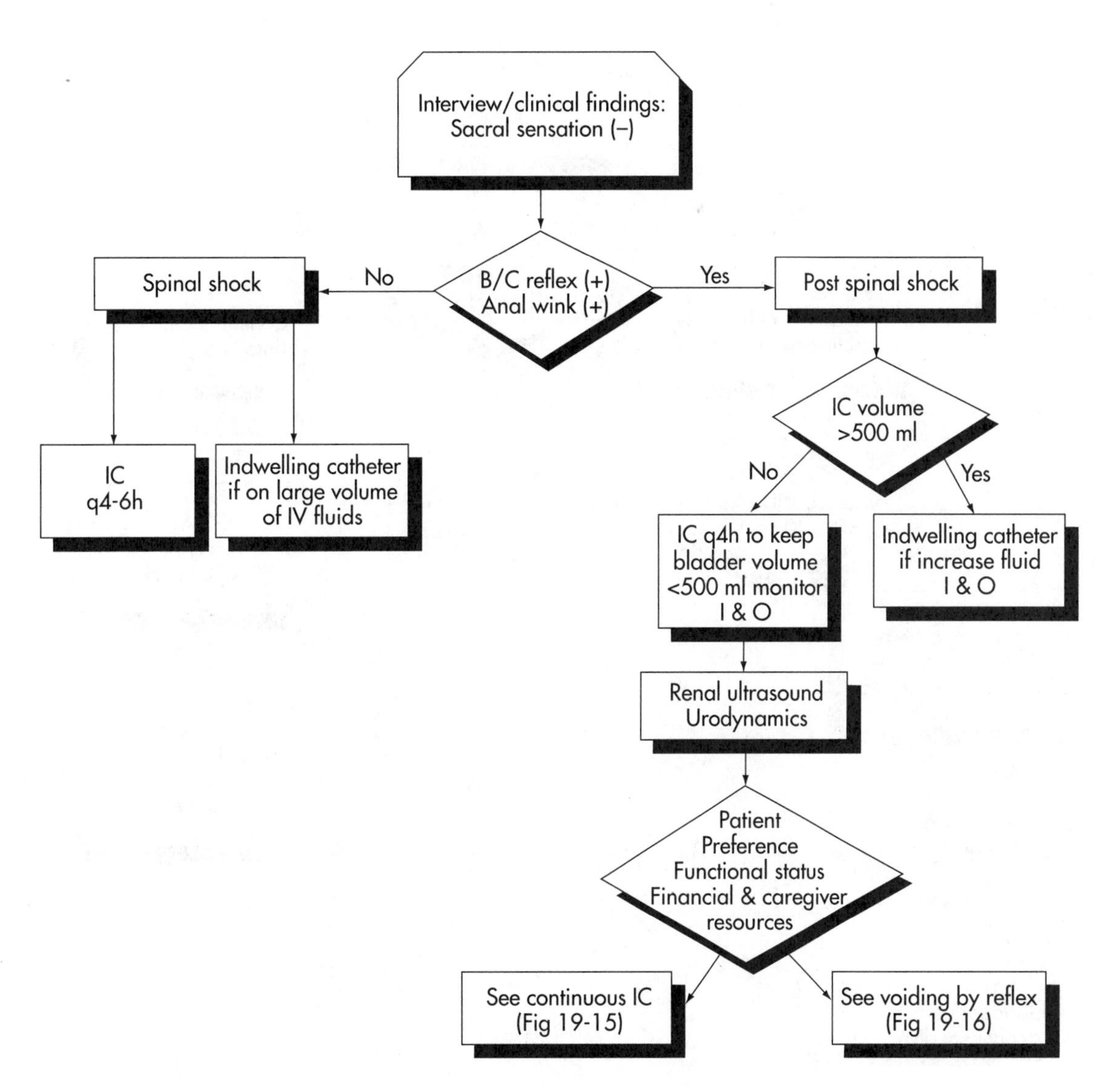

Figure 19-14 Algorithm for reflex bladder. (Copyright 2000, Rancho Los Amigos National Rehabilitation Center, Downey, CA.)

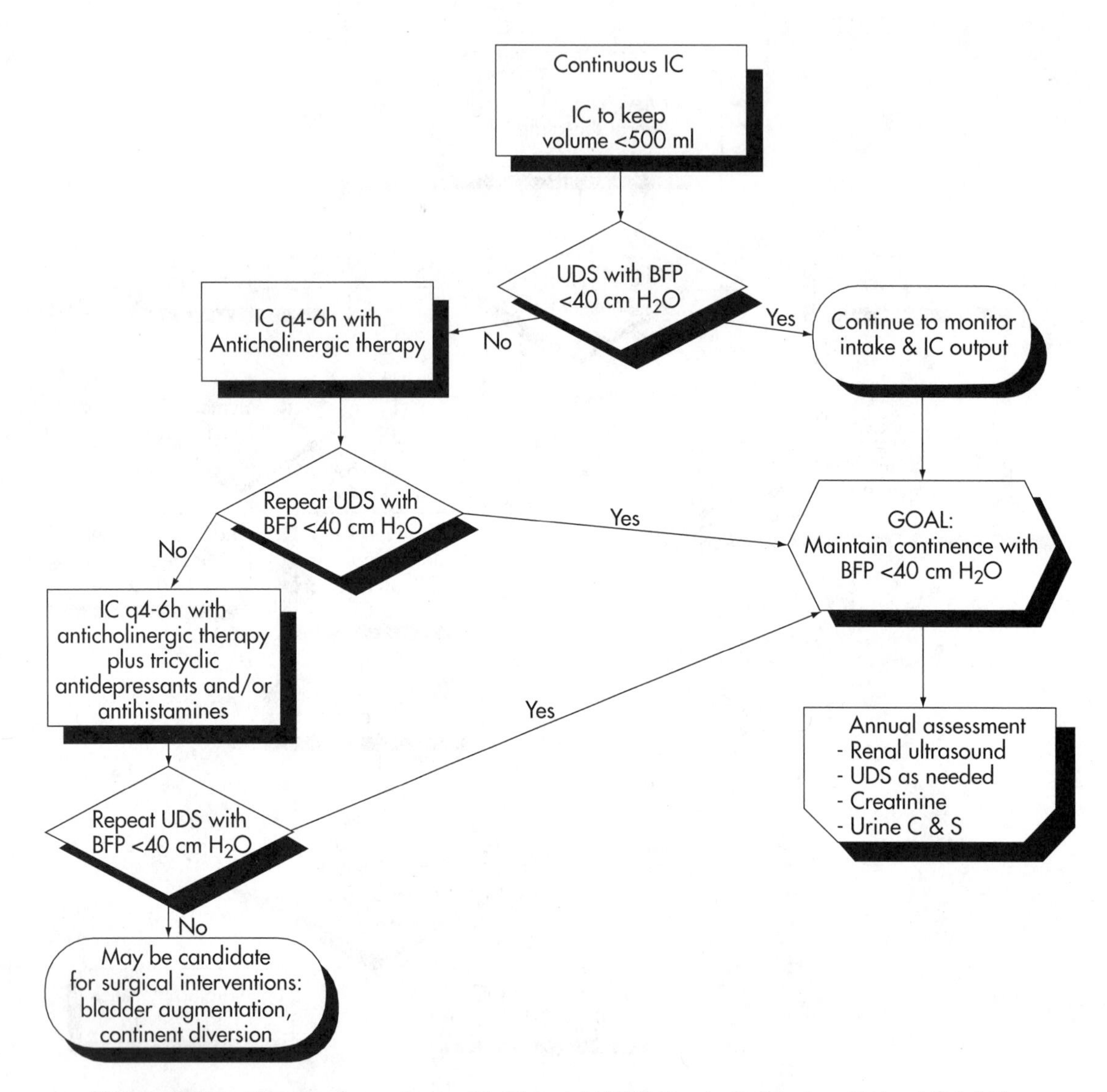

Figure 19-15 Algorithm for continuous IC. (Copyright 2000, Rancho Los Amigos National Rehabilitation Center, Downey, CA.)

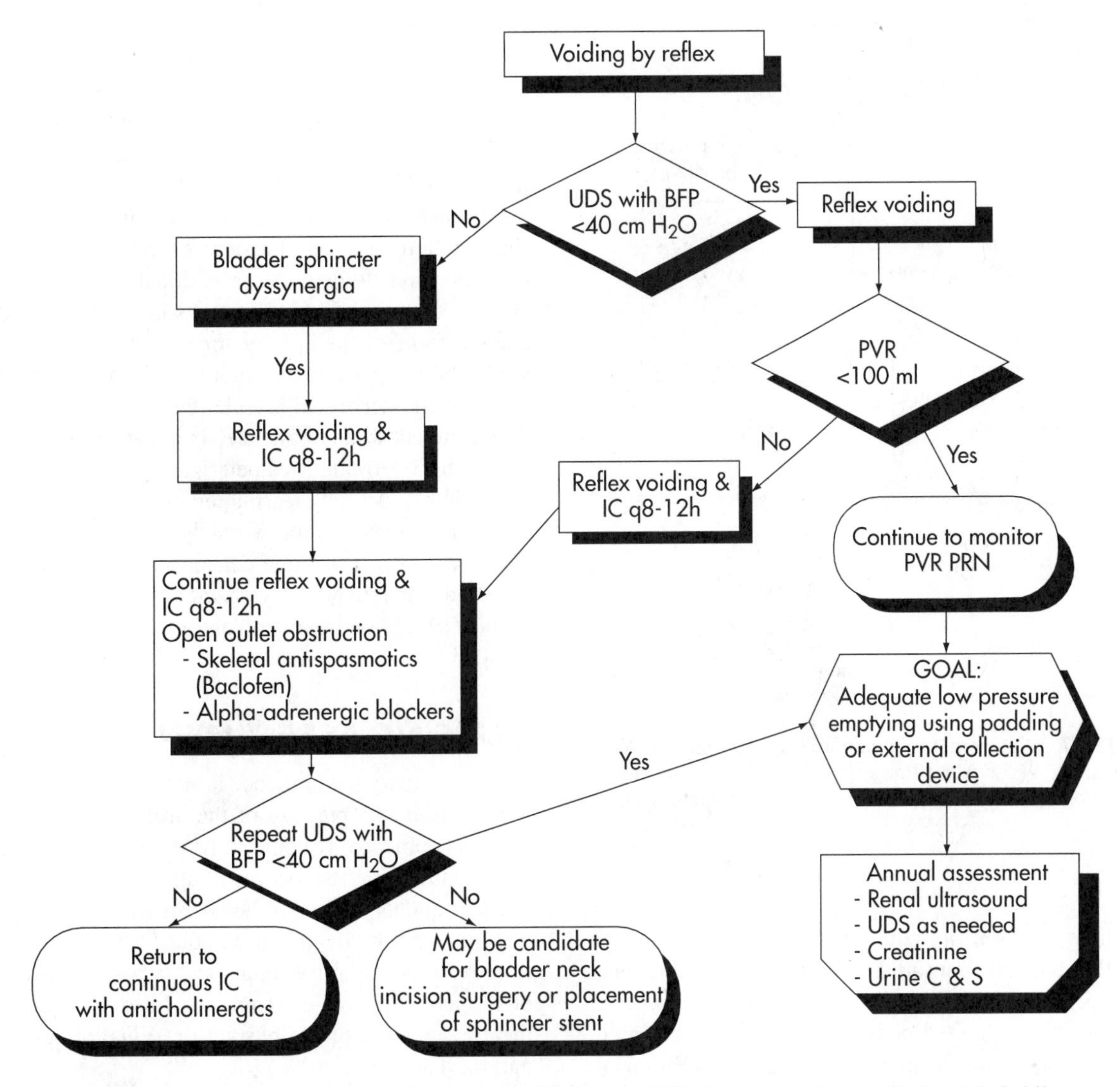

Figure 19-16 Algorithm for voiding by reflex. (Copyright 2000, Rancho Los Amigos National Rehabilitation Center, Downey, CA.)

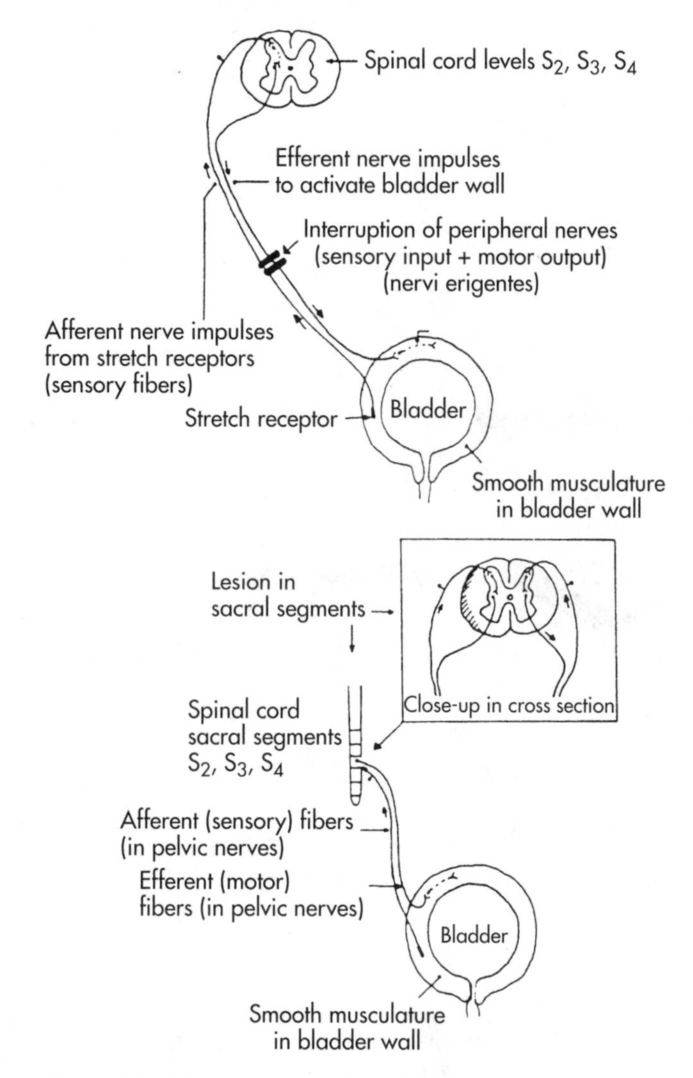

Figure 19-17 Autonomous (nonreflex) neurogenic bladder. (From Pires, M., & Lockhart-Pretti, P. [1992]. Nursing management of neurogenic incontinence. Skokie, IL: Rehabilitation Nursing Foundation.)

The client with sensory paralytic bladder is able to void volitionally, but the sensation of bladder fullness and emptiness is absent. Findings from the CMG demonstrate the absence of uninhibited contractions with an increased bladder capacity. Because of the lack of the sensation of emptiness, the presence of residual urine is variable, as is the presence of the bulbocavernosus reflex and perineal sensation.

The client senses no fullness, pain, or temperature but is able to initiate voiding unless the bladder has become markedly atonic because of prolonged periods of retention and overdistention. A loss of bladder wall tone may develop because of the large volumes of urine that collect in the bladder between voids. This urinary retention can lead to overflow incontinence. Because persons with sensory paralytic bladder retain motor control, they can avoid incontinence by utilizing a timed voiding program (Giroux, 1988). See Figure 19-20 for a treatment algorithm for sensory paralytic bladder.

Motor Paralytic Bladder

The motor paralytic bladder occurs when the efferent or motor side of the micturition reflex arc is damaged. Figure 19-21 demonstrates areas where damage may occur, and Table 19-4 lists the possible causes.

Voluntary control of urination is variable and sensation is normal. The bulbocavernosus reflex is absent. The CMG demonstrates no uninhibited contractions with increased bladder capacity. Residual urine is markedly increased.

Because sensory nerves are intact, the client will sense fullness and emptiness. Motor loss, however, will be partial or complete. When the onset of a motor paralytic bladder is slow and left untreated, the detrusor muscle may stretch and lose tone, resulting in large residual urine volumes. The client may complain of difficulties in initiating voiding, decreased force of the urinary stream, and a need to strain to void. These signs and symptoms result from loss of motor function and decreased muscle tone. The person may experience overflow incontinence, but distention may be prevented by intermittent catheterization. Persons with motor paralytic bladder may learn to empty the bladder by using a Valsalva maneuver and Credé's methods (if permitted) (Giroux, 1988). The same concerns about Credé's methods as noted previously apply to motor paralytic bladder. See Figure 19-22 for treatment algorithm for motor paralytic bladder.

NURSING ASSESSMENT

Because urinary incontinence is a symptom and not a condition in itself, the purpose of the urological nursing assessment is to objectively confirm the incontinence, identify factors contributing to or resulting from incontinence, to identify clients who may need further evaluation or those who may initiate treatment without further assessment, and to make a presumptive diagnosis, if possible. Components of the assessment should include history, physical assessment, estimation of the postvoid residual volume, and urinalysis (Fantl et al., 1996).

Subjective

History

It is important to remember that incontinence carries a social stigma. Not only are many persons embarrassed and reluctant to report incontinence, but often they define the problem of incontinence differently. Awareness and sensitivity to the emotional issues clients associate with incontinence are crucial. Furthermore, terminology used in the nursing assessment may need to be pragmatic. Rather than asking, "Are

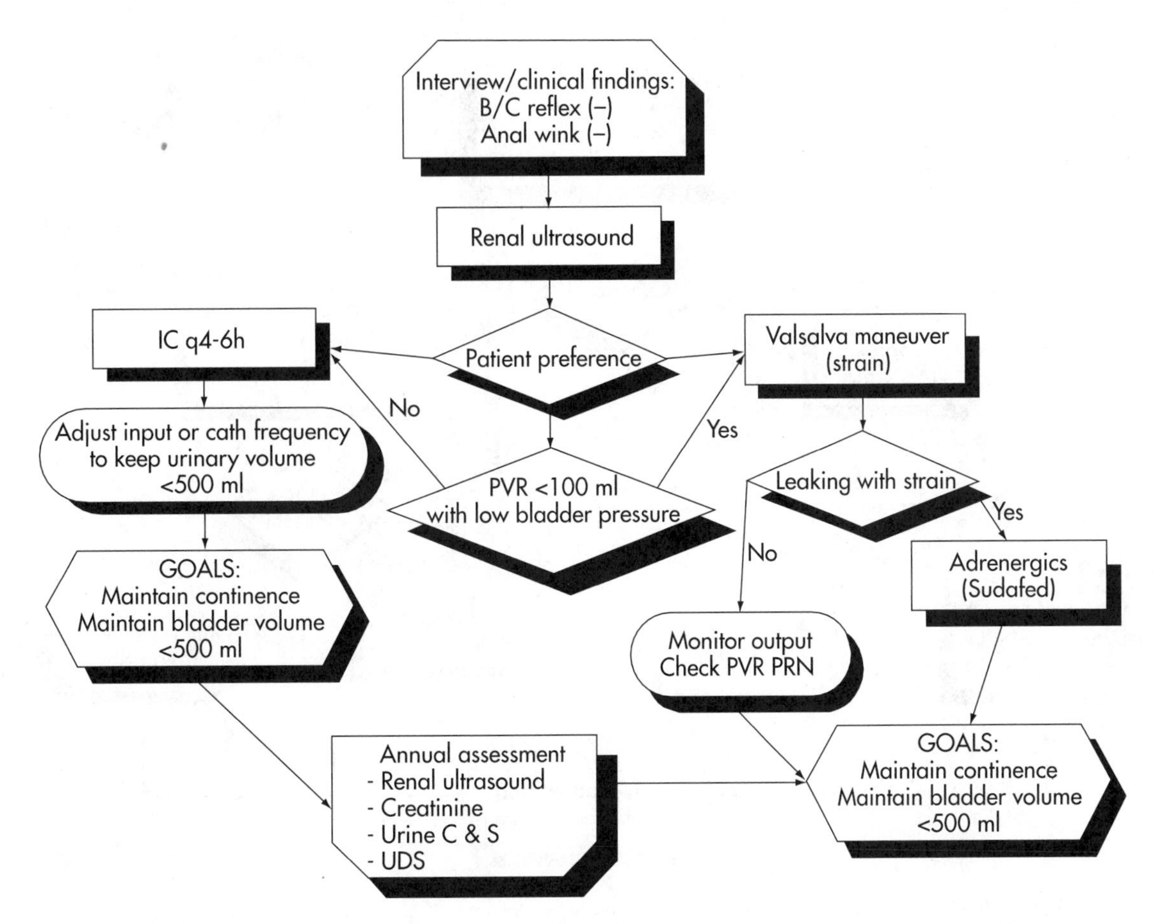

Figure 19-18 Algorithm for areflexic bladder. (Copyright 2000, Rancho Los Amigos National Rehabilitation Center, Downey, CA.)

you incontinent?" or "Do you have bladder control difficulties?" it may be more useful to ask, "Do you have trouble making it to the bathroom in time?" or "Do you lose urine (pass water) unexpectedly?" or "Do you wear pads to catch your urine?" (Wyman, 1988). For persons with neurological impairments, important questions include: "Do you know when you have urinated (passed water)?" and "Can you start or stop your urinary stream?"

The first part of the history focuses on the characteristics of the urinary incontinence in an effort to determine the type (i.e., stress, urge, overflow, neurogenic, functional, or mixed) (Fantl et al., 1996). The characteristics of onset, duration, frequency, and precipitating circumstances of the urinary incontinence are related to the type of incontinence. For instance, urinary leakage that occurs with sneezing, coughing, lifting, bending, laughing, or exercising is suggestive of stress incontinence; whereas leakage that occurs with hand washing or difficulty reaching the bathroom on time is suggestive of urge incontinence. The amount of urine lost with each episode suggests the type of incontinence. A sudden brief spurt of urine may denote stress incontinence; however, a prolonged steady stream is associated with urge

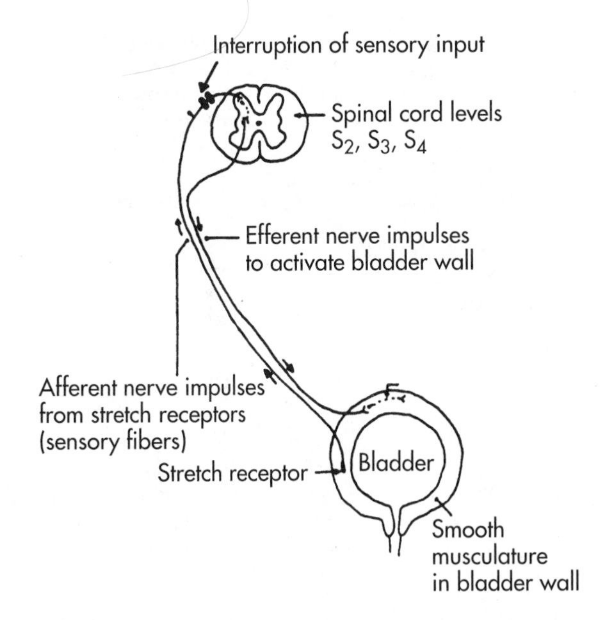

Figure 19-19 Sensory paralytic bladder. (From Pires, M., & Lockhart-Pretti, P. [1992]. Nursing management of neurogenic incontinence. Skokie, IL: Rehabilitation Nursing Foundation.)

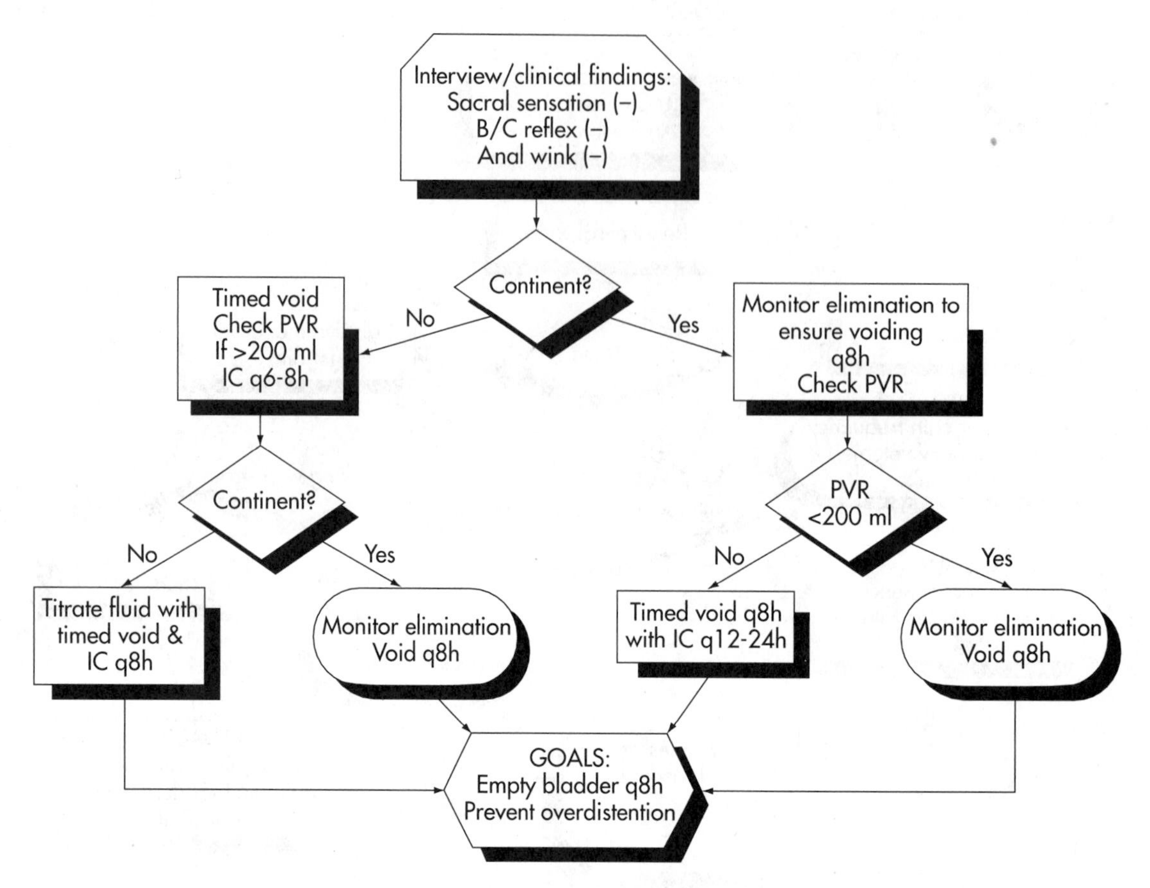

Figure 19-20 Algorithm for sensory paralytic neurogenic bladder. (Copyright 2000, Rancho Los Amigos National Rehabilitation Center, Downey, CA.)

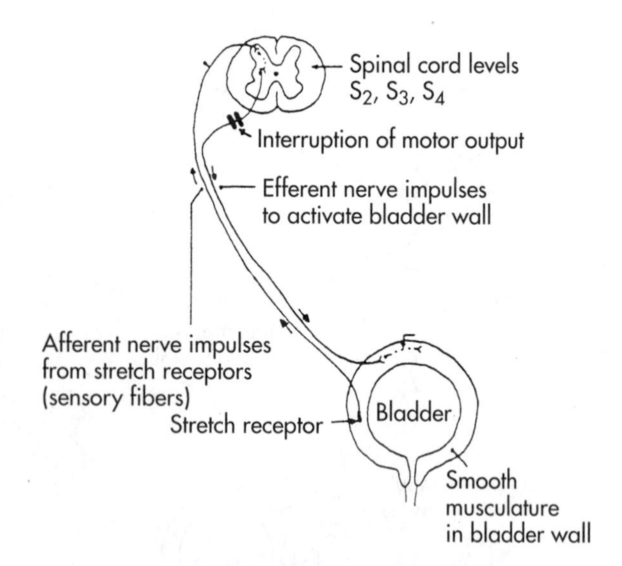

Figure 19-21 Motor paralytic bladder. (From Pires, M., & Lockhart-Pretti, P. [1992]. Nursing management of neurogenic incontinence. Skokie, IL: Rehabilitation Nursing Foundation.)

incontinence, and continual dribbling is associated with overflow incontinence (Wyman, 1988).

Timing of the incontinence is another variable to note in the history. Bladder voiding records are helpful supplements to the history for many clients.

A voiding record, or diary, is a tool to determine the frequency, timing, amount of voiding, and other factors associated with urinary incontinence (Figure 19-23). The person or the caregiver is instructed to document each occurrence in the voiding diary for several days before the incontinence evaluation. These records may provide clues to deciphering the underlying cause of a client's urinary incontinence, as well as setting a baseline to evaluate the efficacy of interventions (Wyman, Choi, Harkins, Wilson, & Fantl, 1988; Guerrero & Sinert, 2001). Usual voiding patterns range from six to eight times during the day and do not exceed two voidings during the night (Abrams, Fenely, & Torrens, 1983). Is the incontinence during the daytime only, or is there enuresis? In children with enuresis it is important to ask if they were ever continent at night or if the enuresis is a new symptom.

Other factors to assess include the presence of concomitant fecal incontinence or other alterations in bowel habits, sensation of bladder fullness before or after voiding, ability to delay voiding once the urge is perceived, symptoms of hesitancy or straining to void, dysuria, or hematuria. It also is important to identify how the person manages the incontinence—for instance, with padding, frequent clothing changes, protective garments, or preventive toileting. Has there been an alteration in sexual function as a result of the incontinence or preceding it? Have there been treatments for incontinence? If so, how

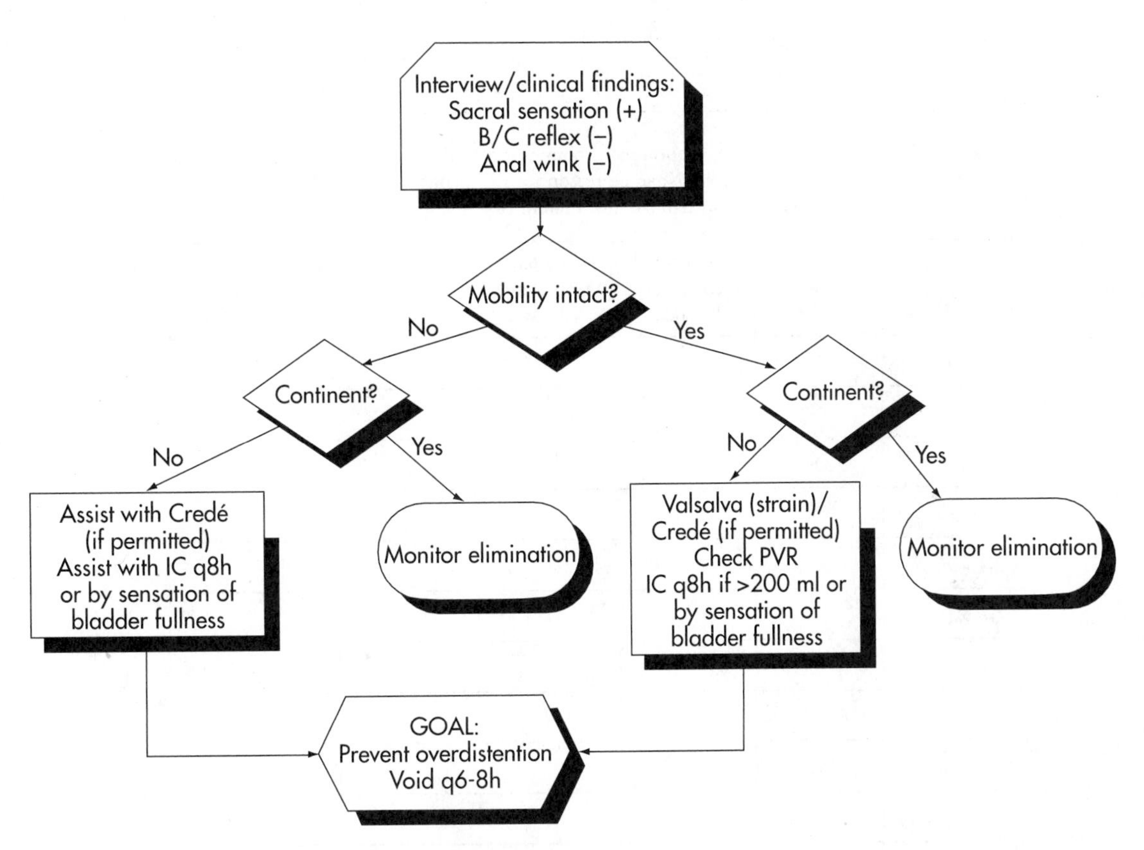

Figure 19-22 Algorithm for motor paralytic neurogenic bladder. (Copyright 2000, Rancho Los Amigos National Rehabilitation Center, Downey, CA.)

successful were they? Has the person had any genitourinary surgery? Review current and past medical problems and any medications used, both prescribed and over-the-counter.

Conditions Associated with Urinary Incontinence

In persons with diabetes, incontinence may be a result of polyuria or from a sensory paralytic bladder causing overflow incontinence from an overdistended bladder resulting from a lack of sensation of the need to void. Neurological disorders with neuropathological lesions in the cortical or subcortical areas, such as cerebrovascular accidents, Parkinson's disease, or traumatic brain injury, may lead to uninhibited neurogenic bladder dysfunction, resulting in urge incontinence. Neurological disorders with neuropathological lesions in the spinal cord, such as multiple sclerosis, spinal cord injury, or tumors, cause reflex neurogenic bladder dysfunction. Autonomous neurogenic bladder may be caused by pathology in the lower part of the spinal canal, such as disk disease or neurological lesions of the peripheral nerves (cauda equina). Persons using diuretics may experience incontinence from a combination of increased urine output and inability to get to the toilet on time.

Perceptions of both client and caregiver, or significant others, about incontinence are important assessments in the clients' history. How does incontinence affect each of their daily lives? What do they expect from the incontinence treatment/management regimen? Are there environmental factors that affect the incontinence such as accessibility of the commode or bathroom, lighting, availability of someone to assist with toileting, or managing clothing? Assessing social factors is important for persons with functional impairments. Social factors include living arrangements, social contacts, and caregiver availability (Williams & Gaylord, 1990). Box 19-1 discusses nursing history for urinary incontinence.

Objective

Physical Examination

The physical examination includes functional physical and cognitive assessments; examination of the abdomen, the genital/pelvic and rectal areas; and neurological and general examinations. The functional assessment evaluates a person's mobility and manual dexterity to determine the ability to reach the toilet and to disrobe in time to be continent (Williams & Gaylord, 1990). A functional assessment of the person's cognitive status provides information about the ability to perceive the need to void, to understand how to reach and use the toilet or toilet substitute, and to participate in the treatment regimen. The Folstein Mini-Mental State Examination is one tool used in standardizing this portion of

NAME: ______________________________

DATE: ______________________________

INSTRUCTIONS: Place a check in the appropriate column next to the time you urinated in the toilet or when an incontinence episode occurred. Note the reason for the incontinence and describe your liquid intake (for example, coffee, water) and estimate the amount (for example, one cup).

Time interval	Urinated in toilet	Had a small incontinence episode	Had a large incontinence episode	Reason for incontinence episode	Type/amount of liquid intake
6-8 AM					
8-10 AM					
10-noon					
Noon-2 PM					
2-4 PM					
4-6 PM					
6-8 PM					
8-10 PM					
10-midnight					
Overnight					

No. of pads used today: ______________ No. of episodes: ______________

Comments: ______________________________

Figure 19-23 Sample bladder record. (From Fantl, J.A., Newman, D.K., Colling, J., DeLancey, J., Keeys, C., Loughery, R., McDowell, B., Norton, P., Ouslander, J., Schnelle, J., Staskin, D., Tries, J., Urich, V., Vitousek, S., Weiss, B., & Whitmore, K. [1996, March]. *Urinary incontinence in adults: Acute and chronic management* [AHCPR Publication No. 96-0682, Clinical Practice Guideline No. 2, 1996 Update]. Rockville, MD: U.S. Department of Health and Human Services, Public Health Service, Agency for Health Care Policy and Research.)

the physical examination (Folstein, Folstein, & McHugh, 1975).

The abdominal examination includes inspection of the skin for scars, which may indicate previous surgeries the client has neglected to report. The abdomen is palpated to identify a distended bladder or suprapubic masses and the presence of any tenderness.

Male genitals are examined to detect abnormalities of the foreskin, penis, and perineal skin; noting the condition of the skin and any swelling, lesions, nodules, or discharge.

For women external genitalia are inspected noting the condition of the skin and signs of atrophic vaginitis or monilial infection. A simple pelvic examination performed by inserting one or two lubricated gloved fingers into the vagina can detect the presence of masses, pelvic prolapse, tenderness, or discharge. During the vaginal examination, ask the woman to squeeze around the examiner's fingers to assess her ability to contract the muscles of the pelvic floor and paravaginal muscle tone.

At this time, provocative stress testing or direct observation of urine loss is performed by having the person relax and cough vigorously while the examiner observes the urethra for loss of urine. If leakage occurs instantaneously, then stress urinary incontinence is suspected. If leakage is delayed or persists after the cough, then urge incontinence or detrusor overactivity is suspected. This test is performed when the client has a full bladder (Fantl et al., 1996). As a rule, if the test initially is performed while a client is in the lithotomy position and no leakage occurs, it is repeated with the person standing (Kadar, 1988). Direct observation of a client's voiding may detect signs of hesitancy or strain, or a slow or interrupted urinary stream. Presence of these symptoms may indicate urinary obstruction or problems with bladder emptying. Ask the person to start and stop the uri-

Box 19-1 Nursing History for Urinary Incontinence

Characteristics of Incontinence
- Onset and duration
- Frequency
- Timing (day, night, or both)
- Precipitating circumstances (cough, sneeze, laugh, exercise, positional changes, hand washing, other)
- Associated urgency
- Amount of leakage
- Type of loss (spurt or stream, or continuous dribbling)
- Use of pads/protective briefs (number of pads or clothing changes per day)

Toileting Patterns
- Diurnal frequency
- Nocturnal frequency

Associated Genitourinary Symptoms
- Awareness of bladder fullness
- Ability to delay voiding
- Sensation of incomplete bladder emptying
- Dribbling after urination
- Obstructive symptoms (hesitancy, slow or interrupted stream, straining)
- Symptoms of urinary tract infection (dysuria, hematuria)

Genitourinary History
- Childbirth
- Surgery (pelvic or lower urinary tract)
- Recurrent urinary tract infections
- Previous incontinence treatment and results (drugs, pelvic floor exercises, surgery, dilatations)

Relevant Medical History
- Acute illness
- Depression
- Diabetes mellitus
- Neurological disease (e.g., cerebrovascular accident, Parkinson's disease, dementia)
- Cardiovascular disease (e.g., hypertension, congestive heart disease)
- Renal disease
- Bowel disorders (constipation, impaction, fecal incontinence)
- Psychological disorders (depression, mental illness)
- Cancer

Medications (Including Nonprescription Drugs)

Client's/Caregiver's Perceptions of Incontinence
- Perception of cause and severity
- Interference with daily activities
- Expectations for cure

Environmental Factors
- Accessible bathrooms
- Distance to bathrooms
- Use of toileting aids

From Wyman, J.F. (1988). Nursing assessment of the incontinent geriatric outpatient population. *Nursing Clinics of North America, 23,* 178-179.

nary stream to observe volitional control and strength of the pelvic muscles.

The rectal examination is conducted to test for perineal sensation (Figure 19-24), sphincter tone with both resting and with active contraction, rectal masses, or fecal impaction. In men the size, consistency, and contour of the prostate is assessed. A bulbocavernosus reflex is attempted during rectal examination for both men and women to determine the status of the sacral reflex arc. This reflex is elicited by squeezing the glans penis or glans clitoris while the examiner's gloved finger is inserted just inside the anus. The examiner notes whether there is anal contraction around the finger and how brisk the contractual response is to the stimulus (Figure 19-25).

A further neurological and general examination may detect conditions such as edema, which may contribute to nocturia, and neurological conditions that may contribute to incontinence (Box 19-2) (Wyman, 1988).

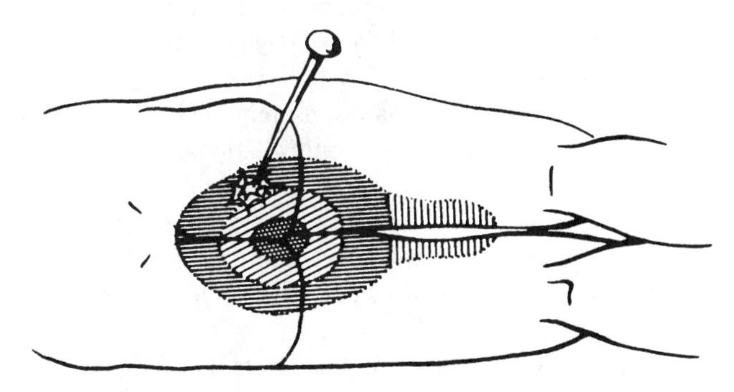

Figure 19-24 Pinprick test for perineal sensation. (Reprinted with permission from Rancho Los Amigos Medical Center, Downey, CA.)

Estimation of Postvoid Residual

Estimation of postvoid residual (PVR) volume is recommended for all persons with urinary incontinence. Catheterization or pelvic ultrasonography is used when a precise measurement of PVR volume is needed (Ireton et al., 1990). Estimation of PVR volume may be accomplished with abdominal palpation and percussion or a bimanual examination; however, the exact amount of volume usually requires catheterization or ultrasound. No clear research is documented in the literature about what are allowable maximum or minimum PVR volumes. The general consensus of the AHCPR Urinary

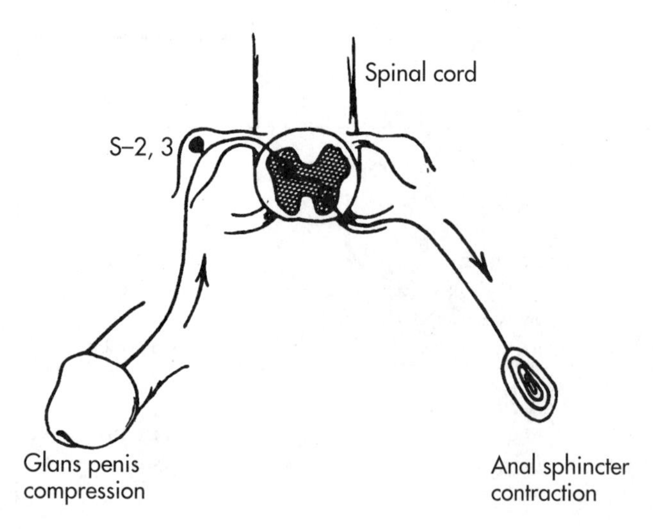

Figure 19-25 Test for the presence of a bulbocavernosus reflex. (Reprinted with permission from Rancho Los Amigos Medical Center, Downey, CA.)

Guideline Panel is that a PVR volume less than 50 ml is considered adequate bladder emptying and more than 200 ml is considered inadequate (Urinary Incontinence Guideline Panel, 1992b). Urethral catheterization in men with prostate obstruction may cause urinary tract infection; therefore, ultrasound measurement is preferable (Fantl et al., 1996).

Urinalysis

Urinalysis is a basic test required to detect conditions that may contribute to urinary incontinence. For instance, hematuria may be a symptom of infection, cancer, or urinary stones; glycosuria and proteinuria indicate further medical work up for diabetes; and pyuria with bacteriuria suggest infection and a specimen for culture. There is no consensus about the relationship of asymptomatic bacteriuria and urinary tract infection in nursing home populations and in those with neurogenic bladder dysfunction. However, no correlation has been found associating asymptomatic bacteriuria with urinary incontinence in noninstitutionalized persons. Until clear data are available about the relationship of asymptomatic bacteriuria and persons in nursing homes, urinary infection is treated first, even before further diagnostic and treatment are initiated or completed (Ouslander, 1989; Hooten, 1999).

Supplementary Tests. Blood tests for blood urea nitrogen (BUN) and creatinine levels are performed for persons with suspected outlet obstruction, noncompliant bladders, or retention. These tests are often part of the routine follow-up in persons with neurogenic bladder dysfunction. Urine cytology is no longer recommended in the routine evaluation of the incontinent client (Fantl et al., 1996).

Further Evaluation

After the basic evaluation, treatment for the presumed type of urinary incontinence should be initiated unless there is an indication for further evaluation (Fantl et al., 1996). See Table 19-5 for the types of clients who may not need further evaluation before initiating treatment.

After the basic evaluation and initial treatment, clients who continue to be incontinent or those who are not appropriate for treatment based on presumptive diagnosis should undergo further evaluation. The objectives of further evaluation are to identify the cause of urinary incontinence by reproducing leakage during testing; to make a differential diagnosis between causes with similar symptoms, but that require different interventions; to detect functional, neurological, or anatomic lesions affecting the lower urinary tract; to obtain specific information necessary to choose the

Box 19-2 Physical Examination for Urinary Incontinence

Cognitive and Affective Status
- Mental status
- Mood
- Motivation

Mobility Status
- Manual dexterity (ability to disrobe for toileting)
- Gait and balance (walking speed, use of assistive devices)

Neurological Examination
- Focal signs
- Signs of Parkinson's disease

Abdominal Examination
- Scars
- Distended bladder
- Suprapubic tenderness
- Mass

Genital Examination
- Skin condition
- Signs of infection
- Bulbocavernous reflex
- Women—atrophic vaginitis, pelvic relaxation, or other abnormality

Rectal Examination
- Sphincteric tone
- Fecal impaction
- Masses
- Men—prostatic size

Stress Test (with Full Bladder)
- Supine and standing

Other
- Signs of congestive heart failure

From Wyman, J.F. (1988). Nursing assessment of the incontinent geriatric outpatient population. *Nursing Clinics of North America, 23,* 178-179.

TABLE 19-5 Management Options after Basic Evaluation

Type of Urinary Incontinence	Characteristics	Management Options
Urge	Detrusor instability with normal PVR; no complicating factors	Behavioral techniques: Bladder training Pelvic muscle rehabilitation Other (e.g., fluid management) Pharmacological interventions: Anticholinergic medications; tricyclic antidepressants as alternative
Stress	With normal PVR; no complicating factors	Behavioral techniques: Pelvic muscle rehabilitation Bladder training Pharmacological interventions: α-adrenergic medications or tricyclic antidepressants Estrogen Combination if needed Surgical techniques: Uncomplicated, nonrecurrent SUI resulting from hypermobility
Mixed (urge stress)	With normal PVR; no complicating factors	Combinations of above, excluding surgical options in most cases.

PVR, Postvoid residual; *SUI,* stress urinary incontinence.

appropriate intervention; and to identify risk factors that may affect the outcome of specific treatments (Fantl et al., 1996).

Specialized Tests

These specialized diagnostic tests usually are completed or ordered by qualified specialists, including advance practice nurses with knowledge, experience, and interest in the management of urinary incontinence in a specific client population. Specialized diagnostic tests include urodynamic tests, endoscopic tests, and imaging tests of both upper urinary tract and lower urinary tract with and without voiding.

Urodynamic tests are designed to evaluate the anatomic and functional status of the bladder. Uroflowmetry is a visual or electronic measure of the rate of urine flow. When an electronic unit is used, it generates an electric flow curve that displays voiding patterns. Uroflowmetry is used when diagnosing bladder emptying problems but is not useful to distinguish between bladder outlet obstruction and detrusor weakness (Urinary Incontinence Guideline Panel, 1992b) or in diagnosing the types of incontinence specific to women (Diokno, Normelle, Brown, & Herzog, 1990).

Cystometry (CMG) is a test of detrusor function. Cystometry can be used to assess bladder sensation, capacity, and compliance and to determine the presence and magnitude of both voluntary and involuntary contractions. A filling CMG measures abdominal and rectal pressure simultaneously to differentiate involuntary detrusor contraction from an increase in intraabdominal pressure that occurs when a client strains to void (Pires & Lockart-Pretti, 1992). A voiding CMG or pressure flow study can measure detrusor contractility and detect outlet obstruction when a person is able to void. Another use of the filling CMG is to determine the leak point pressure. That is, the intravesical pressure is measured at the moment fluid leakage begins during urinary straining or involuntary detrusor contraction. This information is useful to determine whether the person has either low or high voiding pressures. Voiding under high pressure may affect the upper urinary tract, especially with reflex neurogenic bladder dysfunction.

Simple cystometry is a test that may become a bladder training procedure as well (Box 19-3). It is performed by using a urethral catheter to fill the bladder by gravity until either an involuntary contraction occurs or until bladder capacity is reached. This test can be conducted at the bedside to answer questions about how the bladder fills. Does the bladder fill appropriately—for example, does the bladder have good compliance, does the pressure in the bladder allow for adequate filling? Results from simple cystometry also can provide answers to questions about how efficiently the bladder stores urine, whether there is sphincter incompetence or detrusor instability, whether the person accurately perceives the urge to void, and whether the person inhibits the urge to urinate. How adequately the bladder is emptied can be assessed by removing the urinary catheter at the "must" urge, then allowing the person to void, then measuring the PVR volume by catheterization.

Urethral pressure profilometry measures resting and dynamic pressures in the urethra. Passive measurements may

Box 19-3 Procedure for Performing a Bedside (Simple) Cystometrogram

Purpose

1. Assess bladder capacity
2. Assess for an indication of detrusor instability
3. Assess for stress incontinence
4. Teach inhibition of the urge sensation

Equipment

1. Intravenous (IV) tubing or cystometrogram set
2. Bottle or bag of sterile water—500-1000 ml
3. Straight urethral catheterization tray

Procedure

1. Verify standing physician's orders.
2. Explain the physician's orders and procedure to client.
3. Before Foley catheterization, set up the IV/cystometry set by placing tubing into bag of sterile water—using sterile technique. Flush tubing with sterile water, removing all air bubbles, and make sure that tip of tubing remains sterile by placing cap back onto tip of tubing.
4. Place the bag of sterile water on an IV pole so that the bag is approximately 2 feet above the client's symphysis pubis.
5. Place the client on the bedpan to measure any leakage during filling.
6. After the client has been catheterized and the flow of urine stops, connect the tip of the IV tubing .into the open end of the Foley catheter using sterile techniques.
7. Completely open the valve on the IV tubing to allow the sterile water to flow into the bladder. Note on the record if there is any leakage of fluid around the catheter. If there is a large amount of leakage, discontinue the procedure.
8. Do not instill more than 500 ml of fluid.
9. Tell the client to tell the nurse when he or she senses the first urge-to-void sensation.
10. When the client senses the first urge to void, shut the valve on the tubing to stop the flow of sterile water into the bladder. Record this amount as the initial (first) urge sensation.
11. Teach the client to take slow, deep breaths to make the urge sensation go away.
12. After the client has been successful in inhibiting this initial urge, open the valve on the tubing to continue the flow of sterile water into the bladder. (Note if there is leakage of fluid around the catheter at 200 ml. If leakage occurs at volumes less than 200 ml, unstable bladder is likely. If 200-300 ml are instilled without leakage, unstable bladder is unlikely.)
13. Tell the client to tell the nurse when he gets the second ("must" or "I can't hold it any more") urge to void.
14. After the client gets the second ("must") urge to void, close the valve on the tubing to stop the flow of sterile water into the bladder. Record this amount as the "must" urge.
15. Again, teach the client to take slow, deep breaths to make the urge go away.
16. After the client has been successful in lessening or inhibiting the urge and it goes away, remove the catheter.
17. With the client's bladder full, perform a stress maneuver by asking the client to cough forcefully 3 times in the standing position with a pad or tissue near the urethral meatus to collect the urine loss. The nurse also can observe for urine leakage in the supine and standing position. If there is leakage with a cough, estimate the amount (i.e., small, moderate, or large). Stress maneuvers with a full bladder are more sensitive for detecting stress incontinence.
18. Allow the client to empty the bladder into the bedpan or bedside commode, or in the bathroom.

be used to help identify intrinsic sphincter deficiency. Dynamic measurements may be used to measure the effect of exertion on urethral closure mechanism. The relative usefulness of the urethral pressure profilometry versus that of abdominal leak point pressure has not been adequately studied (Fantl et al., 1996).

EMG is performed on the striated urethral sphincter using needle, wire, or surface electrodes to determine the integrity of and function of its innervation. When CMG and EMG are used together, the results are helpful in diagnosing detrusor-sphincter dyssynergia (DSD), which often is seen in reflex neurogenic bladder dysfunction (Blaivas, 1990).

The most useful endoscopic test in evaluating urinary incontinence is cystourethroscopy. This procedure may be helpful in identifying bladder lesions and urethral diverticula, fistulas, strictures, or intrinsic sphincter deficiency. Cystoscopy is not recommended in the basic evaluation of urinary incontinence. However, cystoscopy may be indicated in the further evaluation when the following situations are present: sterile hematuria, or pyuria, when urodynamics fail to duplicate symptoms, new onset of irritative voiding symptoms, bladder pain, recurrent cystitis, or suspected foreign body (Fantl et al., 1996).

Imaging tests sometimes used with persons who have urinary incontinence include upper urinary tract imaging by intravenous pyelogram or, more commonly, ultrasonography of the kidneys. Although these procedures are not routine evaluations of urinary incontinence, they are an important part of routine follow-up in clients with neurogenic bladder dysfunction or those with outlet obstruction who have high bladder pressures. Upper urinary tract imaging can help identify dilation of the ureters and kidney pelvis.

Lower urinary tract imaging with and without voiding is helpful for examining the anatomy of the bladder and the urethra. Nonvoiding cystourethrography can identify mobility or fixation of the bladder neck, funneling of the bladder neck and proximal urethra, and degree of cystocele. The voiding com-

TABLE 19-6 Diagnostic Test Options for Urinary Incontinence*

Mechanism	Associated Factors	Diagnostic Test Options
Urge Incontinence		
Unstable bladder or detrusor instability (DI)	No neurological deficit	Simple or multichannel CMG with or without EMG
Detrusor hyperreflexia, Detrusor sphincter dyssynergia	With neurological lesion such as stroke, supraspinal cord lesions, multiple sclerosis	Simple cystometry or multichannel
Detrusor hyperactivity with impaired contractility	Elderly, usually also associated with obstructive or stress symptoms	Multichannel CMG with or without EMG Videourodynamics
Stress Incontinence		
Hypermobility of bladder neck (female)	Detachment of bladder neck with concomitant hypermobility of the urethra	Provocative stress test (direct visualization) Tests for bladder neck hypermobility Simple or multichannel CMG (to exclude DI) UPP or leak point pressure Videourodynamics
Intrinsic sphincter deficiency	Postoperative (after prostatectomy or antiincontinence surgery), trauma, aging, radiation, congenital (epispadias)	Same as above
Neurogenic sphincter deficiency	Neurogenic, sacral, or infrasacral lesion (e.g., myelomeningocele)	Same as above EMG
Overflow Incontinence		
Overflow from underactive or acontractile detrusor	Neurogenic (low spinal cord lesion, neuropathy, postradical pelvic surgery), idiopathic detrusor failure	Elevated PVR volume Uroflowmetry Voiding CMG (pressure flow) with EMG Cystourethroscopy
Overflow from outlet obstruction	Male: prostate gland disease, urethral stricture Female: postoperative	Same as above Videourodynamics

From Fantl, J.A., Newman, D.K., Colling, J., DeLancey, J., Keeys, C., Loughery, R., McDowell, B., Norton, P., Ouslander, J., Schnelle, J., Staskin, D., Tries, J., Urich, V., Vitousek, S., Weiss, B., & Whitmore, K. (1996, March). *Urinary incontinence in adults: Acute and chronic management* (AHCPR Publication No. 96-0682, Clinical Practice Guideline No. 2, 1996 Update). Rockville, MD: U.S. Department of Health and Human Services, Public Health Service, Agency for Health Care Policy and Research.

CMG, Cystometrogram; *EMG,* electromyogram; *PVR,* postvoid residual; *UPP,* urethral pressure profilometry.

*The urodynamic tests listed here are not recommended for routine use but are options for clients who require further evaluation.

ponent of the cystourethrogram can identify urethral diverticulum, obstruction, and vesicoureteral reflux (Fantl et al., 1996). Table 19-6 provides a list of diagnostic test options.

NURSING DIAGNOSES

Based on the above assessment data, the rehabilitation nurse will make an appropriate nursing diagnosis for the client with altered urinary elimination. Potential diagnoses are as follows (Gordon, 2000):

- Altered urinary elimination pattern (transient incontinence)
- Risk for urinary urge incontinence
- Urge incontinence (uninhibited neurogenic bladder)
- Stress incontinence (overflow incontinence or autonomous neurogenic bladder)
- Reflex urinary incontinence (reflex neurogenic bladder)
- Functional urinary incontinence
- Total incontinence
- Urinary retention (sensory paralytic bladder)

GOALS

Short-term goals are established with the client and vary according to the type of bladder dysfunction and lifestyle issues. Goals that may be established are as follows:

- Client achieves an acceptable level of urinary continence
- Client and family follow a bladder management program consistent with lifestyle
- Client verbalizes knowledge of medications and their side effects related to bladder management program

- Client demonstrates, as applicable, ability to care for indwelling catheter, intermittent catheterization program, external collection device, and perineal/periurethral skin
- Client achieves complete bladder emptying by using appropriate bladder management technique
- Client verbalizes signs and symptoms of urinary retention and actions to take
- Client verbalizes signs and symptoms of urinary tract infection, follows measures to prevent or reduce infection, and what and actions to take should it occur (McCourt, 1993)

INTERVENTIONS

There are three categories of treatment for urinary incontinence: behavioral, pharmacological, and surgical. The AHCPR Urinary Guidelines Panel (1996a, 1996b) suggests that the least invasive and least dangerous procedure appropriate for the person should be the first choice. For many types of urinary incontinence, behavioral techniques meet these criteria. However, individual preferences must be respected (Fantl et al., 1996). For instance, a person may choose a more invasive treatment for the sake of expediency. When the risks, benefits, and outcomes are understood clearly and the client provides informed consent, the person's wishes may supersede this general guideline.

Treatment categories, notably behavioral techniques, generally fall within the scope of the independent realm of rehabilitation nursing. Pharmacological and surgical treatments require nurses' collaboration with physicians and reflect the interdependent and dependent realm of nursing practice. It is exciting to consider the possibility of nurses in advanced practice providing the first line of treatment for persons with urinary incontinence. These techniques are discussed in the following sections.

Behavioral Techniques

Bowel Management

Although not always considered a behavioral technique, rehabilitation nurses will naturally include bowel management as a primary intervention for persons with urinary incontinence. It is difficult to retrain the bladder until the bowel also is retrained. In fact, constipation may be a major contributing factor to urinary incontinence, and restoring regular bowel elimination often alleviates urinary urgency and lack of control. An effective method of restoring regular bowel elimination is to remove any impaction, increase intake of fiber and fluids, and promote mobility or exercise. A special bowel recipe for constipation has assisted in lowering the incidence of constipation for many clients (Chapter 20).

The behavioral techniques delineated in the AHCPR Urinary Guidelines are low-risk interventions intended to decrease frequency of urinary incontinence in most individuals when techniques are provided by knowledgeable health care professionals. Behavioral therapies can be divided into caregiver-dependent techniques for clients with cognitive and motor deficits and those requiring active client participation in rehabilitation and education techniques. Behavioral techniques will be addressed in the order of those requiring passive involvement to those requiring more active client participation. These behavioral techniques include toileting assistance (scheduled voiding, habit training, prompted voiding), bladder training, and pelvic floor exercises, which may be enhanced by biofeedback, vaginal cone retention, or electrical stimulation. In addition, educating the person or the caregiver and providing positive reinforcement for effort and progress is undertaken. These techniques are best offered to persons who are motivated to avoid use of protective garments, external devices, or medications or who shun more invasive treatment methods. (Chapter 11 provides information on client education regarding readiness to learn and planning with clients and family or caregivers.) Behavioral techniques have no reported side effects and do not limit future options (Fantl et al., 1996).

Toileting Assistance. Toileting assistance interventions include routine or scheduled toileting, habit training, and prompted voiding. Scheduled toileting or timed voiding is defined as scheduled toileting on a planned basis. It is the practice of toileting a person using a bedpan/urinal, commode, or toilet at regular intervals, such as every 2 or 3 hours. The goal is to keep clients dry by telling them to void at regular intervals. Within a rehabilitation setting, a timed voiding program is often the precursor to habit training. Habit training is recommended for clients for whom a natural voiding pattern can be determined (Fantl et al. 1996). By keeping a voiding record of the client's continence and incontinence episodes, the nurse can then establish a habit training schedule. Habit training is toileting scheduled to match the client's natural voiding habits. By having the client void at a predetermined time, the person is often able to reduce episodes of urinary incontinence. Success often depends on the caregiver, not the person with incontinence (Pirés & Lockart-Pretti, 1992).

Prompted voiding is defined as a scheduled voiding program that reinforces the person for remaining dry rather than for wetness. Prompted voiding is recommended in clients who can learn to recognize some degree of bladder fullness or the need to void, or who can ask for assistance or respond when promoted to toilet. Clients who are appropriate for prompted voiding may not have sufficient cognitive ability to participate in other, more complex behavioral therapies. The three major components of prompted voiding are:

- Monitoring: client is checked by the caregiver on a regular basis and asked to report verbally if wet or dry
- Prompting: client is asked (prompted) to try to use the toilet
- Praising: client is praised for maintaining continence and for trying to toilet (Fantl et al., 1996)

The goal is to teach the person responsibility for wetness and toileting behavior. Caregivers learn to give a positive response when the client voids in the toilet or is dry. Three steps are followed. With prompted voiding, a caregiver checks with a client at regular intervals, specifically asking the person to state whether the clothing is wet or dry. After the person responds, the caregiver offers the prompt to use the toilet. The person who remains dry or voids using the toilet receives praise; one who becomes wet receives a neutral response. Prompted voiding requires a consistent approach by educated caregivers. When properly conducted, prompted voiding has been useful for assisting persons with cognitive impairments and those who reside in nursing home settings.

Bladder Training

Bladder training, sometimes termed bladder retraining (Box 19-4), is defined as a voiding program that uses distraction or relaxation techniques so a client may consciously inhibit the urge to void. Bladder training is strongly recommended for managing urge and mixed incontinence. Bladder training is also recommended for managing stress incontinence (Fantl et al., 1996). The goal of bladder retraining is to enable the person to resist or inhibit the urge sensation and thus be able to postpone voiding (Smith & Newman, 1992).

Three components to bladder retraining are an education program, scheduled voiding with systematic delay of void-

Box 19-4 Procedure for Bladder Retraining

Purpose

1. Improve the client's pattern of voiding
2. Restore normal bladder function
3. Teach the client how to redevelop control of his/her voiding

Equipment

1. Bladder records
2. Bladder retraining teaching tool

Procedure

1. Send the client's bladder records to complete 1 to 2 weeks before the client's evaluation visit.
2. At the time of evaluation, analyze the client's history, symptoms, and bladder records and determine if bladder retraining will be a part of the treatment regimen.
3. Initiate bladder retraining if the client is mentally and physically capable of toileting as indicated by the nursing assessment and/or a Mini-Mental test and if she has frequency, urgency, urge, or functional incontinence. Frequent toileting would be every 3 hours or more often or a schedule that interferes with and limits a person's lifestyle.
4. Always explain the rationale for the instructions in detail.
5. Teach the client to eliminate or reduce from her diet products containing caffeine or aspartame (NutraSweet).
6. Teach the client to have a daily fluid intake of 48 to 64 oz of caffeine-free liquids.
7. If the client has nighttime frequency, nocturia, or enuresis, teach the client to stop drinking fluids 2 hours before bedtime or to stop after 6 PM.
8. Teach the client relaxation techniques for inhibiting or diverting the urge sensation.
9. Teach these relaxation techniques during the bedside cystometrogram (CMG):
   - When the client gets the first (initial) urge to void, teach the client to take slow, deep breaths through the mouth until the urge sensation lessens or goes away.
   - As the CMG continues, when the client gets the second ("must") urge to void again, instruct the client to take slow, deep breaths until the urge sensation disappears.
10. If a bedside CMG is not performed, teach the client to do the following when a strong urge occurs:
    - Sit and relax.
    - Take slow, deep breaths in and out of the mouth until the urge sensation goes away.
    - Concentrate only on the deep breathing until the urge sensation goes away.
11. Determine the client's average current voiding pattern from the symptoms and the bladder record.
12. Then increase this interval by 15 minutes at a time, teaching the client to use relaxation techniques if the client gets the urge to void sooner.
13. Teach the client not to empty her bladder before she gets the urge to void.
14. Teach the client first to use relaxation techniques at home—when the client is relaxed and knows that the bathroom is readily accessible—so as to avoid anxiety-producing situations.
15. Gradually increase the client's voiding interval as she meets with success.
16. Also, teach the client to use the relaxation technique for diverting the urge to void in common instances when the urge occurs—for example, the "key in the lock" syndrome. Teach the client that if she gets the urge to void when trying to unlock a door, she should stop and use the relaxation technique.
17. Inform the client that at first these techniques may not work but that she should keep attempting to attain the control that these techniques teach.
18. Teach the client never to rush to the bathroom.
19. Have the client keep bladder records to monitor voiding patterns and to record improvement. The client may not notice significant changes in voiding for 6-8 weeks.
20. Schedule follow-up visits according to the client's needs and reinforce the bladder retraining teaching.
21. Provide encouragement to the client at each visit and do not allow her to get discouraged by setbacks that can occur during a cold or an acute illness, during a menstrual period, or if she becomes anxious or fatigued.

ing, and positive reinforcement. An education program contains information about the physiology and pathophysiology of the lower urinary tract, as well as an educational program for urge control. Bladder training also may be incorporated with a bedside CMG to teach the person how to inhibit the urge to void (Pires & Lockart-Pretti, 1992). The person begins a scheduled voiding pattern, with ideal intervals every 2 to 3 hours, with the exception of sleep time. A goal-oriented bladder record helps provide immediate positive feedback to encourage progress to the next interval level. For instance, an initial goal may be to void every 2 hours; using inhibition techniques, the person may progress gradually to 3-hour voiding intervals. Nurses can obtain or create their own relaxation tapes to assist clients who are learning how to relax as a technique for inhibiting the urge to void. Bladder retraining has been used to manage urinary incontinence resulting from bladder instability; however, recent evidence suggests bladder retraining may be useful in managing stress incontinence as well (Fantl, Wyman, Harkins, & Hadley, 1990).

Pelvic Muscle Rehabilitation

Pelvic muscle exercises, also called Kegel exercises, improve urethral resistance through active contraction of the pubococcygeus muscle. Contraction of the pubococcygeal muscle exerts a closing force on the urethra and, over time, improves muscle support to the pelvic structures and strengthens the voluntary periurethral and pelvic musculature. Components of the pelvic muscle exercises are locating and identifying the correct muscles, engaging in active exercise on a regular basis, and using the muscles to control continence (Pires & Lockart-Pretti, 1992).

The first step in pelvic muscle reeducation is for the client to gain an awareness of the pelvic muscles. This may require some concentration but is essential to the next step, which is understanding how to manipulate this muscle group in exercises. Pelvic muscle exercises are performed by "drawing in" or "lifting up" the perivaginal muscles and the anal sphincter, as if attempting to control urination or defecation but without contracting abdominal, buttock, or inner thigh muscles. Even though most persons associate Kegel exercises with women, both sexes benefit from improvements in both fecal and urinary incontinence.

Kegel exercises (Box 19-5) are performed by holding the muscles in contraction for a count of 10 and then relaxing for a count of 10; repeat for 10 minutes three times daily for a total of 30 to 80 exercises per day. An individual can perform these exercises when in any position; the muscle con-

Box 19-5 Patient Teaching: Pelvic Muscle (Kegel) Exercises

How to Find the Pelvic Muscle

To find the muscle, imagine you are at a party and the rich food you have just consumed causes you to have gas. The muscle that you use to hold back gas is the one you want to exercise. Some persons find this muscle by voluntarily stopping the stream of urine. If you are a woman, another way to find the muscle is by pulling your rectum, vagina, and urethra up inside. Try to think about the area around the vagina.

Exercising the Muscle

Begin by emptying your bladder, then try to relax completely. Tighten this muscle and hold it for a count of 10 or 10 seconds; then relax the muscle completely for a count of 10 or 10 seconds. You should feel a sensation of closing between your legs and lifting of the area around the vagina (in women).

When to Exercise

Do 10 exercises in the morning, 10 in the afternoon, and 15 at night—or else you can exercise for 10 minutes, 3 times a day. Set a timer for 10 minutes, 3 times a day. Initially you may not be able to hold this contraction for the complete count of 10; however, you will build slowly to 10-second contractions over time. The muscle may start to tire after 6 or 8 exercises. If this happens, stop and go back to exercising later.

Where to Practice These Exercises

These exercises can be practiced anywhere and anytime. Most persons seem to prefer exercising lying on their bed or sitting in a chair. Women can try doing these exercises during intercourse. Tighten your pelvic muscles to grip your partner's penis and then relax. Your partner should be able to feel an increase in pressure.

Common Mistakes

Never use your stomach, legs, or buttock muscles. To find out if you also are contracting your stomach muscles, place your hand on your abdomen while you squeeze your pelvic muscle. If you feel your abdomen move, then you also are using these muscles. In time you will learn to practice effortlessly. Eventually work these exercises in as part of your lifestyle; tighten the muscle when you walk, when you sneeze, or when you are on the way to the bathroom.

When Will I Notice a Change?

After 4 to 6 weeks of constant daily exercise, you will begin to notice fewer urinary accidents, and after 3 months you will see an even bigger difference.

Can These Exercises Hurt Me?

No! These exercises cannot harm you in any way. Most clients find them relaxing and easy. If you get back pain or stomach pain after you exercise, then you probably are trying too hard and using stomach muscles. Go back and find the pelvic muscle and remember this exercise should feel easy. If you experience headaches, then you also are tensing your chest muscles and probably holding your breath.

tractions are not visible to anyone else and require no equipment and thus can be performed in any environment.

Teaching women pelvic muscle exercises may prevent urinary incontinence. Teaching exercises to strengthen pelvic muscles may decrease the incidence of urinary incontinence. Pelvic exercises are strongly recommended for women with stress incontinence. Pelvic muscle exercises are also recommended for men and women in conjunction with bladder training for urge incontinence. Pelvic muscle exercises may also benefit men who develop urinary incontinence after prostatectomy (Fantl et al., 1996) or women who have had multiple surgical repairs.

Many persons have difficulty identifying the correct muscle group to use to benefit from pelvic muscle exercises. Several techniques have been developed to assist persons with urinary incontinence to learn correct pelvic muscle exercises. They include vaginal weight training, biofeedback, and electrical stimulation (Burgio, Locher, Roth, & Goode, 2001).

Vaginal Weight Training

Vaginal weight training is accomplished by using vaginal cones, which may be a useful adjunct to pelvic muscle exercises in women. The woman is given a set of cones that are the same size and shape but increase in weight from 20 to 100 g. The goal of the program is for the woman to be able to retain the weighted cone for 15 minutes, twice a day. The woman starts with the lowest weight and progresses to the next weight when she can retain the lower level weight for 15 minutes. The woman must stand and retain the weight for the exercises to be effective (Burgio et al., 2001). The sustained contraction required to retain the weighted cone increases the strength of the pelvic muscles. The weight of the cone is assumed to heighten the proprioceptive feedback to the desired pelvic muscle contraction. Vaginal weight training is recommended for stress urinary incontinence in premenopausal women (Fantl et al., 1996).

Biofeedback

Biofeedback is a group of strategies and methodologies that use electronic or mechanical instruments to display information to individuals about their neuromuscular activity. The aim of biofeedback in those with urinary incontinence is to alter bladder dysfunction by teaching clients to change the physiological responses that affect bladder control (Burgio & Engel, 1990). Methods of biofeedback include surface electrodes and sensors inserted either vaginally or rectally. When the proper muscle contraction is accomplished, this information is displayed so that the client can either hear or see it. Auditory or visual display of proper muscle contraction forms the core of biofeedback procedures (Schwartz, 1995). Available biofeedback systems range from stationary to portable and include home training devices. Biofeedback is best used in conjunction with other behavioral techniques such as PME and bladder training.

Success of biofeedback is dependent largely on the skill of the health care provider. The provider must have comprehensive knowledge about evaluation techniques, anatomic and physiological relationship of symptoms to types of bladder dysfunction, and behavioral principles that guide the procedure (Fantl et al., 1996). This is an area appropriate for rehabilitation nurses to expand their practice because a knowledgeable nurse meets and exceeds these criteria. Pelvic muscle rehabilitation and bladder inhibition using biofeedback therapy are recommended for clients with stress, urge, and mixed urinary incontinence (Fantl et al., 1996). Studies have demonstrated reductions in urinary incontinence associated with neurological disease and in frail elderly persons using a combination of biofeedback and behavioral techniques such as bladder training (McDowell et al., 1999)

Electrical Stimulation

Electrical stimulation of the pelvic floor produces a contraction of the levator ani, external urethral and anal sphincters, accompanied by reflex inhibition of the detrusor. This activity depends on a preserved reflex arc through the sacral micturition center. Nonimplantable pelvic floor electrical stimulation uses vaginal or anal sensors or surface electrodes (Vodusek, Plevink, Vrtacnik, & Janez, 1998). Minimal adverse side effects occur with this treatment; pain and local discomfort are the most prominent reactions. Electrical stimulation has been used to manage bladder and dysfunction in persons with neurological and nonneurological impairments. Electrical stimulation also has been used to inhibit detrusor overactivity by modifying the sacral micturition reflex arc (Tanagho, 1990). Pelvic floor electrical stimulation has been shown to decrease incontinence in women with stress urinary incontinence and may be effective in men and women with urge and mixed incontinence (Fantl et al., 1996).

Pharmacological Treatment of Incontinence

Several medications have been beneficial in treating urinary incontinence. They can be categorized into two main groups: medications for incontinence resulting from urethral sphincter insufficiency and medications for incontinence resulting from detrusor overactivity.

Medications used to treat urethral sphincter insufficiency are α-adrenergic agonist agents and estrogen supplementation therapy. α-Adrenergic agonist agents increase urethral resistance by stimulation of urethral smooth muscle acting on α-adrenergic receptors in the urethra. Phenylpropanolamine (PPA), or pseudoephedrine, is the first-line pharmacological therapy for women with stress incontinence who have no contraindications for its use, particularly hypertension. The recommended dose for PPA is 25 to 100 mg in sustained-release form, administered orally, twice daily. The usual dose of pseudoephedrine is 15 to 30 mg, orally, 3 times daily (Fantl et al., 1996).

Estrogen replacement in postmenopausal women may restore urethral mucosal coaptation and increase vascularity, tone, and the α-adrenergic response of the urethral muscle, thus increasing bladder outlet resistance and decreasing stress incontinence. Estrogen (oral or vaginal) may be considered as an adjunctive pharmacological agent for postmenopausal women with stress or mixed incontinence. Conjugated estrogen is usually administered either orally (0.3-1.25 mg/day) or vaginally (2 g or fraction/day). Progestin (e.g., medroxyprogesterone 2.5-10 mg/day) may be given continuously or intermittently. Combined PPA and oral or vaginal estrogen is recommended in the treatment of postmenopausal women with stress incontinence when initial single medication therapy has proven inadequate. Imipramine is recommended as an alternative pharmacological therapy for stress incontinence when the first-line agents have proven unsatisfactory (Fantl et al., 1996).

Medications used to treat detrusor overactivity are anticholinergic and antispasmodic agents. The purpose of these medications is to relax the bladder and increase bladder capacity. Anticholinergic medications include oxybutynin, dicyclomine hydrochloride, and propantheline. Tricyclic antidepressants include imipramine, doxepin, desipramine, and nortriptyline. Medications not as well documented but considered useful are calcium-channel blocking agents (e.g., terodiline) (Fantl et al., 1996).

Anticholinergic agents are the primary pharmacological therapy for clients with detrusor instability as well as those with uninhibited and reflex neurogenic bladder dysfunction. Oxybutynin is the anticholinergic agent of choice. The recommended dosages are 7.5 to 30 mg administered 3 to 5 times per day, but higher doses (15-60 mg qid) may be required. Tricyclic agents should only be used after careful evaluation of the client. The usual oral doses are 10 to 25 mg initially administered 1 to 3 times per day. Less frequent administration is usually possible because of the long half-life of these drugs. The daily total dose is usually 25 to 100 mg (Fantl et al., 1996).

Often, these medications are used to decrease urinary frequency in clients with urge incontinence or uninhibited bladder. In this situation the PVR volume is checked on instituting or adjusting these medications to ensure that emptying has not been compromised. In persons with reflex bladder who void with high pressures or when bladder emptying is incomplete, anticholinergics may be used as an adjunct to intermittent catheterization with the goals of normalizing bladder pressures and establishing continence between catheterizations.

Intermittent catheterization every 6 hours is the preferred method of management of urinary retention and overflow incontinence that result from autonomous, sensory, or motor paralytic bladder. Although sterile technique commonly is practiced when the client is hospitalized, clean technique generally is considered safe in the home or community environment.

Surgical Treatment of Urinary Incontinence

Surgical treatment of urinary incontinence should be considered only after a comprehensive clinical evaluation, including an estimation of the surgical risk, confirmation of the diagnosis and severity, correlation of anatomic and physiological findings with the surgery planned, and an estimation of the impact of the surgical procedure on the quality of the person's life (Fantl et al., 1996).

In addition to the surgeries listed in Table 19-7, several surgical procedures are available for the care of neurogenic bladder dysfunction. These surgeries are indicated in persons with reflex neurogenic bladder when conservative bladder management has failed to maintain a low-pressure, nonrefluxing system. They include transurethral spincterotomy, placement of a sphincter stint, augmentation enterocystoplasty, continent diversion, and neurostimulators.

Transurethral spincterotomy is a surgery that has been useful in managing DSD in males when medications to reduce spasticity of the bladder neck and sphincter have been ineffective and bladder outlet obstruction contributes to high bladder pressures. The indications for transurethral spincterotomy include DSD, bladder wall trabeculations, persistent high voiding pressure, hydronephrosis, repeated urinary tract infections, vesicoureteral reflux, urolithiasis, and severe autonomic dysreflexia.

The procedure consists of visualizing the posterior urethra and making an incision at the 12 o'clock position. This procedure permanently opens the sphincter. These men now will void reflexively with low bladder pressures but will require external condom collection devices

TABLE 19-7 Surgical Management of Urinary Incontinence

Type of Urinary Incontinence	Cause	Treatment
Stress	Hypermobility	Retropubic suspension, needle endoscopic suspension
Stress	Intrinsic sphincter deficiency	Sling (mostly female), artificial sphincter, urethral bulking
Urge	Refractory detrusor instability	Augmentation cystoplasty
Overflow	Obstruction	Relieve obstruction
	Nonobstructive	Intermittent catheterization, other

(Perkash, 1993). A newer procedure developed to open the sphincter, is placement of a sphincter stent. The stent is a wire mesh prosthesis that is placed at the external sphincter and bulbous urethra (Revas, Abdill, & Chancellor, 1996).

In augmentation enterocystoplasty, a short section of small intestine is removed and sutured into place over the bladder (detubuarized), which has been bivalved in the sagittal plane, creating a large, low-pressure urinary reservoir. If limited hand function prevents independent urethral catheterization, a continent stoma can be created by bringing an intussuscepted limb of bowel through the anterior abdominal wall and creating a continent stoma, which can be catheterized more easily. Continent diversions generally are reserved for those persons who have undergone prior cystectomy or those with severe urethral dysfunction (Bennett & Bennett, 1993).

There are many subtypes of continent diversions. Most generally consist of creating a neobladder from detubuarized small intestine and creating an efferent nipple valve to form the continent stoma, as previously described, and creating an afferent nipple valve to form a nonrefluxing attachment for the ureters to pass into the neobladder (Bennett & Bennett, 1993).

New developments in neurourology that are generating excitement are neuromodulation and neurostimulation. Several types of neuroprosthesis are in use or under investigation, including external stimulators that restore micturition. These spinal nerve stimulators consist of an electrical pulse generator with electrodes placed either intradurally or extradurally at the S2-S3 spinal segments. The next frontier of neuroprosthetics is the application of myoplasty, transposed skeletal muscle, coupled with neurostimulation, to restore function to dysfunctional smooth muscle structures of the bladder and sphincters (Chancellor & Revas, 1996). Neuromodulation is used to correct the problems of urge incontinence and involves stimulation of the sacral nerve. The technique of neuromodulation is minimally invasive and may be used when more conservative treatment measures have failed (Buback, 2001).

NURSING OUTCOMES

The nursing interventions and outcomes related to urinary continence and urinary elimination are listed in Table 19-8 (McCloskey & Bulechek, 2000; Johnson, Maas, & Moorhead, 2000).

SUMMARY

Managing bladder elimination problems is an integral component of rehabilitation nursing practice. As described in this chapter, most incontinence can be remedied. Many of the treatments fall within the independent realm of nursing practice. The incontinence that cannot be cured can be controlled through appropriate management techniques and selection of appropriate products. Nurses are an important resource to persons with incontinence in assisting with the selection and management of techniques and products. Other treatments require collaboration with physicians and are within the interdependent scope of nursing practice; however, nursing care is essential to the successful outcomes of the treatments.

CRITICAL THINKING

You have been asked to expand the parish nursing program at a Catholic church. The congregation is 50% Anglo and 50% Latino. The Anglo segment of the congregation consists of generally older couples and many widows. The Latino segment is multigenerational with the majority younger couples with elementary school–aged children. Design a health promotion and education program for elderly women in your parish regarding urinary incontinence. How would this program compare with or differ from one in an institutional rehabilitation setting? What are some barriers (social, language, cultural, age- or gender-based, economic, and other) that you would potentially encounter? What are essential components for the program? What resources, such as online, corporate, professional organization, and other, would be useful? As you are designing this program, clearly identify the roles and responsibilities of the rehabilitation nurse.

TABLE 19-8 Suggested Nursing Intervention Classifications and Nursing Outcome Classifications for Bladder Elimination and Continence

Nursing Interventions Classification	Nursing Outcomes Classification
Urinary Bladder Training	Urinary Continence
Urinary Catheterization	Urinary Elimination
Urinary Catheterization: Intermittent	Knowledge: Treatment Regimen
Urinary Elimination Management	Self-Care: Toileting
Urinary Habit Training	Quality of Life
Urinary Incontinence Training	
Urinary Retention Care	

Data from Johnson, M., Maas, M.L., & Moorhead, S. (2000). *Nursing outcomes classification (NOC)* (2nd ed.). St. Louis: Mosby; McCloskey, J.C., & Bulechek, G.M. (2000). *Nursing interventions classification (NIC)* (3rd ed.). St. Louis: Mosby; and North American Nursing Diagnosis Association. (2001). *Nursing diagnosis: definitions and classification 2001-2002* (4th ed.). Philadelphia: Author.

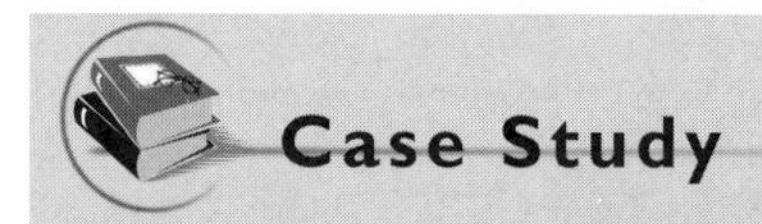

Case Study

Mr. S is a 17-year-old with T1 paraplegia secondary to a gunshot wound. Initially he presented in spinal shock, and during his acute care phase, his bladder was managed with an indwelling catheter. He was transferred to a spinal cord injury center 10 days after his injury. An intermittent catheterization program was instituted on an every-4-hour schedule. The rehabilitation nurses did the catheterization for the first few days. They instructed Mr. S in the technique of intermittent catheterization, using a sterile, no-touch catheterization system. He also was instructed in how to regulate his fluid intake. He takes 100 ml/hour for the 12 waking hours of the day and about 400 ml of fluid with each meal. He became independent in self-catheterization after 4 days. Within 10 days of his rehabilitation stay, Mr. S started to experience lower extremity spasticity and some leaking of urine just before his scheduled catheterization. The appearance of spasticity and some reflex voiding indicated the resolution of spinal shock.

Mr. S was scheduled for urodynamic testing and his CMG-EMG showed evidence of DSD from uncoordinated bladder and sphincter contractions. The results of his urodynamic studies showed that he was voiding with pressures that exceed 40 cm H_2O. After a discussion with his urologist, he was started on an anticholinergic, oxybutynin chloride (Ditropan), to reduce his detrusor hyperreflexia. Because of his lower extremity spasticity, he had already been placed on baclofen (Lioresal) by his physiatrist. Mr. S's nurse explained to him that the oxybutynin chloride will decrease his bladder contractility and lower the pressure in his bladder. He also was told that the baclofen will decrease the spasticity in his external urinary sphincter as well as his lower extremities. Mr. S was told that he could choose to try to urinate reflexively if low bladder pressures could be maintained. He was told this would require wearing an external condom collection device and a leg bag. His other choice was to increase the dose of the oxybutynin chloride to further reduce bladder contractility. This would mean emptying his bladder every 6 hours by intermittent catheterization, which he would continue to do at home using clean technique. He would remain dry between catheterizations and not require any external devices.

Mr. S was very concerned about his body image and did not like the idea of using external collection devices. He chose intermittent catheterization and anticholinergic medication. However, Mr. S had difficulty maintaining a consistent fluid intake and sticking to his catheterization schedule. His intermittent catheterization volumes were more than 500 ml at least once a day. After a week of high volumes, Mr. S experienced a severe pounding headache and was diaphoretic above his level of injury. His nurse took his blood pressure and found that it was 150/90 mm Hg. His usual blood pressure is 100/76 mm Hg. She assisted him with the catheterization and found that his bladder volume was 600 ml. His symptoms resolved as soon as his bladder was empty. Because of his level of injury, Mr. S is prone to autonomic dysreflexia. He was started on an alpha blocker, prazosin hydrochloride (Minipress), and his nurse worked with him on strategies to maintain his fluid restriction and catheterization schedule. For the remainder of his rehabilitation, Mr. S remained dry between catheterizations and had no further episodes of dysreflexia.

Mr. S's nurse reinforced the need to maintain his fluid restriction and catheterization schedule at home and worked with him on problem-solving techniques such as more frequent catheterizations if more fluid has been taken in. Because of the delicate balance of his bladder with medications, Mr. S will have repeat urodynamic testing at 3 and 6 months postdischarge. If there are no problems, he will need yearly routine urodynamic testing along with cine or voiding cystourethrography, ultrasonographic scans of the kidney, and a nuclear scan to determine renal plasma flow.

REFERENCES

Abrams P., Blaivas J.G., Stanton, S.L., & Andersen, J.T. (1988). The standardization of terminology of lower urinary tract function. *Scandinavian Journal of Urology and Nephrology, 114*:5-9.

Abrams, P., Fenely, R., & Torrens, M. (1983). *Urodynamics*. New York: Springer-Verlag.

American Urological Association. (2000). *Understanding urinary incontinence*. Available: http://www.drylife.org.

Bates, P., Bradley, W.E., & Glen, E. (1979). The standardization of terminology of lower urinary tract function. *Journal of Urology, 121*, 551-554.

Bennett, C.J., & Bennett, J.K. (1993). Augmentation cystoplasty and urinary diversion in patients with spinal cord injury. *Physical Medicine and Rehabilitation Clinics of North America, 4*, 377-389.

Blaivas, J.G. (1990). Diagnostic evaluation of incontinence in patients with neurogenic disorders. *Journal of the American Geriatrics Society, 38*, 306-310.

Brandeis, G.H., Baumann, M.M., Hossain, M., Morris, J.N., & Resnick, N.M. (1997). The prevalence of potentially remediable urinary incontinence of frail older people: a study using the Minimum Data Set. *Journal of the American Geriatric Society, 45*:179-184.

Buback, D. (2001). The use of neuromodulation for treatment of urinary incontinence. *Association of Operating Room Nurses Journal, 73*(1), 176-178, 181-187, 189-190.

Burgio, K., Locher, J., Roth, D., & Goode, P. (2001). Psychological improvements associated with behavioral and drug treatment of urge incontinence in older women. *Journal of Gerontological, Behavioral, Psychological Science and Sociology Science, 56*(1), 46-51.

Burgio, K.L., & Engel, B.T. (1990). Biofeedback-assisted behavioral training for elderly men and women. *Journal of the American Geriatrics Society, 38*, 338-340.

Burkhart, K. (2000). Urinary incontinence in women: Assessment and management in the primary care setting. *Nurse Practitioner Forum, 11*(4), 192-204

Chancellor, M.B., & Revas, D.A. (1996). Neuromodulation and neurostimulation in urology. *Topics in Spinal Cord Injury Rehabilitation, 1*(5), 18-35.

Consortium for Spinal Cord Medicine. (1997). *Acute management of autonomic dysreflexia: Adults with spinal cord injury presenting to health-care facilities*. Washington, DC: Paralyzed Veterans of America.

Diokno, A.C., Normelle, O.P., Brown, M.B., & Herzog, A.R. (1990). Urodynamic tests for female geriatric urinary incontinence. *Urology, 36*, 431-439.

Doughty, D.B., & Waldrop J. (2000). Introductory concepts. In D.B. Doughty (Ed.) *Urinary and fecal incontinence: Nursing management* (2nd ed., pp. 29-45). St. Louis: Mosby.

Erickson, R.P. (1980). Autonomic dysreflexia: pathophysiology and medical management. *Archives of Physical Medicine and Rehabilitation, 61*, 431-440.

Fantl, J.A., Newman, D.K., Colling, J., DeLancey, J., Keeys, C., Loughery, R., McDowell, B., Norton, P., Ouslander, J., Schnelle, J., Staskin, D., Tries, J., Urich, V., Vitousek, S., Weiss, B., & Whitmore, K. (1996, March). *Urinary incontinence in adults: Acute and chronic management* (AHCPR Publication No. 96-0682, Clinical Practice Guideline No. 2, 1996 Update). Rockville, MD: U.S. Department of Health and Human Services, Public Health Service, Agency for Health Care Policy and Research.

Fantl, J.A., Wyman, J.F., Harkins, S.W., & Hadley, E.C. (1990). Bladder training in the management of lower urinary tract dysfunction in women: A review. *Journal of the American Geriatrics Society, 38,* 329-332.

Folstein, M.F., Folstein, S.E., & McHugh, P.R. (1975). Mini-Mental state, a practical method for grading cognitive state of patients for the clinician. *Journal of Psychiatric Research, 12,* 189-198.

Giroux, J. (1988). Alterations in bladder elimination. In P.H. Mitchell, L.C. Hodges, M. Muwaswe, & S.C.A. Wallack (Eds.), *AANN's neuroscience nursing phenomena and practice.* Norwalk, CT: Appleton & Lange.

Gordon, M. (2000). *Manual of nursing diagnosis* (9th ed., pp. 195-209). St. Louis, Mosby.

Gray, M. (1992). *Genitourinary disorders.* St. Louis: Mosby.

Gray, M.I. (2000). Physiology of voiding. In D.B. Doughty (Ed.). *Urinary and fecal incontinence: Nursing management* (2nd ed., pp. 1-27). St. Louis: Mosby.

Grimby, A., Milsom, I., Molander, U., Wiklund, I., & Ekelund, P. (1993). The influence of urinary incontinence on the quality of life of elderly women. *Age and Ageing, 22,* 82-89.

Grimby, A., & Svanborg, A. (1997). Morbidity and health-related quality of live among elderly ambulant elderly citizens. *Aging, Clinical and Experimental Research, 9,* 356-364.

Guerrero, P., & Sinert, R. (2001). *Urinary incontinence. Emergency medicine/genitourinary* [On-line]. Available: http://www.knowledge.emedicine.com, eMedicine.com.inc.

Guttmann, L., Frankel, H.L., & Paeslack, V. (1965). Cardiac irregularities during labor in paraplegic women. *Paraplegia, 3,* 144-151.

Guyton, A.C., & Hall, J.E. (1996). *Textbook of medical physiology* (9th ed., pp. 405-421). Philadelphia: WB Saunders.

Hampel, C., Weinhold, D., Brekan, N., Eggersman, C., & Thuroff, J.W. (1997). Prevalence of overactive bladder and epidemiology of urinary incontinence. *Urology 50* (Suppl. 6A), 4-14.

Hooton, T. (1999). Uncomplicating urinary tract infections. Proceedings of the 39th Interscience Conference on Antimicrobial Agents and Chemotherapy. Medscape, Inc.

Ireton, R.C., Krieger, J.N., Cardenas, D.D., Williams-Burden, B., Kelly, E., Souce, T., & Chapman, W.H. (1990). Bladder volume determination using a dedicated portable ultrasound scanner. *Journal of Urology, 143,* 909-911.

Jeter, K.F., Faller, N., & Norton, C. (1990). *Nursing for continence.* Philadelphia: WB Saunders.

Jirovec, M.M. (2000). Functional incontinence. In D.B. Doughty (Ed.), *Urinary and fecal incontinence: Nursing management.* (2nd ed., pp. 145-158). St. Louis: Mosby.

Johnson, M., Maas, M., & Moorhead, S. (2000). *Nursing outcomes classification (NOC)* (2nd ed.). St. Louis: Mosby.

Kadar, N. (1988). The value of bladder filling in clinical detection of urine loss and selection of patients for urodynamic testing. *British Journal of Obstetrics and Gynecology, 95,* 698-704.

Kuric, J., & Hixon, A.K. (1996). *Clinical practice guideline: Autonomic dysreflexia.* Jackson Heights, NY: Eastern Paralyzed Veterans Association.

Kurnick, N.B. (1956). Autonomic hyperreflexia and its control in patients with spinal cord lesions. *Annals of Internal Medicine, 44,* 678-686.

Lapides, J., & Diokno, A.C. (1976). Urine transport, storage, and micturition. In J. Lapides (Ed.), *Fundamentals of urology.* Philadelphia: WB Saunders.

Maloney, C., & Cafiero, M.R. (1999). Urinary incontinence: noninvasive treatment options. *Advance for Nurse Practitioners, June,* 37-42.

McCloskey, J.M., & Bulechek, G.M. (2000). *Nursing interventions classifications (NIC).* (3rd ed., pp. 685-692). St. Louis: Mosby.

McCourt, A. (1993). *The specialty practice of rehabilitation nursing: A core curriculum.* (3rd ed., pp. 94-107). Skokie, IL: Rehabilitation Nursing Foundation.

McDowell, B.J., Engberg, S., Sereika, S., Donovan, N., Jubeck, M.E., Weber, E., & Engberg, R. (1999). Effectiveness of behavioral therapy to treat incontinence in homebound older adults. *Journal of the American Geriatric Society, 47*(3), 309-318.

National Kidney and Urologic Diseases Advisory Board. (1994). Barriers to rehabilitation of persons with end-stage renal disease or chronic urinary incontinence. Workshop summary report. March 7-9, 1994. Bethesda, MD.

Nygaard, I.E., Thompson, F.L., Svengalis, S.L., & Albright, J.P. (1994). Urinary incontinence in elite nulliparous athletes. *Obstetrics and Gynecology, 84,* 183-187.

Ouslander, J.G. (1981). Urinary incontinence in the elderly. *Western Journal of Medicine, 135,* 482-491.

Ouslander, J.G. (1989). A symptomatic bacteriuria and incontinence [Letter]. *Journal of the American Geriatrics Society, 37,* 197-198.

Perkash, I. (1993). Long-term urologic management of the patient with spinal cord injury. *Urologic Clinics of North America, 20,* 423-434.

Peschers, U., Jundt, K., & Dimpfl, T. (2000). Differences between cough and Valsalva leak-point pressure in stress incontinent women. *Neurological Urodynamics, 19*(6), 677-681.

Pires, M., & Lockhart-Pretti, P.A. (1992). *Nursing management of neurogenic incontinence: An independent study module.* Skokie, IL: Rehabilitation Nursing Foundation.

Rathe, R., & Klioze, A. (2000). Basic clinical skills. *Integrated medical curriculum.* Gainsville, FL: University of Florida.

Resnick, N. (1996). Geriatric incontinence. *Urologic Clinics of North America 23*: 55-71.

Resnick, N.M., & Yalla, S.V. (1985). Management of urinary incontinence in the elderly. *New England Journal of Medicine, 313,* 800-805.

Revas, D.A., Abdill, C.K., & Chancellor, M.B. (1996). Current management of detrusor sphincter dyssynergia. *Topics in Spinal Cord Injury Rehabilitation, 1*(5), 18-35.

Schwartz, M.S. (1995). *Biofeedback: A practitioner's guide.* New York: Guilford Press.

Shaw, C., Tansey, R., Jackson, C., Hyde, C., & Allan, R. (2001). Barriers to help seeking in people with urinary symptoms. *Family Practice, 18*(1), 48-52.

Siroky, M.B., & Krane, R.J. (1982). Neurologic aspects of detrusor-sphincter dyssynergia, with reference to the guarding reflex. *Journal of Urology, 127,* 953-957.

Skelly, J., & Boblin-Cummings, S. (1999). Promoting seniors' health-confronting the issue of incontinence. *Canadian Journal of Nursing Leadership, 12*(3), 13-17.

Smith, D.A., & Newman, D.K. (1992). *Behavioral management of urinary incontinence: An independent study module* (p. 10). Skokie, IL: Rehabilitation Nursing Foundation.

Steeman, E., & Defever, M. (1998). Urinary incontinence among elderly persons who live at home: A literature review. *Nursing Clinics of North America, 33,* 441-455.

Tanagho, E.A. (1990). Electrical stimulation. *Journal of the American Geriatrics Society, 38,* 352-355.

Tannenbaum, C., Perrin, L., Dubeau, C., & Kuchel, G. (2001). Diagnosis and management of urinary incontinence in the older patient. *Archives of Physical Medicine Rehabilitation, 82*(1), 134-138.

Teasdale, T., Taffet, G., Luchi, R., & Adam, E. (1988). Urinary incontinence in a community-residing elderly population. *Journal of the American Geriatrics Society, 36,* 600-606.

Urinary Incontinence Guideline Panel. (1992a). In *Urinary incontinence in adults: Quick reference guide for clinicians* (AHCPR Publication No. 92-0041). Rockville, MD: Agency for Health Care Policy and Research, Public Health Service, U.S. Department of Health and Human Services.

Urinary Incontinence Guideline Panel. (1992b). *Urinary incontinence in adults: Clinical practice guidelines* (AHCPR Publication No. 92-0038). Rockville, MD: Agency for Health Care Policy and Research, Public Health Service, U.S. Department of Health and Human Services.

Vickrey, B.G., Shekelle, P., Morton S. Clark, K, Pathak, M., & Kamberg C. (1999). *Prevention and management of urinary tract infections in paralyzed persons.* Evidence Report/Technology Assessment No. 6. (Prepared by Southern California Evidence-Bases Practice Center RAND under Contract No. 290-97-0001.) (AHCPR Publication No. 99-E008). Rockville, MD: Agency for Health Care Policy and Research.

Vodusek, D.B., Plevnik, S., Vrtacnik, P., & Janez, J. (1998) Detrusor inhibition on selective pudendal nerve stimulation in the perineum. *Neurology Urodynamics, 6,* 389-393.

Voelker, R. (1998). International group seeks to dispel incontinence "taboo." *Journal of the American Medical Association, 280*(11), 7.
Wagner, T., & Hu, T.W. (1998). Economic costs of urinary incontinence in 1995. *Urology, 51,* 355-361.
Williams, M.E., & Gaylord, S.A. (1990). Role of functional assessment in the evaluation of urinary incontinence: National Institutes of Health Consensus Development Conference on Urinary Incontinence in Adults. Bethesda, MD, October 3-5, 1988. *Journal of the American Geriatrics Society, 38,* 296-299.
Wyman, J.F. (1988). Nursing assessment of the incontinent geriatric outpatient population. *Nursing Clinics of North America, 23,* 169-187.
Wyman, J.F., Choi, S.C., Harkins, S.W., Wilson, M.S., & Fantl, J.A. (1988). The urinary diary in evaluation of incontinent women: A test-retest analysis. *Obstetrics and Gynecology, 71,* 812-817.
Yarnell, J., Richards, C., & Stephenson, T. (1981). The prevalence and severity of urinary incontinence in women. *Journal of Epidemiology and Community Health, 35,* 71-74.

APPENDIX 19A: AUTONOMIC DYSREFLEXIA

Pathophysiology of Autonomic Dysreflexia

Autonomic dysreflexia occurs after the phase of spinal shock in which reflexes return. Individuals with injuries above the major splanchnic outflow have the potential of developing autonomic dysreflexia.

The major splanchnic outflow is T6 through L2 (the level of the second lumbar vertebra). Intact sensory nerves below the level of the injury transmit impulses to the spinal cord, which ascend in the spinothalamic and posterior columns. Sympathetic neurons in the intermediolateral gray matter are stimulated by these ascending impulses. Sympathetic inhibitory impulses that originate above T6 are blocked as a result of the injury. Therefore, below the injury, there is a relatively unopposed sympathetic outflow (T6 through L2) with a release of norepinephrine, dopamine-beta-hydroxylase, and dopamine.

The release of these chemicals may cause piloerection, skin pallor, and severe vasoconstriction in the arterial vasculature, which can cause a sudden elevation in blood pressure. The elevated blood pressure may cause a headache. Intact carotid and aortic baroreceptors detect the hypertension.

Normally two vasomotor brainstem reflexes occur in an attempt to lower the blood pressure. (Parasympathetic activity originating from the dorsal motor nucleus of the vagus nerve—cranial nerve X—continues following a spinal cord injury.) The first compensatory mechanism is to increase parasympathetic stimulation to the heart via the vagus nerve to cause bradycardia. However, this bradycardia cannot compensate for the severe vasoconstriction. According to Poiseuille's formula, pressure in a tube is affected to the fourth power by change in radius (vasoconstriction) and only linearly by change in the flow rate (bradycardia). The second compensatory reflex is an increase in sympathetic inhibitory outflow from vasomotor centers above the spinal cord injury. However, the inhibitory impulses are unable to pass below the injury, and above the level of injury there may be profuse sweating and vasodilation with skin flushing (Erickson, 1980; Kurnick, 1956).

From Consortium for Spinal Cord Medicine. (1997). *Acute management of autonomic dysreflexia: Adults with spinal cord injury presenting to health-care facilities.* Washington, DC: Paralyzed Veterans of America. Reprinted by permission.

Signs and Symptoms

An individual may have one or more of the following signs or symptoms when he or she is having an episode of autonomic dysreflexia. Symptoms may be minimal or even absent, despite an elevated blood pressure. Some of the more common symptoms are:

- A sudden and significant increase in both the systolic and diastolic blood pressure above their usual levels, usually associated with bradycardia. **An individual with SCI above T6 often has a normal systolic blood pressure in the 90 to 110 mm Hg range.** Therefore, a blood pressure of 20 mm to 40 mm Hg above baseline may be a sign of autonomic dysreflexia (Guttman, Frankel, & Paeslack, 1965).
- Pounding headache.
- Profuse sweating above the level of the lesion, especially in the face, neck, and shoulders, or possibly below the level of the lesion.
- Goose bumps above or possibly below the level of the lesion.
- Flushing of the skin above the level of the lesion, especially in the face, neck, and shoulders, or possibly below the level of lesion.
- Blurred vision.
- Appearance of spots in the client's visual fields.
- Nasal congestion.
- Feelings of apprehension or anxiety over an impending physical problem.
- Minimal or no symptoms, despite an elevated blood pressure.
- Cardiac arrhythmias, atrial fibrillation, ventricular contractions, and atrioventricular conduction abnormalities.

Causes

Autonomic dysreflexia has many potential causes. It is essential that the specific cause be identified and treated in order to resolve an episode of autonomic dysreflexia. Following are some of the more common causes (Kuric & Hixon, 1996):

- Bladder distention
- Urinary tract infection
- Bladder or kidney stones
- Cystoscopy, urodynamics, or detrusor sphincter dysinergia
- Epididymitis or scrotal compression
- Bowel distention
- Bowel impaction

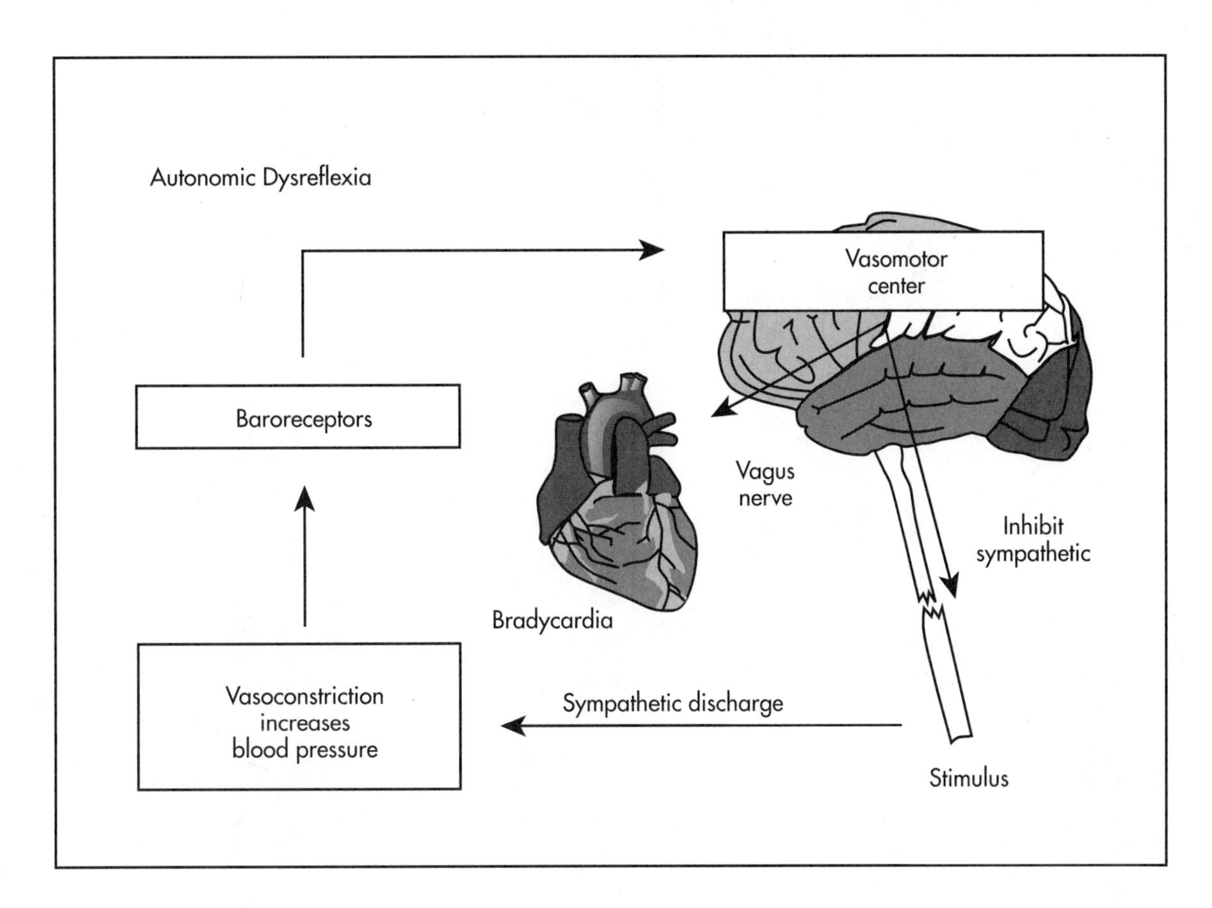

- Gallstones
- Gastric ulcers or gastritis
- Invasive testing
- Hemorrhoids
- Gastrocolic irritation
- Appendicitis or another abdominal pathology or trauma
- Menstruation
- Pregnancy, especially labor and delivery
- Vaginitis
- Sexual intercourse
- Ejaculation
- Deep vein thrombosis
- Pulmonary emboli
- Pressure ulcers
- Ingrown toenail
- Burns or sunburn
- Blisters
- Insect bites
- Contact with hard or sharp objects
- Constrictive clothing, shoes, or appliances
- Heterotopic bone
- Fractures or other trauma
- Surgical or diagnostic procedures
- Pain
- Temperature fluctuations
- Any painful or irritating stimuli below the level of injury

Treatment Recommendations

NOTE: *Pregnant women should be referred to an appropriate consultant.*

1. Check the individual's blood pressure.
2. If the blood pressure is not elevated, refer the individual to a consultant, if necessary.
3. If the blood pressure is elevated and the individual is supine, immediately sit the person up.
4. Loosen any clothing or constrictive devices.
5. Monitor the blood pressure and pulse frequently.
6. Quickly survey the individual for the instigating causes, beginning with the urinary system.
7. If an indwelling urinary catheter is not in place, catheterize the individual.
8. Before inserting the catheter, instill 2% lidocaine jelly (if readily available) into the urethra and wait several minutes.
9. If the individual has an indwelling urinary catheter, check the system along its entire length for kinks, folds, constrictions, or obstructions and for correct placement of the indwelling catheter. If a problem is found, correct it immediately.
10. If the catheter appears to be blocked, gently irrigate the bladder with a small amount of fluid, such as normal saline at body temperature. Avoid manually compressing or tapping on the bladder.
11. If the catheter is draining and the blood pressure remains elevated, proceed with step 16.

Summary of Treatment Recommendations

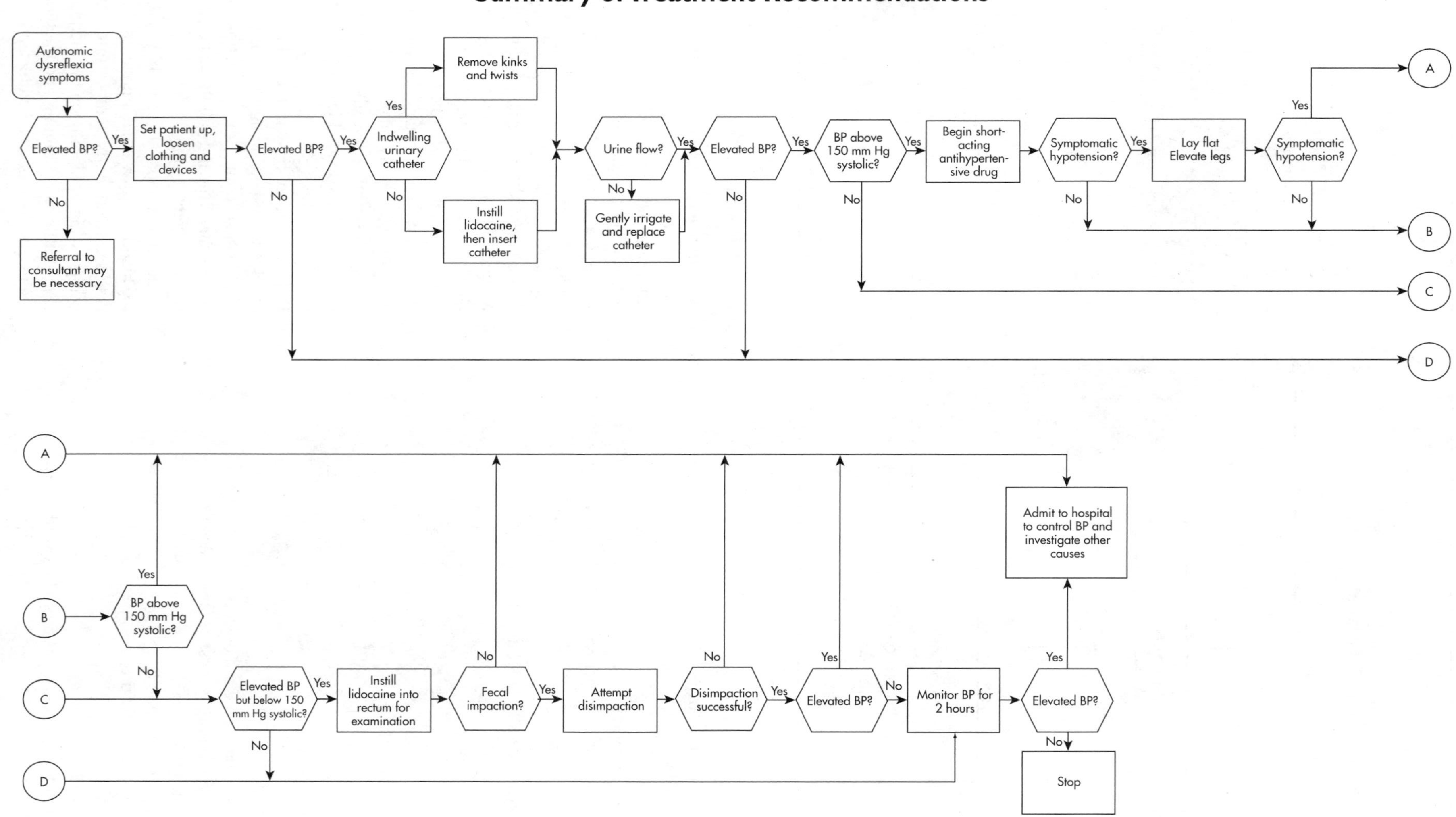

12. If the catheter is not draining and the blood pressure remains elevated, remove and replace the catheter.
13. Prior to replacing the catheter, instill 2% lidocaine jelly (if readily available) into the urethra and wait several minutes.
14. If the catheter cannot be replaced, consider attempting to pass a coude catheter, or consult a urologist.
15. Monitor the individual's blood pressure during bladder drainage.
16. If acute symptoms of autonomic dysreflexia persist, including a sustained elevated blood pressure, suspect fecal impaction.
17. If the elevated blood pressure is at or above 150 mm Hg systolic, consider pharmacologic management to reduce the systolic blood pressure without causing hypotension before checking for fecal impaction. If the blood pressure remains elevated but is less than 150 mm Hg systolic, proceed to step 20.
18. Use an antihypertensive agent with rapid onset and short duration while the causes of autonomic dysreflexia are being investigated.
19. Monitor the individual for symptomatic hypotension.
20. If fecal impaction is suspected, check the rectum for stool, using the following procedure: With a gloved hand, instill a topical anesthetic agent such as 2% lidocaine jelly generously into the rectum. Wait approximately 5 minutes for sensation in the area to decrease. Then, with a gloved hand, insert a lubricated finger into the rectum and check for the presence of stool. If present, gently remove, if possible. If autonomic dysreflexia becomes worse, stop the manual evacuation. Instill additional topical anesthetic and recheck the rectum for the presence of stool after approximately 20 minutes.
21. Monitor the individual's symptoms and blood pressure for at least 2 hours after resolution of the autonomic dysreflexia episode to make sure that it does not recur.
22. If there is poor response to the treatment specified above or if the cause of the dysreflexia has not been identified, strongly consider admitting the individual to the hospital to be monitored, to maintain pharmacologic control of the blood pressure, and to investigate other causes of the dysreflexia.
23. Document the episode in the individual's medical record. This record should include the presenting signs and symptoms and their course, treatment instituted, recordings of blood pressure and pulse, and response to treatment. The effectiveness of the treatment may be evaluated according to the level of outcome criteria reached:
    - The cause of the autonomic dysreflexia episode has been identified.
    - The blood pressure has been restored to normal limits for the individual (usually 90 to 110 systolic mm Hg for a tetraplegic person in the sitting position).
    - The pulse rate has been restored to normal limits.
    - The individual is comfortable, with no signs or symptoms of autonomic dysreflexia, of increased intracranial pressure, or of heart failure.
24. After the individual with spinal cord injury has been stabilized, review the precipitating cause with the individual, members of the individual's family, significant others, and care givers. This process entails adjusting the treatment plan to ensure that future episodes are recognized and treated to prevent a medical crisis or, ideally, are avoided altogether. The process also entails discussion of autonomic dysreflexia in the spinal cord injury individual's education program, so that he or she will be able to recognize early onset and obtain help as quickly as possible. It is recommended that an individual with a spinal cord injury be given a written description of treatment for autonomic dysreflexia at the time of discharge that can be referred to in an emergency.

20 Bowel Elimination and Regulation

Aloma R. Gender, MSN, RN, CRRN

A 56-year-old married housewife is discussing concerns with her mother's home health nurse. "I want to keep my mother at home with me. She had a stroke that affected movement in her left arm and leg 8 months ago. I provide most of her physical care, which I don't mind doing, but she is either incontinent of her bowels or goes through periods of constipation. I'm afraid to take her out of the house for fear of an accident. When she is constipated, she has a lot of pain. I'm afraid that I will need to put her in a nursing home because caring for an incontinent parent is too much for me."

Fecal incontinence affects many persons with disabilities and chronic illness. A humiliating and devastating condition, fecal incontinence can lead to social isolation and low self-esteem (Bentsen & Braun, 1996). A study of 6959 individuals in Wisconsin reported anal incontinence was present in 2.2% of the population (Nelson, Norton, Cautley, & Furner, 1995). Many elderly persons are placed in long-term care facilities prematurely because of the burden of caring for an incontinent adult at home (Seidel, Millis, Lichtenberg, & Dijkers, 1994). Other persons with disabilities limit their activities outside of the home for fear of incontinence (Stiens, Bergman, & Goetz, 1997). In a study of 115 persons with spinal cord injury, researchers found that for 54%, bowel management was a source of emotional upset because of the frequency of fecal incontinence and the time needed for toileting (Glickman & Kamm, 1996).

Disorders of regularity, such as constipation or diarrhea, cause considerable difficulties for many; the estimated prevalence of constipation ranges from 2% to 34% of the population (Cheskin, Kamal, Crowell, Schuster, & Whitehead, 1995). Managing altered bowel elimination is a key responsibility for a rehabilitation nurse. Effective bowel training programs can control incontinence and prevent constipation and diarrhea. The development of an effective program requires knowledge of normal and altered bowel physiology, an in-depth assessment of bowel function, and accurate identification of the causative and contributing factors (Doughty, 2000).

ANATOMY AND PHYSIOLOGY

Normal Bowel Function

Bowel elimination is the process by which the body excretes waste products. Undigested dietary matter passes through the gastrointestinal (GI) tract, after nutrients and water have been extracted for use by the body. The alimentary tract (Figure 20-1) provides the body with a continual supply of water, electrolytes, and nutrients through digestion and absorption. Digestion of food occurs in the stomach, duodenum, jejunum, and ileum; absorption occurs in the small intestine and the proximal half of the colon. A myriad of autoregulatory processes keeps food moving along the GI tract at an appropriate pace for digestion and absorption and to provide the body with nutrients. Defecation of undigested or unabsorbed food involves complex integration of voluntary regulation by the central nervous system, as well as involuntary intrinsic reflex mechanisms (Heitkemper, 2000). Any interruption of these mechanisms may result in impaired bowel function. In this section, normal function of the GI tract is discussed in relation to those functions that affect bowel elimination: secretion, innervation, functional movements, and defecation (Guyton & Hall, 1996).

Secretion

Secretory glands located throughout the GI tract serve two primary functions. First, digestive enzymes are produced from the mouth to the end of the ileum. The appropriate amount of enzymes and electrolytes are formed and secreted in response to food in the alimentary tract for proper digestion. Second, glands located from the mouth to the anus produce mucus to protect and lubricate the walls of the tract and to ease the passage of food and partially digested products.

Innervation

The GI tract is composed of several layers of smooth muscle fibers, which are arranged in bundles. In the longitudinal muscle layer (Figure 20-2), the bundles extend longitudinally down the intestinal tract and the circular muscle layer bundles (see Figure 20-2) extend around the gut. The muscle fibers within each bundle are electrically connected so signals can transmit from one fiber to the next.

The smooth muscle undergoes almost continual but slow electrical activity that produces tonic and rhythmic contractions. Tonic contractions maintain a steady pressure on the contents of the GI tract whereas rhythmic contractions regulate phasic functions, such as mixing of food and peristalsis (Guyton & Hall, 1996). The internal anal sphincter, a circular smooth muscle (Figure 20-3), maintains a state of tonic contraction and safeguards against small amounts of fecal material escaping into the anal canal.

Intrinsic Neural Control. In addition, the GI tract has its own enteric nervous system that lies entirely in the wall of the gut, beginning in the esophagus and extending to the anus. It is composed of two plexuses: (1) the outer or myenteric (motor) plexus located between the longitudinal and circular muscle layers (see Figure 20-2); and (2) the inner layer, which is called Meissner's plexus, or submucosal (sensory) plexus in the submucosa (see Figure 20-2). The myenteric plexus is far more extensive and controls GI movements; the submucosal plexus controls local intestinal secretion and absorption. The enteric nervous system allows the gut to continue to function in isolation from its extrinsic nerve supply; however, signals from the brain through the autonomic nervous system can alter the degree of activity of the intrinsic nervous system (Guyton & Hall, 1996).

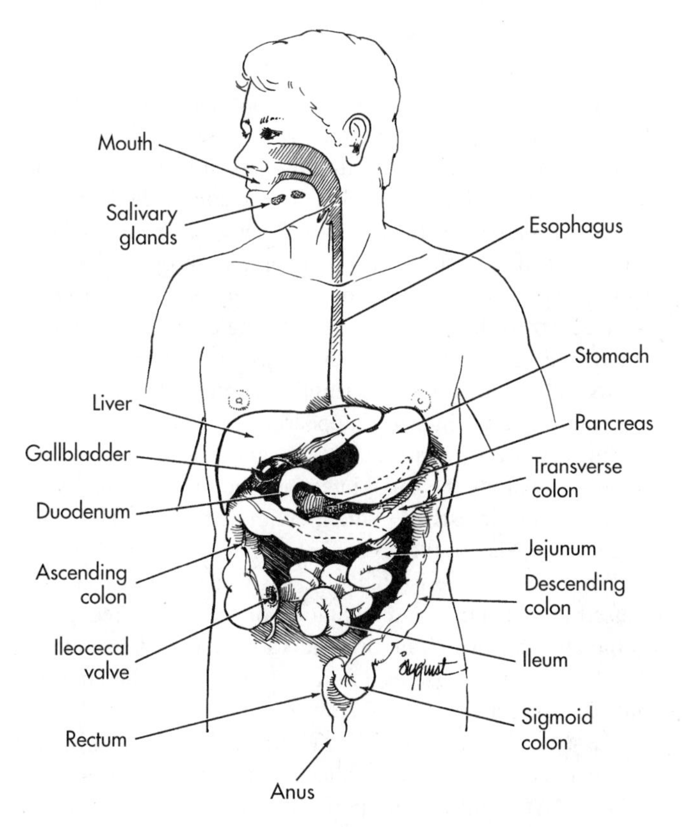

Figure 20-1 The alimentary tract.

Extrinsic Neural Control. Although the primary mediator for peristaltic activity is the intrinsic, or enteric, nervous system, the extrinsic innervation plays an important modulating role (Heitkemper, 2000). Extrinsic innervation includes both parasympathetic and sympathetic activity of the autonomic nervous system that may alter the overall activity of the gut or specific parts.

The parasympathetic cranial supply is transmitted almost entirely by the vagus nerve and provides extensive innervation to the esophagus, stomach, pancreas, first half of the large bowel, and to a lesser extent the small bowel. The parasympathetic sacral fibers originate in S2, S3, and S4 segments of the spinal cord and pass through the nervi erigentes to the distal half of the large bowel (Figure 20-4). The sigmoid, rectal, and anal regions of the large intestine are abundantly supplied with parasympathetic fibers that function to facilitate the defecation reflexes. The postganglionic neurons of the parasympathetic system are located in the myenteric and submucosal plexuses. Stimulation of the parasympathetic nerves cause increased activity of the entire nervous system. The sympathetic fibers originate in the spinal cord between spinal cord segments T5 and L2 and innervate essentially all the GI tract, not only the oral and anal areas as with the parasympathetic system. Stimulation of the sympathetic nervous system generally results in decreased activity of the GI tract, with effects opposite to parasympathetic stimulation. Strong stimulation can totally halt movement of food through the GI tract.

Functional Movements of the GI Tract

The two basic types of movement in the GI tract are mixing and propulsive. Mixing keeps the intestinal contents blended thoroughly by contracting small segments of the gut wall. The propulsive movement of peristalsis moves food along the GI tract at a rate for digestion and absorption. The usual stimulus for peristalsis is a large amount of food collecting in the gut and stimulating the intestinal wall 2 to 3 cm above this point; a contractile ring forms and initiates peristalsis. Some mixing and propulsion occur simultaneously.

The Oral Cavity. The ingestion of food begins with proper chewing of food for digestion because digestive enzymes act only on the surfaces of the food particles. The rate of digestion is highly dependent on the total surface area exposed to intestinal secretions. Grinding food into a fine consistency prevents excoriation of the GI tract and increases the ease with which food is emptied from the stomach into the small intestine (Guyton & Hall, 1996).

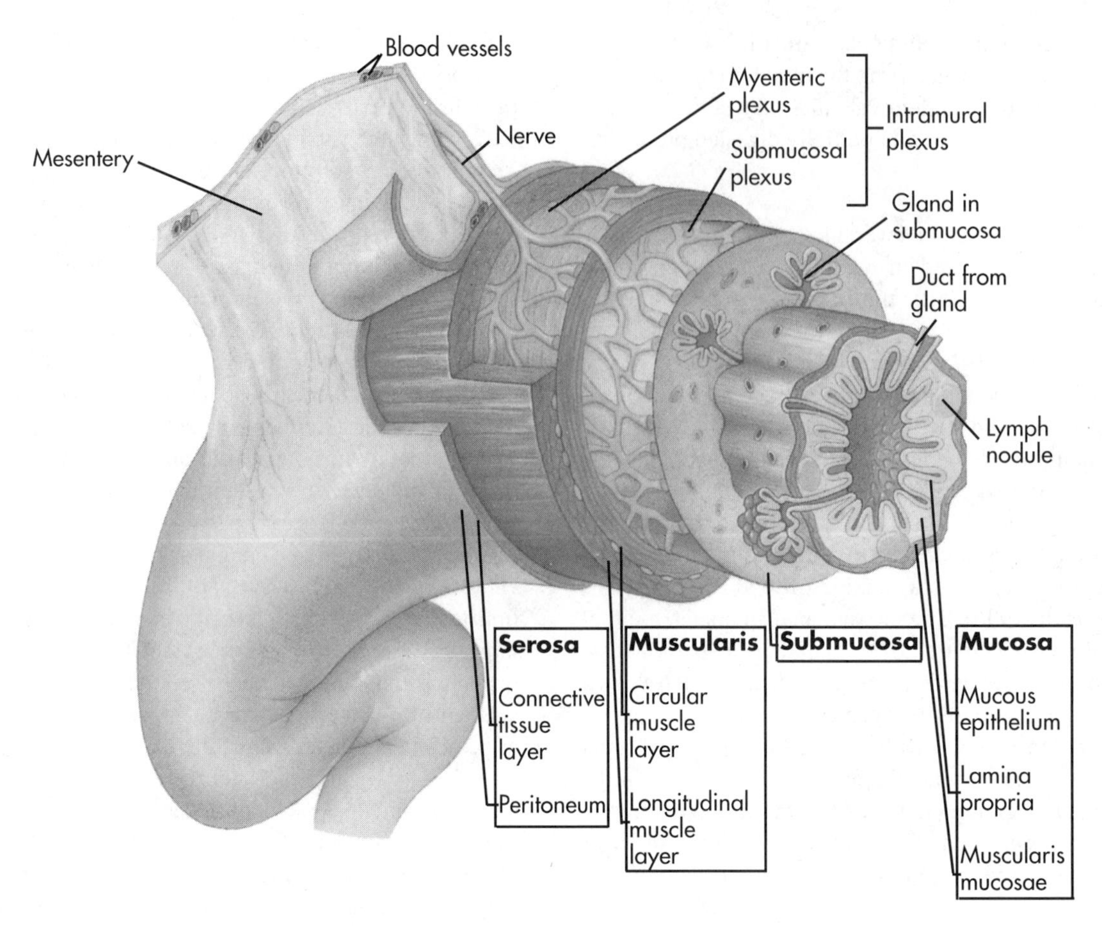

Figure 20-2 Wall of the gastrointestinal tract. (From Thibodeau, G.A., & Patton, K.T. [1999]. *Anatomy & physiology* [4th ed.]. St. Louis: Mosby.)

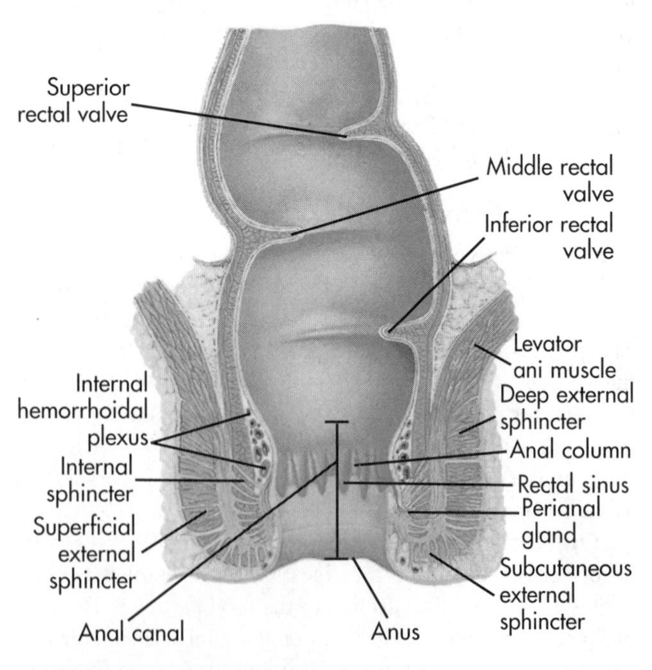

Figure 20-3 Anatomy of rectum, anus, and anal sphincters. (From Thibodeau, G.A., & Patton, K.T. [1999]. *Anatomy & physiology* [4th ed.]. St. Louis: Mosby.)

The Stomach. The stomach has three motor functions: (1) mixing of food with gastric secretions until it forms chyme, which is a semifluid mixture; (2) storage of large quantities of food until it can be accommodated by the lower portion of the GI tract; and (3) slow emptying of food into the small intestine at a rate suitable for proper digestion and absorption by the small intestine (Guyton & Hall, 1996).

The Small Intestine. The mixing contractions of the small intestine occur when chyme is present. The chyme elicits localized, concentric ringlike contractions spaced at intervals along the intestine, appearing as a chain of sausage. As one set of contractions subsides, another occurs at a different point along the small intestine, chopping and progressively mixing intestinal contents with secretions. The contractions depend on the myenteric plexus.

Propulsive or peristaltic activity is a series of waves caused by distention and excitation of the stretch receptors in the gut wall, which in turn elicit a local myenteric reflex. The longitudinal muscles contract, followed by the circular muscle as peristalsis spreads toward the anus.

Passage of chyme from the pylorus to the ileocecal valve, between the small and large intestine, normally requires 3 to 5 hours. After meals this peristaltic activity is greatly in-

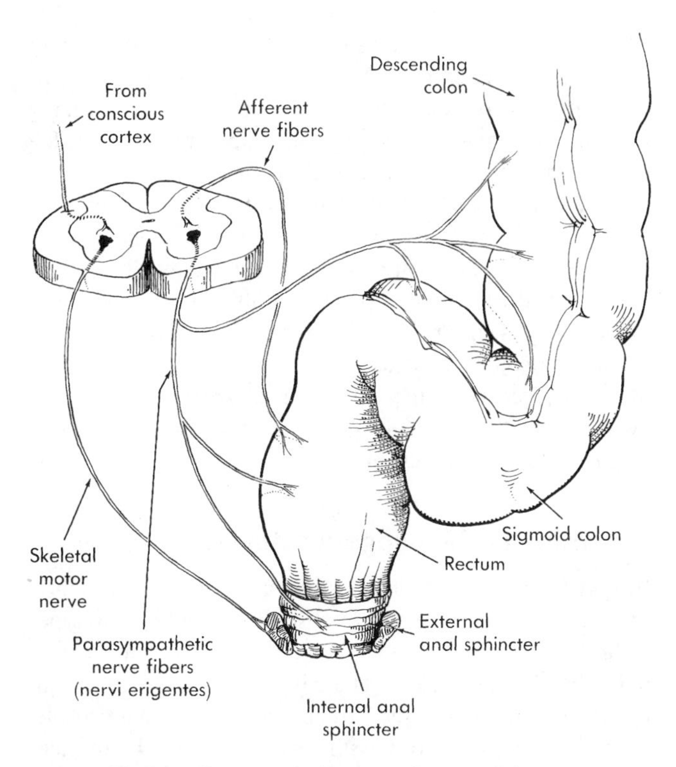

Figure 20-4 Afferent and efferent pathways of the parasympathetic mechanism for defecation reflex. (From Guyton, A.C., & Hall, J.E. [2000]. *Textbook of medical physiology* [10th ed.]. Philadelphia: WB Saunders.)

creased because of the distention of the stomach and duodenum from chyme, which causes gastrocolic and duodenal reflexes (Beddar, Holder-Bennett, & McCormick, 1997). These reflexes stimulate the myenteric plexus to increase peristalsis and secretions in the small intestine. The small intestine can increase peristalsis significantly with irritation or overdistention, a mechanism called peristaltic rush. The waves travel the entire length of the small intestine quickly and can sweep contents of the small bowel into the colon within a few minutes, thus relieving irritation or distention.

The ileocecal valve has the principal function of preventing backflow of fecal contents from the colon into the small intestine. The wall of the ileum has a thickened area, the ileocecal sphincter, just preceding the ileocecal valve. The ileocecal sphincter remains mildly constricted at all times and slows the emptying of small intestine contents into the cecum except after meals when the gastrocolic reflex intensifies peristalsis. This resistance to emptying prolongs retention of intestinal contents to facilitate digestion and absorption. Approximately 1500 ml of chyme empties from the ileum into the cecum every day (Guyton & Hall, 1996).

The Large Intestine. The colon is 5 feet of tubular muscle lined with mucous membrane extending from the ileum to the anal canal. It is divided into the cecum; ascending, transverse, and descending colon; sigmoid colon; and rectum and anus (Figure 20-1). The colon functions to absorb water and electrolytes from the intestinal contents and to store fecal material until expulsion. The colon is normally sluggish.

Colonic mucus contains many bicarbonate ions and is secreted by the parasympathetic nerves to protect the lining of the colon from acids formed in the feces and to bind fecal material. A client's extreme emotional reaction may overstimulate the parasympathetic nerves, causing overproduction of stringy mucoid stools with little or no feces. The colon absorbs large quantities of water (as much as 2.5 L) and up to 55 mEq of sodium and 23 mEq of chloride daily (Berger & Williams, 1992).

Fecal elimination is accomplished by moving the chyme along the colon and into the rectum and anal canal by muscular actions called (1) haustral shuffling, (2) haustral contractions, and (3) peristalsis. Haustral shuffling moves chyme back and forth and aids in absorption of water. Haustral contractions (also called segmentation) propel contents along the colon. When one haustra (pouch-like section of colon) is distended completely, it contracts and empties its contents into the next (Berger & Williams, 1992).

Peristalsis in the colon occurs in mass movements about 15 minutes to 1 hour after a meal and can be strongest after the first meal of the day. A distended or irritated portion of the colon, most often the transverse or descending colon, constricts, forcing the fecal material en masse down the colon to the rectum where the person feels an urge to defecate. Stimulation of the gastrocolic and duodenocolic reflexes transmits when the stomach and duodenum are distended through the myenteric plexus; however, irritation in the colon initiates mass movements. For example, a person with ulcerative colitis has mass movements most of the time; others may have them after ingesting hot or cold liquids.

Sigmoid Colon, Rectum, and Anal Canal. Feces enter and remain in the sigmoid colon and the rectum until just before defecation. The adult rectum is 4 to 6 inches long; the distal anal canal is 1.5 inches long. Vertical and transverse folds of tissue help retain feces in the rectum. Each vertical fold contains an artery and a vein; permanent dilatation of the vein may occur with hemorrhoid conditions (Berger & Williams, 1992). The anal canal contains an internal and external sphincter (Figure 20-3). The internal sphincter is inside the anus and is a continuation of the circular muscle layer, which is smooth muscle and thus involuntarily controlled by the autonomic nervous system. When sensory nerves in the rectum are stimulated by the fecal mass, the person feels the need to defecate (Heitkemper, 2000).

Defecation

Reflexes and voluntary control govern defecation. The internal and external anal sphincters, normally in a state of tonic contraction to prevent continual dribbling, relax with presence of feces. The defecation reflex itself is extremely weak. It is fortified by signals transmitted into the sacral portion of the spinal cord (S2-4), then reflexively sent back to the descending colon, sigmoid, rectum, and anus by the parasympathetic nerve fibers. The signals intensify the peristaltic waves and convert weak movements into a powerful process. The afferent signals entering the spinal cord initiate other concurrent activities associated with defecation. Taking a deep breath, closing the glottis, the Valsalva maneuver, and raising the levator muscles around the rectum aid in defecation, as does a squat position that straightens the anorectal angle (Heitkemper, 2000).

Somatic control also is necessary for voluntary defecation because the conscious mind controls the external sphincter by inhibiting its action to defecate or further contracting if inconvenient. Maintained voluntary inhibition can disrupt the defecation mechanism until more feces enter the rectum. Repeatedly ignoring the urge to defecate can result in an abnormally enlarged rectum and loss of rectal sensitivity, as in children with encopresis who develop megacolon. Eventually, perception of the need to defecate becomes dulled, creating constipation and seeping diarrhea (Guyton & Hall, 1996).

Altered Bowel Elimination

Incontinence

When motor and sensory pathways of the autonomic nervous system or somatic nervous system are compromised, voluntary bowel control is altered. Impairment of cerebral control and anal sphincter or sensation results in fecal incontinence. Damage to the central nervous system (CNS) interrupts nervous pathways between the brain, spinal cord, and GI system, causing neurogenic bowel. Three of the five categories of neurogenic bowel dysfunction are seen commonly in rehabilitation practice: uninhibited, reflex, and autonomous neurogenic bowel; less often, motor paralytic and sensory paralytic neurogenic bowel are seen.

Motor and sensory tests can classify bowel dysfunction, necessary to determine the appropriate bowel program. (1) Saddle sensation is a perianal sensation elicited in response to a pinprick or light touch. Sensation indicates intact sensory function at the sacral spinal cord level; this awareness of the urge to defecate helps establish bowel control. (2) The bulbocavernosus reflex test is used for clients with spinal cord injuries to determine whether an intact reflex arc is present at the level where the bowel, bladder, and genitalia are innervated. Positive results indicate an upper motor neuron (above T12) or reflexic injury with reflex activity in these areas. With a lower motor neuron (T12 or below) or areflexic injury, reflex activity in the bladder, bowel, or genitalia is improbable. A person generally will not have a positive bulbocavernosus reflex while in spinal shock, but this reflex may appear before spinal shock fully subsides (Zejdlik, 1992). Spinal shock is a transient condition with decreased synaptic excitability of neurons, lasting from hours to weeks, and is manifested by absence of somatic reflex activity and flaccid paralysis below the level of damage. Hypotension, bladder paralysis, and interference with defecation may occur because of autonomic nervous system involvement, especially in higher level lesions. Reflex activity may return earlier with incomplete lesions. (3) The bulbocavernosus reflex is elicited by inserting a gloved, lubricated finger into the client's rectum while gently squeezing the clitoris or glans penis. The nurse observes for a visible contraction of the external anal sphincter and a palpable contraction of the bulbocavernosus and ischiocavernosus muscles. A positive response will be immediate and brisk or slow and weak; no contraction is a negative result. The test is performed weekly until positive or until a permanent areflexic injury is confirmed. (4) The anal "wink" reflex is similar to the bulbocavernosus test. It is elicited by a pinprick to the skin adjacent to the external anal sphincter. A visible "wink" contraction of the sphincter is a positive response (Figure 19-24 illustrates this test).

Uninhibited Neurogenic Bowel

In cortical and subcortical lesions above the C1 vertebral level, as seen in stroke, multiple sclerosis, and certain types of brain trauma and tumors, bowel function is classified as uninhibited (Figure 20-5). There is damage to the upper motor neurons located in the cerebral cortex, internal capsule, brainstem, or spinal cord, with sparing of lower motor neurons located in the anterior gray matter throughout the entire length of the spinal cord. Bowel sensation is intact, as is saddle sensation, and the bulbocavernosus reflex and anal reflex are intact or increased. Sensory impulses travel through the sacral reflex arc to the brain, but the brain is unable to inter-

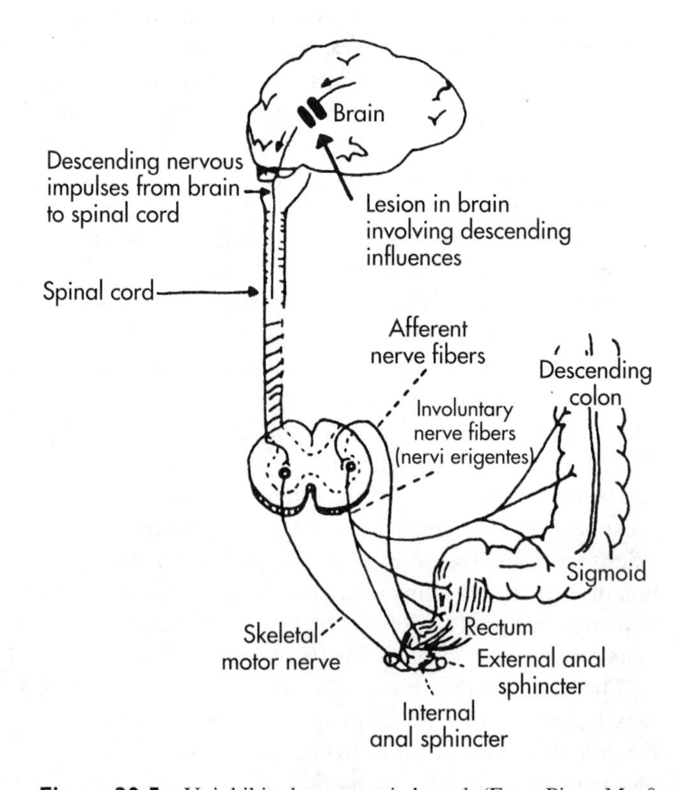

Figure 20-5 Uninhibited neurogenic bowel. (From Pires, M., & Lockhart-Pretti, P. [1992]. *Nursing management of neurogenic incontinence.* Glenview [IL]: Association of Rehabilitation Nurses.)

pret the impulses to defecate. As a result of decreased cerebral awareness of the urge to defecate, there is decreased voluntary control of the anal sphincter. Involuntary elimination occurs when the sacral defecation reflex is activated. Because sensation is not impaired, the incontinence is accompanied by a sense of urgency and often occurs in close proximity with the gastrocolic reflex (Beddar et al., 1997).

Reflex Neurogenic Bowel

Reflex neurogenic (automatic) bowel function (Figure 20-6) occurs with spinal cord lesions above the T12 to L1 vertebral level that involve the upper motor neurons and sensory tracts but spare the lower motor neurons. Tetraplegia, high thoracic paraplegia, and multiple sclerosis are associated; other causes include tumor, vascular disease, syringomyelia, and pernicious anemia. In most instances bowel sensation and saddle sensation are diminished or absent. The bulbocavernosus reflex and anal reflex are increased.

Interruptions of the nerve pathways between the brain and spinal cord may be complete or incomplete. In a complete lesion, and many incomplete, the person has no voluntary control of defection or of the anal sphincter and fecal incontinence occurs without warning from a mass reflex. The sacral nerve segments of S2-4 are intact so it is possible for a client to develop a stimulus-response type of bowel control using the mass reflex. Because the intact spinal reflex arc functions when feces accumulate in the rectum and create distention, the bowel can empty by reflex. The parasympathetic innervation through the sacral segments of the spinal cord maintains anal sphincter tone so that fecal incontinence between mass reflex emptying is not a problem.

Autonomous Neurogenic Bowel

Autonomous (flaccid or nonreflex) bowel function (Figure 20-7) occurs with spinal cord lesions at or below the T12 to L1 vertebral level. Lesions in this area affect the lower motor neurons and usually are associated with paraplegia, spina bifida, tumor, and intervertebral disk disease. Sensation is diminished to absent, as are the bulbocavernosus and anal reflexes. Although nerve pathways between the brain and spinal cord are interrupted, the extent of neural compromise depends on whether the injury is complete or incomplete. As with reflex bowel function, the person has neither cerebral control of defecation nor voluntary control of the anal sphincter. Unlike reflex bowel function, however, the lesion directly involves the S2-4 segments, the activity of the spinal reflex arc is destroyed or unable to be accessed, and no reflex emptying of the bowel occurs. Both the internal and external anal sphincters lack tone, offering little or no resistance in the rectum, resulting in frequent fecal incontinence with oozing stool.

Motor Paralytic Bowel

A motor paralytic bowel occurs with damage to the anterior horn cells of S2, S3, and S4 ventral roots, such as with poliomyelitis, intervertebral disk disease, trauma or tumor (Figure 20-8). Saddle sensation is intact, but the bulbocavernosus reflex and anal reflex are absent. Incontinence is rare except in widespread disease (Cannon, 1981).

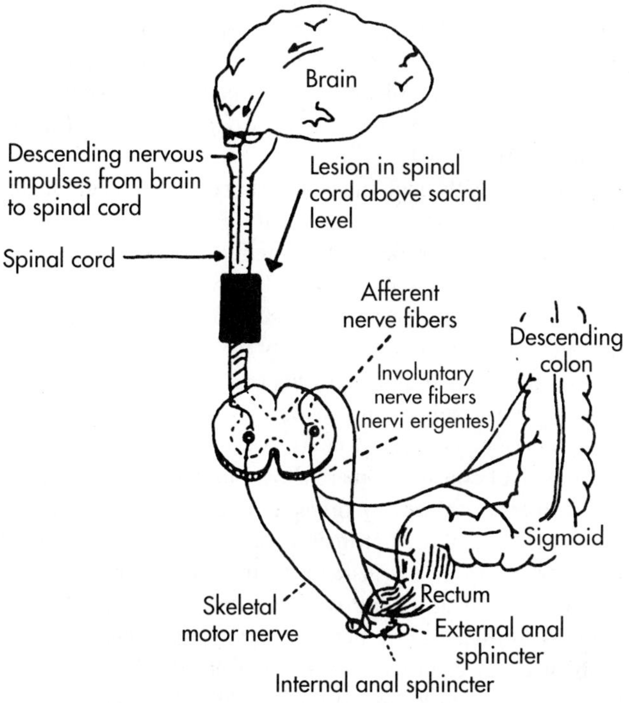

Figure 20-6 Reflex neurogenic bowel. (From Pires, M., & Lockhart-Pretti, P. [1992]. *Nursing management of neurogenic incontinence.* Glenview [IL]: Association of Rehabilitation Nurses.)

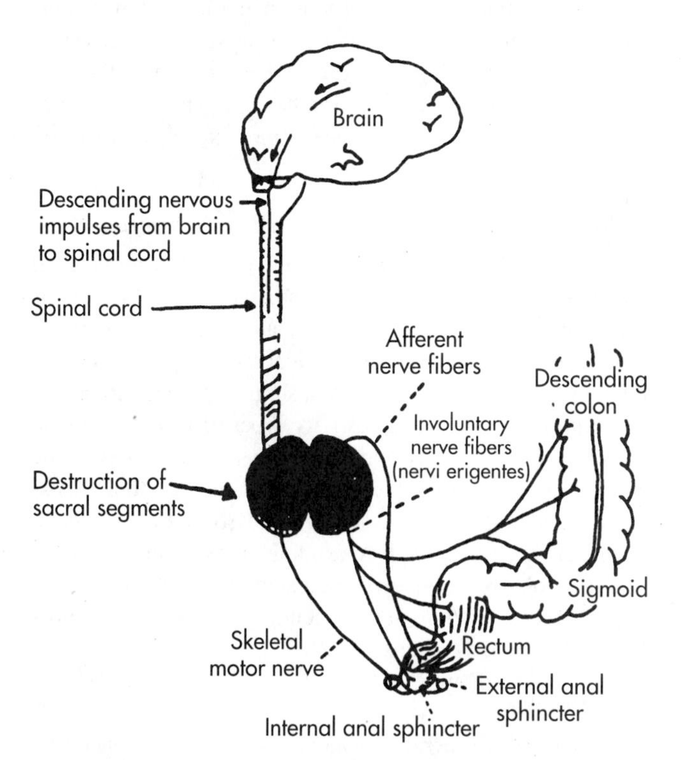

Figure 20-7 Autonomous (nonreflex) bowel. (From Pires, M., & Lockhart-Pretti, P. [1992]. *Nursing management of neurogenic incontinence.* Glenview [IL]: Association of Rehabilitation Nurses.)

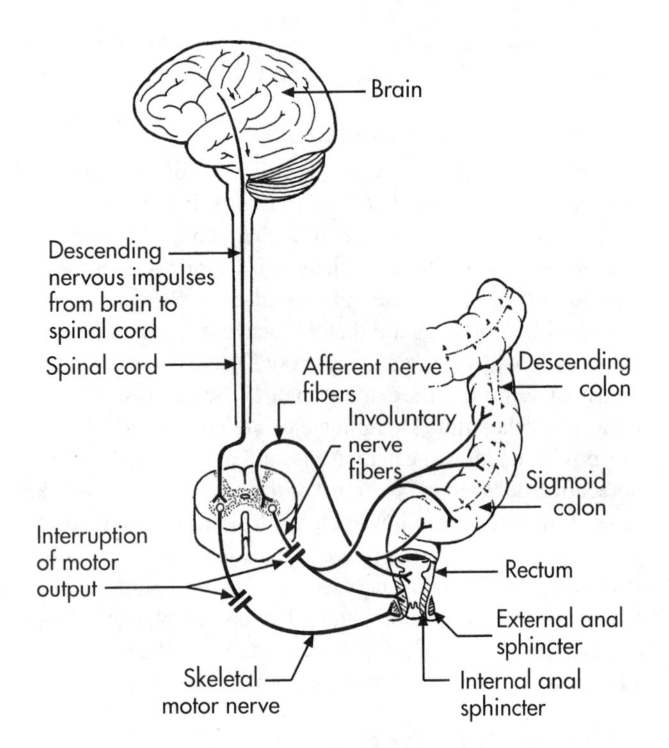

Figure 20-8 Motor paralytic bowel. (From Pires, M., & Lockhart-Pretti, P. [1992]. *Nursing management of neurogenic incontinence.* Glenview [IL]: Association of Rehabilitation Nurses.)

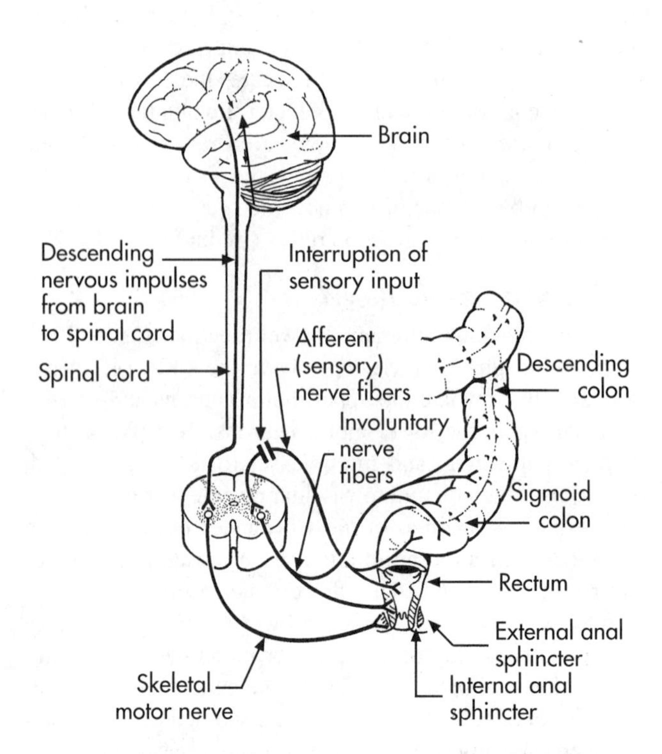

Figure 20-9 Sensory paralytic bowel. (From Pires, M., & Lockhart-Pretti, P. [1992]. *Nursing management of neurogenic incontinence.* Glenview [IL]: Association of Rehabilitation Nurses.)

Sensory Paralytic Bowel

Damage to the dorsal roots of S2, S3, and S4 or dorsal horns of the spinal cord results in a sensory paralytic bowel (Figure 20-9); diabetes mellitus and tabes dorsalis can cause this damage. Saddle sensation is diminished or absent. The bulbocavernosus reflex and anal reflex may be normal, decreased, or absent. Incontinence is rare except in advanced stages (Cannon, 1981).

Other Factors Contributing to Incontinence

Diseases of peripheral nerves supplying the external anal sphincter may result in fecal incontinence. Bowel problems also may arise from disease of the anal sphincter or weakness of the diaphragm, the abdominal muscles, or muscles of the pelvic floor, or as a result of a surgical ostomy after cancer, trauma, or other diseases. Two types of bowel diversion ostomies are ileostomy and colostomy (Figure 20-10). The stoma site determines the consistency of the stool. Ileostomies result in frequent, liquid stools because almost no water has been absorbed. Ascending colostomies also have liquid stools, but transverse colostomies have more solid, formed feces, as does the descending and sigmoid colostomy (Berger & Williams, 1992).

Constipation

Constipation is a condition, not a disease, experienced by most persons at some time during life (Waldrop & Doughty, 2000). Individuals define constipation differently ranging from frequent bowel movements, reduced number, or fewer than the person thinks he or she should have; others define it as difficult movements that require undue straining. Often it is both. Connell, Hilton, Irvine, Lennard-Jones, and Misiewicz (1965) studied frequency of bowel movements and found that 98% of the population moved their bowels between three times a day and three times a week. Based on this study most experts define constipation as defecation of twice a week or less (Abyad & Mourad, 1996; White & Williams, 1992).

Transit time through the colon can be measured clinically by the radiopaque colonic transit time study. The client swallows small capsules containing radiopaque markers followed with either direct radiographic examination of the abdomen or radiographs of the feces on successive days. A person with normal bowel motility passes 80% of the swallowed markers within 5 days, whereas constipated individuals experience delayed transit time of the markers through the colon (Abyad & Mourad, 1996). Characteristics or symptoms of constipation are shown in Box 20-1.

Etiology. A variety of factors contribute to constipation, including those intrinsic to an existing physiological disorder and those extrinsic or environmental. Intrinsic factors may be neuropathic or myopathic in origin. Neuropathic disorders affect nerve pathways to cause motility problems and disordered defecation and lead to constipation. Major neurological disorders that affect GI function are diabetic neuropathy, stroke, spinal cord lesions, Parkinson's disease, multiple sclerosis, or cerebral palsy. In diabetes mellitus, damage to the efferent autonomic nerves

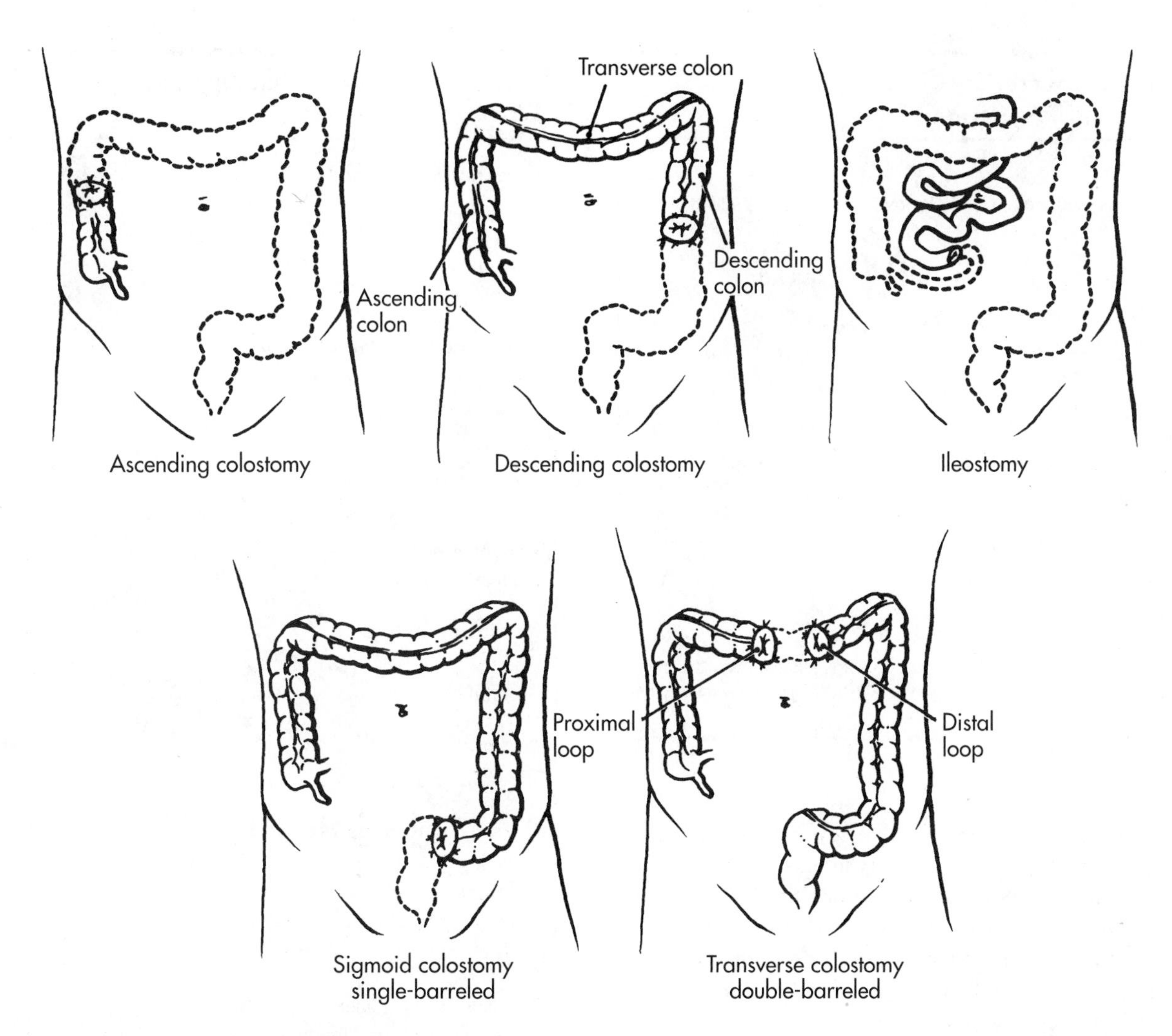

Figure 20-10 Ostomy types. (From Lewis, S.L., Collier, I.C., Heitkemper, M.M., Dirksen, S.R. [2000]. *Medical-surgical nursing: Assessment and management of clinical problems.* [5th ed.]. St. Louis: Mosby.)

leads to diminished intestinal motility and weak smooth muscle contraction (Waldrop & Doughty, 2000). In Parkinson's disease, there is degeneration within the autonomic nervous system, and outlet obstruction with paradoxical puborectalis contraction may occur during straining. This prevents normal straightening of the anorectal angles accentuating the flap valve action and preventing onward passage of feces (Edwards, Quigley, & Pfeiffer, 1992) and possibly delayed colonic transit time (Edwards, Quigley, Hofman, & Pfeiffer, 1993). Myopathic or specific muscle disorders, such as muscular dystrophy may also affect GI motility (Waldrop & Doughty, 2000).

Extrinsic factors that may cause constipation include reduced fiber and fluid intake, decreased activity and mobility, toileting habits, and pharmacological agents. Insufficient fiber intake decreases the amount of water, resulting in small, hard stools that fail to stimulate the enteric nervous system sufficiently to elicit strong peristaltic contractions. Transit time is thus prolonged and more water is absorbed from the stool. Inadequate oral fluid intake will cause more reabsorption of water from the stool and cause constipation. Poor toileting habits or suppressing the normal defecation reflex prolong exposure of the stool to the rectal mucosa and cause further dehydration of the feces. Children, too busy playing, may ignore the urge to defecate and become constipated (Waldrop & Doughty, 2000). Many medications adversely affect intestinal motility through stimulation of the sympathetic nervous system, inhibition of the parasympathetic nervous system, or direct effect on absorption or secretion within the GI tract. Box 20-2 lists various medications that may contribute to constipation.

Diarrhea

Diarrhea means an increase in fecal water content accompanied by increased frequency of defecation (Bisanz, 1997). When something interferes with the absorption of solid wastes from the small intestine or causes the bowel to secrete rather than absorb liquid, or when something speeds the passage of waste through the bowel leaving insufficient time to absorb fluid, diarrhea results. The greatest hazard of diarrhea is the loss of water and electrolytes needed for normal cell function. Severe dehydration and electrolyte imbal-

Box 20-1 Characteristics or Symptoms of Constipation

No stool
Decreased frequency of bowel movements (e.g., fewer than 3 times a week)
Hard, formed stools
Severe flatus
Reported feeling of rectal fullness
Decreased bowel sounds
Distended abdomen
Palpable mass in left lower quadrant
Headache (in the absence of other causes)
Straining and pain on defecation, probably related to hemorrhoids
Anorexia
Nausea and/or vomiting
Diarrhea caused by fecal impaction
Generalized fatigue

Hogstel, M.O., & Nelson, M. (1992). Anticipation and early detection can reduce bowel elimination complications. *Geriatric Nursing, 13,* 28-33.

Box 20-2 Medications That May Cause Constipation

Anticholinergic Medications
Antihistamines
Antispasmodics
Tricyclic antidepressants
Antipsychotics

Cardiovascular Medications
Calcium-channel blockers
β-adrenergic antagonists
Diuretics
Antiarrhythmics

Central Nervous System Depressants
Anticonvulsants
Antiparkinsonian drugs

Narcotic Analgesics
Opiates
Barbiturates

Antineoplastics
Vinca alkaloids

Cation-Containing Medications
Antacids
Sucralfate
Calcium, iron, barium

Others
Bile acid-binding agents (e.g., cholestyramine)
Nonsteroidal antiinflammatory drugs (e.g., ibuprofen, naproxen)
Oral hypoglycemics
Chronic laxative use (bisacodyl and anthraquinones)
Parasympatholytics
Acetylsalicylic acid

From Doughty, D. (2000). *Urinary and fecal incontinence: Nursing management.* (2nd ed.). St. Louis: Mosby.

ance can cause cardiac arrhythmias, severe hypotension, renal failure, and death, especially in infants and very young children, elderly persons, and those debilitated by extreme illness. Otherwise, diarrhea is not severe or life-threatening, although it may be chronic, recurring, or an acute symptom lasting for a short time. It does signal that something has disrupted normal function of the GI tract.

Etiology. Diarrhea may be classified as acute (lasting less than 2 to 4 weeks) (Tobillo & Schwartz, 1998) or chronic. Several pathological processes may cause diarrhea. One disorder allows increased volume of water and electrolytes to be secreted into the lumen of the bowel. Common causes are infectious agents of bacteria or protozoa or a virus in the GI tract, usually at the terminal ileum or large intestine. The mucosa of the infected area of the bowel becomes irritated and increases the rate of secretion that increases bowel motility. The large amounts of fluid are intended to flush the infectious agent and the peristalsis to move the fluid toward expulsion. Diarrhea can be an important mechanism for ridding the intestinal tract of debilitating infections (Guyton & Hall, 1996).

Disorders that reduce absorption of water and electrolytes into the intestinal epithelial cells directly increase the volume of stool and its liquidity. Common causes include ingestion of sorbitol and other hyperosmolar medications, and fat malabsorption syndromes. Lactose intolerance (Waldrop & Doughty, 2000), often a response to milk products and chocolate, is more common among African Americans and Asians (Doughty, 1992). Motility disorders within the bowel are a third cause of diarrhea. Increased motility occurs with inflammatory bowel disease, diabetes mellitus, irritable bowel syndrome, and infectious diarrheas. Decreased motility of the bowel may lead to constipation with seepage of liquid stool that may be misinterpreted as diarrhea (Waldrop & Doughty, 2000).

Finally, diarrhea may result from mixed disorders caused by alterations in secretion or absorption in addition to disordered motility. Examples are laxative abuse, which increases intestinal motility and reduces absorption, infection with *Clostridium difficile* after antibiotic therapy, and acquired immune deficiency syndrome–related diarrhea (Waldrop & Doughty, 2000).

FACTORS ASSOCIATED WITH ALTERED BOWEL ELIMINATION PATTERNS

Life Span Issues

Control of bowel function is a basic human need that is the subject of varying levels of concern throughout a person's life. Children learn early that successful control of bowel function gains them praise and signifies that they are maturing. They learn that control of elimination is valued and that lack of control can be humiliating. Patterns of elimination change throughout the life span. Infants from birth to 1 year of age lack neuromuscular maturity to control their bowels; toddlers are physically ready for bowel control at 18 to 24 months, although cognitive and psychosocial readiness may be achieved later. Daytime control usually occurs at 30 months. Constipation can be common among preschool and school-aged children because of fevers, dietary changes, or emotional and environmental changes. A characteristic individual elimination pattern usually is established at this time. As children mature into adolescence and then young and middle-aged adulthood, other developmental tasks become primary and bowel function receives little thought. Bowel patterns vary with dietary intake, lifestyle, exercise, and emotional state. Irregular meals, changing schedules, and increased stress all affect elimination.

Bowel function reemerges as a concern for some elders who believe a regular or routine bowel habit is essential to maintain health (Ross, 1993). Belief in a daily bowel movement stems from the theory of autointoxication, developed in the early 1900s by Sir Arbuthnot Lane (Ross, 1993). This theory postulated that fluids in the colon were in a constant interchange with the blood current, and that without regular elimination, a person could contract self-poisoning and a variety of diseases and illnesses. Many people brought up during this era were led to believe that regular catharsis, such as laxatives, was necessary for good health (Brocklehurst, 1980). Today advertisements continue to promote products that prevent constipation and imply benefits from a daily bowel movement. Despite the heightened awareness of bowel function and habits, most people decline to think or talk about the subject until faced with a problem in controlling or regulating function.

Clinical Manifestations

The ability to control bowel function may be compromised by a variety of neuromuscular disorders noted previously and altered whenever the CNS has been impaired. Incontinence may become as devastating a problem as the disability itself. Disorders of regularity cause considerable difficulties for some. Constipation persists among elderly persons because of improper diet, inactivity, difficulty chewing resulting from loss of teeth or poor denture fit, medications taken for chronic diseases, decreased mobility, diminished thirst sensation, or loss of colon and abdominal tone (Berger & Williams, 1992). Constipation not only causes discomfort, when neglected it may lead to an impacted stool or possible bowel obstruction. Clients in rehabilitation who have oncology, pulmonary, or pain management problems may be at risk for diarrhea or constipation.

NURSING PROCESS

Subjective Assessment

A client's individualized bowel program must be built from a comprehensive nursing assessment combined with knowledge of normal and impaired bowel function. This is the foundation for successful management.

History

The history elicits a detailed description of the present illness, the perceived bowel problem, bowel function between the time of injury and the present, past bowel routine, dietary factors, medication usage, beliefs about bowel function, and lifestyle goals.

Current Elimination Pattern. The client, or family member if client is unable, should be asked to describe, in their own words, the bowel elimination pattern since their injury or illness. Data include frequency, level of continence, volume and consistency of stool (Doughty, 1992), and time of last bowel movement. If the disability is not recent in onset, clients can describe their bowel care techniques and factors associated with bowel incontinence, such as time of day, frequency, and relationship to eating (Stiens et al., 1997). For persons with cancer, the current history of bowel patterns is more important (Bisanz, 1997). Ask about a client's sensory awareness of rectal filling and the ability to delay and control defecation (Doughty, 1992).

Past Bowel Routine. Questions about former bowel habits include time of day of evacuation, frequency, volume and consistency of stool and the time needed to complete bowel care (Stiens et al., 1997), and personal habits to stimulate defecation. Note reliance on laxatives or enemas, as well as the premorbid pattern, and any incidence of diarrhea or constipation (Lincoln & Roberts, 1989). In most cases, premorbid bowel function and patterns will lay the groundwork for developing a workable rehabilitation bowel regimen by taking advantage of well-established patterns (Stiens et al., 1997).

Dietary Factors. The client's diet and appetite should receive careful attention. Assessment of preonset habits should include food preferences, usual meal routine, amount and type of fluid intake, cultural practices, and number of servings of fiber per day (raw fruits, vegetables, whole grains, bran) (Doughty, 1992). Foods that caused diarrhea, excessive flatus, or constipation before the onset of disability are likely to cause the same response now.

Medication Usage. Clients take many medications that may have undesirable side effects. Antibiotics destroy normal bowel flora and may result in diarrhea. Propantheline (Pro-Banthine) and oxybutynin chloride (Ditropan), used in the management of urinary incontinence, can cause constipation. Ask about previous and current use of laxatives, stool softeners, suppositories, or enemas as part of the nursing history.

Relevant Medical History. A premorbid bowel disorder can complicate a postinjury program. Irritable bowel syndrome or laxative dependency prolong transit time and decrease responsiveness of the gut to bowel medications (Stiens et al., 1997). Any historical report of sphincter disturbances, ulcerative colitis, diverticulitis, spastic colon, diabetes, prolapse, or hemorrhoids should be noted and explored.

Lifestyle Goals and Beliefs about Bowel Function. Clients can identify their bowel management goals in light of their schedules for work or school, available assistance after discharge, and the time to complete a bowel care regimen when at home (Stiens et al., 1997). If the disability is not recent, ask clients to describe the effect of their bowel program on their current lifestyle and any changes they would like made (Doughty, 1992). Beliefs about bowel management can be ascertained throughout the history-taking process.

Objective Assessment

Physical Examination

The overall physical condition of the client must be assessed with special notation made of the cause of the disability, the neurological status, and any other factors that might affect bowel function or ability to participate. The three common neurogenic bowel dysfunctions discussed previously have specific interventions that are described in more detail later in this chapter. The level of neural dysfunction of the bowel is assessed using the motor and sensory tests described earlier. Inspect the abdomen for distention, visible peristalsis, masses, or bulges. Auscultate for normal, hyperactive, or hypoactive bowel sounds and percuss any unexpected dullness, such as over the lower quadrant, which may indicate a mass of feces (Beddar et al., 1997). Abdominal palpation notes muscle tone, contractility (Doughty, 1992), tenderness, and impacted stool (Bisanz, 1997). A rectal examination assesses sphincter tone, strength of the anal sphincter (Beddar et al., 1997), presence and consistency of stool in the rectum (Hogstel & Nelson, 1992), and any rectal excoriations or lesions. Cognitive and communication abilities influence whether a client understands the staff when questioned about the need to toilet. Clients who need assistance to reach or correctly use call buttons or signals, such as clients with speech, language, visual, or auditory impairments may not be able to notify staff or participate fully in a bowel program.

Persons with a stroke or brain injury may suffer from dysphagia, which makes chewing and swallowing difficult. Individuals with facial paralysis or who have lost a great deal of weight after their disability may be left with ill-fitting dentures that now affect their ability to chew food properly. The client's endurance level is considered because those who tire easily may require small, frequent meals rather than struggle to complete a large meal.

Clients' abilities to turn in the bed and ambulate or transfer from bed to toilet or commode may require them to make adaptations, such as bedside rails to pull up on, so they can perform the bowel program with the greatest degree of independence. Hand dexterity for inserting suppositories, performing digital stimulation (Doughty, 1992), or completing wiping and personal hygiene associated with toileting activities relate to bowel program success.

Environmental Assessment

A new, unfamiliar environment may affect a person's ability to call for help or use the toilet or commode. Use of restraints or pain can also be a factor (Beddar et al., 1997). Assess family and social support because family members or attendants will need to help a person with tetraplegia, whereas a person with paraplegia may require only assistive devices and equipment. An elderly client may find degenerative joint disease makes getting to the toilet difficult. A couple may decide that an attendant rather than the spouse will provide assistance.

Nursing Diagnoses

From the assessment data, the rehabilitation nurse makes appropriate nursing diagnoses for the client with altered bowel elimination. Potential diagnoses are as follows (Gordon, 2000):

1. Bowel incontinence related to: environmental factors (e.g., inaccessible bathroom); cognitive impairment; abnormally high abdominal or intestinal pressure (from gas); laxative abuse; dietary habits; immobility; general decline in muscle tone (e.g., abdominal, perineal, bowel sphincter); impaction; incomplete emptying of bowel. Classifications of bowel impairment are:
   - Uninhibited
   - Reflex neurogenic
   - Autonomous neurogenic
   - Motor paralytic
   - Sensory paralytic (McCourt, 1993)
2. Constipation related to: habitual denial/ignoring of urge to defecate; inadequate toileting (timeliness, positioning for defecation, privacy; irregular defecation habits); insufficient physical activity; abdominal muscle weakness; mental confusion; emotional stress; depression; obesity; hemorrhoids.
3. Perceived constipation related to: cultural or family health beliefs; faulty appraisal; impaired thought processes.
4. Intermittent constipation pattern related to: low-roughage diet; low fluid intake; absence of routines

(time); decreased activity level; routine use of enemas, laxatives.

5. Risk for constipation related to: dietary factors (dehydration, insufficient fiber intake, poor eating habits, change in usual foods and eating patterns, decreased motility of GI tract, inadequate dentition or oral hygiene, insufficient fluid intake); functional factors (insufficient physical activity, inadequate toileting, positioning for defecation, privacy, irregular defecation habits, abdominal muscle weakness, habitual denial or ignoring of urge to defecate, recent environmental changes); psychological factors (depression, emotional stress, mental confusion); pharmacological factors.
6. Diarrhea related to: laxative abuse; tube feedings; travel (e.g., bacteria in food and water); alcohol abuse; high stress or anxiety.

Goals

Short-term goals are established with the client and vary according to disability, type of bowel dysfunction, and lifestyle. Goals that may be established are to:

1. Achieve control on a regular basis (a bowel movement every 1 to 3 days) at a planned time and place without the need for laxatives or enemas
2. Establish a bowel program that permits evacuation in the least amount of time possible with no incontinent episodes after the program (Steins et al., 1997)
3. Normalize stool consistency (Doughty, 1992)
4. Eliminate or minimize involuntary bowel movements
5. Plan a diet that includes the appropriate amount of fluid and fiber
6. Incorporate exercise into daily program
7. Help the client to achieve the highest level of independence possible with the program
8. Assist client to problem solve when the bowel program does not perform as planned and to choose appropriate interventions to achieve goal
9. Help the client with an uninhibited neurogenic bowel to plan and regulate bowel elimination at a time when there is likely to be a response
10. Help the client with a reflex neurogenic bowel to stimulate reflex activity that moves feces into the rectum for predictable elimination
11. Assist the client with an autonomous neurogenic bowel to maintain firm stool consistency and keep the distal colon empty
12. Avoid complications of diarrhea, constipation, and impaction by maintaining adequate nutrition, hydration, and activity (McCourt, 1993)

Long-term goals must minimize associated impairments, disabilities, and handicaps, considering instead the person's life goals and role expectations, particularly cultural, sexual, and vocational roles. The entire process requires knowledge of the individual and derivation of his or her person-centered goals (Stiens et al., 1997).

Interventions

Basic Components of a Bowel Program

Rehabilitation nurses are aware that certain factors common to all bowel programs influence efficiency. In addition, specific nursing interventions exist for bowel management in incontinence, constipation, and diarrhea for particular types of neurogenic bowel. Both the problem and the causes enter into the choice of interventions and proper evaluation of results. Certain tenets are foundational to all bowel programs, a "clean" bowel to start, timing, proper diet and fluid intake, physical exercise, privacy, positioning, use of medications as indicated, and client and family education.

A "Clean" Bowel. The bowel must be free from impacted feces. Manual disimpaction, cleansing enemas, or laxatives may be used to free the bowel from an impaction. Laxatives are given 8 to 12 hours before results. Examples of laxatives or enemas that may be used are milk of magnesia, milk of magnesia with cascara, magnesium citrate, Fleet's Enema, oil retention enema, or bisacodyl enema. Clients with loss of sphincter function are not able to retain enemas (Doughty, 1992) and those with pelvic floor dystonia, such as in Parkinson's disease, will not have effective results from laxatives or enemas (Edwards et al., 1992). For children with myelomeningocele who have impacted feces, Coffman (1986) recommends a cleansing enema of lactated Ringer's solution. Persons with cancer benefit from oil retention or milk and molasses enemas because these types ease the stool removal in a nonirritating, noncaustic way, unlike a soap suds or tap water enema (Bisanz, 1997).

Because laxatives increasing the motility of the small bowel and colon, routine use produces unpredictable results and can create bowel dependence (Doughty, 1992). Enemas are not used routinely because they stretch the colon walls and result in loss of elasticity; continued use causes the bowel to respond poorly to reflex stimulation and become dependent. Therefore, after impacted feces have been removed and the bowel training program started, no laxatives or enemas are given unless:

1. The client becomes impacted or severely constipated.
2. There is medical necessity, such as bowel preparation for tests or surgery. (Clients with spinal cord injury have their routine bowel program the night before with manual removal in the morning, rather than the usual preparation.)
3. Recommendations based on evaluations are that this is the best program for the client.

Timing. Scheduling the time of day for a bowel program is important for effectiveness. Timing also accommodates the clients' previous or preferred routine to fit with discharge plans and their future lifestyle. Venn, Taft, Carpentier, and Applebaugh (1992) conducted a research study of 46 stroke clients and discovered that when their premorbid time for elimination was used as the scheduled time of day for their bowel training program, a significantly higher number were able to establish effective bowel regimens. For children and adolescents, a regular routine for toileting needs to be planned around school times (Coffman, 1986); for an adult, around work hours. For example, defecation may be attempted every morning but evaluated and modified according to the client's physical condition and response. Some find an every-other-day routine satisfactory; others manage good evacuation with a 3-day routine.

A key is a consistent time habit for elimination. Clinical experience has demonstrated that for prompt bowel response to stimulation (a bowel movement within 30 minutes), the stimulation method must take place at the same hour every time. The gastrocolic reflex also aids the bowel routine, ideally after any meal, but a hot cup of coffee or tea or an evening snack may produce the gastrocolic reflex at a more convenient time.

Diet and Fluid Intake. The client's preonset dietary habits are evaluated before implementing a bowel program. Physical condition and personal preferences are incorporated as much as possible into a diet high in nutrients and containing a variety of foods. High fiber is important because dietary fiber traverses the small intestine without being digested by the endogenous secretions. Fiber functions by binding water in the intestine in the form of a gel to prevent overabsorption from the large bowel. This action ensures that the fecal content is both bulky and soft and also that its passage through the intestine is not delayed. Delayed transit time of the fecal contents generally results in constipation. Dietary fiber is beneficial in the management of both constipation and diarrhea. Its bulking action helps alleviate diarrhea, and its softening action helps prevent constipation.

The chief sources of dietary fiber are whole-grain cereals and breads, leafy vegetables, legumes, nuts, and fruits with skins. By simply replacing white bread with whole grain bread, the fiber content of the diet can be increased greatly. At least five to nine daily servings of vegetables and fruits, two raw, are recommended. Granola, bran, and wheat germ are excellent sources of fiber and easily added to soups, cereals, meat loaf, baked goods, and other foods. Fiber is introduced into the diet gradually to allow the GI tract time to adapt. Too rapid an increase in fiber may produce distressing side effects such as flatulence, distention, or diarrhea.

Unless fluid intake is restricted for medical reasons, clients should drink 2 to 3 quarts of liquid daily to maintain soft stool consistency. Drinking hot coffee, hot water, or prune juice every morning for breakfast is helpful to some who are initiating a bowel movement. Prunes and prune juice stimulate intestinal motility and therefore act as natural laxatives. Large quantities of prune or other fruit juices, however, may result in loose stools. Setting the table with two or more types of fluid at each meal may increase total intake. Popsicles or ice also may help (Smith, 1988).

Exercise. Physical activity is vital to a successful bowel program. Prolonged bed rest has an adverse effect on bowel motility and tends to cause fecal retention. The client who can be out of bed and involved in physical activities increases muscle tone and has return of bowel function more quickly. In a study of stroke clients, Munchiando and Kendall (1993) discovered that as the number of hours spent in bed increased, the number of days needed to establish a bowel program also increased.

Physical status and type of disability determine exercise capabilities. Encouraging the client to perform activities of daily living (ADLs) with minimum assistance from others helps compensate for the decreased activity level as a result of physical disability. Exercise tapes may be used to guide activities that can be performed while the client is in a wheelchair (Smith, 1988). When subjected to extended periods of bed rest for medical reasons, the client must be urged to continue to carry out as many activities as possible. Turning in bed, lifting the hips, bathing, performing range of joint motion exercises, and carrying out other self-care activities aid in preventing decreased bowel motility and constipation.

Privacy. The act of elimination, in most cultures, is performed in private. Privacy and modesty are particularly important to clients who are from Mexican-American or Native American heritage (Hoeman, 1989). Privacy facilitates relaxation, which in turn facilitates the act of defecation. Privacy also ensures that others will not detect embarrassing sounds or notice odors. Clients in any institution have little privacy; the more dependent the client, the less the privacy. Clients benefit psychologically when privacy is incorporated into the bowel program. Whenever possible, the nurse should assist the client out of bed and onto a toilet where the bathroom door may be closed. If a portable commode must be used, safely roll it into a bathroom or other secluded area.

Positioning. Whenever possible, the client should assume an upright sitting position to defecate. This normal physiological position allows gravity to assist in peristalsis and stool expulsion. Unless absolutely necessary, avoid bedpans and never use them with a client who does not have sensation in the buttocks or sacral area. If a bedpan is unavoidable, position the client carefully to limit the sacral pressure exerted by the bedpan. Elevate the head of the bed, support the back and legs with pillows, and bridge the hips and legs, as necessary. To avoid excessive pressure and potential skin breakdown, never allow anyone to remain on the bedpan or sit on a toilet or commode for longer than 25 minutes. Five to 20 minutes may be necessary for defecation to occur, and when necessary a client can be evaluated and supervised for a longer time (Hogstel & Nelson, 1992). As soon as the client receives medical approval to get out of bed, bedpans should be abandoned. Clients with impaired skin integrity involving the buttocks or who do not have buttock or sacral sensation (i.e., clients with spinal cord injuries [SCI]) evacuate on an incontinence pad in bed. Positioning the client on the right side after inserting a suppository or for manual removal aids elimination because gravity assists evacuation of the descending colon in that position. A squat position with the knees slightly higher than the hips and feet flat on the floor helps to increase abdominal pressure and thus facilitate stool passage. It also straightens the angle between the rectum and anal canal to promote rectal emptying (Heitkemper, 2000). This position is especially important for persons with Parkinson's disease because of their difficulty with voluntary contraction and dystonia of the pelvic floor and anal sphincter muscles (Edwards et al., 1992). If balance is a problem, use armrests and a back support (Wald, 1991).

For those persons with weak abdominal muscles, an abdominal binder increases abdominal pressure as the person bends at the waist, the abdominal muscles to push out the stool (Hogstel, 1992). Abdominal massage also may stimulate and hasten the defecation process. Persons with all types of disabilities and ages find it helpful to massage the abdomen in the direction of the bowel from right groin upward, across and down to the left groin. Breathing techniques can increase intraabdominal pressure. Slow, deep breaths with each inspiration are held for 5 seconds and then combined with abdominal muscle contractions to bear down or perform a Valsalva maneuver. A child can be taught this maneuver by having them blow up a balloon (Doughty, 1992), cough, or blow bubbles (Smith, 1990).

Suppositories and Medications. The rehabilitation nurse develops protocols in collaboration with the physician or nurse practitioner that specify ranges and guidelines for suppositories and medications so the nurse can make adjustments according to the individual client's response. Suppositories are used to initiate reflex emptying of the bowel. To have an optimum effect, the suppository must come in contact with the bowel wall. Before inserting a suppository, the rectum should be checked for stool. If stool is present, enough should be removed to ensure proper placement of the suppository against the bowel wall. The suppository should be stored at room temperature before insertion, because refrigeration delays action and temperatures higher than 90°F (32.2°C) cause the suppository to melt. Table 20-1 summarizes the three types of suppositories commonly used in rehabilitation settings.

Minienemas, such as the Therevac SB, which is a 4-ml solution of docusate and glycerin, may be used to soften and lubricate the stool and initiate evacuation (Dunn & Galka, 1994). Stool softeners and bulk formers are often prescribed to aid in the establishment of a bowel program. For example, dioctyl sodium sulfosuccinate (Colace), 100 mg, 2 to 3 times per day, may be used initially and the dosage adjusted according to the consistency of the stool. When hard stools accompanied by constipation or frequent soft, pasty stools are a problem, bulk-forming laxatives can be given to alter the consistency by making stools soft and bulky. Whenever a mild laxative is needed, senna tablets and granules assist in moving the stool to the lower bowel so that a suppository or digital stimulation can completely empty the bowel.

The nurse should remember that the terminal goal of any bowel program is continence and control without the need for medication. Should medication be needed, consideration must be given to providing medications that will be covered by the client's insurance carriers on an outpatient basis.

Digital Stimulation. Digital stimulation is a technique used to induce reflex contraction of the colon and relaxation of the anal sphincter muscle (Munchiando & Kendell, 1993), resulting in elimination. To perform digital stimulation, the index finger is gloved, lubricated, and gently inserted ½ to 1 inch into the rectum. To stimulate the inner sphincter to relax, the finger is gently rotated in a clockwise motion against the anal sphincter wall. It may take from 30 seconds to 2 minutes for relaxation of the sphincter to occur. While feces pass, the rectal wall is moved gently to one side. When no more stool is expelled, digital stimulation is resumed and the process repeated until the bowel is evacuated. The client should be instructed to take slow, deep breaths during this process.

In successful bowel programs, digital stimulation may replace the suppository after a reflex-response defecation pattern is established. However, digital stimulation also may be used to trigger a bowel movement if a suppository has been less than successful or to ensure complete emptying of the colon after a bowel movement. In persons with SCI who are susceptible to dysreflexia, dibucaine hydrochloride (Nupercainal) lubricant can lower the incidence of dysreflexia during stimulation. The rehabilitation nurse should be aware that children may be unwilling to use a digital stimulation technique for their bowel program (Doughty, 1992).

Education. The details of client education should parallel the individualized bowel program. Education should begin early during hospitalization to give the client sufficient time and opportunity to discover and clarify problems or concerns. Teaching should include an explanation of the disability and how it affects bowel control, including basic anatomy and physiology of the GI tract. The rationale behind a routine bowel program and importance of diet, fluid intake, exercise, timing, and positioning are other educational elements. If medication is used for the program, explain the purpose, precautions, and techniques of suppository insertion or digital stimulation. Decide where the bowel program will take place when the client is at home and assure that client and caregiver practice safe and proper positioning. Discussion of potential problems encountered with a bowel program includes the client and family explaining the steps they would take if diarrhea, constipation, or an accident occurred. They also verbalize their rationale for adjustments in the program and when they would consult with their physician or rehabilitation nurse. Cultural or familial beliefs regarding bowel movements or diet are important and adaptations in the program made to meet their needs. It is essential to detect confusion and correct erroneous information. During the educational experience, the client and family need encouragement, reassurance, and emotional support, as well as information.

Bowel Incontinence

The primary nursing intervention for a client with a diagnosis of bowel incontinence is to establish a bowel training program (McCloskey & Bulechek, 2000). Any changes in a bowel program should not be made before at least a 5- to 7-day trial, and then only one change at a time. Daily changes in a program only modify a program blindly without any learning about the response to the previous bowel program. Accurate documentation of the results of any bowel program is vital because some aspects in management of bowel control is on a trial-and-error basis for many clients. The effectiveness of the program can be evaluated only if accurate records are kept (Figure 20-11).

	Date:		
Suppository =	/ Type		
	Time		
	Inserted by:		
Digital stim	Time		
Manual removal	Time		
Evacuation	Time		
Stool	Amt.		
	Consistency		
	Place		
	Initials		
Normal evacuation	Time		
	Amt.		
	Consistency		
	Place		
	Initials		
Accidents	Time		
(Chart in red)	Place		
	Consistency		
	Initials		
Accidents	Time		
(Chart in red)	Place		
	Consistency		
	Initials		
Enema	Time & initials		
Initials R.N., L.V.N.			

Figure 20-11 Bowel record. (Courtesy San Diego Rehabilitation Institute, San Diego, CA.)

Uninhibited Neurogenic Bowel. In general, the following measures should be taken in establishing a bowel program for a client with an uninhibited neurogenic bowel.

1. Select the time of day for the bowel program according to past habits and for future convenience.
2. Follow a consistent schedule. Assist client to toilet 30 minutes after meals to take advantage of gastrocolic reflex. Start with a daily program and progress to every other day (Munchiando & Kendall, 1993).
3. Provide a nutritious diet with adequate fiber.
4. Give fluids adequate to stimulate reflex activity and to promote soft stool (2000 to 2400 ml/24 hours unless contraindicated).
5. Begin the program with an empty colon.
6. Obtain a physician's order for stool softeners in the early stages of the program.
7. Give a daily suppository to initiate the defecation reflex. Venn et al.'s (1992) research study suggests that if a spontaneous bowel movement occurs within 4 hours before the scheduled time, the suppository may be held back for that day. Table 20-1 provides more detail about suppositories.

Usually the effects of softeners will not be seen for 3 days. Stool softeners should be used on a routine rather than an as-needed basis. Softeners that may be used include the following:

1. Docusate sodium (Dialose; usually one 2 times daily)
2. Docusate calcium (Surfak; usually one 2 times daily; good to use if sodium intake is restricted)
3. Dioctyl sodium sulfosuccinate (Colace; usually one 2 times daily; available in liquid form)
4. Dioctyl sodium sulfosuccinate (Doxinate; usually one 2 times daily).

Softeners with a laxative component may be used when additional softening or peristaltic stimulus is needed. They should be given approximately 12 hours before desired re-

TABLE 20-1 Suppositories

Suppository (Strength)	Action	Time When Results Expected	Disadvantages
Glycerin	Draws fluid from the bowel creating a volume which distends the bowel and initiates reflex peristalsis	Approximately 30 minutes	Abdominal cramping possible
Sodium bicarbonate and potassium bitartrate (CEO-Two)	Activated in water before insertion; suppository releases carbon dioxide, which distends bowel and initiates reflex peristalsis	30-45 minutes	Use of petroleum lubricants negates effectiveness of suppository Abdominal cramping possible
Bisacodyl (Dulcolax)	Contact suppository that stimulates sensory nerve endings in colon and results in reflex peristalsis	15-60 minutes	Abdominal cramping possible

One suppository is the usual dose. Suppositories are given within a half hour after a meal or after a hot drink.

sults and also used on a routine basis. Those that may be used include the following:

1. Docusate sodium and phenolphthalein (Dialose Plus; usually one to two every day)
2. Casanthranol and docusate sodium (Peri-Colace; usually one to two every day)
3. Standardized senna concentrate (Senokot; usually one to two every day)

If combining softeners and softener/laxatives, it is preferable to combine like products (i.e., Dialose with Dialose Plus, Colace with Peri-Colace). Bisacodyl tablets may be used if all other measures are unsuccessful in preventing constipation or impaction. A maximum of two tablets may be given at one time approximately 12 hours before desired results.

Bulk producers may be used for the client who lacks bowel tone, who needs additional softening of the stool, or who has small, infrequent stools. They are not appropriate for the impacted client. They may be used to "form up" stools if the client is on a liquid or tube feeding diet or has an "irritable bowel." Bulk producers that may be used include:

1. Psyllium hydrophilic mucilloid (Metamucil) or psyllium and senna (Perdiem): 1 teaspoon mixed in 200 ml of water or juice and followed by a glass of water
2. "Organic" bulk products of the client's choice, such as alfalfa tablets
3. Calcium polycarbophil (Mitrolan): one to two tablets chewed 1 to 4 times per day

When the client's condition improves so that the diet, fluid intake, and physical activity are well tolerated, these medications may be unnecessary.

Digital stimulation in place of a suppository is used in some rehabilitation settings. Because clients with uninhibited bowel function have intact sensation, digital stimulation may be painful. Document accurately because, depending on the client's condition, it may take a week or longer to establish a satisfactory pattern. Verbal and nonverbal efforts by the client to communicate the need to eliminate are important in those with absence of functional speech. Educate and alert all staff to notice behaviors—something as subtle as a client's restlessness may indicate awareness of rectal sensation. Munchiando and Kendall (1993) discovered that it took longer to establish a bowel program in clients with right-sided hemiplegia, probably as a result of expressive aphasia and difficulty communicating the urge to defecate. Evaluate program effectiveness daily and weekly with only one change at a time. Gradually increase client and family participation in the program and decision making. Guidelines for changes in the program to every other day or every third day include the following:

1. Client has small or no results every other day
2. Client's stool is not hard on daily program
3. Client is well controlled on every program (i.e., results within 1 hour, no constipation or accidents for at least a week).

By complying with the basic components of a bowel program, continence and control can be achieved by the time of discharge and suppositories and medications discontinued.

Reflex Neurogenic Bowel. An upper motor neuron or reflex neurogenic bowel is characterized by fecal retention and requires a scheduled evacuation plan to avoid incontinence and impaction (Stiens, 1995). Recent studies have shown that many clients with traumatic SCI have GI problems after their rehabilitation program that result in severe constipation, difficult evacuation, pain with defecation, or urgency with incontinence (Han, Kim, & Kwon, 1998). Lengthy programs that last longer than 3 hours have also been reported (Stiens, 1995). All of these problems lead to a decreased quality of life and affects ADL functioning. It is imperative, given these findings, that the rehabilitation nurse take responsibility to design an appropriate bowel program with adequate education (Han et al., 1998).

During the acute stage of SCI, spinal shock is responsible for tonic paralysis of the GI tract and flaccid tone of the anal sphincter. Manual removal may be used until spinal shock subsides. In general, the following measures should be taken to establish a bowel program for a client with a reflex neurogenic bowel:

1. After bowel sounds are present, physical activity increases, and oral fluid and food, including high fiber of 30 g/day (Stiens et al., 1997) is tolerated, administer a suppository daily to trigger reflex elimination. Administration time should be consistent with the establishment of preonset habits and anticipated future lifestyle. The suppository is inserted 15 to 30 minutes ahead of the planned evacuation time (Venn et al., 1992). Following a regular schedule is important even if stool elimination does not occur each time. Missed bowel care sessions can contribute to excessive build up of stool in the colon. The stool then becomes less plastic and more difficult to eliminate. Distention of the colon can occur with a decrease in effectiveness of peristalsis (Stiens et al., 1997). If a Bisacodyl suppository is chosen, rehabilitation nurses should be aware that it is prepared with either a vegetable oil base or a polyethylene glycol polymer base. Glycol bases have been reported to produce quicker elimination (Stiens, 1995). A clinically significant research study by Stiens with a single subject T2 SCI client 10 years after injury, showed that using a glycol-based Bisacodyl suppository reduced total bowel program time to 46 minutes as compared with 86 minutes for the oil-based suppository. Total bowel program time included insertion of the suppository until transferring off of the toilet. Dunn and Galka (1994) found that the Therevac SB minienema cut the time needed for bowel care by as much as an hour or more when compared with Bisacodyl suppositories.
2. After a reliable bowel pattern is observed, suppository administration may be decreased to every other day or every third day as long as the stool consistency remains soft. Be alert for signs of fecal impaction or constipation that may develop with infrequent elimination.

3. Have client evacuate on the toilet if possible and bear down if abdominal muscles are strong. The client should lean forward and massage the abdomen in a clockwise manner (Zejdlik, 1992). Digital stimulation may be used alone or in addition to a suppository when the suppository has not produced results within 15 to 20 minutes.
4. Stool softeners, bulk agents, and stimulant laxatives may be necessary to assist elimination when abdominal muscles are weak or paralyzed. Oral senna agents are stimulant laxatives that may facilitate movements in 6 to 8 hours (Stiens et al., 1997). Harsh cathartics must be avoided. The need for medications should decrease as activity increases.
5. Documentation of progress remains important to detect reliable patterns of elimination and to initiate appropriate changes.

For individuals with spinal cord lesions above the T6 vertebral level (above the splanchnic outflow), autonomic dysreflexia is a potential problem. Autonomic dysreflexia (hyperreflexia) is an abnormal hyperactive reflex activity as a result of an interrupted spinal cord. It is set off most often by stimuli arising from a distended bladder, but rectal distention, stimulation, and passage of feces also may precipitate this sympathetic response. This syndrome constitutes a medical emergency that can result in death if not treated promptly. Chapter 19 contains specific information regarding autonomic dysreflexia. Nupercainal ointment applied to the rectum 10 minutes before suppository insertion or digital stimulation is helpful in preventing symptoms in susceptible individuals.

Autonomous Neurogenic Bowel. Management of autonomous neurogenic bowel is difficult. Lower motor neuron loss results in absence of the spinal reflex activity. An atonic bowel with diminished propulsive forces and tone results. A program of suppositories and manual removal can be effective in evacuating stools (Zejdlik, 1992).In general, the following measures should be taken in establishing a bowel program for the client with an autonomous neurogenic bowel.

1. Develop a stool consistency that is firm yet not hard by providing dietary fiber and using bulk-forming agents such as Metamucil and Citrucel.
2. Have the client evacuate on a toilet and perform the Valsalva maneuver (see the discussion on defecation). Massaging the abdomen and leaning forward will augment the effectiveness of the bowel program.
3. If these measures are not successful, manual removal of the stool with a generously lubricated gloved finger can be performed
4. After removal of stool from the lower rectum, administer a suppository as high as possible against the rectal wall. This stimulates the colon to empty stool into the rectum for manual removal. When a client is active, any stool in the rectum may be expelled when intraabdominal pressure is increased. Therefore, a daily program is recommended (Zejdlik, 1992).
5. Assess stool consistency. Loose stools will leak through a flaccid sphincter. Hard stools are difficult to remove manually and can lead to impaction and atony of the colon over time (Rauen & Aubert, 1992).

Children with neurogenic bowels should follow the same routine as adults. Incontinence occurs because of the inability to control the external sphincter. By maintaining the bowel in an empty or near-empty state, continence can be achieved (Gleeson, 1990). The goal for a person born with myelomeningocele, for example, is a soft, formed stool on a daily basis, at the same time each day. This can be achieved through a high-fiber diet, adequate water intake, and habit training (Rauen & Aubert, 1992). Stool softeners, suppositories, and digital stimulation also may be needed (Smith, 1990). When suppositories are used, children with neurogenic bowels may need to have the buttocks closed with paper tape, after suppository insertion, to facilitate absorption (Gleeson, 1990).

In infants with neurogenic bowels, stool consistency must be monitored for signs of constipation. If constipation is present, dietary regulation is the first step before decreasing milk and dairy products and increasing fluids, vegetables, and fruits. Senna concentrate syrup may be added if stool continues to be hard. Bowel continence in children may take months to establish; therefore, parents need encouragement and support. Illnesses, changes in medication, and emotional changes can lead to irregular bowel patterns. Patterns may also alter after the child reaches adolescence (Gleeson, 1990).

Table 20-2 provides a summary overview of the types of neurogenic bowel dysfunctions previously discussed. A successful bowel routine for the client with incontinence resulting from any type of neurological bowel dysfunction requires effort and consistency for the client and the nurse.

Ostomies

A bowel program cannot be established with an ileostomy or ascending colostomy. A bag or pouch must therefore be worn at all times. With regular irrigation, a person with a descending and sigmoid colostomy and sometimes a transverse colostomy can regain a regular bowel pattern. Regulating the diet with selected foods at specific times can also lead to a predictable elimination pattern.

The rehabilitation nurse usually collaborates with an enterostomal therapist to establish a routine program including supplies, skin care, and education of the client. Members of the United Ostomy Association are instrumental in visiting clients and explaining how to live with an ostomy (Berger & Williams, 1992).

Constipation

Constipation is one of the most common complications in persons with neurogenic bowel dysfunction. Interrupted defecation mechanisms can result in a sluggish movement of feces

TABLE 20-2 Neurogenic Bowel Dysfunction

Diagnosis	Level of Lesion	High-Risk Populations	Pattern of Incontinence	Bowel Program
Uninhibited	Brain	Cerebrovascular accident, multiple sclerosis, brain injury	Urgency: poor awareness of desire to defecate	Consistent habit and time according to premorbid history; physical exercise; high fluid intake; high-fiber foods; stool softener, suppository as needed
Reflex	Spinal cord above T12 to L1 vertebral level	Trauma, tumor, vascular disease, syringomyelia, multiple sclerosis	Infrequent, sudden, unexpected	Consistent habit and time, physical exercise, high fluid intake, high-fiber foods; suppository program, digital stimulation, stool softener as needed
Autonomous	Spinal cord at or below T12 to L1 vertebral level	Trauma, tumor, spina bifida, intervertebral disk	Frequent; may be continuous or induced by exercise or stress	Consistent habit and time, physical exercise continuous, high fluid intake, high-fiber foods and bulk agents as necessary for firm stool consistency; suppository program, Valsalva maneuver, manual removal

through the bowel (Zejdlik, 1992). Constipation is also common in clients with cancer as a result of using opioids for pain relief (Bisanz, 1997). Opioids decrease motility and secretion in the GI tract (Mancini & Bruera, 1998). Other diseases that affect constipation are diabetes, Parkinson's disease, and hypothyroidism (Mancini & Bruera, 1998). Clients with diabetes have impaired GI motility, particularly of the colon, and a delayed or absent gastrocolic reflex (Haines, 1995).

To assist the client with constipation to achieve elimination of soft bulky stools on a regular basis, the rehabilitation nurse develop a program of constipation/impaction management (McCloskey & Bulechek, 2000) incorporating diet, fluid intake, exercise, timing, and medication.

Diet and Fluid Intake. The most important dietary factor when considering constipation is the amount of fiber ingested. Authorities disagree about the amount of dietary fiber that constitutes a high-fiber diet. Six to 10 grams of dietary fiber per day have been found to be successful in managing constipation in a majority of subjects (Abyad & Mourad, 1996; Hull, Greco, & Brooks, 1980). Other sources cite the need for 30 to 40 g (Friedman, 1989). The amount of fiber may be individualized according to client need.

In adding fiber to the diet, the rehabilitation nurse must be cognizant of the person's likes and dislikes and especially of ability to chew because many high-fiber foods require adequate mastication. This consideration is extremely important with persons whose residual deficits affect either the innervation or muscle function of the face, mouth, and throat. If the person is unable to handle high-fiber foods adequately, then supplementing the diet with unprocessed bran or adding bran to cooked vegetables and fruit should be considered. As stated previously, fiber binds water in the intestine in the form of a gel. This prevents the overabsorption of water in the large intestine and ensures that the feces are bulky and soft. Fiber also adds weight to the stool, speeds up slow passage, and slows down rapid transit.

The highest source of fiber is minimally processed cereal. Other sources of fiber are legumes such as peas, beans, and millet; root vegetables such as potatoes, parsnips, and carrots; and fruits and leafy vegetables. Bran is one of the most concentrated sources of natural food fiber available. It is the outer layer or covering of the wheat kernel. Miller's bran is the richest source of fiber available, containing 44% dietary fiber (Brunton, 1990). Recipes for adding fiber to the diet are shown in Box 20-3.

Fiber should be introduced gradually into the diet to avoid untoward effects such as abdominal discomfort, flatulence and diarrhea (Brunton, 1990). Bran is considered superior to other bulk laxatives because it is most effective in increasing fecal weight (Iseminger & Hardy, 1982). Bran, however, can bind orally with and reduce the intestinal absorption of many drugs such as cardiac glycosides, sali-

Box 20-3 Fiber Supplement Recipes

Power Pudding*

½ cup prune juice
½ cup applesauce
½ cup wheat bran flakes
½ cup canned or stewed prunes
¼ to 1 cup per day for desired results

Bran Formula

1 cup unprocessed miller's bran
1 cup applesauce
¼ cup prune juice
1 tablespoon per day and increase daily dose by 1 tablespoon each week until desired results

*From Neal L.J. (1995). Power-pudding: natural laxative therapy for the elderly who are homebound. *Home Healthcare Nurse 13*(3):66-71.

cylates, nitrofurantoin, and coumarin derivatives and should therefore be taken separately from them (Brunton, 1990).

Adequate fluids are essential to avoid and manage constipation. It is often necessary for the nurse to be creative in assisting the client to meet the necessary fluid intake. The nurse also must be fully aware of all aspects of the client's rehabilitation plan, including bladder rehabilitation and therapy schedules, so as not to jeopardize but rather to enhance and facilitate the comprehensive plan for rehabilitation.

Exercise. Diet alone is not sufficient to alleviate constipation. Physical activity is essential and can be accomplished easily in rehabilitation settings by incorporating therapy sessions as a means of achieving needed exercise. The activity of physical movement or even ambulating a short distance can be sufficient to stimulate defecation.

Timing. The timing of the bowel program should be considered when establishing the therapy schedule. Ignoring the urge to defecate is a major cause of constipation, and the individual should not be given the impression that defecating is less important than any other part of the rehabilitation plan. For diabetics, a daily toileting time in the morning, when colonic activity is maximal, may help avoid constipation (Haines, 1995).

Medications. Although laxatives are beneficial for treating acute constipation, they are not recommended for chronic problems. An exception would be cancer clients who are taking narcotics. They may need to add a senna derivative, such as Senokot S, plus a stool softener, to their plan to offset the opiate effect on the GI tract. As narcotic doses increase so should the amount of Senna or stool softener to prevent constipation (Bisanz, 1997).

Diarrhea

When a client experiences diarrhea, an investigation for impacted feces is conducted before other action. If the bowel is impacted, then the basic components of bowel management should be explained and the nursing interventions for the client with constipation should be instituted. If diarrhea is treated without assessing for impaction, then a more complex problem could arise—namely, bowel obstruction.

Diarrhea management (McCloskey & Bulechek, 2000) is most easily obtained by treating or eliminating the cause. If it is the result of disease, then the pathological condition should be managed. As stated previously, if antibiotics are the cause, then other antibiotics should be tried. Yogurt can be beneficial in managing the diarrhea. Foods may also cause diarrhea and offending foods can be discovered and eliminated. Some foods help treat diarrhea in children, such as bananas, rice, milk products, or applesauce. Monitor nutritional content in the process of juggling the diet.

Electrolyte imbalance is a potentially serious problem when diarrhea occurs. The client should drink 2 to 3 quarts of fluid a day and also supplement for fluid lost. Excessive use or an excessive dosage of laxatives or the initial phase of dietary supplementation with bran can lead to diarrhea. The following medications may cause diarrhea as a side effect.

1. Broad-spectrum antibiotics
2. Adrenergic neuron blocking agents (reserpine)
3. Bile acids
4. Quinidine
5. Cholinergic agents and cholinesterase inhibitors
6. Prokinetic agents

Whenever diarrhea or incontinence occurs, the potential for skin breakdown exists. Meticulous perianal hygiene, thorough yet gentle, is essential after each episode. Commercial spray cleansers, such as Peri-Wash or Hollister Skin Cleanser, contain substances that emulsify the stool and aid in its removal. The skin also needs protection from exposure to stool. If the skin is denuded, protective powder such a Stomahesive may be applied and then a petroleum-based protective ointment. If a candida infection has caused redness and itching, a medicated antifungal powder or ointment can be prescribed (Lincoln & Roberts, 1989).

Collaboration with the Health Care Team and Community Resources

Although the rehabilitation nurse is the primary team member involved in planning and implementing a successful bowel program with the client and family, other members of the interdisciplinary team may offer important input for the successful management of impaired bowel elimination. The physician, dietitian, occupational, physical, or recreational therapist, speech pathologist, psychologist, pharmacist, and social worker or case manager collaborate with the nurse to plan interventions based on individual needs.

The physician or nurse practitioner prescribes treatments and medications and attends to any active medical problems. The dietitian assists the rehabilitation team in meeting the nutritional and fiber needs of the client. The physical therapist assists the client with an appropriate exercise program and transfer techniques. The occupational therapist designs adaptive devices to help the individual in managing the bowel program. Also, the occupational therapist and physical therapist perform a home evaluation to determine if any bathroom modifications or adaptive equipment are needed to carry out the bowel program at home. The speech pathologist assists with helping clients communicate their needs and, along with the nurse and occupational therapist, assists with feeding and swallowing if a problem is present.

Recreational therapists, or activity coordinators in long-term care settings, assist with toileting goals during activities and community outings. The psychologist assists with any self-esteem or body image issues related to incontinence. The pharmacist is a resource on medication effectiveness, side effects, and interactions. The social worker or case manager assists with discharge planning and discusses with the family any care needs that may be necessary regarding implementing a bowel program at home.

The rehabilitation nurse, along with the case manager, plays a major role in coordinating the discharge plan and community referrals. Supplies and equipment needs related to the client's bowel program must be considered and arranged well in advance. A bedside commode, raised toilet seat, or grab bars may need to be ordered for the home and can be coordinated with the appropriate therapy department. Clients with SCI may require an assistive suppository inserter to be independent in their program. Gloves and lubricant as well as prescriptions for medications need to be arranged. Each client's needs are different and require different community services. But, there are basic considerations when any client with impaired bowel elimination is discharged. The nurse should give attention to the following items:

1. Cost and availability of supplies and equipment needed at home
2. Location of supplier and availability and cost of delivery service
3. Availability of support groups
4. Location of the bathroom in the home
5. Family or agency assistance needed at home to carry out the bowel program

Outcomes

The following are outcome criteria to be used to evaluate the effectiveness of a bowel management program.

1. Evacuation of stool is predictable
2. Control of passage of stool is maintained
3. Regular evacuation of stool occurs at least every 3 days
4. Stool is soft and formed
5. Ease of stool passage occurs
6. Aids are used appropriately to achieve continence
7. Able to get to and from toilet as independently as possible
8. Diarrhea is not present
9. Constipation is not present
10. Ingests adequate amount of fluid
11. Ingests adequate amount of fiber
12. Knows relationship of intake to evacuation pattern
13. Skin is intact
14. Exercises an adequate amount
15. Describes correct administration of medication
16. Describes how to obtain required medication and supplies
17. Recognizes symptom onset of constipation (Johnson, Maas, & Moorhead, 2000).

Remember to assess both the problem and the causes in the context of the intervention to adequately evaluate the intervention's effect. Assessing both the problem and causes assists with problem solving when a problem does not improve after an intervention is administered. For example, if a potential cause (i.e., low fluid intake) of a problem (i.e., constipation) changes for the better (i.e., drinking 1000 ml of fluids per day) and the problem still exists, it may be there are additional causes that were not identified (i.e., poor bowel habits); or maybe the intervention was not strong enough (i.e., need to increase fluid intake to 1500 ml). It is also possible that a problem may not have changed because the cause was incorrect. Assessing both the problem and its sources for change assists with problem solving and with implementing the appropriate bowel management plan.

IMPLICATIONS FOR BOWEL REGULATION AND ELIMINATION

Return to Work, Education, Community, Independence

Regulation of bowel elimination and prevention of incontinence, diarrhea, and constipation are key to achieving a high quality of life for persons with chronic illness and disability. Incontinence limits a person's social activities and may lead to premature placement in long-term care facilities. Incontinence "accidents" and lengthy sessions for managing bowel programs will affect a person's desire to attend school or ability to maintain a job. Self-esteem and body image suffer when bowel programs are unsuccessful.

Implications for Practice, Research, Administration, Professional Education

Control of bowel incontinence and prevention of constipation and diarrhea have been under the purview of the rehabilitation nurse for years. Rehabilitation nurses are now practicing in a variety of settings where this same knowledge base can be used, such as include home health care, outpatient clinics, assisted living, day hospitals, long term acute care hospitals, specialized day care programs, subacute rehabilitation, long-term care, as well as the traditional comprehensive inpatient rehabilitation unit or hospital. Nurses in all settings should receive education on the management of bowel elimination problems.

Research Needs

There is still a need for more research on bowel training methods. Early research on bowel elimination began in the 1960s. It focused primarily on the effects of enemas versus suppositories in achieving control and decreasing nursing time and hospital costs. These studies demonstrated the superiority of suppositories in terms of client comfort and control.

Studies that followed focused on the effects of dietary fiber in preventing constipation and on studying the transit time of food in the GI tract. Recent research on bowel management has been conducted on comparing various bowel training methods for effectiveness and timeliness. More research is needed in this area. The nurse is in the best position to initiate future studies to validate rehabilitation nursing practice in the area of bowel elimination.

CRITICAL THINKING

R.S. is a 30-year-old computer analyst with a T6 paraplegia. He is 4 years postinjury from a motor vehicle accident. R.S. attends the outpatient SCI clinic and presents to the RN with the following concern: His bowel program consists of a daily Bisacodyl suppository 30 minutes after breakfast. It has been taking 70 minutes for evacuation to occur after insertion of the suppository and another 15 minutes for post-toilet management. He is often late to work or finds it necessary to get up earlier than he would like to complete his bowel program. He would like to find a way to shorten his bowel management time. What questions should the RN ask to evaluate his current bowel program? What recommendations for changes in the program might the nurse suggest?

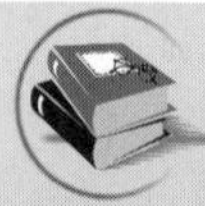

Case Study

Assessment

N.S. is an 80-year-old woman with a right hemisphere stroke. She is a widow and has been living alone. Her 50-year-old daughter will be taking her home to live with her after the mother's rehabilitation stay. Her daughter works as a high school teacher full time.

Upon admission to the rehabilitation unit, the RN notices weakness in both left upper and lower extremities. N.S. is alert and oriented with some slurred speech. An in-depth history is taken. N.S. denies any past bowel problems except for occasional constipation, for which she took milk of magnesia. She usually empties her bowels daily or every other day at 9 AM. Since her stroke 4 days ago, she has been incontinent and has felt a sense of urgency. Her last bowel movement was the day before admission.

Upon physical examination, the nurse noted no abdominal distention, visible peristalsis, masses, or bulges. Normal bowel sounds were auscultated. Percussion and abdominal palpation were normal. A rectal examination revealed a small amount of soft stool. A strong anal reflex was present, as was sensation. No rectal excoriations or lesions were present.

N.S. has full dentures. A bedside swallowing examination conducted by the speech pathologist was normal. A history of prior dietary patterns revealed that N.S. usually had tea, cereal, and fruit for breakfast, a sandwich with whole grain bread and fruit for lunch, and a full dinner of salad, meat, potatoes, and vegetables. Less than three glasses of fluid, other than tea, were usually consumed in a day.

N.S. stated that she wanted to be as independent as possible because she would be home alone when her daughter was working. She expressed that she did not want to be a burden on her daughter. Current medications revealed none that would cause a problem with either constipation or diarrhea.

Nursing Diagnosis and Goals

A nursing diagnosis of bowel incontinence as a result of uninhibited neurogenic bowel was made. The nurse explained to N.S. and her daughter how a stroke can affect bowel function. The short-term goals mutually established with N.S. and her daughter were to:

1. Achieve control without accidents on the toilet daily at 9 AM with the use of stool softeners and daily suppositories
2. Avoid any complications of constipation or diarrhea
3. Plan a diet that includes the appropriate amount of fluid
4. Incorporate exercise into daily program.

The long-term goals were to:

1. Achieve control without accidents on the toilet on a daily or every third day basis at 9 AM without the need for suppositories or medications
2. Demonstrate the techniques of bowel management and assume responsibility for the program
3. Verbalize problem-solving capabilities and appropriate interventions to achieve goals when the bowel program does not perform as planned
4. Avoid complications of diarrhea, constipation, and impaction by maintaining adequate nutrition, hydration, and activity

Interventions

Interventions for establishing bowel control were initiated by the nurse in consultation with N.S. Because N.S.'s usual time was 9 AM after breakfast, it was decided to place her on a bowel program at this time of the morning and delay the start of physical therapy treatment until 10 AM. Her therapy schedule was adjusted accordingly. In exploring N.S.'s usual diet, good fiber was present in the cereal, fruits, whole grain bread, and vegetables. Her fluid intake, however, was not sufficient. The importance of six to eight glasses of fluid per day was explained and this was recorded as an intervention and also discussed with the dietitian. It was felt that good exercise and mobility would be accomplished through increasing wheelchair endurance, therapy, activity, and beginning to perform her own activities of daily living.

A stool softener (Surfak, one 2 times daily) was initiated

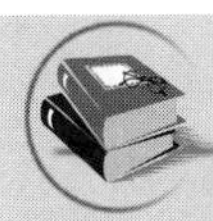

Case Study—cont'd

along with a bisacodyl suppository every day 30 minutes after breakfast. The RN explained the purposes of each. Evacuation was planned to take place on the toilet in the bathroom where a squat position and privacy would be maintained.

Implementation and Evaluation

The next day N.S. had good results on the toilet after a suppository. N.S. maintained this program for 5 days without accidents. On the sixth day the RN noticed that her stools were becoming too soft. Surfak was decreased to one a day at bedtime after agreement with N.S. On the eighth day N.S. had no results, but on the ninth day a good bowel movement was achieved. Again on the tenth day there were no results. The RN decided to change N.S.'s program to every other day with her concurrence.

On the twelfth day, N.S. began to have a bowel movement on her own without the need for a suppository. This occurred again on the fourteenth day. The RN placed her suppository on an as-needed basis "if no bowel movement in 2 days." On the sixteenth day the nurse decided to discontinue the remaining daily Surfak. N.S. remained continent with a daily or every-other-day bowel movement.

Fluid intake of six to eight glasses each day was achieved. A planning team conference determined that N.S. would be ready for discharge by the nineteenth day after her admission. She was doing well in ambulation and needed minimum to moderate assistance in activities of daily living.

Teaching and Discharge Planning

Teaching continued with N.S. and her daughter. The nurse proposed problem-solving situations. She asked, for example, what they would do if N.S. did not have a bowel movement in 3 days after she was home. N.S. replied that she would use a suppository. Because there was a history of occasional laxative use, N.S. and her daughter were instructed that if a suppository did not achieve results, a bisacodyl tablet could be taken at bedtime on a one-time basis followed by a suppository in the morning after breakfast.

On the day of discharge, the RN told N.S. to feel free to call her if any questions or problems arose after discharge. N.S. had been informed where to purchase over-the-counter stool softeners or suppositories if needed. It was also explained that plastic wrap could be used in place of expensive latex gloves for use with suppository insertion, if needed.

REFERENCES

Abyad, A., & Mourad, F. (1996). Constipation: Common sense-care of the older patient. *Geriatrics, 51,* 28-36.

Beddar, S.A.M., Holder-Bennett, L., & McCormick A.M. (1997). Development and evaluation of a protocol to manage fecal incontinence in the patient with cancer. *Journal of Palliative Care, 13,* 27-38.

Bentsen D., & Braun J.W. (1996). Controlling fecal incontinence with sensory retraining managed by advanced practice nurses. *Clinical Nurse Specialist, 10,* 171-176.

Berger, K.J., & Williams, M.B. (Eds.). (1992). *Fundamentals of nursing collaborating for optimal health.* Norwalk: Appleton & Lange.

Bisanz, A. (1997). Managing bowel elimination problems in patients with cancer. *Oncology Nursing Forum, 24,* 679-686.

Brocklehurst, J.C. (1980). Disorders of the lower bowel in old age. *Geriatrics, 35,* 47-54.

Brunton, L.L. (1990). Agents affecting gastrointestinal water flux and motility, digestants, and bile acids. In A.G. Gilman, T.W. Rall, A.S. Nies, & P. Taylor (Eds.), *The pharmacological basis of therapeutics* (8th ed.). New York: Pergamon Press.

Cannon, B. (1981). Bowel function. In N. Martin, N. Holt, & D. Hicks (Eds.), *Comprehensive rehabilitation nursing.* New York: McGraw-Hill.

Cheskin, L.J., Kamal N., Crowell, M.D., Schuster, M.M., & Whitehead W.E. (1995). Mechanisms of constipation in older persons and effects of fiber compared with placebo. *Journal of American Geriatric Society, 43,* 666-669.

Coffman, S. (1986). Description of a nursing diagnosis: Alteration in bowel elimination related to neurogenic bowel in children with myelomeningocele. *Issues in Comprehensive Pediatric Nursing, 9,* 179-191.

Connell, A.M., Hilton, C., Irvine, C., Lennard-Jones, J.E., & Misiewicz, J.J. (1965). Variation of bowel habit in two population samples. *British Medical Journal, 2,* 1095-1099.

Doughty, D. (1992). A step-by-step approach to bowel training. *Progressions, 4,* 12-23.

Doughty, D.B. (2000). *Urinary & fecal incontinence. Nursing management* (2nd ed.). St. Louis: Mosby.

Dunn K.L., & Galka, M.L. (1994). A comparison of the effectiveness of Therevac SB and bisacodyl suppositories in SCI patients' bowel programs. *Rehabilitation Nursing, 22,* 32-35.

Edwards, L., Quigley, M.M., Hofman, R., & Pfeiffer, R.F. (1993). Gastrointestinal symptoms in Parkinson disease: 18-month follow-up study. *Movement Disorders, 8,* 83-86.

Edwards, L.L., Quigley, E.M.M., & Pfeiffer, R.F. (1992). Gastrointestinal dysfunction in Parkinson's disease: Frequency and pathophysiology. *Neurology, 42,* 726-732.

Friedman, G. (1989). Nutritional therapy of irritable bowel syndrome. *Gastroenterology Clinics of North America, 18,* 513-524.

Gleeson, R.M. (1990). Bowel continence for the child with a neurogenic bowel. *Rehabilitation Nursing, 15,* 319-321.

Glickman, S., & Kamm, M.A. (1996). Bowel dysfunction in spinal-cord-injury patients. *The Lancet, 347*(June 15), 1651-1653.

Gordon, M. (2000). *Manual of nursing diagnosis.* (9th ed.). St. Louis: Mosby.

Guyton, A.C., & Hall, J.E. (1996). *Textbook of medical physiology.* (9th ed.). Philadelphia: WB Saunders.

Haines, S.T. (1995). Treating constipation in the patient with diabetes. *The Diabetes Educator, 21,* 223-232.

Han, T.R., Kim, J.H., & Kwon, B.S. (1998). Chronic gastrointestinal problems and bowel dysfunction in patients with spinal cord injury. *Spinal Cord, 36,* 485-490.

Heitkemper, M.M. (2000). Physiology of defecation. In D.B. Doughty (Ed.), *Urinary & fecal incontinence. Nursing management* (2nd ed., pp. 313-323). St. Louis: Mosby.

Hoeman, S.P. (1989). Cultural assessment in rehabilitation nursing practice. *Nursing Clinics of North America, 24,* 277-289.

Hogstel, M.O., & Nelson, M. (1992). Anticipation and early detection can reduce bowel elimination complications. *Geriatric Nursing, 13,* 28-33.

Hull, C., Greco, R., & Brooks, D.L. (1980). Alleviation of constipation in the elderly by dietary fiber supplementation. *Journal of American Geriatric Society, 28,* 410-414.

Iseminger, M., & Hardy, P. (1982). Bran works! *Geriatric Nursing, 3,* 402-404.

Johnson, M., Maas, M., & Moorhead, S. (2000). *Nursing outcomes classification (NOC)* (2nd ed.). St. Louis: Mosby.

Lincoln, R., & Roberts, R. (1989). Continence issues in acute care. *Nursing Clinics of North America, 24,* 741-754.

Mancini, I., & Bruera, E. (1998). Constipation in advanced cancer patients. *Support Care Cancer, 6,* 356-364.

McCloskey J.C., & Bulechek, G. M. (2000). *Nursing intervention classification (NIC)* (3rd ed.). St. Louis: Mosby.

McCourt, A.E. (Ed.). (1993). *The specialty practice of rehabilitation nursing; A core curriculum* (3rd ed.). Skokie, IL: Rehabilitation Nursing Foundation.

Munchiando, J.F., & Kendall, K. (1993). Comparison of the effectiveness of two bowel programs for CVA patients. *Rehabilitation Nursing, 18,* 168-172.

Nelson, R., Norton, N., Cautley, E., & Furner, S. (1995). Community-based prevalence of anal incontinence. *Journal of American Medical Association, 274,* 559-561.

Rauen, K.K., & Aubert, E.J. (1992). A brighter future for adults who have myelomeningocele-one form of spina bifida: A comprehensive overview of this complex disease. *Orthopaedic Nursing, 11,* 16-27.

Ross, D.G. (1993). Subjective data related to altered bowel elimination patterns among hospitalized elder and middle-aged persons. *Orthopedic Nursing, 12,* 25-32.

Seidel, G.K., Millis, S.R., Lichtenberg, P.A., & Dijkers, M. (1994). Predicting bowel and bladder continence from cognitive status in geriatric rehabilitation patients. *Archives of Physical Medicine and Rehabilitation, 75,* 590-593.

Smith, D.A. (1988). Continence restoration in the homebound patient. *Nursing Clinics of North America, 23,* 207-218.

Smith, K.A. (1990). Bowel and bladder management of the child with myelomeningocele in the school setting. *Journal of Pediatric Healthcare, 4,* 175-180.

Stiens, S. (1995). Reduction in bowel program duration with polyethylene glycol based bisacodyl suppositories. *Archives of Physical Medicine and Rehabilitation, 76,* 674-677.

Stiens, S.A., Bergman, S.B., & Goetz, L.L. (1997). Neurogenic bowel dysfunction after spinal cord injury: Clinical evaluation and rehabilitative management. *Archives of Physical Medicine and Rehabilitation, 78,* 86-101.

Tobillo, E.T., & Schwartz, S.M. (1998). Acute diarrhea. *Advance for Nurse Practitioners, October,* 39-76.

Venn, M.R., Taft, L., Carpentier, I.B., & Applebaugh, A. (1992). The influence of timing and suppository use on efficiency and effectiveness of bowel training after a stroke. *Rehabilitation Nursing, 17,* 116-121.

Wald, A. (1991). Approach to the patient with constipation. In T. Yamada (Ed.), *Textbook of gastroenterology* (Vol. 1). New York: JB Lippincott.

Waldrop, J., & Doughty D.B. (2000). Pathophysiology of bowel dysfunction and fecal incontinence. In D.B. Doughty (Ed.), *Urinary & fecal incontinence. Nursing management* (2nd ed., pp. 325-352). St. Louis: Mosby.

White, M., & Williams, J. (1992). A good start to a full life: Managing continence in children with spina bifida and hydrocephalus. *Professional Nurse, 7,* 474, 476-477.

Zejdlik, C.P. (1992). *Management of spinal cord injury.* Boston: Jones and Bartlett.

Muscle and Skeletal Function

21

Gail L. Sims, MSN, RN, CRRN
Rhonda S. Olson, MS, RN, CRRN

I was young and working as a nursing assistant in a long-term care facility. Every day I assisted Ella with her needs. She was a kind, gentle, and courageous elderly woman with rheumatoid arthritis who required complete assistance with activities of daily living. Her hands and legs, in fact her entire body, were deformed from arthritis. As the staff helped her to transfer, she would exclaim in fear, "Now dears, be careful; don't hurt me!" We tried to be careful, but still she cried out in pain. She would talk about how terrible the pain was, how it made life so difficult, and how she worried about when her medication would finally arrive. The truth is, I never understood the meaning of her pain until I had to begin living with chronic, unrelenting daily pain. As nurses, we can never understand the exact meaning of the client's pain experience, but enduring it ourselves gives us a better idea of the dark storm of pain.

Rehabilitation nurses assist clients who experience musculoskeletal dysfunction and live or work in a variety of settings. Understanding general and specific information about the musculoskeletal system, relating it to principles of rehabilitation, and applying them to practice enhance care. This chapter outlines anatomy and physiology, clinical problems, the nursing process, and uses a case study for developing plans of care with clients who have musculoskeletal disorders. Although children and young adults experience musculoskeletal conditions and injuries suitable for rehabilitation nursing practice, adult problems form the larger portion of content in this chapter (Healthy People 2010, 2000).

The Neuman Systems Model is appropriate for rehabilitation nursing in that it approaches the nurse-client relationship holistically (Kain, 2000). Neuman (1995) describes three levels of stressors applicable to the acute and chronic pain and the fatigue common to individuals with musculoskeletal disorders. The model also describes the client's interaction with the interpersonal and extrapersonal environment in the pursuit of independent function. Nursing interventions focus on primary, secondary, and tertiary prevention with individuals and their families who are at risk by providing education, assessing health beliefs, and increasing preventive behaviors with appropriate exercise, dietary, and medication regimens (Hoeman, 1996). Rehabilitation nurses have a major role in primary prevention of osteoporosis and prevention of secondary musculoskeletal complications of stroke.

MUSCULOSKELETAL FUNCTION

Anatomy and Physiology

The musculoskeletal system is one of the body's largest systems, accounting for more than 50% of the body's weight. It is a dynamic system made up of bones, muscles, joints, and supportive structures that interact to provide movement and support body structures.

Bones

The skeletal system consists of the 206 bones of the axial and appendicular skeletons. The 80 bones in the axial skeleton include the hyoid bone and the bones of the skull, spinal column, and thorax. The remaining 126 bones form the appendicular skeleton bones of the upper and lower extremities, pectoral girdle, and pelvic girdle. The four types of bones are long (femur and humerus), short (carpals), flat (skull), and irregular (vertebral). Bones are made up of cells, fibers, and ground substance; they contain crystallized minerals that provide rigidity. The three types of bone cells can grow, repair, and remodel. Osteoblasts, or bone-forming cells, lay down new bone. Osteocytes maintain mineral content and organic elements. Osteoclasts resorb bone during growth and repair.

Bones function to support body tissues, giving form to the body; they protect the vital organs and connect muscles and joints for movement. Hematopoiesis occurs in the marrow of the skull, vertebrae, ribs, sternum, shoulders, and pelvis. Mineral homeostasis is accomplished through the storage of calcium, phosphate, carbonate, and magnesium, minerals necessary for normal cellular function. Factors that influence bone formation include serum levels of calcium, phosphorus, and alkaline phosphatase, and calcitonin; vitamin D levels; growth and sex hormones; glucocorticoids; infection; inflammation; activity; and weight bearing.

Muscles

Three major types of muscle are visceral (smooth, involuntary), cardiac, and skeletal (striated, voluntary). Approximately 350 skeletal muscles function to maintain posture and provide movement that occurs through contraction and work production. Muscle contractions also are classified into nine types.

- Tonic: partial and continuous, helps maintain posture
- Isotonic: provides continuous tension within the muscles as they shorten or lengthen during activities
- Isometric: increases tension within the muscle and is static
- Twitching: isolated, jerking response to a stimulus
- Tetanic: sustained, produced by a rapid succession of stimuli
- Spasms: involuntary movements created by stimulation of a motor unit
- Treppe: stronger twitching resulting from regular, repeated stimuli
- Fibrillation: synchronized contraction of individual muscle fibers
- Convulsive movements: abnormally occurring, uncoordinated contractions of various muscle groups

Cartilage

Cartilage is a firm gel composed of strong but flexible and avascular fibers. Three types of cartilage exist in the body. Fibrous cartilage composes the intervertebral disks. Articular is a type of the spongy, elastic hyaline cartilage found at the ends of bones. Because articular cartilage does not contain any blood vessels, lymph tissue, or nerves, it is insensitive to pain and does not repair itself easily after injury. Elastic or yellow cartilage, such as the external ear and epiglottis, has fewest fibers.

Ligaments. Ligaments are tough, flexible bands of fibrous tissue that connect the ends of bones. Ligaments provide stability and limit movement to prevent injury to joints such as the knees.

Tendons

Tendons are dense fibrous tissue occurring where muscles insert into bones. Fibrous tendons sheath each muscle in complex joints, such as the wrist or ankle. Synovial fluid lubricates and adds stability to the sites. Synovial fluid is a plasma from blood vessels and thus can nourish the joint.

Joints

Joints provide flexibility to the skeletal system. They are categorized by the amount of movement and by the type of connective tissue they contain. Synarthroses or fibrous joints do not allow movement, but contain sutures that hold the bones tightly together, such as is found in the skull. Amphiarthroses or cartilaginous joints allow limited movement and are connected by a ligament in locations such as intervertebral joints and the symphysis pubis. Diarthroses or synovial joints allow free movement and are found in hips, knees, shoulders, and elbows.

Aging, injuries, and disease affect the musculoskeletal system throughout the life span and can affect function temporarily or for life. Degenerative changes in bone mass, muscle strength, and elasticity of cartilage in the joints are all natural responses to the aging process; however, acute injuries and chronic diseases occur at any age, and congenital conditions often produce musculoskeletal problems.

Scope of Problems in Musculoskeletal Dysfunction

Arthritis is among the most common conditions and the leading cause of disability in the United States, affecting more than 43 million persons (Centers for Disease Control and Prevention [CDC], 1999; Elders, 2000). Estimated medical care costs for individuals with arthritis are $15 billion annually (Healthy People 2010, 2000). The most current estimate of the financial impact of arthritis in the United States was nearly $65 billion in 1992 (Healthy People 2010, 2000; Yelin, 1995).

Osteoporotic fractures are a common fall-related injury involving mainly the hip, spine, and forearm. The most recently reported medical cost of osteoporotic fractures was more than $6 billion in 1989 (CDC, 1996). Hip fractures are the most serious and lead to the highest number of health problems and deaths (CDC, 1999). In 1996, total hospital admissions for hip fracture in persons older than 65 years was 340,000; with increased aging in the population, the figure may reach 500,000 by the year 2040 (Brainsky et al., 1997).

Prevention and treatment of musculoskeletal conditions also improves quality of life. Arthritis and other rheumatic disorders, osteoporosis, and chronic back conditions have a tremendous impact on public health and quality of life. Health-related quality-of-life measures for persons with arthritis and rheumatic diseases are determined by (1) healthy days in the past 30 days; (2) days without severe pain; (3) ability days without activity limitations; and (4) difficulty in performing personal care activities (Healthy People 2010, 2000).

The National Arthritis Action Plan (NAAP) developed strategies in 1998 to reduce the burden of arthritis in three main areas:

1. Surveillance, epidemiology, and prevention research
2. Communications and education
3. Programs, policies, and systems (National Center for Chronic Disease Prevention and Health Promotion, 2000a)

The NAAP brings organizations from public health, arthritis, and other interested groups together at the national, state, and local levels and sponsors a network of professionals and trained volunteers.

CLINICAL PROBLEMS RELATED TO MUSCULOSKELETAL DYSFUNCTION

Rehabilitation nurses encounter clients with musculoskeletal disorders ranging from acute fractures and multiple traumas to chronic disorders, such as rheumatoid arthritis and fibromyalgia. The many clinical problems and potential complications resulting from musculoskeletal disorders require expertise from many members of the rehabilitation team.

Arthritis Disorders

The more than 100 types of arthritic disorders (Arthritis Foundation, 2001) have three general classifications: degenerative, inflammatory, and metabolic disorders (Figure 21-1). The different origins of arthritic disorders determine appropriate nursing interventions.

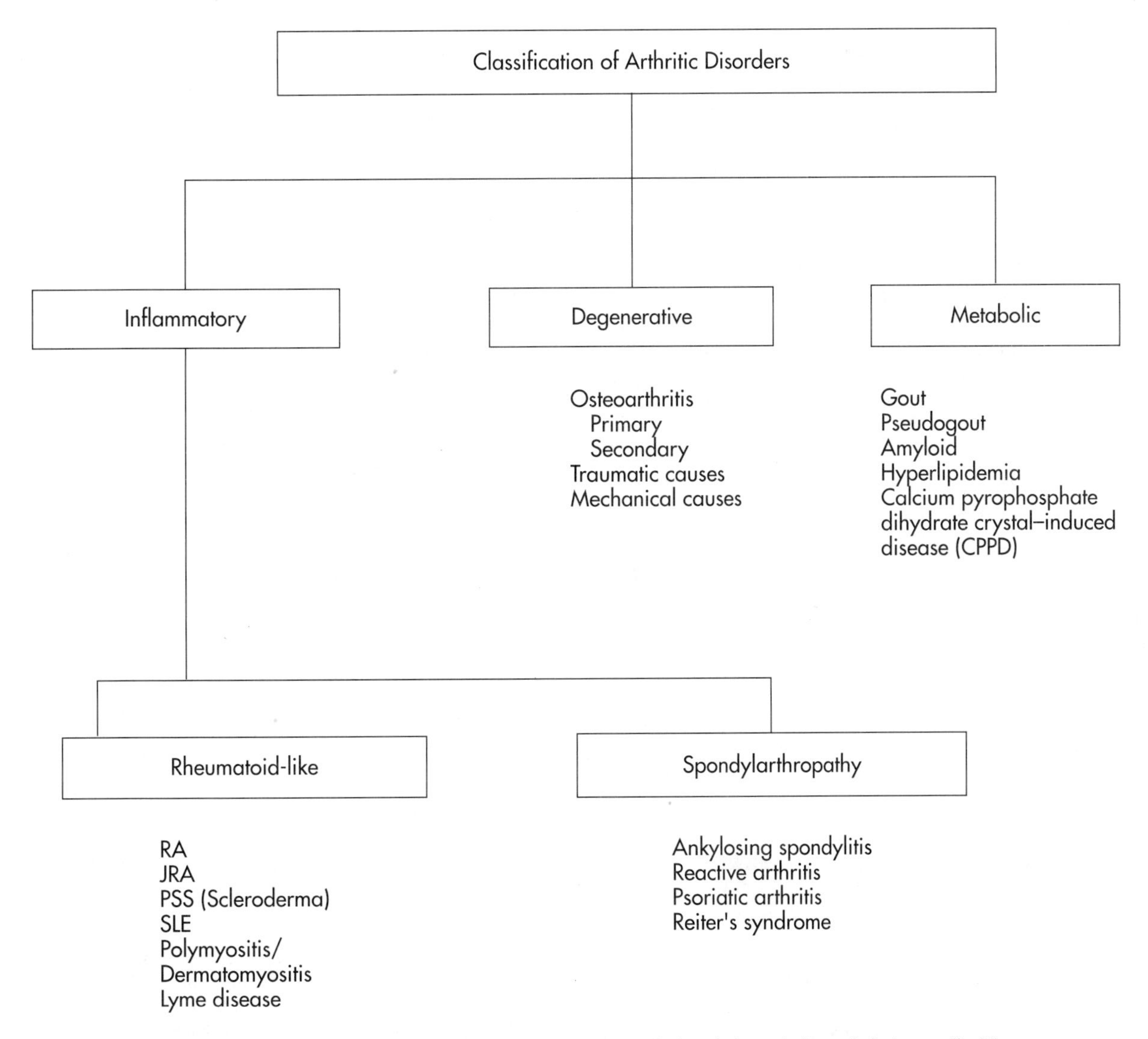

Figure 21-1 Classification of arthritic disorders. (From National Association of Orthopaedic Nurses [1996]. *Core curriculum for orthopaedic nursing.* [3rd ed.]. Pitman, NJ: National Association of Orthopaedic Nurses.)

Degenerative Joint Disorders

Osteoarthritis, or degenerative joint disease (DJD), is caused by loss of cartilage in the synovial joints that can be diagnosed with radiological and clinical evidence (Latman & Walls, 1996). Primary osteoarthritis (idiopathic) is most common and is distributed throughout the central and peripheral joints of the body. The etiology of primary degenerative joint disease is unknown. Age is a factor, and there may be a genetic component. Secondary osteoarthritis is attributed to earlier trauma to the involved joint and to long-term mechanical stressors (Phipps, Sands, & Marek, 1999). Mechanical stressors include obesity, athletics, repetitive tasks, infection, endocrine disorders such as acromegaly or hyperparathyroidism, neurological disorders associated with pain, skeletal deformities, and hemophilia (bleeding at the joints). Secondary osteoarthritis usually is limited to the specific joints that were subjected to stress.

Osteoarthritis is an active process with anabolic and catabolic activity. Characteristic pathological changes include eroding of articular cartilage, thickening of underlying subchondral bone, and forming of osteophytes or bone spurs. Symptoms include a slow, uneven, and variable course involving mild to severe flare-ups. Joint involvement is generally unilateral, and systemic symptoms are rare. Pain and disability result from secondary effects, which include synovitis, joint capsule distention, bony proliferation, and damage to surrounding articular structures. Crepitus, palpable grating, swelling, inflammation, deformity, pain, limited mobility, and instability of the involved joint such as hips and knees are frequent complaints (Kee, 2000). Osteoarthritis, rheumatoid arthritis (RA), and juvenile rheumatoid arthritis (JRA) differ in symptoms (Table 21-1) that ultimately determine the activity performance, long-term goals, and quality of life.

Inflammatory Disorders

One classification of arthritis disorders is characterized by inflammation; rheumatoid-like and spondylarthropathies are pertinent. A history of symmetrically involved peripheral joint inflammation precedes RA. The client often experiences persistent joint pain and tenderness, accompanied by restricted function. Serological tests are positive for rheumatoid factor, antinuclear antibodies, or elevated sedimentation rate, and biopsy of the synovial membrane or subcutaneous nodule reveals histology changes (Dalgas, Logigian, & Liang, 1994). Fatigue often accompanies the pain and is related to depression and sleep disturbance (Belza, Henke, Yelin, Epstein, & Gilliss, 1993).

RA, characterized by inflammation, begins in the synovial membrane within the joint. Edema within the inflamed tissue causes stiffness. Continued inflammation leads to thickening of the synovium, particularly where it joins the articular cartilage. Pannus (granulation tissue) forms at these junctures, invades subchondral bone, and interferes with normal nutrition of the articular cartilage, causing necrosis. Pannus formation leads to adhesions between the joint surfaces, and fibrous or bony union (ankylosis) develops. Destruction of cartilage and bone, in addition to some weakening of tendons and ligaments, may lead to subluxation or dislocation of joints.

The hands often are affected early, with progression to the classic fusiform tapering of fingers and ulnar deviation. Other joints commonly involved are the wrists, ankles, elbows, and knees, with shoulder and hip problems occurring

TABLE 21-1 Three Types of Arthritis

	Osteoarthritis	Rheumatoid Arthritis	Juvenile Rheumatoid Arthritis
Onset	Women >40 years	Any age, but usually women 20-50 years	<16 years
Types of disease	Degenerative; localized	Inflammatory, systemic	Inflammatory, systemic
Signs/symptoms	Morning stiffness lasting less than 1 hour; stiffness at end of day	Morning stiffness lasting longer than 1 hour; improves with activity	Decreased activity level; joint pain and stiffness
Joints affected	Weight bearing; lower extremities	Multiple joints; symmetrical involvement	One or more joints; large joints
Treatment	Mobilization of joints; moderate exercise	Immobilization of joints in acute flare-ups; functional splints to maintain function	Rest periods and self-pacing; use of casting controversial; recommend no longer than 48 hours
Medications	NSAIDs; Hyaluronan, Hylan G-F; intraarticular steroid injections	Steroids, antimalarials, MTX, gold, penicillamine with NSAIDs, Enbrel, Remicade	NSAIDs and DMARDs; (MTX, gold, penicillamine)

Adapted from Krug, B. (1997). Rheumatoid arthritis and osteoarthritis: A basic comparison. *Orthopedic Nursing, 16,* 73-76; Driscoll, S., Noll, S., & Koch, B. (1994). Juvenile rheumatoid arthritis. *Physical Medicine and Rehabilitation Clinics of North America, 5,* 763-783.
NSAIDs, Nonsteroidal antiinflammatory drugs; *MTX,* methotrexate; *DMARDs,* disease-modifying antirheumatic drug.

later. If unarrested, eventually RA may affect all joints and severely limit function. Involvement of the temporomandibular joint may hinder opening the mouth. Subluxation or dislocation of involved cervical vertebra may result in paralysis or death (Phipps et al., 1999).

Although joint involvement is the most obvious problem, the inflammatory process of RA affects all connective tissue. Systematic manifestations include pulmonary, cardiac, vascular, ophthalmological, and hematological systems. The course and severity are unpredictable and marked by periods of exacerbation and remission. Physiological and psychological stressors can contribute to exacerbations. A few individuals may have malignant rheumatic disease, which is marked by rapid progression, unremitting joint destruction, and diffuse vasculitis.

Several theories have been proposed for the etiology of RA; the most probable is an autoimmune process that perpetuates the inflammation. Genetic predisposition is related to a certain human leukocyte antigen (HLA) that leads to synovial microvascular injury (Yocum, 1994). Another proposal is that the disease occurs as an altered immune response to an unknown antigen, such as with Epstein-Barr virus, bacteria, or mycoplasma. Yet another theory is prolonged exposure to some environmental factors may trigger the immune response producing the rheumatoid factor (RF) (autoantibodies). The autoantibodies attack the host tissue (self-antigen) on the blood and synovial membranes to form immune complexes (Phipps et al., 1999).

Juvenile arthritis is the fifth most common chronic illness in children. It fluctuates in a cyclic pattern, suggesting microbial or other environmental factors contribute to its occurrence (Michet, 1998). Symptoms include arthralgias and systemic signs of sepsis, such as fever. Serology results help in accurate diagnosis necessary for establishing an effective interdisciplinary treatment plan (Simmons, Nutting, & Bernstein, 1996). Problems arise when a child is unable to maintain sufficient physiological function and experiences delays in growth and development, including educational potential. The family, teachers, and health care providers are challenged to cope with the demands of the illness (Hartley & Fuller, 1997).

Progressive systemic sclerosis or scleroderma is a complex, multisystem connective tissue disease affecting the skin and internal organs, mainly the lungs and gastrointestinal tract. The impact on the musculoskeletal system occurs when myositis or erosive arthropathy causes joint retraction induced by skin fibrosis (Generini, Fiori, Moggi Pignone, Matucci Cerinic, & Cagnoni, 1999). Klyscz, Rassner, Guckenberger, and Junger (1999) state that aggressive physical therapy significantly improves joint mobility and reduces edema of the skin.

Systemic lupus erythematosus (SLE) is a multisystem, autoimmune, inflammatory disorder with unknown etiology. Possibly hyperactive helper T-cells cause polyclonal B-cell secretion of pathogenic autoantibodies and form immune complexes that deposit in sites such as the kidney (Balow, Boumpas, & Austin, 2000). Genetic, hormonal, and environmental factors of SLE are important considerations under investigation (D'Cruz, 2000; Tsao, 2000).

The initial manifestation of SLE is often a transient arthritis that responds to treatment. Joint deformity and contractures may develop, whereas multisystem involvement is characterized by remissions and exacerbations and leads to myriad clinical manifestations ranging from the characteristic butterfly facial rash, weakness and fatigue, to glomerulonephritis and pericarditis.

Tick-borne *Spirochaeta Borrelia burgdorferi* causes Lyme disease when transmitted to human beings by lxodes ticks (Melski, 2000); deer are reservoirs. Early symptoms range from headache and polyarthritis to carditis or encephalitis. When resistant to treatment, is undiagnosed, or is reemerging, the disease produces muscle weakness, paralysis, and various neurological manifestations (Hoeman, 1996). Arthralgia, known as "Lyme arthritis," is a late manifestation that usually affects the knee joints (Dressler, 1997). Pain related to muscle and joint tenderness and impaired mobility resulting from arthritic symptoms are associated problems. Serological testing confirms diagnosis, although the antibodies may not be detected until 4 to 6 weeks after the initial infection. It is difficult to distinguish Lyme disease from septic arthritis on the basis of laboratory findings. Exposure to an endemic area and clinical findings may help determine the accurate diagnosis (Bachman & Srivastava, 1998).

Spondylarthropathies (SPA), also known as spinal arthritis, consist of a group of inflammatory arthropathies (see Figure 21-1) with unknown etiology. Common features include inflammatory arthritis involving the back, an increase of a specific HLA (HLA-B27), frequent inflammation of tendon-ligament insertion, and extraarticular manifestations, such as iritis or skin lesions. More difficult to recognize than osteoarthritis or rheumatoid arthritis, SPA are sometimes referred to as seronegative spondyloarthropathies because the rheumatoid factor is uniformly absent (Parker & Thomas, 2000).

Ankylosing spondylitis usually begins with dull aching and stiffness in the back during the teenage years. The disease progresses to increased pain and restricted movement in the back, ribcage, and neck. Later postural abnormalities develop, such as flexion of the neck and back and flexion contracture of the hips. Increased severity determines impairment.

Diagnosis is based on symptoms of tenderness to palpation of the sacroiliac joints, reduced chest expansion, calcifications (syndesmophytes) between vertebrae, and fusion of sacroiliac joints. Radiographic evidence reveals what is known as "bamboo" spine. Laboratory tests may not be specific, although erythrocyte sedimentation rate (ESR) may elevate or mild anemia present. Although new bone formation occurs, this ankylosis makes the spine osteoporotic, increasing risk of spinal fracture; joint replacement may be indicated when the hips are severely affected. Lower extremity weakness (cauda equina syndrome) and bowel and bladder dysfunction may occur in advanced cases.

The joints of the spine and the sacroiliac joints, areas where the spine attaches to the pelvis are common sites for manifestation of Reiter's syndrome. Defining characteristics are inflammation of the joints, urinary tract, and eyes. Recently identified are ulcerations of the skin and mouth. Reiter's syndrome is the most common type of inflammatory polyarthritis in young men, affecting men between the ages of 20 and 40 years (Matsen, 2000; Barth & Segal, 1999).

The gene called HLA-B27, important in defense against infection, is found in approximately 75% of those with Reiter's syndrome. When an infectious agent, such as *Salmonella, Shigella, Campylobacter,* or *Yersinia* infects the intestinal tract, genetic predisposition may produce the inflammatory response. Similarly, inflammation of the urinary tract may be caused by specific organisms, but no specific agent has been identified (University of Washington, 2000).

Fragments of infectious agents are found in affected joints. An immune or inflammatory reaction causes the arthritis, although the reason for the joint involvement is not yet known. Symptoms such as mild synovitis with soft tissue swelling, mild flexion contractures (flexor tendinitis), asymmetrical joint inflammation, low back pain, oral or genital lesions, and sacroiliitis of the pelvis and lower spine are characteristics of Reiter's syndrome (Halverson, 1997). These symptoms could be misdiagnosed as fibromyalgia or genital herpes. Other common features include diarrhea and painless lesions of the soles of the feet and palms of the hands. These areas may appear similar to psoriasis.

Metabolic Disorders

Arthritic problems also may be caused by metabolic disorders, such as gout. Gout is a clinical syndrome caused by the deposition of urate crystals in the synovial fluid, joints, or articular cartilage. Nearly all (95%) of the approximately 20 million persons in the United States with gout are men older than 30 years (Edwards, 2000). More than half develop first symptoms in the great toe. Obesity, high-purine diet (e.g., organ meats or sardines), regular alcohol consumption, and diuretic therapy have been implicated as contributing factors (Emmerson, 1996).

Gout initially is asymptomatic, except for elevated urate levels. Then sudden acute attacks of the second stage produce severe pain in one or more joints, including the great toe. Deposits of urate crystals surrounded by inflammation form fibrotic tissue, giant cells, and local necrosis, tissue inflammation and damage may occur. During the third stage, (intercritical period) the client is free of symptoms before attacks. Finally, with chronic gout, joints show urate crystals have formed to replace bony structures. Joint spaces narrow and degenerative changes occur as cartilage is destroyed.

Gout is diagnosed by detailed history and physical examination because it may mask symptoms of other inflammatory arthritis such as rheumatoid arthritis, pseudogout, or septic arthritis (Wise & Agudelo, 1998). The presence of tophi (monosodium urate crystals), urate deposits in the skin and tissue around a joint or in the external ear in synovial fluid, is a classic diagnostic indicator of gout. Serum uric acid, urinary uric acid, and sedimentation rate levels are elevated; albuminuria and leukocytosis occur. The joints initially appear normal on radiographic examination. Renal studies are significant in determining adequate kidney function because colchicine, a drug used to treat acute episodes, has toxic effects.

The client with acute attacks of gout experiences severe joint pain, difficulty in ambulating, and swelling of the affected extremity. Modifications in lifestyle may be necessary during this initial phase. As the individual with gout experiences chronic symptoms, the pain and deformity of joints threatens performance of activities of daily living (ADLs) and may require modifications to the work environment. Hospitalization may be required for episodes of renal dysfunction, cardiovascular lesions, or tophic monosodium urate crystal deposit–related infection. Complications may include thrombosis, hypertension, and chronic pain, all of which disrupt normal living patterns, family-related activities, or work involvement, and may create financial burdens. Rapid diagnosis and appropriate interventions may reduce the stressors to the client and family, including education about dietary factors that contribute to gout.

Gout in elderly persons differs from that found in middle-aged men. Elderly clients present a more equal gender distribution, polyarticular symptoms involving upper extremity joints, fewer acute gouty episodes, but a more chronic clinical course, and an increased incidence of tophi. In elderly persons long-term use of diuretics, renal insufficiency, low-dose aspirin regimens, and alcohol consumption contribute to elevated uric acid levels and thus to gout.

Fibromyalgia

Fibromyalgia syndrome (FMS) is a nonmalignant, chronic musculoskeletal disorder that causes widespread pain, tenderness at specific body sites, and muscular stiffness. These signs must be present to make a definitive diagnosis. Similar to arthritis, fatigue and sleep disturbances are common symptoms. Specific, symmetrical trigger points or pressure points painful to touch are hallmark signs of fibromyalgia; 11 of the 18 pressure points are diagnostic (Cimoch, 2000).

Although not classified as an arthritis disorder, FMS (previously fibrositis or fibrosis), has become an accepted diagnosis in the International Statistical Classification of Diseases and Related Health Problems (Smith, 1998). The generalized pain syndrome is associated with other disorders such as rheumatic arthritis, SLE, polymyosis (chronic acquired inflammatory disorder of the skeletal muscle), and polymyalgia rheumatica resulting from its destructive, inflammatory nature. Etiology is unknown, possibly resulting from normal aging, genetic predisposition, or environmental influences. The incidence rate of FMS is 85% to 90% in females (Smith, 1998).

FMS often is diagnosed by exclusion when other disease processes are ruled out. Commonly FMS is misdiagnosed, resulting from an array of symptoms and lack of current information among health providers. Clients may seek medical advice for what they believe are flulike symptoms or fatigue from daily stresses, only to be viewed as having inadequate coping strategies or told the symptoms are "all in their head." Further complicating diagnosis are those who remain symptomatic for several years, undergoing diagnostic tests and exploratory surgery unnecessarily. Subjective data and FMS criteria are significant in the assessment process.

FMS research hypothesizes the possibility of viruses, bacteria, neuroendocrine dysfunction and amplification, and psychoendocrine dysfunction and amplification as causes (Smith, 1998). Self-help groups and resources for information such as the Fibromyalgia Network provide valuable information about research and offer education and help with coping strategies to individuals, family members, and providers.

Spinal Stenosis

Spinal stenosis, a narrowing of the spinal canal or intervertebral foramina at any level, creates pressure on nerve roots, leading to neurological symptoms. When nerve roots are inflamed, clients experience pain that radiates into muscles innervated by involved nerves; lumbar levels 4-5 and lumbar levels 3-4 are involved most often. Spinal stenosis occurs as a result of aging, degenerative disk disease, spondylosis, osteophyte formation, or congenital conditions. Smoking, sedentary lifestyle, and extensive motor vehicle driving are risk factors.

Traumatic Injuries

Traumatic injuries may be acute with short-term problems, or create long-term impairment, especially without appropriate rehabilitation. Most orthopedic trauma occurs after falls, motor vehicle accidents, or crushing injuries. Musculoskeletal injuries range from simple bone fractures, dislocations, and sprains to complex and multiple trauma. Falls, crushing injuries, motor vehicle accidents, and gunshot wounds, especially when resulting in injury to the brain or spinal cord, are the most common forms of complex trauma. Multiple fractures and internal bleeding may be fatal.

Fractures

Fractures may occur as a result of a severe blow to the body or from minimal injury to weakened bones related to osteoporosis or metastatic cancer. Highest incidence rates occur from trauma in young men between 15 and 24 years of age and after falls related to osteoporosis in elderly women (National Center for Chronic Disease Prevention and Health Promotion, 2000b).The hip, wrist, and vertebrae are the most common locations of fractures in elderly persons. Pelvic fractures are associated with a lack of weight-bearing activity and with calcium leaving the bone matrix and causing it to become porous and at risk for pathological fracture. Pelvic fractures may be complicated by hemorrhage, hypotension, or coagulation. Hip fractures pose a serious problem, especially in the elderly population because 95% of all hip fractures occur in persons older than 50 years. More than 250,000 hip fractures occur annually, costing in excess of $7 billion (Cifu, 2001). Half of all older adults hospitalized for hip fractures do not return home or live independently after sustaining this type of catastrophic injury (National Center for Chronic Disease Prevention and Health Promotion, 2000b).

Use of alcohol may correlate with reduced bone mineral density in men and postmenopausal women. Alcoholism is linked with higher than normal fracture rates and osteopenia, which is a bone volume below the normal level (Felson, Zhang, Hannan, Kannel, & Kiel, 1995). Osteoporosis and prior hip fractures along with advanced age, poor prefracture function or unsteady gait, and cognitive impairment are risk factors. Caucasian women with decreased estrogen levels and those who reside in institutions or have a sedentary lifestyle are at risk (Young, Brant, & German, 1997). Preexisting conditions, such as a syncope episode, transient ischemic attack, or stroke, elevate risk; having several factors creates a challenging rehabilitation course and less potential for recovery. Falls can have a devastating effect on quality of life, especially for elderly clients. Fractures often result in severe loss of function and immobility with deep vein thrombosis; medication for pain contributes to confusion and further falls. The interdisciplinary team takes the client's history of falls, cognitive status, activity limitations, and medications into account and evaluates any need for modifications in the environment. The intent is to provide a safe situation without impeding the client's movement. Restraint-free environments are regulated with guidelines for clinical practice that preserve the client's dignity, rights, and respect.

Persons who incur multiple fractures from trauma, acts of violence, or severe injuries test the experience and resources of the entire interdisciplinary team; spiritual leaders and psychologists often are involved. In some instances, clients may attempt to hide the nature of traumatic fractures or mask pain because of psychological factors, such as fear of further trauma, preexisting personality disorders, or learned behaviors. They also may have a long-term course of care and risk for complications from interventions to repair the fractures.

Simple fractures, knee and ankle ligament damage, and meniscus tears may occur after a fall, sports injury, or motor vehicle accident. Minor injuries are treated as outpatient surgery or in clinics with primary care follow-up visits. Short-term therapy to restore range of motion and function may be part of a home health care plan.

Rehabilitation nurses may teach self-care and mobility skills to clients while they are using crutches, have an upper extremity cast, or are recovering from surgery. Rehabilitation nurses have roles in primary prevention of traumatic injuries; education programs for consumer awareness include the following.

- Use of safety devices, such as seat belts, car seats, helmets, and air bags
- Sports safety gear, diving precautions, safe activity in play
- Restraint-free environment, including medications
- Abuse or neglect
- Home safety and fall prevention
- Violence in the home or community

Amputations

Almost 148,000 amputations are performed in the United States each year. This high number is related to longevity of persons with cardiovascular disease or diabetes mellitus, the underlying cause in 86% of amputations (Amputee Coalition of America, 1999-2000). Malignancy, birth defects, and traumatic injury are other causative factors. Diabetes-specific risk factors depend on time since onset and are aggravated by obesity, hyperglycemia, and minor injury to tissues of the foot. Similarly, bypass surgery affects outcomes for clients with advanced lower-extremity vascular disease; foot or leg amputation increases as narrowed arteries permit less oxygenated blood to reach the tissues (Feinglass et al., 1999). A last resort in severe cases of peripheral vascular disease, surgical removal of an extremity is performed to alleviate pain, eliminate infection (necrotic tissue or gangrene), and restore function.

Older adults with diabetes mellitus experience complications that may include visual impairment, neuropathy, delayed wound healing, and renal insufficiency. Additional medical problems and their complexity influence how an elderly client adapts to amputation and the prosthesis. Impaired eyesight can make multiple medication administration, including insulin and blood glucose monitoring, difficult and potentially unsafe. Neuropathy can impair sensation of fingers necessary for preparing injections and manipulating oral medications. Pressure areas may be ignored because of poor eyesight and lack of sensation. Preexisting cardiac and respiratory conditions may limit endurance, which may prevent the client from being a candidate for any prosthesis.

The residual limb may not heal properly, which may delay the preparation of the limb for prosthetic application. In turn, delayed healing limits mobility and increases risk for other complications, such as urinary tract infections, decubitus ulcers, and respiratory infections. Community reentry is difficult when caregivers cannot assist in transfers and wheelchair mobility; a client may need assisted living housing. The result of experiencing an amputation along with comorbidities can have a devastating effect on the client's quality of life and lead to social isolation and depression.

The objective of an amputation is to preserve healthy tissue with sufficient blood flow, maintain functional length of the extremity, and remove infected or ischemic tissue. Types of amputations based on their body location are defined in Box 21-1. Although any amputation affects function and body image, young persons and those with upper extremity amputations tend to adjust more easily to the amputation. Clients are more likely to use their prostheses when they gain function and accept the cosmetic design; new prosthetic devices appear very natural.

Traumatic Amputation

Most amputations after trauma are caused during motorcycle or pedestrian accidents; 4% involve firearms. They are major sources of permanent impairment and functional limitation, affecting the quality of life for adolescents and young working adults. One fourth of those with lower limb amputation after trauma report severe residual limb pain, phantom limb pain, and wounds at the closure site. Length of the residual limb and level of amputation greatly affect quality of life, ambulation with a prosthesis, and return to work (Pezzin, Dillingham, & Mackenzie, 2000).

Postoperatively, the traditional soft dressing (elastic bandage) remains in use to help shape the residual limb and reduce edema; then "shrinkers" further shape the limb in preparation for a temporary prosthesis. Recent findings support using a plaster cast socket on the healed wound (Vigier et al., 1999). The rigid cast shapes the limb and reduces

Box 21-1 Types of Amputations

Below-the-knee amputation
Above-the-knee amputation
Amputation of the foot and ankle (Syme's amputation)
Amputation of the foot between metatarsus and tarsus (Hey's amputation or Lisfranc's amputation)
Hip disarticulation—removal of the limb from the hip joint
Hemicorporectomy—removal of half of the body from the pelvis and lumbar areas
Amputation of hand or partial (specific digits)
Amputation of arm—above the elbow or below the elbow
Shoulder disarticulation—removal of the limb from the shoulder joint

Adapted from Phipps, W., Sands, J., & Marek, J. (1999). *Medical-surgical nursing: Concepts & clinical practice* (6th ed.). St. Louis: Mosby.

edema, allowing rapid application of a temporary prosthesis. Shortened hospital stay reduces cost, and mobility lessens complications. Similar techniques are effective with above-the-knee amputation.

Total hip disarticulation is a radical form of surgery in which the entire femur is removed; this is performed only when alternatives fail. Roughly 4% of disarticulations result from malignancy, 20% from infection, 20% from vascular disease, 10% from trauma, and 2% from congenital abnormalities. The prosthetic limb of choice since 1957 is the Canadian hip disarticulation version, which has been refined as the Otto Modular endoskeletal version (Zaffer, Braddom, Conti, Goff, & Bokma, 1999). It has the advantage of lighter weight, improved cosmetic appearance, and flexibility. The prosthesis design has total contact suction suspension and an auxiliary custom-shaped pelvic belt offering independent ambulation, improved function overall, and cosmetic appearance.

Successful ambulation using a prosthetic device depends on multiple factors. The residual limb tissue must be able to support the body weight, and the person must be able to balance and adjust to the gait pattern. Cardiac function, metabolic requirements, and energy consumption are components that give younger clients more success, especially with lower limb amputations. An aggressive inpatient rehabilitation program, followed by an outpatient clinic program, provides support, training, and education and helps with motivation for clients who are capable of achieving independent function and return to employment. Elderly persons benefit from intensive therapies and nursing interventions in hospitals paced to their endurance or from gait training as an outpatient. Goals may be modified to wheelchair mobility only when ambulation is unsafe or falls have occurred.

Muscular Dystrophies

Adults of all ages are affected by muscular dystrophies, except for Duchenne's dystrophy (DD), which affects 1 in 3500 male babies at birth. DD is the most common dystrophy, and those affected by it rarely live beyond 25 years of age (Phipps, Sands, & Marek, 1999). Muscular dystrophies are characterized by muscle wasting and specific symptoms; these are categorized by phenotype, method of inheritance, and rate of progress as illustrated in Table 21-2.

Muscular dystrophies are caused by a defect of the intracellular metabolism of the muscle fibers with defects in creatine metabolism and intracellular enzymes in the glycolytic system. Altered striation of muscle fibers leads to hypertrophy or atrophy and when replaced with fat and connective tissue cause fatty infiltration and fibrosis. Diagnosis is based on history and physical examination, muscle biopsy, electromyography, and serum muscle enzyme levels. Creatine kinase levels are elevated during infancy but may elude detection in children who have limited symptoms without onset of muscle weakness.

Postpolio Syndrome

Another chronic disorder of the musculoskeletal system, postpolio syndrome (PPS) is a collection of symptoms that emerge in 28.5% to 64% of persons who experienced acute poliomyelitis (Jubelt & Agre, 2000). Of undetermined origin, PPS appears after an average of 35 years of functional stability, and incidence increases with aging. It may be the result of excessive long-term metabolic stress on motor neurons. New nerve terminals, and eventually the motor neurons themselves, are lost. Degenerating motor units possibly are those that were affected by poliomyelitis or are aging motor neurons associated with stress from muscle overuse. Inflammation of the spinal cord is found frequently on autopsy, supporting theories of persistent poliomyelitis virus infection, an autoimmune syndrome, or a degenerative response.

Symptoms of PPS include generalized fatigue, lack of energy occurring with minimal activity (the "polio wall"), difficulty concentrating, muscle or joint pain, and muscle atrophy. The weakness is usually gradual, asymmetrical, and can be proximal, distal, or patchy. Deterioration is more rapid than in normal aging. Strength of several muscle groups declines, notably in the upper and lower extremity flexor muscles of shoulders, elbows, wrists, hips, or knees, but not in the extensor muscle groups used in weight bearing (Klein, Whyte, Keenan, Esquenazi, & Polansky, 2000).

Repetitive Motion Injuries

Injuries associated with repetitive motion can occur from an acute incident or overuse during recreational activities, exercise, and job-related tasks. Muscle strain, actually a tearing of muscle fibers, may present with tenderness, edema, or discoloration of the skin. With continued use, muscle fibers continue to tear and add to less elastic scar tissue that tends to tighten. Excessive stretching before elasticity is restored may cause reinjury, turning a minor injury into a chronic problem such as contractures. Electrolyte imbalance may occur during any aggressive exercise or recreation without adequate nutrition and fluid intake, causing muscle cramps.

Dance Injuries

All forms of recreational and professional dance, including ballet, classical, and aerobic dance, may cause repetitive motion injuries. Dance-related injuries produce degenerative problems of the hips and knees, stress fractures, tendonitis of the foot and ankle, and toe fractures. Inadequate conditioning may injure the abductor muscles. Snapping and clicking noises at the hip rarely cause pain; they are the result of the iliofemoral ligament rubbing over the head of the femur or the iliotibial band rubbing over the greater trochanter. Degenerative changes of the greater trochanter can occur if the condition persists.

Toe injuries, such as hyperextension of the great toe, are common in dancing because of improperly fitted footwear and techniques. The "turnout" technique produces external

Table 21-2 Muscular Dystrophies

Onset	Symptoms	Progression	Inheritance
Duchenne Muscular Dystrophy (DMD)			
Early childhood—about 2 to 6 years	Generalized weakness and muscle wasting affecting limb and trunk muscles first; calves often enlarged	Disease progresses slowly but will affect all voluntary muscles; survival rare beyond late 20s	X-linked recessive (females are carriers)
Becker Muscular Dystrophy (BMD)			
Adolescence or adulthood	Almost identical to Duchenne's dystrophy but often much less severe; can be significant heart involvements	Slower and more variable than Duchenne's dystrophy with survival well into mid to late adulthood	X-linked recessive (females are carriers)
Emery-Dreifuss Muscular Dystrophy (EDMD)			
Childhood to early teens	Weakness and wasting of shoulder, upper arm, and shin muscles; joint deformities are common	Disease usually progresses slowly; frequent cardiac complications are common	X-linked recessive (females are carriers)
Facioscapulohumeral Muscular Dystrophy (FSH or FSHD)			
Childhood to middle age	Generalized weakness and muscle wasting affecting face, feet, hands, and neck first; delayed relaxation of muscles after contraction; congenital myotonic form is more severe	Progression is slow, sometimes spanning 50 to 60 years	Autosomal dominant
Oculopharyngeal Muscular Dystrophy (OPMD)			
Early adulthood to middle age	First affects muscles of eyelid and throat	Slow progression with swallowing problems common as disease progresses	Autosomal dominant
Distal Muscular Dystrophy (DD)			
40-60 years of age	Weakness and wasting of muscles of the hands, forearms, and lower legs	Slow progression but not life-threatening	Autosomal dominant

Adapted from Muscular Dystrophy Association. (1999). *Neuromuscular diseases in the MDA program* [On-line]. Available: http://www/mdausa.org/disease/40list.html.

rotation of the entire lower extremity, including the knee and lower leg. Required in all types of dance, it may cause tendonitis (Petrucci, 1993). "Knuckling down" of the toes occurs when the toes collapse inside the pointe shoe, leaving the dancer's weight on the interphalangeal joints (knuckles) of the hallux rather than on the first and second digits. The ankle, knee, hip, and spine become off balance, causing acute injuries, such as sprained ankles and knees or ligament injuries. Avascular necrosis of the growth plates of the metatarsals may occur.

Exercise Injuries

Several types of musculoskeletal injuries are associated with exercise. When bones are subjected to repeated stressors or forces in excess of normal activities, they initially thicken at the cortex. When stress ends, the thickening gradually disappears and returns to normal, without residual effect. Repeated contact with hard surfaces can cause lower extremity injuries; over time, impact and shock may cause stress fractures. Tendonitis of the foot and ankle usually involves the flexor hallucis longus or the Achilles tendon.

Sports Injuries

Participation in sports activities, whether for fitness, recreation, or competition, is associated with health benefits. However, it also brings an inherent risk of injury; repetitive activity and overuse are common causes (Ballas, Tytko, & Cookson, 1997; Sevier & Wilson, 1999; Pink & Tibone,

2000). Running, an activity enjoyed by nearly 10 million persons in the United States (American Sports Data, 2001), results in lower extremity injuries for 45% to 70% of runners annually. The primary cause is overuse resulting from training errors, such as running too far, too fast, and too soon. Common injuries from running include patellofemoral pain syndrome with dull aching behind or around the knee, stress fractures, tibial stress syndrome (shin splints), adductor and hamstring strain, iliotibial band syndrome, and plantar fasciitis (burning heel pain). Stress fractures are of particular concern because they may cause long-term morbidity if not treated appropriately (Ballas et al., 1997). Although many running injuries can be prevented, walking may be an alternative with low risk for musculoskeletal injury (Colbert, Hootman, & Macera, 2000). Proper footwear and stretching, especially the Achilles tendon, may prevent or alleviate plantar fasciitis.

The motions of swimming, tennis, golf, and sports with throwing, such as baseball, may result in upper extremity injury. Swimmers are highly vulnerable to shoulder injury; 66% report problems. *Swimmer's shoulder* is a global term for the multiple injuries that may occur as the swimmer pulls the body over the arm and the shoulder undergoes continuous revolutions. Reporting pain before inflammation masks the inciting symptoms helps with diagnosis (Pink et al., 2000). Lateral epicondylitis (tennis elbow) affects approximately half of all tennis players, whereas medial epicondylitis affects golfers. Muscle tendon units that allow wrist flexion and extension, as well as grasping, begin at the elbow so that repeated grasping, gripping, or twisting causes tendon inflammation. Elbow pain that worsens with repetitive gripping or wrist motion is characteristic of epicondylitis (Ciccotti, 1998). A cycle of inflammation and scar formation can become chronic without proper care (Sevier & Wilson, 1999). When the cycle is chronic or complicated, clients experience mild to moderate weakness and pain severe enough to limit daily activities, work, and recreation (Ciccotti, 1998).

Injuries differ across the life span and with gender. The musculoskeletal system of children and adolescents is growing actively; their level of skill and conditioning differs from that of adults (Hutchinson & Nasser, 2000). For older persons, age-related changes in strength, flexibility, and coordination play a role in increased risk for injury, severity of injury, and subsequent rehabilitation time (Lindsay, Horton, & Vandervoort, 2000). Women may be more likely than men to sustain athletic injury, particularly in jumping and cutting action sports, such as basketball, soccer, and volleyball. Increased risk of serious knee injuries, such as to the anterior cruciate ligament, may have relationships with anatomical or hormonal differences (estrogen, progesterone, and relaxin) and with knee instability or length of sports participation (Hewett, 2000).

As Ferrara and Peterson state, "participation in sports activities for people with disabilities continues to gain in popularity" (2000, p. 137). However, injury rates and problems appear to be similar for athletes regardless of their disabilities. Lower extremity injuries are more common among athletes who are ambulatory (e.g., with amputations, visual impairments, or cerebral palsy), whereas upper extremity injuries and carpal tunnel syndrome are found more among athletes who use a wheelchair in sports (Dec, Sparrow, & McKeag, 2000; Ferrara & Peterson, 2000).

Sports or exercise programs that include training for strength and flexibility, as well as promote gradual increases in activity, tend to prevent injuries. Early treatment is important. Rehabilitation nurses play a role in preventing injury and long-term disability or dysfunction. Simply educating athletes and coaches about the difference between soreness and pain may help minimize damage and facilitate return to the sport. Nonetheless, complications from an injury may develop later. For instance, athletes who had a knee injury earlier in life have an increased incidence of osteoarthritis of the knee later (Ivanhoe Newswire, 2000).

Job-Related Musculoskeletal Injuries

In 1994 the U.S. Department of Labor's Bureau of Labor Statistics indicated nearly two thirds of workplace injuries and illnesses were disorders associated with repeated trauma to the upper body, leading with sprains and strains (U.S. Department of Labor, Bureau of Labor Statistics, 1995). In November 2000, the U.S. Occupational Safety and Health Administration released federal ergonomic standards to prevent work-related musculoskeletal disorders, which account for the greatest amount of lost work time and represent the most expensive workers' compensation claims in hospitals (Hospital Employee Health, 1996). Ergonomic-related workplace injuries are caused by repeated irritation to areas such as the wrists, elbows, and shoulders.

Carpal tunnel syndrome, often related to long hours working on computers, is twice as common in individuals with diabetes. Repeated trauma, metabolic changes, or edema within the carpal tunnel compresses a median nerve producing numbness and tingling in its distribution. A weakened abductor pollicis brevis muscle lessens thumb abduction. Problems occur in ADLs, both at home and in the workplace, because of gradual muscle wasting.

Ganglion cysts can develop as a result of light repetitive motion activities such as writing, typing, knitting, and crocheting, or as a result of sudden onset of extreme pulling or pushing of heavy objects. The cyst emerges gradually, although it can occur rapidly to limit movement and cause pain during certain activities. Surgical removal of a ganglion cyst may be required to restore function in job or other activities.

Secondary Complications

Several primary diagnoses may have secondary musculoskeletal complications. Shoulder pain, other complications after a stroke and spinal cord injury, and steroid myopathy are discussed.

Musculoskeletal Problems Associated with Stroke

Pain. A variety of musculoskeletal problems may occur in clients who have had strokes. Pain in an upper extremity associated with hemiplegia may be caused by glenohumeral joint subluxation, spasticity of shoulder muscles, nerve impingement related to improper positioning, soft tissue trauma, complex regional pain syndrome (CRPS), rotator cuff tears, and shoulder-hand syndrome (Dekker, Wagenaar, Lankherst, & de Jong, 1997). Precipitating factors including immobilization of the upper extremity, trauma to the joint, rotator cuff tears, spasticity of the shoulder muscle, and glenohumeral joint subluxation cause injury to central or peripheral neural tissue (Dursun, Dursun, Ural, & Cakci, 2000).

Hemiplegic Shoulder Subluxation. Shoulder subluxation results from the loss of normal muscle tone in the supraspinatus and deltoid muscles (Ikai, Tei, Yoshida, Miyano, & Yonemoto, 1998) allowing downward scapular rotation as the humerus slides down the slope of the glenoid fossa. From 40% to 80% of persons who have new strokes experience hemiplegic shoulder pain (Dekker, Wagenaar, Lankhorst, & de Jong, 1997). Diagnosis is clinical or radiological. The client sits with the shoulder unsupported. Palpation reveals a gap greater than one finger's breath between the inferior aspect of the acromion and the superior aspect of the humeral head. Symptoms include pain with limited range of motion, impaired performance of ADLs, and reduced recovery of function in the arm.

Treatment is to position the upper extremity and support the shoulder with strapping techniques (strapping replaces slings) to prevent complications. A client who has weakened shoulder musculature and needs moderate to maximal assistance in transfers is at risk for glenohumeral joint subluxation. If the patient is incorrectly transferred, such as being pulled under the axilla of the arms, the humeral head may displace inferiorly in the absence of muscular support.

Complex Regional Pain Syndrome. Partial or sustained brachial plexus dysfunction may precipitate shoulder-hand syndrome (Liss & Liss, 2000), also known as CRPS and previously called reflex sympathetic dystrophy. A multisymptom syndrome affecting one or more extremities, CRPS affects any area of the body, often after a stroke. Pain, swelling, stiffness, discoloration, and pain and dysfunction with severity or duration out of proportion to those expected from the injury are characteristic (Wong & Wilson, 1997). Problems associated with CRPS include pain, stress, edema, and vasomotor instability. Medical management includes pharmacological agents (corticosteroids and vasodilators), regional blocks (guanethidine or reserpine), sympathetic blocks (Stellare block), peripheral nerve block (lidocaine/novocaine), or sympathectomy. A national nonprofit organization, the Reflex Sympathetic Dystrophy Syndrome Association, provides information to clients and family members.

Conditions, such as hemiparesis with an unstable knee or preexisting osteoarthritis, may aggravate affected degenerative joints and limit range of motion during neurological recovery. Altered gait patterns predispose clients to falls. Clients who walk in a flexed, rotated posture and sit in a flexed position for extended periods may develop lower back pain, possibly lumbosacral radiculopathy (nerve root damage). Improper positioning eventually creates thoracic kyphosis and kyphoscoliosis, and ambulating with a cane or a hemiwalker predisposes clients to develop carpal tunnel syndrome in the unaffected upper extremity (Liss & Liss, 2000).

Musculoskeletal Problems Associated with Spinal Cord Injury

Secondary complications after spinal cord injury (SCI) include muscle spasticity, contractures, and overuse syndrome in the upper extremities with functional limitations, including altered joint range of motion. Complications, such as knee flexion contractures and footdrop, are preventable. Hypercalcemia, more common in younger clients with SCI, causes calcium to leave the body through the urinary tract, producing increased risk of renal calculi and imbalance in bone remodeling. Heterotopic ossification (HO), a formation of new bone at the joints, may follow SCI or traumatic brain injury. The buildup of bone deposits can cause contractures and limit range of motion, further impaired by pain. Range of motion and weight-bearing exercises help prevent HO, and clients who can tolerate weight bearing, even in a standing frame, benefit from doing so.

Muscle spasticity is more prevalent at higher levels of SCI involvement. These sudden involuntary movements may raise safety concerns for injury to the client or caregiver during transfers or during treatments such as intermittent catheterization. Spasms may be severe enough to cause tissue trauma, bone contusions, and fractures, or lead to contractures. Spasticity management clinics in rehabilitation facilities provide services to prevent complications of severe muscle spasms, including contractures. Approaches to the management are based on early mobilization and minimizing of problems associated with disuse. Intrathecal baclofen pumps and other antispasticity medications, such as Botox injections, are used.

Overuse Syndrome. Overuse syndrome of the shoulders can occur after several years of using a wheelchair (Dec et al., 2000). Important activities, such as weight shifts and other position changes that protect skin integrity, transfer techniques requiring extreme stress on the shoulder joints, and adaptations for independent functioning of ADLs, can produce secondary shoulder injuries. Obesity, insufficient muscle strength, and neurological impairment associated with SCI may contribute to shoulder dysfunction. Problems occur when the individual is no longer able to perform activities and maintain quality of life because of the new limitations of shoulder overuse.

Steroid Myopathy

Steroid myopathy is a secondary complication of glucocorticoid treatment for systemic autoimmune diseases, such as SLE and RA. Corticosteroid use remains controversial and is restricted to relief of acutely inflamed joints with close monitoring for muscle deterioration. Although useful, many toxic effects occur (Frauman, 1996). Muscular atrophy and weakness with the use of adrenocorticosteroids (glucocorticoid) therapy is well documented in the literature; low doses are less likely to cause side effects. Early signs of proximal muscle weakness, as with hip and thigh muscle atrophy, are recognized when the individual begins to have difficulty getting out of a low chair or climbing stairs (Braith, Welsch, Mills, Keller, & Pollock, 1997). Muscle function studies are essential for the client who is at risk of steroid myopathy, especially if symptoms of decline emerge.

FACTORS RELATED TO MUSCULOSKELETAL DYSFUNCTION

Osteoporosis

Osteoporosis, skeletal deformities, age, gender, and ethnic background may influence musculoskeletal dysfunction and affect rehabilitation negatively. The normal aging process, along with obesity, previous trauma, and genetics, can increase the likelihood of complications. Osteoporosis results when bone resorption (osteoclasts) exceeds bone formation (osteoblasts), an imbalance begun when peak bone mass is not achieved during adolescence. An inactive adolescent lifestyle can predispose to obesity and also to osteoporosis later in life. Ironically obesity offers some protection by weight placing additional stress on the weight-bearing joints, thus putting persons with small, thin frames at a disadvantage. A family history of osteoporosis may indicate a genetic predisposition; deficiencies in calcium with vitamin D intake and smoking contribute (Goss, 1998; Taft, Looker, & Cella, 2000; Hightower, 2000).

Osteoporosis, more effectively prevented than treated, is 5 times more common in women, especially those who are postmenopausal because of decreased estrogen. Senile osteoporosis occurs in men and women older than 70 years and is related to the aging process and a chronic lack of calcium. Disuse osteoporosis occurs with disabilities related to immobility. With decreased muscle action and diminished weight-bearing activities, bone is lost (Goss, 1998).

No Food and Drug Administration–approved treatment exists for the 5.6 million men in the United States who are at risk for osteoporosis. Although oral medications are prescribed for men with lowered testosterone after orchiectomies, they also are underused (Kessenich, 2000). Colon-Emeric, Yballe, Sloane, Pieper, and Lyles (2000) found physicians recommended, rather than prescribed, supplements of bisphosphonate (aldondronate and risedronate) and calcium with vitamin D for men after their hip fractures. Their clinical efficacy remains unproved in men.

The mechanism in aging men may be declining testosterone and estrogen levels; certainly excess alcohol or caffeine intake, inactivity, and lower consumption of and reduced ability to absorb calcium contribute (Kessenich, 2000). Aging women have a gradual decrease in ovarian production of estrogen with resulting increased risk of fractures. The exact mechanism and role of estrogen are unclear, but surgically induced menopause, such as removal of the ovaries, causes greater bone loss than natural menopause. Gradual decline in ovarian estrogen production is less influential on bone loss than abrupt interruption of estrogen (Sullivan & Sharts-Hopko, 2000).

Goss (1998) states that women of European or Asian decent tend to have a greater degree of osteoporosis (N = 6 million to 7 million); African-American women follow (N = 300,000), and they have fewer total joint replacements (Healthy People 2010, 2000). The Total Hip Replacement (THR) National Institutes of Health Consensus Development Conference Statement (1994) found disparities in access to care, treatment selections, and client knowledge and referrals that affected THRs. Caucasians received artificial joints and fixation devices at 4.2 per 1000 compared with 1.7 in 1000 for African-Americans. Individuals with higher incomes were 22% more likely to have THR surgeries.

Other Musculoskeletal Problems

Vertebral compression fractures, a complication of osteoporosis, are painful and limit function. The fractures are diagnosed through x-rays or computed tomography (CT). Thoracic lumbar sacral orthosis may be used to support the spinal column and maintain proper positioning for optimal healing.

Other common musculoskeletal difficulties include scoliosis (Figure 21-2), kyphosis, lordosis, genu varum (bowing

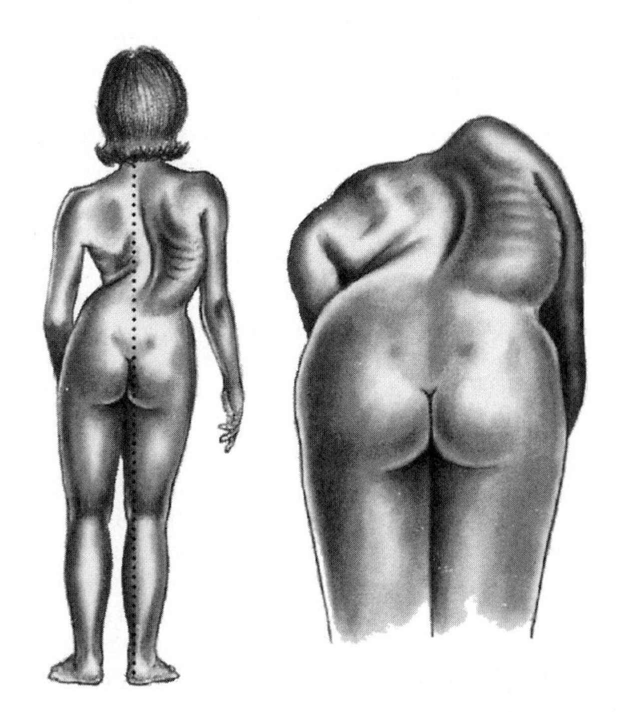

Figure 21-2 Abnormal spinal curvatures associated with scoliosis. (From Thompson, J.M., McFarland, G.K., Hirsch, J.E., & Tucker, S.M. [1998]. *Mosby's clinical nursing.* [4th ed.]. St. Louis: Mosby.)

of the knees), and genu valgum ("knock-knees"). Lordotic (concave) extreme curvature of the spine and kyphotic (convex) excessive curve of the thoracic spine can cause impairments in cardiovascular function, respiratory status, anemia, and altered ambulatory ability. Muscle mass deformities, asymmetries, and masses may be evident.

ASSESSMENT

Comprehensive assessment includes physiological and biopsychosocial aspects, such as the person's perception of the situation, current lifestyle, and support system. Chapter 14 details more about integrating musculoskeletal and neuromuscular assessment. Rehabilitation nurses initially examine baseline functional capacities, a specific dysfunction, or generalized complaints of pain and stiffness. Musculoskeletal assessment can be challenging; some diagnoses are formed entirely by subjective data or by exclusion, as with fibromyalgia. Function may be impaired apart from a client having a painful or limiting condition.

Subjective Assessment

A comprehensive history emphasizes identifying data, source of history, chief complaints, present illness, history, current health status, allergies, environmental hazards, use of safety equipment, exercise and leisure activities, sleep patterns, diet, current medications, and family and psychosocial history. Physical examination includes all body systems. Clients may describe specific areas of discomfort, general and rather vague complaints, short-term acute discomfort, or a long history of chronic pain and fatigue. Subjective assessment of pain is determined using age-specific tools appropriate for the client's condition. Pain intensity scales specifically for adults and children are presented in Chapter 24. Scales for standardized assessment of persons with cognitive impairments using their facial expressions, posture, and guarding are being developed by nurse researchers (McCaffery & Pasero, 1999). Research findings show fewer pain medications prescribed for elderly clients with cognitive impairments, and they routinely receive fewer (Wynne, Ling, & Remsburg, 2000).

History of trauma, strain, muscle weakness, limitation of joint movement, crunching, creaking, or giving way of weight-bearing joints accompanied by pain and stiffness are indicators of a musculoskeletal disorder (Mangini, 1998). Rheumatic fever and Lyme disease manifest with joint pain, fever, rashes and skin changes, eye symptoms, sleep disorders, or fatigue; generalized aches of the joints and muscles may signal acute viral infections. Any evidence of previous trauma may be indicative of reinjury, rather than a new onset of an acute injury, information pertinent in work-related injuries. Limitations in performing ADLs that affect social function, finances, and psychological or spiritual health are important initial assessments.

Psychological assessment includes adjustment to changes in body image, self-concept, and relationships with family members, friends, and coworkers. An assessment of the family member's role and function before and after the disability are important because roles may change after a catastrophic injury or illness. Depression is a complication that can be recognized and treated early. Chapter 12 discusses roles, responsibilities, and coping in detail. Additional resources may assist with financial management and other home or maintenance functions.

Objective Assessment

Establish a baseline through observation of a client's gait, stance, height, posture, and proportions, and screen for abnormalities. Chapter 14 discusses further examination. When muscular weakness is evident, details of the problem and the evaluation are important to understanding the source. Weakness may be acute or chronic and may fluctuate with activity or result from fatigue; it may limit movement to perform ADLs, such as combing hair or brushing teeth. Numbness or tingling in the affected area is investigated to determine the presence of peripheral nerve damage. Distal weakness is often the result of neuropathy leading to difficulty with fine motor actions, such as clothing management or altering gait pattern. Flaccid paralysis results from denervated muscles and may present with visible atrophy, as in stroke or spinal cord injury. Limitation of joint range of motion frequently is accompanied by pain and joint stiffness; Heberden's nodes and Bouchard's nodes appear with osteoarthritis, whereas subcutaneous nodules and ulnar drift and present in RA (Figure 21-3). In RA, stiffness is most severe in the mornings and lessens with use. In contrast, stiffness worsens with increased use in osteoarthritis (Mangini, 1998).

Postacute Assessment

After surgery of the hips, knees, or shoulders or after amputations, a client has a postoperative stay and then transfers to a rehabilitation unit or a skilled facility or goes directly home, depending on the situation. The rehabilitation nurse's assessment is essential in preventing complications. Drains frequently are removed from the surgical site in the acute hospital, necessitating continued monitoring of the operative site in all settings. Early signs of postoperative hemorrhage include decreased blood pressure, increased pulse, and anxiety. The surgical site may present with increased edema, firmness on palpation, or evidence of bleeding.

Circulation, sensation, and movement (CSM) are monitored by observing skin color, temperature, and sensation; level of pain; presence of pulses; and swelling. CSM checks and documentation are essential in the monitoring of extremities with casts, splints, and elastic dressings. Compartment syndrome, a result of trauma, occurs when pressure from bleeding or edema within a limited anatomical space compromises circulation, viability, and function of the tissues within that space. Compartment syndrome also results

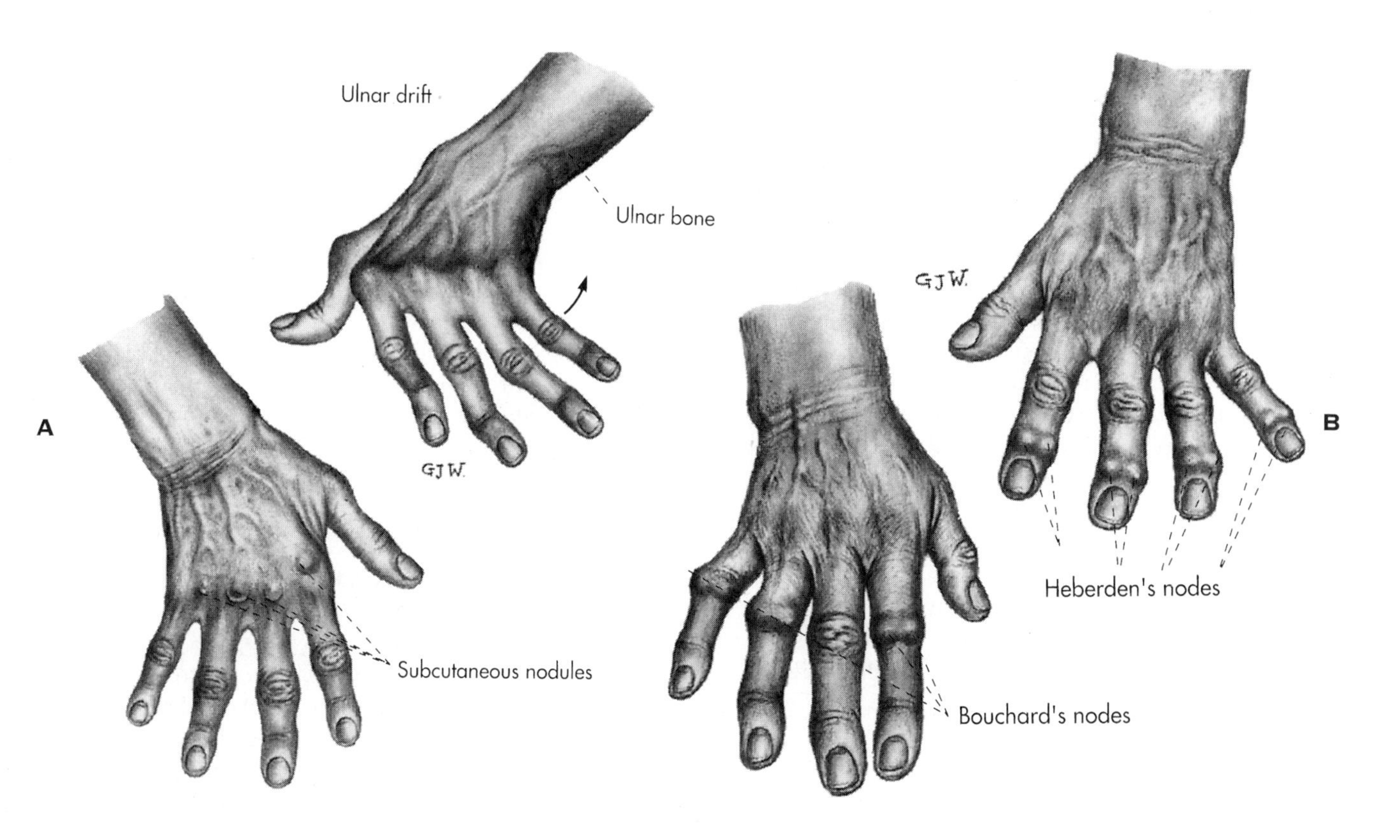

Figure 21-3 **A,** Joint involvement with rheumatoid arthritis. **B,** Osteoarthritis. Herberden's nodes and Bouchard's nodes. (From Mourad, L.A. [1991]. *Orthopedic disorders.* St. Louis: Mosby.)

from external pressure of a cast or tight dressing, especially in the lower legs, forearm, and hand. Undetected, this syndrome can cause loss of function, deformity, and possible amputation. Any new immobilization device, including a cast or splint, may press on a bony prominence and irritate the skin or form blisters that become infected. Skin breakdown delays healing and increases costly hospital stays.

Severe anemia is a complication of musculoskeletal surgery that may lead to myocardial ischemia and increased risk of cardiopulmonary complications during the acute phase of physical rehabilitation (Diamond, 2000). Episodes of desaturation may be evident in oxygen and cardiopulmonary responses to self-care and therapy sessions. Poor endurance and reduced exercise tolerance may limit progress in therapy, lead to extended hospital stays, and create additional risk of complications.

Fat embolism syndrome (FES) is a rare but potentially fatal occurrence that may result from fractures of the pelvis, femur, and tibia, or multiple trauma, or follow total hip or total knee arthroplasty. Fat globules released into the bloodstream from the bone marrow and surrounding tissue travel to the lungs and block the capillaries and arterioles. Symptoms of FES include hypoxia, tachypnea, tachycardia, petechiae, fever, lipuria, and chest pain; neurological symptoms are altered mental status with restlessness, confusion, and lethargy. Diagnostic tests for FES include arterial partial pressure of oxygen, infiltrates found on chest x-ray, arterial blood gases, and lowered hemoglobin and platelet counts.

Laboratory Tests and Diagnostic Studies

Understanding the significance of laboratory tests and diagnostic studies helps in assessing for complications of various conditions. Determining baseline values and monitoring for changes in laboratory test results, radiological studies, and fluid analysis are part of rehabilitation nursing assessment of a client's progress and response to treatment. Results of a variety of laboratory values and their interactions are included in the musculoskeletal assessment as discussed below.

Blood studies provide useful data about musculoskeletal problems in several ways. Red blood cell count reflects the actual number of formed cells and the specific volume of blood; when abnormal, the body is responding or lacks response to certain processes, such as postoperative anemia after hip replacement in elderly persons. White blood cell count and differential detect inflammation and infection. Culture and sensitivity identify the source of infections in surgical wounds, urine, blood, or respiratory secretions.

C-reactive protein is used to measure the clinical severity of osteoarthritis in the hip and knee. The ESR is elevated with RA and other types of inflammation. RF and other proteins coat the erythrocytes and make them heavier; rapid settling of red blood cells is the result of the level of fibrinogen (Corbett, 1998). A negative RF does not rule out RA because some individuals do not show a titer in the presence of active disease or do not appear positive until after the onset of active disease.

Immunoglobulins (gamma globulins) are inflammatory proteins that possess known antibody activity. Immunoglobulin G and immunoglobulin M antibodies are significant in inflammatory and infectious diseases such as hepatitis and rubella. Approximately 25% of clients with chronic hepatitis develop arthritis and 40% have arthralgia related to this inflammatory process (Corbett, 1998).

Electrolyte levels are significant in musculoskeletal dysfunction and monitored throughout the entire postoperative phase of recovery, especially for elderly clients. Hypernatremia results from fluid retention and may be an early sign of congestive heart failure, dehydration, or renal insufficiency.

Potassium levels help indicate renal output. Soft tissue trauma can cause massive cell destruction with transient hyperkalemia and symptoms such as palpitations, sinus tachycardia, and premature ventricular tachycardia. Hyperkalemia can lead to potentially fatal cardiac arrhythmias, such as ventricular fibrillation. Potassium-sparing diuretics, diets high in potassium, and overuse of salt substitutes also produce hyperkalemia. On the other hand, clients recovering from musculoskeletal surgeries, especially elderly clients, may develop hypokalemia when they do not receive adequate oral intake. Cardiac arrhythmias, muscle weakness, and even paralytic ileus may occur. Potassium supplements can be administered through intravenous fluids or tube feedings.

Calcium levels affect musculoskeletal conditions. Hypercalcemia occurs with immobilization, lack of weight bearing, and conditions such as metastatic bone disease when bone calcium is lost. Hypocalcemia often occurs in conjunction with hyperkalemia.

Blood urea nitrogen (BUN) and serum creatinine are two renal function studies that detect levels of dehydration, increased protein metabolism, and renal impairment. In the case of renal insufficiency, the BUN and creatinine elevate together in a 10:1 ratio.

Alkaline phosphatase (ALP) and creatine kinase (CK) are significant in bone disease and muscular damage. Increases in ALP indicate new bone formation and healing fractures. Healthy carriers of X-linked Duchenne muscular dystrophy also have elevated CK levels. Uric acid levels, when persistently elevated in men older than 30 years who have recurrent monoarthritis, may indicate gout. Joint aspiration fluid of urate crystals is the definitive diagnosis.

Radiographic studies including radiographs, fluoroscopy, and tomography can detect fractures and other changes in bone texture and contour (Corbett, 1998). Fluoroscopic studies are not commonly used in evaluation of musculoskeletal disorders. Tomography, in conjunction with computer scanning techniques (CT scan) shows three-dimensional cross sections to detect masses, abscesses, and areas of tissue trauma. MRI uses magnetic forces to produce images.

Dual-energy x-ray absorptiometry (DEXA) is an accurate, sensitive, and painless measure of bone mineral density (BMD). It is the gold standard in testing for osteoporosis (Taft, Looker, & Cella, 2000).

Diskography is used to evaluate the integrity of intervertebral disk space and determine specific levels of vertebral involvement. This test is more uncomfortable because it requires contrast medium and saline to be injected into the disk space to reproduce the back or leg pain associated with the pathological condition.

Scintigraphy, such as bone scan, determines uptake of radionuclide in areas called "hot spots" of osteoblastic and osteolytic processes in the bones. Analysis of joint fluids can be beneficial in the diagnosis of gout and infectious arthritis. Aspirated fluid is analyzed for gram stain, white blood cell count with differential, urate crystals, culture, and sensitivity.

Pediatric Assessment

Infants, young children, and adolescents experience musculoskeletal conditions, such as muscular dystrophy, JRA, and fractures, as well as sequela from congenital conditions of myelomeningocele and cerebral palsy. Pediatric assessment differs greatly because of the need for age and developmentally appropriate techniques and subjective data gathered from parents. Observation, including play and pediatric pain assessment, may replace extensive hands-on assessment. Observing a child's body posture, facial expression, and vocalizations of discomfort while at rest or during movement may provide information about pain. Chapters 24 and 29 provide details about pain and pediatric rehabilitation.

Conditions such as JRA are assessed through history, physical examination, and developmental and functional assessments (Driscoll, Noll, & Koch, 1994). Physical impairments may slow fine and gross motor development and result in functional disability. Symptoms, duration of the disease, joint involvement, degree of pain, stiffness, and fatigue are noted. Systemic symptoms such as weight loss, slowed growth, rash, and shortness of breath are important details. Additional information about the child's support system, home, school, and recreational activities help the rehabilitation nurse determine level of functioning and quality of life for the child, as well as the immediate family members.

Assessment of muscular dystrophy in children follows the same age-appropriate techniques as for JRA. Specific assessment involves observation of posture, respiratory function, cardiac status, ability to ambulate with or without specific devices, and functional level in the home, school and at play. Refer to Chapter 29 for more details regarding pediatric assessment.

NURSING DIAGNOSES

After conducting a thorough assessment of the client with a musculoskeletal disorder, the rehabilitation nurse identifies appropriate nursing diagnoses. Table 21-3 identifies suggested diagnoses common to the rehabilitation of individuals with musculoskeletal disorders.

TABLE 21-3 Nursing Diagnoses

Nursing Diagnosis*	Suggested Nursing Interventions Classification (NIC)	Suggested Nursing Outcomes Classification (NOC)
Pain, acute and chronic	Pain management	Pain control
Activity intolerance (pain and fatigue)	Energy management	Energy conservation
Self-care deficit	Self-care assistance	Self-care: ADLs Self-care: instrumental ADLs
Impaired physical mobility	Exercise therapy: joint mobility Exercise promotion: strength training Exercise therapy: ambulation	Joint movement: Active muscle function Ambulation: walking Ambulation: wheelchair
Disturbed body image	Body image enhancement	Adjustment to changes in physical appearance and body function

Data from Johnson, M., Maas, M.L., & Moorhead, S. (2000). *Nursing outcomes classification (NOC)* (2nd ed.). St. Louis: Mosby; McCloskey, J.C., & Bulechek, G.M. (2000). *Nursing interventions classification (NIC)* (3rd ed.). St. Louis: Mosby; and North American Nursing Diagnosis Association. (2001). *Nursing diagnosis: definitions and classification 2001-2002* (4th ed.). Philadelphia: Author.
ADLs, Activities of daily living.
*Other possible nursing diagnoses include reactive depression, anxiety, social isolation, knowledge deficit, impaired skin integrity, altered sexuality patterns

GOALS

The goal of individuals with musculoskeletal conditions is directed toward achieving and maintaining maximal independence, comfort, and safety. Specific goals are set mutually with the client and family. A young man with a below-the-knee amputation may set a realistic, long-term goal of independently performing all tasks of daily living and functioning at work or school with his prosthesis. A woman with PPS may set goals to coordinate tasks of a caregiver and be independent using a power wheelchair. A child with JRA who has minimal pain and stiffness may desire to participate actively in school and play with other children.

Broad Outcome Goals

Several broad outcome goals for individuals with various musculoskeletal disorders are listed below.

- Control pain
- Manage energy to initiate and sustain activity
- Achieve and maintain maximum independence in ADL/instrumental ADLs
- Perform ADLs and mobility tasks safely
- Maintain joint function and prevent deformities
- Control depression
- Maximize strength and endurance in arthritis cases

Health Promotion/Prevention

Rehabilitation nurses in all practice settings work to assist individuals to achieve national goals of health promotion and health prevention. Healthy People 2010 (2000) lists the following goals for persons with musculoskeletal disorders.

- Decrease the number of cases of osteoporosis and reduce the incidence of osteoporotic fractures by 20%
- Decrease the rate of amputations in persons with diabetes mellitus by 55%
- Prevent illness and disability related to arthritis and other rheumatic conditions
- Decrease injury resulting from overexertion and repetitive motion by 50%

Additional opportunities for health promotion and prevention include promoting ergonomic work environments, maintaining healthy body weight, and encouraging moderate physical exercise. Several programs, such as the Arthritis self-management program (ASMP) (Arthritis Society, 2001) move toward these goals. The ASMP is a 6-week health promotion program designed to help individuals with arthritis gain a better understanding of the disease, take an active role in arthritis care, and cope with chronic pain. Such programs are opportunities for rehabilitation nurses to become involved in community action and as referral resources for clients.

Decreasing Osteoporotic Fractures

Short-term goals in decreasing osteoporotic fractures are to decrease falls and help prevent such fractures. Long-term prevention involves collaborating with the client and family to establish healthy dietary habits, nutritional supplements of calcium and vitamin D, and an exercise regimen to maintain muscle strength and balance. Glucocorticoids are thought to be the most frequent cause of drug-related osteoporosis and may contribute to bone loss in lupus (Cunnanae & Lane, 2000).

Decreasing the Rate of Amputations

Short-term goals to reduce the amputation rate in diabetic clients are individual. Dietary and medication regimens are balanced with activities to provide safe management of blood sugars. Programs such as The Bureau of Primary Health Care's Lower Extremity Amputation Prevention involve standardizing screening techniques for improving clients' detection of impaired sensation in the feet and assigning risk categories based on findings (LEAP Program, 2000). Education about avoiding trauma, performing proper foot inspection, and early intervention with making referrals to podiatrists for examination and preventive treatment are key factors in decreasing the rate of amputations. Tight control of blood sugars early in the disease course is also crucial; the Diabetes Control and Complications Trial reported a 60% reduction in nerve damage (McCarren, 1993).

Reducing Pain

The short-term goals of reducing pain and limitations in activity for adults with arthritis and other rheumatic conditions focus on measures for managing pain and discomfort using combinations of medications, diet, and exercise. Exercise goals are established to maintain joint range of motion, strength, and overall mobility. Long-term goals require a program designed to minimize the effects of pain and joint stiffness and prevent complications or further disability. A self-paced regimen of exercise and rest periods is one way for clients to accomplish ADLs and maintain the highest level of wellness possible for the greatest number of days. Alternative and complementary interventions are important to these clients and discussed further in Chapter 13.

Decreasing Injury Rates

Short-term goals for clients with conditions where fatigue is a problem, such as with multiple sclerosis, include maximizing function, planning individual activities for the most efficient energy expenditure, and using assistive devices appropriate for the functional level of the client. Long-term goals include maintaining an active lifestyle of optimal level of wellness but avoiding overexertion. Modifications in work or school and leisure activities can enable a satisfying lifestyle within realistic goals.

Short-term goals for workplace prevention of overuse and repetitive motion injuries include use of proper body mechanics when lifting, recognition and control of ergonomic hazards, and early detection and treatment of musculoskeletal injuries. Long-term goals are to institute ergonomic approaches in the design stage of work processes and to prevent disability, as well as to increase public awareness and provide education about interventions.

Other Health Promotion/Prevention Goals

Many goals for health promotion and health prevention are addressed in community and workplace education programs. Typically, programs provide information about developing ergonomic work environments, maintaining healthy body weight, and performing moderate physical activity. Analyses of work sites and education about use of proper body mechanics in the workplace are conducted by many industries through employee wellness programs, often led by rehabilitation or occupational health nurses.

Nurses are involved in community wellness offering programs for management of stress, weight, and exercise with content about safety and prevention. Persons with actual or potential musculoskeletal disorders benefit from education and monitoring to avoid complications, such as falls, injuries, or fractures; prevent secondary disabilities, such as contractures; and ways to avoid injuries associated with work, exercise, and recreation. Rehabilitation nurses particularly are able to design, present, and evaluate educational programs designed to address these types of wellness programs in the community. Musculoskeletal injuries associated with obesity and sedentary lifestyles may be reduced through education and counseling about lifestyle and healthy choices shared by rehabilitation nurses.

REHABILITATION NURSING INTERVENTIONS

Rehabilitation nurses have opportunities to use traditional as well as creative interventions when working with clients to meet their challenges posed by musculoskeletal disorders. Interventions are planned based on the nursing diagnoses and directed toward meeting goals mutually established by the client, family, and rehabilitation team.

Pain, Acute and Chronic

Persons with a nursing diagnosis of acute or chronic pain require traditional and alternative treatment strategies and creativity in collaboration with the client and interdisciplinary team. Pain may be specific to sites and diseases or nonspecific and invisible, as with fibromyalgia. Information about a client's experiences in coping with pain helps individualize a plan for pain management, often involving a combination of interventions.

The following section discusses traditional pharmacological methods of pain management followed by alternative, nonpharmacological approaches.

Pharmacological Pain Management

Although nonsteroidal anti-inflammatory drugs (NSAIDs) do not affect the progression of the rheumatoid disease process; they do reduce inflammation by inhibiting two isoforms of cyclooxygenase, COX-1 and COX-2. Celecoxib (Celebrex) and rofecoxib (Vioxx) are two medications known to block COX-2, but not COX-1 (Abramowicz, 2000a). COX-1 maintains prostaglandin synthesis in the stomach, kidneys, and platelets, whereas COX-2 maintains prostaglandin production in inflamed tissues (Gremillion & Vollenhoven, 1998). They have less gastrointestinal toxicity than aspirin or naproxen and are administered singly or in conjunction with NSAIDs for treatment of RA.

Disease-modifying anti-rheumatic drugs (DMARDs) have no immediate analgesic effects, but can control symptoms and may delay progression of the disease. DMARDs such as hydroxychloroquine sulfate (Plaquenil) or sulfasalazine (Azulfidine) are often used for treating mild symptoms; methotrexate (Rheumatrex) when symptoms are more severe. The DMARDs have slow onset and require close monitoring for side effects of nausea, anorexia, and diminished renal function. Many physicians use NSAIDs early in the treatment of RA, adding the DMARDs for maintenance; new regimens start DMARDs for RA earlier.

Oral corticosteroids such as cortisone and prednisone are prescribed for acute episodes of pain and inflammation. They are used in combination with an NSAID and less frequently with DMARDs, Enbrel, Remicade, gold salts, and intraarticular steroids (Berard, Solomon, & Avorn, 2000). Corticosteroids must be used with caution because of side effects such as fluid retention and gastrointestinal irritation. Steroids must be discontinued gradually and never stopped abruptly.

Osteoarthritis pain is managed with a regimen similar to that for RA. Treatment usually starts with acetaminophen and moves to NSAIDs, the drug of choice, when acetaminophen alone is not effective (Berard et al., 2000). Alternative medications have been substituted for drugs that cause gastrointestinal (GI) irritation and renal and liver toxicity. COX-2 inhibitors (Celebrex and Vioxx) reduce pain and inflammation and protect the GI tract. Capsaicin products are applied topically and, when used consistently, can relieve joint discomfort by blocking substance P, a neurotransmitter for pain. Cortisone injections into the intraarticular joint space may provide pain relief for weeks to months, but are to be used sparingly and with caution. Knee osteoarthritis has been successfully treated with hyaluronate solutions, such as hyaluronan (Hylagen), hylan G-F 20 (Synvisc), and sodium hyaluronate (Supartz), in a series of three to five injections (Kee, 2000; Reuters Medical News, 2001).

NSAIDs have elevated blood pressure in persons with otherwise normal blood pressures (Kozuh, 2000). The action of NSAIDs is believed to inhibit arachidonic acid metabolism, resulting in decreased prostaglandin formation. Prostaglandins allow for normal renal functioning and systemic vasoconstriction. Many antihypertensive agents affect renal blood flow, such as thiazides, loop diuretics, beta blockers, alpha blockers, and angiotensin-converting enzyme inhibitors. Calcium channel blockers in combination with NSAIDs have little or no effect on blood pressure. Screening blood pressure, prescribing appropriate antihypertensives, and monitoring medication effectiveness and side effects are important in evaluating treatment outcomes for arthritis.

Rehabilitation nurses may have an advocacy role in assuring adequate assessment and interventions for clients with arthritic conditions. A large study found elderly residents of nursing homes who had comorbid conditions and multiple medications received fewer analgesics for their RA than did elderly persons residing in their homes; the residents were less likely to receive appropriate medication regimens for chronic diseases such as arthritis (Berard et al, 2000).

Traditional Nonpharmacological Pain Management

Many nonpharmacological agents have been used to treat musculoskeletal conditions. Application of heat and cold are used in conjunction with the treatment of inflamed joints and injured muscles after assessment is completed. A newly acquired strain or sprain is treated with cold compresses to reduce swelling and discomfort. Heat applications, when appropriate, can provide increased range of motion and muscle relaxation. Therapists in rehabilitation may apply heat at the beginning of a session, and then apply cold compresses at the conclusion to reduce inflammation and discomfort in the exercised area. The application of heat or cold can be achieved by hydrocollator packs, paraffin baths, moist heat electric pads, and warm soaks in the tub, bath, or shower.

Functional electrical stimulation (FES) has reduced pain and subluxation in persons with hemiplegia and shoulder pain after stroke because of the electrical therapy's strong sedative effect on sensory nerves and muscle fibers. FES may speed up the rate of motor recovery. More research is needed for evidence of the positive effects of this modality (Chantraine, Baribeault, Uebelhart, & Gremion, 1999).

Biofeedback techniques are used to encourage relaxation and to reduce stress and tension associated with musculoskeletal disorders such as fibromyalgia (Smith, 1998).

Alternative Approaches

Rehabilitation nurses assist clients by becoming familiar with underlying principles, proper practices, and research findings about alternative medicine and related therapeutics. Alternative therapies such as acupuncture are of great interest to clients with musculoskeletal conditions. Magnetic therapy is another modality that has been examined for management of chronic pain with musculoskeletal conditions, such as backache, arthritis, carpal tunnel syndrome, sports injuries, and PPS (Whitaker & Adderly, 1998; Vallbona, Hazlewood, & Jurida, 1997). Glucosamine is a dietary supplement refined from shark cartilage that has proven effective in relieving arthritis pain for many clients. Studies are in progress to evaluate the supplement and effect on modification of joint deterioration (Blot, Marcelis, Devogelaer, & Manicourt, 2000).

Herbal preparations, such as ginger, may reduce smooth muscle tone and treat nausea in persons with RA (Blumenthal et al., 1998). A combination of massage and aromatherapy using lavender oil *(Lavendula angustifolia)* was found to benefit persons with arthritis by reducing muscle tension and pain. *Lavendula* has analgesic, antispasmodic, and relaxing properties with no evidence of adverse reaction (Brownfield, 1998). Clients must be assessed for developing sensitivity, however.

T'ai Chi has been used for reducing pain associated with musculoskeletal conditions and eliminating stress (Ryan, 2000). The precise movements and slow motion exercises are used to develop balance, alignment, coordination, and relaxation. Research supports T'ai Chi as improving range of motion, preserving bones and joints, reducing tension, and increasing strength and balance (Lumsden, Baccalo, & Martire, 1998).

Surgical Interventions

Several different surgical interventions are used to relieve pain, stabilize joints, and correct deformities. Procedures for DJD, THR, and total knee replacements have become common; more than 800,000 persons throughout the world undergo THR annually. THR improves quality of life and functional recovery for many healthy adults (Knutsson & Engberg, 1999). The rate of functional recovery for older persons with hip fractures depends on their preoperative condition and other medical disorders (Young, Brant, & German, 1997). THR most frequently is performed for persons with osteoarthritis, RA, traumatic arthritis, avascular necrosis, hip fractures, benign and malignant bone tumors, arthritis associated with Paget's disease, ankylosing spondylitis, or JRA.

Surgical techniques, rehabilitation approaches, the selection of prosthetic designs, and materials for specific client groups vary among physicians. Techniques of surgical repair are based on the location of the fracture, bone quality, displacement, and type (simple or comminuted). Femoral neck fractures are treated by either internal fixation using screws or pins or by prosthetic replacement. Prosthetic replacement is used for older clients with displaced fractures to minimize complications. Intertrochanteric fractures are treated using internal fixation such as screws. Endoprosthesis replacement is performed to remove the femoral head (hemiarthroplasty) or by replacing the acetabular cup and the femoral head (total hip arthroplasty). Prosthetic devices are either cemented in place or may be press-fitted or porous-coated to allow the bone to grow into the prosthesis (Kain, 2000). Figure 21-4 illustrates cemented and cementless hip prosthetic devices.

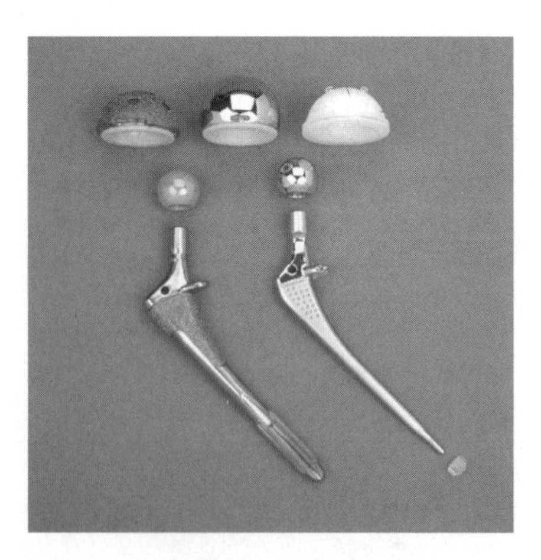

Figure 21-4 Hip Prostheses. *Left:* porous ingrowth acetabular cup and femoral stem, ceramic femoral head. *Middle:* bipolar head for hemiarthroplasty (component fits on top of femoral head component. Used with either cemented or uncemented femoral stems. *Right:* cemented femoral stem and cemented acetabular cup. (Courtesy Zimmer, Inc., Warsaw, IN.)

Fixation techniques are controversial; reports note osteolysis and loosening of cemented and cementless bone in growth sockets. Because of the high cost of revisions, cup fixation has become a major concern (Weber, Schaper, Pomeroy, Badenhausen, Smith, & Suthers, 2000).

Persons who have weight-bearing and hip precautions need close monitoring after hip surgery. Although weight bearing is restricted to reduce the distraction force on the prosthesis, those clients with cemented prostheses usually are allowed to bear weight as tolerated. Walkers and canes allow clients to apply part of their weight on their upper extremities and maintain proper balance and posture. Hip flexion, adduction, or rotation must be avoided after total hip arthroplasty; flexion is limited to 90 degrees for 2 to 3 months. Pillows or abduction splints are used whenever a client is in supine position until the hip capsule is healed to prevent adduction of the operative limb (Figure 21-5).

Another complication from hip replacement surgery is

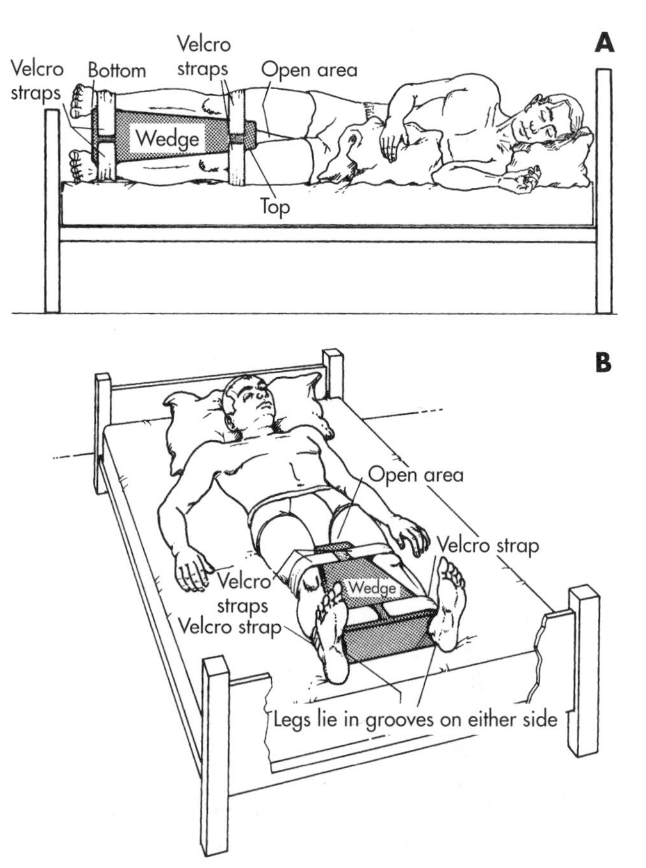

Figure 21-5 **A,** A client who has a hip fracture or hip replacement surgery is positioned on his uninvolved side. His affected hip is slightly flexed. A foam wedge (or pillows) is used to keep his legs apart and abduct the hip joints. Note the 90-degree angle limit of flexion at the hip. **B,** The same client viewed from the front illustrates the use of the foam wedge (or pillows) between his knees and legs. These supports keep the hip joints abducted. The top or affected knee must be supported firmly and steadily; it must not fall off of the wedge. His knees must not be allowed to touch one another. (From Hoeman, S.P. [1990]. *Rehabilitation/restorative care.* St. Louis: Mosby.)

infection at the incision site characterized by a dull ache or unusual or persistent pain. Early signs include fever, redness, swelling, or drainage at the surgical site and increased pain. Infections may be treated with intravenous antibiotic administration and sterile wound care techniques. Because more than half of the infections occur at least 3 months after joint replacement and more than 2 years postoperatively, discharge instructions must include ways to avoid infection and the necessity of antibiotic treatment. Instances of systemic bacterial infections have been documented.

Prophylactic antibiotics may be recommended before dental procedures based on a joint statement issued by the American Dental Association and the American Academy of Orthopaedic Surgeons (1997). The statement defines clients at risk for complications as those with immunocompromised status, such as with RA and SLE, type 1 diabetes mellitus, hemophilia, malnourished status, or previous joint replacement and those within the first 2 years after joint placement.

Client education programs may help to prevent postoperative complications, reduce pain levels, and promote recovery for progress during therapy (Sedlak, Doheny, & Jones, 2000) and improve the quality of life pre- and postoperatively (Knutsson & Engberg, 1999). Clients, families, and the rehabilitation team are responsible for adhering to precautions and being aware of the time span they require.

Total knee replacement often is needed bilaterally and is completed during a single surgical event. Bilateral knee x-rays shown in Figure 21-6 demonstrate the condition of

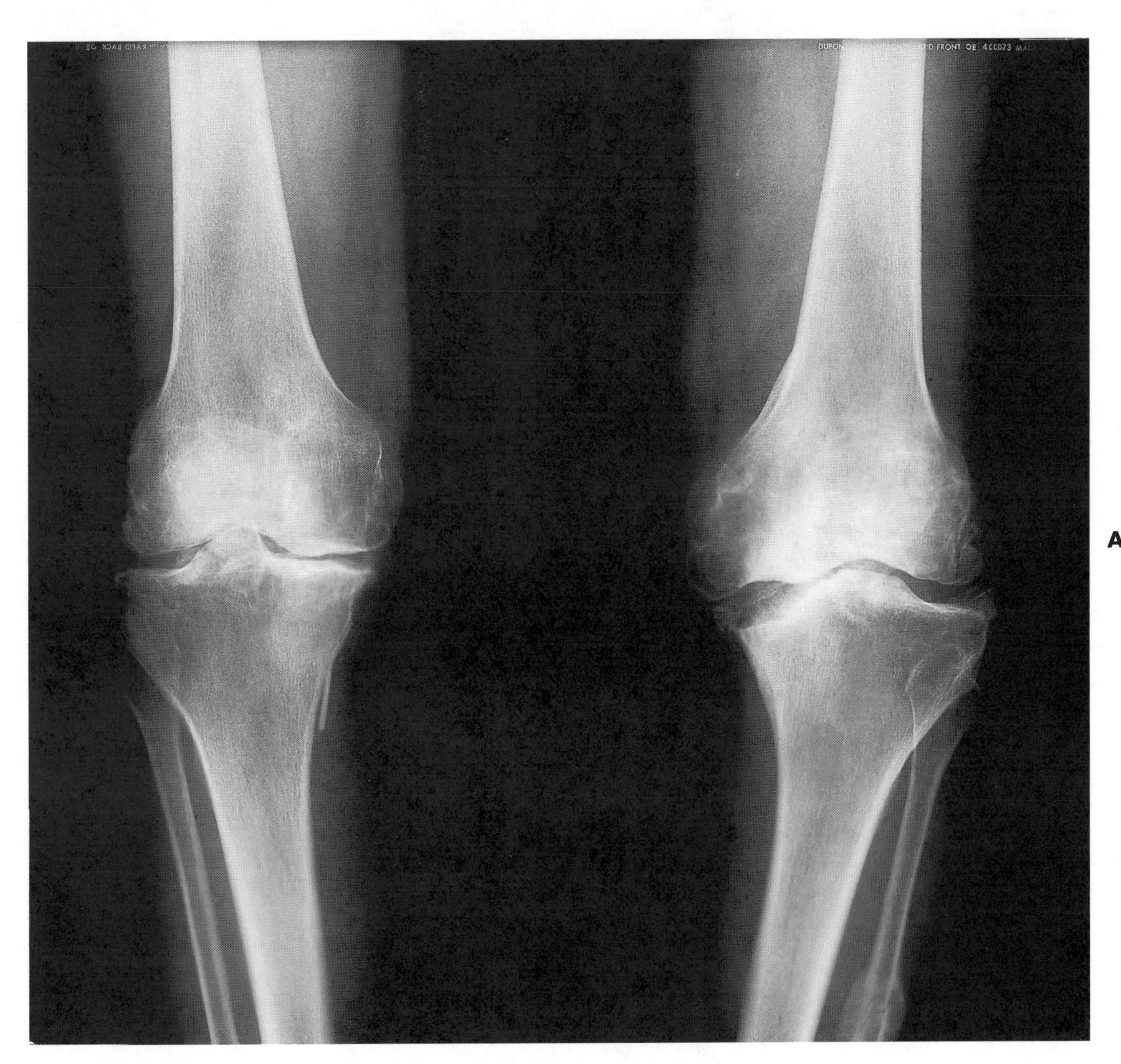

Figure 21-6 **A,** Radiograph of osteoarthritis of the knee. (Courtesy Stryker Howmedica Osteonics, Allendale, NJ.)

Continued

B

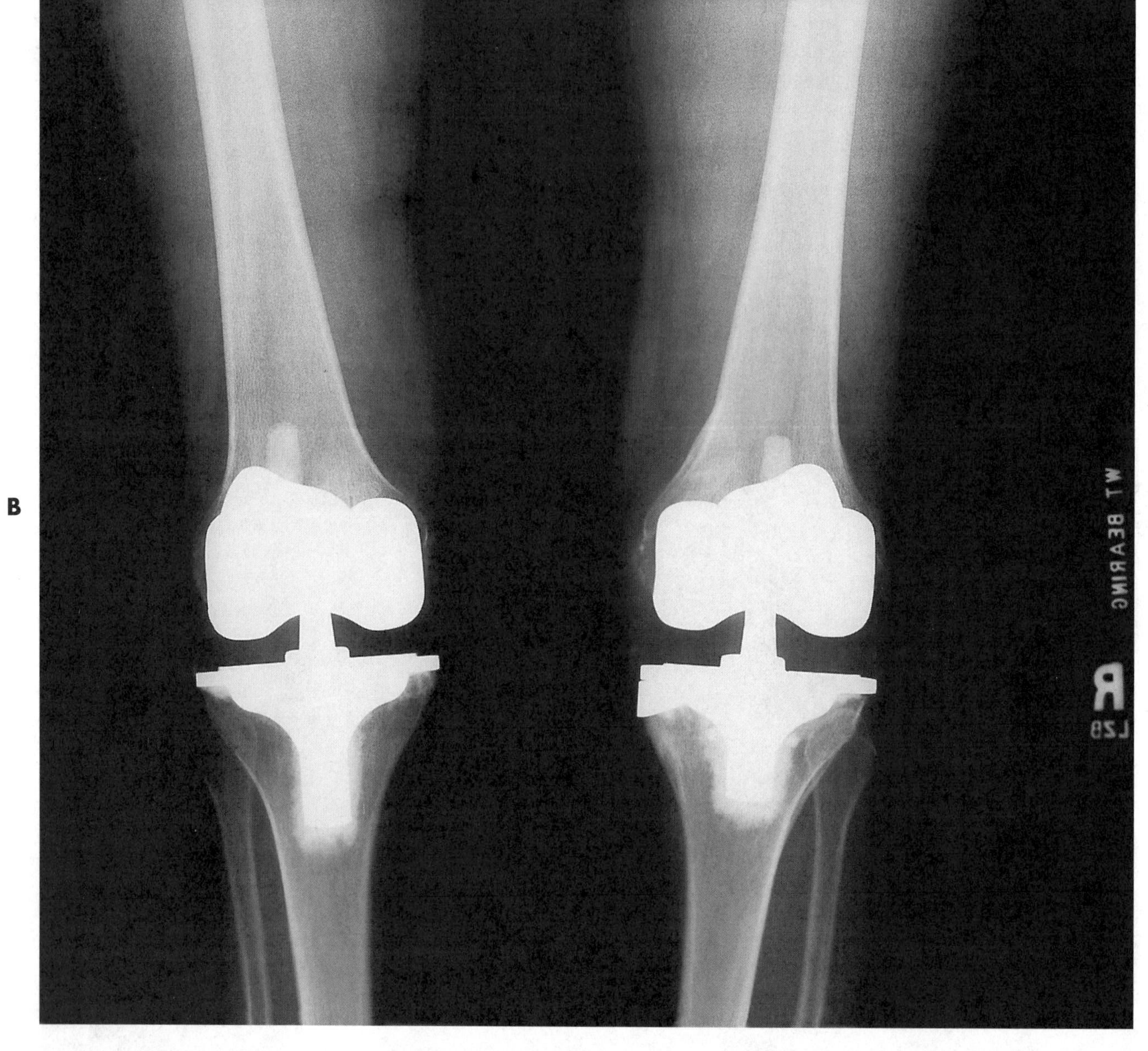

Figure 21-6, cont'd **B,** Radiograph of Duracon PS Total Knee System implants. (Courtesy Stryker Howmedica Osteonics, Allendale, NJ; and Anthony Hedley, MD, St. Luke's Medical Center, Phoenix, AZ.)

the joints before *(A)* and after *(B)* surgery with internal prosthetic implants. Mobilization may be more challenging, but improved ambulatory function in these weight-bearing joints can improve quality of life in a short period. Continuous passive motion (CPM) machines sometimes are used in the immediate postoperative phase of total knee replacement surgery, but do not replace joint range of motion exercises or ambulation during therapy. The CPM machine is complementary to therapy programs to increase the degree of movement. Findings from studies of surgeries for various types of DJD will be beneficial in weighing the risks versus benefits for clients at greater risk because of their premorbid or coexisting conditions.

Some surgical procedures may be performed in attempts to relieve pain or correct deformities. For example, fusion of bony joints may be a last resort for severe pain and defomity. Surgeries are performed for fractures and tumors. Phipps et al. (1999) provide the following definitions:

- Laminectomy—removal of a portion of the lamina, the posterior arch of the vertebra to access the disk and spinal canal
- Discectomy—removal of all or part of a herniated intervertebral disk
- Foraminotomy—widening of the intervertebral foramen to allow free passage of the spinal nerve
- Spinal fusion—stabilization of two or more vertebrae by inserting bone grafts, with or without hardware to gain vertebral stability

TABLE 21-4 Energy Conservation Technique

Technique	Example
Take your time	Plan ahead; stay with schedule
Rest breaks	Rest 10 minutes for every hour of activity; 30-45 minutes after meals
Sit down	Adapt activities to perform from sitting position
Avoid extreme temperatures	Do outdoor activities on cool days; use a fan when cooking or ironing; keep water and juices in the refrigerator; use an electric blanket
Avoid extra movements	Plan ahead all items needed for an activity; make bed while still in it; put clothing in easy to reach locations; put underwear inside pants to put on together
Keep frequently used items in easy reach	Avoid bending, reaching, and stooping; keep items at arm level
Ask for help	If an activity is exhausting, get assistance with the task
Analyze your activities	Watch for stress signals (chest pain, shortness of breath, sweating, fatigue); start small and build up; use a rolling cart and work in a circle
Use good posture	Sit and stand straight; do not cross your legs
Use correct body mechanics	Use two hands; use smooth movements that flow; slide or roll objects; push objects instead of pulling on them

Adapted from Romanik, K. (1994). *Around the clock with C.O.P.D.: Helpful hints for respiratory (chronic obstructive pulmonary disease) patients.* East Hartford, CT: American Lung Association.

- Decompression—release of pressure or impingement on spinal nerve roots by removal of osteophytes, bone, or soft tissue

Client and family education, including discussions about pharmacological and nonpharmacological agents occurs before interventions. Fusion after trauma to the spine may be performed in an emergency situation to prevent complications of cord compression. Explanations detail intended results, side effects, precautions, and possible complications or risk of paralysis for clients as part of their informed consent in weighing the potential benefits of increased function and decreased pain. The rehabilitation nurse encourages dialogue about previous pain management strategies and activities that may aggravate pain. Clients may take analgesics before exercise or certain activities during therapy that may increase discomfort so they manage the pain, reduce anxiety, and participate fully. Education and full information build trust in relationships and increase possibilities for improved outcomes.

Activity Intolerance

The nursing diagnosis of activity intolerance is defined as abnormal responses to energy-consuming body movements involved in required or desired daily activities (Gordon, 2000). Activity intolerance may be related to pain, discomfort, or muscle weakness; energy management, relaxation techniques, and stress reduction may increase a client's tolerance for activities.

Energy Management

Energy management is defined as regulating energy use to treat or prevent fatigue and optimize function (McCloskey & Bulechek, 2000). After assessing a client's physical limitations, perception of fatigue, and feelings about the situation, the rehabilitation nurse seeks potential sources of fatigue. Chronic and disabling conditions can cause pain and fatigue; medication regimen, nutritional intake, and sleep patterns may contribute. Clients with reduced independence in ADLs may need assistance from a caregiver and use of adapted or assistive devices to conserve energy, such as utensils with built-up handles. Clients who are able to walk independently at home may combat fatigue by using a wheelchair to move through the community.

Clients who experience extreme fatigue work with the rehabilitation nurse to schedule their physical activities and find other ways to reduce demands for oxygen supply to vital body functions. Conditions such as RA cause clients to experience variations in energy and pain levels. Planning for rest periods may pace a client until the component steps of activities can be relearned and better endured. Performing activities during periods when the client has the most energy and arranging commonly used items in convenient places on shelves and in kitchen cabinets helps conserve strength. Table 21-4 explains several energy conservation techniques recommended for those clients who have conditions that produce variations in energy and pain levels.

Treatment recommendations regarding energy management for PPS have changed over the years (Table 21-5). After the polio epidemic of the 1950s, clients were told to exert maximal energy by training hard, being as active as possible, trying to blend into society, making the best of their situation, and managing in society. Society considered institutionalization appropriate because the clients were not viewed as peers (Ahlstrom & Karlsson, 2000). Some clients responded by overly achieving, trying to fit in, and minimizing the impairments created by polio. In the current culture, persons with PPSe are accepted and included in society and

TABLE 21-5 Interventions for Postpolio Syndromes

Symptoms	Treatments
Generalized fatigue	Energy conservation; weight-loss program; lower extremity orthoses
Muscle weakness	Strengthening exercises; physical activity pacing with rest periods; avoid overuse of weakened muscles
Bulbar muscle weakness (respiratory failure and dysphagia)	Noninvasive positive-pressure ventilation at night and as needed; tracheostomy and permanent ventilation may be necessary; instruct on swallowing techniques
Pain and joint instability	Reduce stress on joints and muscles through lifestyle changes; weight loss; avoid overworking muscles; return to use of assistive devices; antiinflammatory medications
Cardiopulmonary conditioning	Upper extremity exercise program; aquatic exercise

Adapted from Jubelt, B., & Agre, J. (2000). Characteristics and management of postpolio syndrome. *Journal of the American Medical Association, 284,* 412-414.

encouraged to conserve or improve existing muscle strength to help maintain independence (Klein, Whyte, Keenan, Esquenazi, & Polansky, 2000). Rehabilitation methods and equipment can improve function, namely orthotic devices made of lightweight material, alterations to the home, ergonomic modifications to work settings, appropriate levels of exercise, and selected physical therapy activities (Gandevia, Allen, & Middleton, 2000).

Relaxation, Prayer, and Stress Management

Progressive muscle relaxation techniques, guided imagery, and stress management are known to reduce pain and muscle spasms, and improve sleep for clients with FMS. Heat therapy, stretching techniques, massage, and relaxation programs help relax muscles and thus reduce spasms. Transcutaneous electrical nerve stimulation, gentle massage, acupuncture, acupressure, spray and stretch treatments, and biofeedback may be effective when used complementary to medications and exercise (Smith, 1998). Assessing and mobilizing clients' strength according to their belief system helps the rehabilitation nurse provide spiritual support (Gruca, 2000). Research findings show that spiritual care, especially prayer, supplements and brings about inner strengthening (O'Brien, 1999). Prayer has been studied as a method for either singly or collectively accessing a power greater than oneself to overcome adversities.

Client and Family Education

Support groups specific to a problem can help clients share problems and solutions for energy conservation because ideas come from those who have dealt with obstacles of pain and fatigue in their own lives. Likewise, rehabilitation nurses can share information gained through their knowledge and experiences during formal or informal educational sessions with clients and caregivers.

Self-Care Deficit

Self-care activities to carry out tasks of daily living include personal hygiene, grooming, dressing, eating, and toileting. Hoeman states that this process allows individuals to function in their immediate environment to meet basic needs. The level of participation must be correlated according to the client's extent of injury, degree of impairment, and length of time since the onset of the disorder. Sensitivity to the client's lifestyle and preferences enables the nurse to individualize self-care goals. Understanding the client's beliefs and readiness to learn can help the nurse prepare to teach techniques to maximize independent functioning. Self-care activities are directed by the client's strengths, abilities, preferences, lifestyles, and participation (Hoeman, 1996).

Performing self-care activities without some level of assistance is related to the amount of muscle stiffness and weakness or pain; client and family education addresses ways for meeting self-care needs. Alternative approaches are attractive to clients with chronic pain. Peck (1998) compared the effects of therapeutic touch (TT) with that of progressive muscle relaxation (PMR) in improving functional ability of elderly clients with RA. Therapeutic touch promoted functional ability better than PMR in this study. Peck also demonstrated TT to be effective in relieving pain for elderly clients with degenerative arthritis (1997); however, results cannot be generalized to other populations (Peck, 1998).

In addition to TT, using analgesics, stretching, and joint range of motion exercises to manage pain before engaging in activity helps to minimize discomfort and maximize functional capacity. An array of assistive devices can aid clients in performing tasks safely and independently. For instance, after THR, clients use an elevated commode seat to avoid hip flexion past 90 degrees and a long-handled, lightweight reacher to grasp items without bending or flexing the hip joint. Other assistive devices help clients to conserve energy during dressing, grooming, or performing personal hygiene while adhering to precautions (Figures 21-7 and 21-8). Clients with limited joint range of motion maximize their independence in dressing and self-care with modifications, such as large buttons or zippers with loop pull tabs, Velcro fasteners, stretchable material, or elastic shoelaces.

Assistive devices also aid in donning and doffing prostheses. Elastic shoelaces, Velcro fasteners, and long-handled

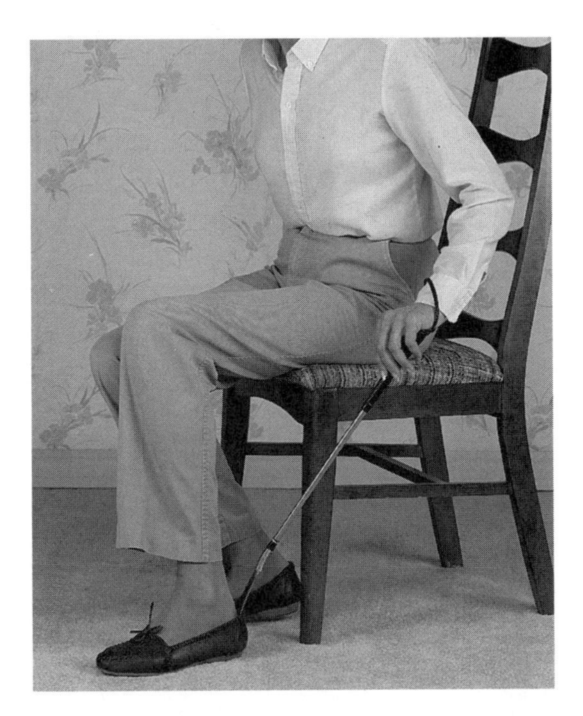

Figure 21-7 Long-handled shoehorn. (Courtesy Sammons Preston, Bolingbrook, IL.)

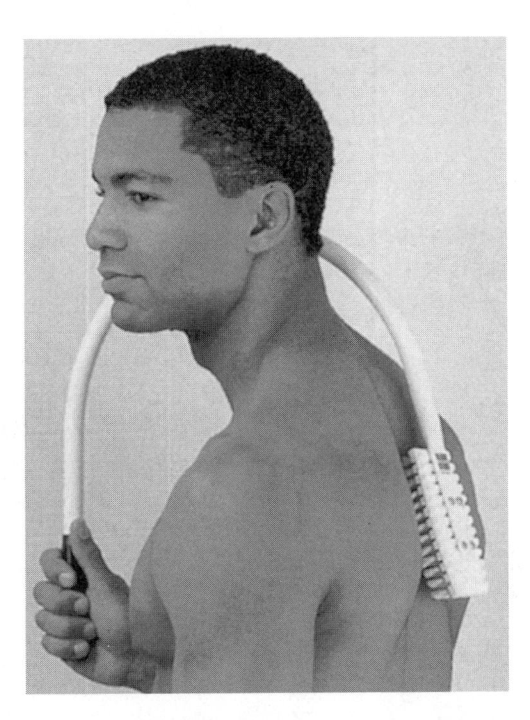

Figure 21-8 Long handles on brushes enable clients to perform their own bathing activities. (Courtesy Sammons Preston, Bolingbrook, IL.)

shoehorns enable clients to put socks and shoes on despite limited fine motor coordination or dexterity. The Utah Arm, an example of a motor-driven upper extremity prosthesis, allows greater independence in self-care and work skills (Figure 21-9). The Boston Elbow is a variation on this prosthesis

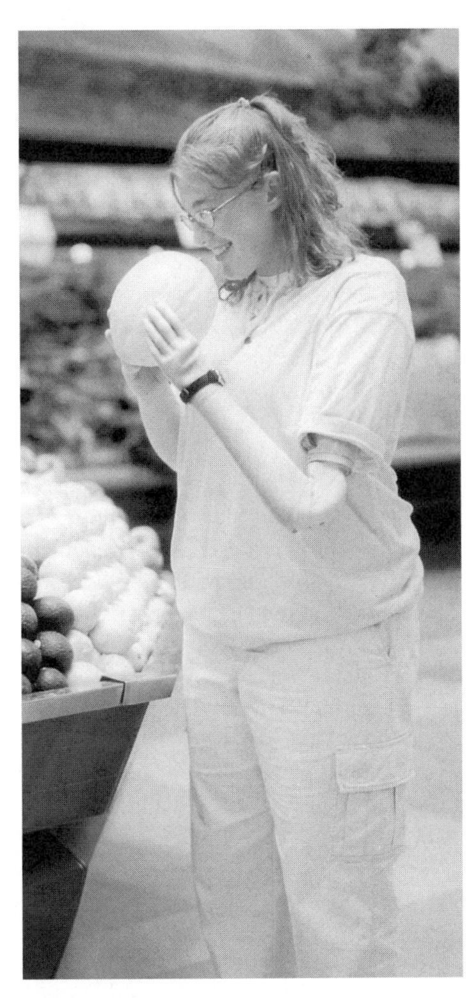

Figure 21-9 The Utah arm is a myoelectric elbow and hand system developed to enable clients with above and below elbow amputations to function independently and with high levels of skill in their daily activities and work. The Utah myoelectric arm features proportional control. (Courtesy 10 MED, Inc., Salt Lake City, UT.)

that features digital control circuitry and computer software for adjustments (Albertson, 1999). Various adaptive devices are introduced to the client and family members as recovery progresses to include independent self-care. The therapist and rehabilitation nurse evaluate a client's readiness to learn, cognitive ability, and strength and endurance when selecting devices or practicing new techniques. Clients may not accept the need for assistive devices initially; they may need time to adjust to an altered body image. A willingness to perform self-care tasks may signal the clients' acceptance and readiness to master self-care and employ assistive devices. Chapter 14 discusses more about assistive devices and adapted equipment.

Impaired Physical Mobility

Impaired physical mobility may be related to muscle weakness, joint swelling or pain, and degeneration of bone or muscle, or absence of an extremity. The impairment may be temporary, as in the case of a fracture or meniscus tear, or long-term, as with osteoarthritis. Rehabilitation is of paramount importance in either instance and at all levels of care. For example, short-term rehabilitation after a fracture—a tertiary intervention—is really primary prevention in that it prevents long-term mobility problems.

Various forms of traction are used to enable a client to mobilize during the healing of a musculoskeletal injury or after reconstructive surgery. Skeletal traction paraphernalia can be attached to a trapeze device on a hospital-style bed or affixed to the individual to promote mobilization. Halo traction is applied to the head of the individual to stabilize the bony structure and promote correct positioning during the healing process (Figure 21-10). The Ilizarov device is a form of external traction shown in Figure 21-11. The external fixation device is designed to lengthen the distance between the approximal ends of a bone by separating them in traction; simultaneously fixing them in alignment as they grow back together. Each institution establishes procedures for care of the pin sites and for specific use of external fixation devices. Literature review findings recommending standardization of an effective method of performing care of a pin site are listed in Box 21-2; appropriate materials and techniques prevent complications (Olson, 1996). The rehabilitation nurse assesses extremities, performs site care, promotes wound healing, ensures safe maintenance of external fixation devices, and encourages optimal mobility for clients while fractures are healing.

Box 21-2 Pin Site Care Protocol for Hospital Use

1. Inspect for signs and symptoms of infection.
2. Cleanse pin sites with antimicrobial soap and normal saline. Use sterile cotton tipped applicator. Rinse with sterile normal saline.
3. If crusting is present: wrap pin site with saline-soaked gauze for 20 minutes. Remove with sterile cotton-tipped applicator soaked in saline, using gentle rolling motion. Avoid vigorous cleaning.
4. Perform pin site care *daily* if there are no signs and symptoms of infection. If crusting or drainage present, perform every shift.
5. Lab test for culture and sensitivity when signs and symptoms of infection noted. Physician will then order systemic or topical antibiotic treatment.

From Olson, R. (1996). Halo skeletal traction pin site care: Toward developing a standard of care. *Rehabilitation Nursing, 21,* 243-246, 257.

Figure 21-10 Halo vest. Note the rigid shoulder straps and encompassing vest. Various vest sizes are available prefabricated. The halo ring, superstructure, and vest are magnetic resonance imaging compatible.

A

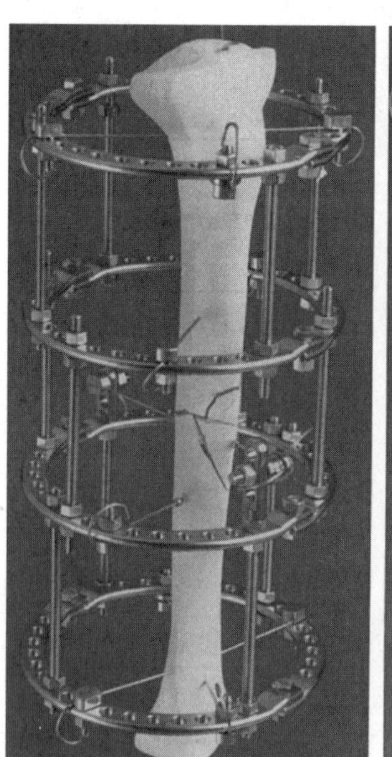

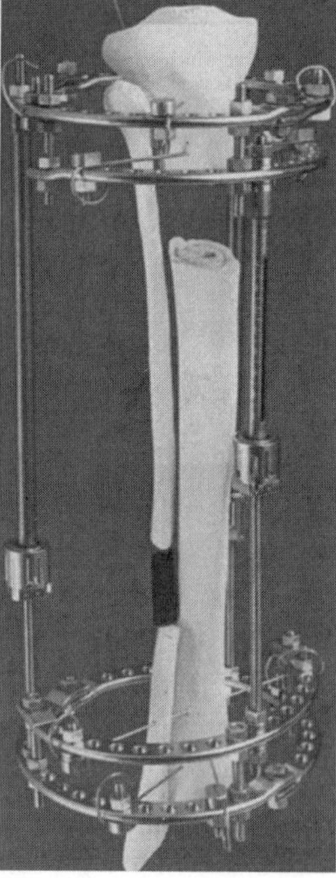

B

Figure 21-11 **A,** Ilizarov device in place to treat comminuted fracture. **B,** Ilizarov device assembly for lengthening of tibia. (Courtesy Smith & Nephew, Memphis, TN.)

Exercise Promotion and Therapy

Exercise regimens tailored to clients' specific conditions also offer opportunities for them to participate in altering the course of their disease, such as by maintaining muscle strength and mobility. An individualized treatment plan targets relief of pain, control of inflammation, maintenance of joint integrity, and maximization of function (Gremillion, 1998); goals must be realistic and acceptable to the client.

Interventions for Specific Conditions

Rheumatoid Arthritis. Exercise programs for clients with RA are based on the severity of the disease and rate of progression, the client's energy, fatigue, and emotional status, along with their knowledge or education and support system. Goals of an exercise regimen are for clients to achieve joint range of motion (JROM), strength, to preserve function, and employ aggressive pain management. For example, in acute-stage inflammation resulting from RA, goals simply are to maintain JROM, strength and endurance, while resting affected joints to reduce pain and inflammation. During the subacute stage of inflammation, efforts change to increase JROM, strength, and endurance. After RA becomes chronic, rehabilitation targets resuming previously independent levels of activity, including work.

Osteoarthritis. Exercise prescriptions for persons with osteoarthritis center on the three principles of daily exercise, general fitness, and exercise progression. Clients are encouraged to participate so they can maintain muscle strength maximize range of motion, and reduce complications from joint deterioration. Moderate activities can be introduced and accomplished gradually, such as walking on smooth surfaces, swimming, stationary bicycling, and low-impact aerobics. Community programs are available for most of these activities (Medical Multimedia Group, 2001).

Joint protection, important during all activities, is augmented through muscle conditioning and controlling movement. Aids to ambulation, such as canes, crutches, and walkers, alleviate stress to weight-bearing joints. Clients should prevent high-impact shock to the joints by wearing good quality shoes, selecting soft walking surfaces, such as grass or cinder rather than cement, and choosing low-impact exercises, such as water aerobics or stationary bicycling. Proper joint alignment protects joints from extra pressure; bracing and orthotic shoe inserts with a heel wedge relieve pain and pressure (Medical Multimedia Group, 2001).

Redesigning daily activities can limit strain on joints. Recommendations include limited standing or stair climbing, frequent rest periods, parking close to destinations, and using assistive devices such as elevated beds, chairs, and commodes. The Americans with Disabilities Act contains provisions to improve access in the community for persons with impairments, such as special automobile license plates that permit parking in reserved locations. Clients and families participate with the interdisciplinary team to identify and activate creative interventions that match client goals, abilities, and lifestyle preferences.

Fibromyalgia. FMS requires a multifaceted treatment approach. Exercise is believed to be the most effective component to reducing pain and strengthening muscles. A structured program of moderate physical activity reduces symptoms of pain, tenderness, muscle stiffness, and sleep disturbance. Exercise begins very slowly and builds over time to prevent overexertion. Low-impact aerobics may avoid overtaxing the muscles and exacerbating pain while preventing muscle atrophy and reducing fatigue and pain (Well-Connected, 1999).

Cardiovascular fitness training or simple flexibility training, water exercise, and group education increased the distance clients with FMS were able to walk, improved their sense of well being, and reduced fatigue (Smith, 1998).

Postpolio Syndrome. Clients with PPS also benefit from exercises to reduce fatigue. Because cardiovascular deconditioning and weight gain occur with aging, exercise is important to the care plan. However, lower aerobic capacity combined with higher body weight may contribute to increasing polio-related symptoms and disability (Stanghelle & Festvag, 1997); and exertion during walking may produce pain of varying intensities (Willen & Grimby, 1998). Thus, although moderate exercises improve muscle strength, individual exercise programs are essential; the balance between disuse and overuse is quite narrow. Aquatic exercise programs may strengthen muscles and improve cardiovascular fitness. Client participation is necessary to establish nutrition regimens that avoid obesity, accommodate appropriate rest and exercise, and foster optimal independence using assistive devices and adaptation techniques as necessary.

Clients who develop new weakness with PPS may benefit from mild to moderate exercise that does not cause them fatigue. The exercises rely on clients exerting both submaximal and maximal strength in combination with repetitions of short duration alternated with short intervals of rest. Bulbar (brainstem nuclei) muscle weakness is a concern and may lead to respiratory failure, dysphagia, and sleep apnea (Jubelt & Agre, 2000). Strengthening muscles used in respiration may improve outcomes, such as with incentive spirometry. Many clients find using noninvasive positive-pressure ventilation during the night provides needed rest and enables them to have more independent respiratory function during the day.

Ambulation Techniques

Safety is an important goal for any client who experiences a musculoskeletal disorder, whether it is a simple ankle sprain, a gouty great toe, or an above-the-knee amputation. Altered gait patterns require the interdisciplinary team to assess mobility and develop a plan to retrain and strengthen muscles, ligaments, and tendons. However, a client's health status, financial situation, acceptance of adaptive and assistive devices, home environment, and available caregivers directly influence the plan for care.

An accessible environment is essential to optimal function in ambulation and requires a detailed home and community assessment. Chapters 9 and 14 contain more information. On-site evaluations conducted during the hospital stay or by community health nurses or therapists at discharge include measurements of doorways, evaluation of stairs, bathrooms, and kitchen areas. Family and caregivers assist in preparing a safe environment. Many clients will use safety devices that notify selected friends or relatives should a problem such as a fall occur; Lifeline is an example of a call-response system. Walkers, crutches, and canes assist clients to ambulate during the initial phase of rehabilitation after hip and knee surgery (Figure 21-12 and Table 21-6), some will advance to walking without a device by discharge. Proper measurement of the device, training, and education ensure safe ambulation; wheelchairs, walkers, and placing stationary chairs for the client to rest in help the transition to home.

Ambulation in the community is a challenge after hospitalization; caregivers need training for assisting clients to make a safe transfer to a car, perform basic wheelchair maintenance, and identify community resources for transportation. Manual wheelchairs and motorized carts are often available in shopping malls, airports, and theaters, but gaining access to events using a wheelchair or scooter requires making phone calls and planning in advance. Successful social experiences promote self-confidence and life satisfaction.

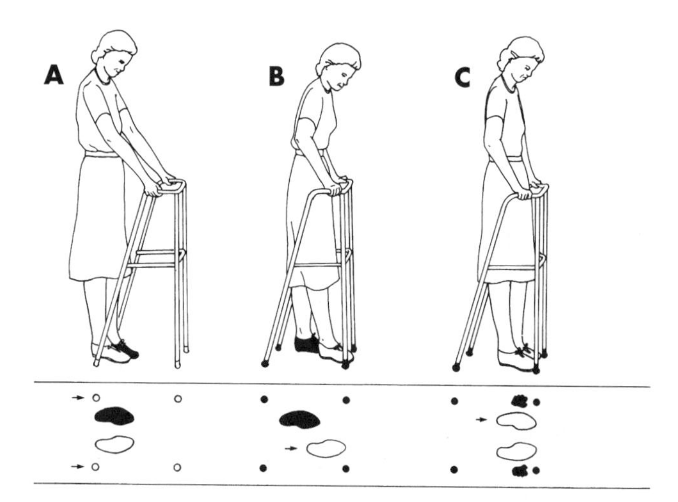

Figure 21-12 **A** to **C,** Technique of walking with a double-support device. (From Hoeman, S.P. [1990]. *Rehabilitative and restorative care in the community.* St. Louis: Mosby.)

Children with muscular dystrophy may be able to maintain functional ambulation after lower limb musculotendinous releases; 70% to 76% of clinics performed this intervention, which allows for ambulation without bracing and less physical therapy. Use of long leg braces has declined in recent years, possibly as a result of earlier surgical interventions or increased costs of orthoses (Bach & Chaudhry, 2000).

After an amputation, the residual limb initially is wrapped with elastic bandages using the figure-eight technique (Figure 21-13). The bandages help control edema and conform the distal site for future prosthetic application. Functional ambulation for persons with amputations was discussed previously in this chapter. Advances in technology have increased prosthesis choices, such as ultralight-weight components of titanium and carbon fiber composites, improved cosmetic appearance, and functional flexibility; enabling some to set realistic goals to walk without assistive devices (Figure 21-14) (Zaffer, Braddom, Conti, Goff, & Bokma, 1999). Many clients conduct activities in their home and community independently as a result, in part, of rehabilitation interventions; impatient stays are especially beneficial (Gauthier-Gagnon, Grise, & Potvin, 1999). Resources for clients who have had an amputation are listed in Box 21-3.

Client and Family Education for Improving Mobility

Goals for exercise, therapy, and ambulation are mutually set from the time of admission to final discharge from the acute rehabilitation unit, but also depend on the client and family

TABLE 21-6 Techniques of Walking with Ambulatory Aids*

Device	Gait
Double-support device (walker)	Walker is advanced first (Figure 21-12, *A*), then the involved extremity (Figure 21-12, *B*), then the uninvolved extremity (Figure 21-12, *C*)
Single-support device (cane, quad cane, single crutch)	Device is held in the hand opposite the involved leg Device and involved leg are advanced first, followed by the uninvolved leg
Crutches	Three-point gait—the same as walker gait Four-point gait—crutch, opposite leg, opposite crutch, other leg Two-point gait—both crutches, both legs (one leg may be non–weight bearing)

From Phipps, W., Sands, J., & Marek, J. (1999). *Medical-surgical nursing: Concepts and clinical practice* (6th ed.). St. Louis: Mosby.
*Climbing up stairs is accomplished by moving the uninvolved leg first, then the device and the involved leg; to descend stairs, the involved leg and the device are moved first, then the uninvolved leg. The device and the involved leg always move together.

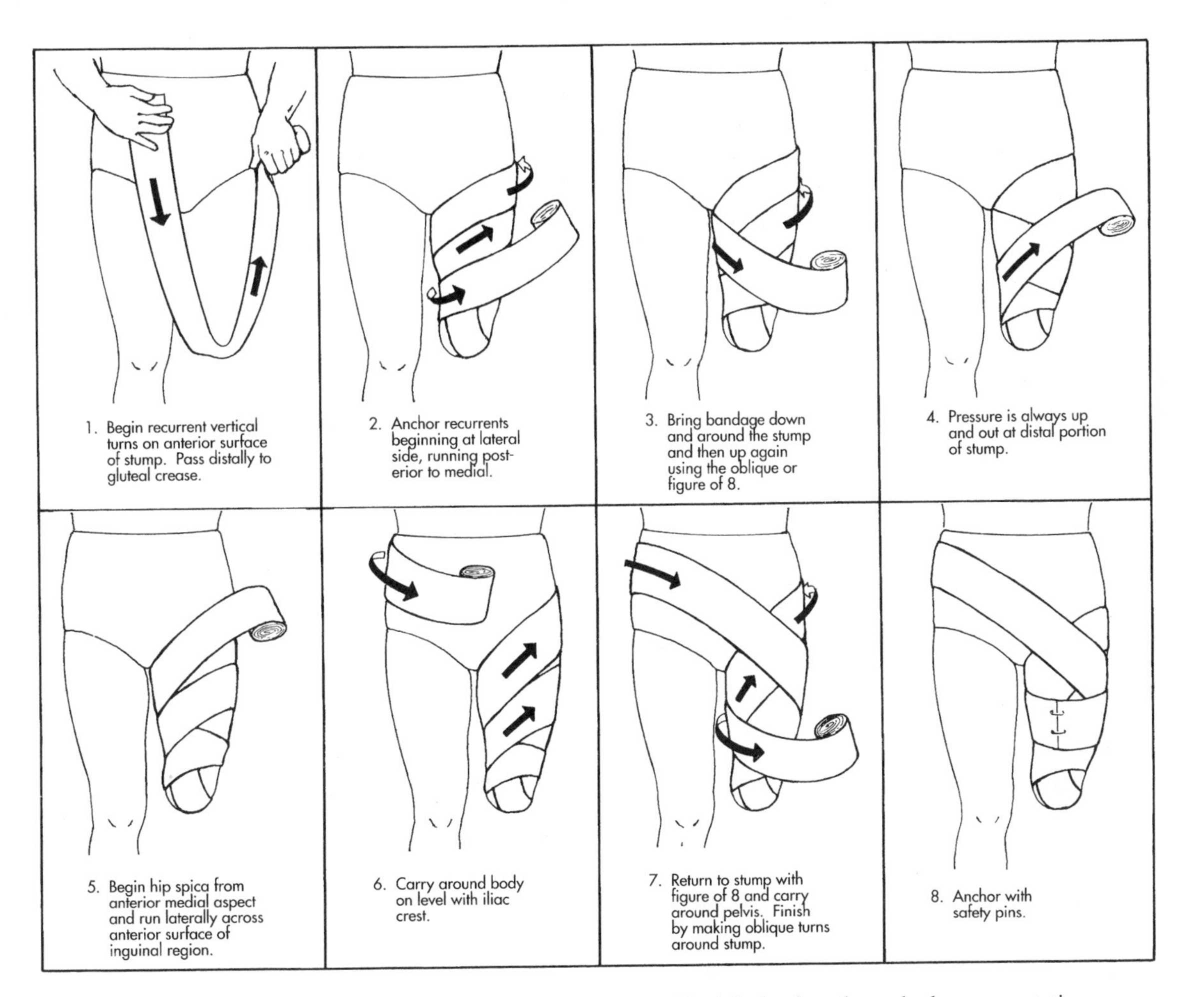

Figure 21-13 Method of wrapping to help shape the residual limb after above-the-knee amputation. (From Mourad, L.A. [1991]. *Orthopedic disorders.* St. Louis: Mosby.)

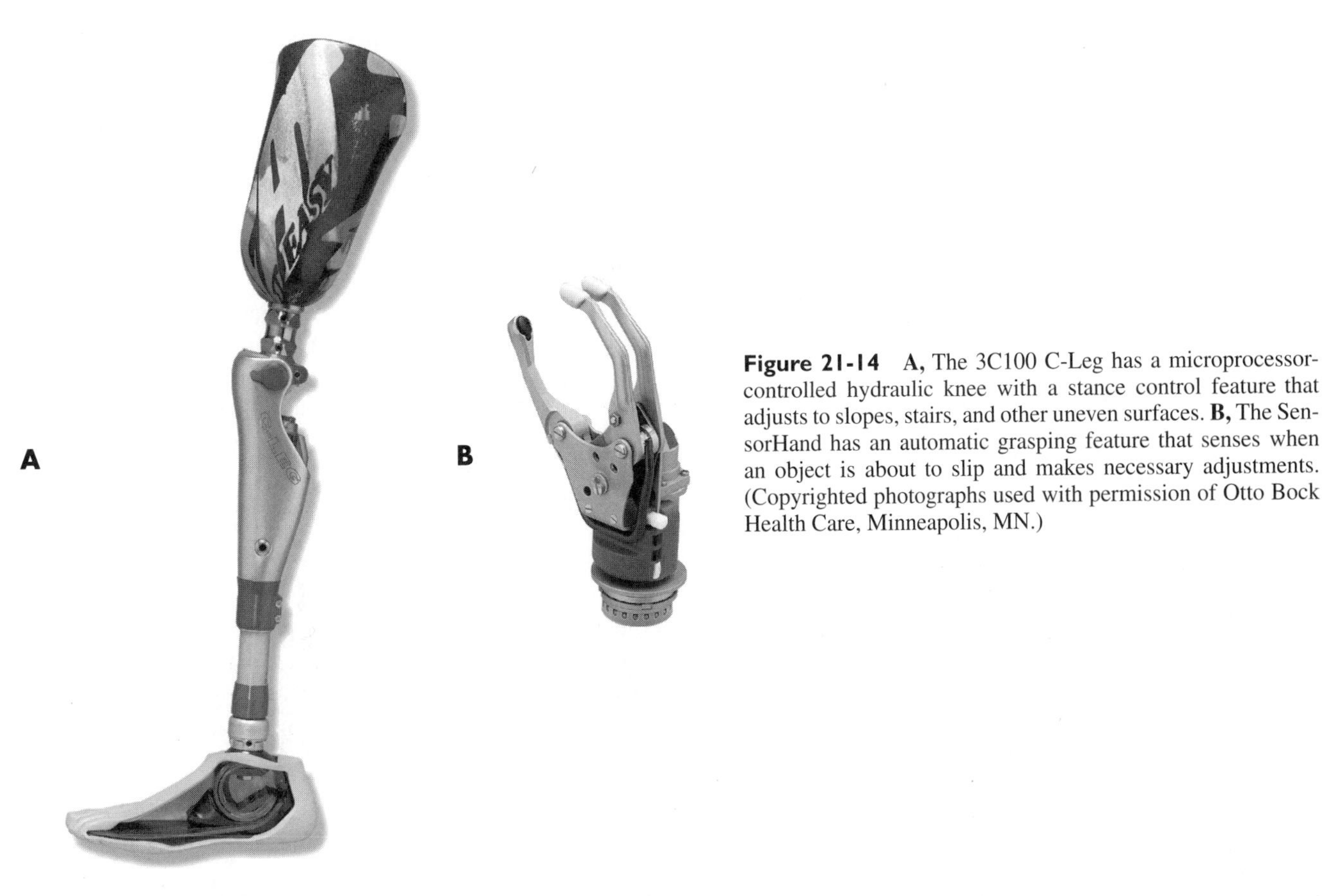

Figure 21-14 **A,** The 3C100 C-Leg has a microprocessor-controlled hydraulic knee with a stance control feature that adjusts to slopes, stairs, and other uneven surfaces. **B,** The SensorHand has an automatic grasping feature that senses when an object is about to slip and makes necessary adjustments. (Copyrighted photographs used with permission of Otto Bock Health Care, Minneapolis, MN.)

Box 21-3 National and World Resources for Amputation

Amputee Coalition of America
900 East Hill Avenue, Suite 285
Knoxville, TN 37915-2568
888-267-5669
http://www.amputee-coalition.org

Amputee Support Group
West Gate Baptist Church
2235 Old Harrisburg Pike
Lancaster, PA 17601
717-898-8384

Amputees in Motion International
PO Box 2703
Escondido, CA 92033
619-454-9300

National Amputation Foundation
73 Church Street
Malverne, NY 11565
516-887-3600

United Amputee Services Association, Inc.
PO Box 4277
Winter Park, FL 32793-4277
407-678-2920

Adapted from DD in site. (Retrieved December 29, 2000.) *The tech knowledge developmental disability resource for Georgia* [On-line]. Available: http://www.arch.gatech.edu/crt/techknow/medconditions/amputation.htm.

readiness to learn and participate. Education about various external fixation devices focuses on preventing complications of infection (Olson, 1996). Preventive care for braces and casts emphasizes maintaining skin integrity, sensation, and circulation. A community health nurse or therapist may visit in the home, especially when a client uses assistive or immobilizing devices.

Body Image Disturbance

Negative feelings or perceptions about characteristics, functions, or limits of body or body part create a disturbance in body image (Gordon, 2000), a common nursing diagnosis for individuals with musculoskeletal disorders. Altered gait patterns, use of assistive devices or wheelchairs, deformities, rheumatoid nodules, loss of height, or a dowager's hump resulting from osteoporosis, easy bruising, or loss of an extremity all may affect body image.

Body image enhancement relates to improving clients' conscious and unconscious perceptions and attitudes toward their body (McCloskey & Bulechek, 2000). The impact of altered body image is significant for a young man who experiences muscle atrophy from spinal cord injury; an actress feels devastation with the effects of multiple trauma on her personal appearance. An elderly adult with diabetes mellitus is affected by an amputation, and again when the residual limb does not heal sufficiently to apply the prosthesis. Rehabilitation nurses conduct ongoing assessments of clients' expectations of body image based on their developmental stage and intervene with anticipatory guidance for predictable changes. Body image is directly related to a person's functional ability. The impact of changes may be reduced by having clients view pictures of persons using assistive devices in daily activities or recreation or handle tools that will be used to enhance their appearance and improve function. Timing is important; and adjustment is influenced by premorbid function, personal and cultural attitudes of the client, family, and community, and the degree or severity of changes. Rapid events after a spinal cord injury may be more traumatic than a gradual change in muscle mass from PPS or RA.

Additional interventions for persons with altered body image include involvement in peer support groups to encourage interactions with others when appropriate; some clients benefit from meeting someone with a similar experience in a private situation. Others become comfortable interacting in a support group after developing trust and rapport with a peer counselor. Professional counseling that focuses on the needs, problems, and feelings of the client and family or significant others to enhance and support coping, problem-solving, and interpersonal relationships may be indicated (McCloskey & Bulechek, 2000).

Pharmaceutical Management of Selected Musculoskeletal Disorders

Advances in pharmacological therapy slow the progression or alleviate symptoms of musculoskeletal disorders. Medications used to manage selected musculoskeletal conditions are discussed in the following section.

Osteoporosis

Medications used for osteoporosis management include alendronate (Fosamax), estrogen (Premarin), raloxifene (Evista) (these three approved for prevention), and calcitonin-salmon (Miacalcin),. Of these four medications, alendronate, calcitonin, and raloxifene are approved for treatment (Taft, Looker, & Cella, 2000). Easily administered and well-tolerated, calcitonin nasal spray (Miacalcin) has received attention for its role in the reducing osteoporotic vertebral fractures in postmenopausal women (Chestnut et al., 2000). Studies of hormone replacement therapy (HRT) and alendronate, used alone or in combination, examine their role in preserving BMD, an indicator of bone mass and risk of fracture. Biphosphonate drugs (alendronate and etidronate) increase bone mass density, whereas HRT and selective estrogen receptor modifiers act

Box 21-4 Alendronate (Fosamax) Guidelines for Administration

Take first thing in the morning
Drink 1 full glass (8 oz) of water with medication; be sure to take with water only
Do not eat or drink anything for 30 minutes to 1 hour after taking medication
Stay in an upright position during this period to minimize esophageal irritation
Do not lie down until after eating a meal after the 1 hour waiting period

Adapted from Herndon, R., & Mohandas, N. (Retrieved June 10, 2000). *Osteoporosis in multiple sclerosis: A frequent, serious, and under-recognized problem* [On-line]. Available: http://www.mscare.com.

to reduce bone loss by stabilizing bone turnover; both decrease the incidence of fractures (Tiras, Noyan, Yildiz, Yildirim, & Daya, 2000; Herndon & Mohandas, 2000). Precautions for the administration of alendronate are listed in Box 21-4.

Lyme Disease

Lyme disease is acquired from the bite of an infected tick, but is prevented if antimicrobial agents are administered within 72 hours (Well-Connected, 2001). Human recombinant outer-surface protein vaccine (LYMErix) is available to persons from 15 to 70 years old who are at high risk for exposure to ticks. Oral antibiotics, such as doxycycline, amoxicillin, and cefuroxime axetil, are effective first-line agents (Abramowicz, 2000b) requiring a 21- to 30-day treatment course. Intravenous antibiotics (usually ceftriaxone or cefotaxime) are administered for persistent or widespread disease (Well-Connected, 2001).

Reiter's Syndrome

Reiter's syndrome requires antibiotic treatment if a bacterium is isolated. When triggered by chlamydia, a 3-month course of doxycycline or a derivative has shortened the initial acute illness (Parker & Thomas, 2000).

Gout

Colchicine is taken at the first sign of an acute attack and may not be beneficial when administered after several days of symptoms. Diarrhea is a dose-related adverse effect. NSAIDs are considered first-line therapy with adequate renal function; corticosteroids are used when NSAIDs are contraindicated; however, the duration of prophylactic therapy using colchicine or NSAIDs is controversial. Prevention through losing weight, increasing fluid intake, eliminating alcohol consumption, eating low-fat and high-carbohydrate foods, and using rest and relaxation to reduce stress is preferable (Escott-Stump, 1992).

Fibromyalgia

Treatment for FMS includes tricyclic antidepressants for sleep and cyclobenzaprine (Flexeril) for muscle relaxation. Tricyclic antidepressants work to increase non–rapid eye movement stage 4 sleep by increasing serotonin levels. Sleep disturbance, myofascial pain, and depression, common in most FMS clients, may improve with tricyclics, such as amitriptyline (Elavil) and imipramine (Tofranil). Cyclobenzaprine (Flexeril) has significantly reduced muscle spasms and pain with FMS (Smith, 1998) and promotes sleep. Initial reports from research using human growth hormone to treat FMS are promising.

Rheumatoid Arthritis and Osteoarthritis

A new treatment for RA that targets white blood cells has demonstrated good response in early trials. The treatment removes B-lymphocytes, which are antibody-forming white blood cells. Normal cells make normal antibodies return to "reboot" the immune system. B-lymphocytes are removed using the new drug, rituximab (Mabthera) in conjunction with prednisone, a steroid, and cyclophosphamide, called Cytoxan. These medications are given intravenously during two separate administrations (Edwards, 2001). Etanercept (Enbrel) and leflunomide (Arava) are new drugs that fight only RA (Goad, 2001) and leave most of the immune system unaffected, targeting the area that causes the uncontrolled inflammation. Enbrel is an injectable medication taken twice weekly. It targets a protein that plays an important role in early inflammation. Arava, taken orally in a tablet, targets white blood cells. Clients who respond well to these medications can experience complete remission without signs of the disease. The drugs are used early in the course of the disease in an attempt to slow the progression. Side effects of Enbrel include redness and itching, pain, or swelling at the injection site. Side effects of Arava include diarrhea, skin rash, liver toxicity, and hair loss. The cost of Arava is almost $3,000 annually; Enbrel costs approximately $12,000 per year. Infliximab (Remicade) is another new medication that may improve joint function (Lipsky et al., 2000). Research will continue to determine the efficacy of these medications for treating persons with RA.

Steroids are used intermittently during acute flare-ups of RA and osteoarthritis. They may be given orally or intravenously, or through intraarticular injection into the affected joint providing relief for 2 to 3 months. New medications used with osteoarthritis of the knee involve a series of three to five injections into the knee joint. The medications hyaluronan (Hylagen), hylan G-F (Synvisc), and sodium hyaluronate (Supartz) work as substitutes for hyaluronic acid that normally is present in the joint space (Kee, 2000; Reuters Medical News, 2001).

Health Promotion and Prevention

Interventions aimed at health promotion and health prevention are important components of rehabilitation in all settings. They range from primary prevention, as with osteoporosis, to tertiary prevention of complications, such as avoiding shoulder subluxation with hemiplegia. Other interventions involve modifying or changing the environment and clients' lifestyle choices.

Osteoporosis

Primary prevention of osteoporosis focuses on a healthy lifestyle throughout the life span. Wellness programs promote weight-bearing exercise and healthy choices in nutrition, and adequate intake of calcium with vitamin D; those with lactose intolerance need special attention. Clients learn the benefits of not smoking and reducing or eliminating consumption of alcohol, caffeine, and carbonated beverages. Those who develop peak bone mass during adolescence can reduce the rate of bone loss later in life, especially with menopause.

Early screening for asymptomatic osteoporosis is now recommended by the National Osteoporosis Foundation. Bone density testing is appropriate for women younger than 65 years who are postmenopausal and have one or more additional risk factors for osteoporosis, and for all women older than 65 years (Taft et al., 2000).

When osteoporosis has developed, secondary interventions include redesigning activities to reduce physical demands of job tasks and using ergonomic principles to change the environment to reduce risk for injury. Ergonomics can be applied in a variety of settings and used in conjunction with physical conditioning, maintaining ideal body weight, and training for body mechanics to prevent or reduce the incidence of fractures related to osteoporosis. Steroid medications or decreased bone density along with limited weight bearing and decreased mobility lead to osteoporosis and fractures that are frequent and very serious among clients with multiple sclerosis (Herndon & Mohandas, 2000). Unfortunately, using drugs for one condition, such as diphenylhydantoin for multiple sclerosis, may contribute to bone loss and increase the risk of osteoporosis. After a fracture occurs, the deconditioning and immobility accompanying the healing process perpetuates bone loss.

Identifying these risks enables the rehabilitation nurse to promote the use of strategies such as low-impact exercises, nutritional supplements, and environmental modifications that promote safe ambulation. Education alone has not motivated individuals to change their behavior. Lifestyle changes in diet and exercise are more likely when the client is experiencing an acute episode such as a fracture, a functional decline, or altered body image. Gaining an understanding of the losses and fears associated with musculoskeletal dysfunction helps rehabilitation nurses provide meaningful and compassionate care.

Amputation

Prevention of amputations for persons with diabetes mellitus begins with blood sugar control. Intensive therapy resulting in clients maintaining tight blood glucose control has reduced the risk of peripheral neuropathy (nerve damage) that leads to amputations after type I and type 2 diabetes (McCarren, 1993; American Diabetes Association, 1999). Teaching the client with diabetes other prevention strategies, such as foot inspection and nail care, can prevent the pain and loss of mobility that accompanies amputation. Foot sensation assessment and skin inspection programs can help individuals of all ages prevent diabetic foot ulcers that can lead to numerous, expensive, and painful surgical interventions. Rehabilitation nurses conduct clinics or education programs in the community concerning wound management, diabetes care, and specialized programs about a balance between diet, exercise, and medication, and preventing complications.

Shoulder Subluxation

Careful positioning and passive range of movement (ROM) exercises can prevent pain associated with shoulder subluxation. Positioning is a key intervention in preventing many of the complications that may occur secondary to stroke. Proper techniques for transferring clients without pulling under the arms and by using wedges and pillows in bed and lap trays on wheelchairs are examples of preventive interventions. Other treatments used to prevent or alleviate shoulder pain include spasmolytic drugs, relaxation techniques, FES, and a plan of care for ROM and active movement with correct positioning to prevent nerve impingement (Hanger et al., 2000; Ikai et al., 1998).

Preventive measures are initiated early to prevent complications of shoulder dysfunction. Once used regularly, slings have been replaced by shoulder strapping. Slings may be contraindicated because they hold the arm in a position of internal rotation and adduction at the shoulder that encourages disuse, tone changes, and muscle shortening. The advantage of shoulder strapping is that because it is in constant use, even while showering, it reduces subluxation while allowing freedom of movement in the upper extremity. A disadvantage is that the material stretches and needs to be reapplied at least every 3 days. One layer of undertape (Hypafix) is applied to clean, dry, intact skin. Nonstretch tape (e.g., Elastoplast Sports tape) is applied in strips over the original layer (Hanger et al., 2000). The skin is inspected with each reapplication. Selection of a device should be done in collaboration with the client, physiatrist, nurse, and occupational therapist.

Repetitive Motion Injury

Workers, including those in health care, are prone to injury from performing repetitive motions in their job tasks. Even moderate exercise routines can strengthen muscles, maintain balance, and improve flexibility and coordination. Sports training programs emphasize warming up and stretching before beginning any exercise or workout or participating in sports or recreational activity. Devices that support and protect vulnerable or involved joints, such as elastic bandages, wrist splints, and knee and back braces prevent injury during repetitive movement, heavy lifting, or twisting when stress is placed on the joints. The devices are not intended to add a false sense of confidence about the capacity of the joint leading clients to overextend their limits with repetitive movements.

Prevention through Ergonomics

Ergonomics is a study of the work or home environment that results in adaptations or modifications for safe, effective, and accessible activity. The underlying principle is that by "fitting the job" to the worker by actions, such as adjusting the workstation, rotating between tasks, or using mechanical assists, stress on the musculoskeletal system can be reduced and ultimately eliminated (Occupational Safety and Health Association, 2000). Many work environments promote healthy living through ergonomic workstation assessment, educational programs, and incentives for participation in health facilities. An important component of the work environmental analysis involves education about positioning, proper body mechanics, periodic rest and stretch breaks, and stress reduction techniques all designed to prevent injuries. The adjustable height lift device pictured in Figure 21-15 illustrates how therapists who perform serial casting may use it to prevent back strain during these lengthy procedures. Many nursing interventions and techniques can be modified to prevent repetitive motion injuries. Creative problem solving is a role for rehabilitation nurses in evaluating work sites, modifying repetitive tasks, adapting routines or procedures, and educating clients during discharge planning; and incorporating ergonomic principles when teaching staff and others.

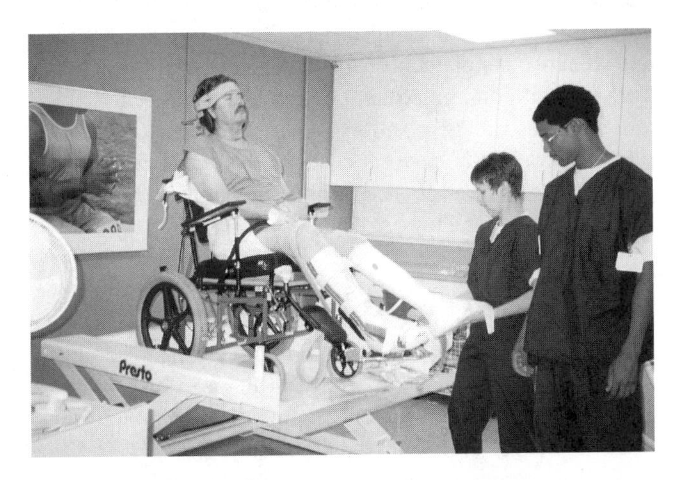

Figure 21-15 Use of a height adjustable platform creates an ergonomic workstation for rehabilitation staff doing frequent casting. (Courtesy the Institute for Rehabilitation and Research (TIRR), Houston, TX.)

Promoting a Healthy Lifestyle

Healthy lifestyle patterns often have roots in a family's social, cultural, or economic models. Those who practice a healthy lifestyle may have more motivation in related areas, such as accepting responsibility for self-care and adhering to therapeutic regimens. Healthy living is not compartmentalized, it occurs in the home, workplace, and with others in the community. Family modeling of regular exercise and activities, healthy choices in diet and maintaining the proper weight, and avoiding alcohol and other substances during a child's life can have a lasting behavioral effect on wellness. Persons with physical impairments may require adjustments in the mode of exercise, activities, or special diets, but overall they can lead a healthy lifestyle to enhance wellness and prevent complications or further disability. Industries can support the concept of healthy lifestyles by offering employee fitness centers on-site or discounts for private clubs, gyms, or community organizations, such as the YMCA. Stress management workshops, along with employee assistance programs, promote conflict resolution and resource management that convey the message of health promotion and wellness. Many musculoskeletal problems result from or are exacerbated by stressors. A proactive approach to employee wellness communicates that the organization values their employees and offers solutions and resources to resolve problems encountered in everyday life. The benefit of these services lies in the prevention of lost hours, a positive work climate, and a constructive and positive environment that nurtures the individual, regardless of a person's acute or chronic impairment.

Healthy lifestyles are promoted in the home through environmental and safety measures to prevent stressors and accidents. Proper body mechanics taught to clients of all ages help prevent musculoskeletal injuries of the back, shoulders, and legs. Proper seating systems are essential for posture and safety for clients who use wheelchairs. Chapter 9 discusses more about vocation and the community and Chapter 14 contains additional information about safety and movement.

OUTCOMES

The broad outcome for clients with musculoskeletal dysfunction is the ability to manage pain and energy to allow maximum independence in ADLs, including mobility. Home safety and use of proper body mechanics are critical elements. Samples of measurable outcome criteria are listed in Table 21-7.

Preventing Complications

In the community, nurses conduct health promotion programs and screening activities at a variety of locations, such as at health fairs, shopping malls, churches, or senior centers. Rehabilitation nurses contribute to the overall health of the community by providing education about restorative care and prevention in these settings. Examples of other venues

TABLE 21-7 Nursing Outcomes

Pain control	Client uses nonanalgesic pain relief measures
	Client uses analgesic relief measures
	Client reports pain controlled sufficiently to allow participation in ADLs
Energy conservation	Client balances activity and rest
	Client adapts lifestyle to energy level
	Client uses energy conservation techniques
Self-care deficit: ADLs	Client performs ADLs at maximum level of independence
Mobility level	Client safely performs mobility skills at maximum level of independence
Body image	Client will adjust to changes in physical appearance
	Client will adjust to changes in body function
	Client will use strategies to enhance appearance and function

Adapted from Johnson, M., Maas, M., & Moorhead, S. (2000). Nursing outcomes classification (NOC) (2nd ed.). St. Louis: Mosby.
ADLs, Activities of daily living.

are speaking at local organizations, such as Rotary Club meetings, writing columns for the newspaper, or providing continuing education about rehabilitation principles or restorative care for colleagues in community health agencies.

Health promotion and prevention of complications improve outcomes. For example, lifetime increased calcium intake and preventive medication (alendronate or estrogen) by persons unable to participate in weight-bearing activities contribute to decreased incidence of osteoporotic fractures. Similarly, foot care and control of blood glucose levels decrease amputations associated with diabetes mellitus.

IMPLICATIONS

Quality of life is one of the most important factors to consider when assisting individuals with musculoskeletal dysfunction. Whether clients experience an acute injury or have a chronic, slowly progressing degenerative illness, their commonly held goal is to attain meaning and satisfaction in their lives. A positive self-concept is related to a person's attitudes and outlook, combined with that of the family, significant others, and the rehabilitation team. An effective nurse-client relationship must include trust and close collaboration to help the client become independent of the health care system. Nurses contribute by conducting ongoing and comprehensive assessments, developing appropriate nursing diagnoses and setting realistic goals with clients, and evaluating a client's progress toward achieving the highest possible level of wellness. Rehabilitation nurses are advocates who learn about available resources, evaluate their worth, educate clients about their operations, and understand how to access their services to help clients meet their goals within the health care continuum.

One function of a healthy community is to encourage agencies and groups to collaborate in promoting wellness and preventing musculoskeletal dysfunction in its members. The economic benefit affects the national and worldwide economy. Rehabilitation nurses are crossing socioeconomic, ethnic, cultural, and religious barriers to collaborate in research and present information at international conferences. They share ideas and information on the World Wide Web and travel to rehabilitation facilities or programs across the world. They share interventions, collaborate on their knowledge, and learn to appreciate the challenges experienced by others. Many nurses provide rehabilitation services—such as during mission trips sponsored by international voluntary organizations—including technology, equipment, and education. Developing countries and persons living in remote areas have great needs for medications, wheelchairs, braces, and many other treatment modalities for managing with musculoskeletal problems. They also need education about preventing problems and promoting health that is specific to their environment and situation. Rehabilitation nurses have an important role in the international scope of practice in the twenty-first century.

Research directions are to uncover the causes of diseases such as RA, to determine the effectiveness of alternate therapies and treatment modalities, such as for fibromyalgia, and to identify methods for preventing complications involving musculoskeletal disorders. Many new medications and dietary supplements are being evaluated, such as COX-2 inhibitors, glucosamine, and chondroitin. Rehabilitation nurses are in positions where they can investigate ways to promote behavioral changes that encourage clients to enhance their wellness and test clinical practices concerning musculoskeletal impairments.

CRITICAL THINKING

You are a rehabilitation nurse in a clinic setting. The physician you work with is not current in RA and osteoarthritis medications and management regimens. Clients are going elsewhere to seek alternative therapies.

1. What would you do to ensure quality care?
2. How would you approach the situation diplomatically while maintaining a professional relationship?
3. Discuss with colleagues to determine available resources.

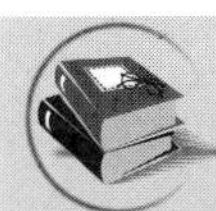

Case Study ~ *A Client Experiencing an Amputation*

Mr. G, a 26-year-old African-American, was admitted to an acute hospital with fever of 107°F. He developed generalized tonic-clonic seizures and mental status changes. Mr. G required intubation for airway support and respiratory distress. Additional admitting medical diagnoses were multisystem failure and purpura fulminans with gangrene to all four extremities. Aggressive wound care did not heal the sites and he eventually required bilateral below-the-knee amputations and removal of all digits of his hands. Nursing diagnoses included impaired mobility, altered body image, self-care deficit, alteration in comfort, potential for contractures, and impaired skin integrity.

Mr. G was admitted to the long-term acute care unit (LTAC) and later transferred to the acute rehabilitation unit for continued medical management, physical and occupational therapies, and wound care. Pertinent medical history included two episodes of pneumonia. As his medical condition improved, Mr. G was extubated and remained stable without ventilatory assistance.

Married and without children, he worked as a car rental salesperson, and his wife was a homemaker. He had a history of social drinking, but no prior drug or tobacco use. He had no known allergies.

Mr. G's physical assessment revealed stable vital signs on admission to the long-term acute facility. His mental status showed no gross focal findings. He was alert and oriented. Sensation appeared grossly intact. He had a tracheostomy with room air mist. His hands were dressed because of multiple middigit amputations. The bilateral below-knee amputations were also covered and dressed, with no evidence of edema.

The physiatrist coordinated the interdisciplinary team in developing a comprehensive plan of care. This client's clinical course was developed using the expertise of the rehabilitation team in occupational therapy, physical therapy, social services, and nutritional and pain management consultation. The plan of care included several aspects of treatment that were developed in collaboration with each discipline. The nursing process was used to outline this complex plan.

Nursing goals included improvement in functional mobility and activities in daily living (ADLs), restoration of positive self-image, prevention of contractures, pain management, and restoration of skin integrity. The nursing team developed a care plan to meet the client's goals of pain management by monitoring pain levels and providing medications to maximize function. Mobility goals were challenging because of the complexity of this client's clinical picture. The abilities to don and doff the prosthesis and ambulate indoors and outdoors were not realistic to accomplish during the inpatient setting. Self-wrapping of the extremities was challenging for him because of the upper extremity involvement, but the wife assisted in this process. Amputations of fingers as well as both lower legs also limited short-term goals to independence at the wheelchair level and independent transfers using a transfer board. Clients with upper extremity amputations have greater difficulty with activities, such as dressing and bathing. If there is unilateral involvement of an upper extremity, all tasks need to be done with the unaffected arm. In cases of bilateral upper extremity involvement, the client must learn to perform ADLs using feet or prosthetic devices. Mr. G learned compensatory strategies for ADLs using his hands, even though the digits were removed. Although deficits can be severe in the first several weeks after upper extremity amputations, prosthetics and compensatory strategies can be learned for performing ADLs independently. This client was determined to regain his strength and return home to his wife. His goals included upper extremity strengthening to facilitate safe transfers and bed mobility.

Nursing interventions included modification of the wound care regimen to promote healing and prevent complications such as infection. Wound care goals included closure of the ends of all residual limbs. Loss of dexterity did not allow Mr. G to participate in desensitization of the lower extremity sites. No further antibiotics were necessary after the completion of Ancef. All potential sites for infection were closely monitored.

The interdisciplinary team established pharmacological and nonpharmacological regimens to help manage Mr. G's pain and promote relaxation. Neuropathic pain limited the client's progress in therapies. Collaboration of the team was essential for the coordination of all activities to maximize the benefits of his analgesic medication. Premedicating him before therapy sessions allowed him to participate in therapies with minimal discomfort. Distractions such as guided imagery helped to take the focus away from the extremity during range of motion exercises. Zoloft was prescribed to elevate mood and combat depression. Xanax was administered 3 times daily as an adjunct to Vicodin to curb anxiety.

Nursing goals included resolution of infection and restoration of skin integrity. Antibiotics in the form of Ancef were continued intravenously for a brief period after admission to complete the series. Heparin 5000 U subcutaneously was given prophylactically to prevent deep vein thrombosis, frequently found after amputations (Burke et al., 2000). Calcium carbonate 500 mg was given to Mr. G orally 3 times daily to prevent hypocalcemia associated with immobility. Nutritional supplements were ordered in conjunction with a high protein diet to promote muscle strengthening and wound healing.

Both nursing staff and respiratory therapists continued to assess pulmonary status throughout the LTAC and acute rehabilitation stay to prevent complications resulting from immobility. Mr. G had no further episodes of pneumonia because of aggressive respiratory management. Respiratory therapy interventions included coordinating tracheostomy weaning. Oxygen saturation was monitored during therapies because of Mr. G's complex medical history. Laboratory studies included complete blood count, electrolytes, arterial blood gases, and cultures to monitor for complications. Prothrombin time/International Numeric Ratio (PT/INR) was obtained during anticoagulation therapy, which was changed to Fragmin subcutaneously daily. An initial chest x-ray and a second comparison were obtained before discontinuing the tracheostomy.

The physical therapist's interventions included the application of a rigid cast to manage edema when wound closures of the bilateral lower extremities progressed. This technique helped to prepare the limbs for the application of temporary prosthetic devices. Mr. G was transferred to the acute rehabilitation unit for aggressive mobilization therapy when his residual limbs were ready to be fitted with temporary prostheses.

Continued

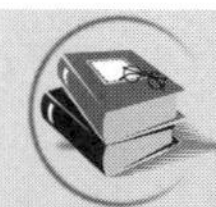

Case Study ~ *A Client Experiencing an Amputation—cont'd*

The occupational therapist developed interventions for upper extremity strengthening and for the retraining of ADLs with minimal hand function. Adaptive devices were designed to enable Mr. G to perform basic hygiene independently. After much practice, Mr. G was able to apply all adaptive devices and use them efficiently. Application of prostheses continued to require assistance because this was a new skill.

The neuropsychologist provided emotional support through the adjustment to altered body image. Because Mr. G was a young man, the staff expected him to continue to grieve over such a tremendous loss, both physically and psychologically. Sexuality issues, including body image, positioning, and modification of techniques, were discussed with the client and his wife. They expressed satisfactory results after a day pass to the home. Mr G's wife was supportive and overly attentive to his needs. She needed coaching from the interdisciplinary team to advise her not to perform tasks for him that he was capable of doing independently. The neuropsychologist met with the client as well as the wife in an effort to support the new roles they were adjusting to in the course of inpatient rehabilitation. Role reversal was discussed with the client and his wife because she had not been accustomed to handling home management duties. She used assistance from a family member as she adjusted to this new role.

Neuman Systems Model applied to this case because of the nurse/client relationship and the holistic approach. There were several interpersonal and extrapersonal stressors this client had to overcome, such as changes in body image, role reversal, loss of employment, and need to pay medical bills. As an African-American, Mr. G was at risk for hypertension and heart disease. Primary prevention focused on teaching to promote healthy dietary habits. Secondary prevention was shared with the client and his wife during discussions of monitoring of blood pressure and cholesterol screening for early detection. Tertiary prevention was covered in teaching about prevention of complications related to his amputations. It accordance with the Neuman Model, these interventions support healthy living and preventive measures.

The client's extended family lived in the immediate area, so they were also involved in frequent visits and family conferences to discuss discharge plans, and they remained supportive throughout his recovery. Although Mr. G experienced periods of low motivation and pain during the course of his rehabilitation, he progressed through an appropriate period of adjustment to his changed body image and changes in functional status. The rehabilitation team encouraged him and shared their experiences in working with clients who had similar levels of musculoskeletal dysfunction.

The outcome for Mr. G and his wife was their discharge to the home 8 weeks after his admission to the LTAC unit after a brief stay of 2 weeks on the acute rehabilitation unit for gait training with preparatory prostheses. He was ultimately discharged at a modified independent level for all tasks at the wheelchair level, except for bathing. His wife provided minimal assistance with tub transfers for safety. He continued to participate in outpatient physical therapy for mobility training and adaptation to definitive prosthetic devices. He continued to require occasional Vicodin for pain, but he no longer needed Zoloft to manage depression. He was referred to a vocational rehabilitation counselor for exploration of future employment opportunities.

Wheelchair van public transportation services were secured at the time of discharge to enable Mr. G to attend outpatient therapies, follow-up physician office visits, and attend social functions in the community. Resources were shared by the social worker to assist with finances during the client's extended hospitalization. Mr. G's wife secured full-time employment to help meet the financial responsibilities of the family toward the end of the rehabilitation stay when it was determined that the client would be able to function independently in the home at the time of discharge. He expressed satisfaction with the progress he had made and discussed plans for his discharge with enthusiasm. He continued to participate in outpatient therapy for several weeks and began to explore options to return to work in the future. His wounds remained closed, which allowed the use of bilateral lower extremity prostheses. He progressed in upper extremity strengthening until he was able to use his prostheses to ambulate short distances using a walker with upper arm supports. He came to our unit on Easter morning to demonstrate his newly acquired skills with the staff. Our team felt the satisfaction of assisting this individual in successfully transitioning home and restoring his independence.

REFERENCES

Abramowicz, M. (2000a). Drugs for rheumatoid arthritis. *The Medical Letter on Drugs and Therapeutics, 42* (July 10), 57-64.

Abramowicz, M., (2000b). Treatment of Lyme disease. *The Medical Letter on Drugs and Therapeutics, 42* (May), 37-40.

Ahlstrom, G., & Karlsson, U. (1999). Disability and quality of life in individuals with postpolio syndrome. *Disability and Rehabilitation, 22,* 416-422.

Albertson, D. (1999). Technology transfer embodies approach to disability: Liberty Mutual Research Center for Safety and Health. *Employee Benefit News, 13,* 47-48.

American Dental Association & American Academy of Orthopaedic Surgeons. (1997). Advisory statement: Antibiotic prophylaxis for dental patients with total joint replacements. *Journal of the American Dental Association, 128,* 1004-1008.

American Diabetes Association. (1999). Implications of the United Kingdom prospective diabetes study. *Diabetes Care, 22* (Suppl. 1), S27-S31.

American Sports Data. (Retrieved February 13, 2001). *State of the sport* [On-line]. Available: http://www.runningusa.org/state/demographics.shtml.

Amputee Coalition of America (1999/2000; retrieved May 27, 2001). *Limb loss research and statistics program update* [On-line]. Available: http://www.amputee-coaltion.org/llrsp/llrsp_update.html.

Arthritis Foundation (Retrieved February 13, 2001.). Available: http://www.arthritis.org.

Arthritis Society. (Retrieved February 10, 2001.). *Arthritis self-management program* [On-line]. Available: http://www.cbnet.ns.ca/cbnet/health/asmp.html.

Bach, J., & Chaudhry, S. (2000). Standards of care in MDA Clinics. *American Journal of Physical Medicine and Rehabilitation, 79,* 194-196.

Bachman, D., & Srivastava, G. (1998). Emergency department presentations of Lyme disease in children. *Pediatric Emergency Care, 14,* 356-361.

Ballas, M.T., Tytko, J., & Cookson, D. (1997). Common overuse running injuries: Diagnosis and management. *American Family Physician, 55,* 2473-2480.

Balow, J., Boumpas, D., & Austin, H. (2000). New prospects for treatment of lupus nephritis. *Seminar on Nephrology, 20,* 32-39.

Barth, W., & Segal, K. (1999). Reactive arthritis (Reiter's syndrome) *American Family Physician, 60,* 499-503, 507.

Belza, B., Henke, C., Yelin, E., Epstein, W., & Gilliss, C. (1993). Correlates of fatigue in older adults with rheumatoid arthritis. *Nursing Research, 42,* 93-99.

Berard, A., Solomon, D., & Avorn, J. (2000). Patterns of drug use in rheumatoid arthritis. *The Journal of Rheumatology, 27,* 1648-1655.

Blot, L., Marcelis, A., Devogelaer, J., & Manicourt, D. (2000). Effects of diclofenac, aceclofenac and meloxicam on the metabolism of proteoglycans and hyaluronan in osteoarthritic human cartilage. *British Journal of Pharmacology 131,* 1413-1421.

Blumenthal, M., Busse, W., Goldberg, A., Gruenwald, J., Hall, T., Klein, S., Riggins, C., & Rister, R. (1998). *Complete German Commission emonographs: therapeutic guide to herbal medicines.* Boston, MA: Integrative Medicine Communications.

Braith, R., Welsch, M., Mills Jr., R., Keller, J., & Pollack, M. (1997). Resistance exercise prevents glucocorticoid-induced myopathy in heart transplant recipients. *Medicine & Science in Sports & Exercise, 30,* 483-489.

Brainsky, G., Lydick, E., Epstein, R., Fox, K., Hawkes, W., Kashner, T., Zimmerman, S., & Magaziner, J. (1997). The economic cost of hip fractures in community-dwelling older adults: A prospective study. *Journal of the American Geriatrics Society, 45,* 281-287.

Brownfield, A. (1998). Aromatherapy in arthritis: A study. *Nursing Standard, 13,* 24-25.

Burke, B., Kumar, R., Vickers, V., Grant, E., & Scremin, E. (2000). Deep vein thrombosis after lower limb amputation. *American Journal of Physical Medicine and Rehabilitation, 79,* 145-149.

Centers for Disease Control and Prevention. (1999). National Arthritis Month. Impact of arthritis and other rheumatic conditions of the health care system—United States, *Morbidity and Mortality Weekly Report, 48,* 349-353.

Centers for Disease Control and Prevention. (1996) Incidence and costs to Medicare of fractures among Medicare beneficiaries aged ≥ age 65 years—United States, July 1991-June 1992. *Morbidity and Mortality Weekly Report, 45,* 877-883.

Chantraine, A., Baribeault, A., Uebelhart, D., & Gremion, G. (1999). Shoulder pain and dysfunction in hemiplegia: Effects of functional electrical stimulation. *Archives of Physical Medicine and Rehabilitation, 80,* 328-331.

Chestnut, C., Silverman, S. Andriano, K., Genant, H., Gimona, A., Harris, S., Kiel, D., LeBoff, M., Maricic, M., Miller, P., Moniz, C., Peacock, M., Richardson, P., Watts, N., & Baylink, D. (2000). A randomized trial of nasal spray salmon calcitonin in postmenopausal women with established osteoporosis: The prevent recurrence of osteoporotic fractures study. *The American Journal of Medicine, 109,* 267-276.

Ciccotti, M.G. (1998). *Elbow epicondylitis and surgery* [On-line]. Available: http://rothmaninstitute.com/sportsmed/elbow2.htm.

Cifu, D. (Retrieved February 24, 2001.). Rehabilitation following hip fracture [On-line]. Available: http://www.pmr.vcu.edu/department/facility/dcifu/hip1/.

Cimoch, P. (2000). *Fibromyalgia (FMS) and chronic fatigue syndrome (CFIDS)* [On-line]. Available: http://content.health.msn.com/content/article/1700.50843.

Colbert, L.H., Hootman, J.M., & Macera, C.A. (2000). Physical activity-related injuries in walkers and runners in the aerobics center longitudinal study. *Clinical Journal of Sports Medicine, 10,* 259-263.

Colon-Emeric, C., Yballe, L., Sloane, R., Pieper, C., & Lyles, K. (2000). Expert physician recommendations and current practice patterns for evaluating and treating men with osteoporotic hip fracture. *American Geriatric Society, 48,* 1261-1263.

Corbett, J. (1998). Laboratory tests and diagnostic procedures in orthopedic nursing practice. *Nursing Clinics of North America, 33,* 685-700.

Cunnanae, G., & Lane, N. (2000). Steroid-induced osteoporosis in systemic lupus erythematosus. *Rheumatic Disease Clinics of North America, 26,* 311-329.

Dalgas, M, Logigian, M., & Liang, M. (1994). Disability issues in rheumatoid arthritis. *Physical Medicine and Rehabilitation Clinics of North America, 5,* 859-866.

D'Cruz, D. (2000). Autoimmune diseases associated with drugs, chemicals and environmental factors. *Toxicological Letter* (March 15), 112-113, 421-432.

Dec, K.L., Sparrow, K.J., & McKeag, D.B. (2000). The physically-challenged athlete. *Sports Medicine, 29,* 245-258.

Dekker, J., Wagenaar, R., Lankhorst, G., & de Jong, B. (1997). The painful hemiplegic shoulder. *American Journal of Physical Medicine and Rehabilitation, 76,* 43-48.

Diamond, P. (2000). Severe anemia: Implications for functional recovery during rehabilitation. Rehabilitation in practice. *Disability and Rehabilitation, 22,* 574-576.

Dressler F. (1997). New aspects in the diagnosis and treatment of Lyme arthritis. *Review of Rheumatology (English Edition), 15,* 207S-208S.

Driscoll, S., Noll, S., & Koch, B. (1994) Juvenile rheumatoid arthritis. *Physical Medicine and Rehabilitation Clinics of North America, 5,* 763-783.

Dursun, E., Dursun, N., Eksi Ural, C., & Cakci, A. (2000) *Archives of Physical Medicine and Rehabilitation, 81,* 944-946.

Edwards, J. (2001, October 30). U.K. researcher targeting arthritis. Philadelphia (AP). pp. 1-3.

Edwards, P. (Ed.). (2000). *The Specialty practice of rehabilitation nursing: A core curriculum* (4th ed.). Glenview, IL: The Rehabilitation Nursing Foundation of the Association of Rehabilitation Nurses.

Elders, M. (2000). The increasing impact of arthritis on public health. *Journal of Rheumatology Supplement, 10*(60), 6-8.

Emmerson, B. (1996). The management of gout. *New England Journal of Medicine, 334,* 1543-1544.

Escott-Stump, S. (1992). *Nutrition and diagnosis related care* (3rd ed.). Philadelphia: Lea and Febiger.

Feinglass, J., Brown, J., LoSasso, A., Sohn, M., Manheim, L., Shah, S., & Pearce, W. (1999) Rates of lower extremity amputation and arterial reconstruction in the United States in 1979. *Journal of the American Public Health Association, 89,* 1222-1227.

Felson, D., Zhang, Y., Hannan, M., Kannel, W., & Kiel, D. (1995). Alcohol intake and bone mineral density in elderly men and women: The Framingham Study. *American Journal of Epidemiology, 142,* 485-492.

Ferrara, M.S., & Peterson, C.L. (2000). Injuries to athletes with disabilities: Identifying injury patterns. *Sports Medicine, 30,* 137-143.

Frauman, A. (1996). An overview of the adverse reactions to adrenal corticosteroids. *Adverse Drug Reactions & Toxicological Reviews, 15,* 203-206.

Gandevia, S., Allen, G., & Middleton, J. (2000). Post-polio syndrome: assessments, pathophysiology and progression. *Disability Rehabilitation, 22*), 38-42.

Gauthier-Gagnon, C., Grise, M., & Potvin, D. (1999). Enabling factors related to prosthetic use by people with transtibial and transfemoral amputation. *Archives of Physical Medicine and Rehabilitation, 80,* 706-713.

Generini, S., Fiori, G., Moggi Pignone, A., Matucci Cerinic, M., & Cagnoni, M. (1999). Systemic sclerosis. A clinical overview. *Advances in Experimental Medicine & Biology 433,* 73-83.

Goad, M. (Retrieved February 24, 2001.). *Costly new drugs curb rheumatoid arthritis* [On-line]. Available: http://www.portland.com.

Gordon, M. (2000). *Manual of nursing diagnosis* (9th ed.). St. Louis: Mosby.

Goss, G. (1998). Osteoporosis in women. *Nursing Clinics of North America, 33,* 573-582.

Gremillion, R., & Vollenhoven, R. (1998). Rheumatoid arthritis. *Rheumatoid Arthritis, 103,* 103-123.

Gruca, J. (2000). Mobilizing your client's spiritual strengths. (2000, October 11-14). Association of Rehabilitation Nurses Annual Educational Conference, Reno, Nevada.

Halverson, P. (1997). The spondyloarthropathies. *Orthopedic Nursing, 16,* 21-25.

Hanger, H., Whitewood, P., Brown, G., Ball, M.C., Harper, J., Cox, R., & Sainsbury, R. (2000). Randomized controlled trial of strapping to prevent post-stroke shoulder pain. *Clinical Rehabilitation 14,* 370-380.

Hartley, B., & Fuller, C., (1997). Juvenile arthritis: A nursing perspective. *Journal of Pediatric Nurses, 12,* 100-109.

Healthy People 2010. (Retrieved November 3, 2000.). *Conference edition.* http://www.health.gov/healthypeople/document/html/volume1/02 Arthritis.htm.

Herndon, R., & Mohandas, N. (2000). Osteoporosis in multiple sclerosis: A frequent serious and under-recognized program. *International Journal of Multiple Sclerosis Care, 2,* 1-9.

Hewett. T.E. (2000). Neuromuscular and hormonal factors associated with knee injuries in female athletes: Strategies for intervention. *Sports Medicine, 29,* 313-327.

Hightower, L. (2000). Osteoporosis: Pediatric disease with geriatric consequences. *Orthopaedic Nursing, 19,* 59-62.

Hoeman, S. (Ed.). (1996). *Rehabilitation nursing: Process and application* (2nd ed.). St. Louis: Mosby.

Hospital Employee Health. (1996). *Preventing musculoskeletal injuries requires proactive approach* (No. 15): Author.

Hutchinson, M.R., & Nasser, R. (2000). *Common sports injuries in children and adolescents* [On-line]. Available: http://www/medscape.com/medscape/OrthoSportsMed/journal/2000/vo4.no4/mos4420.hutc/mos4420.hutc-01.html.

Ikai, T., Tei, K., Yoshida, K., Miyano, Y., & Yonemoto, K. (1998). Evaluation and treatment of shoulder subluxation in hemiplegia. *American Journal of Physical Medicine and Rehabilitation, 2*), 421-426.

Ivanhoe Newswire. (2000). *Soccer injury increases risk of arthritis* [On-line]. Available: http://www.ivanhoe.com/sportsmedicine/soccerinjury increaseriskofarthritis.shtml.

Johnson, M., Maas, M., & Moorhead, S. (2000). *Nursing Outcomes Classification. (NOC)* (2nd ed.). St. Louis: Mosby.

Jubelt, B., & Agre, J. (2000). Characteristics and management of postpolio syndrome. *JAMA, 284,* 412-414.

Kain, J.H. (2000). Care of the older adult following hip fracture. *Holistic Nursing Practice, 14,* 24-39.

Kee, C. (2000). Osteoarthritis: Manageable scourge of aging. Nursing Clinics of North America, 35(1), 199-208.

Kessenich, C. (2000). Update on osteoporosis in elderly men. *Geriatric Nursing, 21,* 242-244.

Klein, M., Whyte, J., Keenan, M., Esquenazi, A., & Polansky, M. (2000). Changes in strength over time among polio survivors. *Archives of Physical Medicine and Rehabilitation, 81,* 1059-1064.

Klyscz, T., Rassner, G., Guckenberger, G., & Junger, M. (1999). Biomechanical stimulation therapy. A novel physiotherapy method for systemic sclerosis. *Advances in Experimental Medicine and Biology, 445,* 309-316.

Knutsson, S., & Engberg, I. (1999) An evaluation of patients' quality of life before, 6 weeks and 6 months after total hip replacement surgery. *Journal of Advanced Nursing, 30,* 1349-1359.

Kozuh, J. (2000). NSAIDs & antihypertensives: An unhappy union. *American Journal of Nursing, 100,* 40-42.

Latman, N., & Walls, R. (1996). Personality and stress: An exploratory comparison of rheumatoid arthritis and osteoarthritis. *Archives of Physical Medicine and Rehabilitation, 77,* 796-800.

Lindsay, D.M., Horton, J.F., & Vandervoort, A.A. (2000). A review of injury characteristics, aging factors and prevention programmes for the older golfer. *Sports Medicine, 30,* 89-103.

LEAP Program. (Retrieved November 3, 2000.). *What is LEAP?* [On-line]. Available: http://www.bphc.hrsa.dhhs.gov/leap.

Lipsky, P., van der Heijde, D.M., St Clair, E.W., Furst, D.E., Breedveld, F. C., Kalden, J.R., Smolen, J.S., Weisman, M., Emery, P., Feldmann, M., Harriman, G.R., & Maini, R.N. (2000). Infliximab and methotrexate in the treatment of rheumatoid arthritis. *New England Journal of Medicine, 343,* 1594-1602.

Liss, H., & and Liss, D.(Retrieved October 19, 2000.). *Musculoskeletal sequelae of cerebrovascular accidents* [On-line]. Available: http://www.rehabmed.net/documents/cva.htm.

Lumsden, D.B., Baccalo, A., & Martire, J. (1998). T'ai chi for osteoarthritis: An introduction for primary care physicians. *Geriatrics, 53,* 84-88.

Mangini, M. (1998). Physical assessment of the musculoskeletal system. *Nursing Clinics of North America, 33,* 643-653.

Matsen, F. (2000). *Reiter's syndrome* [On-line]. Available: http://www.orthop.washington.edu/bone%20and %20joint%20source/izzzzzzz1_1.html.

Melski, J. (2000). Lyme borreliosis. *Seminars in Cutaneous Medical Surgery,* 19(1), 8-10.

McCaffery, M., & Pasero, C. (1999). *Pain: Clinical Manual* (2nd ed.). St. Louis: Mosby.

McCarren, M. (1993). Intensive therapy reduces the risk of diabetic eye, kidney, and nerve disease. *Diabetes Forecast, 46,* 48-51.

McCloskey, J., & Bulechek, G. (2000). *Nursing Interventions Classification (NIC)* (3rd ed.). St. Louis: Mosby.

Medical Multimedia Group. (Retrieved October 30, 2000.). *A patient's guide to knee problems. Osteoarthritis* [On-line]. Available: http://www.sechrest.com/mmg/knee/degen/degen.html.

Michet, C. (1998). Update in the epidemiology of the rheumatic diseases. *Current Opinion of Rheumatology, 10,* 129-135.

Muscular Dystrophy Association. (1999). *Neuromuscular diseases in the MDA program* [On-line]. Available: http://www/mdausa.org/disease/40list.html.

National Center for Chronic Disease Prevention and Health Promotion. (Retrieved October 19, 2000a.). Available: http://www.cdc.gov/nccdphp/arthritis/index.htm.

National Center for Chronic Disease Prevention and Health Promotion. (Retrieved October 19, 2000b.) Available: http://www.cdc.gov/ncipc/factsheets/fallcost.htm.

Neuman, B. (1995). *The Neuman Systems Model* (3rd ed.). Norwalk, CT: Appleton and Lange.

Occupational Safety and Health Association. (Retrieved November 20, 2000.). *Ergonomics standard regulatory text* [On-line]. Standard 1910.900. Available: www.osha-slc.gov/ergonomics-standard/regulatory/regtext.html.

O'Brien, M. (1999). *Spirituality in nursing: Standing on holy ground.* Boston: Jones and Bartlett.

Olson, R. (1996). Halo skeletal traction pin site care: Toward developing a standard of care. *Rehabilitation Nursing, 21,* 243-246.

Parker, C., & Thomas D. (2000). Reiter's syndrome and reactive arthritis. *Journal of American Osteopathic Association, 100,* 101-104.

Peck, S. (1998). The efficacy of therapeutic touch for improving functional ability in elders with degenerative arthritis. *Nursing Science Quarterly, 11,* 123-132.

Peck, S. (1997). The effectiveness of therapeutic touch to decrease pain in elders with degenerate arthritis. *Journal of Holistic Nursing, 15,* 176-198.

Petrucci, G. (1993). Prevention and management of dance injuries. *Orthopaedic Nursing, 12,* 52-60.

Pezzin, L., Dillingham, T., & Mackenzie, E. (2000). Rehabilitation and the long-term outcomes of persons with trauma-related amputations. *Archives of Physical Medicine and Rehabilitation, 81,* 292-300.

Phipps, W., Sands, J., & Marek, J. (1999). *Medical-surgical nursing: Concepts and clinical practice* (6th ed.). St. Louis: Mosby

Pink, M.M., & Tibone, J.E. (2000). The painful shoulder in the swimming athlete. *Orthopedic Clinics of North America, 31,* 247-261.

Reuters Medical News. (Retrieved February 1, 2001.). *Smith & Nephew's injectable osteoarthritis wins FDA approval* [On-site]. Available:http://orthopaedics.medscape.com/reuters/prof/2001/01/01.31/20010130rglt005.html.

Romanik, K. (1994). *Around the clock with C.O.P.D.: Helpful hints for respiratory (chronic obstructive pulmonary disease) patients.* Connecticut: American Lung Association.

Ryan, T. (2000). *The therapeutic effects of Tai Chi.* (2000, October 11-14). Association of Rehabilitation Nurses 26th Annual Educational Conference, Reno, NV.

Sedlak, C., Doheny, M., & Jones, S. (2000). Osteoporosis education programs: Changing knowledge and behaviors. *Public Health Nursing, 17,* 398-402.

Sevier, T.L., & Wilson, J.K. (1999). Treating lateral epicondylitis. *Sports Medicine, 28,* 375-380.

Simmons, B.P., Nutting, J.T., & Bernstein, R.A. (1996). Juvenile rheumatoid arthritis. *Hand Clinic, 12,* 573-589.

Smith, W. (1998). Fibromyalgia syndrome. *Nursing Clinics of North America, 33,* 653-669.

Stanghelle, J., & Festvag, L. (1997). Postpolio syndrome: A 5 year follow-up. *Spinal Cord, 35,* 503-508.

Sullivan, M., & Sharts-Hopko, N. (2000). Preventing the downward spiral. *American Journal of Nursing, 100,* 26-32.

Taft, L. B., Looker, P.A., & Cella, D. (2000). Osteoporosis: A disease management opportunity. *Orthopaedic Nursing, 19,* 67-76.

Tiras, M., Noyan, V., Yildiz, A., Yildirim, M., & Daya, S. (2000). Effects of alendronate and hormone replacement therapy, alone or in combination, on bone mass in postmenopausal women with osteoporosis: A prospective randomized study. *Human Reproduction, 15,* 2087-2092.

Total Hip Replacement National Institutes of Health Development Conference. (September 12-14, 1994). (Retrieved October 19, 2000.). Available: http://text/nln.nih.gov/nih/cdc/www/98text.html.

Tsao, B. (2000). Lupus susceptibility genes on human chromosome 1. *International Review of Immunology, 19,* 319-334.

United States Department of Labor, Bureau of Labor Statistics. (1995). *Survey of occupational injuries and illnesses.* Washington, DC: Author.

University of Washington Orthopedics. (Retrieved October 30, 2000.). *Reiter's syndrome* [On-line]. Available: http://www.orthop.washington.edu/bond%20andjoint.

Vallbona, C., Hazlewood, C., & Jurida, G. (1997). Response of pain to static magnetic fields in postpolio patients: A double-blind pilot study. *Archives of Physical Medicine and Rehabilitation, 78,* 1200-1203.

Vigier, S., Casillas, J., Dulicu, V., Rouhier-Marcer, I., D'Athis, P. & Didier, J. (1999). Healing of open stump wounds after vascular below-knee amputation: Plaster cast socket with silicon sleeve versus elastic compression. *Archives of Physical Medicine and Rehabilitation, 80,* 1327-1330.

Weber, D., Schaper, L., Pomeroy, D., Badenhausen, Jr., W., Curry, J., Smith, M., & Suthers, K. (2000). Cementless hemispheric acetabular component in total hip replacement. *International Orthopaedics (SICOT), 24,* 130-133.

Well-Connected. (1999). *What are lifestyle and therapeutic methods for treating and managing fibromyalgia?* [On-line]. Available: http://content.health.msn.com/content/dmk/dmk_article_5462093.

Well-Connected. (Retrieved February 11, 2001.). *How are Lyme disease and ehrlichiosis treated?* [On-line]. Available: http://content.health.msn.com/content/dmk/dmk_article_5462485.

Whitaker, J., & Adderly, B. (1998). *The pain relief breakthrough: The power of magnets to relieve backaches, arthritis, menstrual cramps, carpal tunnel syndrome, sports injuries, and more.* Boston: Little, Brown, & Co.

Willen, C. and Grimby, G. (1998). Pain, physical activity, and disability in individuals with late effects of polio. *Archives of Physical Medicine and Rehabilitation, 79,* 915-919.

Wise, C., & Agudelo, C. (1998). Diagnosis and management of complicated gout. *Bulletin of Rheumatological Disease, 47,* 2-5.

Wong, G., & Wilson, P. (1997). Classification of complex regional pain syndromes: New concepts. *Hand Clinics, 13,* 319-325.

Wynne, C., Ling, S., & Remsburg, R. (2000). Comparison of pain assessment instruments. *Geriatric Nursing, 21,* 20-23.

Yelin, E.H., (1995). The impact of arthritis. *Arthritis Care and Research, 8,* 201-202.

Yocum, D. (1994). Immunopathogenesis of RA: What happens in the rheumatoid joint? *The Journal of Musculoskeletal Medicine, 11,* 47-55.

Young, Y., Brant, L., & German, P. (1997). A longitudinal examination of functional recovery among older people with subcapital hip fractures. *Journal of the American Geriatric Society, 45,* 288-294.

Zaffer, S., Braddom, R., Conti, A., Goff, J., & Bokma, D. (1999). Total hip disarticulation prosthesis with suction socket. *American Journal of Physical Medicine and Rehabilitation, 78,* 160-162.

BIBLIOGRAPHY

DD in site. (Retrieved December 29, 2000). *The tech knowledge developmental disability resource for Georgia* [On-line]. Available: http://www.arch.gatech.edu/crt/techknow/medconditions/amputation.htm.

Fibromyalgia Association. (Retrieved October 30, 2000). Available: http: w2com/fibro3.html.

22 Neuromuscular Disorders

Leslie Jean Neal, PhD, RNC, CRRN

Ms. G was a 32-year-old African-American woman with multiple sclerosis. Before her diagnosis she had been independent and held a midlevel position in a big company. She had lived alone and enjoyed the company of many friends. After her diagnosis, her parents moved in with her so they could be close at hand and monitor her health.

On admission to home health, Ms. G was incontinent of bladder and constipated. She used a wheelchair and required assistance with all of her activities of daily living (ADLs). Her short-term memory was failing, but she was otherwise cognitively intact.

On assessment it was clear that Ms. G's parents managed all of her care. They responded to my questions throughout the first visit, and they appeared to resent any implication that Ms. G might be able to manage her health care without their involvement. When asked, Ms. G indicated that her goal of our partnership was to be able to go to the shopping mall with her friends but without her parents.

I used rehabilitation principles and interventions to teach Ms. G how to manage her incontinence, resolve her constipation, and compensate for her short-term memory loss. Helping Ms. G's parents to understand that she needed to control and direct her care was a more difficult matter, but Ms. G and I were rewarded when she visited the shopping mall in her wheelchair without her parents and when she made arrangements with her employer to work at home from a computer on a part-time basis. My work with Ms. G is memorable because I feel that I made a significant difference in the quality of her life.

Jackson and Kelsey (1999) conducted a literature review of the needs of neurology clients and their caregivers before discharge from an inpatient facility. The authors found that clients' families are most concerned with the well-being of the client and less concerned with the needs of the family or of the household. According to the literature, clients were most concerned with disability management, including the potential effects on vocational and financial status. Many and varied psychosocial consequences of disability are discussed in the literature, according to Jackson and Kelsey, and include concerns about isolation, uselessness, and anger. Loss of independence; cognitive, sensory, and perceptual abilities; and the ability to communicate clearly contribute to a loss of confidence.

Caregivers, according to the literature review, were affected by changes in their lifestyle and overall health, consequences of caring for a person with deteriorating health. Emotions, such as depression, frustration, stress, and fatigue cloud the caregivers ability to remain loving and keep the peace, tasks they feel are important to perform. Caregiver stress relates to fear and anxiety about the future, fear that health care professionals will abandon them, and concerns about finances (Jackson & Kelsey, 1999).

This chapter discusses several neuromuscular disorders—Huntington's disease (HD), Parkinson's disease (PD), multiple sclerosis (MS), Guillain-Barré syndrome (GBS), myasthenia gravis (MG), amyotrophic lateral sclerosis (ALS), and spinal cord injury (SCI)—that have a significant impact on the client, family, and caregiver. With the exception of GBS, these diseases are only manageable, not curable. Rehabilitation nurses play a key role in assisting clients, families, and caregivers to adjust to the lifestyle and functional changes and to promote everyone's successful adaptation to these alterations.

Although the anatomy and physiology principles that pertain to these diseases are described, the reader is encouraged to see Chapter 15 for further discussion of neurology. Because the diseases discussed in this chapter share many common traits, part of the discussion will be grouped, and tables will be used throughout the chapter to list information specific to a particular disease. Issues related to each disease, including statistical information, such as the prevalence and incidence of each disease, will be discussed specific to each disease.

ANATOMY AND PHYSIOLOGY RELEVANT TO NEUROMUSCULAR DISORDERS

The nervous system is divided into the peripheral nervous system (PNS) and the central nervous system (CNS). The CNS includes the brain and the spinal cord, whereas the PNS includes the spinal and cranial nerves. Ascending pathways carry impulses to the CNS, and efferent pathways carry impulses away from the CNS. Efferent pathways stimulate skeletal muscle and effector organs (Huether & McCance, 2000).

The somatic nervous system and the ANS make up the functional component of the PNS. The somatic system regulates voluntary motor ability while the autonomic system controls the internal environment of the body through involuntary regulatory mechanisms. The ANS comprises the sympathetic and the parasympathetic nervous systems (Huether & McCance, 2000). The CNS, PNS, and ANS function together in an integrated way (Copstead & Banasik, 2000).

Nervous tissue is made up of two basic types of cells: neurons and supporting cells (neuroglia in the CNS; Schwann cells in the PNS). Neurons detect threats to homeostasis and initiate change to maintain the steady state. Each neuron is specialized in its function. Glucose fuels neurons. Neurons are composed of a body, dendrites, and an axon. The axon of the neuron may or may not be covered with a membrane called a *myelin sheath.* This sheath insulates the axon and allows neural transmission to occur rapidly (Huether & McCance, 2000).

Mature nerve cells in the CNS are not capable of dividing (although recent research indicates that this theory may not be completely true), so when injury occurs, it is typically accompanied by permanent loss of function. Myelinated nerves in the PNS may regenerate after injury depending on the location, type, and severity of the injury (Huether & McCance, 2000).

Neurotransmitters are chemicals that transmit impulses from one cell to another. Among them are acetylcholine, dopamine, norepinephrine, serotonin, and histamine. Deficiencies or excesses in neurotransmitters contribute to pathology (Huether & McCance, 2000).

The spinal cord facilitates the transmission of impulses between the brain and spinal nerves that innervate organs and muscles. Spinal reflexes regulate responses to pain, muscle tone, and urination. Gray matter in the spinal cord is involved in the integration and processing of impulses and responses, whereas the white matter consists of myelinated axons that transmit impulses. The ventral roots of the spinal cord contain motor neurons that travel to the skeletal muscles. The dorsal roots of the spinal cord convey sensory information. "The points at which sensory neurons enter the cord and at which motor neurons exit represents the separation of the central and peripheral nervous systems" (Copstead & Banasik, 2000, p. 980).

LIFE SPAN ISSUES

During the third week of embryonic development the nervous system begins to develop. Beginning at this time, neurons multiply quickly and begin to make synaptic connections. Stimulation appears to cause division of neurons specific to a particular function. The size of the brain increases until puberty and then remains steady until middle adulthood. Neurons are lost gradually as adults age, without significant loss of function within a typical life span. However, older age is directly correlated to neurological impairment and excessive neuronal loss, and degeneration is associated with dementia. The secretion and metabolism of neurotransmitters are also altered by age. Dopamine and norepinephrine decrease in particular. Additionally, nerve fibers in the ANS decline in quantity, and motor nerve fibers and the myelin sheath in the PNS degenerate (Copstead & Banasik, 2000).

Changes in posture and fluidity of movement occur with age. Bradykinesia, rigidity, and tremor may be signs of age or of PD (to be discussed later in this chapter). Visual changes, such as decreased acuity and pupillary response time, may occur. These changes combined with hearing loss may lead to confusion and disorientation.

Additionally elderly persons may be more sensitive to cold temperatures than to heat and less sensitive to pain. Sensitivity to taste, smell, and tactile sensation also tends to diminish. Changes in mental status should be carefully evaluated as to their source because medications, dehydration, depression, and changes in the ability to hear and see may account for confusion and may not be related to a disease process (Smeltzer & Bare, 2000).

ASSESSMENT

Nursing assessment of the client with a neurological impairment includes the health history, review of systems, physical examination, selected tests and procedures, and environmental assessment. The neurological assessment begins when the examiner first encounters the client because the level of consciousness, physical appearance, behavior, affect, facial expression, and ability to communicate can all be noted during the greeting phase of the encounter. Should the client be an unreliable source for the information to be elicited during the health history, this first encounter will signal the nurse to consider exploring the history with a reliable family member and proceeding directly to the objective phases of the assessment.

Health History

Neurological dysfunction may be a primary complaint or may be secondary to other problems. Thyroid disease, diabetes mellitus, cancer, infection, pernicious anemia, hypertension, and substance abuse may contribute to neurological

Box 22-1 Health Patterns and Neurological Dysfunction

Health Perception–Health Management Pattern
- Daily activities
- Drug use
- Safety practices
- Previous hospitalizations

Nutrition-Metabolic Pattern
- Diet recall
- Difficulty chewing, swallowing

Elimination Pattern
- Incontinence
- Constipation
- Hesitancy, urgency, retention

Activity-Exercise Pattern
- Weakness
- Poor coordination
- Reduced independence

Sleep-Rest Pattern
- Problems sleeping
- Use of sleep-inducing medications

Cognitive-Perceptual Pattern
- Changes in memory
- Vertigo
- Temperature insensitivity
- Numbness, tingling, pain
- Difficulty communicating

Self-Perception–Self-Concept Pattern
- Effect of neurological problem on self-concept

Role-Relationship Pattern
- Changes related to neurological dysfunction

Sexuality-Reproductive Pattern
- Satisfaction
- Dysfunction
- Need for counseling
- Alternative methods

Coping–Stress Tolerance Pattern
- Coping pattern
- Needs being met

Value-Belief Pattern
- Culturally-specific beliefs, perceptions that may influence treatment

Adapted from Lewis, S.L., Collier, I.C., Heitkemper, M.M., Dirksen, S.R. (2000). *Medical-surgical nursing: assessment and management of clinical problems* (5th ed.). St. Louis: Mosby.

dysfunction. Additionally hospitalizations and surgeries will offer clues to whether the client has a history of neurological impairment (Lewis, Collier, Heitkemper, & Dirksen, 2000).

A thorough medication history is integral to any health assessment. Mood elevators, tranquilizers, narcotics, and sedatives are particularly influential in causing neurological symptoms such as dizziness and drowsiness. Additionally medications are a cue to health status. Clients receiving antiepileptic medication or antispasmodics are likely to have neurological dysfunction (Lewis et al., 2000). The client should be questioned regarding the use of over-the-counter medications as well as prescription drugs because ephedrine has recently been implicated in brain attacks.

Exposure during the perinatal period to toxic substances, including alcohol, viruses, drugs, tobacco, and radiation, can adversely affect embryonic neurological development. Alterations from the norm of success at developmental tasks during growth may indicate neurological dysfunction (Lewis et al., 2000). Exposure to these elements from birth may also contribute to neurological dysfunction. A family history of stroke, seizures, and brain or spinal tumors is also worth documenting for future reference during the assessment.

It is important that the nurse ask key questions related to health patterns while obtaining the client's history. Box 22-1 contains possible alterations in health patterns related to neurological impairment.

Risk factors associated with neurological disease include increasing age, sex (male), heredity, hypertension, cigarette smoking, diabetes mellitus, carotid artery disease, heart disease, and polycythemia. Additionally use of drugs and alcohol and certain climactic conditions and socioeconomic factors may contribute to brain attacks and injury (Wilson & Giddens, 2001).

Any changes in function noted by the client or others should be investigated. Any history of neurological disease, trauma, or chronic disease should also be explored in depth.

Physical Examination

A simple but thorough tool can be used to guide the neurological assessment (Neal, 1997). The tool consists of a mnemonic device ("Is anybody home?") that helps the clinician to remember to include the many parts of the neurological assessment (Box 22-2).

The clinician uses a variety of instruments while conducting the neurological assessment. However, perhaps the most important instrument the clinician uses is the power of observation. Looking at the client while observing for alterations in affect, appearance, and appropriateness will provide clues to neurological dysfunction that may be substantiated as the assessment continues.

Diagnostic Tests and Procedures

A number of tests and procedures can be performed to determine and evaluate neurological function. Table 22-1 includes a brief description of these tests and procedures.

Environmental Assessment

The environmental assessment is an important part of the assessment of any client, but it can be particularly crucial in clients with a neuromuscular disorders related to safety issues. The environmental assessment includes the tangible environment, such as the home or other setting in which the client lives. However, the environment also refers to the client's support system and the client's ability to obtain resources, such as food, medicine, and equipment. The setting in which the client resides should be assessed for clear pathways; cleanliness; adequate light and stair railings; and accommodations for bathing, eating, and sleeping.

Box 22-2 Is Anybody Home?

I: Intellect, including thought processes and reasoning, judgment, and simple calculations
S: Sensation, including touch, pain, temperature

A: Appearance, appropriateness, affect
N: Nerves, cranial
Y: Yak, yak; communication and use of language
B: Balance
O: Orientation
D: Deep tendon reflexes
Y: Yesterday; short- and long-term memory

H: Health history
O: Observe for alterations between assessments
M: Muscle strength and motor ability
E: Energy level and emotional state

From: Neal, L.J. (1997). Is anybody home? *Home Healthcare Nurse, 15*(3), 158-167.

Whether the client with a neuromuscular disease has a solid support system and a caregiver must be assessed carefully. The client may have members of his or her religious congregation who can visit to bring food or clean the home on a short-term basis. On a long-term basis, these persons may be able to provide social interaction rather than continued food and services. Family members may be very young, aged, or frail and unable to provide the physically demanding services needed by the client with a neuromuscular disease. Again, in the short-term, family members may be able to assume the burden of personal care services but may find themselves worn down and debilitated by the time and attention required. Family dynamics may also preclude comfortable interaction between the client and family caregivers.

Financial status may prevent another barrier to obtaining the environmental support needed by the client. If family members work outside the home, a full-time hired caregiver might be necessary. Additionally food, medicine, equipment, and supplies can be costly and may not be reimbursable by insurance.

Narayan and Tennant (1997) suggest that the following factors should be considered when assessing the client's environment:

- Food and fluids/eating
- Elimination/toileting
- Hygiene/bathing/grooming
- Clothing/dressing
- Resting/sleeping
- Medications
- Shelter
- Safety and security
- Fire/burn prevention
- Crime/injury prevention
- Caregiver
- Communication
- Family/friends/pets
- Self-esteem and self-actualization

TABLE 22-1 Neurological Tests and Procedures

Test/Procedure	Rationale/Purpose
Computed tomography	X-ray beam scans head in layers to provide images of the brain; distinguishes differences in densities
Positron emission tomography	Computer imaging of organ function; allows measurement of blood flow, brain metabolism, and tissue composition
Magnetic resonance imaging	Uses a magnetic field to show images; gives information about intracellular chemical changes
Single photon emission computed tomography	Three-dimensional imaging; contrasts normal and abnormal tissue
Cerebral angiography	X-ray film of cerebral circulation using contrast dye
Electromyography	Needle electrodes in skeletal muscles measure changes in electrical potentials
Nerve conduction studies	Stimulation of a peripheral nerve to record muscle action potential or sensory action potential
Lumbar puncture and cerebrospinal fluid examination	Spinal tap to remove cerebrospinal fluid for analysis

From Smeltzer, S.C., & Bare, B.G. (2000). *Medical-surgical nursing.* Philadelphia: JB Lippincott.

PATHOPHYSIOLOGY OF SELECTED NEUROMUSCULAR DISEASES

It is important to have background knowledge of the pathophysiology of the neuromuscular diseases to be discussed in this chapter before beginning to design realistic goals and a plan for clients with these diseases. The diseases are described in an order that should help the reader logically understand the differences and similarities among the diseases and begin to comprehend why these diseases share many goals, interventions, and outcomes.

Huntington's Disease

HD is a degenerative neuromuscular disease. Its prevalence is 5 per 100,000 persons, and it is not race or sex specific (Huether & McCance, 2000). It is genetically acquired but typically does not present itself until approximately 40 years of age. The gene abnormality has been isolated to chromosome 4 (Copstead & Banasik, 2000). Children of a parent with HD have a 50% chance of acquiring the disease. Once the disease is diagnosed, clients usually survive for 10 to 15 years and may die of infection, choking, falls, pneumonia, or heart failure (Smeltzer & Bare, 2000).

Glutamine, used in protein synthesis, builds up to abnormal levels in the brain and destroys brain cells (Smeltzer & Bare, 2000). The degeneration occurs in the basal ganglia and in the cerebral cortex. The basal ganglia normally control movement, and the cerebral cortex is involved with thought, judgment, perception, and memory. The cerebellum is also affected, and consequently balance and coordination are disrupted. The neurotransmitters acetylcholine and γ-aminobutyric acid (GABA) are lost, and this contributes to dysfunction in motor and mental capability. An excess of dopamine also occurs relative to the deficiency of GABA and acetylcholine, and this contributes to chorea, or nonfluid, writhing, twisting, involuntary movements (Huether & McCance, 2000). Chorea and dementia characterize the manifestations of the disease (Carter et al., 1999). Dopamine is an inhibitory neurotransmitter, whereas acetylcholine is an excitatory neurotransmitter. Consequently an excess of dopamine relative to acetylcholine deficiency results in involuntary and abnormal movement.

Purposeful movement is lost as the disease progresses. All of the muscles in the body are involved in involuntary movement. Speech, chewing, swallowing, and gait become disorganized and difficult. Eventually the person also displays dementia but will also be irritable and may act out violently. Hallucinations, paranoia, and impaired judgment evolve with the disease, whereas emotional changes such as impatience, anger, and suicidal tendencies tend to decrease later on. Diagnostics related to HD include:

- Clinical presentation of symptoms
- Family history
- Neurological examination
- Ruling out other causes of symptoms
- Imaging studies
- Magnetic resonance imaging (MRI) scan
- Computed tomography (CT) scan: shrinkage of brain in some cases
- Genetic marker: 28 or fewer CAG repeats

Parkinson's Disease

PD also affects the basal ganglia and is related to a deficiency rather than an excess of the neurotransmitter dopamine. It affects approximately 1% of Americans (130 to 150 per 100,000 [Huether & McCance, 2000]) and like HD usually presents in persons older than 40 years. PD occurs in both sexes and in persons of all races (it is slightly more likely in men [Huether & McCance, 2000]). PD may be idiopathic in that the cause is unknown or it may occur as a consequence of infection, trauma, or drug or other toxicity (Copstead & Banasik, 2000; Young, 1999).

Enzymes required to metabolize dopamine are deficient in the basal ganglia. Consequently, dopamine levels are reduced, and the classic triad of symptoms, rigidity, tremor, and bradykinesia, appears (Figure 22-1). Recently a fourth symptom has been added to this classic triad: impaired postural righting reflexes (Imke, 2000). Interestingly the brains of some clients with PD present on autopsy with amyloid plaques and neurofibrillary tangles characteristic of Alzheimer's disease. However, the dementia that occurs in PD (30% to 50% of all cases) may occur in clients with or without the plaques or tangles (Copstead & Banasik, 2000).

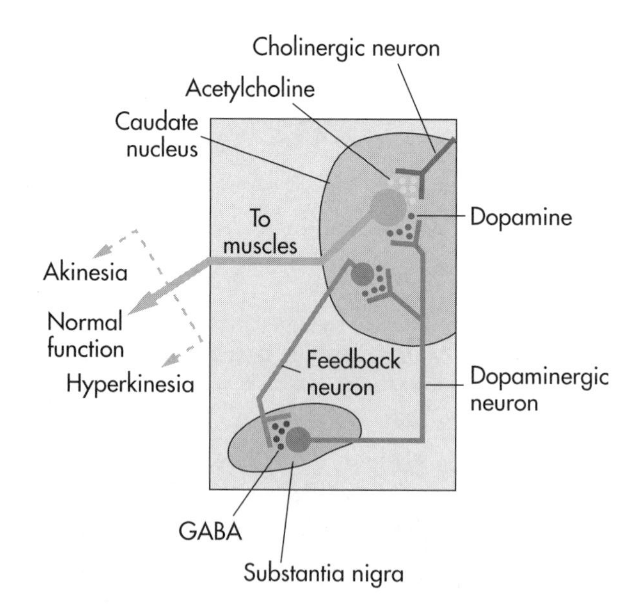

Figure 22-1 Dopaminergic synaptic activity is mediated by dopamine. Cholinergic synaptic activity is mediated by acetylcholine. A balance between the two kinds of activity produces normal motor function. A relative excess of cholinergic activity produces akinesia and rigidity. A relative excess of dopaminergic activity produces involuntary movements. Neurons in the caudate nucleus contain γ-aminobutyric acid *(GABA)* and possibly control dopaminergic neurons in the substantia nigra through a feedback pathway. (From Huether, S.E., & McCance, K.L. [2000]. *Understanding pathophysiology* [2nd ed.]. St. Louis: Mosby.)

The deficiency of dopamine results in a relative excess of acetylcholine, the opposite of what occurs in HD. This deficiency of dopamine allows acetylcholine to contribute to sustained, excitable activity and is manifested in the classic triad mentioned above. Additionally clients with PD typically display dysarthria, dysphagia, and postural disturbance. Reduced arm swing, foot drag, a hoarse voice, and a flat affect are also characteristic (Figure 22-2). Initially one side of the body is affected but eventually both sides are involved. Imke (2000) reports that clients often remark that their handwriting has become illegible (micrographia), an important clue to the clinical diagnosis.

One current theory regarding the pathophysiology of PD is that free radicals add to the damage done to neurons. Reduced levels of ferritin in clients with PD support this theory because ferritin is normally used to protect neurons from free radicals. Another theory is that PD is genetic. This is supported by the fact that 15% to 20% of persons with PD have a relative who demonstrates parkinsonian symptoms. This theory is currently the focus of intensive study. Additionally it is thought that certain persons may experience accelerated aging of dopaminergic neurons, which causes the disease (National Institute of Neurological Disorders and Stroke, 2001).

The onset of PD is insidious, and medications and treatments may contribute to the client's safety risk (Huether & McCance, 2000). Diagnostics related to PD include:

- History
- Medication review
- Neurological examination
- Review of systems
- Positron emission tomography (PET) scan
- Two of the three classic symptoms: bradykinesia, rigidity, and tremor

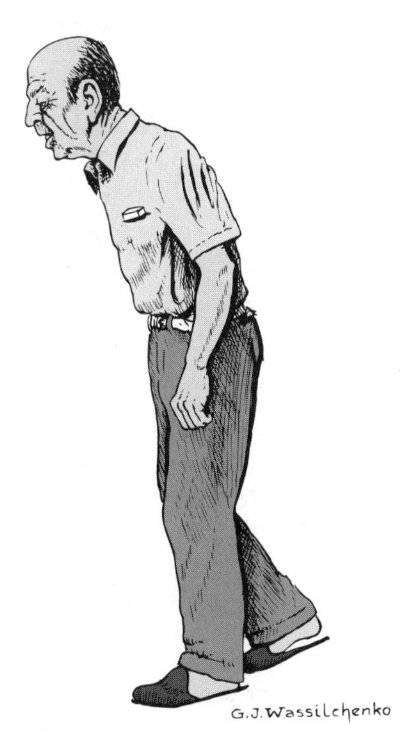

Figure 22-2 Characteristic shuffling gait of a client with Parkinson's disease. (Modified from Rudy, E.B. [1984]. *Advanced neurological and neurosurgical nursing.* St. Louis: Mosby.)

Myasthenia Gravis

MG is a disease of impaired transmission of acetylcholine across the neuromuscular junction. It affects 5 to 10 per 100,000 persons (Bullock & Henze, 2000). Persons with pathological changes of the thymus appear to be more likely to contract the disease and men are more likely than women to experience thymic changes, particularly tumors (Huether & McCance, 2000).

It is a chronic autoimmune disease and is associated with other autoimmune diseases. Acetylcholine receptors cease to be recognized as "self"; thus autoantibodies (immunoglobulin G) are produced against the acetylcholine receptors and block the binding of acetylcholine. This immune response eventually destroys receptor sites for acetylcholine and results in diminished nerve transmission (Huether & McCance, 2000). Muscle weakness and fatigability result.

There are three types of MG: ocular (more prevalent in men and muscle weakness is restricted to the eyes), generalized (typically includes the proximal muscles with occasional remissions), and bulbar (includes muscles affected by cranial nerves IX, X, XI, and XII). Generalized and bulbar MG may be rapidly progressive or fulminating. However, generalized MG may also be slowly progressive.

The onset of MG is usually insidious, and the client presents with fatigue. A history of frequent upper respiratory tract infections is also common. The symptoms of muscle weakness manifest in ptosis, speech slurring, dysphagia, and facial droop. Neck, shoulder, and hip flexor muscles may also be affected. Eventually all muscles are affected, and ventilatory support is needed (Huether & McCance, 2000).

Profound muscle weakness occurs with myasthenic crisis and causes quadriparesis or quadriplegia. This is a condition requiring emergency respiratory support. A cholinergic crisis occurs related to toxicity from the administration of anticholinesterase drugs used to treat MG (Table 22-2). Smooth-muscle hyperactivity occurs related to an accumulation of acetylcholine and excessive parasympathetic nerve activity. Clinically the crisis resembles myasthenic crisis with added parasympathetic nerve–like symptoms (Huether & McCance, 2000). Diagnostics related to MG include:

- Tensilon test: administration of Tensilon immediately improves muscle strength
- Electromyography (EMG)
- Antiacetylcholine receptor antibody titers
- History
- Neurological examination
- MRI
- Mediastinal tomography

TABLE 22-2 Comparison of Myasthenic Crisis and Cholinergic Crisis

	Myasthenic Crisis	Cholinergic Crisis
Causes	Exacerbation of myasthenia following precipitating factors or failure to take medication as prescribed or dose of medication too low	Overdose of anticholinesterase drugs resulting in increased acetylcholine at the receptor sites, remission (spontaneous or after thymectomy)
Differential diagnosis	Improved strength after intravenous administration of anticholinesterase drugs; increased weakness of skeletal muscles manifesting as ptosis, bulbar signs (e.g., difficulty in swallowing, difficulty in articulating words), or dyspnea	Weakness within 1 hour after ingestion of anticholinesterase; increased weakness of skeletal muscles manifesting as ptosis, bulbar signs, dyspnea; effects on smooth muscle include pupillary miosis, salivation diarrhea, nausea or vomiting, abdominal cramps, increased bronchial secretions, sweating, or lacrimation

From Lewis, S.L., Collier, I.C., Heitkemper, M.M., & Dirksen, S.R. (2000). *Medical-surgical nursing: Assessment & management of clinical problems.* (Sihor). St. Louis: Mosby.

Multiple Sclerosis

MS is a demyelinating disease of the CNS. It usually presents between the ages of 20 and 50 years and is twice as prevalent in women as in men. It is most common in Caucasians and occurs in 30 to 80 per 100,000 persons in the United States. Prevalence appears to increase with increased distance from the equator. It is considered to have a probable genetic link because 15% of clients with MS have a relative with MS (Huether & McCance, 2000). A hypersensitivity response to a slow-growing virus followed by recurring inflammatory reactions may be responsible (Huether & McCance, 2000). Another prevailing theory is that an autoimmune response against myelin causes the disease. In any case, the cause of MS remains largely unclear.

Repeated inflammatory responses leave behind plaques and lesions in the myelin. The demyelination or destruction of the myelin sheath of axons in the CNS most frequently affects the optic and oculomotor cranial nerves and the cerebellar, corticospinal, and posterior column systems (Figure 22-3). Consequently, clinical manifestations although typically individualized, include abnormalities of vision and eye movement, motor skills, coordination, and gait, as well as spasticity and sensory disturbances, such as pain and paresthesia (Copstead & Banasik, 2000). Fatigue is the symptom most commonly identified by individuals with MS. Dysphagia and dysarthria are other common symptoms. Approximately 50% of clients with MS have some dysphagia and/or dysarthria (Brown, 2000).

In 1996 (Lublin & Reingold, 1996) a new classification system for MS was devised. These categories have since been modified and include newly diagnosed or a probable diagnosis of MS, relapsing-remitting MS, primary-progressive MS, secondary-progressive MS, and progressive-relapsing MS (Holland & Halper, 1999; Multiple Sclerosis Nurse Specialists Consensus Committee, 2000). Table 22-3 differentiates the forms of MS.

Most clients are initially diagnosed with relapsing-remitting MS. Clinical manifestations relate to the portion of the CNS that is affected. Many persons develop cognitive disturbances or psychosocial problems related to MS (Huether & McCance, 2000). Furthermore, complications from MS may be debilitating and include bowel and bladder management difficulties, impaired skin integrity, and contractures.

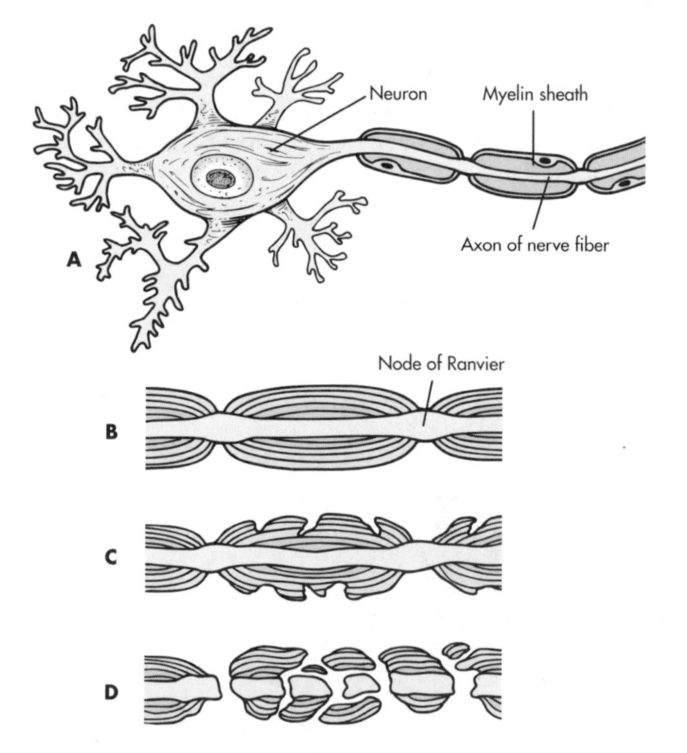

Figure 22-3 Pathogenesis of multiple sclerosis. **A,** Normal nerve cell with myelin sheath. **B,** Normal axon. **C,** Myelin breakdown. **D,** Myelin totally disrupted; axon not functioning. (From Lewis, S.M., Collier, I.C., Heitkemper, M.M., & Dirksen, S.R. [2000]. *Medical-surgical nursing: assessment and management of clinical problems* [5th ed.]. St. Louis: Mosby.)

Gulick's (1998) 10-year longitudinal study of clients with MS found that over time there is "a slow but signifi-

TABLE 22-3 Classifications of Multiple Sclerosis

Category	Definition
Newly diagnosed	Clients are reacting to diagnosis
Relapsing remitting	No disease progression between exacerbations*
Primary progressive	Progressive functional decline without distinct relapses*
Secondary progressive	Starts with relapsing remitting and becomes progressive
Progressive relapsing	Progressive disease, acute exacerbations with progression

*Exacerbation: Relapse or "an episode of new or worsening MS symptoms that lasts more than 24 hours and is not related to metabolic changes or steroid withdrawal" (Multiple Sclerosis Nurse Specialists Consensus Committee, 2000).

cant increase in three symptom complexes: motor (extremity weakness, tremors, balance difficulties, spasms, falling, and knee locking), brain stem (double vision, dysphagia, blurred vision, and forgetfulness), and elimination (urinary frequency and difficulty reaching the toilet during the daytime and nighttime) and an overall downward trajectory in all ADL functions: fine and gross motor (eating, bathing, transfer, dressing, travel, walking), socializing/recreation (indoor and outdoor activities), communication (writing, phoning, reading), and intimacy" (p. 144). Subjects ranked the symptoms.

According to Ransohoff (2000) there has been a change in the way health care professionals view MS. Previously the prevailing theory was that active disease did not occur during periods of remission. Recent research indicates, however, that MS is a continuous process (Figure 22-4). Some clients produce new lesions without evidence of disease activity (Ransohoff, 2000). Diagnostics related to MS include:

- History, including sexual history
- Neurological examination
- Urodynamic studies
- MRI
- Electrophoresis of the cerebrospinal fluid
- Evoked potential studies

Guillain-Barré Syndrome

GBS, or acute infectious polyradiculoneuritis, affects the PNS. It is an inflammatory disease that affects approximately 1 person per 100,000 in the United States (Worsham, 2000). It appears to affect slightly more men than women and more Caucasians than African-Americans, and it is more prevalent in persons older than 45 years. However, it occurs all over the world and does not appear to be correlated with seasonal or climactic changes (Copstead & Banasik, 2000).

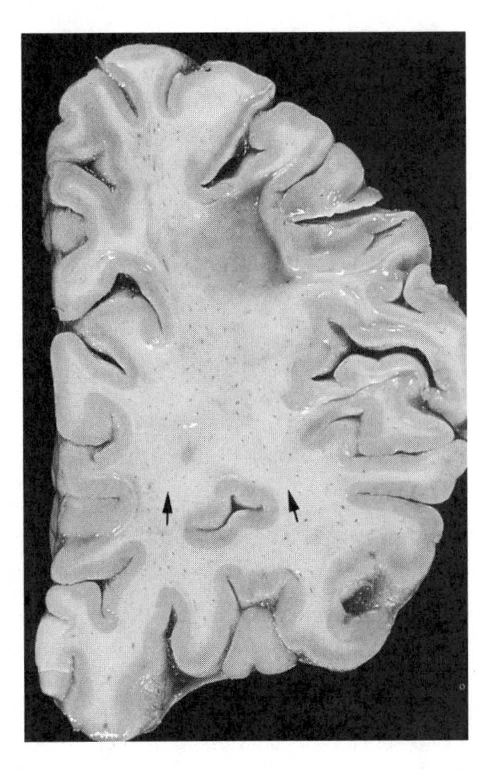

Figure 22-4 Chronic multiple sclerosis. Demyelination plaque at gray-white junction and adjacent partially remyelinated shadow plaque *(arrows)*. (From Damjanov, I, & Linder, J. [1996]. *Anderson's pathology* [10th ed.]. St. Louis: Mosby.)

The inflammatory reaction that occurs in GBS seems to be an allergic or hypersensitivity reaction because its onset tends to occur shortly after a febrile illness, surgery, trauma, or vaccination. Although the etiology may be viral, the cause is unknown (Bullock & Henze, 2000).

Whereas MS affects the myelin of the nerves in the CNS, GBS affects the myelin of the nerves of the PNS, the Schwann cells (Worsham, 2000). An antimyelin antibody has been identified as the cause of an antimyelinating process that occurs in the segmental peripheral nerves and the anterior and posterior spinal nerve roots. Sensitized leukocytes destroy the myelin. The inflammatory response further contributes to nerve degeneration and demyelination (Bullock & Henze, 2000).

Ascending weakness is the primary initial symptom and begins in the lower extremities. It is postulated that muscle weakness, tingling, and numbness begin in the lower extremities because signals to and from the lower extremities have the farthest to travel and may be most vulnerable to interruption (Worsham, 2000). Eventually, proximal and distal muscles and the muscles of the neck, trunk, and chest are affected, as well as those innervated by the cranial nerves. Some individuals develop paresthesia and pain in the neck and back. However, sensory involvement tends to be less severe than motor involvement and most commonly involves proprioceptive and vibratory changes in function. Sympathetic and parasympathetic nervous system dysfunction results in blood pressure changes (orthostatic hypotension or hypertension), bradycardia, bowel and bladder problems, and diaphoresis (Lewis et al., 2000). Most clients with GBS recover spontaneously. Recovery and remyelination tend to occur in a descending fashion, opposite to the onset of the disease (Worsham, 2000). However, some (7% to 22%) are left with disability. Complete flaccid paralysis may develop and lead to the need for ventilatory support (Copstead & Banasik, 2000; Bullock & Henze, 2000). Diagnostics related to GBS include:

- History to rule out other causes
- Neurological examination
- CSF studies: CSF protein rise
- Electrodiagnostic studies of nerve conduction

Amytrophic Lateral Sclerosis

ALS affects approximately 1.5 of every 100,000 persons (Polak & Boynton de Sepulveda, 2000). It is more common in men than in women (although after menopause, the incidence equalizes) and usually occurs after the age of 40 years. It occurs all over the world and involves the upper and lower motor neurons (Huether & McCance, 2000).

The disease primarily involves the brainstem, spinal cord, and cerebral cortex and specifically affects the motor neurons in these areas. Progressive muscle weakness and wasting lead to death within 3 to 5 years after diagnosis (Bullock & Henze, 2000). A genetic alteration of chromosome 21 has been detected in 50% of clients with familial ALS. The genetic defect causes the inhibition of the function of an enzyme that normally kills free radicals. Consequently, glutamate toxicity occurs and causes nerve degeneration. Degeneration occurs without inflammation. Additionally demyelination occurs in motor neurons secondary to the death of the neurons with subsequent scarring (Huether & McCance, 2000).

Although immunological factors are suspected, the etiology of ALS is unknown. Viruses or toxins are considered possible causes (Copstead & Banasik, 2000). A recent study found a virus in the spinal cords of 15 of the 17 ALS clients studied, providing support for the theory of a viral cause (Polak & Boynton de Sepulveda, 2000).

Most clients present with upper body weakness and wasting, whereas some present with symptoms in the lower extremities. Dysarthria and dysphagia occur, eventually followed by altered respiratory function (Copstead & Banasik, 2000). The ability to move the eyes and maintain continence usually remains until late, and muscle involvement is typically asymmetrical. Fasciculations of the tongue, hands, and upper extremities are early signs of brainstem involvement. Bulbar palsy, or paralysis or paresis of muscles innervated by the cranial nerves, may either be of the flaccid or spastic type. Neuronal involvement is typically confined to motor function, whereas sensation and intellectual function remain intact (Bullock & Henze, 2000). Diagnostics for ALS include:

- History
- Physical examination
- EMG
- Muscle biopsy

Spinal Cord Injury

Every year 10,000 to 12,000 persons experience SCIs. Males aged 16 to 30 years are most commonly affected (80%) (Farnan, 2000). This is related to their tendency to participate in high-risk activities. Elderly persons are also likely to have SCIs related to degenerative vertebral disease and an increased risk for falls (Huether & McCance, 2000). The Spinal Cord Injury Association (SCIA; http://www.spinalcord.org/resource/factsheets) lists the incidence of SCI related to high-risk activities:

- Motor vehicle accidents: 44%
- Acts of violence: 24%
- Falls: 22%
- Sports: 8%
- Other: 2%

According to the SCIA, the risk from falls becomes greater than the risk from motor vehicle accidents after the age of 45 years, whereas the risk from violence and sports decreases as individuals age.

SCI occurs as a result of contusion, compression, transection, or compression of the spinal cord. Flexion with associated ligamental tearing and dislocation is the most unstable SCI. Significant neurological impairment typically ensues. Hyperextension is the most common cause of SCIs (Copstead & Banasik, 2000). SCIs may result from hyperflexion, lateral flexion, rotational movement, or vertical compression. The degree of damage to the cord in a vertebral injury relates to the extent of bony involvement or cord compression (Bullock & Henze, 2000) (Figure 22-5).

The actual damage to the spinal cord results from ischemia or reduced blood flow and from the inflammatory response that follows the injury. The gray matter of the cord enlarges and becomes hemorrhagic and eventually necrotic, followed by the formation of scar tissue. The white matter becomes hemorrhagic and severely edematous (Bullock & Henze, 2000).

Blood flow to the spinal cord is compromised because there is interference with the body's compensatory response, autoregulation, which usually serves to maintain blood flow to tissues. The reduced blood flow also contributes to the ischemia. In addition, free radicals released from these areas begin to destroy tissue (Copstead & Banasik, 2000). These processes lead to necrosis and are progressive for several hours after injury. However, it is preferable to intervene within 60 to 90 minutes (Copstead & Banasik, 2000).

Swelling of the spinal cord increases dysfunction and

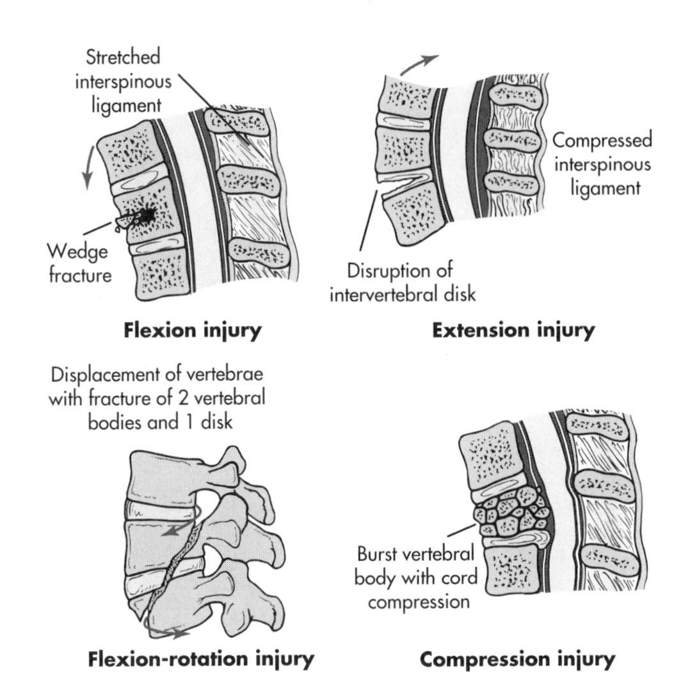

Figure 22-5 Mechanisms of spinal injury. (From Lewis, S.M., Collier, I.C., Heitkemper, M.M., & Dirksen, S.R. [2000]. *Medical-surgical nursing: assessment and management of clinical problems* [5th ed.]. St. Louis: Mosby.)

TABLE 22-4 Categories of Spinal Cord Injuries

Complete (All Motor and Sensory Function Is Lost)
Cervical cord injury: quadriplegia
Thoracic cord injury: paraplegia
Incomplete (Varying Loss)
Central cord syndrome: usually related to hyperextension injury; motor weakness in upper and lower extremities with greater loss in upper extremities; loss of pain and temperature sensation varies
Anterior cord syndrome: related to dislocation or subluxation, herniation, flexion injuries, compression of arteries; seen in persons older than 40 years; loss of motor function, touch, pain, temperature sensation below level of injury; vibratory sense, touch, position sense retained
Brown-Sequard syndrome: injury to one side of the spinal cord; ipsilateral paralysis, proprioceptive loss, loss of touch, vibratory sense; contralateral loss of pain and temperature below level of lesion

Data from Bullock, B.A., & Henze, R.L. (2000). *Focus on pathophysiology.* Philadelphia: JB Lippincott.

may be life-threatening if it involves the diaphragm and vegetative functions (Huether & McCance, 2000). The inflammatory response eventually subsides, and the site of injury is replaced by scar tissue.

Spinal shock refers to the alteration in function of the spinal cord that accompanies the injury. It is temporary and affects the function and reflexes below the site of the injury. Flaccid paralysis, loss of spinal reflexes and sensation, decreased thermoregulatory ability, and bowel and bladder dysfunction may result. Spinal shock may occur when the injury occurs, or it may appear a week or so later. It typically lasts for 7 to 10 days if no infection is present. The resumption of reflex responses and a change from flaccidity to spasticity signal the resolution of spinal shock (Copstead & Banasik, 2000).

Functional loss after recovery from spinal shock is reflective of the level of the injury and the cord involvement (Figure 22-6). Injuries are categorized as complete or incomplete (Table 22-4).

Beck, Harris, and Basford (1999) conducted a retrospective study of clients with thoracic SCI after discharge from a rehabilitation unit. They concluded that "it is difficult to predict the functional outcomes of persons with acute traumatic thoracic SCI, and it is also difficult to predict their discharge deposition. Multiple factors can impede the person's return home" (p. 131). However, they found that the severity of the impairment, the level of the injury, and comorbidities were not related to discharge disposition.

Autonomic Dysreflexia

Clients with SCI are at risk of experiencing dysreflexia. This is an acute emergency condition characterized by a rapid rise in blood pressure, headache, bradycardia, diaphoresis, and nausea. Clients with injuries above the T6 (thoracic) level become dysreflexic in response to otherwise harmless stimuli, such as constipation, a distended bladder, or tactile stimuli. Interventions must be prompt and appropriate (discussed later in this chapter) to avoid an increase in intercranial pressure or a cerebral vessel rupture (Smeltzer & Bare, 2000). Diagnostics related to SCI include:

- Neurological examination
- X-rays
- Electrocardiograph monitoring
- CT scan

NEUROMUSCULAR DISEASE IN CHILDREN

Although neuromuscular diseases of children will not be discussed in detail in this chapter, it is important to mention those that are most common. Muscular dystrophy, cerebral palsy, and spina bifida are the most common neuromuscular diseases of children. The last two diseases are discussed at length in Chapter 29. Muscular dystrophy is a congenital disease that causes severe muscular weakness. *Cerebral palsy* is an umbrella term for a group of disorders that do not progress but do affect the brain and motor activity. A recent study (Ruess, Paneth, Pinto-Martin, Lorenz, & Susser, 1996)

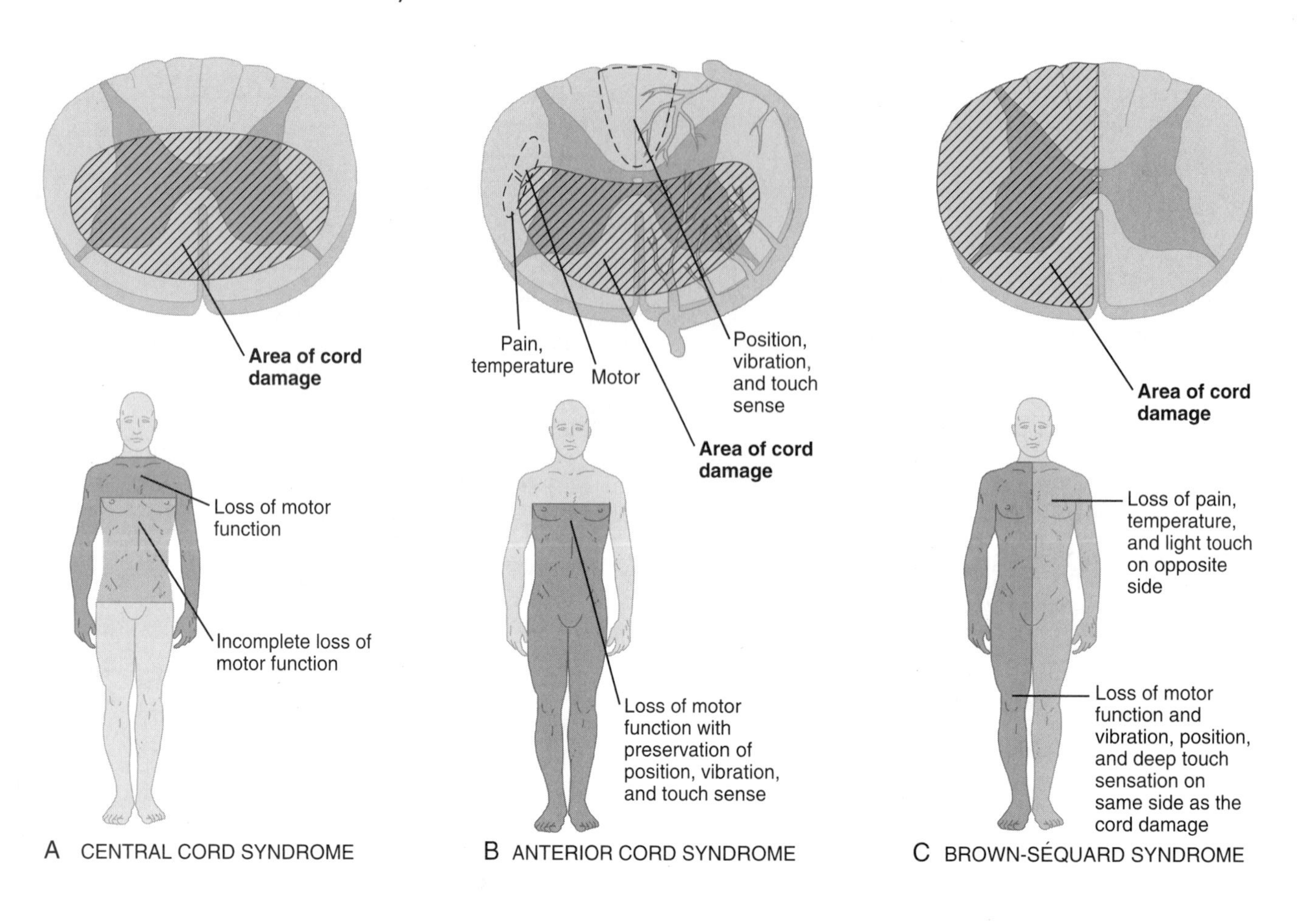

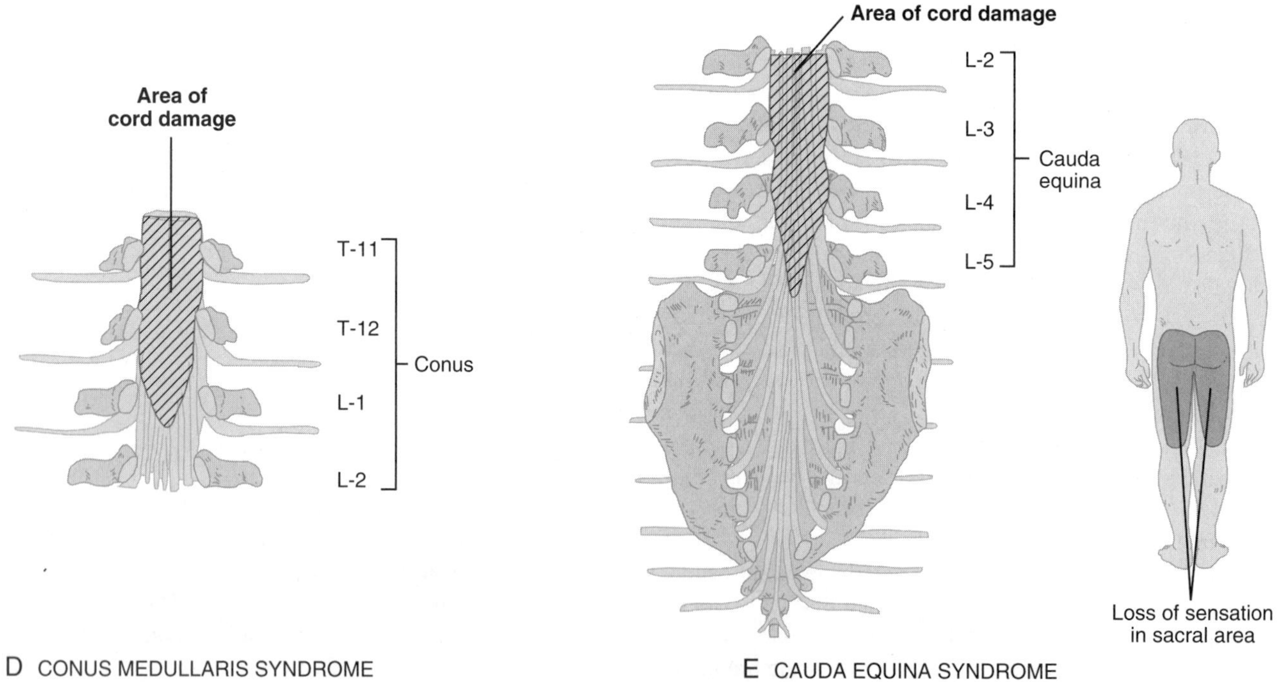

Figure 22-6 Patterns of injury leading to paralysis. **A,** Central cord syndrome. **B,** Anterior cord syndrome. **C,** Brown-Séquard syndrome. **D,** Conus medullaris syndrome. **E,** Cauda equina syndrome. (From Black, J.M., Hawks, J.H., & Keene, A.M. [2001]. *Medical-surgical nursing: clinical management for positive outcomes* [6th ed.]. Philadelphia: WB Saunders.)

found that low levels of thyroid hormone correlate with cerebral palsy in preterm neonates. Spina bifida refers to a defect in which the neural tube protrudes through the spinal cord and vertebrae. Motor disturbances, including gait abnormalities, sphincter disturbances, and muscle weakness, are common resulting dysfunctions.

NURSING DIAGNOSES

The neuromuscular diseases discussed in this chapter (other than SCI) share several common characteristics (Box 22-3). Therefore many of the same nursing diagnoses, nursing interventions, and desired outcomes apply (Table 22-5).

GOALS

The goals for Healthy People 2010 (http://www.health.gov/healthypeople) are relevant to a discussion of neuromuscular disease and include:

- To increase quality and years of healthy life
- To eliminate health disparities

The ideal goal for the client with a neuromuscular disease is to enhance the quality and length of life as much as possible. These clients and their caregivers cope with disability and an altered lifestyle, so interventions are always guided by the goal of enhancing quality of life and prolonging health to the maximum extent possible given the disease.

Health disparities are evident in the incidence and prevalence of these diseases. It is unknown whether increased prevalence by ethnicity, geographical location, or sex are related more to genetic differences or to disparities in the health of groups and individuals because of the inability to obtain adequate food, nutrition, or health care. In any case individuals and groups should have equal access to health care services regardless of socioeconomic status, race, or ethnicity.

More specifically the primary goals of nursing for clients with neuromuscular disease pertain to comfort measures and to maintaining maximum function. Other than the possibility of a functional recovery with GBS, there is no known cure for any of the other diseases discussed in this chapter. Each disease involves functional loss that is typically progressive. Self-care to the client's maximum ability, reduced caregiver strain, client comfort, and safety are key goals.

Regarding MS, Halper (2000) comments that "the focus of care . . . has changed from one of maintenance and crisis intervention to a more positive and proactive approach" (p. 1). Nursing care of clients with MS and other neuromuscular diseases "is a collaborative effort whose goal is self-awareness and self-responsibility; its activities involve supporting a great deal of self-care by clients, families, and care partners" (p. 1).

Box 22-3 Shared Characteristics of Degenerative Neuromuscular Diseases

Usually progressive
Etiology typically unknown
Brain degeneration (some cases)
Neuromuscular changes with regard to:
- Coordination
- Speech
- Swallowing
- Ambulation
- Cognition
- Fatigue
- Weakness
- Tremors
- Self-care agency
- Bowel and bladder management
- Respiration

Diagnosis is typically made after ruling out other possibilities
Usually no known cure
Palliative measures:
- Provide comfort
- Maintain function
- Teach self-care
- Support client/family
- Administer medication

Consider hospice care
Suggest genetic counseling
Prevent rehospitalization
Obtain adaptive equipment and durable medical equipment
Refer to nutritionist or physical, occupational, or speech therapist

PLANNING

Breathing

The risk for aspiration and respiratory failure inherent in these diseases requires long-term planning. Assessment of breathing patterns and swallowing should be incorporated into every assessment of the client. The additions to the interdisciplinary team of a respiratory therapist, should ventilatory support be required, and of a speech pathologist for the evaluation and treatment of dysphagia should be anticipated.

Dysreflexia

Autonomic dysreflexia is relevant to the client with SCI. The client and caregiver should be knowledgeable about precautions to avoid this emergency condition and how to manage it effectively should it arise. Planning should include awareness of the triggering stimuli and an understanding by the client and caregivers of potential solutions that can be instituted immediately (Travers, 1999).

Pain

Planning for the client with pain or paresthesias should include short- and long-term alternatives. The nature of pain

TABLE 22-5 Suggested Nursing Diagnoses, Nursing Interventions Classifications, and Nursing Outcomes Classifications for Degenerative Neuromuscular Diseases

Nursing Diagnoses	Suggested Nursing Interventions Classification (NIC)	Suggested Nursing Outcome Classification (NOC)
Breathing pattern, ineffective (ALS, MG)	Respiratory monitoring	Normal breathing pattern
Aspiration, risk for (ALS, MG, MS)	Aspiration precautions	No aspiration
Dysreflexia, autonomic (SCI)	Dysreflexia management	No dysreflexia
Swallowing, impaired (ALS, MS)	Aspiration precautions, swallowing therapy	No aspiration
Chronic pain/sensory disturbance	Pain management	Comfort
Injury, risk for	Surveillance: safety	Safety
Activity intolerance	Energy management	Energy conservation
Fatigue	Energy management	Activity tolerance
Imbalanced nutrition: less than body requirements	Nutrition management	Nutritional status
Disturbed thought processes	Cognitive stimulation, emotional support	Cognitive orientation
Communication, impaired verbal	Active listening	Communication
Anticipatory grieving	Counseling	Quality of life
Chronic sorrow	Emotional support	Hope
Fear	Active listening	Mood equilibrium
Anxiety	Touch	Fear control
Constipation, risk for	Constipation/impaction management	Bowel elimination
Incontinence, bowel	Bowel incontinence care, bowel training	Bowel management
Incontinence, urinary	Urinary incontinence care, bladder training	Bladder management
Mobility, impaired physical	Exercise therapy, positioning	Mobility
Skin integrity, impaired risk for	Skin surveillance	Intact skin
Sexual dysfunction	Sexual counseling	Sexual function
Self-care deficit: all ADL	Self-care assistance	Self-care
Caregiver role strain	Caregiver support	Caregiver well-being

Data from Johnson, M., Maas, M.L., & Moorhead, S. (2000). *Nursing outcomes classification (NOC)* (2nd ed.). St. Louis: Mosby; McCloskey, J.C., & Bulechek, G.M. (2000). *Nursing interventions classification (NIC)* (3rd ed.). St. Louis: Mosby; and North American Nursing Diagnosis Association. (2001). *Nursing diagnosis: definitions and classification 2001-2002* (4th ed.). Philadelphia: Author.

ALS, Amyotrophic lateral sclerosis; *MG,* myasthenia gravis; *MS,* multiple sclerosis; *SCI,* spinal cord injury.

and paresthesias related to neuromuscular disease, although chronic, is often intermittent. A thorough and ongoing assessment of pain will provide the data necessary to plan interventions and to keep interventions effective.

Injury

The risk of injury is high for all clients discussed in this chapter because of alterations in mobility, muscular strength, balance, and cognition. The site of care must be a safe environment, and careful consideration must be given to appropriate equipment to enhance mobility and reduce the risk of injury.

Activity Intolerance

Clients with neuromuscular disease are typically easily fatigued and unable to negotiate previous levels of activity without frequent rest periods. Rest periods need to be built into planning for these clients, as do methods for participating in ADLs while conserving energy. A qualitative study of clients with MS discovered five themes associated with the experience of clients with fatigue:

- Fatigue as an ever-present, ongoing experience
- The pervasive impact of fatigue on life
- The exacerbation of symptoms with increasing fatigue
- Fatigue as a paralyzing force
- The "undertow effect" of severe fatigue (Stuifbergen & Rogers, 1997, p. 5).

According to researchers, self-care strategies need to be directed to reducing the impact of fatigue on the lives of clients. Nurses should recognize that managing chronic fatigue is different from managing acute fatigue.

Altered Nutrition

Despite decreased levels of activity clients may not be consuming enough food and fluids to meet the demands of the body. Energy with which to eat may be compromised. Dysphagia and the risk of aspiration often require feeding tube placement to ensure that clients receive sufficient calories for energy. A nutritionist should provide input during the planning phase of the nursing process and should be included as needed as the client's condition deteriorates.

Altered Thought Processes

Long-term planning for the potential eventuality of altered thought processes should be considered by the interdisciplinary team. Clients with MS, HD, or PD may develop cognitive changes. All clients with HD develop dementia. Approximately 65% of clients with MS experience some cognitive loss (Halper, 2000), and about 30% of clients with PD do as well (Copstead & Banasik, 2000).

Communication

Impaired verbal communication related to muscular weakness and paralysis reduces the client's ability to participate in his or her own care. Planning should include the input of a speech pathologist and adaptive equipment to enhance and maintain whatever form of communication is possible for the client.

Psychosocial Status

Clients with neuromuscular disease are likely to experience changes in the opportunities for social interaction, in roles, and in relationships. Whether clients can continue to be employed and for how long they can work in an office or at home may be significant to their views of themselves. Loss of hope and feelings of helplessness may contribute to higher than normal rates of suicide compared with the general population (Holland & Halper, 1999).

Clients may be fearful and anxious, confused, and in a state of denial about the disease. The fact that these diseases are incurable may precipitate feelings of grief and loss among clients. Limits on mobility and energy are likely to restrict activities and may contribute to the exclusion of the client from previously enjoyable pastimes. Considerations related to fertility and the effects of the disease on pregnancy and childbearing may be devastating.

Planning regarding psychosocial issues should pervade all communication among interdisciplinary team members. Interventions related to any of the other problem areas are likely to affect or be affected by the client's perceptions of himself and his situation. Considerations about how each intervention will be received by the client in the context of his views about his care and his goals for care are vital to the nursing process.

Bowel and Bladder Management

Clients with neuromuscular diseases may be at risk for constipation and/or may become incontinent of bowel and bladder. Some clients, such as those with MS, may retain urine at times. Behavioral techniques may be appropriate to incorporate early in planning. However, medications and procedures, such as digital stimulation for clients with SCI and intermittent catheterization for clients with MS, will likely be added later. The urologist and the enterostomal nurse may be added to the team at any point from initiation of the plan because they can help guide short- and long-term care planning.

Mobility

Muscular weakness, paresis, and paralysis are characteristic features of all of the diseases discussed in this chapter. Physical therapy is an integral component of the care plan because the goals are to maintain and optimize client mobility. The rehabilitation nurse as well as the other team members, including the caregiver, follow the plan of the physical therapist and recommend alterations to the plan as needed.

Skin Integrity

Frequent assessments of the client's skin must be incorporated into the plan of care. Careful positioning is vital to the maintenance of skin integrity, and arrangements must be included for the caregiver to provide this properly and frequently. The caregiver's sleep time and daily activities must be considered because outside assistance may be needed to help with positioning when the caregiver is unavailable.

Self-Care Deficit

It is important that maximal participation in self-care activities be made possible for each client with a neuromuscular disease. However minimal that participation may be, it is crucial to assisting clients to maintain some control over their care during a time when others are so involved in their lives. Caregivers and family members must be included in planning regarding how to help the client participate, and nurses are obliged to teach them why client self-care is necessary.

Involvement in self-care is a component of the client's perception of the illness. A qualitative, ethnographic study (Quinn, Barton, & Magilvy, 1995) explored how clients with MS adapt to their illness. Metaphors, such as the term "roller coaster" (p. 22) to describe the ups and downs of daily living with the disease, appeared to help clients understand the disease and its meaning for them. "Being in a prison" (p. 22) is how one person described the limits imposed by the disease. The study found that participants told stories of personal growth and empowerment as a result of the challenges they faced and weathered related to the disease. Another study by Armer, McDermott, and Schiffer (1996) found that clients with MS who perceived themselves as having less personal control reported a "higher degree of life changes" (p. 109) associated with the disease.

Sexual Dysfunction

Sexual dysfunction may be an early sign of disease in many clients. After careful assessment of the extent of the problem, planning to either include suggestions for improved function or include a sex therapist on the team must take place. The nature of the problem may convince some professionals that sexual dysfunction is a low priority for planning. However, clients may consider it very important, and therefore it is the client's perception of the problem that determines the order of the problem among the priorities.

Gulick (1998) studied clients with MS over a period of 10 years and found that sexual dysfunction is relevant to a decline in intimacy. A decrease in social support may reduce "opportunities to confide" (p. 145), and both of these are also related to the level of intimacy. Neurological impairment as well as fatigue, and in some cases spasticity, can affect libido and the ability to perform sexually.

Caregiver Role Strain

Watson, Modeste, Catolico, & Crouch (1998) hypothesized that caregiver burden would increase as the self-care deficit increased in clients who had formerly received rehabilitation care. Their findings supported the hypothesis specifically with regard to deficits of social cognition. "The more severe the deficits in the client's cognition and self-care capacity, the higher the burden score for the caregiver" (p. 260).

Neuromuscular diseases tend to be progressive and degenerative. The stress, both physically and emotionally, is placed on the caregiver. Planning should incorporate time to instruct caregivers regarding strategies for maintaining their emotional and physical health and for locating acceptable respite care for the client.

The possible genetic component of some of the diseases discussed in this chapter (MS, ALS, HD) supports the need for lifelong planning by clients and their families. Consideration of the likelihood of a genetic component may reduce the incidence of these diseases, particularly HD. Long-term planning may also include the need for institutionalization, such as nursing home placement or full-time home health care.

Short-term planning often includes the need for reliable support systems of skilled and support professionals, as well as durable medical equipment and adaptive equipment. A realistic assessment of the caregiver's capabilities both in the short and long-term will help the nurse, client, and family to design a realistic plan. The interdisciplinary team must be involved in the planning and should also include the physician; physical, occupational, and if needed, speech therapists; a nutritionist; and community resources as appropriate.

The environment to which the client will be discharged must be considered in planning. Goals or the planning designed to achieve the goals may be unrealistic depending on the site of care. The home setting may be more or less adaptable to the plan, as might be the economic resources of the client and caregiver to carry out the planning.

INTERVENTIONS

The neuromuscular diseases discussed in this chapter share many of the same interventions. All of the interventions discussed are only as effective as the strength and collaborative capacity of the interdisciplinary team that plans and performs them. Always, the director of the team is the client and/or the family, and their needs as individuals and as a group must be considered when designing interventions that meet the client's needs. The planning phase of the client's care should include the setting for care so that interventions can be performed and adapted to the site of care. Additionally, community resources such as support groups for both the client and the caregiver and organizations that provide services and equipment might be included during the planning and interventions stages. Representatives of community resources can be invited to participate in care planning and conferencing because their input enhances the ability of each team member to view care in realistic terms. Interventions common to the diseases described in this chapter will be discussed; Table 22-6 lists disease-specific interventions.

Breathing

Maintenance of an effective airway is the most important of all nursing interventions. A through and ongoing assessment of breathing patterns and factors that could disrupt them is integral to timely and appropriate intervention. Proper management of the dysphagia and muscular weakness associated with these diseases will help prevent or forestall respiratory complications.

The nurse monitors the client's vital signs for changes in respiratory function. Oxygen therapy and positioning may be needed to assist breathing as early interventions. Eventually, many of these clients may require mechanical ventilation to assist or assume respiratory function. Interventions specific to clients with difficulty breathing include:

- Maintaining a patent airway
- Assessing respiration frequently
- Monitoring arterial blood gases
- Providing chest physiotherapy as needed
- Referring to the respiratory therapist
- Assisting with mechanical ventilation if needed
- Offering emotional support
- Assessing cough
- Suctioning as needed

Most clients with ALS eventually develop difficulty breathing. However, according to Sivak, Shefner, & Sexton

TABLE 22-6 Interventions and Research Specific to Neuromuscular Disease

Disease	Interventions
Parkinson's disease	Clinical trials of new medications Pallidotomy Deep brain stimulation (Imke, 2000) Trials of pramipexole compared to levodopa (there is less likelihood of wearing off and dyskinesias with pramipexole) (Holloway, 2000)
Multiple sclerosis	New approaches to the management of fatigue (Chan, 1999): physiological, education, modification, compensation, participation in physical exercise ABC approach: Avonex, Betaseron, Copaxone Transplantation of cells that produce myelin (Halper & Holland, 1998)
Guillain-Barré syndrome	Plasmapheresis Intravenous immunoglobulin
Amyotrophic lateral sclerosis	Multidisciplinary clinics
Spinal cord injury	Central nervous system cell research Nerve cell replacement Axon regeneration Axon remyelination Functional electric stimulation Omentum transposition

(1999), respiratory difficulty may go unrecognized if the person is still able to propel a wheelchair or exercise. A headache or mental "fuzziness" may indicate respiratory changes.

Dysreflexia

The following interventions are recommended for clients with autonomic dysreflexia or clients with SCIs of T6 or above. The goals of care are to discover and remove the stimulus and thereby reduce blood pressure high enough to threaten life.

- Raise the head of the bed
- Lower the client's legs
- Loosen clothing, vascular devices, and appliances
- Monitor blood pressure every 2 to 3 minutes
- Contact the physician if blood pressure is approximately double baseline
- Attempt to alleviate cause
- Empty bladder if distended
- Relieve fecal mass, applying a topical anesthetic 5 minutes before the mass is removed
- Check rectum 20 minutes after removal of mass
- Examine and relieve skin
- Remove any other trigger or stimulus
- Give nifedipine (Procardia) or other antihypertensive as ordered if no relief
- Monitor client for rebound hypertension (Travers, 1999)

Swallowing and Nutrition

Dysphagia places the client with neuromuscular disease at increased risk of aspiration. Initially positioning and alterations of the consistency of foods may suffice. Later, placement of an enteral feeding tube may become appropriate.

A diet that promotes energy is high in calories. Small, frequent meals allow the client to conserve energy while consuming the calories and nutrients needed to meet metabolic demands. Adequate fluid intake to prevent dehydration may be oral initially and may require alternative methods as the disease progresses. Water administered through the client's enteral feeding tube will ensure adequate fluid intake. Interventions specific to clients with dysphagia and altered nutrition (less than body requirements) are listed below. Many drugs may contribute to dysphagia by causing dry mouth. A saliva substitute or sips of water before and after meals can help (Brown, 2000). A barium swallow can help diagnose and assess swallowing problems. Behavioral therapies, such as sensory enhancement and postural techniques, can be effective interventions (Brown, 2000). Other interventions specific to dysphagia and altered nutrition include:

- Assessing for gag reflex
- Noting drooling and difficulty controlling secretions
- Monitoring fluid and electrolytes
- Providing a balanced diet that can be chewed and swallowed easily
- Referring to a dietitian
- Providing thick liquids or semisolid food
- Maintaining an upright position during meals
- Massaging the neck and facial muscles before eating
- Monitoring calorie count and weekly weights
- Scheduling medications so peak action minimizes chewing difficulty
- Referring to a speech pathologist

Injury

The key to preventing injury in a client with a neuromuscular disease is surveillance. This includes not only clients' physical environment for safety hazards but also their cognitive ability related to the identification of potential hazards and their understanding of the existence of real hazards in the environment. Clients may be in denial about the disease or be unrealistic about their ability to negotiate potential safety hazards. Additionally, caregivers may overestimate the client's ability to recognize a safety hazard and be able to avoid it.

Teaching the client and the caregiver about the potential for injury to the client is the primary intervention. The plan for teaching will need to be modified as care continues and as the client's awareness or mobility declines. The following list provides interventions specific to risk for injury related to sensory deficit and inadequate self-protective abilities.

- Assess environment for safety hazards
- Teach client and caregiver how to avoid injury
- Provide supportive devices such as padded side rails if ordered and if permitted in care setting

Activity Intolerance/Impaired Physical Mobility

Energy conservation measures, physical and occupational therapy, strength training, and pain control all serve to enhance activity tolerance and physical mobility. The client's ability to breathe without difficulty also contributes to active participation in activities. Participation in activities requiring energy should occur when energy levels are highest. Scheduled rest periods can be helpful to conserve energy (Halper, 2000).

Because these neuromuscular diseases are incurable (although GBS may be curable, recovery may be prolonged), therapeutic exercises are important to maintaining and maximizing strength, to preventing muscle atrophy, and to decreasing the risk of complications related to immobility, such as deep vein thrombosis. Exercise is recommended for clients with MS and PD. However, it is stressed that moderation should be practiced because overdoing exercise can further compromise the muscular system, increase pain, and contribute to overwork and stress. Endurance programs, aerobic and aquatic exercise, and inpatient rehabilitation programs have been shown to be effective with MS clients. Multiple Sclerosis Society chapters often offer exercise groups (Chan, 2000).

The physician and the physical therapist should be consulted to help determine the best exercises for the individual, the appropriate intensity, and the duration of the workout. It is recommended that clients exercise in a safe environment, use grab bars to stabilize balance, and proceed slowly. MS clients in particular should avoid exercising during the heat of the day and should be aware of the outside temperature and their body temperature (www.clevelandclinic.org).

Clients with HD are also encouraged to maintain fitness as much as possible. Walking is recommended even if the client's coordination is poor. Padding, assistive devices, and sturdy shoes can help prolong the ability to walk for as long as possible (National Institute of Neurological Disorders and Stroke, www.ninds.nih.gov/patients/Disorder/HUNTING).

The following interventions are specific to clients with activity intolerance and impaired physical mobility (Figure 22-7):

- Assess sensory and motor status regularly
- Ensure good pulmonary function
- Perform range-of-motion frequently
- Use assistive devices as needed to minimize fatigue and to prevent contractures
- Assist with ambulation if possible
- Teach and assist with therapeutic exercises
- Teach ways to assist with mobility
- Assess tremor if appropriate
- Position properly
- Administer medication to enhance motor function
- Refer to physical and/or occupational therapist

Communication

Difficulties with verbal communication provide another valid reason to refer to the speech pathologist. These specialists are trained to conduct thorough assessments of communication problems and recommend and implement strategies to improve communication. Specific interventions for clients with impaired verbal communication follow:

- Provide opportunity for the client to communicate without pressure
- Instruct the client to take deep breaths before speaking
- Use assistive devices to enhance communication: flash cards, pictures, computer technology
- Massage neck and facial muscles to enhance relaxation
- Refer to the speech pathologist

Psychosocial Issues

It is important that the nurse acknowledge to the client that psychosocial issues may arise. The client and family may be reluctant to voice concerns for fear that their feelings are unusual or unjustified. Clients and their significant others might benefit from speaking to the nurse in private and as a group. However, the nurse will find that a thorough assessment of the client's concerns should occur

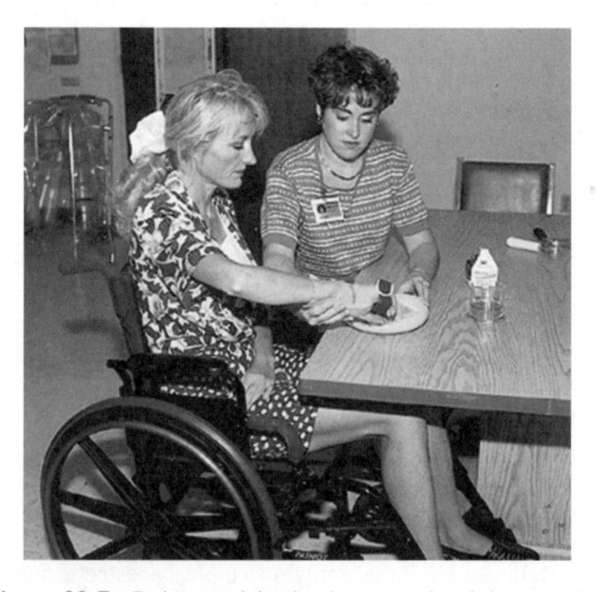

Figure 22-7 Patient participating in occupational therapy using mobile arm supports and upper-extremity orthotics. (From Lewis, S.M., Collier, I.C., Heitkemper, M.M., & Dirksen, S.R. [2000]. *Medical-surgical nursing: assessment and management of clinical problems* [5th ed.]. St. Louis: Mosby.)

initially because confidentiality is paramount. Some specific interventions for clients with psychosocial concerns follow:

- Provide information about the anticipated pattern of illness
- Provide information about treatments as they become available and appropriate
- Affirm client's symptoms and concerns
- Encourage client and family to express concerns
- Recruit community resources as appropriate
- Recruit neighbors and congregation members to provide support
- Recommend support groups and associations/societies
- Provide pain relief
- Provide interventions for sufficient rest

Bowel and Bladder

Alterations in neurological function, dysphagia, altered nutrition, and decreased mobility contribute to bowel and bladder problems among clients with neuromuscular diseases. Behavioral techniques and medications can supplement interventions related to motor and sensory loss, reduced bulk in the diet, inadequate fluid intake, and decreased gastric motility. Interventions specific to bowel and bladder management follow.

Constipation

- Encourage mobility to increase peristalsis
- Maintain adequate fluid intake
- Provide high-fiber foods
- Consider advising the client to use Power Pudding (Neal, 1995)
- Administer tool softeners as ordered
- Instruct client and caregiver in regular bowel program

Urinary Retention (MS)

- Administer medications as ordered
- Teach client/caregiver intermittent catheterization techniques
- Use reflex stimulation as an alternative method
- Maintain adequate fluid intake
- Instruct client/caregiver in signs/symptoms of urinary tract infection

Urinary Incontinence

- Administer medications as ordered
- Instruct client/caregiver in prompted/timed voiding
- Maintain fluid intake
- Consider intermittent or continuous catheter urinary drainage

Skin Integrity

Impaired mobility and altered nutrition as well as a susceptibility to infection related to the disease process interact to alter the integrity of the skin. Vigilance to prevent pressure ulcers from developing is key because healing of wounds once they occur is also compromised by the aforementioned alterations in health status. Interventions related to the prevention and care of the skin follow:

- Inspect skin frequently for signs of breakdown
- Position and turn client frequently
- Provide optimal nutritional (protein and fluids) intake
- Keep skin clean and dry

Self-Care Deficit

A guiding principle of rehabilitation nursing is that clients will be taught and encouraged to participate to the best of their ability in self-care management. Often it is deemed easier by the caregiver to perform ADLs for the client, and caregivers may not recognize that participation in self-care is therapeutic. Very debilitated clients can assist with self-care in some form even if their participation is limited to communicating choices about how someone else will perform their care.

Instruction of clients and caregivers and the use of assistive devices to maximize self-care ability are the key interventions. Assistive or adaptive devices such as special eating utensils, dicem, and plates with guards can significantly increase clients' abilities to feed themselves.

Rehabilitation nurses play a vital role in assisting clients with chronic diseases and disabilities to adjust to their illnesses. Davidhizar (1997, pp. 33-35) concluded after a search of the literature that nurses can best help these clients by complying with the following:

- Assess client for psychological and adjustment problems
- Encourage clients to express feelings
- Do not make promises or give false assurances
- Communicate empathy for the client's feelings
- Be aware of cultural differences in the way clients cope
- Inform clients about the disability and the treatment
- Encourage a positive body image
- Encourage the use of role modeling and mentoring
- Build a network of support
- Promote the use of a variety of coping techniques
- Guide toward seeking employment
- Cultivate a positive and realistic outlook on life

Sexual Dysfunction

Clients with sexual dysfunction frequently require the service of a trained sex counselor. It is best to provide the client and significant other a safe and confidential environment in which to express their concerns, explain that these concerns are not unexpected in light of the client's condition, and provide resources for seeking counseling. Special aids, pain medications, lubricants, and prosthetics may enhance comfort and confidence (Holland & Halper, 1999).

TABLE 22-7 Pharmaceutical Management of Neuromuscular Disease

Medication	Use	Disease
Corticosteroids	Treat exacerbations	MS, MG, GBS
Immunomodulators	Treat exacerbations	MS, MG
Cholinergics	Urinary retention	MS
Anticholinergics	Urinary frequency	MS
Anticholinergics	Tremor	PD
Muscle relaxants	Spasticity	MS, SCI
Antispasmodics	Urinary retention	MS, SCI
Dopaminergic	Bradykinesia, tremor, rigidity; maintain mean arterial pressure	PD, SCI
Antihistamine	Tremor, rigidity	PD
MAO inhibitor	Bradykinesia, tremor, rigidity	PD
Anticholinesterase	Prolong acetylcholine	MG
Antipsychotics, antichorea	Reduce psychosis, chorea	HD
Antidepressants	Reduce depression	All
Methylprednisolone	Improve blood flow, reduce edema	SCI
COMT inhibitors	Inhibit breakdown of levodopa	PD
Antioxidants	Slow disease progression	PD
Methotrexate	Immunosuppression	MS
T-cell receptor peptides	Inhibit immune system attack	MS
Monoclonal antibodies	Suppress abnormal immune response	MS
Stool softeners	Constipation	All
β-Agonist/GABA antagonists	Spasticity	MS
Riluzole	Reduce release of glutamate from cells	ALS
GM-1 ganglioside	Increased functional recovery	SCI

MS, Multiple sclerosis; *MG,* myasthenia gravis; *GBS,* Guillain-Barré syndrome; *PD,* Parkinson's disease; *SCI,* spinal cord injury; *HD,* Huntington's disease; *ALS,* amyotrophic lateral sclerosis; *SCI,* spinal cord injury; *MAO,* monoamine oxidase; *COMT,* catechol-O-methyltransferase; *GABA,* γ-aminobutyric acid.

Caregiver Role Strain

The stress and strain on caregivers of clients with neuromuscular diseases is great. Permission giving allows the caregiver to express frustration and stress without guilt or fear of betrayal. Some caregivers may require professional counseling if stress is impairing their ability to provide safe care for the client. Specific suggestions for obtaining rest and respite are most helpful to caregivers and include, but are not limited to, the following:

- Requesting the assistance of neighbors or members of the caregiver's congregation
- Hiring a companion or aide to sit with the client for brief periods or care for the client at night
- Reserving respite space at a local nursing home so the caregiver can take a vacation

Disease-Specific Interventions

In addition to the aforementioned interventions, Table 22-6 lists interventions and research specific to the neuromuscular diseases discussed in this chapter.

Pharmaceutical Management

According to the Multiple Sclerosis Nurse Specialists Consensus Committee (2000) there are several considerations when medicating clients with MS. These considerations appear to apply to all of the clients discussed in this chapter:

- Determine contraindications
- Instruct clients in anticipated outcomes and adverse or side effects of drug therapy
- Encourage clients to attend follow-up visits so that the effectiveness and tolerance of treatments can be evaluated

Table 22-7 lists medications currently used to treat the neuromuscular diseases discussed in this chapter.

OUTCOMES

To achieve the desired outcomes (see Table 22-5) for clients with neuromuscular disease, careful planning, appropriate intervention, and the continued involvement of all pertinent interdisciplinary team members are necessary. As the goals of care are set with the client and/or caregiver and evaluated as realistic and attainable by all involved, outcomes should reflect successful achievement of these goals. It is difficult to predict outcomes related to a population of clients. It is preferable to design goals and measure outcomes on the basis of the individual's clinical presentation and disease process. Table 22-8 lists the desired outcomes for the goals and interventions that have been discussed in this chapter.

TABLE 22-8 Desired Outcomes in Neuromuscular Disease

Nursing Diagnosis	Desired Outcome
Breathing	Arterial blood gases within normal range Lungs clear to auscultation No respiratory distress Normal chest x-ray film
Dysreflexia	No occurrence Prompt and appropriate intervention
Impaired communication	Communication
Swallowing/altered nutrition	Maintenance of adequate body weight
Injury	No injury
Activity intolerance/fatigue	Energy conservation and activity tolerance
Psychosocial issues	Contentment
Constipation	Bowel elimination
Incontinence	Bowel and bladder management

EVALUATION

The outcomes listed above are ideal. As stated earlier the client, caregiver, and interdisciplinary team design goals that are realistic for the client in the context of his or her environment and resources. Satisfactory achievement of these goals as outlined and agreed on by the team constitutes a successful outcome. Ongoing modification of the plan and the goals is necessary so that efforts to accomplish goals remain realistic.

IMPLICATIONS FOR CLIENTS WITH NEUROMUSCULAR DISEASE

During early stages of disease, many clients will be able to continue work and their normal activities. Clients with SCI will stabilize at a level of paralysis and be able to adapt their future lifestyle to the injury. All clients with neuromuscular disease need to plan for the long-term. The ability to work, attend school, participate in the community, and be independent will depend largely on the client's motivation and emotional resources; support system, both professional and nonprofessional; and adaptive and assistive equipment. Many persons with disabilities currently remain in work settings that are adapted to meet their needs. Others work from home. However, the ability to continue these activities changes as the client's condition deteriorates.

Care planning, as mentioned earlier, must be ongoing, and goals and interventions must be modified as the client's status changes. Goals and desired outcomes should remain realistic to avoid frustration and hopelessness.

IMPLICATIONS FOR POLICY

A new presidential administration took office this year, and the Congress is divided evenly along party lines. A new legislature has implications for changes in health care. Persons with neuromuscular disease require many medications to deal with the complications of their disease and frequent physician visits, home health stays, and hospitalizations. Many persons eventually require a nursing home stay. Inpatient and outpatient rehabilitation may or may not be reimbursed by insurance. Changes in health care policy are needed to help persons with chronic illnesses afford their medications and appropriate treatment. It is hoped that the new president and Congress will develop and implement plans that reduce costs for the chronically ill and thus reduce the burden on clients and caregivers.

IMPLICATIONS FOR LONG-TERM CARE AND RESEARCH

Persons with chronic illness are living longer (Feder & Moon, 1999) and many are being cared for in the home setting (Mackin & Forester, 1999). There are implications for rehabilitation nursing practice related to this increase in chronically ill clients at home. Rehabilitation nurses need to move into the home and community settings in greater numbers to meet the needs of these clients. Rehabilitation nurses possess the skills and experience most needed by clients living with chronic illnesses in the home setting.

The prevalence of neuromuscular disease has implications for research because recent studies indicate correlations with climatic conditions, geographical regions, sex, and genetics. Clinical research that investigates the relationships between and among these variables will certainly impact prevention, treatment, and recovery. Research that explores the quality of life of clients and caregivers may help persons cope with and better understand these diseases and how to adapt to them. Studies of various interventions and their effects will undoubtedly contribute to improved outcomes and may influence increased length of life after diagnosis. Pharmacological research studies continue to result in improved medications to help persons manage symptoms and prevent complications. Much work remains to be done toward eventual eradication of these diseases or, at least, improved management of them. Rehabilitation nurses are in a unique position to participate as principal investigators and as members of research teams to explore the possibilities.

CRITICAL THINKING

Considering the common characteristics of many neuromuscular diseases, develop one nursing approach for each of the following issues related to the client's response to the diagnosis of an incurable neuromuscular disease: fear, reduced sense of control, inability to return to work, and dependence on others.

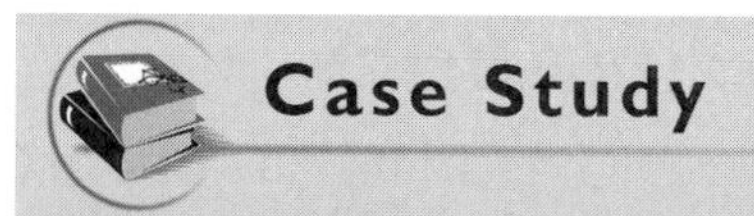

Case Study

Mr. J is a 75-year-old man diagnosed with PD 23 years ago. No longer able to operate his watch repair shop because of his hand tremors, he and his wife sold the business and lived on business profits, payments from a preexisting disability insurance policy, and their investments. Within 2 years he developed increased tremors of the hands and tongue, "pill rolling" with his fingers, and a shuffling gait. He refused medication, embarking instead on his own regimen of nutrition; vitamins; herbal remedies; and a tonic of honey, water, and cider vinegar. Always self-disciplined, he performed daily exercise. His wife prepared his diet and joined him in activities to "keep mentally alert." Although he had difficulty walking and slurred speech, little changed for 6 more years. The Js traveled and met with friends, and Mr. J continued to drive their car.

At 62 years of age, things changed dramatically. He began L-dopa concurrent with his own regimen. Mr. J used a cane, a wheelchair, or an Amigo cart in public. The Js moved to a one-level ranch-style house accessible for Mr. J's wheelchair; he walked "on good days." After his urinary frequency, difficulty turning in bed, and nightmares began interrupting sleep for both Mr. and Mrs. J, he slept in a separate bedroom. Larger and more frequent doses of L-dopa did not control periods of bradykinesia, cogwheeling, and rigidity. "Freezing," which impaired self-care with ADL and drooling, caused him embarrassment and anxiety. He contacted a physician who would prescribe anti-PD drugs in combinations and newly released medications.

At 70 years of age, Mr. J took a "drug holiday," a decision not supported by his wife or physician, both of whom described Mr. J as "demanding and stubborn" concerning his health regimen. He was rushed to the hospital after experiencing dyskinesia, hypotension, pain, confusion, nausea, and incontinence. Mrs. J was depressed and anxious about how she would continue to care for him. He returned home unable to perform bathing or dressing but able to walk "on good days." Although he could feed himself, everything was slowed, including his speech. His overall health status was excellent, except for dental care needs because he had not visited a dentist for 15 years. He played games for stimulation, but fewer friends came to visit, and Mrs. J became his main contact. Ironically Mr. J drove the car to his biweekly physical therapy sessions.

Mrs. J continued care for her husband until he fell during the night several times. Unable to assist him off the floor, she called 911 for help. The Js refused visiting nurse services as "charity care," so Mrs. J hired the first of three "helpers" who were to assist Mr. J with his personal care, meals, and exercises three times a week. When the third helper left, Mrs. J, who had experienced a mild stroke earlier the same year, decided that Mr. J should move to a nursing home. The Js' long-term care policy covered most costs. Mrs. J would visit regularly, and Mr. J would receive therapy, medical supervision, and assistance with ADLs. Reluctantly Mr. J agreed to a trial stay in the nursing home, provided he came home on Saturdays.

After a month at the nursing home, Mr. J was functioning at a higher level: walking more, sleeping through the night, and experiencing fewer speech problems. Mrs. J began to attend local social activities and rejoined her bridge and garden clubs. Mr. J came home on Saturdays but increasingly objected to returning to the nursing home on Saturday nights. He began to complain about the nursing home food and being lonely for his own home. When Mrs. J stated she could not take care of him at home, he accused her of "putting him away." However, both Mr. and Mrs. J are reluctant to have help in the home, especially live-in help. They state they want privacy and are fearful and distrustful of outsiders.

This week Mr. J informed his wife that he is coming home. He arranged a driving assessment and plans to resume driving. Although he has difficulty with ambulation, he insists the reflexes required for driving are intact. Mrs. J sought advice from a cousin whose husband lived at home after a stroke and as a result has hired an independent rehabilitation nurse as case manager. Eventually the Js worked with the nurse to write a health contract identifying their goals and responsibilities based on the following nursing diagnoses and process.

Nusing Diagnosis	Assessment	Interventions	Outcomes
Ineffective coping due to denial and anger	Inability to adjust to changes; unrealistic expectations from self and others; lack of control over disease process; lack of problem-solving; fear of abandonment by spouse	Write health contract, elicit Mr. J's perception and appraisal, then institute reframing and decision-making techniques; discuss methods for coping with loss and change; remove barriers to self-care; evaluate marriage relationship	Adherence to written contract, empowerment for decision-making, and improved interpersonal relationships
Knowledge deficit	Stress from rejection or denial of disease process and drug therapy; lack of acknowledgement of wife's health condition	Empower client by educating about disease trajectory; inform of local PD support groups; educate regarding wife's health condition; educate about medications and drug holidays, assistive devices, speech therapy, and relaxation techniques	Revise regimen; recognize wife's role and responsibilities; use assistive devices and techniques to reduce stressors; verbally describe treatment program. (Refer to Chapter 11 for discussion of education and teaching)

OT, Occupational therapist; *PT,* physical therapist; *ROM,* range of motion.

Nusing Diagnosis	Assessment	Interventions	Outcomes
Caregiver role strain; potential for breakdown of trust in the marriage relationship	Caregiver has history of stroke, restricted socialization, primary responsibility for client's care and safety	Arrange respite care when Mr. J returns home; educate about services and support groups; teach relaxation techniques and interpersonal skills; ensure safety in home; inform community emergency services; evaluate relationship	Reduced stress from daily responsibilities; resumption of club activities; use of personal relaxation techniques; monitoring of health status
Altered health status (dental)	Regular checkups and overall excellent health status apart from signs and symptoms of PD, except for dental caries, reddened gums with bleeding, chipped teeth, and malocclusion resulting in damage to lips and oral mucosa	Provide information about dentist skilled in working with clients who have conditions such as PD	Dental appointments for preventive and restorative care
Alterations in urinary pattern; frequency, incontinence	Refer to Chapter 19 for discussion of bladder elimination		
Impaired mobility; potential for altered skin integrity	Reduced ability to initiate movements voluntarily or to move from bed to chair or commode; rigidity, tremor bradykinesia, cogwheeling, "pill rolling," and shuffling gait; potential for injury, falls, damage to skin	Teach ROM exercises; teach exercises specific for coping with immobility due to PD (e.g., position "nose over toes" to rise from chair, stepping over imaginary mark to initiate walking, or rocking side to side to move legs); evaluate need for special mattress and trapeze bar in bed; observe for edema; consider occupational and/or physical therapy consultations for ambulation, fine motor movements (refer to Chapter 14 for discussion of mobility)	Prevent complications or further immobility, maximize comfort and sense of control; adherence to regimen
Disturbed sleep pattern; safety issues	Inability to sleep through the night; nightmares, falls	Negotiate use of side rails or other devices, bedside urinal; relaxation and ROM before bedtime; medications as ordered	Establish rest and sleep patterns with minimal interruptions (refer to Chapter 27 for discussion or sleep and rest)
Social isolation; potential for reduced satisfaction with quality of life	Physical, social, and spiritual isolation; reduced stimulation and access to information or contact with others; caregiver has responsibility for all interactions	Institute community programs such as day care centers, senior center, van transportation, attendant services, church programs, Meals on Wheels, partners for "thinking games," support groups, exercise or therapy programs; respite for wife; obtain realistic evaluation of ability to drive	Encourage maximum stimulation and independence in social interaction; reduced stressors in marriage relationship; improved quality of life

Other problems for nursing diagnosis and process: (1) Impaired communication, slurred speech; (2) self-care deficit, ADL; (3) threats to community re-entry, driving, refusing attendant services; (4) potential for altered nutritional status, family dysfunction, financial problems, and chronic condition for caregiver

WEBSITE RESOURCES

Amyotrophic lateral sclerosis: www.lougehrigsdisease.net.
Huntington's disease: www.hdsa.org.
Multiple sclerosis: www.nmss.org.
Myasthenia gravis: www.myasthenia.org.
Parkinson's disease: www.pdf.org.
Spinal cord injury: www.aascin.org, www.alsa.org, and www.fscip.org.

REFERENCES

Armer, J.M., McDermott, M.P., & Schiffer, R.B. (1996). Psychological characteristics of MS patients: Determining differences based upon participation in a therapy regimen. *Rehabilitation Nursing Research, 5*(3), 102-111.

Beck, L.A., Harris, M.R., & Basford, J. (1999). Factors influencing functional outcome and discharge disposition after thoracic spinal cord injury. *SCI Nursing, 16*(4), 127-131.

Brown, S.A. (2000). Swallowing and speaking: challenges for the MS patient. *International Journal of MS Care* [On-line], *2*(3). Available: http://www.mscare.com/a0009/page_02.htm.

Bullock, B.A., & Henze, R.L. (2000). *Focus on pathophysiology.* Philadelphia: JB Lippincott.

Carter, R.J., Lione, R.A., Humby, T., Mangiarini, L., Mahal, A., Bates, G.P., Dunnett, S.B., & Morton, A.J. (1999). Characterization of progressive motor deficits in mice transgenic for the human Huntington's disease mutation. *Journal of Neuroscience 19*(3), 3248-3257.

Chan, A. (2000). Review of common management strategies for fatigue in multiple sclerosis. *International Journal of MS Care, 1*(2), 13-19.

Copstead, L.E.E., & Banasik, J.L. (2000). *Pathophysiology* (2nd ed.). Philadelphia: WB Saunders.

Davidhizar, R. (1997). Disability does not have to be the grief that never ends: helping patients adjust. *Rehabilitation Nursing, 22*(1), 32-35.

Farnan, C.M. (2000). Spinal cord injuries. *Advance for Nurses, February 28,* 19-20.

Feder, J., & Moon, M. (1999). Can Medicare survive its saviors? *Caring, XVIII*(9), 30-33.

Gulick, E.E. (1998). Symptom and activities of daily living trajectory in multiple sclerosis: a 10-year study. *Nursing Research, 47*(3), 137-146.

Halper, J. (2000). The evolution of nursing care in multiple sclerosis. *International Journal of MS Care, 2*(1), 13-20.

Halper, J., & Holland, N. (1998). Part I: new strategies, new hope: meeting the challenge of multiple sclerosis: treating the person and the disease. *American Journal of Nursing, 98*(10), 26-31.

Holland, N., & Halper, J. (1999). Primary care management of multiple sclerosis. A guide for nurse practitioners. *ADVANCE for Nurse Practitioners, March,* 27-32.

Holloway, R. (2000). Pramipexole vs Levodopa as initial treatment for Parkinson disease. *Journal of the American Medical Association, 284,* 1931-1938.

Huether, S.E., & McCance, K.L. (2000). *Understanding pathophysiology* (2nd ed.). St. Louis: Mosby.

Imke, S. (2000). Parkinson's: a medical management update. *The Parkinson Report, 19*(3), 1-7.

Jackson, G., & Kelsey, A. (1999). The needs of neurology patients after discharge. *Professional Nurse, 14*(7), 467-470.

Lewis, S.M., Collier, I.C., Heitkemper, M.M., & Dirksen, S.R. (2000). *Medical-surgical nursing: assessment and management of clinical problems* (5th ed.). St. Louis: Mosby.

Lublin, F.D., & Reingold, S.C. (1996). Defining the clinical course of multiple sclerosis: results of an international survey. *Neurology, 46,* 907-911.

Mackin, A.L., & Forester, T.M. (1999). Home health at the crossroads. *Caring, XVIII*(9), 12-15.

Multiple Sclerosis Nurse Specialists Consensus Committee. (2000). *Multiple sclerosis: best practices in nursing care* [Monograph]. Columbia, MD: Medicalliance.

Narayan, M., & Tennant, J. (1997). Environmental assessment. *Home Healthcare Nurse, 15*(11), 798-805.

National Institute of Neurological Disorders and Stroke. (2001, March 15). Available: http://www.ninds.nih.gov/health_and_medical/pubs/parkinson_disease_htr.htm.

Neal, L.J. (1995). Power pudding: Natural laxative therapy to the elderly who are homebound. *Home Healthcare Nurse, 13*(3), 66-71.

Neal, L.J. (1997). Is anybody home? *Home Healthcare Nurse, 15*(3), 158-167.

Polak, M., & Boynton de Sepulveda, L. (2000). Care of the patient with amyotrophic lateral sclerosis. *Advance for Nurses, May 8,* 15-16.

Quinn, A.A., Barton, J.A., & Magilvy, J.K. (1995). Weathering the storm: metaphors and stories of living with multiple sclerosis. *Rehabilitation Nursing Research, 4*(1), 19-26.

Ransohoff, R. (2000). A fundamentally new view of multiple sclerosis. *International Journal of MS Care, 2*(2), 2-5.

Ruess, M.L., Paneth, N., Pinto-Martin, J.A., Lorenz, J. M., Susser, M. (1996). The relation of transient hypothyroxinemia in preterm infants to neurologic development at two years of age. *New England Journal of Medicine, 334*(13), 821-827.

Sivak, E.D., Shefner, J.M., & Sexton, J. (1999). Neuromuscular disease and hypoventilation [Review]. *Current Opinion in Pulmonary Medicine 5*(6), 355-362.

Smeltzer, S.C., & Bare, B.G. (2000). *Medical-surgical nursing.* Philadelphia: JB Lippincott.

Stuifbergen, A.K., & Rogers, S. (1997). The experience of fatigue and strategies of self-care among persons with multiple sclerosis. *Applied Nursing Research, 10*(1), 2-10.

Travers, P.L. (1999). Autonomic dysreflexia: a clinical rehabilitation problem. *Rehabilitation Nursing, 24*(1), 19-23.

Watson, R., Modeste, N.N., Catolico, O., & Crouch, M. (1998). The relationship between caregiver burden and self-care deficits in former rehabilitation patients. *Rehabilitation Nursing, 23*(5), 258-262.

Wilson, S.F., & Giddens, J.F. (2001). *Health assessment for nursing practice* (2nd ed.). St. Louis: Mosby.

Worsham, T.L. (2000). Easing the course of Guillain-Barré syndrome. *RN, 63*(3), 46-50.

Young, R. (1999). Update on Parkinson's disease. *American Family Physician, 59*(8), 2155-2167.

BIBLIOGRAPHY

Muscular Dystrophy Association. (2000). *The ALS Newsletter* [On-line]. Available: http://www.madausa.org/publications/als/.

Sexuality Education and Counseling

23

Susan B. Greco, MSN, RN, CRRN

In my role as client educator I conduct sexual education seminars for rehabilitation hospitals. A few staff members usually attend, and clients show a great interest in learning how to participate as fully as possible in sexual activities. One person in particular stands out, a woman in her early 20s. She had been a newlywed of less than a year at the time of her thoracic spinal cord injury (SCI). She and her husband were from a Christian background and enjoyed their sexual relationship. I gave them a schedule for SCI education classes, explaining that I was teaching the next day but that during the course educators of various disciplines would speak on their areas of expertise. That evening I entered her room to find the couple conversing intently. I asked if they were taking the SCI course. "Yes, but we have a request; first teach us right here about sexual function, then we will be ready to listen to whatever else you want to teach us in class." I would have preferred to follow the schedule beginning with physiology and changes related to SCI. However, I gathered my materials used for the sexuality class, returned to the room, and began at what was usually the end of the program. They were great learners, and I enjoyed my time with them.

Only a few persons have not wanted the class on sexuality, usually women who lost their partners. Both young and old are interested. One woman older than 70 years had fallen and fractured a hip. Married to a younger man, she believed her only learning need was how to have intercourse without violating her postsurgical hip precautions; she was a most appreciative learner.

My thinking concerning sexuality has been expanded in rehabilitation by staff responses to hypersexual and inappropriate behavior by persons with brain injury. Their shocked response and difficulty in finding an approach fueled my desire to learn more about the cognitive influence on sexual activity and how to manage client behavior in a facility.

Many have expressed their confusion about sexual activity when one of the couple has become ill or experienced mental or physical changes. With universal relief, they learned that in most cases, after the person is medically stable, sexual activity will not worsen the condition, and they can resume sexual activities. It seems they awaited permission and answers to sexual questions from providers, but no team member initiated information or addressed sexual questions unless the client or partner asked.

SEXUALITY AND SEXUAL FUNCTION

Human beings are sexual beings. The common response after an ultrasonograph—"Is it a boy or girl?"—has profound effects throughout the life span. Sexuality is vital to being and to rehabilitation nursing practice. The concept of human sexuality encompasses how one thinks, feels, and acts as a sexual being; needs and drives; roles and expression of maleness or femaleness; interactions; identity; and development and function (National Guidelines Task Force, 1991). Who and what we are is incorporated into our sexuality, inseparable from ourselves. Expressing sexuality through intimate involvement with another is a developmental task of adolescence and young adulthood.

A holistic view of sexuality embraces biology, psychology, sociology, relationships, and spirituality. Biological factors dictate sexual development from conception to birth, reproductive ability after puberty, and certain sex differences in behavior; they also elicit physical responses, such as with sex organs or pulse rate. Sexual desire, functioning, and satisfaction have physical and psychological components. The psychosocial dimension, the sense of gender identity, is shaped by information and attitudes transmitted by parents, peers, teachers, and society. Because sexual behavior is a product of biological and psychosocial forces, it sheds light on why and how persons act, not only what they do (Malek & Brower, 1984). Ultimately sexuality is a construct of one's body image and self-concept. Maslow (1954) identified the sexual drive as a basic human need that varies with culture, life stage and status, physical and emotional well-being, and available opportunities. Essential to reproducing the species, sexuality certainly has affected lives throughout history. Positive nonreproductive purposes of sex include:

- Strengthening of pair bonding
- Fostering intimacy between partners
- Providing pleasure
- Bolstering self-esteem
- Reducing tension and anxiety
- Demonstrating masculinity or femininity (Reinisch, 1990)

The World Health Organization (1975) defined sexual health as "an integration of somatic, emotional, intellectual, and social aspects of sexual being, in ways that are positive, enriching, and that enhance personality, communication, and love." Three basic tenets are (1) the ability of a person to enjoy sexual and reproductive behavior in accordance with personal and social ethics; (2) freedom from fear, guilt, shame, and false information, which impair a sexual relationship and inhibit sexual response; and (3) freedom from organic disease and disabilities that present barriers to sexual and reproductive functions (World Health Organization, 1975).

Cultural Influences

Culture defines usual and acceptable sexuality and sexual performance, as well as variations of sexual pleasuring. Common threads forbid incest and advocate privacy during sexual relations (Woods, 1988). Some permit premarital intercourse, especially for men; others tolerate it if with intent to marry; extramarital sex is generally condemned (Monga & Lefebvre, 1995). Culture also defines whether help can come from outside the family and by whom; educators must learn the client's cultural norms before offering advice or education.

The Social Organization of Sexuality survey about sexual activities was based on interviews with 3500 Americans aged 18 to 59 years. In contrast to the Kinsey Reports, researchers found that Americans were largely monogamous: 83% had 0 to 1 partners per year, men had 6 in a lifetime, and women had 2. Marriage meant the most sex and greatest likelihood for orgasm among couples, 94% of whom were faithful to their spouses. Adultery is the exception, with 75% of men and 85% of women in intact marriages being faithful. Only 2.7% of men and 1.3% of women reported homosexual sex (Elmer-Dewitt, 1994).

Changes in thinking result from active research in the rehabilitation of persons with sexual impairments and new practices, such as drugs and treatments for erectile dysfunction (ED) (who has not heard of Viagra?), successes with infertility, and information about orgasm with complete and incomplete SCI. Educators providing sexual content must remain current with research findings and practice guidelines.

Sexual Response

Sexual response follows a natural progression for all ages. Masters, Johnson, and Kolodny (1986) gave a classic description of changes during sexual response: excitement, plateau, orgasm, and resolution. The physiological processes of sexual response are not simply mechanical movements but are part of psychosexual involvement and identity of the whole person. Two basic physiological reactions occur during human sexual response: vasocongestion and increased neuromuscular tension or myotonia, followed by resolution. Just after orgasm, hyperventilated breathing with a rapid pulse (100 to 160 beats/minute) and a rise in blood pressure occur but recede as the body relaxes (Masters, et al., 1986). Resolution is longer after considerable excitement without orgasm; lingering pelvic heaviness is due to continued vasocongestion, and sleep or masturbation usually bring relief.

PHYSIOLOGY OF SEXUAL RESPONSE

Overview

Psychological desire precludes initiating and performing sexually; vascular, hormonal, and neurological systems must connect synergistically and work in balance in either gender. The limbic system and hypothalamus help facilitate and inhibit erection. Psychogenic stimuli can both facilitate and inhibit; psychic stimulation can affect the tactile stimulation necessary for a reflex erection. Messages from the brain descend in the lateral columns near the pyramidal tracts of the spinal cord. Spinal centers for erection are in sympathetic preganglionic fibers (T11 to L2) and parasympathetic fibers (S2 to S4); the systems act synergistically to produce erections. Nitric oxide is involved in the nonadrenergic, noncholinergic neurotransmission in men, leading to smooth muscle relaxation in the corpus cavernosum. Penile erection occurs as blood rushes in from an intact vascular system (Yarkony & Chen, 1995).

Male sex organs also receive somatic innervation as sympathetic fibers (T11 to L3) synapse on the sympathetic chain ganglia and then onto the pelvic plexus via the hypogastric nerve. This efferent and afferent innervation to the testes, prostate, seminal vesicles, and vas deferens allows seminal emission by causing contraction of the prostate while closing the bladder neck. Parasympathetic innervation, responsible for erections, is via the pelvic nerves that are formed by the preganglionic fibers originating in the intermediolateral nuclei (sacral spinal cord S2 to S4). The fibers innervate the penis, prostate, seminal vesicles, and vas deferens. The pudendal nerve, a mixed motor and sensory nerve, supplies motor innervation to the pelvic floor (S2 to S4), and the sensory dermatomes are from S2 to S5 (Horn & Zasler, 1990). Somatic neural stimulation (S2 to S5) is necessary for sensation and contraction of the bulbocavernous and ischiocavernous skeletal muscles during erection and ejaculation. Distally the pudendal nerve becomes the dorsal nerve of the penis and carries the messages for somatic neural stimulation (Monga, Bernie, & Rajasekaran, 1999) (Figure 23-1). Other important components are the arteries that bring blood to the penis via the internal pudendal artery to the penile artery and the venous drainage, which comes from variable areas of the penis. Neurotransmitters also help norepinephrine act on smooth muscle to cause detumescence via sympathetic nerve fibers; acetylcholine acts on parasympathetic fibers.

Male Erectile Function

Erections in neurologically intact men can begin through both reflexogenic and psychogenic pathways (Figure 23-2). Reflexogenic erections occur when tactile genital stimulation is conveyed to the sacral spinal cord via the pudendal nerve. Activation of the sacral parasympathetic outflow via the pelvic nerve to the cavernosal nerve leads to relaxation of the corporal smooth muscle and erection. Reflex erections are poorly maintained without constant tactile stimulation and require intact S2 to S4 nerve roots. Psychogenic erections are activated by stimuli from the brain, mental images, or nontactile sensory stimulation, including thoughts, sights, sounds, tastes, and smells, and travel via the thoracolumbar sympathetics (T10 to L2) to the sex organs (Figure 23-3). The phenomenon of psychogenic erections in paraplegics with complete motor neuron lesions and abolished reflexogenic erections indicates that pathways exist for erection from the sympathetic outflow (Yarkony & Chen, 1995).

Male erection requires neurological innervation of a competent vascular response in a sequence of events. Relaxed smooth muscles allow the corpora cavernosa to fill with excess arterial blood while blocking blood drainage via the veins. Chemical factors during the process include hormones, neurotransmitters, and substances released locally from endothelial or smooth muscle components of the erectile tissue. Nitric oxide, released from the nerve endings and vascular endothelium, facilitates smooth muscle relaxation; it effects a second

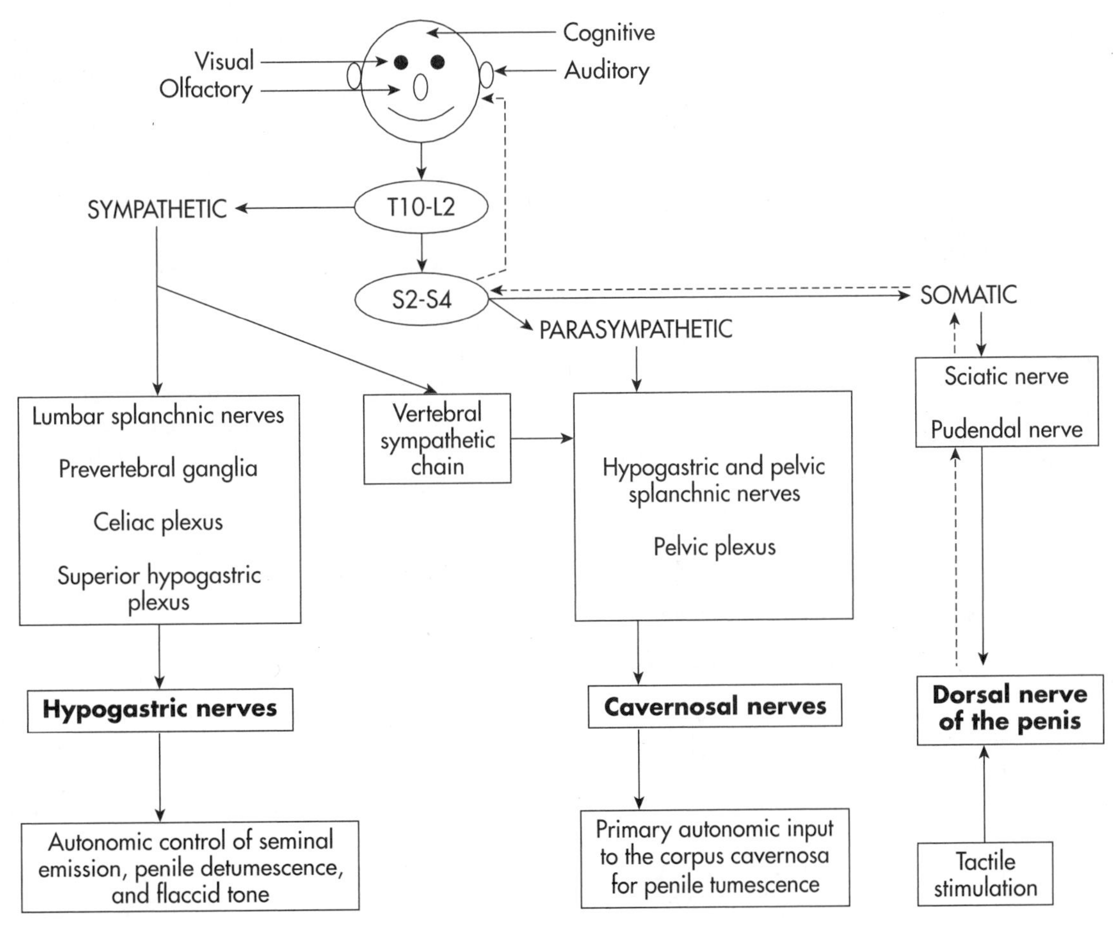

Figure 23-1 Innervation of the penis. (From Monga, M., Bernie, J., & Rajasekaran, M. [1999]. Male infertility and erectile dysfunction in spinal cord injury: A review. *Archives of Physical Medicine and Rehabilitation, 80*[October], 1332.)

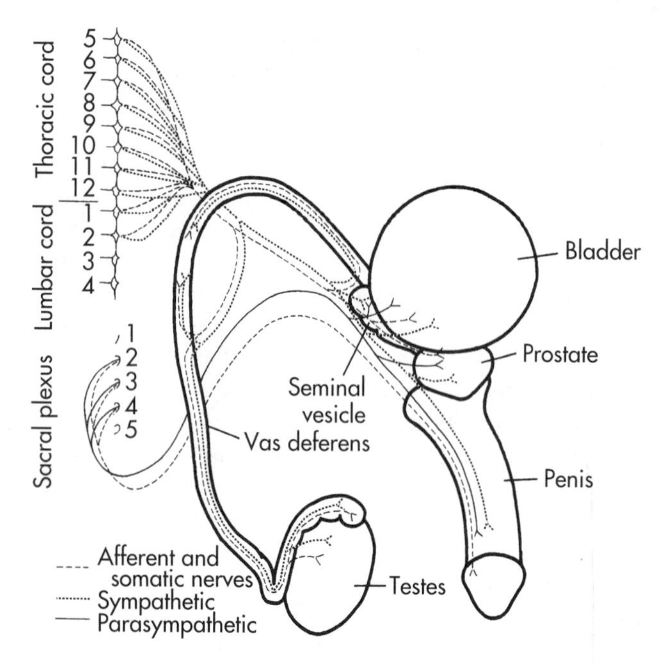

Figure 23-2 Reflexogenic erections and psychogenic pathways in male reproductive organs. (From Woods, N.F. [1984]. *Human sexuality in health and illness* [3rd ed.]. St. Louis: Mosby.)

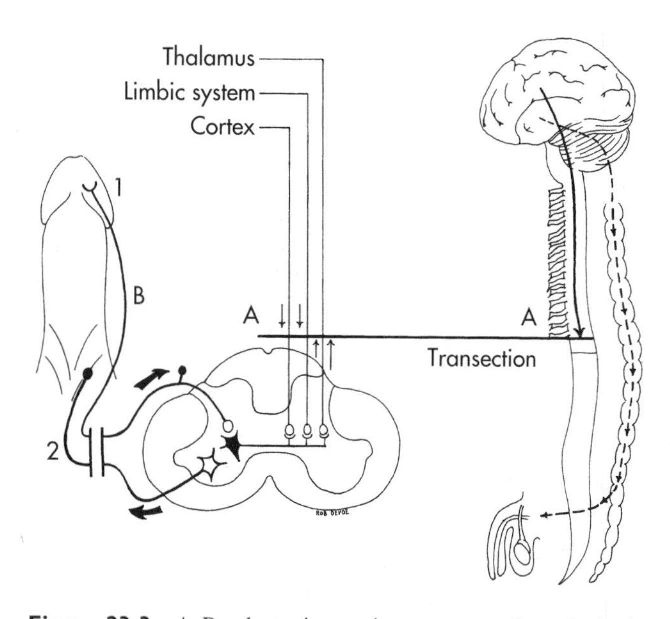

Figure 23-3 *A,* Psychogenic erection: messages from the brain are blocked at the level of the lesion but may bypass the lesion via the autonomic nervous system. *B,* Reflexogenic erection: sensory nerve *(1)* relays message to the spinal cord and synapses with the nerve that carries information to the genitals *(2)* and produces erection. (From Woods, N.F. [1984]. *Human sexuality in health and illness* [3rd ed.]. St. Louis: Mosby.)

messenger, cyclic guanosine monophosphate (cGMP) (Burnette, 1998). Research with another smooth muscle relaxant second messenger, cyclic adenosine monophosphate (cAMP), is in developing oral therapeutics. Any action that affects blood vessels, nerves, or chemical substances supplying the genital region may influence erectile response (Burnette, 1999).

Male Ejaculation Function/Orgasm

Semen arriving at the prostatic urethra is dependent on intact hypogastric sympathetic nerve function, whereas true ejaculation results from pudendal nerve activity and contraction of the pelvic floor muscles. Diseases affecting the peripheral or autonomic nervous system can impair erectile capacity, and almost any pathological process involving the spinal cord may lead to ejaculation dysfunction. True ejaculation is rare in men with SCIs, especially with complete quadriplegia (Horn & Zasler, 1990); it is more common with lower motor neuron lesions and more caudal lesions (Yarkony & Chen, 1995).

Neurophysiology does not explain why some with a complete SCI experience orgasm but others do not, although orgasm is a separate entity from ejaculation, and a number of women with complete and incomplete SCIs have had documented orgasms. Self-report and laboratory studies of men and women with SCIs indicate almost half experience orgasm, without relationship to level or completeness of injury (Tepper, 1999).

Female Sexual Physiology

The sensory pathways from the clitoris and vagina are in the pudendal nerves. The pelvic nerves innervate the vagina, clitoris, and fallopian tubes via the hypogastric and uterine plexus and receive mixed autonomic innervation. Clitoral swelling and reflex vaginal secretions are triggered by parasympathetic activity (S2 to S4). Psychogenic lubrication involves both the thoracolumbar sympathetics and sacral parasympathetics. The ovaries and uterine smooth muscle are innervated by the sympathetic nervous system (T10 to L2) sympathetic pathways. the female sympathetic nerve supply is mixed and carried by the preganglionic splanchnic nerves and the postganglionic fibers to the ovarian plexus. When the somatic pudendal nerves activate, the vaginal wall and pelvic floor musculature contract (Boone, 1995) (Figure 23-4). The autonomic nervous system is not as critical to fertility in women with SCI; those fecund before injury may become pregnant.

Brain Structures' Effect on Sexuality

The brainstem maintains arousal and alertness in sexual function; the reticular activating system prepares information processing so that behavior keeps its driving force. Libido and potency may require specific activation within certain limbic and cortical structures, initiated by externally or internally generated stimuli. The brainstem also carries motor and sensory messages via the spinal tracts, which allow participation in sexual activity.

An intact thalamus probably aids erection, and lesions in the thalamus are associated with hypersexuality. Limbic and paralimbic structures are intrinsic actors, especially the hippocampus (may help produce erection), amygdala (associated with hypersexuality), septal complex (associated with erection and a pleasurable sexual sensation), and several hy-

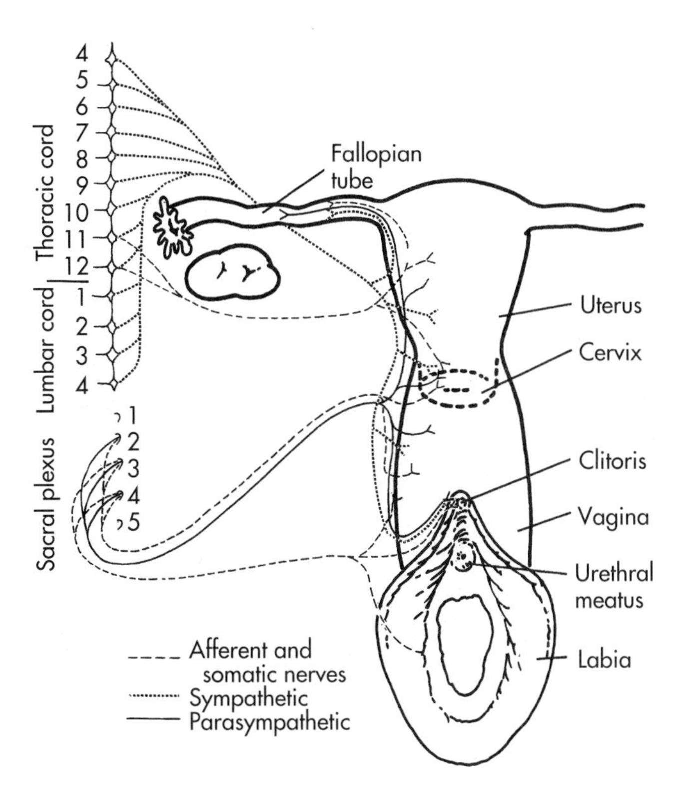

Figure 23-4 Neurological bases of female sexual response. (From Woods, N.F. [1984]. *Human sexuality in health and illness* [3rd ed.]. St. Louis: Mosby.)

pothalamic nuclei (damage can disturb sexual behavior). Temporal lobe epilepsy has been associated with disturbances in sexual function (Horn & Zasler, 1990).

Other higher brain centers affect sexual function; damage to the frontal cortex may produce disinhibited, sexually inappropriate verbal behavior, devoid of true sexual arousal or, more rarely, increased promiscuity with full arousal but difficulty with erection or emission. Injury to the dorsolateral convexities of the frontal lobe produces a more apathetic and akinetic effect. Initiation is impaired, but the client can be led step by step through erection and copulation. Frontal injury may affect attention and impair the ability to fantasize.

Problems in the left-brain hemisphere can affect sexual function. Language problems, as with aphasias, may impede comprehension of verbal requests or directions for sexual activity. Motor apraxia may impair motor movement. The right hemisphere is more active during orgasm; damage may produce impulsiveness, denial, and occasionally euphoria. Visual-perceptual problems make aligning the body with a partner difficult and hamper interpretation of nonverbal cues or expressing emotional communication (Horn & Zasler, 1990).

Hormonal Influence on Sexual Function

Hormones influence sexual activity from conception. Brain injury or stroke can affect structures that regulate hormone balance, such as with secondary hypogonadism or with damage to the pituitary. In the 20% who develop temporal lobe epilepsy after brain injury, 40% to 58% of men are impotent or hyposexual, and up to 40% of women have menstrual abnormalities with reproductive endocrine dysfunction (Horn & Zasler, 1990).

Present in both men and women, testosterone is the most important biological determinant of the sex drive in both; deficiencies reduce sexual desire, and excess heightens sexual interest.

The ovaries and testes manufacture estrogens. In women estrogen maintains vaginal elasticity, lubrication, and condition of the lining and preserves breast texture. Excessive estrogen in males can reduce libido, affect erection, and enlarge the breasts.

The hypothalamus, through gonadotropin-releasing hormone, controls secretion of two hormones made in the pituitary gland that act on the ovaries and testes. Luteinizing hormone stimulates the testes to manufacture testosterone and the ovaries to ovulate. Follicle-stimulating hormone promotes production of sperm cells in the testes and prepares the ovary for ovulation. No direct or individualized relationship exists between hormone levels and sexual ability or behavior, although deficient testosterone reduces sexual interest in both sexes (Reinisch, 1990).

Deficits

Effects from interventions for cancer, surgery, radiation, chemotherapy, or medications can disrupt the hormonal supply and may affect sexual function. Surgery for prostate, testicular, bladder, colon, or rectal cancer in men may cause impotence or inability to ejaculate. Radiation or chemotherapy on the gonads in either sex can affect hormone levels and libido. In women with cervical, vulvar, breast, or ovarian cancer the treatments that eliminate estrogen and testosterone can cause reduced libido and vaginal lubrication, as well as produce the effects of early menopause.

Neurological dysfunction affecting the brain, spinal cord, or peripheral nerves may affect sexual function. Any alteration of the circulatory system can deter erection dependent on intact blood flow. Those with cardiac and pulmonary problems may lack the endurance required for sexual activity or have limited desire.

SEXUALITY THROUGHOUT THE LIFE SPAN

Maturation

The process of puberty toward sexual and reproductive maturity is marked by various highly individualized physical, psychological, and social changes. The process begins before birth and unfolds as hormones effect changes to stimulate physical development and intensified sexual feelings and fantasies in the brain, combining to cause spontaneous erections, increased vaginal lubrication, and tendency for masturbation (Reinisch, 1990).

Tanner's (1962) classic grouping visually documented physical changes of puberty into measures of developmental stages for each sex. For boys the first changes of puberty, between 9 and 15 years of age, are internal as testicles begin to mature and produce increased amounts of testosterone, in turn causing growth of the prostate gland and other internal organs related to male reproduction. Girls begin to develop sexually at an earlier age, with changes appearing in a different order, beginning some time between 8 and 11 years of age. Internal changes are initiated by hormones, particularly estrogen. In a study of girls aged 3 to 12 years who visited pediatricians, African-American girls were found to be more advanced than white girls with respect to all secondary sexual characteristics, as well as menses onset (Herman-Giddens et al., 1997). Puberty normally is completed by the early 20s.

Children develop socially and in their relationships with same-sex and opposite-sex friends. Children with impairments are at risk for social isolation and sexual exploitation. All children need information about appropriate sexual behavior and context, as well as age-appropriate content on sexual exploitation, how to avoid it, and how report it to parents or others.

Aging

Sexual changes occur with aging. Male testosterone declines and may alter libido, with fewer viable sperm. Muscle tone decreases, the testes become more flaccid, and the diameter of the testicular tubules narrows, predisposing benign prostatic hypertrophy. Weakened prostate contractions reduce the volume and viscosity of the seminal fluid and decrease ejaculation force; the postejaculation refractory period increases at 12- to 24-hour intervals. Although erection requires longer, more intense, direct stimulation, it can be maintained longer and may satisfy a partner. Mulligan and Moss (1991) questioned male veterans, aged 30 to 99 years, and found that sexual interest remained but lessened with age. Vaginal intercourse was uniformly preferred sexual contact regardless of age, availability of a partner, or current sexual activity level. All forms of sexual activity—kissing, petting, oral sex, partner masturbation, self-masturbation, as well as intercourse—were less prevalent among these older persons. For those in nursing homes, all sexual activity is reduced.

The onset of menopause and associated hormone deprivation directly affects women's interest in sex and performance. The lowered estrogen levels during menopause result in gradual atrophy of the uterus and vagina, concurrent with reduced firmness and size of genital tissues. The vaginal mucosa thins, the canal shortens, and lubrication decreases with fewer, less active Bartholin's glands; a friable vagina may make intercourse painful. The excitement level of the sexual response is slowed, the plateau stage lasts longer, and orgasm takes longer. Longer times may enhance a woman's sexual experience both physically and emotionally, but orgasmic capacity is decreased. Estrogen deficiency may cause pain during normal uterine contractions during orgasm. With pelvic relaxation and tissue atrophy, a woman may have urinary stress incontinence, adversely affecting the couple.

RELATIONSHIP FACTORS THAT MAY AFFECT SEXUALITY

Relationship factors affect the quality of sexual relationships and responses, but strong relationships overcome many obstacles to a satisfactory sexual relationship. Conversely disability may further stress a marginal relationship, leading to separation. Often an impairment gives partners a focus on factors that maintain relationships, such as love, communication, maintaining trust, intimacy, affection, romance, timing, sensory stimulation, fantasy, and self-concept.

"Love is patient, love is kind. It does not envy, it does not boast, it is not proud. It is not rude, it is not self-seeking, it is not easily angered, and it keeps no record of wrongs. Love does not delight in evil but rejoices with the truth. It always protects, always trusts, always hopes, always perseveres. Love never fails" (I Cor. 13:4-8a; the Bible). Effective communication is a cornerstone of interpersonal and sexual intimacy that occurs in a committed, intimate, and caring relationship within a safety net of trust and support. Communication is essential when one partner has impaired or altered functions. With sensory loss, partners must find ways to share feelings of pleasure, lack of sensation, or pain or discuss potential incontinence beforehand. Partners share when they are fatigued, discomforted, or frustrated. Communication adds stability and satisfaction that may suffer when a person is unable to use or understand language; concepts are difficult to convey without words. Some couples find the sexual relationship conveyed their love when language could not.

Trust necessary for intimacy develops over time as partners learn to rely on each other's words, commit to value and honor each other, and mutually solve problems. Love is a choice to build security into a relationship (Smalley & Trent, 1988). Intimacy builds commitment through crises, boredom, and fatigue, not only joy, prosperity, and excitement.

Affection may be transmitted when spoken, by touch, or other direct behavior. Consistent, gentle touching is a powerful messages of security, emotional bonding, and romance, superseding sexual activity for some (Smalley & Trent, 1989). Without words of affection, caring is questioned. Persons with sexual impairments may find fulfillment in intimacy, communication, meaningful touch, affection, and eye contact with caring partners.

Romance helps set the stage for a positive sexual experience and demonstrates value in togetherness. Taking time for romance affords a chance for preparation, relaxation, and enjoyment, limited only by one's imagination, privacy, and safety (Dobson, 2000).

Timing and mood for sexual activities occur day or night, when both partners feel rested and relaxed. Impairments affect timing; function improves with arthritis after morning stiffness subsides, and incontinence is less likely after bowel programs for those with SCI. With cardiac or pulmonary dysfunction, schedule sexual activity before a heavy meal accompanied by alcohol.

The brain is the central coordinating center for sensory stimulation or fantasy. Sexual desire begins in this great sense organ fueled by sights, sounds, tastes, smells, or touches. For some, fantasy is a powerful producer of sexual desire, as well as a means of expression. Sexual fantasies can enhance psychological and physiological sexual responses by counteracting boredom, focusing thoughts and feelings, boosting self-image, and imagining the partner who suits all needs (Masters et al., 1986). Stimulating the senses enhances psychological sexual desire, and partners may sense or emit natural body scents or pheromones during arousal. An odor may relax and arouse one person while repelling another; some scents may enhance the sexual experience.

Arousing touch includes massage with body oils, creams, or lotion; light touch to sensitive areas; kissing; or licking. Hot or cold applications, rubbing, textures, or vibrators enhance sexual arousal and increase sensory input. Some individuals with sensory impairment report enhanced sexual feelings, almost orgasmic, from touch in areas of intact sensation (Woods, 1988). Sight is a powerful sensory tool. For instance, positioning a person to see what is occurring, lighting the room, and strategically placing mirrors allow the brain to enjoy what the eye can see when the body is impaired. The technique of sensate focus (Masters et al., 1986) encourages partners to explore each others' bodies without leading to intercourse or orgasm. Concentration on touching all areas and telling the partner what is pleasuring helps restore focus on the other. Chapter 24 has more content about sensation and perception.

ALTERATIONS IN SEXUAL FUNCTION

Physiological Alterations

Clients with chronic disease or disability involving the neurological, musculoskeletal, respiratory, cardiovascular, or digestive systems are at risk for altered sexual function. Fatigue with arthritis or cardiac or pulmonary conditions and positioning for lower extremity spasticity necessitate adjustments for both partners. Many fear that sexual activity may cause harm or adverse effects. Table 23-1 discusses functional complications that may affect sexuality.

Effects of Medication

Analgesic drugs that depress the central nervous system affect sexual function similar to alcohol. Addictive narcotic drugs produce ED, retarded ejaculation, low libido in men, and low sexual interest and orgasmic dysfunction in women. Many clients with neurological involvement take medication to manage health problems or control neurological symptoms, only to find effects on sexual function. Diazepam decreases the hypertonic response of spasticity but also reduces sexual desire, and like baclofen (Lioresal) it can contribute to problems with ejaculation or orgasm (Table 23-2).

Antihypertensive drugs may contribute to impotence (Reinisch, 1990). Tranquilizers reduce sexual desire; diazepam and alprazolam (Xanax) cause difficulty with ejaculation and orgasm. Carbamazepine and phenytoin, antiseizure medications used by clients who have posttraumatic seizure disorder after a head injury, can affect ejaculation. Some medications used to reduce excess body fluid cause reduced sexual desire and erection problems in men and painful intercourse from vaginal dryness in women (Reinisch, 1990). Diuretics, exogenous hormones, H_2 blockers, tricyclic antidepressants, and antihypertensive medications all have links to loss of sexual function (Boone, 1995); some street drugs, cocaine, amphetamines, barbiturates, and opiates may cause ED (Morley, 1993).

Psychosocial Alterations

Psychosocial alterations, social isolation, role changes, and issues with partnership or self-esteem, along with physical problems of chronic, disabling conditions, may affect sexuality.

Social isolation is a major barrier for persons with brain injury and their families (Davis & Schneider, 1990) and for children mainstreamed in schools. Friends move ahead in school or on to work, making it difficult to meet the persons of opposite sex and build social skills or reduce barriers to sexual activity. Children who learn social skills become comfortable and in turn make others comfortable with their disability.

Researchers questioned persons (n = 192) aged 32 to 79 years after stroke, as well as 94 of their spouses. Clients (57%) and spouses (65%) reported diminished libido compared with before stroke; 79% of clients and 84% of spouses practiced sexual intercourse before stroke, which decreased to 45% and 48%, respectively, after stroke; 33% of the clients and 27% of spouses reported cessation of sexual intercourse. Men (75%) reported decreased erection capacity, and women (46%) reported decreased vaginal lubrication; 55% reported decreased orgasm. Nearly half of clients and a third of spouses were dissatisfied, primarily because of inability to discuss sexuality, unwillingness to participate in sexual activity, and functional disability. Altered sexual functions were not related to gender, marital status, etiology, or lesion location. Findings support psychosocial factors playing crucial roles in sexual drive, activity, and satisfaction after stroke, stronger influences than medical factors (Korpelainen, Nieminen, & Myllyla, 1999). Some persons feel unworthy after impairment and drive their partners away.

Self-concept includes all the beliefs concerning the ideal self, the value of self or self-esteem, and internal feelings

TABLE 23-1 Relationship of Chronic Diseases to Sexual Dysfunction

Factors Related to Preparation for Sexual Activity	Diseases/Condition	Effects
Impaired mobility	Neurological conditions: SCI, stroke, Parkinson's disease, multiple sclerosis, cerebral palsy, amyotrophic lateral sclerosis, muscular dystrophy, brain injury, Guillian-Barré syndrome, chronic pain, cancers Musculoskeletal conditions: rheumatic disease, fractures, limited range of motion, amputations	Hypertonia affects most positions for intercourse; hand function deficits affect manual stimulation of partner; transfers to bed, chair, etc.; dressing/undressing; personal hygiene; insertion/application of birth control devices; coordination of motion/apraxia or ataxia; balance/positioning; no pelvic movement
Increased or decreased sensation	Neurological conditions or peripheral nerve damage in musculoskeletal injuries	No/decreased sensation in genital area or other erogenous zones Cervical SCI—most of skin surface may be affected CVA—decrease to affected side of body or painful touch to upper extremity or shoulder Brain injury—may be defensive to areas of altered sensation
Pain/discomfort	Neurological, musculoskeletal, respiratory, cardiovascular, digestive dysfunction or cancer in any system	Affects libido, limits positions, limits movement, depression
Bowel/bladder incontinence	Effects from neurological/urological deficits/cancer surgeries Incontinence types: stress; urge; overflow; neurogenic bladder, reflexic or hyporeflexic; neurogenic bowel, reflexic or hyporeflexic	Incontinence, increased risk of infection For females the steady stretch from the penis in the vagina can activate bowel reflexes and initiate bowel emptying; fecal odor can decrease libido Urine smell and wetness can damage surfaces like mattresses Determine who will provide assistance with bowel/bladder management before sexual activity
Fatigue	Brain injury, stroke, rheumatic disease, multiple sclerosis, cancer, respiratory disease, cardiovascular disease, deconditioning	Decreased libido, depression, ADLs take so much energy there is none left for sex, scheduling/pacing issues
Changes in libido	Hypersexuality (sexual addiction); brain dysfunction, especially in thalamus, limbic system, bitemporal injury, or disinhibition from frontotemporal damage; hyposexuality; brain injury; stroke; depression; stress/anxiety; Parkinson's disease; affective disorders	Partners have difficulty fulfilling the multiple requests for sex or partners miss the sexual sharing in their relationship Disinhibition can lead to problems of STDs, undesired pregnancy, relationship problems, especially if multiple partners In facility settings overt sexual behavior distresses staff Alcohol is physically inhibiting, but in some is psychosocially disinhibiting and lowers testosterone levels

SCI, Spinal cord injury; *CVA,* cerebrovascular accident; *ADLs,* activities of daily living; *STDs,* sexually transmitted diseases.

about body parts and body image. Cosmetics, clothes, and jewelry, as well as input from the environment or genetics, are external factors. Knowledge of self related to positive or negative views or gender identity develops early in life as individuals interact with others; in adolescents and adults homosexuality is a function of self-concept. Adjustment to changes with chronic or disabling conditions varies but always challenges body image and self-concept (Hirsch, Seager, Seldor, King, & Staas, 1990). Having a positive body image before impairment tends to allow more effective coping with body changes than a negative image. Independence in self-care and social roles eliminates barriers and promotes a positive self-concept.

Partnership issues arise when a spouse becomes disabled, especially when cognition is impaired, and the partner and usually the entire family sense the lost contribution to the relationships (Crewe, 1992). When one partner serves dual caregiver and provider roles, such as after SCI, the burdens can lead to burnout and imbalance in the relationship. Too often a partner becomes preoccupied with tasks or finan-

TABLE 23-1 Relationship of Chronic Diseases to Sexual Dysfunction—cont'd

Factors Related to Preparation for Sexual Activity	Diseases/Condition	Effects
Female genital sexual function: dysfunction, excitement disrupted, insufficient vaginal lubrication, orgasm decreased or absent	Diabetes; alcoholism; drug use; medications like antihistamines can increase dryness; neurological disturbances; hormone deficiencies; postmenopausal and cancer treatments, which result in lack of estrogen; pelvic disorders (i.e., infections, trauma, scarring from surgery)	Dysparunia (painful intercourse), decreased satisfaction with the sexual experience, altered spontaneity due to need to apply lubricants Vaginal atrophy and friability can result from lack of estrogen
Male genital sexual function: erectile dysfunction (impotence), premature ejaculation, delayed or absent ejaculation, orgasm	Diabetes, alcoholism, neurological dysfunction (particularly spinal cord injury and multiple sclerosis), prostrate surgery, infection or injury to sex organs, hormone deficiencies, circulatory problems	Impotence/inability to maintain an erection firm enough for coitus at least 25% of the time; may affect 1 of 10 men in the United States; may have physiological and/or psychological component SCI, once spinal shock subsides, reflex erections occur if injury at T11 or above; paraplegics with no S2-S4 reflex connection have psychogenic erections via the sympathetic pathway, T10-L2; ejaculation is rare in men with SCI (reports of from 10% to 32%), but orgasm has been shown to be present in approximately 50% of sexually active men and women
Female fertility	SCI during initial onset when menses ceases Damage to endocrine system Brain injury or disease that affects ovarian endocrine dysfunction Polycystic ovaries, hypogonadism Alcohol detrimental to unborn child Some medications contribute to birth defects	All women should know that generally fertility is unchanged once menses resumes, unless there is damage to the endocrine system or ovarian function Birth control options can be affected by the disease/injury (i.e., with an increased risk of deep venous thrombosis in persons with SCI who smoke, the birth control pill may not be the best option)
Male fertility	SCI Endocrine dysfunction—decreased serum testosterone levels Alcoholism	Semen has lowered volume and sperm counts overall and progressively slower sperm motility, impaired sperm membrane integrity, and poor oocyte-penetrating capabilities of the sperm (Yarkony & Chen, 1995) Retrograde ejaculation can occur, altering fertility; retrograde ejaculation contributes to infertility Decreased libido Erectile dysfunction Altered secondary sex characteristics

SCI, Spinal cord injury; *CVA,* cerebrovascular accident; *ADLs,* activities of daily living; *STDs,* sexually transmitted diseases.

cially unable to continue participating in activities that brings zest to life. Communication and problem-solving skills to bridge the strains of financial, health, and physical needs are vital issues for couples dealing with disability. Married women who experience SCI are vulnerable, with six of seven eventually divorcing (Smith, 1990).

A survey of clients 9 years after SCI (n = 407 selected from the National Spinal Cord Injury data bank) revealed 68% remained married, as compared with 75% of the general population. However, those with SCI who had married twice or more had double the divorce rate compared with those in first-time marriages (Divorce Trends in Spinal Cord Injury, 1990). Other findings were that marriages after injury resulted in more satisfaction with the sex life, living arrangement, and social life. The mitigating factor in this research may have been the survey sample, which contained 79% employed persons (Smith, 1990). Physical, psychological, cognitive, and behavioral alterations that affect sexuality also have profound effects on clients who are homosexual and require information and counseling about sexual func-

TABLE 23-2 Sexual Problems Resulting from Medication

Sexual Problem	Medication
Reduced desire and sexual function	Tranquilizers, SSRIs, most drugs listed below can reduce desire for sex in men and woment
Erectile dysfunction	Diuretics, exogenous hormones, H_2 blockers, tricyclic antidepressants, antihypertensives, street drugs
Ejaculation problems	Diazepam (Valium), methyldopa (Aldomet), ranitidine (Zantac), phenytoin, baclofen (Lioresal), cimetidine (Tagamet), carbamazepine
Priapism	Hydralazine (Apresoline), prazosin (Minipress), labetalol (Trandate)
Gynecomastia	Methyldopa (Aldomet), hydrochlorothiazide and spironolactone (Aldactazide), raudixin, rauzide, reserpine (Serpasil), spironolactone
Menstral changes	Hydrochlorothizide and spironolactone (Aldactazide), spironolactone (Weiss, 1991; Sullivan & Lukoff, 1990)
Drowsiness, decreased vaginal lubrication	Antihistamines
Impaired arousal/anaorgasmia	Alprazolam (Xanax), amitriptyline (Elavil), amphetamines, fluoxetine (Prozac), haloperidol (Haldol), molindone (Moban), nortriptyline (Pamelor), thiothixine (Navane), doxepin, paroxetine (Paxil), sertraline (Zoloft), and similar drugs of the same class (Goodwin & Agronin, 1997)

tion. Nurse educators and counselors either provide information or refer to other professionals.

Cognitive and Behavioral Alterations

Cognitive function must be intact, and behavioral alterations must be managed for clients to participate in sexual activity satisfactorily. Cognitive impairments or alterations occur with brain injury, stroke, multiple sclerosis, Parkinson's disease, and other neurological diseases. Of particular concern are attention, memory, executive function, communication, mood, social perceptiveness, higher cognitive skills, and behaviors that affect sexual function or sexuality.

Deficits in attention affect the ability to attend to a task for a required time. A doorbell or telephone ringing can break attention to or concentration on sexual activity, but persistent partners can help refocus attention. When inattention disrupts concentration, the partner may fantasize or use sexual play or psychogenic means to maintain erection. When one partner is egocentric, focusing on self needs, it detracts; equal contributions by persons focused on the other create balance in a sexual relationship.

Executive function impairments affect the quality of reasoning, planning, organization, and judgment. Sexual function is a high-level social skill that requires planning, preparation, and anticipation. In a sexual scenario this translates to understanding nonverbal and verbal signals, knowing what is expected of each partner, anticipating what comes next, and selecting the best approach, all of which are difficult for those with impaired executive function. Similarly, when a partner lacks social perceptiveness skills to express personal feelings or show love through actions, words, and nonverbal communication, the entire intimate relationship, not only sexual, is threatened. Truly understanding and comprehending how one is perceived may be altered by brain injury, causing other relationship problems.

Effective communication sharing hopes, dreams, values, and critical needs maintains and enhances intimacy but requires high-level communication skills. With altered communication, such as after stroke or brain injury, couples may have a signal to initiate sexual intimacy when they cannot communicate verbally.

Mood disturbances, often depression after chronic or disabling conditions, can adversely affect libido and sexual performance. Depression may decrease libido or, alternatively with euphoria, increase libido. The cycle in which depression leads to decreased sexual activity and, in turn, to depression alters sexual function. Irritability occurs more frequently in persons with brain injury, stroke, or neurological diseases. An irritable person does not make the best partner because incorrect perception of a behavior may elicit an irritable response, disrupting the sexual encounter.

Disinhibition differs greatly from depression but can change the nature of the sexual encounter for some spouses. Sexual function has social and cultural rules that vary greatly in practice among couples. For instance, a verbal interaction may carry over into sexual relations, becoming a turnoff for some partners. Children need to learn the social rules to overcome their inherent disinhibition, by learning to differentiate public from private behavior. For some who are without a partner, sexual disinhibition can cause problems in the community; the person relearns that sexual activity is only performed in private and among consenting adults.

ASSESSMENT OF SEXUAL FUNCTION

A holistic assessment for sexual function considers impaired or altered sexual function and sexuality in relation to the relationship, as well as work, home maintenance, and recreation. Sexuality and sexual response may not be a priority early in a client's rehabilitation process; later sexual function may be a major concern. At various stages in the process, rehabilitation nurses are responsible to address the topic and assess, educate, and counsel clients; assessment of sexual function is an interdisciplinary process. Rehabilitation nurses integrate data from assessment with information from other team members to provide sexual education or counseling as a therapeutic intervention. The sexual assessment obtains a sexual history, identifies physical and psychosocial strengths and limitations, determines the client's sexual values, and assists with performing diagnostic tests.

The following guidelines prepare clients for an assessment environment:

- Provide privacy and ensure confidentiality through site selection
- Establish trust and rapport
- Convey sexual health as part of personal health
- Ask about cultural or ethnic needs
- Evaluate language and understanding
- Assess general level of sexual knowledge
- Individualize teaching and counseling
- Proceed logically with information
- Allow time and encourage questions
- Validate and empower client
- Reassess through feedback

Clients are informed that they can refuse to answer any questions. Sociocultural factors, such as sex as a taboo topic or age and gender, may be barriers that dissuade clients from answering questions. Never cause clients or partners to come into conflict with their moral or ethical views. A referral to someone from the same religious or cultural background may be in order. Questions proceed from less to more sensitive areas. A life cycle chronology provides a logical unfolding of events, as well as a progression from less to more threatening topics. The impact of any questions can be softened by making a general statement and then proceeding with the question. For instance, the nurse can make a general statement about sexual activity as a normal form of sexual release and then ask the client's opinion about this practice. Or ask about the ideal rather than the real to facilitate communication such as, "Statistically, persons near your age have intercourse from three times a week to once a month. How often do you have intercourse?"

Sexual History

The purpose of the sexual history is to identify problems and misconceptions, as well as areas requiring education and counseling regarding sexual issues (Box 23-1).

Sexual Physical Examination

Findings from the physical examination guide content of sexual education and counseling. External genitalia are inspected in both male and female clients. Women may have a pelvic examination and complete breast inspection. Assess both for sexually transmitted diseases (STDs) using urine cultures or wet pap smears. A neurological examination of the genital area is useful to determine rectal sphincter tone; normal sphincter tone indicates both the lumbar and sacral segments of the spinal cord are intact, allowing strong reflex erections in the male. Ask the client to contract the rectal sphincter voluntarily; ability to do this implies preservation of efferent motor fibers in the pyramidal tract system essential for ejaculation.

Pain and temperature presence in the saddle area (S2 to S4) mean sensory awareness of orgasm. Sensation from the testes enters the spinal cord at the T9 level, so if squeezing the testicle elicits a pain response, psychogenic erections are likely because their pathway is through the T11 to T12 spinal nerves via the sympathetic nervous system (Figure 23-2).

Assess the bulbocavernosus reflex manually by compressing the penis while palpating the perineum or anus for a reflex contraction, present in approximately 70% of neurologically intact males. In female clients press on the clitoris to contract the rectal sphincter. In both, contraction of the anal sphincter is a positive response that indicates an intact reflex arc, allowing reflex erections in males. Eliciting contraction of the anal sphincter, the anal wink reflex indicates an intact sacral reflex arc and potential for strong reflex erections (Zasler & Horn, 1990).

Diagnostic Tests

Because the urinary tract and genital organs share much innervation, tests of bladder function (urodynamics) help estimate the neurological integrity of the genital system. Urodynamic testing identifies a person's reflexic versus areflexic neurological status and sphincter dyssynergia. If reflexes are present, reflex erections are possible; if not, psychogenic erections may be tried. Efferent neurological pathways can be assessed by nocturnal penile tumescence testing, a measure of penile erection during sleep conducted in a sleep laboratory or at home. The test provides a reliable report of all nighttime penile activity for frequency, quality, duration, and amplitude of any nighttime erections. If erections occur during sleep, the clinician has some information about the motor and autonomic efferents involved in penile erection.

Another method to evaluate erection potential is intracavernosal injection of pharmacological agents. When all physical components of erection are present, vasodilators such as papaverine, phentolamine, or prostaglandin E1 are injected into the corpus cavernosum of the penis, leading to erection. Failure of the injection to produce erection suggests the vascular system to the penis is not intact and functioning, leading to impotence.

Tests conducted in selected rehabilitation centers are penile biothesiometry (skin vibration sensitivity) and dorsal somatosensory-evoked potential testing. Biothesiometry provides information on the sensory afferents by measuring the vibration perception threshold of the penis. A small electromagnetic test probe is placed on the penis and allowed to

Box 23-1 Sexual History Form

Name ______________ Age ____
Marital/partnership status (includes quality, duration)
____
Occupation ______________ Highest education ______
Religion ______________ Interests/hobbies ______
____

Medical History

Psychological/psychiatric problems ______
Behavioral/emotional problems ______
Cognitive dysfunction ______
Renal insufficiency ______
Diabetes ______
Neurological conditions ______
Hereditary disorders ______
Hypertension ______
Endocrine disorders ______
Sexually transmitted diseases ______

Current Medications

Antihypertensives ______
Antipsychotics ______
Antihistamines ______
Alcohol ______
Analgesics ______
Narcotics ______
Recreational drugs ______

Premorbid Sexual Function

Description of sexual activities preferred ______
Frequency of sexual activity ______
Partner who generally initiates sexual activity
______
Sexual preferences of the client ______

Specific Concerns of the Couple

Importance of sex in the relationship ______
Physical issues that affect sexual function
Transfers ______
Ability to dress/undress ______
Monoplegia/hemiplegia/hemiparesis ______
Paraplegia/quadriplegia ______
Range-of-motion limitations ______
Hypertonicity ______
Hypotonicity ______
Endurance ______
Balance ______
Decreased sensation versus hypersensitivity ______
Presence and location of pain ______
Presence of bowel and/or bladder incontinence
______
Presence of genitourinary or gastrointestinal collection devices and their position
______
Difficulty with vision, hearing, oral motor control, memory, communication ______
General and genital hygiene and cleanliness ______

Sexual Response Issues

Female
- Menstrual history ______
- Sexual interest ______
- Frequency of sexual interaction ______
- Vaginal lubrication ______
- Sensation present ______
- Orgasmic capacity ______
- Fertility/birth control ______
- Pregnancy ______

Male
- Sexual interest ______
- Presence of morning erections ______
- Presence of erections with manual stimulation ______
- Process for ejaculation ______
- Sensation present ______
- Type of ejaculation and volume ______
- Fertility/birth control ______

vibrate gently. Vibration testing evaluates only the function of the sensory nerves; sensory nerve deficits occur with diabetes or with a history of alcohol abuse. Somatosensory-evoked potential testing specifically localizes the anatomic lesion in peripheral, sacral, or suprasacral nerves. Impaired dorsal nerve activity adversely affects the ability to sustain penile erection (Zasler & Horn, 1990).

Penile arteriography and/or corpus cavernosography (radiographs taken of the penis after a special dye has been injected) can identify involved blood vessels and Doppler analysis (ultrasonography) evaluates arterial blood flow (Leslie, 1990). Diagnostic testing in women is not as sophisticated or available, but changes in vaginal hemodynamics can be measured through photoplethysmography and heat electrode techniques. The technology can be incorporated in biofeedback programs to address orgasmic or arousal problems (Reinisch, 1990).

NURSING DIAGNOSES

Nursing diagnoses related to sexual function that are accepted by the North American Nursing Diagnosis Association include the following (Table 23-3).

1. *Sexual dysfunction or altered sexuality patterns:* Expression of concern regarding sexuality with reported difficulties, limitations, or changes in sexual behaviors

TABLE 23-3 Nursing Diagnoses, Interventions, and Outcomes Related to Sexual Function

Nursing Diagnosis	Nursing Interventions Classification (NIC)	Nursing Outcomes Classification (NOC)
Sexual dysfunction or altered sexuality patterns	Sexual counseling, anticipatory behavior guidance, sexual management, anxiety reduction, body image enhancement, role enhancement, self-esteem enhancement, coping enhancement Teaching: sexuality, safe sex, fertility (preservation, reproduction technology enhancement, birth control)	Sexual functioning, child development for children and adolescents, sexual identity acceptance, self-esteem, body image, psychosocial adjustment to life change, social interaction skills, role performance Risk control: unintended pregnancy, sexually transmitted diseases Abuse recovery
Activity intolerance	Exercise promotion Strength training Energy management Body mechanics promotion Pain Management Therapy	Activity tolerance Endurance Energy conservation Cardiac pump effectiveness Respiratory status: Gas exchange Meets physiological mobility level
Body image disturbance, low self-esteem	Counseling, body image enhancement, coping enhancement, emotional support, pain management, self-esteem enhancement, socialization enhancement, support system enhancement Teaching: urinary, bowel incontinence care related to preparation for sex	Body image, psychosocial adjustment to life change, self-esteem, acceptance of health status, social involvement, social interaction skills, development commensurate with age, bowel/bladder managed during sexual activity
Altered sexual role performance, support system deficit, social isolation	Role enhancement, caregiver support, complex relationship building, normalization promotion, socialization enhancement, self-awareness enhancement, self-esteem enhancement, mutual goal setting, values clarification, socialization enhancement	Adjustment to life change, social interaction skills, social involvement, social support, well-being, leisure participation
Knowledge deficit: sexual health	Teaching: sexuality, safe sex Sexual counseling, health education, health system guidance, preconception, counseling	Knowledge: Sexual functioning Information processing: memory Communication: receptive ability Cognitive ability

Data from Johnson, M., Maas, M.L., & Moorhead, S. (2000). *Nursing outcomes classification (NOC)* (2nd ed.). St. Louis: Mosby; McCloskey, J.C., & Bulechek, G.M. (2000). *Nursing interventions classification (NIC)* (3rd ed.). St. Louis: Mosby; and North American Nursing Diagnosis Association. (2001). *Nursing diagnosis: Definitions and classification 2001-2002* (4th ed.). Philadelphia: Author.

or activities. Sexual dysfunction describes perceived problems in sexual function viewed as unsatisfying, unrewarding, or inadequate. The related factors that may contribute to this nursing diagnosis are injury, illness, or medical treatment; altered body structure or function; knowledge or skill deficit regarding sexual function and effects of disability; values/cultural conflict; lack of privacy; ineffective or absent role models; lack of or impaired relationship with significant other; conflicts with sexual orientation or variant preferences; fear (pregnancy); physical or psychosocial abuse; or values conflict (Gordon, 2000).

2. *Activity intolerance, particularly level III or IV:* Abnormal responses to energy-consuming body movements involved in required or desired activities. Related to sexual function cues, signs of activity intolerance include dyspnea with sexual activity, fatigue, heart rate changes and failure to return to baseline within 3 minutes, muscle weakness, discomfort, and pain. Rehabilitation clients experience activity intolerance because of deconditioning, long-term immobility, changes with aging or cardiovascular or pulmonary conditions, or alterations in sympathetic nervous system control.
3. *Body image disturbance and low self-esteem:* Negative self-evaluation or feelings about self or self-capabilities, which may be directly or indirectly expressed. Body image disturbance involves negative feelings or perceptions about characteristics, functions, or limits of the body or body parts, as well as verbalized actual or perceived changes in body structure and or function accompanied by feelings of helplessness, hopelessness, and/or powerlessness in relation to the body and fear of rejection or reaction of

others. Related factors for body image disturbance are seen as repeated self-negating verbalizations; an inability to deal with the situation; repeated verbalizations focusing on past strength, function, or appearance; and negative talk about the body's functions or characteristics. For persons with stroke or brain injury, signs include changes in the ability to estimate the spatial relationship of the body to the environment and refusal to verify actual change in body or loss of a part; not touching, looking at, or using a body part or extension of the body's boundary to incorporate environmental objects may herald body image disturbance due to altered perception.

4. *Altered sexual role performance/support system deficit/social isolation:* Feelings of aloneness attributed to interpersonal interaction below level desired or required for personal integrity. Support system deficit involves insufficient emotional and/or instrumental help from others. Sexual role performance is related to a change in physical capacity or in the usual patterns of responsibility. Related factors for these nursing diagnoses include impaired mobility; therapeutic isolation; altered thought processes to include depression or anxiety; inability to use or understand language; fear of embarrassment, rejection, discovery, environmental hazards, or violence; incontinence; body image disturbance; disfigurement; sensory losses of sight or hearing; insufficient or absent social network to provide instrumental assistance (i.e., transportation, household assistance, community resources, loss of employment, or sociocultural dissonance) (Gordon, 2000).
5. *Knowledge deficits:* Inability to state or explain information or demonstrate a required skill related to disease management procedures, practices, and/or self-care health management (i.e., alternative methods to achieve sexual gratification, parenthood, or need for birth control information). The client may not be aware of alternatives to traditional sexual activities, and the disabling condition may result in motor or sensory impairments that interfere with the ability to perform sexual activities in the usual manner. The client may not be aware of ability or lack of ability to produce children. An inability to use or understand language can have a profound effect on ability to learn. Related factors for this nursing diagnosis include onset of disability; low readiness for reception of information; lack of interest or motivation to learn; cognitive limitations, particularly memory loss; inadequate recall, understanding, or misinterpretation or misconception of information; psychomotor limitations; inability to use materials or information resources due to, for example, cultural or language barriers; change in health status; and a new or complex treatment program.

GOALS

Realistic goals for the client, mutually established with the client and partner, may include the following:

1. Maintains or restores function as a sexual being within own and partner's value systems, expresses sexual interest, attains and maintains sexual arousal through orgasm, and demonstrates ability to use appropriate assistive devices
2. Has endurance to complete sexual activity
3. Maintains or restores positive self-esteem, including improving body image
4. Has overcome social isolation, has developed a social support system, has managed sexual role changes, has become knowledgeable concerning building social interaction, and reports healthy intimate relationships
5. Is knowledgeable concerning sexual options; compensation strategies for pain, medical complications, and incontinence; alternative positions/activities and devices; fertility and birth control or infertility and interventions; prevention of STDs; and professionals to contact for further information or interventions

CARE PLANS

A care plan is individualized, proactive, based on assessment, and developed with the client and partner. The focus is on education and/or counseling that incorporates techniques for everyday functioning as taught and practiced in rehabilitation therapy and nursing units. For example, transfers from the wheelchair to the bed or undressing are not sexual activities but are needed to prepare for sexual activity.

INTERVENTIONS

Education for Client and Partner

Rehabilitation nursing roles in sexual counseling are education and counseling. Sexual education offers suggestions about interventions and provides information to a client and partner (or to a client through the course of daily interactions) about sexual options, positions for sexual activities, management or relief of pain, management of bowel and bladder function, psychosocial aspects of human sexuality, effects of medications on sexual function, prevention of STDs, and birth control methods. A session on human sexuality included in education programs reaches groups who experience altered sexual function, similar to community support groups for men experiencing impotence. Composed of clients at similar adjustment stages or with diagnoses that risk similar sexual problems, groups may mix clients and partners segregate by sex. Either way, groups focus on education and management strategies.

Even if they do not lead a group or class on sexual health, rehabilitation nurses provide sexual information during daily contact. Essential knowledge about sexuality and function is only effective when nurses also are comfortable with their own sexuality, with discussing sexual topics with clients, with a client's "need to know" apart from sexual preferences and practices, and with not discussing sexuality when a client so chooses. Preparation for sexual counseling begins with self-education and knowledge about the following topics:

- Human sexual response, variety and prevalence of sexual behaviors, and anatomy and physiology of sexual function
- Types of sexual dysfunction and other deficits that affect sexual function (i.e., paralysis, especially potential experiences for clients counseled)
- Relationship of age, life events, pathologies, behavior problems, or pharmaceuticals with sexual function
- Signs of fertility in females and appropriate effective contraception methods
- Benefits of abstinence and assertive communication skills to resist peer pressure and social pressure of sexual activity
- Professional responsibility for holistic care

Compensation Strategies for Sexual Dysfunction or Altered Sexuality Pattern

Alternative Techniques

Clients may learn to compensate for sexual dysfunction in all areas of deficit, but when intercourse is not an option, strategies for satisfying sexual activities are especially important. Physical impairment usually does not reduce interest in sex or capacity for sexual functioning, except when intercourse is too difficult or impossible. Many clients report difficulty in finding sexual partners and thus masturbate to orgasm; in one survey 63% of men and 42% of women reported masturbation in that year (Elmer-Dewitt, 1994). Options with a partner, manual sexual stimulation, and orogenital stimulation (cunnilingus and fellatio) may be options. Concerning cunnilingus, educate clients never to blow air forcibly into the vagina, as fatal air embolism may result for the woman and/or fetus, if pregnant. Clients with sensory loss may find fulfillment from pleasing a partner by performing manual or orogenital sexual stimulation. However, assess clients' feelings about the topic because some may find it incomprehensible or taboo to discuss, despite its relatively common practice in the United States (Reinisch, 1990).

Strategies to compensate for ED involve the partner. When a man has ED, his female partner positions the soft penis into her vagina and contracts vaginal (pubococcygeal) muscles; this action holds the penis in the vagina ("stuffing technique") (Griffith & Trieschmann, 1983). Or a woman in the dominant position performs a rotary or circular motion; this is useful also for impotence, regardless of underlying pathophysiology. ReJOYn, available from a pharmacy, is a stiff latex device that fits around the penis while being held in place by straps around the testicles. Lubrication makes the device, used as an adjunct to "stuffing," comfortable for women, and it allows for intercourse with a flaccid penis.

Vacuum entrapment systems or pumps are external devices that can produce or maintain erection (Figure 23-5). The man lubricates the flaccid penis and places it into a clear acrylic tube that is held tightly against the body. Then he uses the pump device to produce a vacuum in the acrylic tube, which encourages blood flow into the penis. When the penis is rigid, a rubber ring is moved from the end of the tube onto the penis and around the base, to hold the blood in the penis. The tube then is removed, and the erection can be maintained for as long as the rubber band can stay in place, about 30 minutes. At orgasm, the rubber ring may prevent ejaculation for some; others report pain or numbness. Potential problems are damage to the penile shaft, damage to internal penile tissue, and infection of or irritation to the urinary tract. Should venous leakage cause failure in erections, partners can try to reduce leakage by performing pelvic floor exercises or using the constriction band once erection occurs. The devices can be purchased at local pharmacies but are intended for use under supervision of a physician or nurse practitioner and in concert with counseling for client and partner including regular evaluations (Doerfler, 1999).

Pharmacological Agents

Techniques to manage impotence include nonhormonal oral medications by prescription, some only through research trials. Sildenafil citrate (Viagra) potentiates the second messenger mechanisms, leading to erection by potentiating the relaxation of smooth muscle. With dose regulation, 69% of men in trials reported successful sexual intercourse while taking this medication. Specific groups reported higher improvement rates: 75% of men with SCI, 56% of men with diabetes, and 84% of men with a psychogenic etiology. Sildenafil cannot be used with nitrate-containing medications, nitroglycerin, amyl nitrate, or isosorbide dinitrate because all have a systemic vasodilatory effect; combining two could be fatal. The drug is used with caution in persons with retinal damage, such as retinitis pigmentosa. Viagra is one of the most frequently prescribed drugs, with more than 3.5 million prescriptions written in the United States during the first 4 months after its release. It has replaced many of the other techniques as the preferred erection aid method. Viagra is taken 20 to 60 minutes before intercourse but can be used only once in 24 hours; the dose is not to be exceeded (Monga et al., 1999). Vasomax, another phentolamine drug, blocks epinephrine and norepinephrine to reduce sympathetic tone and relax arterial and corporal smooth muscles, allowing for erection. Available in Mexico, it is undergoing trials in the United States (Albaugh, 1999).

L-Arginine, the precursor of nitric oxide, has been found effective for ED in a small study; 40% of participants had no

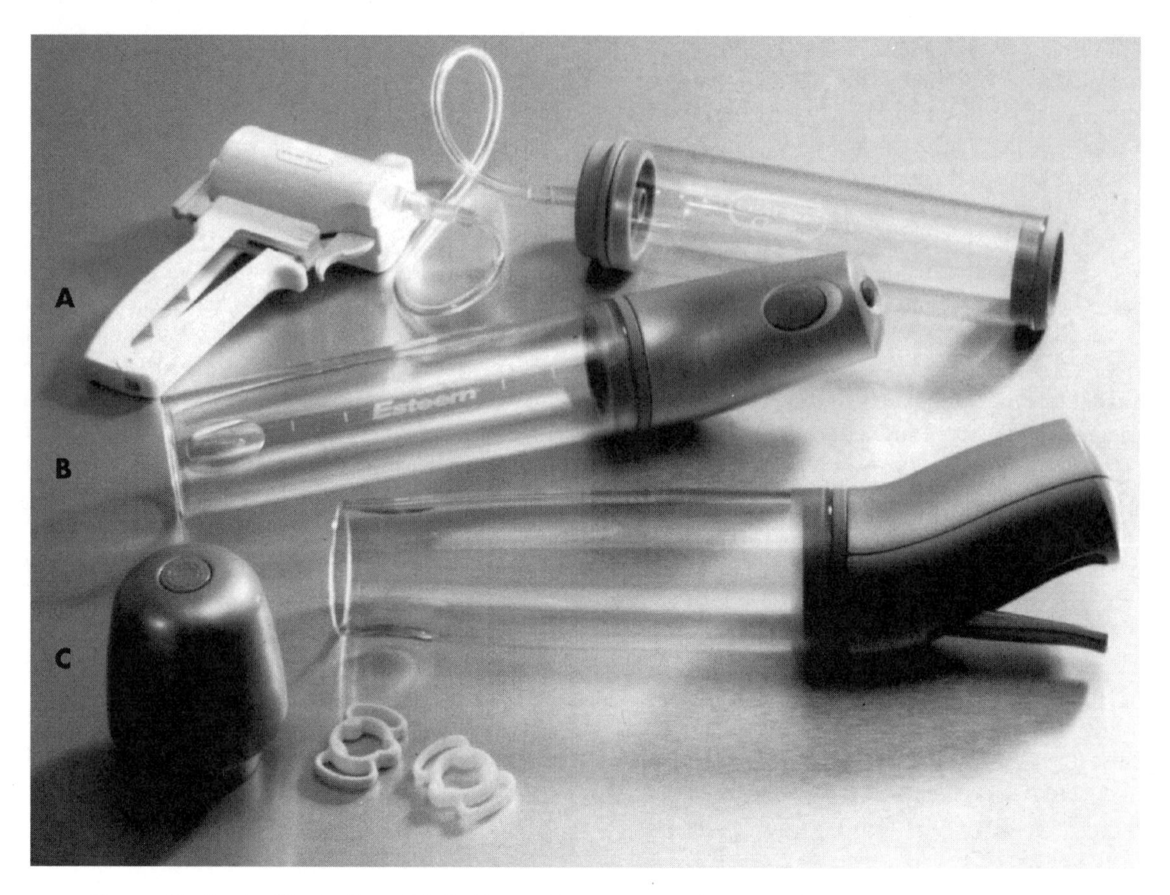

Figure 23-5 **A,** Classic ErectAid. **B,** Esteem battery-operated system. **C,** Manual system. (Courtesy Timm Medical Technology, Eden Prairie, MN.)

apparent side effects. Apomorphine (Spontane) an experimental dopaminergic agonist, produces erectile responses in men. It is held in the mouth until absorbed buccally; swallowing the drug decreases its effectiveness. Client reports of successful intercourse were 64% in a small sample and 59.6% in a larger sample, with nausea as the most common side effect. Levodopa, another dopamine agonist, has been used to achieve erection in a high percentage of men, but results during intercourse have not been measured. Phentolamine, a drug used for penile injection, is now available in oral form for research trials. It has produced erection in 42% to 69% of men without any serious side effects. Limaprost, a peripherally active vasodilator in oral form similar to prostaglandin E1, has been found effective in persons with mild ED but requires further testing (Burnette, 1999).

Testosterone injections help increase libido and even improve erectile function in persons with borderline low serum testosterone levels (Zasler & Horn, 1990). If testosterone levels are not low, there is no benefit to testosterone injections. A history of prostate cancer or heart, kidney, or liver disease contraindicates testosterone therapy.

Medications that relax smooth muscle and allow for an increase in penile blood flow can be prescribed for penile intracavernosal injection. Papaverine and phentolamine were the vasoactive agents first used in self-injection programs; now prostaglandin E1 has led to triple-drug therapy (Trimix) that reduces doses of the other two drugs. Cavernosal fibrosis is a concern with long-term use in a small percentage of men; fibrosis may adversely alter erectile ability. The injections affect erection only but do not increase ability to ejaculate or experience orgasm. Priapism occurs in 3% to 10% of men, who must be counseled to seek treatment if the condition persists longer than 4 hours. Oral Brethine (terbutaline 5-mg tablets × 2) can be an initial antidote, but without results clients should go to the hospital emergency department. Findings suggest that up to 95% of persons with SCI can be successfully treated with a self-injection program (Boone, 1999). Alprostadil (Caverject or Edex) is another injectable medication; it relaxes the arterial smooth muscle and allows the penile sinusoids to fill with blood (Albaugh, 1999).

The medicated urethral system for erection (MUSE) was released in 1997 for the treatment of ED. A pinhead-sized pellet of alprostadil is placed in the male urethra. A 65% success rate of erection has been reported in men, including those with SCI. To prevent hypotension and syncope, especially in men with SCI, a venous constrictor band can be placed at the base of the penis before inserting the MUSE to prevent systemic absorption of the prostaglandin. Once the MUSE is inserted, the penis must be rubbed for 10 seconds to help with absorption of the medication, and the penis must be held upright to keep the medication from falling out.

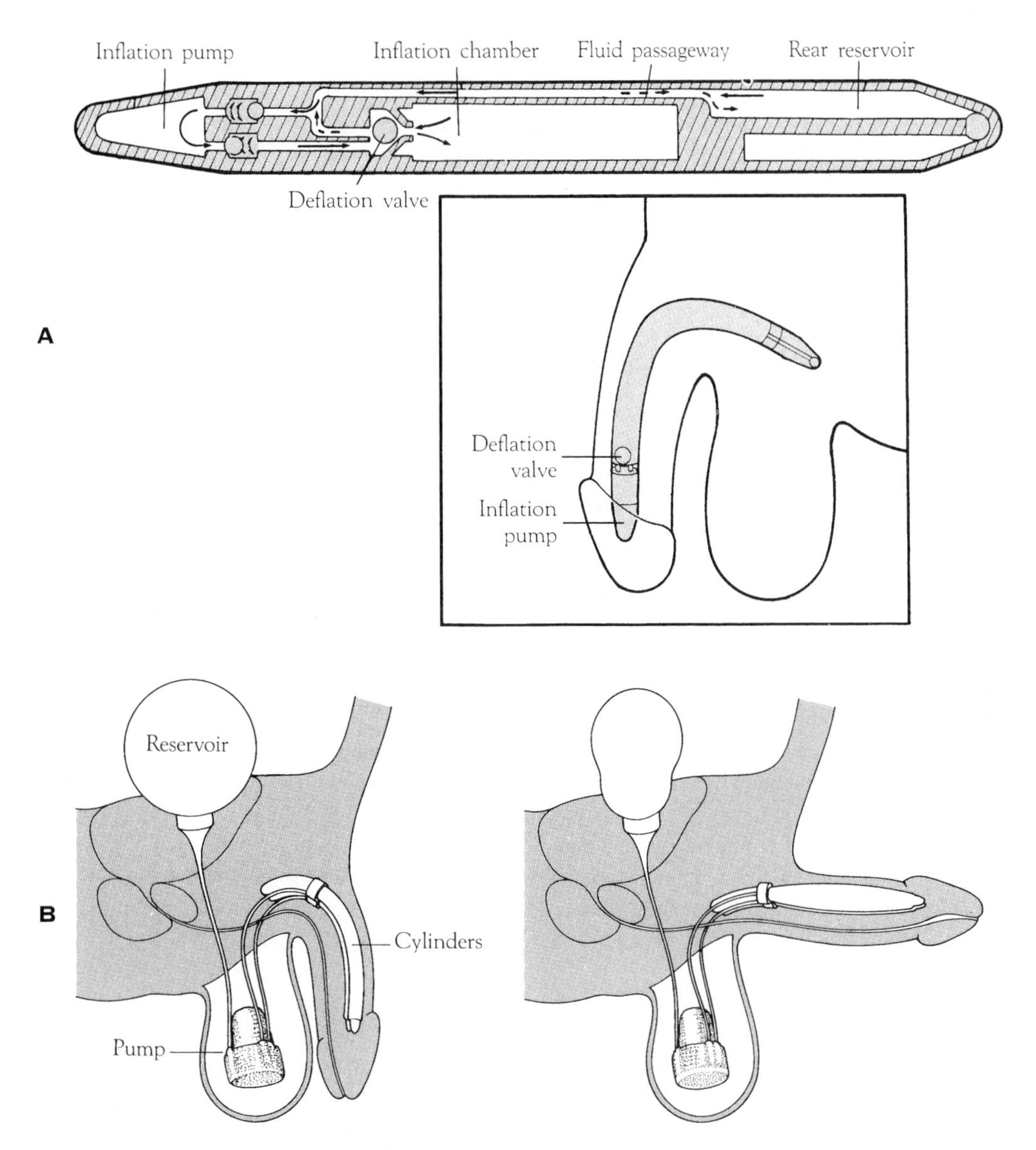

Figure 23-6 **A,** One-piece inflatable penile prosthesis. **B,** Scott inflatable penile prosthesis. (From Thompson, J.M., McFarland, G.K., Hirsch, J.E., & Tucker, S.M. [1998]. *Mosby's clinical nursing* [4th ed.]. St. Louis: Mosby.)

Penile Implants

Penile implants are options for some men impotent as a result of SCI, diabetes, arterial ischemia, extensive pelvic surgery, or long-term use of drugs, such as antihypertensives. Implantation may diminish the ability to achieve partial erection, but presurgical sperm count and sensations during intercourse will remain as before surgery. Penile implants or prostheses can be hydraulic inflatable, noninflatable semirigid, or malleable. Inflatable prostheses are three-piece devices with two cylinders implanted in the corporal bodies of the penis, a pump placed in the scrotum, and a fluid reservoir located behind the abdominal wall (Figure 23-6).

Noninflatable implants are either semirigid or hinged malleable. The semirigid implant is a rodlike silicone form that is surgically inserted into the penis, which then is always erect but positioned down to be concealed by clothing. The hinged-malleable implant has springs that interlock when the penis is pulled straight outward and then lock into a rigid position when pressed toward the body (Figure 23-7). When the process is reversed, the springs unlock for a more natural position in clothing. Both prostheses require a 3-day hospital stay to recover from surgery, but with few mechanisms or replacement parts, they are maintenance free (Leslie, 1990). However, semirigid devices caused penile erosion in 20% of men with SCI, suggesting that implants may be reserved until options are exhausted. All parties need full information that a prosthetic device does not enhance

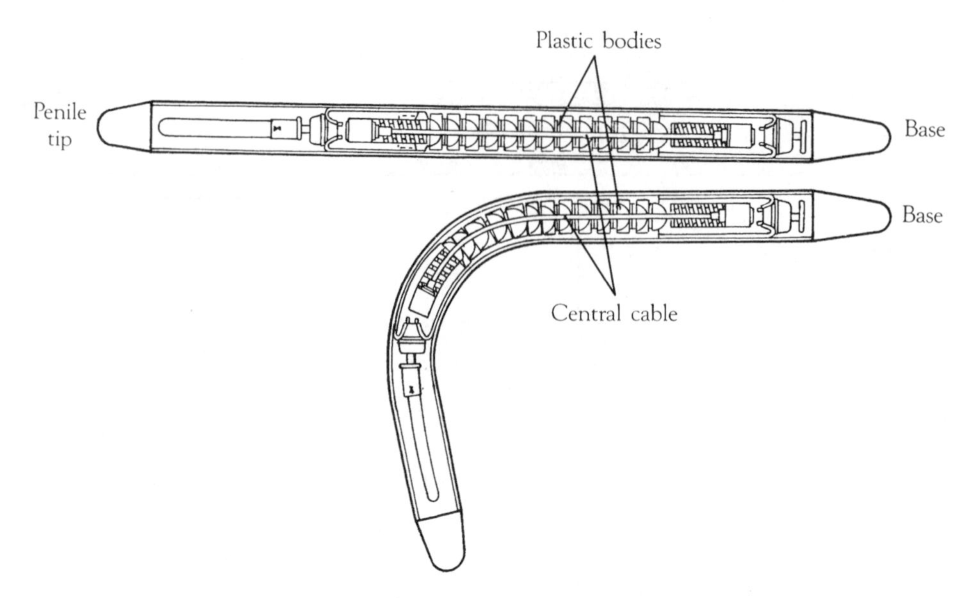

Figure 23-7 One-piece prosthesis with a central cable that shortens the plastic bodies to produce erection. (From Gray, M.L. [1992]. *Genitourinary disorders.* St. Louis: Mosby.)

orgasm. Also, should the device require removal, all other treatment options are eliminated because permanent damage occurs to the erectile cylinders of the penis. The Vocare system uses functional electrical stimulation (FES), primarily for bowel and bladder emptying and continence, but it can initiate erection in persons with neurological impairment. A thoughtful screening process goes into selecting candidates because there is loss of reflex function, and thus reflex erection, after the placement.

Clients who cannot tolerate or do not want penile implant surgery may decide to use an artificial penis, a device strapped onto the groin that simulates natural erection. Some use a vibrator to intensify stimulation in the genital area to facilitate erection or ejaculation. Because rough handling damages genital tissues and structures, a vibrator is used gently with a water-soluble lubricant and is halted immediately on discomfort or irritation. Vibrator stimulation may enhance sexual function for some; however, those who become dependent on intense stimulation may find it difficult to achieve orgasm from less stimulating touch. Electrovibration is used to collect sperm for fertility treatments because it increases the possibility of antegrade ejaculation.

About 5% of all persons with impotence may be candidates for some form of penile vascular surgery, microscopic reconstruction of the arterial blood supply, or removal of veins that drain blood from the penis too rapidly. Surgery is successful for 60% to 65% of candidates (Leslie, 1990). For men having problems with premature ejaculation, the "squeeze" technique delays ejaculation. A man must be aware of preejaculation to signal either himself or his partner to compress behind the glans or at the base of the penis; this squeeze inhibits the ejaculatory reflex, and intercourse can be resumed (Masters et al., 1986). Some clients will accept and try these approaches as appropriate, whereas others will have concerns, prohibitive beliefs, or be unwilling to try new approaches. Sexual activity is an individual choice, and clients choose which activities they wish to learn about or practice.

Compensation for Motor Dysfunction

Persons with central nervous system injury, including SCI above T12 or L1, multiple sclerosis, stroke, cerebral palsy, spina bifida, or brain injury experience hypertonicity. Not only do they have difficulty attaining and remaining in a position, but involuntary movements may be embarrassing, inconvenient, or even a safety hazard during sexual activity. Medications to relieve or reduce the spasticity also reduce libido (Nygaard, Bartscht, & Cole, 1990). Steady stretching of a hypertonic muscle and avoiding jerking movements may relieve an isolated spasm, but it also may interfere with sexual activity. For persons with hemiplegia, positioning the affected side downward helps by allowing the unaffected side to move freely. Those with hypotonicity find careful positioning can defend against subluxation at involved joints. Pillows or other supports prevent further stretching of ligaments, and joints are supported in proper alignment at all times.

A client's inability to move the lower body places the responsibility for motor movement on the partner. Waterbeds allow one partner to initiate movement of the water as though the other person were moving also. Waterbeds have hazards for those with limited head control while lying prone or for transfers (in or out) with paralysis. A person with apraxia, motor planning dysfunction, may not be able to initiate the thrusting motor movement but can participate in the movement once initiated by the partner. The partner must be willing to assume the dominant role in motor movement, which may be difficult for some women. Clients with ataxia, uncoordinated muscle movement, need guidance to find a position sufficiently stable for them to perform the motor components of coitus. With motor perseveration that interferes with a client moving from one activity to another, the partner can redirect the activity verbally or physically.

In the individual with SCI, especially complete injury at the T6 level or above, sexual activity may elicit autonomic dysreflexia or hyperreflexia, notably in certain positions that provide greater stimuli below the level of injury. Should symptoms of dysreflexia occur, the couple is taught to cease sexual activity so that symptoms subside or to seek help as indicated. In general, the client sits upright, monitors blood pressure, and takes prescribed medications. Mecamylamine hydrochloride (Inversine) may prevent dysreflexia symptoms but may reduce desire and lead to erection problems. Refer to Chapter 19 for complete information about autonomic dysreflexia.

Compensation for Sensory Dysfunction

Persons who have lost sensation to the genital area include those who have experienced SCI (complete or that affects sensation), those with diabetes or multiple sclerosis, and a few with heightened or diminished sensation on the affected side after stroke or brain injury. Persons with SCI report a wide variety of sexual sensations ranging from anesthesia to orgasm, and some report heightened pleasurable sensation similar to sexual orgasm in other areas of the body, especially intact areas generally considered erogenous zones, such as the breasts, ears, eyes, neck, lower abdomen, groin, inner thighs, and back above the level of the spinal cord lesion (Woods, 1984). Literature about SCI has information concerning true versus pseudoorgasm, with true orgasm being experienced by those with a neurologically intact nervous system and pseudoorgasm being related to emotional components. In the last few years research studies have demonstrated orgasm in a number of women with complete and incomplete SCIs. Self-report and laboratory studies of orgasm indicate that almost half of all persons with SCI experience orgasm unrelated to the level or completeness of injury. Most report that a relationship with a trusted sexual partner was the pathway to achieving pleasure and orgasm and also added emotional and spiritual aspects to the experience (Tepper, 1999). Sensory amplification involves thinking intensely about a physical stimulus and mentally amplifying that sensation; in some instances this technique facilitates orgasm.

Sensory stimulation may enhance sexual enjoyment; especially for men viewing the activity may compensate for decreased genital sensation. Light the room, place mirrors, and position for visualization; use the senses to promote fantasy through pleasant sounds, music, or the noises and words uttered during sexual activity to increase sexual desire or release. Touching intact areas of sensation; rubbing or caressing with various textured items or lotions; or smelling pleasant odors in the environment, on the person, and from sexual activity can be a powerful precursors to sexual pleasure. The taste of the partner is unique, and the special taste during sexual excitement brings sexual pleasure to some. Treat hypersensitivity to touch with a topical anesthetic or avoid that area when possible (Grana, 1995).

Box 23-2 Pain Control for Sexual Activity for Persons with Rheumatic Disease

- Practice muscle relaxation techniques and mental imagery to promote comfort and tranquility
- Practice range-of-motion exercises without resistance to promote comfortable movement
- Apply moist heat to painful joints 10 to 15 minutes before sexual activity to reduce swelling and promote increased range of motion
- Rest after completing bathing and grooming activities
- Position pillows under affected painful limbs for support; always remove the pillows after sexual activity to prevent contractures
- Schedule pain medications and arrange for sexual activities around the period of maximum drug effectiveness and when less fatigued, when possible
- Explore massage, vibration, or self-hypnosis to relieve pain and use effective techniques before sexual activity
- Explore alternative styles of sexual expression to convey caring, concern, and love (Malek & Brower, 1984)
- Use a warm waterbed, an electric blanket over the client, or a bed warmer under the sheets to ease pain or stiffness; use a moist heating pad for a particularly painful joint
- Precede sex by a warm bath or massage and mild exercise
- Try cold rather than hot applications, especially for inflamed joints; some may have better relief from these
- Understand that frequent sexual activity may reduce pain of arthritis by stimulating adrenal glands to increase production of the body's own natural antiinflammatory and pain-reducing corticosteroids (Reinisch, 1990)
- Be aware that joint injections of corticosteroid for pain relief at joints impacted by sexual activity may help

Pain Control

Persons with chronic pain, with rheumatic diseases, or after joint replacement surgery may experience pain that inhibits sexual activity. Rehabilitation team members can suggest techniques to control pain during sexual activity. Malek and Brower (1984) suggest alleviating the pain of rheumatoid arthritis during sexual activities by avoiding fatigue, engaging in anticipatory planning, and managing activity. These suggestions also apply to clients with other conditions involving painful muscles and joints (Box 23-2).

Couples develop techniques to alert a partner that a particular activity or position is painful. The "hand riding" technique signals distress when one person places a hand on the partner's hand. Painful intercourse is referred for a thorough gynecological examination to rule out or identify organic causes and suggest corrections. Without a physical cause, referral to a certified sex therapist may be appropriate because psychosocial conditions can contribute to painful intercourse (Reinisch, 1990).

Women, particularly those who are postmenopausal or those with neurological or vascular compromise, may experience discomfort during intercourse because of accompanying changes and a tendency to vaginal and urinary tract infections. For vaginal lubrication use only water-soluble lubricants that can be flushed from the body easily, such as KY Jelly (reapply frequently), and longer lasting lubricants including KY Longlasting, Vagisil, KY Silk-e, ViAmor, Astroglide, and Lubrin inserts. Some lubricants are applied three times per week for consistent vaginal moisture, Replens is one. Estrogen creams have the best restorative value to vaginal and external orifices but cannot be used by all women, especially those with estrogen-dependent cancers. Oil-based lubricants (Vaseline, baby oil, etc.) are not recommended because they increase risk of infection, particularly for women. Also they rapidly destroy the effectiveness of latex condoms, diaphragms, and cervical caps.

Continence Management

Because the autonomic nervous system regulates sexual function and influences bowel and bladder control, activation of one set of neurons can activate the others. A partner is advised when potential for incontinence exists to prevent embarrassment and allow for preparation. Use protection for bed covers, rinse items in white vinegar while washing to eliminate any urine odor, and use incense or cologne to mask odor if no one is sensitive or allergic. Prepare by emptying the bladder and limiting liquid intake and schedule sexual activity soon after completing an established bowel program. A man with an indwelling urinary catheter holds it in place with nonstick tape near the base of the penis or sheathes it in a condom. Apply lubricant to smooth the presence of the catheter or tape. Women tape an indwelling catheter to the abdomen or remove it before sexual activity and replace it afterward. Suprapubic or ileoloop appliances need not be removed but are taped to the abdomen. Urinary flow to any catheter cannot be obstructed for long periods without increasing the risk for urinary tract infection. The newer continent internal urinary storage pouches require no special preparation; catheterizing before sexual activity will ensure they are empty.

Medication Management

Medications and other ingested substances can affect sexual performance. It is possible that medication taken for the treatment of hypertension, heart disease, anxiety or stress, depression, psychiatric illness, sleeplessness, convulsions, gastrointestinal disorders, or arthritis may affect sexual functioning. Symptoms may not develop immediately; the onset may occur later in the course of drug therapy. Clients who develop sexual dysfunction discuss the effects and potential for a different dosage or an alternative drug with a physician or nurse practitioner. Clients who go against medical advice by experimenting with dosages or deleting medications may jeopardize their health. A woman who intends or suspects pregnancy is referred to her obstetrician, and medications are evaluated to prevent birth defects (Reinisch, 1990).

Reproduction Issues

Fertility and infertility are major issues during childbearing years, especially after an accident or illness. *Healthy People 2010* objectives concerning family planning apply to all, regardless of disability. Guidelines include reducing unintended pregnancies, postponing sexual activity among adolescents, increasing education and counseling, and reducing the prevalence of infertility (U.S. Department of Health and Human Services, 2000). Some form of birth control and permanent sterilization are options for persons who do not want to become parents or who are cognitively unable to decide or to parent. Birth control information shared with all fertile clients and partners is essential. A common misperception is that no precautions are needed and that disability results in infertility. Clients able to impregnate or become pregnant need correct information before sexual activity. Conversely clients whose impairments contribute to infertility need information and resources in their community to provide services for childbearing or adoption when desired.

Fertility instruction includes information on sexual anatomy, the physiology of contraception, and birth control devices or methods. A contraceptive method is chosen based on accurate information about failure rates, reversibility, safety, and personal health status. The nurse obtains feedback from the couple about previous (preinjury or preillness) birth control practices, as well as their preparation to meet future birth control needs. Referral to a gynecologist or urologist may be required for the birth control method of the couple's choice. Birth control pills do not protect from STDs and may reduce the effectiveness of antibiotics (ampicillin and tetracycline). Antibiotics also can reduce the effectiveness of the pill, as can anticonvulsants (phenytoin and primidone). This is important for adolescents who take antibiotics for acne or those with brain injury who take anticonvulsants for prophylaxis or treatments. Table 23-4 and related material provide a brief discussion of birth control methods, including effectiveness, availability, and advantages and disadvantages for certain disability groups.

Pregnancy and Disability. Women with chronic illnesses or traumatic injuries generally maintain fertility and childbearing options. Although women with chronic illness or traumatic injury, including rheumatic disease, SCI, multiple sclerosis, or brain injury, can deliver healthy infants, mother and infant have increased risks during pregnancy, labor, and delivery. Regardless of diagnosis, pregnant women with chronic illness need supervision by a team of obstetricians and physicians knowledgeable about their disability. The needs of women with multiple sclerosis differ from those of women with rheumatic disease or cancer. For example, women with multiple sclerosis or rheumatic disease risk exacerbation postpartum. Not only are mothers closely mon-

TABLE 23-4 Birth Control Methods and Disability

Method	Effects	Advantages	Contraindications
Oral contraceptives	Alters hormone patterns to suppress ovulation; cervical mucosa and endometrium resist sperm	2%-3% failure rate due to irregular use	Those with a history of blood clots, such as after SCI, multiple trauma, stroke, or coronary artery disease; those with hypertension, diabetes, gallbladder disease, or irregular menses
Norplant	Levonorgestrel released steadily into the bloodstream through small implanted tubes; drug inhibits ovulation, thickens mucosa to inhibit sperm motility	No estrogen; <1% failure rate in 5 years	No research regarding persons with disabilities; not used with breast cancer, liver disease, uterine bleeding problems, breast-feeding, or pregnancy
Depo-Provera (DMPA-depotmedroxy-progesterone acetate)	Hormone that regulates the menstrual cycle; one injection intramuscularly prevents pregnancy for 12 weeks by keeping the ovaries from releasing eggs and thickening cervical mucosa to keep sperm from joining with eggs	Failure rate is 3 per 1000 in 1 year; can be used while breast-feeding	Not used if planning to become pregnant within 18 months; not used with unexplained vaginal bleeding, with serious liver disease, after a heart attack stroke, breast cancer, or with severe high blood pressure long-standing or complicated diabetes
Intrauterine device (IUD)	Appears to act by preventing implantation of ovum; monthly check required for string placement	5% failure rate with Para Guard; 2% fail with Progestasert; reversible	Some women with disabilities are unable to check the string; those with decreased sensation in saddle area may not notice pain or bleeding
Male condom	Only latex protects from HIV and hepatitis B; use new condom for each encounter and discard after use; may use spermicide in addition to condom	10% failure due to improper use or product failure; 2%-3% failure with proper use; high failure rate with nonlatex condoms	Allergies to latex may develop; oil-based lubricants destroy latex; partner may have to apply condom for male client
Diaphragm	Barrier to sperm; placed over female cervix; may be used with various spermicides; must be used each time	As low as 2% failure when correctly sized, placed, and used; 10%-19% failure in some studies	Use during menstruation may lead to toxic shock; allergies to latex or spermicide may develop; with limited saddle sensation, client may not notice dislodgment; partner may have to insert, remove, or apply
Spermicidal foams, jellies, creams, dissolving tablets, suppositories NOTE: Mountain Dew and Coke are not spermicides	Chemical attacks sperm, while base forms mechanical barrier; renew application with each encounter	Protects against many STDs when ingredients include nonoxynol-9 or octoxynol; 18%-21% failure rate when used alone; increased effectiveness when used with condom or diaphragm	Douche may wash away spermicide prematurely; partner may need to apply; difficult for those with impaired hand function, balance or flexibility
Sponge	Soft, round polyurethane sponge fits over cervix; sponge contains spermicide that is activated when moistened with water before insertion; for a second encounter, reapply spermicide	10%-20% failure rate	Do not use during menses or 3-4 weeks postpartum to avoid toxic shock syndrome; partner may need to insert and remove

STDs, Sexually transmitted diseases; *HIV,* human immunodeficiency virus.

Continued

TABLE 23-4 Birth Control Methods and Disability—cont'd

Method	Effects	Advantages	Contraindications
Withdrawal (coitus interruptus)	Removal of penis from vagina before ejaculation; man determines timing unless woman controls movement	23% failure rate; cooperation, communication, and timing are essential	Enjoyment may be decreased or partner may miscalculate
Natural methods: rhythm, fertility awareness techniques, calendar, basal body temperature cervical mucus test	Abstinence during at-risk times as determined by different methods; abstinence during fertile times and ovulation is required (approximately 10 days/month)	Inexpensive, reversible, no chemicals or hormones; 2%-10% failure rate for those with regular cycles and proper use; 24% failure rate overall; 40% failure rate with cervical mucus test alone; promotes awareness of bodily functions in women	Persons not cognitively able to calculate and those who do not adhere to schedules are not candidates
Permanent sterilization: vasectomy or tubal ligation	Vasectomy: vas deferens is cut to block sperm ejaculation Tubal ligation: fallopian tubes are blocked or cut to prevent ova from reaching the uterus or from fertilization in the tubes	Vasectomy is effective and popular; failure rate is 160 per 100,000 Tubal ligation is effective and popular; failure rate is 276-326 per 100,000	Permanent; very difficult to reverse Ethical issues may arise when used with vulnerable populations Both are surgical techniques and require some recovery time

STDs, Sexually transmitted diseases; *HIV,* human immunodeficiency virus.

itored, but their infants must be monitored by a team of professionals with expertise in their condition.

Medication management is addressed early, before pregnancy if possible. Baclofen for spasticity is tapered gradually to prevent seizures from sudden withdrawal. Anticonvulsant drugs, such as phenytoin or carbamazepine, are evaluated and managed carefully. A mother receiving antiseizure drugs has double the risk (4% to 6% versus 2% to 3%) of bearing an infant with special needs; however, injuries from falls during grand mal seizures have more potential to injure mother and fetus. Diazepam raises the potential for fetal cleft palate and infant withdrawal after birth. Nonsteroidal antiinflammatory drugs (NSAIDs) are withdrawn in the client with rheumatic disease. As with all pregnant women, smoking and using alcohol, caffeine, and some artificial sweeteners are discouraged.

SCI and Pregnancy. Complications of concern for a pregnant woman with SCI include urinary tract infections, anemia, decubitus ulcers, thromboembolic phenomenon, hypotension, unattended birth, and autonomic hyperreflexia (Monga & Lefebvre, 1995). Interventions may vary with physicians but typically include preventive measures, including prophylactic antibiotics against urinary tract infection, weight control to retain movement and transfers, and skin inspection twice daily to avoid pressure ulcers. The team must adhere strictly to preserving skin integrity, especially during labor and delivery. Should a pressure area develop, the resulting nutritional catabolic state or anemia is treated aggressively to avoid inhibiting fetal growth. Attention to decreased gastrointestinal motility with pregnancy may prevent constipation and maintain bowel programs (Craig, 1990).

SCI Labor and Delivery. Vaginal checks for signs of premature labor begin earlier in women with SCIs, but uterine contractions can be monitored at home using tocodynamometry. Hospitalization is recommended from 10 days to 3 weeks before the due date if premature labor threatens. Terbutaline prevents premature labor in selected instances (Sipski, 1991). A client with diminished sensation needs assistance to monitor contractions. Those with injury above the T10 level are educated that increased vaginal discharge, ruptured membranes, increased leg spasticity, difficulty breathing, back or convulsive abdominal pains, and autonomic hyperreflexia may be signs of labor.

Uterine contraction and cervical dilation travel via sympathetic nerves entering the spinal cord between T10 and L1. In later stages of labor, impulses from the perineum travel via the pudendal nerves, entering the spinal cord at S2 to S4. Thus women with lesions below T12 may have uterine sensation but perineal anesthesia. Episodic hypertension may be the first sign of uterine contractions because the uterus contracts during labor by intermuscular communication without a connected nerve supply. The hypertension of autonomic dysreflexia can be differentiated from toxemia by the episodic nature of the hypertension that follows uterine contractions and the onset of labor and is not present in toxemia. With lesions at the T10 to T11 level, uterine contractions may be stronger, but the abdominal muscles used for pushing are affected and may necessitate cesarean section (Sipski, 1991). Induced labor is contraindicated for women with lesions at the T6 level or above.

Autonomic dysreflexia may occur during labor and delivery (Box 23-3 lists interventions; refer to Chapter 19 for full description and management information). Breast-feeding is

Box 23-3 Autonomic Dysreflexia: Interventions during Labor and Delivery

- Differentiate from toxemia of pregnancy (i.e., blood pressure rises associated with uterine contractions)
- Monitor blood pressure frequently
- Use Reserpine 2 weeks before due date to prevent dysreflexia
- Avoid external restraints
- Use anesthetic ointments during insertion of an indwelling catheter and during vaginal examinations, enemas, and the like
- Position upright to decrease symptoms and shorten labor
- Use an epidural anesthetic, as suggested in the literature; a spinal anesthetic may be used as well
- Use medications as prescribed for blood pressure control
- Know that when dysreflexia is uncontrolled by medications and anesthesia, prompt delivery by cesarean section may be the most expedient method of management

Data from Nygaard, I., Bartscht, K.D., & Cole, S. (1990). Sexuality and reproduction in spinal cord injured women. *Obstetrical and Gynecological Survey, 45,* 727-732; Sipski, M. (1991). The impact of spinal cord injury on female sexuality, menstruation and pregnancy: A review of the literature. *Journal of the American Paraplegia Society, 14*(3) 122-126; Yarkony, G.M. & Chen, D. (1995) Sexuality in patients with spinal cord injury. *Physical Medicine and Rehabilitation: State of the Art Reviews Sexuality and Disability, 9*(2), 325-344.

not contraindicated in women with SCI, but with lesions at T6 they may have decreased milk supply after 6 weeks because of the lack of sensory input when breast-feeding.

Infertility. Many conditions contribute to infertility: erectile or ejaculation dysfunction, decreased sperm quality and quantity, altered thermoregulation to the testicles from autonomic nervous system dysfunction in men, and genitourinary infection or hormonal irregularities in both sexes. Infertility treatment has grown in many rehabilitation centers as results have improved. Specific programs offer education for couples with disabilities who are infertile but wish to bear children. Couples who have had successful unprotected intercourse for 1 full year during the woman's most fertile time in each cycle without pregnancy benefit from fertility evaluation. Refer to an accessible clinic with expertise on infertility management for couples with disabilities; many conduct research on each aspect of the cause for infertility. One example of research concerns sperm retrieval and quality, and applications of findings for families with disabilities. Sperm collection uses electrovibratory stimulation applied directly to the penis or electroejaculation techniques. The semen is washed and used for artificial insemination or in vitro fertilization. Vibroejaculation used at home requires little sperm preparation of the semen. In research, approaches to improve sperm quality for men with SCI include bladder management, early treatment of urinary tract infection, and reduced scrotal temperatures. With the introduction of micromanipulation techniques, using one sperm to unite with one ovum and microsurgery to obtain sperm samples, even men with SCI and poor semen quantity have increased reproductive potential (Rutkowski et al., 1999).

Interventions for Activity Intolerance

The plan of care for activity intolerance involves the client and partner in active therapy; they identify deficits in activity level. They then receive instruction in how to perform the desired activity, make adaptations, and modify the environment to accommodate it. Rehabilitation activities that build strength and endurance for activities of daily living and community living can include those to enable sexual activity once the client returns home (McCloskey & Bulechek, 2000).

Positions for Sexual Activity

A nurse may encourage clients to experiment with positions that are comfortable and appropriate for them, that is, those that enhance comfort and facilitate sexual activity. Couples often welcome information about alternate positions, as well as encouragement to experiment. Assistive devices or adapted equipment, such as side rails, bed loops, or an overhead trapeze, may ease changing positions and be safe for those with difficulty in bed mobility. Loss of range of motion in the joints, particularly the hips, limits movements during sexual activity and restricts favorite positions. Pillows are for positioning; those shaped like an armchair back can position the person with high SCI to see what is transpiring. Some persons are more comfortable in a recliner or other chairs than in a bed. Helping couples select positions that place the least stress on involved body parts manages pain, reduces potential for injury or complications, and allows the most sexual pleasure.

Specific disabilities preclude certain positions. For example, clients who have cardiac problems should avoid positions that place undue stress on the arms for sustained periods. The supine position is less stressful physically, as long as breathing is not restricted. The side-by-side position and face-to-face position create less worry about compromising cardiac function. Sexual activity for the client with cardiac problems is resumed based on the cardiologist's recommendations; generally, a few weeks after heart surgery and 3 to 8 weeks after myocardial infarction. Energy requirements range between 3 and 6 METs (metabolic equivalent units), that is, from light to moderately heavy activity. Chapter 31 discusses more about specific activity levels following myocardial infarction. Refer to Box 23-4 for guidelines for sexual intercourse following myocardial infarction.

Common Positions and Precautions

Persons with disabilities may use variations of the four basic positions; all provide access for genital-to-genital contact, cunnilingus, and fellatio.

- Face-to-face, man above (or missionary position)
- Face-to-face, woman above
- Face-to-face, side-lying (provides for freedom of movement for both partners)

Box 23-4 Guidelines for Sexual Intercourse after Myocardial Infarction

- Familiar surroundings are important in diminishing psychological stress
- A comfortable temperature, neither too cold nor hot, can decrease heart stress
- Prepare gradually for the increased activity of intercourse through foreplay; gradually prepare the heart
- Positions must be comfortable, relaxing, and not restrict breathing; usual positions are most comfortable
- Person on the bottom position causes less stress because person on the bottom is not supporting the body
- Orogenital sex and masturbation cause no undue strain, so they may be used for sexual expression
- Intercourse is best performed when the couple is rested; morning is an ideal time for couples at home
- Delay sexual activity for at least 3 hours after eating a heavy meal or drinking alcohol
- Take medications such as nitroglycerin before intercourse, if required to prevent chest pain; if chest pain occurs, stop sexual activity and follow regimen; if chest pain persists, contact the physician
- Notify physician if a rapid heart rate persists longer than 15 minutes after intercourse
- Sex with a new partner may increase stress to the heart

Seidl et al., 1991; Tardif, 1989.

- Rear entry, which is possible from a side-lying or sitting position or when the woman is kneeling or lying prone; hand stimulation is possible for both partners, and penetration into the vagina may be regulated (Reinisch, 1990)

Some precautions are sensible in sexual positioning for clients who have been immobile for long periods or who cannot bear weight on their lower extremities. Weight of a partner on a client's osteoporotic bones may be sufficient to cause fractures; others with recent orthopedic injuries and concomitant neurological injuries may require bracing for bone stabilization. Until the physiatrist or orthopedist determines a brace can be removed safely during sexual activity, the person wears it, even if the brace is removed in bed otherwise. A brace also can dictate positions because undue pressure is not applied to any area of the body that is braced. Persons with heterotropic ossification may have limited joint motion and painful joint areas; they benefit from positioning that allows them maximum functional mobility without pain.

Avoiding complications and providing a comfortable sexual activity are goals when experimenting with positions. Persons with rheumatic disease, for example, select positions that place the least stress on the involved joints. Although clients with restricted joint motion must limit movements during sexual activity, experimenting with several positions may yield one that permits both comfort and flexibility. Many (70%) persons with arthritic hip joint problems report sexual difficulties (Reinisch, 1990). Women whose arthritis affects the hip joint find the spoon position, side lying with the man behind the woman, more comfortable. Recommended for men with hip joint problems is a position with the couple lying facing and side by side; the woman wraps her upper leg around the man's upper hip or both legs around his hips. Alternatively the man lies supine while the woman sits astride his hips with her knees, lower legs, and feet on either side of his body. Her knees provide support, and she can put her hands on the bed to control her weight on his pelvis (Reinisch, 1990). Pillows all around help support the weight and cushion painful joints.

Those with multiple sclerosis who experience fatigue and spasticity consider scheduling and positioning that is the most comfortable and least tiring. Persons with SCI may need encouragement to experiment with various positions. Usually the person with SCI takes the bottom position because of the motor dysfunction and lack of movement. Pillows placed under a woman's hips make this a comfortable position, but the couple may experiment with prone or side-lying positions. Couples are educated to manage autonomic dysreflexia, should it occur.

Psychosocial Interventions

Body Image Disturbance and Low Self-Esteem

Body image and self-esteem may be affected adversely by altered sexual abilities. Nurses assess the client's body image expectations based on developmental stage and provide anticipatory guidance about predictable changes, such as with a congenital condition, injury, disease, or surgery. Children or adolescents may draw pictures that reflect their body image perceptions. They need to learn how their impairment affects sexuality and effective strategies to accept their appearance. Sexuality is more than sexual activities, and the groundwork is laid in early developmental stages.

Nurses can find ways to enhance a client's life satisfaction through rehabilitation interventions because success with bowel and bladder retaining, success with transfers, and independence in activities of daily living improve self-concept. Self-esteem thrives in a therapeutic environment with trusting relationships between nurses who communicate acceptance and include clients as worthwhile and unique apart from the impairment. The sooner a client returns to meaningful work and resumes roles in the family and community, the greater the self-esteem and role balance. All factors that build self-concept contribute positively to the sexual relationship. On the other hand, a decrease in sexual abilities and performance has a negative impact. Men anxious about sexual problems may voice concern about their ability to satisfy their partners. When role changes become necessary for sexual activities, rehabilitation nurses can support and encourage couples, including educating them about compensation strategies, fertility clinics, and other options, as appropriate.

Interventions for Sexual Role Performance/Support System Deficit/Social Isolation

Social Isolation

A client whose self-concept is threatened may avoid contact with others and become socially isolated. Involving the client in social interaction as early as possible, complimenting efforts to appear attractive, discussing individual sexual concerns, and accepting concerns as a matter of course may help maintain or restore self-concept. As children grow, they need the same interventions as adults to develop a social network. Planning involves assessing whether altered body image contributes to increased social isolation. Reducing the impact of physical changes with accessories, such as scarves, manageable clothing, wigs, or cosmetics as appropriate may help some to feel more comfortable in public and avoid social isolation. Peer counseling with someone who has similar alterations in body image helps some to find support (McCloskey & Bulechek, 2000).

In a facility clients are encouraged to eat with others in the dining room, participate in groups in therapy departments and on nursing units, join in education programs, and attend social skills or support groups. Some support groups have special meetings for "survivors" or former clients to help clients meet their social needs. Some clients gain socialization by serving others, many volunteer in their community. Nurses who can identify community resources help clients and families to obtain needed services, and along the way, clients meet others, some with similar interests, and may find ways to work, attend school, or become involved in activities. Community resources include spiritual institutions, such as churches, synagogues, mosques, temples; special-interest groups; schools; community education classes and programs; sports programs; and volunteer opportunities. All are places to meet others.

Social isolation also restricts opportunities to meet that special someone and build a strong interpersonal or sexual relationship. Tips concerning fostering relationships include:

- Do not believe that no one will love you because you have a disability
- Do not build your life in search of romance; use activities to meet others
- Be a friend first
- Keep up on current events
- Be patient in your search for connection with others
- Be open about your disability
- Know that regardless of your disability, lovemaking is possible (National Information Center for Children and Youth with Disabilities, 1992).

Building and Maintaining Relationships

Information concerning building and maintaining relationships is an essential component of education programs for clients and their partners. High levels of subjective quality of life and life satisfaction are possible for couples with SCI. One study found the three most frequent problems in these relationships were sex, communication, and recreation, and men with SCI expressed less affection to their wives than other husbands. Suggestions were emphasizing sexual rehabilitation, encouraging positive communication patterns, and encouraging mutually enjoyable activities (Yim et al., 1998; Masters et al., 1986) offer ideas for communicating about sex (Box 23-5).

Box 23-5 Communicating about Sex

- Talk with your partner about how and when it would be most comfortable to discuss sex. This will let your partner know you are interested in feedback about your sexual interaction.
- Consider the possibility of using books or other media sources to initiate discussions. One disadvantage is that books do not always suit the personal style of the couple, so choose one that is not offensive.
- Use "I" language as much as possible when talking about sex together and try to avoid putting blame on your partner for your own patterns of response (or lack thereof).
- Remember that if your partner rejects a type of sexual activity that you think you might enjoy, he or she is not rejecting you as a person.
- Be aware that sexual feelings and preferences change from time to time.
- Do not neglect the nonverbal side of sexual communication because these messages often speak louder than words.
- Do not expect perfection.

Talking about sex with your partner is not something to do once and then put aside. Like all forms of intimate communication, this topic benefits from the ongoing dialogue that permits a couple to learn about each other and resolve confusion or uncertainties over time. One area where men and women differ is communication. In general, men process and remember in conversation mainly through the left side of the brain, and focusing on the literal words and factual data, they miss the underlying emotions. Women, however, store nonverbal and emotional communication, perceiving the tone of voice as well as the emotional or pictorial messages. One technique to reconcile the differences is using word pictures or analogies that bridge both sides of the brain, enabling a couple to be open to intimacy (Smalley & Trent, 1988). For example, couples learn to build an analogy, "I'll love you until I've drained the Pacific Ocean by removing the water one bucket at a time." Relationships are nurtured by the daily sharing of our feelings, needs, hopes, and dreams and by active listening when a partner shares. Effective social interaction skills incorporate elements of disclosure, receptiveness, cooperation, sensitivity, assertiveness, confrontation, consideration, genuineness, warmth, poise, relaxation, engagement, trust, and compromise (Johnson, Maas, & Moorhead, 2000). Building trust and honor is a choice for a lifelong commitment, to understand each other's needs, to develop the skills to meet those needs, and for a desire to resolve conflicts and promote harmony. After an illness or injury partners who commit to each another choose to accept each other as unique, complete persons who are loved, and to look for ways to comfort and nurture.

Affection and Romance

Privacy for a hug or kiss and to express affection with meaningful touch are encouraging during hospitalization and rehabilitation. Most persons retain some areas of intact sensation, making meaningful touch effective. Eight to 10 meaningful touches a day keep fires of a relationship burning. Verbal communication, verbal communication with signals such as gestures or facial movements, and sign language are all means of communicating feelings (Spica, 1989). Romance is a shared emotional experience of special times in which couples focus on how valuable each is to the other, but couples may require careful planning and conversation to rediscover romance and to build it into their lives. They are encouraged to schedule intimate times together despite the pressures of life with a chronic condition or disability (Smalley & Trent, 1988).

Sexual role performance can be enhanced by sexual education and by introducing role models who have overcome a similar problem. Roles are discussed with the partner, and compensation strategies for role performance are included in the education program (McCloskey & Bulechek, 2000).

Interventions for Knowledge Deficit

Comprehensive Sexuality Education

According to the Sex Information and Education Council of the United States, comprehensive sexuality education should address facts, data, and information; feelings, values, and attitudes; and the skills to communicate effectively and to make responsible decisions (Haffner, 1990). The goals of sexuality education are to:

1. Provide information about human growth and development, human reproduction, anatomy, physiology, masturbation, family life, pregnancy, childbirth, parenthood, sexual response, sexual orientation, contraception, abortion, sexual abuse, and STDs, including the human immunodeficiency virus (HIV) and acquired immunodeficiency syndrome (AIDS).
2. Develop values. As a result of sexuality education, clients may question, explore, and assess attitudes, values, and insights about human sexuality. Understanding family, religious, and cultural values helps clarify personal values, increases self-esteem, provides insight about relationships with members of both sexes, and defines personal responsibility to others.
3. Develop interpersonal skills. Participating in sexuality education can help clients develop skills in communication, decision making, assertiveness, peer refusal skills, and the ability to create satisfying relationships.
4. Develop responsibility. Providing sexuality education helps to develop a concept of responsibility extending to sexual relationships. Informed, responsible persons are able to consider abstinence, resist pressure to become prematurely involved in sexual intercourse, properly use contraception, take other measures to prevent sexually related health problems such as teenage pregnancy and STDs, and resist sexual exploitation or abuse (Haffner, 1990).

The Rehabilitation Nurse's Role as Counselor. Counselors become aware of their personal value systems, including biases and beliefs about appropriate and inappropriate sexual behavior; all rehabilitation team members ideally understand their own sexuality. Nurses are never to negate their own beliefs, but while acknowledging their validity should be aware of what they can or cannot acceptably teach. Should conflicts interfere with counseling or education, the nurse refers clients to other health professionals. All persons providing counseling or education have limitations and at times refer to others qualified in specific areas or able to provide the counsel or education the client wants or needs.

A therapeutic relationship based on trust and respect enhances counseling; clients are more open when assured of privacy and confidentiality. The individual is of primary importance; certainly group classes are useful in rehabilitation and for sharing basic information; however, each client's needs are worth private discussion. Timing is important when opening the door for sexuality discussions. Clients and partners learn that sexuality is an important part of life that is affected by their current physical condition or functional ability. Holistic care means the rehabilitation nurse is poised to provide information and support at the time sexual function problems are discovered, observed, or expressed. Communication is on the client's level, using language they understand and discussing sexuality with ease and confidence. Communication skills include active listening, techniques to elicit feelings, strategies for showing acceptance, goal setting, and problem solving. Compassion, a sense of humor, patience, perceptiveness, ingenuity, and flexibility are strengths in counseling relationships. It is helpful to preface questions with a statement that tells clients they are not alone in experiencing sexual difficulties (e.g., "Some persons with SCI experience problems with ejaculation, is that something you have had a problem with since your injury?"}. Moving from a less sensitive to a more sensitive topic keeps the information flow from disruption.

Effective counseling begins with a willing, available listener who spends quality time listening to a client express needs as a sexual being. Empathetic and active listening is a foundational technique for counseling, guiding a client through problem solving toward being comfortable in discussing sexuality and eliciting specific needs relative to self and family members. Counseling is an opportunity for clients to express grief and anger about altered body image and function and for their partners to learn to accept the changes. Guilt expressed during counseling may relate to the cause, or beliefs about the cause, of the illness or accident (McCloskey & Bulechek, 2000).

Counseling the Sexual Partner. Partners need counsel about how to react to changes in body image, in preparation for what can happen during sexual intercourse, and to understand effects of medications and certain disabilities on sexual function. This counsel can help alleviate a partner's anxiety about engaging in sexual acts (Kroll & Klein, 1991). Both the client and partner may need to dispel myths and correct misconceptions about sexual options. The nurse can confirm that a particular sexual practice is acceptable and not harmful, but responses must be appropriate to clients' lifestyles, beliefs, and needs. The couple makes final decisions and sets the guidelines for their comfort. Successful coping strategies used in the past will help place events in proper perspective and assist to identify strengths and previous successes. When couples can reframe a situation knowing that things have changed but are not necessarily worse than before, they may adjust to altered sexual ability more readily (Kroll & Klein, 1991).

All too often in Western culture, sexual acts are taken seriously, without humor. In a trusting relationship, humor can serve as a form of tension release and a means of dealing with problematic or potentially embarrassing situations. Counselors anticipate a client's reactions to surgeries, procedures, or impairments and supply information before events occur, strategies that may alleviate threats to self-esteem or perceived loss of control. A nurse counselor builds expertise with counseling clients who have similar disabilities, as well as gaining knowledge for comprehensive health assessment and improving competency in intervening with person of various developmental levels and cultural or religious values.

The PLISSIT Model. The PLISSIT model developed by Annon (1976) helps nurses evaluate their role and level of comfort in sexual counseling. The acronym PLISSIT defines possible levels of involvement for nurses: permission, limited information, specific suggestions, and intensive therapy. With increased comfort and experience, a nurse may use more complex levels while choosing to refer at any time. The nurse gives the client permission to discuss concerns and problems related to sexuality—permission to be a sexual being. For instance, when a client is queried concerning sexuality during an admission assessment, the door is open for any questions or discussion by the client. The nurse may give permission by reassuring that sexual practices of the client are appropriate and healthy and that worrying about sexual function is common, or the nurse may give permission to experiment with new forms of sexual expression.

Clients should not leave the rehabilitation setting without limited information concerning how their illness or accident has or has not affected their sexual function. Part of the basic education for clients, information must answer their questions about sexual function.

The nurse can offer specific suggestions to address specific concerns. For example, clients with total hip replacements need specific suggestions about positions for sexual function that are not contraindicated. Specific suggestions include strategies for direct problem solving or referrals for medical interventions. Suggestions may help clients to rethink a problem and make changes to alleviate the concern. Clients can practice the suggestions and evaluate progress and problems.

Intensive therapy uses the referral process to meet the needs of a client whose problems cannot be solved using the first three levels. This level of intervention is required by some clients and especially appropriate for those with significant psychosocial sexual dysfunction (Annon, 1976). Rehabilitation nurses who are uncomfortable with any of these levels refer clients to team members who are skillful and knowledgeable in specific areas for counseling and education. Other team members who may be skilled in sexual counseling include the clinical nurse specialist, nurse practitioner, psychologist, social worker, rehabilitation counselor, therapy staff, gynecologist, physiatrist, urologist, and sex therapist. The team approach offers opportunity for individual or group counseling and the resources of a number of health care professionals. Couples who require a higher level of expertise can contact professional organizations such as the Society for Sex Therapy and Research (New York) and the American Association of Sex Educators, Counselors, and Therapists (Washington, DC). They publish national directories of qualified sex therapists. Local medical societies, psychological associations, certified psychiatric or mental health nurses, mental health associations, and other nurses working in rehabilitation centers or as members of a sexual management team may be helpful in identifying qualified sex therapists in an area.

Many rehabilitation facilities have initiated sexual education programs after educating members of the team for sexual counseling. Information is gathered from professionals with expertise, literature reviews, conferences and seminars, and other resources. Planned, structured opportunities allow health care providers to become desensitized to hearing sexual terms and concepts, to evaluate their values and cultural practices through role-playing and small-group discussion, and to consider personal feelings and beliefs about sexual behavior for themselves and others.

Counseling for Children. Although sexual counseling is primarily directed toward adults and older persons, sexual counseling is not an adults-only activity. When children and adolescents require sexuality information and counseling, parents are involved in setting up any individualized or group sexual education programs. Understandably parents may be anxious concerning sexual education for their children. More often they allow sexual education that does not teach simply "how to do it," but rather, material emphasizing sex roles, understanding of the body, and socialization skills. Programs on sexual abstinence, especially in younger teens, have been well received by parents and teens. Research findings indicate that students who understand their sexuality and the responsibilities that go with it are less likely to encounter sexual troubles than students who are uninformed. Parents have legal and ethical rights to retain primary responsibility for transmitting values and building morality in their children (Johnson & Kempton, 1981). When teaching sexual information in the rehabilitation setting or any setting, it is imperative to receive permission from parents before providing information to teenagers or children.

Rehabilitation nurses and case managers who work with pediatric and adolescent clients may become the providers of sexual education when parents are unable or unwilling to do so. In group homes, where young persons with chronic, disabling, or developmental delays live, staff members may impart sexual information through daily contacts and as part of the fabric of daily life, as well as in formal classes.

Sexual education programs for youth and adolescents include content on responsible sexual behavior such as social skills, how to avoid being sexually exploited, appropriate body exposure, privacy of sexual behavior, responsibility of sexual behavior including abstinence, and how to prevent pregnancy (Johnson & Kempton, 1981). Children with disabilities will mature sexually. They need to be prepared for the changes that will occur in their bodies. Social skills concerning sexuality are very important for children with disabilities. Children in some settings, where personal assistance with bowel/bladder management and assistance with dressing are provided, are more vulnerable to sexual exploitation. Children and adults with cognitive dysfunction should be taught appropriate social behavior concerning sexuality, including what constitutes proper touching.

The following information might be shared with parents of children with disabilities to enhance sexual education:

1. Parents should demonstrate acceptance of the child's body
2. Parents and siblings will provide the first experience with love and socialization
3. Social relationships with siblings and friends should be encouraged
4. Children need to understand the difference between private and public behavior
5. Children need to learn the role behaviors of the same-sex parent in daily interactions (Selekman & McIlvain-Simpson, 1991)
6. Sexuality information is presented related to a child's age (Table 23-5)

Prevention of Sexually Transmitted Diseases

STDs are at near-epidemic levels in the United States. Uncomfortable or painful, inconvenient, embarrassing, anxiety producing, and sometimes fatal, many STDs persist or leave residual damage, as with chlamydia and gonorrhea. Tenacious herpes virus, found in up to 30% to 40% of single, sexually active persons, and syphilis, at a 40-year high, are among STDs that increase cervical cancer risk. Any symptoms of genital infection need immediate diagnosis and treatment for protection of all involved parties. Sexually active persons, especially those not in monogamous relationships or who change partners, need to recognize symptoms and have annual tests. Early diagnosis and treatment may prevent some long-term complications. Preven-

TABLE 23-5 Age-Related Sexual Information for Children and Adolescents

Ages 5 to 7 Years	Ages 8 to 11 Years	Ages 12 to 18 Years
Correct name of body parts and their functions	Girls learn about menses; boys learn about nocturnal emissions	Health maintenance (regular examination of breasts or testicles by self-examination and primary care provider)
Differences and similarities between boys and girls	Signs and variations of puberty	Sexuality as part of the total self, to include communication, love, dating, and intimacy
Elements of reproduction and pregnancy	Sexuality as part of the total self	Masturbation becomes a private practice
Qualities of good relationships (love, friendship, communication, and respect)	Information on reproduction and pregnancy	Importance of values in guiding one's behavior
Decision-making skills; all decisions have consequences	Importance of values in decision making	How alcohol and/or drugs influence decision making
Beginning social responsibility, values, and morals	Communication within family unit about sexuality	Intercourse and other ways to express sexuality
Masturbation may be found pleasurable	Masturbation	Birth control and the responsibilities of childbearing, reproduction, and pregnancy
Ways to avoid and report sexual exploitation	Abstinence from sexual intercourse	Pros and cons of condoms in disease prevention
	Avoidance and reporting of sexual abuse	
	Sexually transmitted diseases, including HIV/AIDS	

From Sexuality education for children and youth with disabilities. (1992). Fostering relationships: Suggestions for young adults. *News digest.* Washington DC: National Information Center for Children and Youth with Disabilities.

HIV, Human immunodeficiency virus; *AIDS,* acquired immunodeficiency syndrome.

tion involves education, counseling, increased abstention, and partner notification.

Teenagers are noted for their risky sexual behavior, exemplified in teen pregnancies. Feelings of invincibility and denial influence risk-taking behaviors, such as unprotected sexual activity. However, with the spread of STDs, including HIV and AIDS, the consequences have escalated from unwanted pregnancy to long-term illness and even death. Recommendations for providing the most effective sex education programs for teenagers include the following:

- Deliver a clear message: Delay sex until you are older, of if you have sex, use a latex condom.
- Focus on setting peer norms: Not everyone is doing it and you do not have to either.
- Teach resistance skills through role-playing and group discussion on how to say no without hurting someone's feelings and how to avoid situations in which you might have to say no. Repetition of the practice builds learning (Hahn, 1995).
- Include special training for teachers. The SHARE program is one abstinence program that can be used in schools for education (refer to Resources). Safer sex guidelines were developed for all persons, although they originated in response to the AIDS epidemic (Box 23-6). The goals are to reduce risks of STDs, as well as unplanned pregnancy, when used properly and every time. Guidelines for safe sex include abstinence until marriage, monogamous sex, and marriage for life.

Box 23-6 Safer Sex Guidelines

1. Delay engaging in sexual intercourse as long as possible. Abstinence is the only completely safe behavior for preventing sexually transmitted diseases (STDs) and pregnancy.
2. Learn proper use of effective birth control methods and regard abstinence as a best practice for birth control.
3. Restrict the number of sexual partners; the fewer sexual partners in a lifetime, the less chance of exposure to any STD.
4. A mutually exclusive sexual relationship (sex with only one partner) lowers the risk for STDs. Avoiding body penetration or exchange of body fluids decreases risk of some STDs.
5. Be selective when choosing sexual partners; learn as much as possible about them, including their sexual history. Never assume that a woman is automatically in a low-risk group for STDs or that a male partner has never had sex with other men; bisexual behavior occurs among some groups.
6. Avoid high-risk sexual behavior until you know with certainty that your partner is not infected with an STD. The most risky behaviors are unprotected anal intercourse and unprotected vaginal intercourse.
7. Any activity that exposes a person to blood, semen, vaginal secretions, menstrual blood, urine, feces, or saliva is high-risk behavior, unless partners are in a mutually exclusive sexual relationship and neither is infected. A condom for oral, anal, and/or vaginal sex, with a spermicide containing nonoxynol-9 or octoxynol added for vaginal or anal intercourse, can help to prevent STDs. If engaging in cunnilingus, a barrier in the mouth, like a dental dam, may add some protection where it covers oral parts (Reinisch, 1990).
8. Condoms do not provide protection when an infectious area is not covered. For example, a herpes sore on the scrotum would not be covered. Condoms do fail on occasion, creating risk. Natural skin condoms do not protect from the AIDS virus, and oil-based products weaken latex condoms, encouraging breakage.
9. Good hygiene, lubrication, and voiding after intercourse decrease some susceptibility to infections.
10. Vibrators, dildos, or other items used for sexual stimulation are not shared with others until thoroughly washed with soap and water. Plenty of lubricant and gentle use prevent skin irritation or breakdown of vaginal or rectal tissues.
11. Those at risk for STDs need to have regular examinations, including testing, by their health care provider (McCloskey & Bulechek, 2000).

EVALUATION

Evaluation of nursing interventions for education or counseling follow the nursing process. Evaluation methods are client demonstrations of learned skills and verbal repetition of the information. Because sexual activity is a private matter, the socially acceptable evaluation is questioning and evaluating the verbal responses. A nurse might ask about achievement of individualized goals, and the client and partner decide how or if they wish to reply. When teaching psychomotor domain skills, such as using devices to promote erections (injections or a vacuum device) or applying birth control devices, clients can perform return demonstrations. Performance criteria, such as correct placement and use of the device or adaptations for impairments, ensure quality. The effectiveness of birth control methods is evaluated readily by the absence of pregnancy and side effects.

Sexual function outcomes for clients include expressing sexual interest; attaining sexual arousal; sustaining penile/clitoral erection through orgasm; using assistive devices safely; adapting sexual techniques as needed; and being able to perform sexually, despite physical impairments (Johnson et al., 2000). Activity intolerance outcomes are evaluated by physiological signs of tolerance to activity. Outcomes include compensated heart rate, respiratory rate, blood pressure, skin color, and ability to speak while sexually active as signs of increased activity tolerance. Those related to sexual activity are best assessed by the couple in private. Outcomes for self-esteem and body image disturbance include expresses self-esteem, challenges negative images of sexual self, expresses willingness to be sexual, and expresses comfort with body and satisfaction with body appearance.

Relationship factors are evaluated by observing interactions between the client and partner. Outcomes for sexual functioning that involve relationship factors include expresses ability to be intimate, reports access to consenting partner, expresses respect/acceptance of partner, and expresses knowledge of partner's sexual capabilities (Johnson et al., 2000).

Knowledge outcomes concerning sexual function include identification of body part and understanding physical/emotional changes of puberty and reproduction for younger clients, understanding of physical/emotional changes with aging for older clients, and knowledge of safer sexual practices and cultural influence on sexual behavior. Key outcomes are all related to evaluation of knowledge. Some research exists on physiological function with observations of actual sexual activity, but most knowledge and data have been gathered through communication techniques (Johnson et al., 2000).

IMPLICATIONS FOR PRACTICE

Increasingly, rehabilitation nurses work in the community as consultants or direct-service providers. Rehabilitation nursing assessment and interventions during hospitalization are instrumental in identifying sexual problems requiring early intervention, discharge planning, and follow-up, especially because a great deal of adjustment to disability will occur in the community. Problems resolved during the hospitalization with team collaboration lay groundwork for decision making and problem solving at home.

Ideally, rehabilitation facilities, nursing homes, and other residences provide privacy for clients and spouses or partners to experiment with techniques. Facilities, personnel, and clients need to know what is provided and allowable. Some inpatient facilities permit sexual activity only for married couples to avoid lawsuits and to protect those incompetent to make rational decisions. Visiting for sexual purposes may be possible only in certain areas and where more privacy can be afforded. Weekend passes from the facility or hospital provide clients and partners opportunities to explore sexual options in the privacy of their own home. Time set aside to discuss the weekend experiences and offer additional information is often overlooked but can be a planned method for intervention and evaluation. Common courtesy dictates that all staff members knock on a client's closed door and wait for permission to enter. Door signs displayed for privacy alert anyone not to enter without permission. Staff and visitors tend to disregard common courtesies for persons in hospitals or other residences, taking liberties with privacy and personal effects that would be unacceptable by any standards elsewhere.

Rehabilitation nurses also need to know community resources and nurses working in various community-based programs including home health care, case management, and specialized programs. Arranging appropriate referrals for clients who require continuing services is part of the team plan. Basic sexuality education and counseling are available from nurses in the community; sexual difficulties related to a disability indicate community nurse collaboration for follow-up appointments with a rehabilitation nurse or team member.

Ideally, sexual assessment is part of assessment in all health care settings, and providers are educated to provide information related to sexual health. The relationship-building component must not be neglected when counseling on sexual health. Behavior, self-determination, and self-concept are essential for improving outcomes and topics for research. Information on sexual function incorporated into the basic curricula for health care providers can address interventions and specific suggestions related to sexual function. More research is needed in all areas of sexual function for enhancement, as well as prevention and treatment, of STDs. Education content needs to include evidence from research because information about sexuality has changed over time. For example, the sexual function of persons with SCIs was believed to be related to category of spinal injury (i.e., complete versus incomplete injury) or level of function. While physiologically true for many activities and abilities, research demonstrates that the ability to experience orgasm is based on the physiology as well as behavioral and relationship issues; a higher percentage of persons experience orgasm than originally believed (Tepper, 1999). What an encouragement to persons with SCIs and a mandate to health professionals to share this information. However, nurses may find, in addition to the wealth of information on legitimate websites, that some of the older literature is very helpful as a foundation for sexual information. Current literature reviews are needed about interventions, especially those related to impotence, fertility, infertility, orgasm, and medications.

Sexual issues are worldwide and affect all persons, including the disabled. Those with impairments are exposed to the negative impact of violence, abusive behavior, STDs, rape, incest, and substance abuse and may be more vulnerable in some situations because of economic, social, or cognitive/behavioral issues. Preventing these negative events is a goal for all persons and a major challenge for the health professional, as well as for societies.

SUMMARY

The ability to function as a sexual being is a basic need of all persons. This need coexists with chronic illness or disability, where sexual concerns may become a major focus. Because sexual concerns are tremendously complex, no simple behavioral or medical approach will suffice to assess or treat individual sexual problems. Ideally a team approach—with members who are comfortable with their own sexuality, knowledgeable about sexuality, and willing to commit a considerable amount of time—is required to plan and implement with the individual experiencing sexual problems.

Rehabilitation nurses frequently deal with clients' sexual problems at their level of comfort, refer to other team members when unable to address the problems expressed, and participate as members of the sexuality management team. It is the responsibility of every rehabilitation nurse to give the client permission to discuss sexual concerns and then to deal with any expressed difficulties appropriately. Clients should leave rehabilitation settings knowledgeable concerning their sexual function, with their questions answered, and prepared to manage their sexual function independently or direct their partner in the process.

CRITICAL THINKING

1. You are providing a client with nursing care when the client reaches out and touches you inappropriately. If the client is cognitively intact, how would you respond? How would you respond if the client cognitively could not distinguish cause and effect, and what should your interventions be?
2. The husband of a married couple is no longer cognitively intact due to stroke. What would you assess and how would you advise the wife on their sexual relationship?

Case Study I

Daniel Lacey is a 57-year-old African-American man who experienced a left middle cerebral artery cerebrovascular accident 3 months ago. Currently he is ambulatory for community distances using a straight cane; his right (dominant) arm is hypertonic and has minimal movement; sensation is diminished on the right side. He has predominantly expressive aphasia and a right visual field cut. He is independent in self-care and in some home maintenance and is bowel and bladder continent. He takes antihypertensive medication regularly, which controls his blood pressure.

Mr. Lacey is unable to return to his previous job as a truck driver. The Laceys have been married for 30 years and have four grown children. He regularly attends a Baptist church. Church attendance and family visits are his primary outings. Mrs. Lacey works full-time and feels she cannot quit her job, especially now that her husband is not working. The Laceys have a strong relationship and premorbidly had a good sexual relationship, especially after the children left home. Mrs. Lacey had a tubal ligation shortly after the birth of her last child. Their usual method of sexual expression is genital intercourse.

During his rehabilitation stay Mr. Lacey attended a group class on sexuality, but because of his communication problem, he did not verbally participate. During his follow-up visit at 3 months, his wife asked physiatrist whether she and her husband could resume their sexual relationship. The physiatrist assured her they could but felt they needed more education than he had time to give. The Laceys were referred to the case manager, a nurse, for further counseling.

The case manager identified the need for education concerning compensation strategies for sexual function as a primary need for this couple, especially as related to their communication problem and Mr. Lacey's motor and sensory deficits. She also noted a need to work with Mr. Lacey concerning issues of self-esteem related to the change in his role of provider.

The nurse did a thorough assessment and reviewed the physical examination completed by the physician. She noted that Mr. Lacey had normal rectal sphincter tone and control of external anal and bladder sphincters. He had normal sensation when his testicles were squeezed, and his bulbocavernosus and anal wink reflexes were normal. Premorbidly Mr. Lacey had normal sexual function.

The nurse identified problems that could be encountered sexually by this couple. She developed the following nursing diagnoses:

1. Knowledge deficit concerning how stroke affects sexual function, positioning for sexual function for a person with hemiparesis, compensation for sensory dysfunction and communication impairment, potential of impotence related to antihypertensive medication
2. Self-concept deficit related to recent change in lifestyle

Goals

After the education provided by the case manager, the Laceys will:

1. Be knowledgeable about basic information on the effects of the cerebrovascular accident on sexual function
2. Discuss information about sexual options, compensation strategies, and devices
3. Begin to participate in sexual activity at a level near their preillness level
4. Experience maintenance or restoration of a positive self-concept including improving body image

The case manager's plan of care included teaching the Laceys the following:

1. Because of his normal sensation and voluntary motor control over bowel and bladder function, sexually Mr. Lacey's body should work like it did before his stroke. It may take some time, 6 to 7 weeks after stroke, to return to previous levels, but it should have returned by this time. If impotence is an issue the physician should be notified, and perhaps the physician may change the antihypertensive medication.
2. Participation in sexual activities would not increase Mr. Lacey's potential for another stroke or harm him.
3. Positions that may increase Mr. Lacey's ability to move and participate include side-lying position with his right side on the bed to free his more mobile side for stroking or caressing his wife. Having his right side downward would also allow his wife to be in his intact field of vision. Positioning could include face-to-face or front-to-back. Another possible position is man on his back, woman on top. For Mr. Lacey, semisitting in a supported position would allow increased visualization. Mrs. Lacey would have to assume the motor movement in this position. To gradually work back into genital intercourse, dual partner stimulation may be initiated as a first step.

Continued

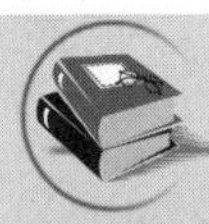

Case Study 1—cont'd

4. Other sexual activities that have been pleasurable should be encouraged, such as kissing, touching sensitive body areas, caressing, licking, hugging, or oral sex.
5. To compensate for diminished sensation on the involved right side, the intact side of the body should be used for rubbing and pleasuring. The couple may wish to use sensate focus activities to redefine the pleasurable areas or activities. Leaving the light on may be helpful with decreased visual fields. Auditory and olfactory stimuli may be increased as compensation.
6. The communication problem is a major barrier to the sexual relationship. The couple may want to discuss using yes/no communication and developing a signal to use for interest in sexual activity and a signal for discomfort, should that occur during sexual activity. Some couples express that with the decreased intimacy resulting from the communication deficit, sexual activity helps maintain the couple's oneness.
7. Working to build self-esteem involves every facet of life, not sexual function in isolation. Mrs. Lacey should allow her husband to be as independent as possible and to contribute as much as possible to family responsibilities and their relationship. Finding an effective method for communication through continued speech therapy would be helpful. The nurse suggests psychological counseling. Medication may be ordered by the physician. This may have the adverse effect of decreasing libido, so caution should be advised. To compensate for lost work status and social isolation, a volunteer position or return to work in a different capacity may be suggested.

Outcome several months later showed that Mr. and Mrs. Lacey increased their understanding of compensation strategies and returned closer to their premorbid rate of sexual activity over a period of time using the compensation strategies. They discovered the pleasurable sensory areas and used increased sensory stimulation. Their intimacy grew through sexual expression, as did Mr. Lacey's self-concept. Frustration with limited communication continues to be a problem, but speech therapy continues.

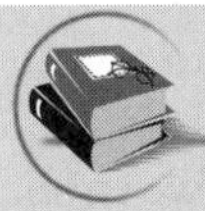

Case Study 2

Pam Delaney is a 27-year-old white woman who experienced a complete SCI at T10 in a motor vehicle accident. She has been married 4 years and has a 2-year-old son. Before the accident she was a speech/language pathologist; her husband Jim teaches history at the local high school. Pam is in an acute rehabilitation hospital. She attends daily group education classes on spinal injury. The team feels she will be independent with transfers, activities of daily living, and home management, including child care on discharge. She will wear a clam shell body brace for 3 months from the date of the accident. The rehabilitation nurse will teach an individualized education program to Pam and her husband on the subject of sexual function. Pam and Jim had a satisfying sexual relationship before the accident, and he has been supportive of her since.

The teaching plan includes the following nursing diagnoses:

1. Sexual dysfunction related to motor and sensory deficit, reduced activity tolerance, and body image disturbance
2. Knowledge deficit concerning the effects of T10 SCI on sexual dysfunction, positioning for sexual function, compensation for sensory loss, special precautions, and birth control issues

Goals

After the education provided by the rehabilitation nurse, the Delaneys will:

1. Be knowledgeable concerning the effects of complete SCI at the T10 level on sexual function
2. Be knowledgeable concerning compensation for sensory loss, positioning, and motion for sexual function, special precautions, and birth control
3. Begin to accept Pam's altered body image and experience beginning return of positive self-concept

The teaching plan included the following information regarding the overview of changes related to sexual function. Pam will have no sensation related to genital sexual function. She will have no ability to move the pelvic area of her lower body or to position her legs without use of her hands. Pam may not experience vaginal lubrication during sexual stimulation. With practice and patience she has a 50% potential of experiencing orgasm. She will experience the same level of fertility as before injury because there was no damage other than the SCI. Brain function is intact and so is sensation above T10. Pam has good hand function and will eventually have good bed mobility skills, as well as the ability to perform all activities of daily living including bowel and bladder programs.

Compensation strategies to be taught:

1. Compensation for sensory loss will include manual stimulation of the woman to the intact areas of function, including the breasts, face, ears, and eyes. Pam can supply manual stimulation to her husband in all areas. Increasing visual stimuli by having lights on may be helpful. Fragrance worn by both partners may be positively stimulating. Using fantasy for both partners may promote sensory appreciation.
2. Positions that will be suggested include face-to-face or front-to-back with the woman on the bottom, or side-lying. Pam should be cautioned to wear her back brace during sexual activity for as long as the physician recommends it for support. Also, both should be cautioned that osteoporosis makes her bones more prone to fractures, her husband's weight should be kept off her legs. They may participate in orogenital intercourse if they desire. Movement may be enhanced for Jim by use of a full-motion waterbed.

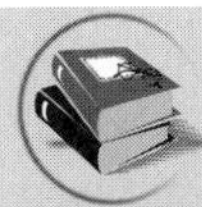

Case Study 2—cont'd

3. Education concerning maintaining relationships should be provided to this couple. Information concerning the value of each to the relationship, honoring each other, and building romance and fun into their time together should be shared. Working together to build self-esteem should be encouraged.
4. To enhance self-esteem, Pam should consider a return to work at a later date. She also should practice child care from her wheelchair and assume that role as soon as feasible. She should be shown dressing and makeup techniques to enhance attractiveness in the wheelchair. Social skills training should be a part of the education. She should go home as soon as possible to help in maintaining relationships. Rehabilitation should continue on an outpatient basis.
5. Pam should be referred to her gynecologist for birth control advice and ordering. She should be instructed that she is fertile. The gynecologist also should be consulted on decisions concerning pregnancy in the future. Referrals should be made to other professionals as required.

Evaluation

Pam and Jim state they understand the information presented. They accept the written information given. An appointment is made with the gynecologist. They are encouraged to call the nurse should they have questions or encounter problems after returning home. More information and counseling may be required at a later date, and appropriate referrals can be made through the outpatient program.

RESOURCES

General

Abstinence education: The SHARE program, provides sexual health and relationship education (1-877-44SHARE)

AIDS Hotline: Program of the Centers for Disease Control, open 24 hours per day (800-342-AIDS)

American Association for Marriage and Family Therapy: 1717 K Street NW, Suite 407, Washington, DC 20006

American Association of Sex Educators, Counselors, and Therapists (AASECT): PO Box 238, Mount Vernon, IA 52314; 319-895-8407; http://www.assect.org (a list of therapists can be obtained by sending a self-addressed, stamped envelope)

American Cancer Society: 1599 Clifton Rd NE, Atlanta, GA 30329; 800-ACS-2345 (227-2345); http://www.cancer.org (click on map for local chapter information)

American Fertility Society: 2140 11th Avenue S, Suite 200, Birmingham, AL 35205-2800

American Mental Health Counselors Association: 800-326-2642

American Paralysis Association: 800-225-0292

CDC National STD Hotline: 800-227-8922

Coalition on Sexuality and Disability: 122 E 23rd St, New York, NY 10010

Eastern Paralyzed Veterans of America and American Association of Spinal Cord Injury Nurses: 75-20 Astoria Blvd., Jackson Heights, NY 11370-1177; 718-803-3782

Edna Gladney Center: 800-452-3639 (a maternity home and infant placement center)

Herpes Resource Center: 800-230-6039

Impotence Information Center: 800-843-4315

Impotence Institute of America: 800-669-1603

Information Center for Individuals with Disabilities: 20 Park Plaza, Room 330, Boston, MA 02116

National Abstinence Clearinghouse: http://www.abstinence.net

National Brain Injury Association: 800-444-6443

National Multiple Sclerosis Society: 800-344-4867

National Spinal Cord Injury Association: 800-962-9629

Paralyzed Veterans of America: http://www.pva.org

Pediatric Projects: 800-947-0947 (projects related to mental health of chronically ill children; disabled, hospitalized children; and their families)

Planned Parenthood Federation of America: 800-829-7732; for local clinics call 800-230-7526

RESOLVE, The National Infertility Association: 1310 Broadway, Somerville, MA 02144; 617-623-0744; http://www.resolve.org/index.htm (sponsors a help line, publications, and support groups for members)

SIECUS—Sex Information and Education Council of the United States: 33 Washington Place, 5th Floor, New York, NY 10003

Spina Bifida Association: 800-621-3141

Spinal Cord Injury Hotline: 800-526-3456

Stroke

American Heart Association Stroke Connection: 800-553-6321

National Institute of Neurological Disorders and Stroke: 800-352-9421

National Stroke Association: 800-787-6537

Women's Health

Association of Women's Health, Obstetric and Neonatal Nurses: 800-673-8499

Older Women's League: 800-825-3615

Websites

Warning: Much on the Internet might be considered pornography and comes at a variety of websites, at times from unexpected sources. The sites listed here have been established by organizations whose goal is to enhance health education, and they contain information related to the issue of sexuality in the client populations they serve. Information must be correct, current, and reliable before being used in education or practice.

http://www.healthatoz.com: 50,000 topics related to health information

http://www.wwwomen.com: health topics specific to women

http://search.info.nih.gov: information from the National Institutes of Health

http://www.healthfinder.gov: information on health from other governmental agencies

http://www.forumone.com: search engine for online discussion groups

http://www.medcareonline.com: information on men's health, women's health, sexuality, pregnancy, reproduction

Search engines (Kuric, 1999)

REFERENCES

Albaugh, J. (1999). Erectile dysfunction: Newer treatment options don't decrease the need for education, counseling. *ADVANCE for Nurse Practitioners, 7*(4), 43-44.

Annon, J.S. (1976). The PLISSIT model: A proposed conceptual scheme for behavioral treatment of sexual problems. *Journal of Sex Education Therapy, 2,* 1-15.

Boone, T.B. (1995). The physiology of sexual function in normal individuals. *Physical Medicine and Rehabilitation State of the Art Reviews Sexuality and Disability, 9*(2), 313-324.

Burnette, A.L. (1998). New options for erectile dysfunction. *Supplement to Clinical Reviews, June,* 3-7.

Burnette, A.L. (1999). Oral pharmacology for erectile dysfunction: Current perspectives. *Urology, 54,* 392-399.

Craig, D.I. (1990). The adaptation to pregnancy of spinal cord injured women. *Rehabilitation Nursing, 15,* 6-9.

Crewe, N.M. (1992). Marital status adjustment to spinal cord injury. *Journal of the American Paraplegia Society, 15,* 14-18.

Davis, D.L., & Schneider, L.K. (1990). Ramifications of traumatic brain injury for sexuality. *Journal of Head Trauma Rehabilitation, 5,* 31-37.

Divorce trends in spinal cord injury: Worth taking the chance. (1990). *Spinal Network Extra, 41.*

Dobson, J. (2000). Solid Answers. *Focus on the Family, February,* 5.

Doerfler, E. (1999). Pearls for practice male erectile dysfunction: A guide for clinical management. *Journal of the American Academy of Nurse Practitioners, 11*(3), 117-123.

Elmer-Dewitt, P. (1994, October 17) Now for the truth about Americans and sex. *Time,* 62-70.

Goodwin, A.J., & Agronin, M.E. (1997). *A woman's guide to overcoming sexual fear and pain.* Canada: New Harbinger Publications.

Gordon, M. (2000). *Manual of nursing diagnosis* (9th ed.). St. Louis: Mosby.

Grana, E.A. (1995). Sexuality issues in multiple sclerosis. *Physical Medicine and Rehabilitation State of the Art Reviews Sexuality and Disability, 9*(2), 377-386.

Griffith, E.R., & Trieschmann, R.B. (1983). Sexual dysfunctions in the physically ill and disabled. In C.C. Nadelson & D.B. Marcotte (Eds.), *Treatment interventions in human sexuality* (pp. 241-277). New York: Plenum Press.

Haffner, D.W. (1990). *Sex education 2000: A call to action.* New York: Sex Information and Education Council of the United States.

Hahn, M.S. (1995). The ticking time bomb: Defusing risky sexual behavior in teens. *ADVANCE for Nurse Practitioners, December,* 42.

Herman-Giddens, M.E., Slora, E.J., Wasserman, R.C., Bourdony, C.J., Bhapkar, M.V., Koch, G.G., & Hasemeier, C.M. (1997). Secondary sexual characteristics and menses in young girls seen in office practice: A study from the Pediatric Research in Office Settings network. *Pediatrics, 99*(4), 505-12.

Hirsch, I.H., Seager, S.W., Seldor, J., King, L., Staas, W.E., Jr. (1990). Electroejaculatory stimulation of a quadriplegic man resulting in pregnancy. *Archives of Physical Medicine and Rehabilitation, 71,* 54-57.

Horn, L.J., & Zasler, N.D. (1990). Neuroanatomy and neurophysiology of sexual function. *Journal of Head Trauma Rehabilitation, 5,* 1-13.

Johnson, M., Maas, M., & Moorhead, S. (Eds.). (2000). *Nursing outcomes classification* (2nd ed.). St. Louis: Mosby.

Johnson, W.R., & Kempton, W. (1981). *Sex education and counseling for special groups* (2nd ed.). Springfield, IL: Charles C. Thomas.

Korpelainen, J.T., Nieminen, P., & Myllyla, V.V. (1999). Sexual functioning among stroke patients and their spouses. *Stroke, 30,* 715-719.

Kroll, K., & Klein, E.L. (1991). *Enabling romance: A guide to love, sex, and relationships for the disabled (and the people who care about them).* New York: Crown.

Kuric, J. (1999). How do I find what I want on the Internet? *SCI Nursing, 16*(4), 137.

Leslie, S.W. (1990). *Impotence: Current diagnosis and treatment.* Lorain, OH: Geddings Osbon, Sr. Foundation.

Malek, C.J., & Brower, S.A. (1984). Rheumatoid arthritis: How does it influence sexuality? *Rehabilitation Nursing, 9,* 26-28.

Maslow, A. (1954). *Motivation and personality.* New York: Harper and Row.

Masters, W.H., Johnson, V.E., & Kolodny, R.C. (1986). *Masters and Johnson on sex and human loving.* Boston: Little, Brown.

McCloskey, J.C., & Bulechek, G.M. (Eds.). (2000). *Nursing interventions classification* (3rd ed.). St. Louis: Mosby.

Monga, M., Bernie, J., & Rajasekaran, M. (1999). Male infertility and erectile dysfunction in spinal cord injury: A review. *Archives Physical Medicine and Rehabilitation, 80,* 1331-1338.

Monga, T.N., & Lefebvre, K.A. (1995). Sexuality: An overview. *Physical Medicine and Rehabilitation: State of the Art Reviews Sexuality and Disability, 9*(2), 299-312.

Morley, J.D. (1993). Management of impotence. *Post Graduate Medicine, 93*(3), 65-72.

Mulligan, T., & Moss, C.R. (1991). Sexuality and aging in male veterans: A cross-sectional study of interest, ability, and activity. *Archives of Sexual Behavior, 20,* 17-25.

National Guidelines Task Force. (1991). *Guidelines for comprehensive sexuality education: Kindergarten-12th grade.* New York: Sex Information and Education Council of the United States.

National Information Center for Children and Youth with Disabilities (NICCYD). (1992). *Sexuality education for children and youths with disabilities. Fostering relationships: Suggestions for young adults. News digest.* Washington, D.C. Author.

Nygaard, I., Bartscht, K.D., & Cole, S. (1990). Sexuality and reproduction in spinal cord injured women. *Obstetrical and Gynecological Survey, 45,* 727-732.

Reinisch, J.M. (1990). *The Kinsey Institute new report on sex: What you must know to be sexually literate.* New York: St. Martin's.

Rutkowski, S.B., Geraghty, T.J., Hagen, D.I., Bowers, D.M., Craven, M., & Middleton, J.W. (1999). A comprehensive approach to the management of male infertility following spinal cord injury. *Spinal Cord, 37*(July), 508-514.

Seidl, A., Bullough, B., Haughey, B., Scherer, Y., Rhodes, M., & Brown, G. (1991). Understanding the effects of a myocardial infarction on sexual functioning: A basis for sexual counseling. *Rehabilitation Nursing, 16,* 255-264.

Selekman, J., & McIlvain-Simpson, G. (1991). Sex and sexuality for the adolescent with a chronic condition. *Pediatric Nursing, 17,* 535-538.

Sipski, M. (1991). The impact of spinal cord injury on female sexuality, menstruation and pregnancy: A review of the literature. *Journal of the American Paraplegia Society, 14*(3) 122-126.

Smalley, G., & Trent, J. (1988). *The language of love.* Pomona, CA: Focus on the Family Publishing.

Smalley, G., & Trent, J. (1989). *Love is a decision.* Phoenix: Today's Family.

Smith, J. (1990). Joy rises, misery falls, communication works. *Spinal Network Extra,* 40.

Spica, M.M. (1989). Sexual counseling standards for the spinal- cord injured. *Journal of Neuroscience Nursing, 21,* 56-60.

Sullivan, G., & Lukoff, D. (1990). Sexual side effects of antipsychotic medication: Evaluation and interventions. *Hospital and Community Psychiatry, 41,* 1238-1241.

Tanner, J.M. (1962). *Growth at adolescence* (2nd ed.). Oxford: Blackwell Scientific.

Tardif, G.S. (1989). Sexual activity after a myocardial infarction. *Archives of Physical Medicine and Rehabilitation, 70,* 763-766.

Tepper, M.S. (1999). *Attitudes, beliefs, and cognitive processes that impede or facilitate sexual pleasure in people with spinal cord injury.* Unpublished dissertation. Philadelphia: University of Pennsylvania.

U.S. Department of Health and Human Services. (2000). *Healthy people 2010.* Washington, DC: Author.

Weiss, R.J. (1991). Effects of antihypertensive agents on sexual function. *American Family Physician, 44,* 2075-2082.

Woods, N.F. (1984). *Human sexuality in health and illness* (3rd ed.). St. Louis: Mosby.

Woods, N.F. (1988). Human sexuality: An overview. In P.H. Mitchell, L.C. Hodges, M. Muwases, & C.A. Wallick (Eds.), *Neuroscience nursing* (pp. 459-469). Norwalk, CT: Appleton & Lange.

World Health Organization. (1975). *Education and treatment in human sexuality: The training of health professionals* (WHO Technical Report Series No. 572). Geneva: Author.

Yarkony, G.M., & Chen, D. (1995) Sexuality in patients with spinal cord injury. *Physical Medicine and Rehabilitation: State of the Art Reviews Sexuality and Disability, 9*(2), 325-344.

Yim, S.Y., Lee, I.Y., Yoon, S.H., Song, M.S., Rah, E.W., & Moon, H.W. (1998). Quality of marital life in Korean spinal cord injured patients, *Spinal Cord,* 826-831.

Zasler, N.D., & Horn, L.J. (1990). Rehabilitative management of sexual dysfunction. *Journal of Head Trauma Rehabilitation, 5,* 14- 24.

SUGGESTED READING

Banja, J.D., & Banes, L. (1993). Moral sensitivity, sodomy laws, and TBI rehabilitation. *Journal of Head Trauma Rehabilitation, 8,* 116-119.

Burling, K., Tarvydas, V.M., & Make, D.R. (1994). Human sexuality and disability: A holistic interpretation for rehabilitation counseling. *Journal of Applied Rehabilitation Counseling, 25,* 10-17.

Cole, T., & Cole, S. (1976). *A guide for trainers: Sexuality and physical disability.* Minneapolis: University of Minnesota Medical School, Multi-Resource Center.

Kerfoot, K.M., & Buckwalter, K.C. (1985). Sexual counseling. In G.M. Bulechek & J.C. McCloskey (Eds.), *Nursing interventions: Treatments for nursing diagnosis* (pp. 127-138). Philadelphia: WB Saunders.

Nay, R. (1992). Sexuality and aged women in nursing homes. *Geriatric Nursing, 13,* 312-314.

Rutkowski, S.B., Middleton, J.W., Truman, G., Hagen, D.L., & Ryan, J.P. (1995). The influence of bladder management on fertility in spinal cord injured males. *Paraplegia, 33,* 263-266.

Sipski, M.L., Alexander, C.J., & Rosen, R.C. (1995). Orgasm in women with spinal cord injuries: A laboratory-based assessment. *Archives of Physical Medicine and Rehabilitation, 76,* 1097-1102.

Smedley, G. (1991). Addressing sexuality in the elderly. *Rehabilitation Nursing, 16,* 9-11.

Smith, M. (1993). Pediatric sexuality; promoting normal sexual development in children. *Nurse Practitioner, 18,* 37-38, 41-44.

Tepper, M.S. (1997). Living with a disability: A man's perspective. In M.L. Sipski & C. J. Alexander (Eds.). *Sexual function in people with disability and chronic illness: A health professional's guide* (pp. 131-146). Gaithersburg: Aspen.

Tepper, M.S. (1997). Providing comprehensive sexual health care in spinal cord injury rehabilitation: Implementation and evaluation of a new curriculum for health professionals. *Sexuality and Disability, 15,* 3.

Whipple, B., Richards, E., Tepper, M., & Komisaruk, B.R. (1996). Sexual response in women with complete spinal cord injury. In D.M. Krotoskie, M.A. Nosek, & M.A. Turk (Eds.). *Women with physical disabilities* (pp. 69-80). Baltimore: Paul H Brookes.

White, M.J., Rintali, D.H., Hart, K.A., Young, M.E., & Fuhrer, M.J. (1994). Sexual activities, concerns and interests of women with spinal cord injury living in the community. *American Journal of Physical Medicine and Rehabilitation, 75,* 276-278.

Zejdlik, C.M. (1992). *Management of spinal cord injury* (2nd ed.). Monterey, CA: Wadsworth Health Sciences Division.

24 Rehabilitation Involving the Senses, Sensation, Perception, and Pain

Pamela M. Duchene, DNSc, RN, CRRN

Imagine a warm summer day. You find yourself drifting in a canoe on a clear pond in New Hampshire. The sky is bright blue, and there are three small white clouds drifting lazily across it. As you take a deep breath, the scent of pine trees is present in the clear air, and somewhere nearby there is a blooming wild rose bush. The water laps against the canoe, making gentle slapping sounds. The warmth of the sun feels like melted butter all over your skin. The taste of the barbecue you had for lunch is still in your mouth. Just as you start to be lulled to sleep by the quiet and peacefulness of the setting, a large black fly lands on your nose for a bite.

The setting above uses all senses. Vision senses record the picture of the sky and clouds. Auditory senses identify the sounds of the water against the canoe. Gustatory senses relay information to the brain about the tastes of the recent meal. Olfactory senses note the smells of pine and roses. The large black fly stimulates sensors for touch, pressure, and pain. The senses provide information about the environment and surroundings and make it possible for persons to communicate, interact, and respond to stimuli. Individual's perceptions of the environment enable them to interpret, predict, and respond to sensory input.

Live each season as it passes; breathe the air, drink the drink, taste the fruit, and resign yourself to the influences of each.
—Henry David Thoreau

In this chapter each of the senses, including the sensation of pain, will be reviewed. Common impairments, nursing interventions and outcomes, as well as rehabilitation strategies and advocacy programs are identified. A case study on multiple sclerosis incorporates sensory dysfunction and low vision.

THE SENSES

The primary method through which we understand, interpret, and respond to the world around us is through the senses: vision, hearing, taste, smell, and touch. Loss of one or more of the senses requires a means of compensation, or there is a risk that the environment could be misinterpreted. For example, older persons who experience loss of olfactory acuity cannot smell the characteristic sulfur odor that emanates from a gas stove leak. For safety they can compensate by using an electric stove. Similarly the visual system requires function of the eyes and their associated systems in conjunction with the cerebrum in order to make sense of the world.

Vision

Healthy People 2010 (U.S. Department of Health and Human Services [USDHHS], 2000) targets a reduction of blindness and visual impairment in those younger than 17 years from 25 in 1000 to less than 20 in 1000. According to the Centers for Disease Control and Prevention, self-reported blindness in either or both eyes resulting in trouble seeing is considered significant vision impairment.

Anatomy and Physiology

The eye has three layers, the fibrous tunic, the vascular tunic, and the nervous tunic. The fibrous tunic, including the cornea (Figure 24-1) and the sclera, functions as a protective barrier to the more fragile components of the eye. This layer causes tearing and blinking in response to foreign bodies and prevents microorganisms and chemicals from penetrating the eye (Stoney & Jackson, 1999).

The middle layer of the eye is the vascular tunic, which includes the iris, the ciliary body, and the choroid. Through constriction and expansion of the iris, the pupil dilates (iris sphincter contraction) and constricts (iris dilator extension).

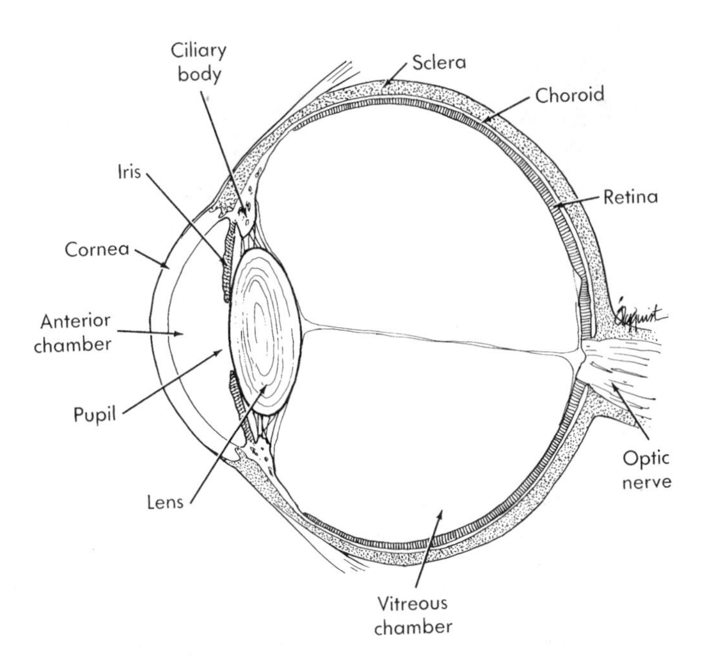

Figure 24-1 Cross-section of the human eye.

The ciliary body contains the ciliary muscle, which changes the shape of the lens and allows accommodation. The choroid provides vascular nourishment and removal of wastes from the outer half of the retina.

The inner layer of the eye is the nervous tunic, which contains the retina, rods, and cones, which communicate light stimulation to the optic nerve fibers. The cones recognize colors and are responsible for fine discrimination and daylight vision. The rods respond to dim light and are responsible for peripheral vision.

The supporting and accessory structures of the eye include the eyelids, conjunctiva, lens, anterior and posterior eye cavities, and the lacrimal apparatus. The eyelids protect the eye from foreign objects. The conjunctiva is a mucous membrane that lines each lid and covers the eyeball surface. The lens is primarily composed of water. Changes in the lens shape occur with changes in the ciliary body. The lens bulges for near vision and flattens for far vision. The anterior cavity of the eye contains aqueous humor, which maintains intraocular pressure and nourishes the iris and posterior aspect of the cornea. The posterior cavity is filled with vitreous humor, which creates stable pressure. The lacrimal apparatus includes the lacrimal glands, lacrimal canals, lacrimal sacs, and nasolacrimal ducts and is responsible for tears.

The iris controls the amount of light entering the eye through the pupil. Light rays travel to the retina, which records images. The chemical and physical changes that take place in the retina create electrical impulses that are conducted along the optic nerve fibers to the occipital lobe of the cortex, where visions are interpreted (Figure 24-2).

Assessment of Vision

The initial assessment of vision includes a history, examination of all eye components, and questions about any specific problems, including symptoms, pain, redness, discharge, and visual acuity changes (Merck, 2000).

Visual Acuity. Visual acuity is assessed through use of a Snellen or other type of eye chart. The client stands 20 feet (6 m) away from the chart. If the client usually wears eyeglasses, the test should be administered with glasses in place. Each eye is assessed separately. A Snellen reading of 20/30 (metric 6/9) means that what someone with normal vision can read at 30 feet (9 m), the client can read at 20 feet (6 m). The glasses should be assessed for cleanliness, scratches, comfort, and the type of problem they are correcting.

Pupil Reaction. To assess equal reaction to light, the nurse uses a penlight. The light is moved from the temporal to nasal side of the client's eye while the client focuses ahead. The nurse assesses whether the pupils constrict at an equal speed. Pupillary reaction to accommodation is tested while the client looks into the distance and then at the nurse's finger, which is held 5 to 10 cm from the bridge of the client's nose. The pupils should converge and constrict symmetrically, with a slightly slower response in older than in younger persons.

Inspection. The eyelids are assessed for lesions, inflammation, foreign bodies, or other problems. The conjunctiva and sclera are assessed for color and characteristics of the blood vessels. Yellowish conjunctiva may be due to jaundice or fat deposits associated with aging. In children the conjunctiva may appear bluish because it is thinner and allows the pigmentation of underlying structures to be apparent. Reddened conjunctiva and sclera are indicative of conjunctivitis, which requires further investigation. The pupil is examined for size, shape, and equality.

Palpation. The area around the lacrimal sacs should be palpated to identify any possible obstructions. Eversion of the eyelids is completed to identify problems with foreign bodies, inflammation, or other issues.

Nursing Diagnosis: Sensory Loss (Vision)

Loss of vision, compensated or uncompensated, may occur due to a variety of factors. Nursing assessment information appropriate to the nursing diagnosis of sensory loss (vision) is included in this section. Nursing diagnoses, nursing outcomes classifications, and nursing interventions classifications are included in Table 24-1.

Refractive Error. Refractive error is a defect of the refracting media of the eye. The most common visual impairment, it occurs when light rays fail to converge into a single focus on the retina, resulting in blurred vision and discomfort. Regardless of the cause of the refractive error, most cases may be corrected by corrective lenses.

Hemianopsia. Hemianopsia is defective vision or blindness of half of the visual field due to brain injury from cerebrovascular disorders, trauma, or tumors. It is not a disorder of the eyes but of the cerebrum. Hemianopsia is classified as homonymous, bitemporal, or attitudinal. *Homonymous hemianopsia* refers to the loss of vision in the temporal field of one eye and the nasal field of the other (Figure 24-3). Left homonymous hemianopsia sometimes occurs after a

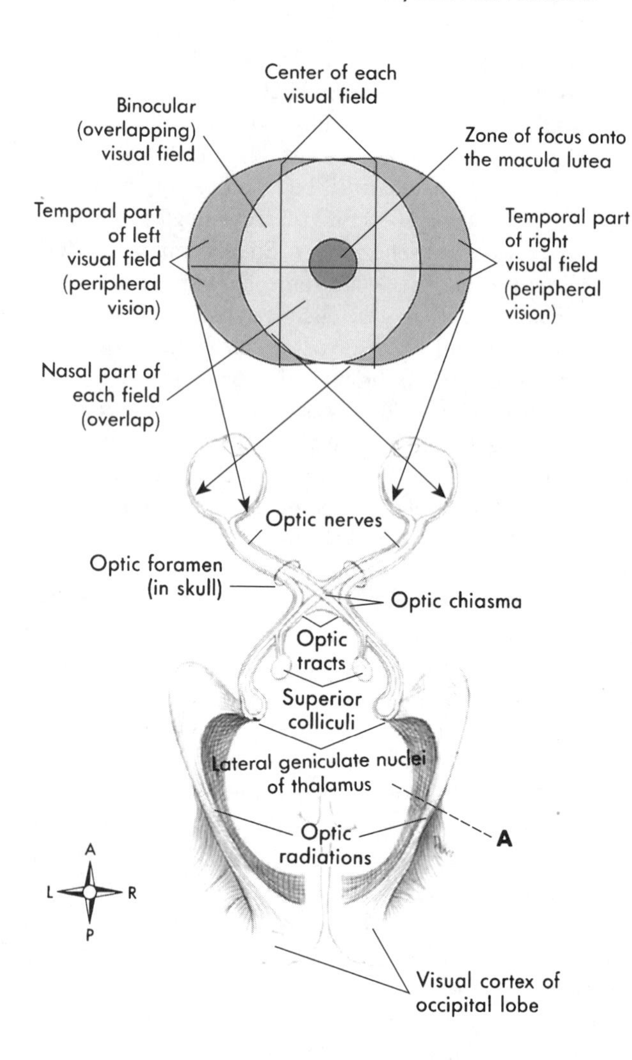

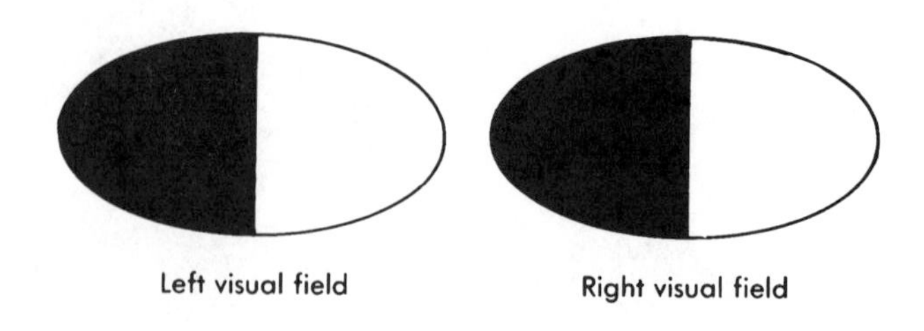

Figure 24-2 Visual fields and neuronal pathways of the eye. Note the structures that make up each pathway: optic nerve, optic chiasma, lateral geniculate body of the thalamus, optic radiations, and visual cortex of the occipital lobe. Fibers from the nasal portion of each retina cross over to the opposite side at the optic chiasma and terminate in the lateral geniculate nuclei. Location of a lesion in the visual pathway determines the resulting visual defect. Damage at point *A,* for example, would cause blindness in the right nasal and left temporal visual fields, as the ovals indicate. (From Thibodeau, G.A., & Patton, K.T. (1999). *Anatomy & physiology* [4th ed.]. St. Louis: Mosby.)

right-sided brain lesion. It is not unusual for persons with left homonymous hemianopsia not to recognize the deficit until it is diagnosed during rehabilitation. This syndrome will be discussed further in the section of this chapter on perception.

Intraocular Disease. Intraocular disease may present with cataracts, glaucoma, or retinal detachment. Cataracts are an opacity or clouding of the lens that blocks the passage of light needed for vision. Cataracts develop slowly with age and may cause blurred vision, obliteration of parts of images, double images, decreased perception of color, or distorted images. The only treatment for cataracts is removal. Intraocular lens implantation is an effective method of visual rehabilitation for persons with cataracts (Apple, 1999). First developed by Dr. Harold Ridley more than 50 years ago, the intraocular lens is implanted in more than 6 million persons annually throughout the world.

Glaucoma. Glaucoma is the third leading cause of blindness. It occurs when a buildup of intraocular pressure (due to a blockage of aqueous humor) gradually destroys the optic nerve. the person may not have symptoms or awareness of the problem. Open-angle glaucoma is due to a reduction in the outflow of aqueous humor and is treated with eyedrops such as pilocarpine and timolol maleate. If eyedrops are ineffective, surgery may be an option. Closed-angle glaucoma presents with acute eye pain and nausea. The iris is displaced in the periphery of the anterior chamber, and the aqueous filtration network is blocked, causing the intraocular pressure to rise quickly, resulting in a surgical emergency.

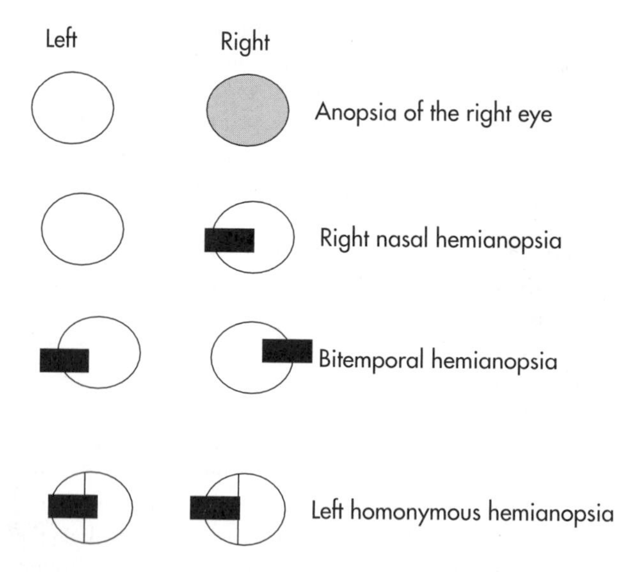

Figure 24-3 Visual alterations with various hemianopsia.

TABLE 24-1 Nursing Diagnoses, Nursing Outcomes Classifications, and Nursing Interventions Classifications for Sensory Loss (Vision)

Nursing Diagnosis	Suggested Nursing Outcomes Classification (NOC)	Suggested Nursing Interventions Classification (NIC)
Sensory loss (vision)	Anxiety control Body image Cognitive ability Cognitive orientation Distorted thought process Energy conservation Vision compensation behavior Neurological status Risk control: visual impairment	Cognitive restructuring Cognitive stimulation Communication enhancement visual deficit Emotional support Environmental management Fall prevention Surveillance: safety Eye care Medication management Self-esteem enhancement
Risk for injury	Knowledge: personal safety Risk control: visual impairment Risk detection Safety behavior: home physical environment Safety behavior: personal Safety status: falls occurrence Safety status: physical injury	Environmental management: safety Home maintenance assistance Risk identification
Communication, impaired verbal	Communication ability Communication: receptive ability Information processing	Communication enhancement: visual deficit Presence Surveillance: safety Touch Decision-making support Learning facilitation Referral Support system enhancement

Data from Johnson, M., Maas, M.L., & Moorhead, S. (2000). *Nursing outcomes classification (NOC)* (2nd ed.). St. Louis: Mosby; McCloskey, J.C., & Bulechek, G.M. (2000). *Nursing interventions classification (NIC)* (3rd ed.). St. Louis: Mosby; and North American Nursing Diagnosis Association. (2001). *Nursing diagnosis: definitions and classification 2001-2002* (4th ed.). Philadelphia: Author.

Retinal Detachment. Retinal detachment is a serious situation occurring when the retina separates from the choroid. The person may report a "shade lowering" over the visual field or may experience blurry vision and light flashes. The rods and cones atrophy and become damaged. Surgical intervention, such as a vitrectomy, is usually required.

Low Vision. Visual deficits that cannot be corrected may result in low vision, a condition that affects 13.5 million Americans (Low Vision Council, 2000). When surgery, medical treatments, or correctional eyeglasses will not fully correct the problem, the rehabilitation strategies listed in Table 24-2 are useful.

Carle Clinic (Urbana, IL) has developed a model program to provide housing for persons with low vision. A home near the central Illinois medical center contains features that facilitate assessing needs and function for persons with low vision so that they can make reasonable changes within their home environments. One modification for low vision is the use of low illumination. In a study of 41 persons with age-related macular degeneration, Kuyk and Elliott (1999) found that clients had fewer mobility incidents and required less time for mobility in an environment with low illumination than in one with high illumination.

Blindness. The distinction between low vision and blindness is not clear. The term *legally blind* is used to indicate a corrected visual acuity in the corrected stronger eye of 20/200 (metric 6/60) or less. *Functional blindness* indicates total blindness or a minimum of light perception or projection.

Rehabilitation efforts revolve around increasing the functional ability of persons with blindness and decreasing the environmental barriers that may be experienced. Communication through writing for persons with blindness has been revolutionized during the past decade with the advent of screen-reading computer programs, such as JAWS and Windoweyes (Quattrociocchi, 2000). JAWS (Henter-Joyce Inc.) enables persons with visual impairments to navigate the Windows environment of the computer system, for word processing or any computer text-based program, as well as e-mail and the Internet. Anything presented on the screen is read aloud by the screen-reading programs. Both programs use shortcut keys to eliminate the need to use a mouse with the computer. There are also programs, such as the Duxbury Translator, that translate written materials to Braille to be printed on a Braille embosser (a Braille version of a printer). Other major developments toward accessibility of written materials are the text-to-speech conversion programs, such

TABLE 24-2 Low Vision Rehabilitation Strategies

Device/Strategy	Use and Comments
Magnifying glass	Hand-held magnifying glass with a strong convex lens may be useful for short focal distances, for close vision, and for reading and writing Must be held, thus limiting its practicality in situations requiring both hands (such as crafts, needlepoint, woodworking, and item assembly)
Telescope	Binoculars and field glasses may be used for magnification of items at a distance Require use of the hands, thereby limiting their use in situations requiring both hands
Light filters	Light filters are used over glasses to limit glare Require application and removal with changes in lighting or when entering or leaving sunlight
Tinted lenses	Used to reduce glare Not removable from the glasses and may limit vision in some lighting situations
Prisms	Glass devices used to change images to a different part of the retina and to promote vision through such redirection Require use of the hands
Microscopes	Similar in use to a telescope but for nearby items Require use of the hands and do not assist with peripheral vision
Reading rectangle	Used to limit the number of words on which the reader is focusing at a single time Must be moved as the reader completes reading a section; assists with focus but requires use of the hands; best suited for reading texts and documents
Large type	Many books, magazines, and documents are available in large type Increases the visibility of the text without requiring the use of magnifying glasses or microscopes; increases the size and weight of magazines and books because more pages are required for the printed information

as the Open Book Ruby Edition and Kurzweil software programs, which scan written documents and present the information through speech output. These programs allow an individual to edit and modify scanned documents.

Methods of reducing barriers to mobility for persons with functional blindness include the standard white cane or guide dog. Canes made of lightweight fiberglass or aluminum and are about 0.5 inch in diameter. Individuals use the cane by moving it in front of them from side to side in an arc to extend the sense of touch by letting them know whether obstacles lie in their path. Guide dogs work with individuals as part of a team, with the dog serving as the individual's eyes. Strategies for reducing barriers for persons with visual impairment are listed in Box 24-1.

Application of Concepts

A critical aspect of rehabilitation nursing is the ability to visualize potentials for persons recovering from or coping with devastating disabilities and chronic illnesses. This characteristic of rehabilitation is true with visual deficits as with other physical disabilities. For example, Ruth experienced a right cerebrovascular accident 1 week before being admitted to an acute rehabilitation unit. She became depressed, chose to remain in her room, and ignored staff members when they entered the room to speak with her. Noting that Ruth did not eat food placed on the left side of her dinner tray, the nurse assessed Ruth's vision and confirmed left homonymous hemianopsia. Because of her disability and the position of her bed, Ruth had been unable to see anyone entering the room. Ruth's bed was turned so she could see the doorway. The nurse and team members taught Ruth visual scanning; not only did her dinner become visible to her, but Ruth began to acknowledge those entering her room, and her depression symptoms decreased.

Hearing

Hearing is a complex phenomenon that requires the integration between the external and internal ear and the cerebrum. Hearing alone does not ensure the person will process and remember what is heard.

Healthy People 2010 (USDHHS, 2000) identifies an objective for newborns to be screened for hearing loss by 1 month, referred for audiological evaluation by 3 months, and involved in appropriate intervention by 6 months of age. *Healthy People 2010* also lists the objective of a hearing examination every decade after the age of 18 years.

Anatomy and Physiology

Figure 24-4 illustrates the major anatomical structures of the ear.

External Ear. The external ear forms the passageway for sounds and contains mechanisms to protect the hearing organ from penetration by microorganisms and foreign objects.

The auditory canal extends approximately 2.5 cm to the tympanic membrane. Sebaceous and other glands in the outer half of the canal secrete cerumen, which has a protective function. Hair follicles are also found in the outer half of the canal. The tympanic membrane receives sound waves from the external ear and canal. Normally the tympanic membrane appears cone shaped, shiny, translucent, and pearl gray.

Box 24-1 Guidelines to Assist an Individual with Visual Impairment

1. Present verbal instructions clearly and succinctly and use touch and other senses to compensate for lack of vision
2. When teaching, break down tasks into smaller component steps and teach one at a time
3. Orient the person to the surroundings and remind staff members and visitors to introduce themselves
4. Maintain personal items such as combs, brushes, and room furniture in the same place and arrangement; do not move equipment or furniture in the room without discussing the new arrangement with the client
5. When speaking with the client, speak directly to him or her using a natural tone of voice; do not assume the person has poor hearing in addition to a visual impairment
6. Encourage involvement of the client in problem solving
7. Assist the person in organizing the life space (e.g., hanging clothing by color, type, or style)
8. Attach or sew tactile symbols to clothing and personal items to help identify color and contents
9. Assist the person in localizing and discriminating sounds
10. Assist the person in learning to detect temperatures and to manipulate objects safely; for example, when pouring a hot beverage, teach the person to wrap the fingers around the upper third of the cup to identify when the beverage is at that level
11. Instruct the person to visualize the meal plate as a clock to assist in communication of the location of the food or other items
12. When assisting a visually impaired person in walking, walk about a half step ahead and have the person grasp your arm lightly but firmly just above the elbow so that the thumb is on the outside and the fingers are on the inside of the arm; both of you should hold your upper arms close to the body so that your movements can alert the individual to curbs, turns, and stops

The middle ear cavity is filled with air and transfers airborne sound pressure fluctuations in the external canal to pressure variations in the fluid-filled inner ear. The sound that vibrates the tympanic membrane is transmitted to the cochlea by the malleus, incus (anvil), and stapes bones. The middle ear also contains the eustachian tube, which opens into the nasopharynx and provides equalization of air pressure between the middle ear and the pharynx. The eustachian tube is usually closed but may open during yawning, swallowing, or chewing. Cranial nerve VII, responsible for control of facial movement, is located within the middle ear.

Inner Ear. As sound vibrations pass through the middle ear, they cause waves of pressure that correspond to incoming sound waves, which transfer the vibrations to the cochlea, which is part of the inner ear. A second function of the inner ear is in maintenance of balance and equilibrium.

The inner ear is a maze formed by a bony labyrinth (vestibule, cochlea, and semicircular canals) and a membranous labyrinth (utricle and saccule). The vestibule, or organ of balance, is the central portion of the bony labyrinth and is

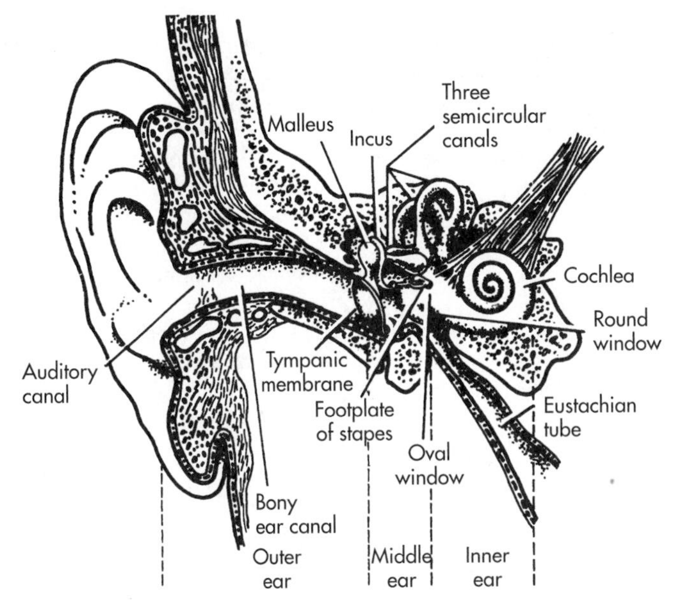

Figure 24-4 The anatomy of the ear has three main areas: the external auditory area, the middle ear, and the inner ear. Obstructions, including earwax, in the auditory canal or fluid in the eustachian tube may reduce hearing. The middle ear contains three small bones (the incus, malleus, and stapes) that vibrate to assist in the transmission of sound during normal hearing. The bones may become stabilized by calcified deposits and produce conductive hearing losses. Inner ear deficits often involve sensorineural losses. These may affect a client's balance and produce ringing in the ears as well as hearing loss. (From Hoeman, S.P. [1990]. *Rehabilitation/restorative care in the community.* St. Louis: Mosby.)

bathed in endolymph fluid. The cochlea contains the organ of Corti, the sense organ of hearing, which is composed of 24,000 hair cells bathed in perilymph. The hair cells become distorted and mechanically bent when sound waves enter the cochlea. As hair cells are displaced along the length of the cochlea, they are transformed into neural activity. Neural impulses travel along to the eighth cranial nerve to the brain to produce the sensation and recognition of sound. The three semicircular canals enlarge into ampullae, which contain receptors from cranial nerve VIII (the acoustic nerve).

Perception of Sound. Sound is carried in waves caught in the outer ear and travels as vibrations to the inner ear canal, causing the tympanic membrane to vibrate and initiate movement of the bones in the middle ear. Vibration of the last and smallest bone, the stapes, passes through the oval window to the inner ear. Perilymph fluid vibrates in harmony with incoming sound waves. These waves communicate vibration to the cochlea, where the hair cells bend and activate nerve impulses, which stimulate the auditory nerve. The auditory nerve conveys the impulse to the auditory cortex in the brain, where the vibration is recognized and sound is perceived.

Assessment of Hearing

Hearing assessment is a part of any rehabilitation nursing admission or initial assessment. Given the essential need for

TABLE 24-3 Methods for Testing Hearing Acuity

Hearing Test Method	Description	Purpose, Comments
Self-assessment	Many questionnaires are available for individuals to identify whether a hearing problem exists; one such method is available through the Miracle Ear website: www.miracle-ear.com/hearing_n_hearing_loss/hearing_assessment_questionnaire.htm	Allows individuals to self-test for possible symptoms of hearing loss; tests are free to administer and can be done at home
Air conduction testing	Acoustic stimulus is presented through earphones to the individual	Detects defects in hearing due to problems in the ear canal, middle ear, inner ear, central auditory pathways, or acoustic nerve (CN VIII)
Tuning fork	Tests for bone conduction of sound through the vibration of the tuning fork tongs	Provides direct stimulation to the inner ear, bypassing the external and middle parts of the ear
Weber's test	After the tuning fork is struck, the vibrating end is placed on the head midline; patient identifies the ear in which the sound is the loudest	Differentiates sensorineural loss from conductive loss: unilateral conductive loss presents as a stronger signal in the affected ear, and unilateral sensorineural loss presents as a stronger signal in the unaffected ear
Rinne's test	Vibrating tuning fork is used by placing it on the mastoid process and then near the pinna; patient is asked to identify the strongest sound	Normally sound is heard by air conduction more loudly than by bone conduction; sensorineural loss presents as a decrease in both air and bone conduction, with air slightly louder; conduction loss presents with air heard less than bone conduction
Audiometry	Audiometer is used to present acoustic stimuli for specific tone frequencies	Allows identification of the hearing threshold for specific frequencies
Speech audiometry	Specific two-syllable words are spoken in conversational English; percentage of words noted correctly are recorded	Assesses speech reception threshold and is an index of the individual's ability to hear under optimal conditions; a score of 90% to 100% is normal
Tympanometry	Sound source probe with a microphone is placed in the ear canal to measure the amount of acoustic energy absorbed by the middle ear	Measures possible hearing impairment resulting from otitis media
Acoustic reflex testing	Tones of various intensities are presented to each ear, and the patient is monitored for a reflex contraction of the stapedius muscle (acoustic reflex)	In neural hearing loss, this reflex decays or adapts
Auditory brainstem response (ABR)	Acoustic stimulation is presented, and electric waveforms are monitored as generated from the brainstem, CN VIII, and other regions	Lesions will present as lost waveforms; testing allows differentiation between sensory and neural hearing loss
Otoacoustic emissions (OAEs)	Sound source is presented in the ear canal, and a microphone records the response	Tests the sounds generated by the outer hair cells within the cochlea; commonly used for hearing testing in infants

Data from Merck. (2000). *The Merck manual of diagnosis and therapy.* Whitehouse Station, NJ: Author.
CN, Central nerve.

communication during rehabilitation, information on the ability of the individual to hear is critical for therapeutic teaching and carryover. The environment in which the hearing assessment is completed should be free from distractions and extraneous noise to the extent possible.

External Inspection. External inspection of the ears includes inspecting the ears for any deviations, moving the ears, and noting any pain or tenderness in the ears or mastoid processes experienced by the client. Use an otoscope to visualize the ear canal, and note redness, drainage, accumulated cerumen, or any abnormalities of the tympanic membrane.

Hearing Acuity. Hearing acuity is a complex phenomenon and requires a multidimensional assessment. The assessment includes differentiation of conductive and sensorineural hearing loss and speech reception and discrimination. Common methods for testing hearing acuity are summarized in Table 24-3.

TABLE 23-4 Nursing Diagnoses, Nursing Outcomes Classification, and Nursing Interventions Classifications for Sensory Loss (Hearing)

Nursing Diagnosis	Suggested Nursing Outcomes Classification (NOC)	Suggested Nursing Interventions Classification (NIC)
Sensory loss (hearing)	Anxiety control Body image Cognitive ability Cognitive orientation Hearing compensation behavior Risk control: hearing impairment	Cognitive restructuring Cognitive stimulation Communication enhancement: hearing deficit Communication enhancement: speech deficit Emotional support Environmental management Exercise therapy: balance Surveillance: safety Developmental enhancement: child Ear care Medication monitoring Self-esteem enhancement
Risk for injury	Risk control: hearing impairment Safety behavior: home physical environment	Environmental management: safety Home maintenance assistance Risk identification Surveillance Presence Referral
Impaired verbal communication	Communication ability Communication: receptive ability Cognitive ability Information processing	Communication enhancement: hearing deficit Presence Surveillance: safety Decision-making support Learning facilitation Referral Support system enhancement

Data from Johnson, M., Maas, M.L., & Moorhead, S. (2000). *Nursing outcomes classification (NOC)* (2nd ed.). St. Louis: Mosby; McCloskey, J.C., & Bulechek, G.M. (2000). *Nursing interventions classification (NIC)* (3rd ed.). St. Louis: Mosby; and North American Nursing Diagnosis Association. (2001). *Nursing diagnosis: definitions and classification 2001-2002* (4th ed.). Philadelphia: Author.

Nursing Diagnosis: Sensory Loss (Hearing)

As many as 28 million Americans have hearing loss (HearingLossWeb, 2000). This projection is expected to increase as the baby boomers age and experience the consequences of noise pollution. Nursing assessment information appropriate to the nursing diagnosis of sensory loss (hearing) is included in this section. Nursing diagnoses, nursing outcomes classifications, and nursing intervention classifications are included in Table 24-4.

Conductive Hearing Loss. Conductive losses are the most common type of hearing deficits and are usually due to frequent or severe otitis media. Risk factors for otitis media include immune deficiencies, day care placement, exposure to tobacco smoke, or craniofacial abnormalities such as a cleft palate. Prenatal exposure to maternal smoking may place an infant at risk for frequent otitis media (Stathis et al., 1999), with the risk a prevalent factor through the age of 5 years. Otitis media, although common, must not be assumed to be easily treatable or well understood. Use current clinical practice protocols. Pulec and Deguine (1999) reported a case of severe otitis media due to tuberculosis occurring in a 5-year-old child. They stated that all causes and unusual diagnoses should be considered when treating otitis media, and they recommended that diagnosis be made on bacteriological smear and culture.

Sensorineural Hearing Loss. Sensory (hair cell) and neural (spiral ganglion cell) factors result in sensorineural hearing loss. Such losses may occur prenatally. According to *Healthy People 2010* (USDHHS, 2000), 1 in 1000 children is born deaf. An additional 3 in 1000 babies are born with a moderate hearing loss (American Speech-Language-Hearing Association [ASHA], 2000). These statistics make hearing loss the most common congenital defect. The inability to hear during infancy affects the development of normal speech and language skills and may adversely affect social, emotional, cognitive, and academic development. It is significant to note that some within the deaf community perceive deafness to be a difference in lifestyle rather than a disability. These individuals would disagree with the perspective that deafness has an adverse impact on development (Feller, 1999) but instead view deafness as an enhancement of vision. Despite such perceptions from those affected by deafness, the National Institutes of Health (NIH) (1993) developed a consensus statement on the need for early identification of hearing impairment in young children. Given that the first 3 years of life are the most crucial in speech and language development and given that most cases of congenital deafness are not diagnosed until after 3 years of age, it is essential that testing be done at a younger age. Universal hearing screening (ASHA, 2000) for newborns is done in only 20% of the hospitals in the United States. Legislation is pending in many states that would require implementation of universal hearing screening for all newborns. The goal of such legislation is early intervention for infants with hearing deficits. Recommended testing of newborns is through the auditory brainstem response (ABR) or otoacoustic emissions (OAEs) (Table 24-3).

Sensorineural hearing loss may be acquired as a result of autoimmune disorders or exposure to ototoxic substances (aminoglycosides, cisplatin, aspirin). It may also be caused by bacterial meningitis, viral infections (congenital rubella, cytomegalovirus, mumps), or bacterial endotoxins and exotoxins. Additionally, sensorineural hearing loss may occur as a result of sound trauma from firearms, engine noise, loud toys, loud music, or head trauma (Merck, 2000). Homoe, Christensen, and Bretlau (1999) note in their study of 740 children that acute otitis media is multifactorial in nature and is determined by multiple genetic and environmental factors. With respect to noise exposure, Hinze, DeLeon, and Mitchell (1999) recommend that dentists wear earplugs to prevent sensorineural hearing loss from the constant and repetitive noise of drills and dental equipment.

Another cause of sensorineural hearing loss is otosclerosis, which is due to ankylosis of the stapes caused by the growth of immature bone through the vascular channels of the ear (Merck, 2000). A common cause of hearing impairment, otosclerosis affects around 10% of adults (University of Washington, 2000). Otosclerosis may be present but does not interfere with hearing function in as many as 90% of those with the disease. Otosclerosis may affect the stapes, inner ear, or both. Cochlear otosclerosis occurs with the spread of otosclerosis to the inner ear and results in sensorineural hearing loss and balance impairment. If the otosclerosis extends to the stapes, surgery may be recommended. Hearing aids may be of benefit.

Sensorineural hearing loss with balance disturbance may be seen with acoustic neuroma. Caused by a tumor, acoustic neuroma occurs in 1 of every 3500 persons between the ages of 30 and 60 years. The precipitating cause of the tumor is unknown (University of Washington, 2000). The tumor is benign and grows on cranial nerve VIII, affecting hearing and balance. Acoustic neuromas grow slowly and cause symptoms that increase in severity with time. Symptoms include unilateral hearing loss, tinnitus, dysphagia, facial numbness, weakness or paralysis, ataxia, headaches, visual loss, and death if untreated. Diagnosis is through symptom presentation and through the ABR test (Table 24-3). Persons with acoustic neuroma may have normal audiological presentations (Magdziarz, Wiet, Dinces, & Adamiec, 2000). According to researchers, persons presenting with unilateral audiovestibular symptoms should be evaluated for acoustic neuroma. Surgical removal is the usual and recommended treatment, with one study demonstrating significant long term preservation of hearing following surgery for acoustic neuroma (Inoue et al., 2000). Most surgeries, however, result in permanent hearing loss.

Implications for Rehabilitation

Marie had severe bunions on her feet. She had the bunion on the right foot removed and experienced a significant amount of postoperative pain. The surgeon explained that she should just "take it easy" for a few days. Unfortunately Marie has a severe hearing deficit. She wears bilateral hearing aids, but they enable her to hear only loud noises and some limited speech. Marie reads lips to a limited extent. Her primary method of communication is through American Sign Language. When the surgeon told her to "take it easy," she guessed at what he said and nodded. The surgeon believed she understood his instructions. Marie believed he had told her to not walk on her foot. She went home and stayed in bed for 7 days, minimizing any out-of-bed activity. After 7 days of bed rest, she experienced severe pain in her right leg. The pain was sharp and increased with flexion of her toes. When her daughter stopped by for a visit, Marie explained her leg pain. Her daughter immediately took Marie to her primary care physician, who diagnosed her leg pain as a deep vein thrombosis. Marie was directly admitted to the hospital for a short stay and was given intravenous heparin therapy. The admitting nurse noticed Marie's speech pattern and bilateral hearing aids and asked whether Marie understood the questions. Marie nodded that she understood. Later in the shift the admitting nurse responded to Marie's call light. Marie's family was visiting and appeared angry that no interpreter was available because Marie speaks only through sign language.

Resources and Technology for Persons with Hearing Loss. Primary concerns for rehabilitation involving persons with hearing losses are communication and safety within the environment. Box 24-2 contains recommended strategies for communicating with persons with hearing impairment. Growth in computer technology has led to a dazzling, confusing, and sometimes misleading array of devices, equipment, and software. These are summarized in Table 24-5.

Box 24-2 Guidelines for Communication with Persons with Hearing Deficits

1. Gain the listener's attention before speaking and wait until the person is ready to listen
2. Talk clearly and distinctly, but do not shout
3. Face the person
4. Stand or sit close to the person
5. Repeat once and then rephrase
6. Identify the topic, and make it clear when the subject changes
7. Use your hands to gesture
8. Confirm comprehension
9. Avoid background noise and distractions

TABLE 24-5 Resources for Individuals with Hearing Loss

Resource	Description	Comments
Alerting devices	Smoke alarms	Must be visual or vibrating
	Wireless X-10 systems for doorbells, telephone, baby alarms, telephone	Provides remote activation of alarm devices through a visual indicator such as a light
Assistive listening devices	Microphones, pickups, headphones, earphones	All enable user to focus on a single desired signal and filter other noises; intent is to allow one signal to be amplified in comparison with the sounds from the remaining environment
Personal assistive listening devices	Pocket talker	Uses a microphone and headphones connected through a small amplifier
	Personal FM system	Similar to the pocket talker but wireless; speaker is given a transmitter and microphone, and listener receives the acoustic equivalent to the electronic signal; ideal for lectures, church, or concerts
	Wireless headphones	Use an input plug into an audio device, such as the television
Group assistive listening devices	Infared systems	Depend on a clear line of sight between transmitter and receiver, portable
	FM systems	Signals are more versatile and portable
	Loop systems	Permanently installed in a room
Hearing aids	Acoustic aid	Amplifies sound and sends the amplified acoustic energy to the eardrum
	Conduction aid	Transmits sound to the inner ear using the bones of the skull
	Implantable hearing aid	Experimental treatment, with the first device implanted in December 1999
Automatic speech recognition (ASR)	Dragon System's Naturally Speaking, IBM's Via Voice, Lernout & Hauspie's Voice Xpress, Philips Dictation, Systems' Free Speech	Application for individuals with hearing loss is to have the microphone pick up the speech of one individual and type the spoken words on a computer screen, providing immediate translation of the spoken word; all have difficulty and depend on the clarity and speed of speech; a goal for this technology is use for situations that require interpreting, including business meetings or classrooms
Telephones	Speech-Adjust-A-Tone	Connects to the telphone; can be adjusted to the level of amplification needed
	Cellular phones	Only the Nokia 51-61 series is compatible with hearing aids that use telecoils
TTYs or TDDs	Text telephones, telecommunications devices for the deaf	Assist those with hearing loss to communicate using standard telephone lines; through the TTY or TTD and Telecommunication Relay Service, communication is possible with persons who use standard voice telephones
Two-way pager	ReachNet, RIM Inter@ctive pager by WyndTell	Provide individuals with hearing loss the ability to communicate anywhere at anytime with anyone, are interactive, and provide a visual typed message
Visual communications	Visual intercom	In experimental stages at present but have a significant potential to augment emergency verbal messages in large, crowded environments, such as airports and amusement parks
Relay service		All require use of either a TTY or TDD and connection to a relay access number for the state. All state relay numbers are toll free and can be obtained at the website: www.hearinglossweb.com
	Standard relay call	TDD user types in the message, which is interpreted by the state relay operator, who types the response of the person called back to the TDD user
	Voice carryover call	TDD user speaks directly, and the state relay operator types the response of the person called; faster than the standard system
	Two-line voice carryover call	TDD user is able to hear the response of the person called, and the state relay operator types in the response to fill in any gaps; requires the cost of a 3-way call

Despite the advances made during the last decade in resources for persons with hearing loss, artificial acoustic devices or aids are not equivalent to an intact auditory system. Box 24-3 contains information written by consumers on the advantages and disadvantages of different hearing aid systems. Rehabilitation nurses need to be familiar with the variety, benefits, and disadvantages of resources for persons with hearing loss. No single system or method will work for all persons requiring assistance with hearing; therefore the more options there are, the more likely individuals will be to find one that meets their needs and lifestyle. Box 24-4 lists high-quality, consumer advocacy– based websites to provide rehabilitation nurses with insights and direction on resources available for those with limited or no hearing.

Box 24-3 Hearing Aid Consumer Tips

Before Buying a Hearing Aid

- Check with a physician and an audiologist for easily correctable causes to hearing impairment

After the Decision to Purchase a Hearing Aid Has Been Made, Consider the Following Points before Making a Purchase

- Digital technology offers improvements over standard hearing aids but is costly; consumer should make sure the added quality is worth the added cost
- Although hearing aids that seem invisible in the ear tend to be visually appealing, they are often more fragile, with a shorter life expectancy and a lower degree of quality than traditional behind-the-ear models
- The hearing aid selected should include strong, preamplified telecoils, positioned for loop and telephone use
- Three aids should be tried before making a selection
- Expect a 90-day return policy and accept no less than 60 days for return
- Determine the refund policy; expect that the audiogram and earmold will not be refunded
- Expect a manufacturer warranty of no less than 2 years

After Fitting the Aid but before Leaving the Store

- Use the distributor's phone to check for quality and function of the device

After Buying the Device

- The aid should be worn continuously
- Signs that the hearing aid is not fitted well include feedback; causes of an ill-fitted hearing aid are cracked tubing, loose earmold, or loose fitting
- Every problem and irritation should be recorded
- At the end of 1 week, the consumer should return to the distributor and review any concerns noted

If a Return of the Hearing Aid Is Necessary

- Expect return of the audiogram because this is a medical record and belongs to the person for whom it was recorded

Cochlear Implants. About 20 years ago, cochlear implants made headlines as a breakthrough for persons with profound hearing impairment. The cochlear implant is considered a prosthetic device used to replace the function of the cochlea. Part of the device is surgically implanted behind the ear to bypass the cochlea. The remainder of the device is external. It is battery operated and contains a microphone, a speech processor, and connecting cables (University of Washington, 2000). The device, implant surgery, and speech therapy may cost as much as $80,000, and these costs often are not covered by health care insurance (Strickland, 1999). The cochlear implant offers miracles for some but not without significant effort and adjustment. Only one in five children who receive the cochlear implant are able to acquire language (Mayer, 1999).

The advent of the cochlear implant led to an extensive uproar and even protesting from the deaf community (Zak, 1996), some members of which perceive implants as a form of genocide because they eliminate deafness (Feller, 1999). The view of the deaf community was that it is healthier for deaf persons to learn to use sign language than to have an expensive, experimental surgery. In 1998 the National Association for the Deaf withdrew their opposition to cochlear implants and at present are reevaluating their position.

According to the NIH (2000), cochlear implants are not for all persons with hearing loss. The NIH consensus statement on cochlear implants presents several factors as keys in the success of cochlear implants: age at onset of deafness (postlingual is optimal), age at implantation (younger than 3 years is ideal), duration of deafness (shorter is better), extent of residual hearing (undetermined), electrophysiological factors (the presence of some surviving spiral ganglion cells is essential), and device factors (effectiveness of the transmitter, receiver, and microphone).

Sign Language. Approximately 2 million Americans with deafness use American Sign Language. In several of the states, American Sign Language is recognized as an official foreign language for which academic credit may be given (Gallaudet University, 1999). The first academic pro-

Box 24-4 Websites for Consumers with Hearing Impairment

- http://www.hearinglossweb.com: provides extensive information and links to other sites for resources for those with hearing loss
- http://www.deafworks.com: DEAFWORKS organization manufactures technology for those with deafness
- http://www.wynd.net: Wynd Communication is a deaf person–owned company specializing in providing accessible communication for persons with hearing loss
- http://www.webcom.com/~houtx/: SayWhatClub website provides a listing of resources for those with hearing loss

gram to promote American Sign Language was at Gallaudet University in Washington, DC. Gallaudet University has served as the hub of education for deaf persons since 1856. Sign language has been used on Gallaudet's campus for more than a century, with the exception of a short period when lipreading was required. It was sign language between Gallaudet's football team members that led to the football huddle when it was discovered that other teams were reading their signs for plays. Given the prevalence of sign language and the need for clear communication, rehabilitation nurses who are unable to sign must know how to access translators.

Computerization and the Internet. Perhaps the most significant opportunity to reduce accessibility barriers for persons with significant hearing loss is through the use of computers and the Internet. The use of company e-mail, for example, can minimize or even eliminate the need for voice communication. The Internet makes it possible for those within the deaf community to communicate in chat rooms, web pages, and e-mail, and it widens communication pathways with every technological advance.

Taste

Taste is a cellular reaction caused by the mixture of food and drink with saliva (Cooper, 1998). Although not a critical sense for survival, taste is a complex sense, and it is influential in nutritional intake. Individuals tend to have a craving or attraction to nutrients in which their bodies are deficient.

Anatomy and Physiology

Taste cells are located within the mouth and throat. Clusters of 50 taste cells form taste buds, which are located around the tongue's papillae. Taste buds function through convergence of synapses, with many of the receptors within taste buds synapsing to a single interneuron. Stimulations of the taste receptors within the taste buds travel through the interneuron by the vagus, glossopharyngeal, and facial nerves to the ventral posterior nucleus (thalamus). From the thalamus, the signals are transferred to the ipsilateral gustatory cortex of the cerebrum. Taste receptors are specific to the four basic sensations of taste. The posterior central aspect of the tongue is sensitive to bitter tastes. The lateral portions of the tongue are sensitive to sour tastes. Salty tastes are noted by the lateral aspects adjacent to the end of the tongue. In the anterior tip of the tongue, sweet tastes are identified (Figure 24-5). Olfactory sensors in combination with gustatory sensors are responsible for the ability to identify specific flavors.

Assessment of Taste. Assessment of taste sensation is a significant portion of the nursing assessment but is typically not completed as a routine inpatient or outpatient admission assessment. Rather, it is a key assessment when indicators are noted that a problem might exist, for example, if the client reports that all foods taste the same or if the client demonstrates a decreased or depressed appetite. Assessment is completed by preparing four distinct taste sensations in liquid forms (salt water, sugar water, lemon juice, and coffee). One at a time, cotton swabs are soaked in each liquid

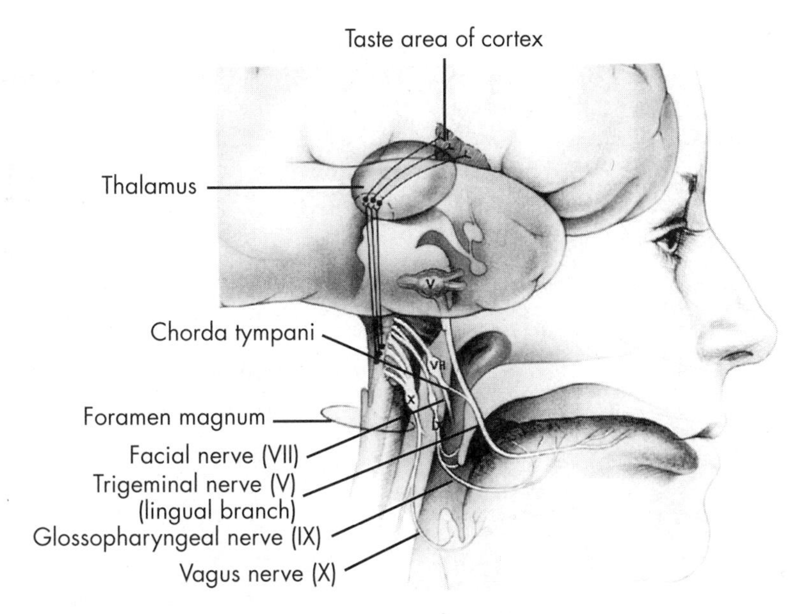

Figure 24-5 Central nervous system pathways for taste from the facial nerve (anterior two thirds of the tongue), glossopharyngeal nerve (posterior one third of the tongue), and vagus nerve (root of the tongue). The trigeminal nerve is also shown. It carries tactile sensations from the anterior two thirds of the tongue. The chorda tympani from the facial nerve (carrying taste input) joins the trigeminal nerve. Nerves carrying taste impulses synapse in the ganglion of each nerve, in the nucleus of the tractus solitarius, and in the thalamus, before terminating in the taste area of the cortex. (From Seely, R.R., Stephens, T.D., & Tate, P.P. [1991]. *Essentials of anatomy and physiology.* St. Louis: Mosby.)

and placed individually on the client's tongue. The client is asked to identify the category of taste sensation for each one.

Assessment includes visualization of the tongue and oral cavity for asymmetrical spots or plaques. The presence of black or darkly pigmented papillae is considered a normal finding in dark-skinned persons (Pehoushek & Norton, 2000).

Nursing Diagnosis: Sensory Loss (Taste)

Taste may be impaired by a variety of problems, including heavy smoking, desquamation of the tongue, oral infection, cerebrovascular accident, aging, and radiation of the head or neck. Intake of amitriptyline or vincristine may alter taste. In some cases zinc supplementation has been demonstrated to correct problems with taste. Testing, in addition to a focused history and physical and examination, should be sufficient to identify the problem (Bromley, 2000). Nursing assessment information appropriate to the nursing diagnosis of sensory loss (taste) is included in this section. Nursing outcomes classifications and nursing interventions classifications are included in Table 24-6.

Implications for Rehabilitation

Although impairments in taste may not be life threatening, they do interfere with the quality of life and may impede adequate nutritional intake (Bromley, 2000). If possible, the cause of the problem should be eliminated. If the cause cannot be alleviated, food flavor and appearance should be enhanced. Older persons may be tempted to add large quantities of sugar and salt to achieve flavor. Rehabilitation nurses should work with clients to encourage the addition of seasonings instead. The taste of foods may be enhanced through smoking cessation, tongue cleaning, and adequate nutrition (Winkler, Garg, Mekayarajjananonth, Bakaeen, & Khan, 1999).

Smell

The sense of smell is complex and involves the detection and perception of different odors. Olfactory accuracy peaks between 30 and 60 years of age. Olfactory stimulation through aromatherapy is a key aspect of complementary medicine. Controversy exists on the validity of aromatherapy for treatment of clinical conditions (Kalish, 1999); however, its significance is evident in the mind-body connection.

Anatomy and Physiology

Olfactory receptors located in the cilia of the nasal passageways are stimulated through the conversion of odors to chemicals that dissolve in the epithelium of the nose. They are transferred through the cilia to the axon to the olfactory bulb and on to the olfactory tract, which leads the signal to the olfactory cortex, amygdala, hippocampus, hypothalamus, and pyriform cortex. Olfactory information is relayed directly to the cerebral cortex without traveling through the thalamus. The olfactory pathway divides in the amygdala-pyriform area, with one pathway projecting through the medial dorsal nuclei to the orbitofrontal cortex and the second pathway projecting to the limbic system. The first pathway is linked with perception of odor and smell, and the second is associated with memory and the emotional response to smells (Figure 24-6).

TABLE 24-6 Nursing Diagnoses, Nursing Outcomes Classifications, and Nursing Interventions Classifications for Sensory Loss (Gustatory and Olfactory)

Nursing Diagnosis	Suggested Nursing Outcomes Classification (NOC)	Suggested Nursing Interventions Classification (NIC)
Sensory/perceptual alterations: olfactory	Anxiety control Body image Electrolyte balance Fluid balance	Environmental management Nutrition management Nausea management Weight management Medication management Surveillance: safety
Sensory/perceptual alterations: gustatory	Anxiety control Body image Electrolyte balance Fluid balance	Electrolyte monitoring Environmental management Fluid management Fluid monitoring Nausea management Nutrition management Surveillance: safety
Imbalanced nutrition: less than body requirements	Nutritional status: nutrient intake Weight control Sensory function: taste and smell	Nutrition management Nutritional monitoring Weight gain assistance Weight management

Data from Johnson, M., Maas, M.L., & Moorhead, S. (2000). *Nursing outcomes classification (NOC)* (2nd ed.). St. Louis: Mosby; McCloskey, J.C., & Bulechek, G.M. (2000). *Nursing interventions classification (NIC)* (3rd ed.). St. Louis: Mosby; and North American Nursing Diagnosis Association. (2001). *Nursing diagnosis: definitions and classification 2001-2002* (4th ed.). Philadelphia: Author.

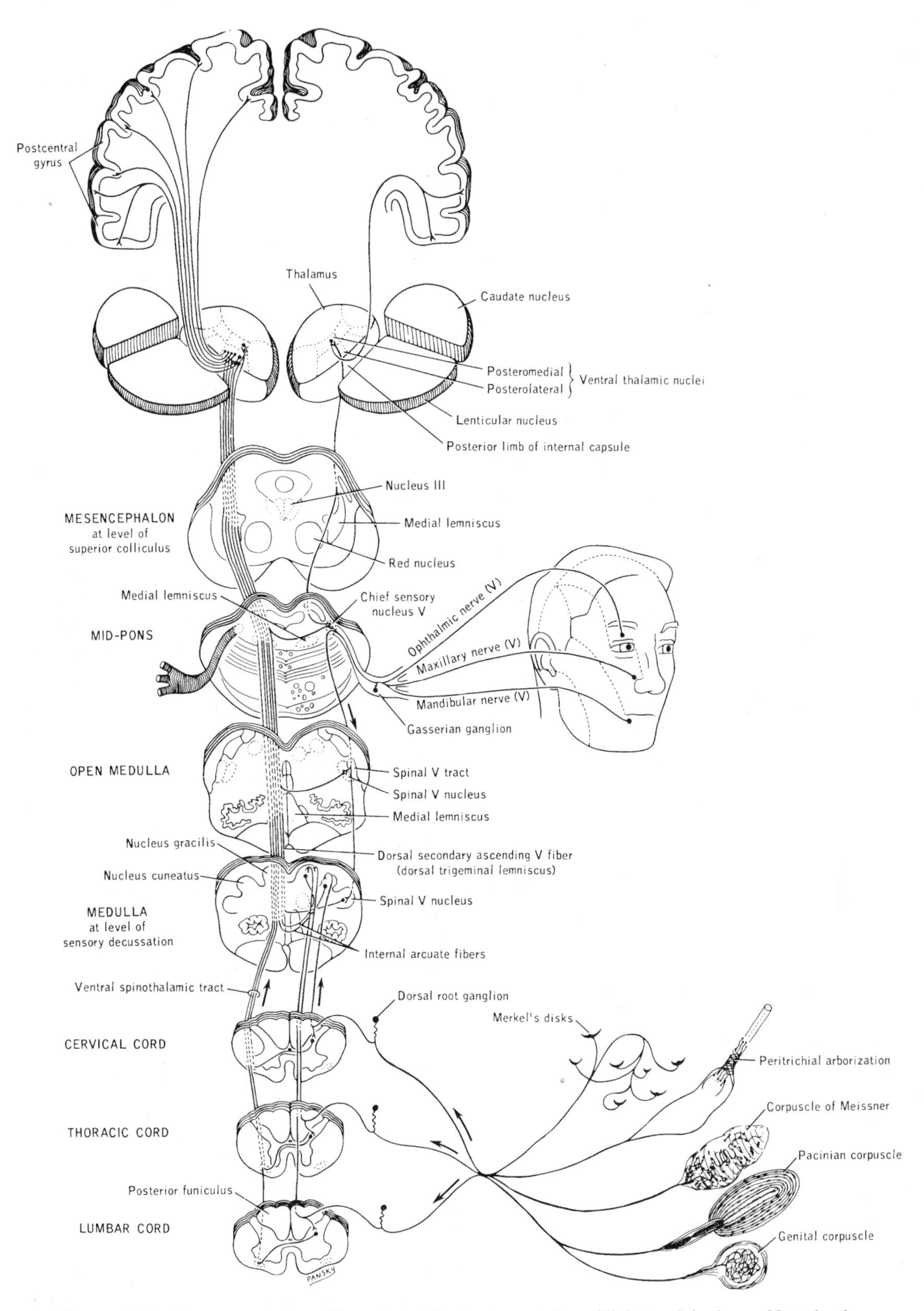

Figure 24-6 Sensory pathways. The pathway for the transmission of light touch is shown. Note that input from the peripheral nerves serving the head and face is at the brainstem level. Touch sensory fibers from the trunk, arms, and legs travel upward in the posterior funiculus and join head and face fibers in the brainstem in the medial lemniscus.

Assessment of Olfactory Sensation

As with gustatory assessment, olfactory assessment is a significant portion of the nursing assessment but is typically not completed as a routine inpatient or outpatient admission assessment. Commercially available systems exist for testing olfaction, including a smell diskette with eight different odorants (Briner & Simmen, 1999). However, when problems exist, the nurse can assess olfactory acuity through a simple, readily available test using coffee, peppermint oil, and lemon juice. The client is asked to close the eyes, and each item is held under the nose for a brief time, during which the nurse asks the client to identify the substance. Examination of olfaction also requires assessment of the upper respiratory tract.

Nursing Diagnosis: Sensory Loss (Smell)

The most common cause of the loss of smell or olfactory acuity is aging, with an estimated 50% of those older than 65 years experiencing moderate to severe loss of smell. Past the age of 80 years, more than 75% of adults have a severe loss of smell (Winkler et al., 1999). The loss of olfaction in the elderly is linked with poor oral conditions (Duffy, Cain, & Ferris, 1999). Other causes of olfactory impairment include sinus infections, allergies, medications, vitamin deficiencies, chemical exposure, radiation, smoking, and cerebrovascular injury. In young adults anosmia (loss of olfaction) may occur after head injury (Bromley, 2000). Nursing diagnoses, nursing outcomes classifications, and nursing interventions classifications are included in Table 24-6.

Implications for Rehabilitation

As with geriatric clients with disorders of taste, the rehabilitation nurse should encourage geriatric clients with anosmia to use seasonings for flavor instead of salt and sugar. Calorie counts for persons with disorders of olfaction should be monitored to ensure adequate intake of nutrients. Routine assessment of weight should be completed because weight gain or loss may by linked with olfactory impairment.

Assessment of the home environment is important to rehabilitation for persons with olfactory disturbance, who may not detect a gas leak, something burning, or spoiled foods.

Touch and Sensation

The concept of therapeutic touch, and that of Reiki imply that energy transfer is possible without physical contact (Narrin, 1996/2000). In reality, however, the sense of touch relies on physical contact (Rosa, Rosa, Sarner, & Barrett, 1998).

Anatomy and Physiology

Touch, pressure, and vibration are components of the somatosensory system. As mechanical stimuli place a force on the skin, the mechanoreceptors located within the skin and subcutaneous tissues are activated. The quality of sensation perceived is a factor of the adequacy of the stimulus, one's threshold for stimulation, the pattern of discharge, and the adaptation rate. There are six types of sensory receptors, which are summarized in Table 24-7.

The receptors change energy from a stimulus to an electrical signal. The signal must be strong enough to evoke action in the afferent fibers. The stimulus is transmitted through afferent fibers to the spinal cord and brain.

The anterolateral spinothalamic tract contains pathways for nondiscriminative sensations such as touch, tickle, itch, pain, and temperature. The information relayed is not specific to intensity and location of the triggering signal. The signal is carried through the spinal cord on the contralateral side of the cord to the thalamus and lower brainstem (Figure 24-6).

The dorsal column medial lemniscal system conveys impulses that are specific with respect to intensity and localization. Information relayed through the dorsal column system includes barognosis, kinesthesia, proprioception, vibration, stereognosis, discriminative touch, tactile pressure,

TABLE 24-7 Types and Function of Sensory Receptors

Receptor Type	Function	Comments
Mechanoreceptors	Touch, flutter, pressure, vibration	Meissner's corpuscle and Merkel's receptors: important for fine discrimination, graphesthesia, sterognosis Ruffini's corpuscle: responds to pressure Pacinian corpuscle: responds to vibration Hair receptors Free nerve endings
Proprioceptors	Position sense	Essential for sense of body schema, limb position, movement, force, or effort
Thermoreceptors	Thermal sense	Identify hot and cold substances
Nociceptors	Pain	Respond to tissue damage or injury
Chemoreceptor	Chemical reactions	Receptors for taste; smell; arterial oxygen; and blood levels of glucose, amino acids, fatty acids, and carbon dioxide
Photic receptors	Vision receptors	Receptors for light; include rods and cones

two-point discrimination, and graphesthesia. The impulses are carried through large, rapidly conducting fibers to the dorsal column of the spinal cord, where the impulse crosses over to the opposite side and continues to the thalamus through the medial lemnisci and the sensory cortex (Figure 24-7).

Assessment of Sensation

In a routine assessment, sensory functions would not be reviewed by the nurse. If, however, issues are noted in pain, paresthesias, or motor deficits, a full sensory examination should be completed. Methods of sensory assessment are identified in Box 24-5.

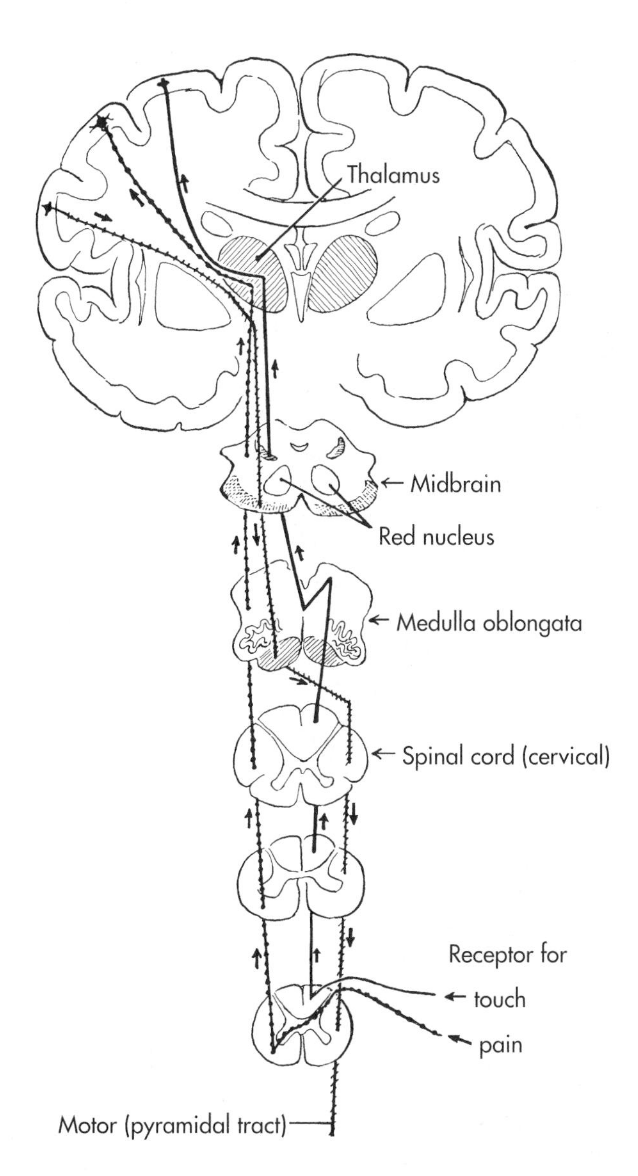

Figure 24-7 Diagram of the main motor and sensory pathways. The perceptions of touch, passive motion, position, and vibration are transmitted through the posterior tract in the spinal cord through the medial lemniscus in the brainstem to the thalamus and through the internal capsule to the cortex (this pathway is represented by the *solid line*). Pain and temperature sensations are transmitted through the anterolateral tract and lateral lemniscus to the thalamus and then through the internal capsule to the cortex *(dotted lines)*. (Courtesy John Muhm, EdD.)

Nursing Diagnosis: Sensory Loss (Tactile)

Many neurological problems affect sensation. A stroke or cerebrovascular accident resulting in hemiplegia results in impaired sensation to one side of the body. Multiple sclerosis may result in paresthesias to affected body areas. Aging may lead to sensory loss. Diabetic neuropathy is a common cause of paresthesias and loss of sensation in the lower extremities. Nursing diagnoses, nursing outcomes classifications, and nursing interventions classifications for sensory loss are included in Table 24-8.

Implications for Rehabilitation

The rehabilitation nurse must expect that any client with neurological impairment may experience sensory losses and impaired sensation and identify risks for the client. Because the sensory system provides the body with warnings for excessive pressure, potential tissue injury, and location of the body in space, impairment of sensation places the client at risk for injury. Clients are taught safety in the environment and how to use environmental clues to compensate for the lack of sensory perception. For example, if proprioceptive and tactile sensation is deficient in the left arm and leg, the client is taught to visually assess the location and safety of the left arm and leg.

Box 24-5 Sensory Assessment Methods

Pain discrimination: a safety pin is opened and placed against the skin; client is asked to identify the location of the stimulus and to describe it and note if it is sharp or dull

Two-point discrimination: with the client's eyes closed, two sharp points (toothpicks) are used to lightly prick the skin; client is assessed to determine the minimum distance at which he or she is able to identify two points

Proprioception: with the client's eyes closed, a single toe or finger is moved by the nurse, and the client is asked to identify the location of the phalange and whether it is up or down

Vibratory sense: with the client's eyes closed, a tuning fork is struck and placed end down on the client's extremity; client is asked to report whether any sensation is felt and to describe it; if the client identifies the vibration, he or she is asked to tell when vibration is no longer perceived

Temperature sense: cold water is placed in one glass container and warm in another; client is asked to identify the temperature (warm or cold) of each item when placed against the skin

Tactile sense: client's eyes are kept closed, nurse uses a cotton swab to gently touch the client's skin in symmetric points, and client is asked to identify when the touch is felt; results are identified as normal, hypesthetic, anesthetic, or hyperesthetic

TABLE 24-8 Nursing Diagnoses, Nursing Outcomes Classifications, and Nursing Interventions Classifications for Sensory Loss (Tactile)

Nursing Diagnosis	Suggested Nursing Outcomes Classification (NOC)	Suggested Nursing Interventions Classification (NIC)
Sensory/perceptual alterations: tactile	Anxiety control Body image Cognitive orientation	Environmental management Exercise therapy: balance Peripheral sensation management Positioning Pressure management Surveillance: safety Touch

Data from Johnson, M., Maas, M.L., & Moorhead, S. (2000). *Nursing outcomes classification (NOC)* (2nd ed.). St. Louis: Mosby; McCloskey, J.C., & Bulechek, G.M. (2000). *Nursing interventions classification (NIC)* (3rd ed.). St. Louis: Mosby; and North American Nursing Diagnosis Association. (2001). *Nursing diagnosis: definitions and classification 2001-2002* (4th ed.). Philadelphia: Author.

Perception

The ability to make sense of the environment through the identification, integration, and interpretation of incoming stimuli is perception. It is difficult to consider perception apart from sensation because perception is the way one interprets sensations, making perception and sensation interrelated phenomena.

Anatomy and Physiology

Perception occurs primarily in the parietal lobes of the cerebral cortex. The right and left parietal lobes tend to process different aspects of perception. Verbal input, through writing and reading, and right/left discrimination are usually processed in the left parietal lobe. Information on space, texture, geography, construction, and body schema is processed in the right parietal lobe.

A highly individualized process, perception of stimuli is influenced by past experiences, age, culture, beliefs, education, attitudes, goals, and expectations. Additionally perception is modified through feedback from others. Perceptual ability is essential for learning and must be present for successful rehabilitation of individuals with or without disabilities.

Assessment of Perception

The rehabilitation nurse assesses perception in conjunction with therapists of other disciplines related to specific issues identified in the routine assessment. For example, a person with left hemiplegia should be assessed for left-sided neglect and homonymous hemianopsia because both are common deficits associated with right cerebrovascular accidents. Assessment of specific perceptual problems is discussed in conjunction with common perceptual impairments identified in the next portion of this chapter.

Nursing Diagnosis: Unilateral Neglect

Many neurological problems affect cognitive-perceptual patterns. Perceptual problems are often experienced by persons with brain injuries or lesions. There are numerous variations of perception that may present, many of which are discussed next. Nursing diagnoses, nursing outcomes classifications, and nursing interventions classifications for unilateral neglect are included in Table 24-9.

Body Image or Schema Problems. These types of problems may result after brain injury because the ability to integrate and make sense of tactile and proprioceptive input may be impaired. Somatosognosia is one type of body image problem in which there is an unawareness of one's body structure and body parts. It typically occurs with lesions of the dominant parietal lobe and often is associated with right-sided hemiplegia. The client may have difficulty imitating movements and following directions such as "move your left leg." The client may have less difficulty responding to simple gestures and instructions identifying specific body parts.

Right and left discrimination is a type of body image or schema deficit that may occur after damage to either the right or left parietal lobe. With this deficit the person is unable to determine the right of left sides of his or her own body and will not be able to follow verbal commands that include references to right and left. Rehabilitation nurses should avoid mention of right or left in directions. Correction for the deficit is best done through the use of environmental cues (other than left and right) or pointing.

Another type of body image or schema is visual spatial neglect, which usually occurs after a parietal lobe lesion of the nondominant hemisphere and usually affects awareness of the left side of the body. The person may be unaware of any stimuli on the affected side, including tactile and environmental stimuli. This disorder creates the potential for serious safety hazards because the person is not aware of objects to the left within the environment. Although the person is being taught how to correct the problem, the rehabilitation nurse should provide modifications to the surroundings to create a safe environment. Therapy revolves around increasing the person's awareness of the left side of the environment and of his or her body. The use of auditory and olfac-

TABLE 24-9 Nursing Diagnoses, Nursing Outcomes Classifications, and Nursing Interventions Classifications for Unilateral Neglect

Nursing Diagnosis	Suggested Nursing Outcomes Classification (NOC)	Suggested Nursing Interventions Classification (NIC)
Unilateral neglect	Body image Body positioning: self-initiated Self-care: ADLs Balance Joint movement: active Joint movement: passive Neurological status Safety behavior: home physical environment Safety behavior: personal Self-care: instrumental ADLs Transfer performance	Body image enhancement Coping enhancement Communication enhancement: visual deficit Environmental management safety Positioning Touch Unilateral neglect management Caregiver support Exercise promotion Exercise therapy: ambulation Exercise therapy: balance Exercise therapy: joint mobility Exercise therapy: muscle control Mutual goal setting Support system enhancement Teaching: individual

Data from Johnson, M., Maas, M.L., & Moorhead, S. (2000). *Nursing outcomes classification (NOC)* (2nd ed.). St. Louis: Mosby; McCloskey, J.C., & Bulechek, G.M. (2000). *Nursing interventions classification (NIC)* (3rd ed.). St. Louis: Mosby; and North American Nursing Diagnosis Association. (2001). *Nursing diagnosis: definitions and classification 2001-2002* (4th ed.). Philadelphia: Author.
ADLs, Activities of daily living.

tory stimulation used on the left side of the body or environment may help provide cues for the person to scan the environment to the left. Placing a radio or tape player on the left side can provide an auditory cue to check that area of the environment. Applying hand cream or perfumed lotions to the left arm will provide tactile stimulation, and olfactory stimulation from the left provides environmental and personal cues to remember the left side of the room and body.

Finger agnosia and anosognosia are two additional types of body image or schema disorders. With finger agnosia, the person is unable to identify specific fingers bilaterally. The problem usually results after a lesion to the parietal lobe of the dominant hemisphere and is linked with aphasia. Anosognosia is a serious problem in which individuals deny the presence of paralysis. Usually parietal lobe of the dominant side is affected. The condition is linked with a poor prognosis because it is difficult to teach individuals to correct deficits that they do not perceive. Treatment may involve discriminative touch and pressure to cue the individual in to the fingers. The rehabilitation nurse should focus on teaching ways to ensure a safe environment.

Spatial Relation Disorders. These types of perceptual deficits may occur after damage to the nondominant hemisphere of the brain and are usually seen in conjunction with left-sided hemiplegia. Spatial relation deficits entail problems in identifying items' distance and relationship in space. Figure-ground discrimination is the inability to distinguish an item from the background, which creates problems in all activities of daily living. For example, it is necessary to be able to distinguish a towel from the wall and a bar of soap from the sink in order to wash the face, and it is necessary to be able to distinguish a slice of bread from a plate in order to eat. Persons with this deficit tend to have less difficulty with items that are defined clearly and contrast in color from the background.

Form constancy, is a type of spatial relation problem in which persons have difficulty identifying similarly shaped but distinct objects from one another. For example, a person with spatial relations problems may not be able to distinguish between a glass and a vase sitting side by side. Likewise, a toothbrush lying near a pencil may be confused. Problems with this deficit can be minimized by controlling the environment and encouraging the person to feel the objects and inspect them closely. Persons with spatial relations problems may show deficits in other visual spatial areas requiring judgment, for example, with direction, depth, and distance. These persons, when mobilized with a wheelchair, have difficulty not running into the wall and getting through doorways due to the inability to gauge distance and depth. When using the stairs or ambulating, they need consistent and constant reminders to learn to compensate for the deficit.

Agnosia. Persons with agnosia are unable to identify familiar items with one sense, although the use of an alternative sense may help them recognize the object. For example, a woman may not be able to find her mirror when looking on a table until she actually feels the mirror with her hands. The fork and spoon may be confused until the person picks up each and recalls the differences. This deficit is corrected by encouraging clients to use more than a single sense in locating and identifying objects. However, correction is not as easy for agnosias involving other senses. For example, with auditory agnosia, the person may not recognize familiar nonspeech sounds such as bells, whistles, and car horns. The difference between the telephone ringing and the doorbell may not be distinguishable to the individual.

Apraxia. Persons with apraxia cannot remember movements they once knew. Although they have sufficient strength, coordination and attention to perform the action, they are unable to do so. For example, a client with ideational apraxia may be capable of shaving, but if he is told to do so, he may not be able to conceptualize the task. If the person has ideomotor apraxia, he may be able to pick up the shaver and shave out of habit. However, if a nurse or therapist tells him to shave, he may be confused as to what is expected.

Implications for Rehabilitation

Perceptual deficits often are viewed by family members as indicators of mental confusion. It is essential that they be assisted in understanding the nature of such problems. Through careful assessment of the patterns of behavior and deficits, treatment plans can be designed to correct many of the problems. General approaches to perceptual programs are presented in the following.

Transfer of Training. The transfer of training approach is based on the belief that learning a skill for one application will carry over to other applications. For example, the practice of scanning for pieces while completing a puzzle can help the client remember to scan the dinner table during meals.

Sensorimotor Approach. With the sensorimotor approach, motor output is controlled, and specific sensory stimulation is offered to influence cerebral sensory organization and processing. Adaptive motor reactions are required in response to carefully controlled sensory stimuli. For instance, the client could be assisted into a standing table for proprioceptive input.

Functional Approach. Probably one of the most common approaches to sensory and perceptual problems, the functional approach, is based on the concept that practicing functional tasks will result in relearning and independence. Methods of compensation and adaptation are incorporated in functional teaching. For example, repeatedly practicing buttoning a shirt with a buttonhook is an example of a functional approach to relearning the skill of buttoning.

Safety Concerns. While the client is relearning functional skills and abilities, the environment must be as safe as possible. For example, the environment around persons with neglect and homonymous hemianopsia must have essential bedside needs (e.g., telephone, call light, and tissues) on the uninvolved side. While the client is learning scanning techniques, colored tape may be used to attract attention to items.

Pain

Physical pain is a normal sensation that indicates the presence of tissue damage. Pain impulses are transmitted to the substantia gelatinosa within the lateral spinothalamic tract of the spinal cord. The impulses ascend to the thalamus of the brain and to the cerebral cortex. Simultaneously, descending fibers from the cerebral cortex moderate the way pain is perceived.

Anatomy and Physiology

According to Wall (1999), a noted British neurophysiologist, the substantia gelatinosa of the spinal cord is the "gate" of the pain experience. According to Wall's gate-control theory of pain, pain impulses are transmitted via small α-delta afferent fibers to the substantia gelatinosa of the spinal cord. Large fibers transmit touch, temperature, and pressure and travel a similar route to the spinal cord. The gate theory holds that if the large fibers are stimulated simultaneously with the small fibers, the pain impulse will be weakened and perceived to a lower degree. Likewise, if one is experiencing pain, the pain perception may be decreased by stimulating the large fibers through touch, temperature change, or pressure. Simultaneously, the descending fibers from the cerebral cortex decrease the pain perception through distraction and relaxation (Figure 24-8).

Assessment of Pain

Although pain is a common experience, there are a variety of widely held myths regarding pain perception. It seems that few have objective opinions about another's pain experience. According to McCaffery and Ferrell (1995), there are a variety of myths about the pain experience, all of which affect the assessment of pain.

Myths. One myth relates to the need for a physical explanation or reason for pain. If none is apparent, it is believed by many that the pain is of a psychological or emotional nature. This is untrue because in some cases the physical reason for pain is undetermined but may become clear at a later date and time. A second myth holds that malingering is common and that individuals will lie about the existence of pain to receive narcotics or sympathy. There is no clinical evidence in support of this myth. Although some persons may malinger, it is not common. In fact, more clients understate their pain than overstate it. Another commonly held myth about pain is that persons in pain always show visible signs of pain that verify the existence of the pain, including restlessness, apprehension, and a drawn expression. As with the other myths, this is also unfounded. Individuals respond differently to pain. It is not unusual for persons who have been in pain for long periods of time to fail to show any emotion, let alone the strong emotion expected to be seen with pain. This failure to demonstrate strong emotion with pain is particularly evident with chronically ill children (McCaffery & Ferrell, 1997).

Until the past two decades, the topic of pain in infancy and childhood was conspicuously absent from the literature or supported by a set of myths. A prevailing notion was that

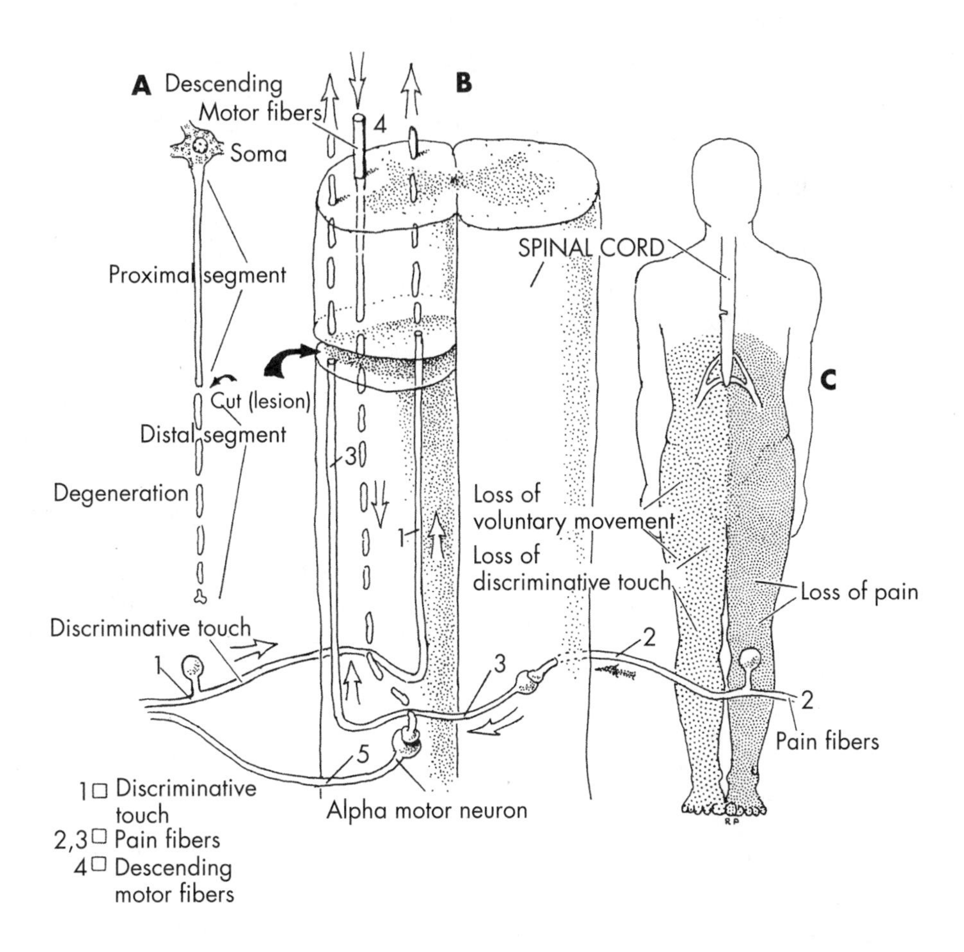

Figure 24-8 Effect of a spinal cord lesion on ascending or descending tracts. Degeneration of ascending tracts occurs above the lesion; descending tracts will degenerate below the lesion.

infants and young children with immature neurological systems could not distinguish pain or realized lesser degrees of pain than did adults. "Growing pains" were just to be outgrown. These ideas, coupled with concern that exposure to pain medication would lead children into addiction, contributed to poor pain management for children. Nurse researchers are credited with instituting many of the changes in this area. However, early studies have centered on acute pain, whereas many children in rehabilitation experience chronic or recurring pain (Hoeman, 1990).

A final myth is that health care professionals are the experts about a client's pain experience. It is imperative that rehabilitation nurses and all health care professionals realize that pain is whatever the experiencing person says it is and exists whenever the person says is does. No one is an expert in describing or identifying another's pain perception (McCaffery & Ferrell, 1997).

Cultural Implications. The pain experience is highly individualized. Persons respond to pain based on their culture, their background, and prior ordeals with pain. Culture affects the way individuals respond to pain. In the United States, under Western medicine, we believe that pain is unnecessary and should be treated. Persons who report having a headache will be asked if they have taken anything for it. If they respond that they have not taken anything, others will assume that they deserve to suffer for not having done anything to help themselves. Another Western expectation of the pain experience is that the affected individual will deal with the pain in a quiet, controlled manner. That is, it is not appropriate for a person in pain to lose control and yell or cry incessantly. The person in pain should not talk about the pain frequently. In contrast, some cultures, such as some Hispanic groups, consider it proper to display strong emotion with pain. Other groups, such as Scandinavians, consider pain to be a character-building experience.

Personal Background and Other Influences on Pain Perception. A person's background also tempers the pain experience. One clear example of this is childbirth. The daughter who hears her mother describe a 40-hour labor involving intolerable pain will dread the onset of labor, anticipating that she also will suffer intolerable pain. An additional way in which the pain experience is modified is through prior pain experiences. The individual who experiences migraine headaches, for example, often recognizes the preceding signs and symptoms and anticipates that the pain experience will equate or surpass prior episodes. Part of the pain experienced with migraines may be due to the fear of impending pain.

Assessment Tools. Because there is little correlation between one's physical appearance or facial expressions and the degree of pain experienced, assessment of pain depends primarily on subjective reporting. The nurse records the client's pain history, including the maximum, minimum, and typical amount of pain experienced. The nurse assesses what the client finds exacerbates the pain and what alleviates the pain. A standardized scale for pain assessment should be used, such as the visual analog scale (Figure 24-9) or the McGill-Melzack pain questionnaire. In addition, with chronic nonmalignant pain, the nurse assesses the client's premorbid and postmorbid lifestyle and the impact on lifestyle that the client perceives pain to have had.

A number of assessment tools are available that are designed specifically for assessing pain in children. The Wong-Baker Faces scale is used for both children and adults (Figure 24-10). The Wong-Baker scale has the advantage of clear visual identification of pain ratings across age, language, and comprehension continuums. Children may benefit from art, play, or music therapy as both assessment and intervention techniques. All approaches with children consider the total family system and family participation in child-centered goals.

Assessment and Management Mnemonics. Regardless of the specific pain assessment scale used, the rehabilitation nurse should use a system to ensure that all parameters of pain are assessed. A common mnemonic for pain assessment is shown in Box 24-6.

Another helpful mnemonic for pain assessment and management was developed by the Agency for Health Care Policy and Research (1994). The ABCs of pain management include:

- **A**sk about pain and assess for the presence of pain regularly and systematically
- **B**elieve what clients state about their pain experience
- **C**hoose appropriate pain control options
- **D**eliver timely, coordinated pain relief interventions
- **E**mpower and enable clients to take control over their pain relief measures

Nursing Diagnosis: Pain

Pain may be classified as chronic nonmalignant, acute, or chronic malignant (Katz, 1998). Acute and chronic malignant pain problems tend to follow a predictable course, whereas chronic nonmalignant pain follows an ill-defined

Categoric scale

0	No pain
1	Mild pain
2	Discomforting pain
3	Distressing pain
4	Horrible pain
5	Excruciating pain

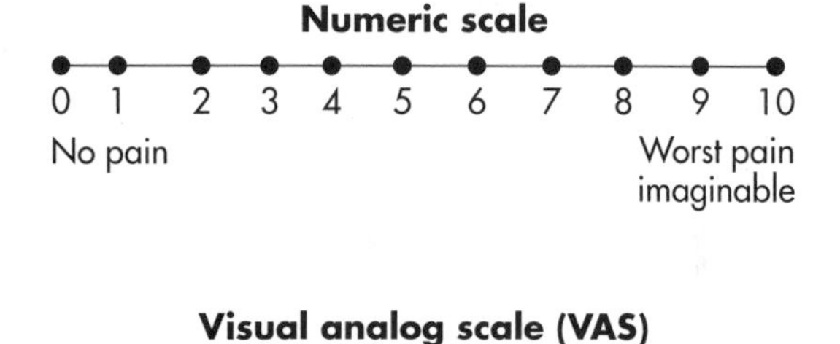

Visual analog scale (VAS)

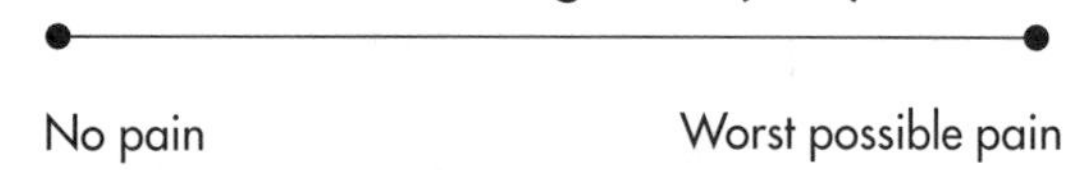

Figure 24-9 Pain intensity rating scales. (From Phipps, W., Sands, J., & Marek, J. [1999]. *Medical-surgical nursing: concepts and clinical practice.* St. Louis: Mosby.)

Box 24-6 PQRST Mnemonic for Pain Assessment

Palliative, provacative pain factors: What makes the pain better or worse?
Quality factors: How does the client describe the pain?
Radiating or region of the pain: Is the pain localized or does it radiate?
Severity of the pain: What is the intensity of the pain?
Temporal factors: When is the pain better or worse; does time of day matter?

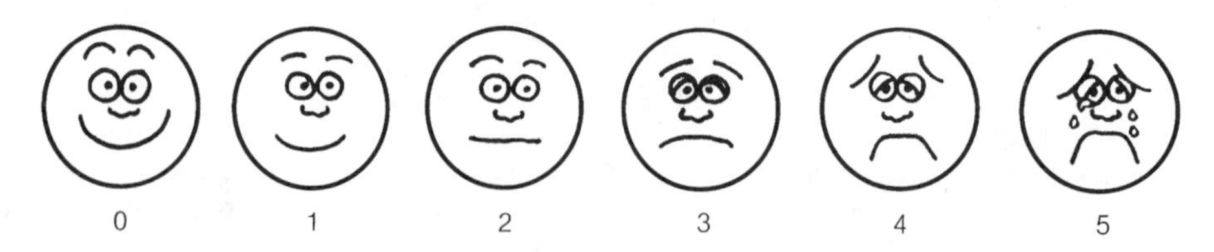

Figure 24-10 Faces pain rating scale. To use, explain to the child that each face is for a person who either feels happy because there is no pain (hurt) or feels sad because there is some or a lot of pain. Face 0 is very happy because there is no hurt. Face 1 hurts just a little bit. Face 2 hurts a little more. Face 3 hurts even more. Face 4 hurts a whole lot, but face 5 hurts as much as you can imagine, although you do not have to be crying to feel this bad. Ask the child to choose the face that best describes his or her own pain. Record the number under the chosen face on a pain assessment record. (From Wong, D.L., Hockenberry-Eaton, M., Wilson, D., Winkelstein, M.L., & Schwartz, P. [2001]. Wong's essentials of pediatric nursing [6th ed.]. St. Louis: Mosby.)

clinical course with an uncertain therapeutic outcome. Nursing diagnoses, nursing outcomes classifications, and nursing interventions classifications for pain are included in Table 24-10.

Pain as the Fifth Vital Sign. Regardless of classification of the type of pain experienced, the most common problem with pain is that of undertreatment and underrecognition. Dr. James Campbell (1995), during his presidential address to the American Pain Society, proposed that pain should be considered the fifth vital sign. According to Dr. Campbell, "Vital signs are taken seriously. If pain were assessed with the same zeal as other vital signs are, it would have a much better chance of being treated properly. We need to train doctors and nurses to treat pain as a vital sign. Quality care means that pain is measured and treated." The Joint Commission on Accreditation of Healthcare Organizations (JCAHO) (1999) reinforced Dr. Campbell's sentiments with an announcement that the JCAHO had revised standards to focus on pain management and assessment in all health care settings. The intent was to reinforce the client's right to pain assessment and management. The JCAHO standards have been endorsed by the American Pain Society.

Chronic Nonmalignant Pain. Although pain is a normal sensation, most persons believe they would be better off without it. Just the opposite is true, however, as demonstrated by the devastation of Hansen's disease, or leprosy. One of the key characteristics of Hansen's disease is the destruction of pain receptors, resulting in anesthesia. The prob-

TABLE 24-10 Nursing Diagnoses, Nursing Outcomes Classifications, and Nursing Interventions Classifications for Pain

Nursing Diagnosis	Suggested Nursing Outcomes Classification (NOC)	Suggested Nursing Interventions Classification (NIC)
Pain	Comfort level Pain control Pain: disruptive effects Pain level Symptom control Symptom severity Well-being	Analgesic administration Anxiety reduction Environmental management: control Heat/cold application Medication administration Medication management Pain management Active listening Animal-assisted therapy Autogenic training Bathing Biofeedback Coping enhancement Distraction Energy management Environmental management Exercise promotion Hope instillation Humor Hypnosis Medication facilitation Music therapy Oxygen therapy Positioning Presence Progressive muscle relaxation Security enhancement Simple guided imagery Simple massage Simple relaxation therapy Sleep enhancement Therapeutic play Therapeutic touch Vital signs monitoring

Data from Johnson, M., Maas, M.L., & Moorhead, S. (2000). *Nursing outcomes classification (NOC)* (2nd ed.). St. Louis: Mosby; McCloskey, J.C., & Bulechek, G.M. (2000). *Nursing interventions classification (NIC)* (3rd ed.). St. Louis: Mosby; and North American Nursing Diagnosis Association. (2001). *Nursing diagnosis: definitions and classification 2001-2002* (4th ed.). Philadelphia: Author.

lem, of course, is that persons with Hansen's disease fail to recognize tissue damage in time to prevent serious injury. Yancey (1977) described a client with Hansen's disease becoming blind because the eye surface did not detect irritation and the client did not perceive the need to blink, resulting in drying of the eyes. However, just as a complete absence of pain is life threatening, the unceasing presence of pain also is intolerable. Such is the case with chronic nonmalignant pain syndrome.

Chronic nonmalignant pain is a disorder of sensation that affects every aspect of an person's life: family, friends, work, and play. Although there is a wealth of literature on the syndrome, there is no consensus as to why some persons develop chronic nonmalignant pain syndrome and others with equivalent or even more physically severe injuries do not. One hypothesis is that a pain cycle develops and results in chronic nonmalignant pain syndrome. In response to injury the person protects and immobilizes the injured area, such as a joint. The immobilization of the area leads to the development of scar tissue around the site and a reduction in synovial fluid production. The joint becomes stiff and difficult to move, leading to increased pain, inflammation, and tendonitis. The person guards and immobilizes the joint to an even greater degree, with resulting weakness and loss of function. To continue guarding the area, the person develops compensatory mechanisms to protect the joint, such as limping and altering the gait. These compensatory mechanisms do not act in the body's favor, and the altered gait leads to back pain, resulting in more extensive guarding of multiple areas. The result is chronic presence of pain without a clear link to a pathophysiological problem.

Chronic nonmalignant pain interferes with vocational and avocational aspects of life. Time off from work due to therapy and medical appointments, illness, and loss of function results in poor attendance and difficulty maintaining a job. Complaints about the amount of pain experienced and restrictions of avocational activities lead to limited family and community involvement. Reductions in activity result in weight gain and decreased energy and endurance levels. As more and more money is spent looking for cures, causes, and relief, finances become exhausted. As the pain continues with no relief in sight, depression becomes a way of life. Persons with chronic nonmalignant pain have little reason to look forward to days filled with more and more pain; less and less function; and constant work, family, and financial problems. Such persons experience difficulties coping with their pain and may develop addictions to alcohol and narcotics. Eventually they reach the end of the medical therapeutic gamut and are depressed, are financially drained, have employment and family problems, and are in constant pain.

Given the pervasiveness of the problem of chronic nonmalignant pain, it is unlikely that any single modality of intervention will be effective in providing relief from the syndrome. Therefore programs having the greatest success provide a variety of interventions and use a comprehensive and multifaceted approach. Comprehensive programs for chronic nonmalignant pain usually involve a variety of disciplines, including but not limited to nursing, physical therapy, medicine, occupational therapy, vocational counseling, therapeutic recreation, and psychology.

Just as in other areas of rehabilitation, client education is a cornerstone of treatment for chronic nonmalignant pain. Self-application of local therapies such as ultrasound, transcutaneous electrical stimulation, and hot or cold packs may be of benefit and should be included in client education programs. A second component of client education for chronic nonmalignant pain is instruction in the use of nonpharmacological methods of pain relief such as biofeedback, relaxation, and self-hypnosis. Clients should be taught the use of work simplification and energy conservation methods but need to be encouraged to increase activity level gradually. The client should receive instructions in posture, body mechanics, and positioning. The program should include an assessment of workplace design and ergonomics.

Chronic Nonmalignant Pain across the Life Span. Persons in two age groups, the very young and the very old, tend to experience subtle discrimination with respect to chronic nonmalignant pain. Although more than 50 million children in the United States experience chronic nonmalignant pain, there is a paucity of health care resources for them. Health care professionals often underestimate the amount of pain experienced by children, and because many children are hesitant to talk to physicians and nurses, their pain may be underreported. The second age group in which persons are undertreated for chronic nonmalignant pain is the geriatric group. Many older person experience chronic nonmalignant pain due to chronic illness and disability, and they assume that it is a normal part of the aging process. Although few children or elderly persons require the comprehensiveness of a chronic nonmalignant pain management program, they will benefit from an open-minded approach toward alleviation and moderation of the pain experienced.

Common conditions for chronic nonmalignant pain in childhood include juvenile rheumatoid arthritis, sickle cell crises, recurrent headaches, recurrent abdominal pain from a variety of conditions, reflex sympathetic dystrophy syndrome, malignancies, and pain after multiple traumas or amputation. The impact of a child's pain on the family is part of the assessment.

Children with chronic, disabling, or developmental disorders must be assessed within the context of their developmental stage. Two variables contribute to difficulty in assessing pain in children: the expression of pain and the experience of pain. A child's experience and expression of pain will differ with the developmental stage, but more importantly, these cannot be equated with adult behaviors or judged using adult terms. A child who has prolonged chronic nonmalignant pain or whose pain worsens gradually may not be able to distinguish changes in pain intensity or determine duration and location of pain. Children may play or sleep through pain as ways of coping with discomfort. In fact, children may not refer to the pain as pain. A child's self-report of having no pain may not be reliable for a variety of reasons. For instance, some children may not be able to associate pain relief measures with improved comfort; others may assign themselves personal responsibility for the pain or believe they deserve punishment. For these reasons, it often is beneficial to ask a child who or what causes the pain and to describe and explain pain using the child's own words (Hoeman, 1990).

Older persons may try to ignore or bear their pain or conversely may complain about pain (Won et al., 1999). Those who are cognitively intact may not require any adaptations for pain assessment. However, impaired or altered sensory function, such as vision or hearing, and reduced sensation and perception may alter the pain experience. An older person may deny pain but guard movement or positioning, change patterns of ambulation, pace level of activity, or avoid painful activities without reporting pain. Often, older persons accept pain as a consequence of aging (Luggen, 1998). Those with cognitive or communication impairments may become frustrated, angry, or contentious because they cannot express or explain their pain. Additionally the elderly client may experience chronic but transient pain and describe it as discomfort, aches, or by such colloquial names as "old friend" or "rheumatiz," thus avoiding the nature of the pain. Older persons are at risk for undertreatment of pain due to their tendency to understate the amount of pain experienced or due an appearance of tolerating pain well (National Cancer Institute of the NIH, 1999). Management of pain experienced by older persons should include involving the client and family and providing them with control over the pain management tools and options selected (Luggen, 1998).

Pain is a multidimensional phenomenon. Even with the use of a comprehensive approach to pain management, the prognosis for persons with chronic nonmalignant pain is a long and hard fight for recovery and return to function, without any guarantees that pain will cease.

Malignant Pain. Pain from cancer may occur due to nerve compression, infection, and release of prostaglandins. Unlike chronic nonmalignant pain, the cornerstone of treatment for malignant pain is pharmacological. The guiding principles of narcotic use for malignant pain are matching dose to client response and giving the medication on a regular and consistent basis rather than on an as-needed basis. The World Health Organization (National Cancer Institute of the NIH, 1999) developed a ladder for pharmacological pain management that indicates the appropriate steps for managing increasing pain. The ladder progresses as noted in Figure 24-11.

Nonmalignant, Intermittent Pain. Pain that occurs on an irregular but severe basis, such as with sickle cell disease, typically is treated as acute pain. Nonpharmacological pain relief methods may be of benefit, but the primary mode of treatment is the use of medications to manage acute episodes.

Another type of nonmalignant pain is phantom limb pain, a natural consequence after the loss of a body part. Typically

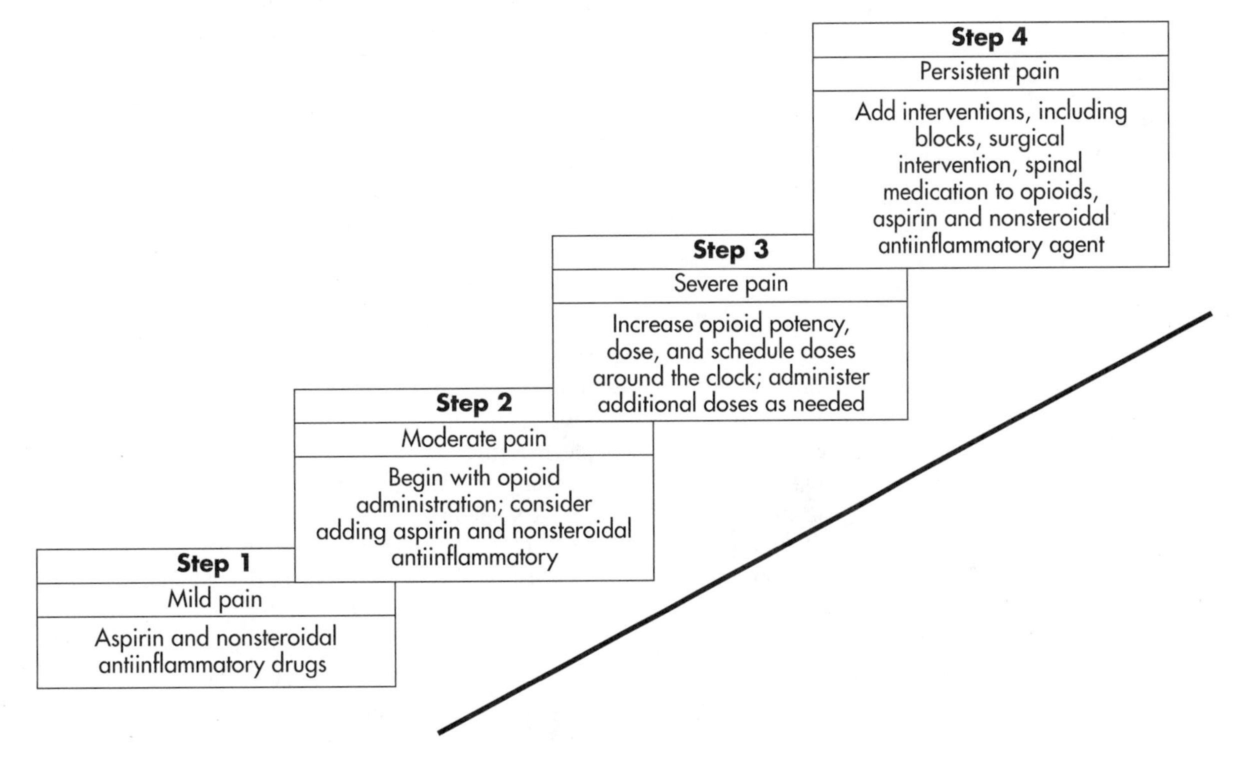

Figure 24-11 Modified, four-step pain ladder. (Modified from the World Health Organization. [1996]. *Cancer pain relief* [2nd ed.]. Geneva: Author.)

TABLE 24-11 Nonpharmacological Pain Management Tools

Method	Comments, Applications
Heat	Use caution in application of heat to prevent burns or tissue injury; temperature of the warm compress should be tested before application, and the site should be reassessed frequently
Cold	Flexible ice packs tend to work well and may assist in decreasing inflammation or swelling, cold treatments should not be applied for longer than 15 minutes and should not be used when peripheral vascular disease is present
Repositioning	Tendency to "fluff and puff" pillows can work well to assist an individual in pain in gaining a position of comfort
Exercise	Avoid exercise during acute pain, with the exception of range of motion; exercise may restore mobilization, coordination, and balance
Massage, pressure, and vibration	Provide physical stimulation and enhance relaxation
Relaxation and imagery	Used to augment other methods of pain relief or during procedures; may provide assistance during times of anxiety and fatigue
Cognitive distraction	Use of music, television, visiting, reading, or a focal point may reduce the focus on pain and provide relief for a limited time
Hypnosis	Used in conjunction with relaxation and visual imagery techniques; most effective when used with individuals whose concentration and motivation are strong
Transcutaneous electrical nerve stimulation	Low-voltage electrical impulse is relayed to peripheral muscle fibers through a device controlled by the person in pain; impulse is believed to function by "closing the gate" and blocking the pain impulse transmission
Acupuncture	Small needles are inserted, and electrical current may be used to block pain impulses; placement of the needles is designed through Eastern vital energy flow theory
Therapeutic touch	Whether through massage or a system such as Reike, can be beneficial in promoting relaxation and through stimulating large afferent fibers that may block transmission of pain impulses
Biofeedback	Tool through which electrical impulses or skin temperature is assessed as an index of relaxation; can be of benefit in educating patients how to relax
Aromatherapy	May be effective for pain reduction through stimulating descending pathways and providing distraction while enhancing relaxation
Herbal medicines	Many varieties; it is imperative that rehabilitation nurses educate patients that such medications do not go through FDA approval and may have harmful or no effects

FDA, Food and Drug Administration.

it does not present problems with therapeutic management, although on occasion individuals experience extreme phantom limb pain. Treatment for severe phantom limb problems usually follows the comprehensive approach used for management of chronic nonmalignant pain.

Implications for Rehabilitation

Because pain is a unique experience for all individuals, it is unlikely that any single solution will be effective for all. Therefore it makes sense that there should be variety of tools available for those experiencing pain. Table 24-11 contains a listing of nonpharmacological tools for pain management. Although many of these nonpharmacological pain management methods work for some individuals, it is important to note that there is a lack of evidence-based practice to validate the methods. They will work for some and not for others; however, it is important for persons in pain to have choices, and it is critical that rehabilitation nurses provide educated options for their clients in pain.

Pain is an example of a normal sensation that is perceived uniquely by individuals. The response to pain is both automatic and learned. Children who touch a hot stove will remove their fingers automatically and will learn not to touch hot stoves. A similar learned response to perception of other sensations occurs. In addition, individuals learn how to organize and process sensory input. Because we are constantly bombarded with sensory stimulation, we must select to which stimuli we will respond. Individuals adapt to different environments and learn alternative methods of organizing and processing sensory input in those environments. For example, the smell of smoke outside on a fall day is processed as an insignificant and pleasant olfactory stimulation. The same smoke smell indoors triggers quite a different response. Consider a hospital setting, with all its associated noises, sights, and smells (e.g., paging, footsteps, medication, food carts, alcohol, and cleansers). Although such an environment is not novel to health care professionals, it is novel to the clients we serve. Even clients with intact neurological systems may have difficulty organizing and processing the sensory input associated with a hospital setting. When clients have impaired sensation and perception, their ability to organize and make sense of their environment may be limited severely.

CRITICAL THINKING

Frank has two great loves in life: food and his work (see Case Study below. He explains to his nurse that, for him, giving up food would be like giving up on life. In short, he would rather die than diet. Frank enjoys tasting different foods and shows a preference for high-fat, high-carbohydrate foods. Frank is aware that his love for food is unhealthy, but he points out that his health will continue to worsen, even if he diets, and then the quality of his life will be low. Would you work with Frank to motivate him toward compliance with a restricted diet? If so, what strategies could you use that incorporate the senses that Frank has that remain intact?

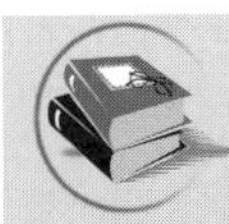

Case Study — *Client with Multiple Sclerosis*

Assessment

Frank is a 56-year-old man admitted for acute rehabilitation after an exacerbation of multiple sclerosis. Frank is weak and uses a power chair for mobility. His rehabilitation progress is complicated by his weight of more than 500 lb. Frank is employed through a government office that services individuals needing medical assistance, and he is able to maintain employment when not hospitalized. His employers (the state government) are accepting of Frank's physical limitations and of his need for medical care.

Frank has many of the complications associated with multiple sclerosis, including severe weakness of the lower extremities with no functional ambulatory ability, paresthesias of the lower extremities and hands, and urinary retention requiring an indwelling catheter. During his admission, Frank has an ophthalmology consultation and receives and additional diagnosis of optic neuritis and severe optic nerve atrophy resulting in a significant loss of vision.

Frank is placed on a rehabilitation program including therapeutic exercise and practice with activities of daily living. Frank is angry with the prognosis of eventual blindness. He refuses to participate in therapy sessions and verbally abuses many of the therapists. The team members are frustrated with his lack of progress, and his response to the new diagnosis of vision impairment threatens even the limited progress Frank has made. The team members suggest transfer to a skilled nursing level of care. During evening care, Frank breaks down emotionally and begins crying. He says that if transferred to a nursing home, he will lose his job, which is the one thing remaining in his life that gives him a purpose to continue to try.

Nursing Diagnosis and Goals

The nursing diagnosis of uncompensated loss of visual acuity due to optic neuritis is made (Gordon, 2000). The nurse works with Frank to establish the following mutual goals:

- Frank will participate in all scheduled therapy sessions for the remainder of his acute rehabilitation stay
- Frank will verbalize his frustrations with his caregivers to enable them to support him as possible and to provide him with an outlet for his frustrations
- Team members will assess the work environment to identify means of providing Frank with necessary adaptations
- Frank will participate in identifying feasible adaptations to his environment
- Team members will work toward a discharge to a facility close to Frank's office, where accessible transportation will be available

Interventions

The interventions for Frank were established with the team members and with Frank. The key to attaining a successful outcome with Frank was cohesive teamwork between the nurses and therapists. To prevent team splitting and friction, twice-daily team meetings were established. A brief meeting of the therapists and Frank's primary nurse was held each morning to assess any changes from the preceding night and to determine the strategy for the day. In late afternoon the therapists met with the evening nurse to review progress made and to discuss any incidents or issues noted. The evening nurse had a strong rapport with Frank and would spend uninterrupted time with Frank during evening care to promote his verbalization of concerns and progress.

Frank received education on the use of his power chair with limited vision. Frank learned to run the chair at slower speeds and to be cautious of objects in his pathway. The long-range plan was to provide a personal care assistant when Frank's vision no longer provided him with any functional acuity.

Frank received education on the use of materials for low vision, including magnifying glasses for writing and reading. He was able to use field glasses for distance vision. The occupational therapist provided him with a modification of the field glasses for use while in his power chair.

Frank's office was assessed and adapted with custom lighting to improve the lighting contrast possible in the room. A special desk lamp was purchased for reading to provide an increased contrast between print and background. Frank also learned to use a reading rectangle for reading focus.

Implementation and Evaluation

After two months of rehabilitation and an exhaustive search for a nursing home capable of meeting Frank's needs for bariatric equipment, visual modifications, and proximity to his work setting, Frank was discharged.

After his discharge, Frank returned to work within a week. The occupational therapist was able to make a visit to Frank's office to assess the efficacy of the completed adaptations. Two weeks after his discharge, two of Frank's nurses visited Frank in his office. Frank reported feeling positive about the adjustment to the new environment, although his missed the therapists and nurses. Although Frank's rehabilitation plan did not have the outcome of increased functional capacity or physical endurance, it was successful in meeting Frank's goal of discharge into the community with return to work.

REFERENCES

Agency for Health Care Policy and Research. (1994). *Management of cancer pain: quick reference guide for clinicians* (AHCPR Publication No. 94-0593). Washington, DC: U.S. Department of Health and Human Services.

American Speech-Language-Hearing Association. (2000). *Newborn and infant hearing screening action center.* Rockville, MD: Author.

Apple, D. (1999). Harold Ridley, MA, MD, FRCS: a golden anniversary celebration and a golden age. *Archives of Ophthalmology, 117,* 827-282.

Briner, H., & Simmen, D. (1999). Smell diskettes as screening test of olfaction. *Rhinology, 37*(4), 145-148.

Bromley, S. (2000). Smell and taste disorders: a primary care approach. *American Family Physician, 61*(2), 427-436.

Campbell, J. (1995, November 11). *Presidential address.* Los Angeles: American Pain Society.

Cooper, N. (1998). The chemical senses. *Exploring biopsychology: topics and perspectives.* Denver: University of Colorado.

Duffy, V., Cain, W., & Ferris, A. (1999). Measurement of sensitivity to olfactory flavor: application in a study of aging and dentures. *Chemical Senses, 24*(6), 671-677.

Feller, L. (1999, August 1). With implant, she doesn't miss a beat. *The New York Times: Sunday Connecticut Weekly Desk.*

Gallaudet University (1999). States that recognize American sign language. *Info to Go, Gallaudet University.* Washington, DC: Author.

Glenn, A. (1997). *H. L. Mencken.* www.chesco.com/~artman/mencken.html.

Gordon, M. (2000). *Manual of nursing diagnosis* (9th ed.). St. Louis: Mosby.

HearingLossWeb. (2000). *Hearing loss web.* www.hearinglossweb.com.

Hinze, H., DeLeon, C., & Mitchell, W. (1999). Dentists at high risk for hearing loss: protection with custom earplugs. *General Dentistry, 47*(6), 600-605.

Hoeman, S.P. (1990, October 5). Chronic pain in childhood. *Keynote presentation of Caring for Persons in Pain Workshop.* Reading, PA: Alvernia College.

Homoe, P., Christensen, R., & Bretlau, P. (1999). Acute otitis media and sociomedical risk factors among unselected children in Greenland. *International Journal of Pediatric Otorhinolaryngology, 49*(1), 37-52.

Inoue, Y., Kanzaki, J., Ogawa, K., Hoya, N., Takei, S., & Shiobara, R. (2000). The long-term outcome of hearing preservation following vestibular schwannoma surgery. *Auris Nasus Larynx, 27*(1), 9-13.

Joint Commission on Accreditation of Healthcare Organizations. (1999). Joint Commission focuses on pain management (On-line Press Release). Available:
http://www.pain.com/news/jcaho_standards_professionals.cfm.

Kalish, R. (1999). Randomized trial of aromatherapy: Successful treatment for alopecia areata. *Archives of Dermatology, 135*(5).

Katz, W. (1998). The needs of a patient in pain. *American Journal of Medicine, 105*(1B), 2S-7S.

Kuyk, T., & Elliott, J. (1999). Visual factors and mobility in persons with age-related macular degeneration. *Journal of Rehabilitation Research and Development, 36*(4), 303-312.

Low Vision Council. (2000). *Making vision rehabilitation a national priority.* Available: http://www.lowvisioncouncil.org/index/html. New York: Low Vision Council.

Luggen, A. (1998). Chronic pain in older adults. A quality of life issue. *Journal of Gerontological Nursing, 24*(2), 48-54.

McCaffery, M., & Ferrell, B. (1995). Nurses' knowledge about cancer pain: A survey of five countries. *Journal of Pain and Symptom Management, 10*(5), 356-369.

McCaffery, M., & Ferrell, B. (1997). Influence of professional versus personal role on pain assessment and use of opioids. *Journal of Continuing Education in Nursing, 28*(2), 69-77.

Magdziarz, D., Wiet, R., Dinces, E., Adamiec, L. (2000). Normal audiologic presentations in patients with acoustic neuroma: an evaluation using strict audiologic parameters. *Otolaryngology–Head and Neck Surgery, 122*(2), 157-162.

Mayer, N. (1999, July 31). "Do you hear mama's voice?" A cochlear implant brings a 5-year-old girl the hope of hearing. *Portland Oregonian.*

Merck. (2000). Ophthalmologic disorders. *Merck manual.* Whitehouse Station, NJ: Author.

Narrin, J. (1996/2000). *Reiki and four building blocks for the future.* Seattle: One Degree Beyond: Next Step © Project.

National Cancer Institute of the National Institutes of Health. (1999). *Supportive care information for health professionals: pain* (On-line). Available: http://cancernet.nce.nih.gov/clinpdq/supportive/Pain (last modified August 1999).

National Institutes of Health. (2000). *Cochlear implants* (Publication No. 00-4798). Washington, DC: Author.

National Institutes of Health. (1993, March 1-3). Early identification of hearing impairment in infants and young children. *NIH Consensus Statement Online, 11*(1):1-24.

Pehoushek, J., & Norton, S. (2000). Black taste buds. *Archives of Family Medicine, 9*(3), 594-595, 597-598.

Pulec, J., & Deguine, C. (1999). Otoscopic clinic: tuberculous chronic otitis media. *Ear, Nose and Throat Journal, 78*(11), 820.

Quattrociocchi, T. (2000). Personal communication on the use and applications of assistive technology for individuals with visual and auditory limitations.

Rosa, L., Rosa, E., Sarner, L., & Barrett, S. (1998). A close look at therapeutic touch. *Journal of the American Medical Association, 279,* 1005-1010.

Stathis, S., O'Callaghan, D., Williams, G., Najman, J., Andersen, M., & Bor, W. (1999). Maternal cigarette smoking during pregnancy is an independent predictor for symptoms of middle ear disease at five years' postdelivery. *Pediatrics, 104*(2), e16.

Stoney, S., & Jackson, W. (1999). Brain function. In T. Nosek (Ed.), *Essentials of human physiology.* Atlanta: Gold Standard Multimedia Inc. and Medical College of Georgia.

Strickland, L. (1999, June 4. Sound barrier: deaf girl from Kosovo gains hearing through Dallas surgery. *Dallas Morning News.*

University of Washington, Department of Neurological Surgery. (2000). *Treatment of acoustic neuroma.* Seattle: Author.

U.S. Department of Health and Human Services. (2000). *Healthy People 2010: understanding and improving health.* Washington, DC: Author.

Wall, P. (1999). Introduction. In P. Wall & R. Melzack (Eds.), *Textbook of pain* (4th ed., pp. 1-12). Philadelphia: WB Saunders.

Winkler, S., Garg, A., Mekayarajjananonth, T., Bakaeen, L., & Khan, E. (1999). Depressed taste and smell in geriatric patients. *Journal of the American Dental Association, 130*(12), 1759-1765.

Won, A., Lapane, K., Gambassi, G., Bernabei, R., Mor, V., & Lipsitz, L. (1999). Correlates and management of nonmalignant pain in the nursing home. *Journal of the American Geriatric Society, 47,* 936-942.

Yancey, P. (1977). *Where is God when it hurts?* Grand Rapids, MI: The Zondervan Corp.

Zak, O. (1996). *Cochlear implants protest in France.* www.zak.co.il/deaf-info/old/ci-france.html.

Communication: Language and Pragmatics 25

Barbara J. Boss, PhD, RN, CFNP, CANP
Billie R. Phillips, RN, MSN

A 58-year-old woman living in a rural community in the South was admitted to the neurology service of a major teaching hospital because of sudden loss of her previously intact ability to understand and use language. Her husband discovered her at home speaking a nonsense language, unable to speak meaningfully or understand speech. Her family brought her to the medical center.

She had an unremarkable medical history, had no diagnosed health problems, was taking no medication, and was well when last seen by her family and neighbor the previous day. Her physical examination findings were completely within normal limits except for a dense Wernicke's aphasia at the time of admission. She did not understand any verbal or written language. She comprehended gestures, facial expression, pantomime, and body language. She initially spoke, but the language made no sense (nonsense language). Soon, however, she realized that her words were not being understood, and she spoke less and relied more and more on gestures, pictures, drawing, and other nonverbal communication. Her frustration increased day by day. She began to say "it is so frustrating," often repeating this phrase several times and shaking her head no. This was the only intelligible language output she recovered.

Because aphasia was her only observable problem, her family could not understand what had happened to her. It was incomprehensible to them that she had had a stroke. They believed that stroke paralyzed individuals and made them bedridden. They viewed her problem as "having lost her mind." Several months later, the family committed her to a state mental institution, believing she had become psychotic. The inability to effectively communicate with the family and thus help this patient drove our interest and commitment to study and develop an expertise in language and pragmatics.

Communication is more than talk. Communication is a rich and complex social activity involving linguistic, cognitive, and pragmatic competence. Linguistic competence is the ability to form and use symbols. Language is the symbolic signal system used by a person to communicate with others. Effective language involves many processes: development of thoughts to be communicated; selection, formulation, and ordering of words; application of rules of grammar; and initiation of muscle movements to produce speech or written output. Speech output also requires control of respiration to produce the required sounds and verbalization. Individuals listen to or look at their language output, evaluate the output, and correct the language when necessary. Language, speech, and writing provide individuals with a well-ordered, rule-bound system of communication. But communication is more than language. Pragmatic competence is the ability to use language appropriately in situational and social contexts and involves all nonlanguage aspects of communication. Cognitive competence is required for communication to be relevant, to be accurate, and to evidence clear thinking. All aspects of communication are active processes, initially learned within the family and deeply influenced by culture.

A working knowledge of the types of communication deficits helps rehabilitation nurses recognize and assess communication deficits experienced by their clients. This knowledge is invaluable in planning appropriate therapeutic interventions to assist with communication and helps the nurse appreciate the prognosis for recovery, which is fundamental to facilitating the client and family in their adaptation and coping.

LINGUISTICS

Linguistic or language competence involves the comprehension and transmission of ideas and feelings by use of conventionalized marks and sounds and the sequential ordering of them according to accepted rules of grammar. This concept involves at least three subcompetencies: phonological competence, semantic competence, and syntactic competence. *Phonology* is the process of recovery of the phonological formation of a word, that is, ordering the sounds used to form the words (e.g., "wa gon" versus "gon wa"). *Semantics* refers to the ability to relate a symbol or sign to an object, that is, applying the correct meaning to words; it is the use of nominal words (substantive words). *Syntax* is the grammatical structure in language production and refers to the rules for interrelating words or ordering statements. Appropriate application of plurality and tense also is involved.

Language Acquisition

Skinner advanced the theory that language is learned through reinforcement by the environment when spontaneous sounds of the infant that resemble adult speech are encouraged by the caretaker (family). Chomsky challenged this traditional theory that human beings innately possess the capability for language acquisition.

Most recent theoretic explanations of language acquisition are multifactorial. Wexler used an innateness/maturational approach to explain linguistic development. Harkness proposed a cultural model that incorporated the innatist view but also focused on experiences within cultural context. Zukow took a socioperceptual/ecological position founded in the belief that the dynamic structure of the social-interactive environment in which the child develops is central to language acquisition. Dent argued for a functionalist approach in which language development is not rooted in the child or the language environment but rather in perceptual systems that detect language-world relationships and guide attention and action. Language development requires attention and memory (Bower, 1998b).

Research in the past 30 years has established a genetic, neuroanatomical, and functional basis for many language disorders, and a few theorists argue against the contribution of the neural system to language development. Recent research on syntactic ability and vocabulary size in 15- to 48-month-old children with unilateral antepartum or perinatal brain injury suggests that both cerebral hemispheres make critical contributions in the earliest stages of language acquisition.

The role of babbling in language development has received recent attention, and research with tracheotomized infants suggests that the audibility of babbling and early language may contribute to later language development (Hill & Singer, 1990; Locke & Pearson, 1990). Locke and Pearson asserted that links between babbling and speech support the role of innate factors and central control mechanisms in language development. Neural capabilities provide the child with control over initial speechlike movements and direct attention to salient linguistic patterns. Masataka (1998) found that infants preferentially focus on their mother baby talk, which he believed provides the perceptual building blocks of babbling. Rovee-Collier (1997) and Hartshorn et al. (1998) have demonstrated that brain mechanisms exist that enable a 3-month-old to learn and remember serial position, an essential capacity for learning language.

Language Development

Language development requires the substitution of a series of sounds or marks for objects, persons, and concepts and is similar across racial, cultural, and socioeconomic groups (Adams, Victor, & Ropper, 1997). The first stage of language development is the infantile languageless phase, in which there is inability to comprehend or produce language. The newborn initially vocalizes reflexively by crying to indicate discomfort. Around 2 months of age, the infant experiments with various sounds and vowel sounds emerge. As early as 3 to 4 months of age, the consonants *b, g, k, n,* and *p* are heard in infant language. Cooing, gurgling, laughing, babbling, and repeating alternating consonant and vowel sounds, such as *dadada,* begin around 4 months of age. Around 8 months the consonants *d, t,* and *w* appear (Wong et al., 1999). Repetition of heard sounds, or lalling, begins between 6 and 9 months and progresses until intonations approximate adult speech at 1 year. By 12 months of age the infant attends to words. By 1 year of age, infants use three to five words with meaning.

In second stage of language development, there is auditory comprehension of language, but oral communication is fragmentary, ineffective, and contextually meaningless. One-word sentences (holophrases) are possible, and 25% of speech is intelligible. Between 12 and 18 months of age, the toddler begins to use words intentionally and demonstrates behavior that indicates developing understanding of words in context.

By 21 months the child says single words with meaning, evidencing the beginning of the third stage of language development: the use of substantive words, called *semantics.* Between 18 and 24 months the child's vocabulary grows from 20 to 100 words and consists primarily of free morphemes, the smallest form of sound that possesses meaning (e.g., "go, bye, me, eat"). Toddlers learn as many as nine new words per day (Bower, 1998b).

By 24 months, the toddler should be using 2- and 3-word combinations to express needs and ideas (e.g., "me go bye-bye"). Between 2 and 3 years of age, the child's vocabulary expands to approximately 300 words, predominantly nouns and verbs, 65% of which are intelligible by the end of the third year. By 3 years of age, the child talks in sentences. All vowels should be mastered by 3 years of age. During the third and fourth years, vocabulary expands rapidly from 900 to 1500 words with increasing use of pronouns, adverbs, and adjectives. Consonant mastery continues to occur in a hierarchical fashion with *s, z, sh, ch,* and *j* being the last sounds to be mastered, at around 7 or 8 years of age. Consonants *m* and *h* are mastered early, and *w* may be substituted for *l* and *r* (e.g. "wice" for "rice" or "wook" for "look"). By 4 to 5 years of age the child uses fully intelligible speech; *f* and *v* are mastered, but *r, l, s, z, sh, ch, yt,* and *th* may still be distorted. By 6 years of age, *r, l,* and *th* are mastered.

The final and highest stage of language development is the ability to apply the rules of grammar to language, called *syntax.*

Linguistic competence does not appear to decline with normal aging. Linguistic disintegration is evidence of a presence of a pathological process.

Three levels of language production/availability (levels of intention) also are described:

1. Automatic language: the basic level of language output consisting of habitual responses such as prayers, social responses, curses, and songs
2. Imitation (language heard before): a higher level of language output that requires the person to hear what is said, process the messages, produce the appropriate response, and evaluate the context of the transmission (e.g., repeat after me, "no ifs, ands, or buts")
3. Symbolic language: the highest level of language produced without the benefit of a model and expression of one's own choice (language or original intention); it involves the use of words with the correct meaning, application or rules for ordering sounds and words, and use of appropriate tense and plurality (e.g., "I want to describe for you how my reading difficulty is affecting my life; this has been very hard to deal with")

Neuroanatomy and Neurophysiology Related to Linguistics

The left hemisphere's mediation of language function in nearly all persons regardless of handedness is well accepted. The primary neuroanatomical structures involved with language competence are Wernicke's area, the angular gyrus, and Broca's area (Figure 25-1). The angular gyrus at the temporoparietal occipital junction is thought to link the visual impression of an object carried via the primary visual cortex and visual association areas of the occipital and posterior temporal lobes to the spoken word carried via the primary auditory cortex and auditory association areas. After the initial linkage is made, when the name if registered by the auditory areas, it is transmitted to Wernicke's area for recognition of the sound patterns of the word. This stimulates the angular gyrus, evoking a visual memory of the seen object.

Brain imaging studies consistently remind researchers and clinicians that this is an oversimplification (Posner & Raichle, 1994). The language network is complex and involves many regions of the brain (Neville & Bavelier, 1998; Neville, Bavelier, Corina, Rauschecker, Karni, Lalwani, Braun, Clark, Jezzard, & Turner, 1998; Peterson, Fox, Posner, Mintun, & Raichle, 1998) (Figure 25-2). For example, in the past several years, the cerebellum, in particular, the neodentate of the dentate nucleus, has been linked to word-selection tasks. Bavelier et al. (1998) have demonstrated that not only the left Broca's area, Wernicke's are, and the angular gyrus, but also the superior temporal lobes bilaterally and the left frontal cortex, increase activity on reading sentences in English. Additionally individual variation was found among subjects. Hirsch and Kim (1997) found that, in learning a second language, adults and children use the same Wernicke's area, but adults who learn a second language use a different region in Broca's area for each language, whereas children use the same region for both languages. Interestingly Nishimura et al. (1999) demonstrated that the secondary region of the auditory cortex is activated when deaf persons interpret sign language, which argues for

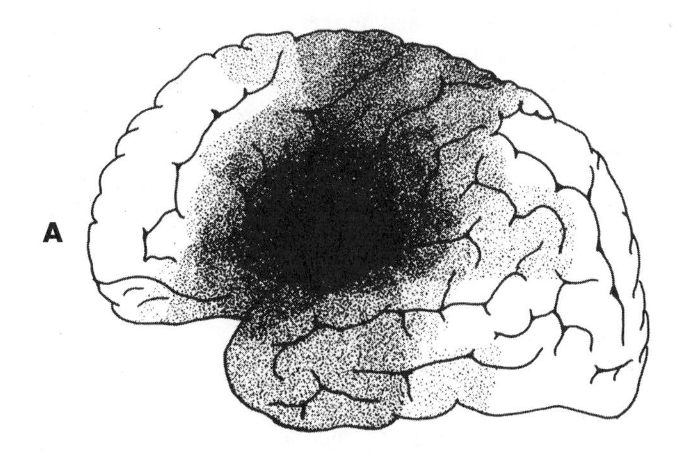

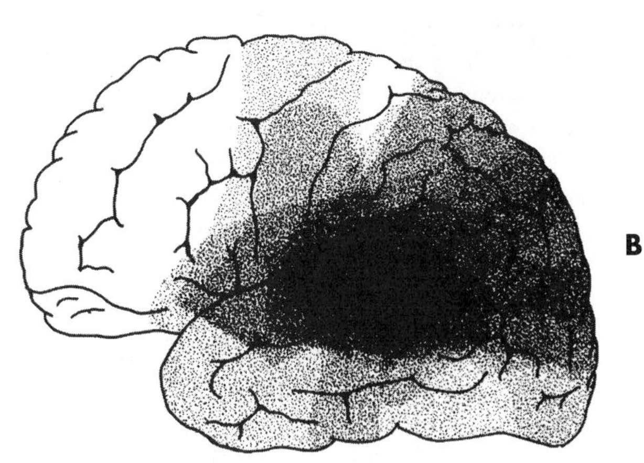

Figure 25-1 Sites of damage causing Broca's or Wernicke's aphasia. **A,** Areas infarcted in 14 clients, all diagnosed as suffering from Broca's aphasia, were determined by radioisotope brain scan (which measures leakage from damaged capillaries in an area of infarct). All 14 lesions were then superimposed, indicating a focus of damage in the posterior part of the left inferior frontal gyrus. **B,** Areas infarcted in 13 clients, all diagnosed as suffering from Wernicke's aphasia, were determined by radioisotope brain scan. All 13 lesions were then superimposed, indicating a focus of damage in the posterior part of the left superior temporal gyrus. (From Kertesz, A., Lesk, D., & McCabe, P. [1977]. Isotope localization of infarcts in aphasia. *Archives of Neurology, 34,* 590.)

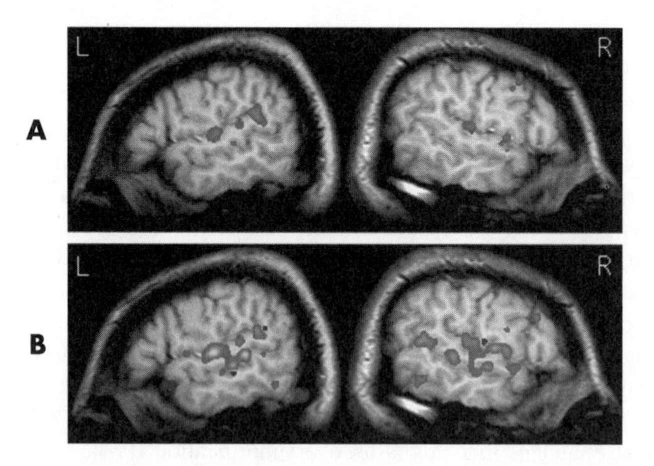

Figure 25-2 Functional magnetic resonance imaging demonstration of the human auditory and visual cortex. Functional magnetic resonance imaging data from a 30-year-old man listening to white noise **(A)** and to spoken words **(B)** were superimposed on T_1-weighted parasagittal slices of his left *(L)* and right *(R)* hemispheres. Both stimuli activate the superior temporal gyrus, but spoken words activate a more extensive area of the gyrus. (From Binder, J.R., Rao, S.M., Hammeke, T.A., Yetkin, F.Z., Jesmanowicz, A., Bandettini, P.A., Wong, E.C., Estkowski, L.D., Goldstein, M.D., Haughton, V.M., et al. [1994]. Functional magnetic resonance imaging of human auditory cortex. *Annals of Neurology, 35,* 662.)

the brain's ability to recruit one area for use by another sensory modality.

Linguistic Deficits

Aphasia is the loss or impairment of a previously established capacity for comprehension and/or formulation of language caused by injury to the brain (Benson & Ardila, 1996). There is a phonetic, semantic, and/or syntactic disintegration at the production and/or comprehension level of communication. The language dysfunction is manifested by incorrect word sounds, incorrect choice of words, or incorrect grammar. For infants and young children, a linguistic deficit is called a *language delay.* For older children a linguistic deficit is referred to as a *developmental language disorder* or *developmental aphasia.* The process underlying linguistic deficits in adults or children is not known.

The history of modern aphasiology dates back to Broca, who correlated the clinical picture of individuals with the location of the anatomical lesion. Despite critics who argued that there was only one type of aphasia—a general disturbance of language produced by injury—this localization approach dominated the field until after World War I, when a holistic view gained predominance. Since the mid-1960s, with improved imaging techniques, most researchers and clinicians have returned to a modified localization viewpoint. Therefore one of the useful classification systems for the aphasias, based on the neuroanatomical localization of the lesions, names the aphasias using anatomical terms (Table 25-1). A linguistic classification of aphasia is given in Table 25-2.

Broca's Aphasia

Broca's aphasia reflects a loss of syntax (agrammatism) due to damage in and around Broca's area. The person has impoverished syntax, short utterances, and a tendency to delete inflections or other grammatical forms. Contradictory research data related to linguistic deficits have led some aphasiologists to suggest agrammatism represents several different deficits. Some persons with Broca's aphasia appear to have a disorder of omission of structural form and simplification of the grammatical structure of speech production but retain the ability to understand syntactic relations and to use this understanding to analyze intended sentences. Other persons appear to have a central disorder affecting appreciation of syntactic relations in all modalities. Still other persons appear to have intact syntactic comprehension; written production is intact, and only verbal output is affected. In addition to the communication deficit, right-sided hemiplegia is present, with little use of the right arm and limited use of the right leg. Usually, facial apraxia and ideomotor apraxia of the left arm to verbal commands also are present.

Wernicke's Aphasia

In contrast, Wernicke's aphasia represents a semantic problem due to damage to Wernicke's area. The person is unable to understand verbal language. Interestingly understanding of axial (truncal, whole body) commands such as "stand up" or "turn around" often is intact. However, extremity commands such as "point to the door" are not understood. Reading comprehension and writing are seriously impaired, although one may be more impaired than the other. Related to language production, the output is fluent, that is, a normal or above normal number of words per minute. There is ease of language production and normal phase length. Articulation is normal, as are melody and inflection qualities. Syntax (grammar) is normal, but semantics are abnormal. Words lack specific meaning, and little information is communicated. Nonspecific words such as *it, thing,* and *us* are used. There is a tendency to use both verbal and semantic paraphasia—that is, substitution of one word for another (e.g., "The car would spit sweetly down the road" instead of "The car sped swiftly down the road")—and to a lesser extent, phonetic or literal paraphasia—that is, a phonetic substitution (e.g., "mesatence is instans" instead of "persistence is essential"), as well as nonsense or nonexistent words, called *neologisms* (e.g., "logper" for "plant") (Boss, 1984a). Repetition and naming are impaired. To communicate with this person, one must depend on facial expressions, gestures, pantomime, and tone of voice. In addition to the communication deficit, sensory loss may be present. If a visual field cut is present, it is usually a superior quadrantanopia caused by involvement of the pathway in the temporal lobe. The person may show a lack of concern, especially early after

TABLE 25-1 Clinical Features of Aphasias

Aphasias	Spontaneous Speech	Auditory Comprehension	Repetition	Naming	Reading	Writing
Broca's	Nonfluent	Preserved	Impaired	Often impaired	Impaired	Impaired
Wernicke's	Fluent, paraphrasic	Impaired	Impaired	Impaired	Impaired	Impaired
Conduction	Fluent, paraphrasic	Preserved	Impaired	Often impaired	Preserved	Impaired
Global	Nonfluent	Impaired	Impaired	Preserved	Impaired	Impaired
Aphemia (apraxia)	Nonfluent	Preserved	Impaired	Impaired	Preserved	Preserved
Pure word deafness	Fluent	Impaired	Impaired	Preserved	Preserved	Preserved
Transcortical motor	Nonfluent	Preserved	Preserved	Impaired	Preserved	Impaired
Transcortical sensory	Fluent, paraphrasic	Impaired	Preserved	Impaired	Impaired	Impaired
Mixed transcortical	Nonfluent	Impaired	Preserved	Impaired	Impaired	Impaired
Anomic	Fluent	Preserved	Preserved	Impaired	Occasional impairment	Often impaired

Adapted from M-M. Mesulam (Ed.), *Principles of behavioral neurology.* Philadelphia: FA Davis. Copyright by FA Davis. Adapted by permission.

TABLE 25-2 Linguistic Classification of Aphasia

Aphasias	Distinguishing Features
Syntactic aphasia (loss of grammatical function of language)	Simplified, concrete, often telegraphic speech Little use of connective speech elements Tense and gender may be used improperly Use of substantive words intact
Semantic aphasia (inability to relate the symbol to the object)	Restriction of vocabulary present Circumlocution is dominant Grammatical form may be intact
Pragmatic aphasia (breakdown in regulating function of language; inability to obtain meaning from stimuli and to use such stimuli as a basis for symbol formation)	Disoriented speech with paraphasia, meaningless neologisms Errors in language are not recognized by person
Jargon aphasia (profusion of phonetically disorganized combinations of language elements without understanding of person)	Babbling, noncommunicative speech Reading and writing impaired
Global aphasia (lack of linguistic ability); inability to form verbal symbols for use or incomprehension	Speechless generally Little response to environmental stimuli Automatic speech and echolalia may be present

sustaining the injury. Paranoid behavior more commonly is seen later, after injury.

Conductive Aphasia

Conductive aphasia, currently recognized as more common than previously thought, involves a striking repetition problem. The language output is fluent. Literal paraphasia is more common than verbal paraphasia or neologism. Naming is impaired mostly due to the literal paraphasia problem. Reading aloud also is impaired. Writing may be less impaired but contains spelling errors, omitted words, and altered letter and word sequencing. Verbal comprehension is relatively intact. The pathology producing conductive aphasia is in the supramarginal gyrus and/or in the area adjacent to the arcuate fasciculus. With conductive aphasia, paresis or a visual field cut also may be present. A cortical sensory loss involving position sense and stereognosis—that is, the ability to recognize forms of objects by touch—is common.

Pure Word Deafness

Pure word deafness manifests as an inability to comprehend verbal language. Repetition also is seriously impaired. Earlier after injury, there may be some degree of paraphasia in the person's language production, but the output is fluent. Reading and writing are intact, and ability to name is adequate. A superior quadrantanopia—that is, loss of vision in one fourth of the visual field—may be present. Pathologically the left auditory association is isolated from receiving auditory input.

Global Aphasia

Global (total) aphasia involves a striking inability to understand verbal and written language and to write. Naming and repetition are seriously impaired, and the person is nonfluent. Global aphasia often is accompanied by right-sided hemiplegia. Persistent global aphasia involves damage to a large area of the frontal and parietotemporal language areas.

Transcortical Aphasias

If repetition is intact despite other language comprehension and/or production deficit, transcortical aphasia is present. There are three types of transcortical aphasias: motor, sensory, and mixed.

When aphasia resembles Broca's aphasia but repetition is intact, transcortical motor aphasia is present. Transcortical motor aphasia often is accompanied by hemiplegia. Hemisensory loss and/or visual field loss may be present. The area of damage may be anterior to Broca's area or to the supplementary motor area (SMA), and its pathways cause a disconnection of the SMA from Broca's area.

When aphasia resembles Wernicke's aphasia but repetition is intact, transcortical sensory aphasia is present. The syndrome often is accompanied by agitation. The area of damage is the border zone of the parietotemporal junction, which is at the end of the arterial supply. Often the middle and lower temporal gyri are damaged also.

When aphasia resembles global aphasia but repetition is intact, the disorder is called *mixed transcortical aphasia* or *isolated speech area.* In this rarely occurring aphasia, the person does not speak unless spoken to and then echoes (repeats) what the other person says. The perisylvian language areas are preserved, but there is extensive damage to the surrounding cortical areas. Grossi et al. (1991) offer evidence of right hemisphere involvement. The syndrome may follow head injury and acute carotid occlusion but most often follows hypoxia.

Anomic Aphasia

Anomic aphasia, a phonologic problem involving a word-finding failure, is the most common type. The person has an inability to find the correct word in spontaneous speech and writing and when asked to name objects. Many other aphasias resolve into persistent anomic aphasia. Some persons with predominant anomic aphasia also lack comprehension of verbal and written language to some degree and display impaired writing, especially when fatigued. Severe anomic aphasia of acute onset typically involves damage in the left temporoparietal junction area. Mild anomic aphasia's site of injury may be the left frontal, parietal, or temporal area; a subcortical area; or even a right-sided cortical injury. Anomic aphasia is associated with head injury, Alzheimer's dementia, and space-occupying lesions, as well as metabolic or toxic encephalopathies, although in the last case, writing usually is more dramatically affected. Four varieties of anomic aphasia are described in Table 25-3.

Language Disorders in Children

Language disorders are considered a major developmental disability in children and may include an inability to assign meaning to words (vocabulary); an inability to organize words into sentences; or an inability to alter the form to tense, possession, or plurality (Paul, 1995). Language and speech (discussed later in the chapter) disorders characteristically are more common in males. A family history of language and learning difficulties often exists. Although there is no single definite cause, an association with chromosomal abnormalities is present. Global language problems, repetitive problems, expressive problems, articulation problems, and phonological problems may be found. Warning signs that a child is having difficulty assigning meaning to words include not speaking first words before 2 years of age, having a vocabulary size that is reduced for age or is not steadily increasing, having difficulty describing characteristics of objects even though able to name them, infrequently using adjectives and adverbs, and using excessive jargon past 18 months of age (Wong et al., 1999). Clinical signs that the child may have an inability to organize words into sentences include not uttering first sentences before 3 years of age; using short and incomplete sentences; omitting words like articles and prepositions; misusing the verb forms for *be, do,* and *can;* having difficulty understanding and producing questions; using easy speech patterns; and reaching plateaus early in language development (Wong et al., 1999). Cues that the child is not able to alter word forms include omitting endings for plurals and tenses, inappropriately using plurals and tense endings, and inaccurately using possession words (Wong et al., 1999).

Concerns about language delay usually emerge around 2 years of age. Global mental retardation is the most common cause of delayed language development. Hearing impairment and specific development language disorders, called *developmental aphasia,* may present as language delays. Affected children have normal cognition and often develop elaborate gestural communication systems to convey their needs and thoughts. Children with infantile autism, in contrast, show a global lack of communication and use neither language nor nonlanguage communication systems. Children with hearing impairment and language disorders may have difficult behavioral problems, in part due to their frustration over their inability to communicate.

TABLE 25-3 Syndromes of Word-Finding Impairment (Anomia)

Impairment	Distinguishing Features
Word-Production Anomia	
Articulatory initiation problem	Failure to name object on request but able to produce name if given a clue
Paraphasic disturbance	Easy initiation of a word but verbal production is so contaminated with literal paraphasia substitutes that response is wrong
Word-evocation anomia	Inability to produce desired name although word is known to person
Word-Selection Anomia	
	Failure to name object on presentation in any sensory modality but can describe use of object and can select appropriate object when presented for name (pure word-finding problem); cannot think of word
Semantic Anomia	
	Inability to name object or point to correct object when name is presented (word has lost its symbolic meaning); both comprehension and use of name are disturbed
Disconnection Anomia	
Modality-specific anomia	Normal naming in all sensory
Category-specific anomia	Normal naming except for a given stimulus category (e.g., color)
Callosal anomia	Inability to make or recognize name of unseen object in left hand, although may recognize object

Dyslexia

Brain imaging studies used to study dyslexia have isolated multiple areas of disruption of brain activity. Persons with dyslexia have a difficult time applying appropriate sounds to the letters that make up written words. On brain imaging studies this network dysfunction includes Wernicke's area, parts of the visual cortex, and a section of the association cortex that integrates sight of printed letters with their corresponding sound (Shaywitz et al., 1998). Nagarajan et al. (1999) have found that the primary auditory cortex yields only weak, disorganized responses in persons with dyslexia, whereas Horwitz, Ramsey, & Donohue (1998) found that the angular gyrus was dysfunctional in their sample of dyslexic men. Dyslexic readers have also been found to have greater activity in the inferior frontal gyrus and Broca's area.

PRAGMATICS

"Pragmatics is that component of communication that transcends language in terms of its isolated words and grammatical structure" (Milton, Prutting, & Binder, 1984). "Pragmatics refers to a system or rules that clarify the use of language in terms of situational or social content" (Sohlberg & Mateer, 1989). Pragmatics is heavily cultural laden. Pragmatics may be viewed as a distinct component of language, or it may be viewed as an umbrella function overlying all other aspects of language. The richness and complexity of a person's communication exists because of the contributions of both the right and left cerebral hemispheres. The right hemisphere is now known to play a major role in the prosody, attitude, emotions, and gestural behaviors involved in language and communicative behaviors. The right hemisphere is dominant for organizing the affective-prosodic component of language and gestural behavior, and the cerebellum may coordinate physical cues through which nonverbal communication occurs (Richardson, 1996).

Pragmatics is a young area of speech and language pathology. Tracking of its development in childhood has not yet been extensively reported. It is known that before children begin to talk they use prosodic features (detailed in the following material) to express themselves. They learn from family and other caretakers how to alter pitch, loudness, tone, inflection, and duration to achieve a desired effect. Thus the quality of the child's cry may be different to indicate different needs. Around 6 months of age, the infant will begin to experiment with inflections heard in other voices. By listening to prosodic features in the language of others, the child learns their meaning. Children imitate rhythm and pacing of vocalization, which results in different dialects. It has been found that the parietal, occipital, and temporal lobes undergo marked development between ages 1 and 7.5 years (Allison, 1992). During this time children perfect their ability to form images. Parietal occipital development is enhanced between the ages of 11 and 13 years, and the temporal lobes mature further between the ages of 13 and 17 years (Allison, 1992). Pragmatics has not been specifically examined in aged persons as yet, but retrieval of visual-spatial memories is known to decrease more than retrieval of language-related memories after age 70 years.

Prosodia

Prosodia, referring to the "melody, pause, intonation, stresses and accents applied to the articulatory line," is the most studied aspect of pragmatics to date. Prosodia imparts affective tone, introduces subtle grades of meaning, and varies emphasis in spoken language. Prosodia is primarily responsible for both the richness and the complexity of communication with its many familial and cultural nuances. Crystal, Lewis, and Monrad-Krohn believe that prosodia, not linguistics, forms the fundamental building blocks for language.

Prosodia was studied first by Monrad-Krohn (1947), who theorized that prosodia has four components: intrinsic, intellectual, emotional, and inarticulate prosodia. "Intrinsic prosodia serves specific linguistic purposes and gives rise to dialectical and idiosyncratic differences in speech quality" (Ross, 1985). Examples of intrinsic prosodia are as follows:

1. Stress differences on segments of word to clarify whether it is a noun or a verb (e.g., the noun *combine* [com' bin] or the verb *combine* [com bin'])
2. Differences in pause structure of a sentence to clarify potentially ambiguous or unclear statements: "the boy and girl with the dog" (said with no pauses and meaning that the dog was with both children) versus "the boy" (pause) "and the girl with the dog" (the four words said together and meaning that the dog was with the girl only)
3. Changing pitch of voice to indicate a question rather than a declarative statement: "Not true?" (high-pitched ending) versus "Not true" (low-pitched ending)

Intellectual prosodia conveys the speaker's attitude about the information being communicated (e.g., "He is smart" with *is* stressed reflects the speaker's acknowledgment that the person possesses the characteristic). Stress placed on *smart* may convey that although the person is smart, the use of the quality may not meet the speaker's approval.

Emotional prosodia contributes emotion to speech and has a large cultural component. Inarticulate prosody is the use of paralinguistic elements such as sighs, grunts, and groans.

The right brain has a role in the emotional aspects of communication. The left ear (right hemisphere) is better at understanding the intonational aspects of speech. The right ear (left hemisphere) is better at linguistic aspects of speech. Right hemisphere brain injury very seriously impairs affective components of prosody and gestures. Persons with right hemisphere damage are unable to insert affective and attitudinal variation into speech and gestural behavior. Affected persons cannot put any emotion into their voices and actions and are aware of this. They speak in monotone and do not use gestures. Right hemisphere damage also disrupts comprehension of the affective components of language. The listener cannot tell the difference between a flat command statement (e.g., "Get the door") and a pleasant request (e.g., "Get the door?"). They cannot insert intonation on request or by imitation.

The linguistic (i.e., intrinsic) component of prosodia can be impaired by either right hemisphere brain injury or left hemisphere brain injury. The basal ganglia most frequently is involved in aprosodia followed by anterior temporal lobe and insular involvement. Schmahmann and Sherman (1998) documented a transient flatness of emotions with cerebellar injury.

Kinesics (Gestures)

Kinesics is the study of limb, body, and facial movements associated with nonverbal communication. When kinesic activity has a semantic purpose—that is, conveys a specific meaning—it often is referred to as *pantomime.* Pantomime conveys specific semantic information. When movements convey an emotional and attitudinal component, they often are referred to as *gestures.* Gestures are movements used to color, emphasize, and embellish speech and are highly reflective of the speaker's cultural background.

Both the right and left hemispheres appear to contribute to kinesic comprehension and production, but the specific neuroanatomy/neurophysiology involved is not yet well understood. Disturbances in performance and comprehension of pantomime are found in persons with left hemisphere injury along with aphasia. Pantomime comprehension deficit is attributed to an inability to comprehend symbols. The deficit, in execution of pantomime, is associated with the presence of ideomotor apraxia. Persons with Broca's aphasia use more pantomime, whereas persons with Wernicke's aphasia use more gestures. Loss of kinesic activity also occurs with right-sided brain injury. Injury to the right frontal inferior area results in complete loss of spontaneous gestural activity without the presence of apraxia.

The development of kinesic comprehension and production has not yet been explicated. It is known that at 9 months of age an infant gives attention to gestures. Layton (1999) and Acredolo and Goodwyn (1996) hold that infants have the ability to gesture and use sign before they have the ability to speak. The expressions of meaning through body movement, or kinesics, are learned through observation initially within the confines of the family and other caretakers. Children learn meanings associated with certain body movements or gestures and how to use movement to accompany language or to substitute for language. One of the earliest gestures learned is that of the hand wave to indicate good-bye and, later, hello. The child also learns that a shoulder shrug can indicate "I don't know." Layton and Acredolo and Goodwyn are studying the effects of teaching the use of simple signs at age 10 and 11 months. The effects of aging in kinesics has not been specifically studied.

Facial Recognition and Facial Expression

Facial recognition (prosopagnosia), a right-sided temporal function, is an inability to recognize previously known faces including one's own or to learn new ones (Haxby et al., 1996). Actually the deficit is not limited to faces but extends to individuals in groups. Minor distinguishing features cannot be recognized.

Facial expressions convey mood and emotional state. They set the stage for the dynamics of communication. The right hemisphere is held to be crucially concerned in the appreciation and production of emotional messages via facial expression. However, recognition of fear in others' faces activates the left amygdala (Morris et al., 1996).

The development of facial recognition begins in the first months of life within the family and progresses as the temporal, parietal, and occipital lobes develop in childhood. The development of facial expression, comprehension, and production has not been specifically examined. Facial recognition declines after 70 years of age.

Pragmatic Deficits

Monrad-Krohn (1947) defined dysprosody as a change in voice quality giving a different accent because of inability to properly stress segments and words. This definition limits dysprosody to a disorder of intrinsic prosodia. Aprosodia for Monrad-Krohn referred to a general lack of prosodia such as found in a person with parkinsonism because of akinesia and masked facies. Mesulam (1990) defined aprosodias as encoding and decoding disorders of affective behavior. Hyperprosodia is the excessive use of prosodia such as often found in persons with mania or persons with Broca's aphasia, who may be able to use few words effectively to communicate.

Ross, Holzapfel, and Freemen (1983) described an anatomical/functional classification model for the aprosodias that mirrors the organization for language presented early (Figure 25-3). Table 25-4 summarizes the characteristics of these aprosodias.

Motor Aprosodia

A motor aprosodia is characterized by flat, monotone speech with loss of spontaneous gesturing. Repetition of affective prosodia (e.g., repeating "I am having company for dinner" in a happy voice) is severely compromised. However, comprehension of affective prosodia and visual comprehension of emotional gesturing are intact. Motor aprosodia is associated with right frontal and anteroinferior parietal damage and occasionally with subcortical right-sided basal ganglia and internal capsule damage. Accompanying clinical findings include moderate to severe left-sided hemiplegia, variable left-sided sensory loss, and transient dysarthria and anosognosia (e.g., inability to recognize the neurological deficits being experienced). Under extreme emotional conditions, persons with motor aprosodia often are able to laugh or cry in a fleeting all-or-none fashion, resembling the pathological affect found in pseudobulbar palsy.

Sensory Aprosodia

In sensory aprosodia, there is severely impaired auditory comprehension of affective prosody, visual comprehension of emotional gesturing, and repetition of affective prosodia. Affective prosodias in speech and active gesturing, however, are intact. In fact, the person may appear somewhat euphoric and overly happy even when talking about serious topics. Sensory aprosodias is associated with right-sided pos-

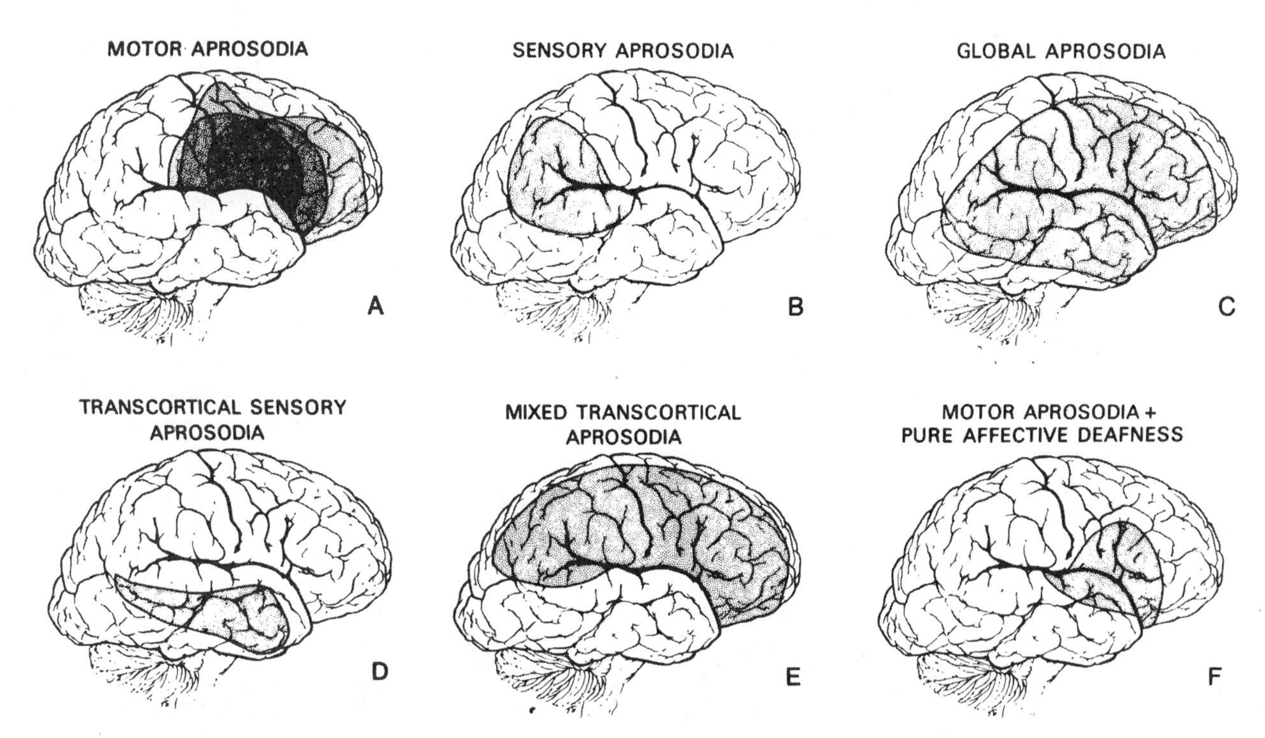

Figure 25-3 **A** to **F,** Right lateral brain templates showing the distribution of infarctions seen on computed tomography scans of 8 of 10 clients with various aprosodias. (From Mesulam, M.M. [1985]. *Principles of behavioral neurology.* Philadelphia: FA Davis.)

TABLE 25-4 The Aprosodias

Aprosodias	Spontaneous Affective Prosody and Gesturing	Affective Prosodic Repetition	Affective Prosodic Comprehension	Comprehension of Emotional Gesturing
Motor	Poor	Poor	Good	Good
Sensory	Good	Poor	Poor	Poor
Global	Poor	Poor	Poor	Poor
Conduction	Good	Poor	Good	Good
Transcortical motor	Poor	Good	Poor	Good
Transcortical sensory	Good	Good	Poor	Poor
Mixed transcortical	Poor	Good	Poor	Poor
Anomic	Good	Good	Good	Poor

From M-M. Mesulam (Ed.), *Principles of behavioral neurology.* Philadelphia: FA Davis. Copyright by FA Davis. Reprinted by permission.

terotemporal and posteroinferior parietal injury. Sensory aprosodias may be accompanied by moderate deficits in left-sided vibration sense, position sense, and stereognosis, as well as a dense left-sided hemianopia.

Global Aprosodia

The person with global aprosodia has severely compromised comprehension and repetition of affective prosodia, severely compromised visual comprehension of emotional gesturing, and an inability to display affect through prosodia and gestures. The person exhibits a very flattened affect. Global aprosodia is associated with a large right-sided perisylvian injury involving the frontal, parietal, and temporal lobes and occasionally with deep right-sided intracerebral hemorrhage. Global aprosodia is accompanied typically by severe left-sided hemiplegia, left-sided hemisensory loss, and left-sided hemianopia.

Transcortical Aprosodias

Descriptions of transcortical motor aprosodia, transcortical sensory aprosodia, and mixed transcortical aprosodia are based on limited data and so must be discussed with caution. Transcortical motor aprosodia appears to manifest as aprosodic-gestural speech with preserved repetition and comprehension of affective prosodia and emotional gesturing. Left-sided hemiparesis without sensory loss may be present. A right-sided basal ganglion injury is thought to produce such an aprosodia. Transcortical sensory aprosodia appears to manifest as a severely impaired comprehension of affective prosodia, whereas emotional gesturing, spontaneous affective prosodia, and its repetition are intact. A right-sided anteroinferior temporal lobe injury is believed to account for this aprosodia. Mixed transcortical aprosodia is believed to manifest as absent gesturing and spontaneous affective prosodia, impaired but present repetition of affective prosodia, and poor comprehension of affective prosodia and emotional gesturing. The lesion is thought to be in the right suprasylvian region and a small portion of the posteroinferior temporal lobe. Severe left-sided hemiplegia and hemisensory loss also are present.

Pure Affective Deafness

Pure affective deafness plus motor aprosodia is thought to be characterized by a flattened voice devoid of affective variation, blunted gesturing, poor comprehension, and repetition of affective prosodia but intact comprehension of emotional gesturing (i.e., visual comprehension is intact). This aprosodia is accompanied by severe left-sided hemiplegia without sensory loss or aphasia. The right-sided inferior frontal, anterior insular, and anteroinferior temporal areas are believed to be the locations of the injury.

Developmental Affective-Prosodic Deficits

Developmental affective-prosodic deficits may occur in children with congenital or very early right hemisphere injury. Acquired motor-type aprosodias after acute right-sided focal brain injury have been documented in school-aged children.

Other pragmatic deficits in the literature are inappropriate reactions to humor and misinterpretation of metaphors. These deficits may arise with right hemisphere injury.

HIGH-LEVEL LANGUAGE SKILLS

Language is a cognitive network, and at the same time many cognitive functions mediated by the left hemisphere are language dependent. Human beings use language when performing cognitive activities. For example, the left hemisphere transfers memory and permanently stores memory in a language format. We form language concepts using symbolic representations and move from literal interpretations to abstract principles and meanings. Human beings think in symbols, that is, in words referred to as internal speech.

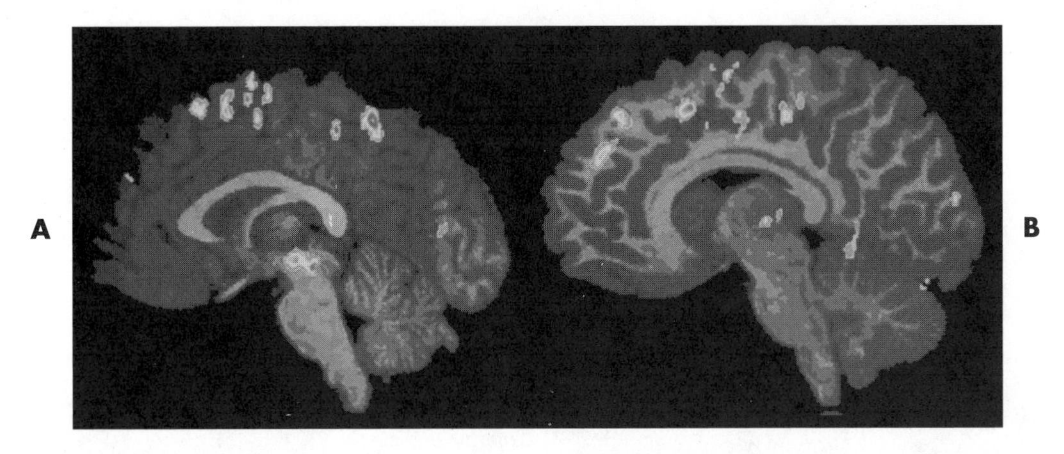

Figure 25-4 Positron emission tomography images in parasagittal planes, demonstrating increased blood flow in the midbrain reticular formation **(A)** and intralaminar nuclei of the thalamus **(B)** as a subject engages in an attention-demanding task (pressing a key as quickly as possible after a visual or somatosensory stimulus). (Reprinted with permission from Kinomura, S., Larsson, J., Gulyas, B., & Roland, P.E. [1996]. Activation by attention of the human reticular formation and thalamic intralaminar nuclei. *Science, 271,* 512. Copyright 1996 American Association for the Advancement of Science.)

Dysfunction in any of the cognitive networks may seriously influence communication.

According to Groher (1977) confused language may result from disorientation in time and space, faulty short-term memory, poor thinking, mistaken reasoning, poor understanding of the environment, and inappropriate behavior. Aphasia may resolve into a more confused language profile. Development of cognitive functions and dysfunctions in cognitive systems are discussed in Chapter 26.

Attention Networks

Dysfunction in attention networks, either arousal or selective attention, produces altered communication patterns. Without arousal—that is, without wakefulness or consciousness mediated by the ascending reticular activating system of the brainstem—communication is tremendously restricted. There is no language and only inarticulate prosody (the most primitive nonverbal output). Reception of communication is limited and at a primary sensory level at best.

The selective attention network facilitates orienting to specific information of interest. Selective orienting of attention may be either overt (movement of the head, eyes, and body to the point of interest) or covert (mental shifting of attention to the source of interest). Evidence supports that the thalami mediate the engage component of selective attention (Figure 25-4). The right-sided parietal area also has been demonstrated to mediate the disengage component of selective attention. With a weak orienting network, a unilateral neglect syndrome develops. When this syndrome is present, the person cannot orient to any sensory stimuli coming from the contralateral left side. This dysfunction will influence any communication embedded in spatial, tactile, auditory, or visual information on which the person cannot focus. Pragmatics is impaired. Cerebellar damage in human beings has been linked to an impaired ability to shift attention quickly from one task to another (Richardson, 1996).

Lack of visual selection attention after 6 weeks of age raises the question of the presence of a visual impairment. Likewise, a dissociation between visual motor behavior and motor behavior during the first 6 months of life may suggest a visual impairment. Failure to "listen" or to pay attention to auditory stimulation in the environment is seen in children with autism. In any of these situations communication is affected at the time as well as in the future.

Recent Memory Network

Memory is the encoding, consolidation, and retrieval of information. The recent memory system transfers short-term memories into permanent (i.e., long-term) memory stores. The encoding and consolidation of information (i.e., recent memory) are mediated by the hippocampi, amygdalae, and probably adjacent temporal lobe and diencephalic areas (Figure 25-5). The left hippocampus and related temporal areas encode and consolidate language-related memories. The right hippocampus and related temporal areas encode and consolidate nonlanguage auditory and visual-spatial memory stores. The amygdalae are believed to participate in transferring the affective component of the experience into a permanent memory store. The recent memory network appears to be functional shortly after birth (Allison, 1992). The hippocampi develop quite early and have reached 40% of maturation by birth, 50% by 1 month, and 100% by 15 months of age (Allison, 1992). The person with a recent memory deficit cannot learn any new information and is disoriented to all new persons, all new places, time, and the current situation. Affected individuals do not remember what they have been told, what they have read, or what they have experienced. The individual's communication appears con-

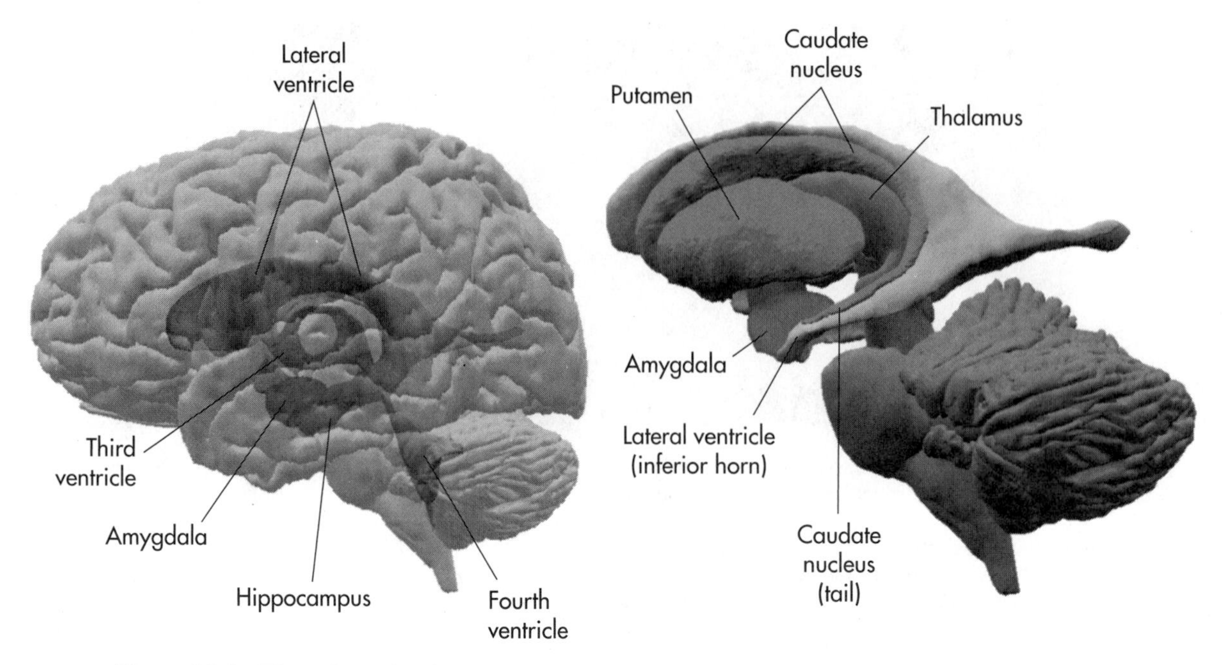

Figure 25-5 Three-dimensional reconstruction showing the spatial relationships between the amygdala, hippocampus, putamen, and caudate nucleus. (Modified from Nolte, J., & Angevine, J.B. [1995]. *The human brain in photographs and diagrams.* St. Louis: Mosby.)

fused and not very meaningful, although syntax and semantics may be intact. The person appears forgetful.

Recent memory decreases with aging but not sufficiently to impair cognitive functioning. This may be related to hippocampal changes.

Remote Memory Network

The remote memory involves pattern recognition and stores long-term memories. These long-term memories are believed to be sorted within the association areas of the parietal, temporal, and occipital lobes. The left hemisphere association areas store memories related to language, mathematics, and abstractions in language format. The right hemisphere association areas store nonlanguage sounds such as music, spatial relationships, and visual experiences. During the time that the parietal, occipital, and temporal lobes undergo marked development between ages 1 and 7.5 years (Allison, 1992), children perfect their ability to form images, use words, and place things in serial order. By about age 10 years, children begin to perform simple operational functions such as weight determination and logical mathematical reasoning. Parietal occipital development is enhanced from 11 to 13 years of age. The temporal lobes mature further between 13 and 17 years of age (Allison, 1992). Dysfunction in the remote memory network of the left hemisphere association areas may produce a loss of comprehension of verbal and/or written language, that is, an aphasia. Some of the deficits that may be produced by dysfunction in the remote memory system of the right hemisphere association areas are aprosody, loss of facial recognition, loss of facial expression, and loss of comprehension of gestures and pantomime. Visual-spatial memory retrieval is more impaired in normal aging than language-related memory retrieval.

Executive Attention Networks

Dysfunction in the executive attention networks—vigilance, detection, and working memory—alters communication patterns. The vigilance network enables a person to maintain a sustained state of alertness for searching and scanning activities. Related to communication, the vigilance network, for example, would help a person scan the environment when there is a competing sound that is not part of the ongoing conversation. Right frontal areas and the locus ceruleus of the brainstem contribute to the vigilance network. The detection network provides target selection among competing complex contingencies, referred to as *object identification,* and realization that the object fills a desire. The anterior cingulate cortex, basal ganglia, and other frontal lobe areas participate in the network. Motivation, self-monitoring, and use of feedback (self-correction) are mediated by this network. One of the striking communication deficits in persons with diffuse traumatic brain injury is their loss of motivation to initiate communication. The apathy blocks their ability to communicate and hinders, if not totally discourages, other persons who may be trying to communicate with them. Akinetic mutism exemplifies a severe detection deficit. Persons with a detection network dysfunctions, because of their impaired ability to self-monitor, cannot recognize their communication deficits and cannot understand what is wrong with the other person. Feedback from others cannot be used, nor can this individual use self-feedback. This detection network dysfunction makes rehabilitation extremely difficult and places most of the change on the other persons in the communication rather than on the affected person.

The working memory network mediated by the anterior cingulate and more lateral areas of the frontal lobes provides the person with temporary storage areas for information, such as instructions needed to process incoming sensory information and guide behavioral responses to that sensory information. Courtney, Petit, Maisog, Ungerleider, and Haxby (1998) have evidence to support that there are at least two distinct types of working memory located in different areas of the prefrontal cortex—one for objects and another for spatial relationships, which is located near eye movement control. The function mediated by working memory has been called *sustained attention* or *concentration over time.* A more complex form is called *tracking,* the ability to maintain focus despite the presence of competing stimuli or the need to engage in alternating tasks. This network enables a person to choose or set goals; to make plans and "think things through"; and to initiate, maintain, and discontinue activities and behaviors. This ability to temporarily hold and interrelate several pieces of information allows for understanding of language and pragmatic communication. Holding newly acquired communication temporarily is essential to interrelate it with previous knowledge to generate a more permanent memory storage. With an inability to goal form or goal select, the person is unable to communicate goals because they do not exist; therefore the person appears indecisive. Communication is one way, with the other person forming goals and making decisions. The person's communication evidences little if any planning and more often reflects ill-conceived needs, wants, and desires that cannot be realized. Often the person acts without any preliminary communication of intentions. The person with a working memory dysfunction is inattentive or distractible. Concentration on the communication, in all of its fullness and complexity, is not possible. The person does not retrieve and register the communication. These persons do not hear, see, or feel the communication. The inattentive behavior is difficult for other persons to deal with and communicate around. There is evidence (Schooler, Neumann, Caplan, & Roberts, 1997) that in schizophrenia there is an inability to clear working memory of irrelevant information and preserve useful visual material no longer in view. These findings help account for the confused language often present in persons with schizophrenia.

The detection and working memory networks develop in early childhood until 6 years of age. At about 7.5 years of age, these frontal areas undergo accelerated development for a few years. These areas continue their maturation between the ages of 17 and 21 years (Allison, 1992).

Concept Formation

Concept formation (image processing, semantic processing) involves the ability to (1) categorize, sort, and analyze relationships between objects and their properties; (2) perform deductive and inductive reasoning; and (3) abstract. Concept formation and storage are accomplished by the memory networks. The same neural areas used for sensory-specific computations are used for higher level thoughts. The differences is these areas are activated from the detection and working memory networks rather than from sensory areas by specific sensory stimuli (Boss, 2000). Related to incidents in one's life, the left prefrontal cortex participates in the acquisition of novel information (learning) while the right prefrontal cortex consistently aids in remembering that material later on (recall) (Nyberg et al., 1996). These areas receive information from specific parts of the brain that deal with content, location, or time of various events. The left hemisphere mediates formation of language concepts. The right hemisphere mediates formation of visual-spatial concepts. Concept formation is fundamental to language development. The ability to form concepts develops throughout childhood, as was previously described in the Remote Memory Network section. Even before 6 years of age, children begin to develop tactics for problem solving. The continuing development of the visual and auditory regions of the cortex permits children from 10 to 13 years of age to perform formal operations such as calculations and to perceive new meaning in familiar objects. The continued development of the visual-auditory, visual-spatial, and somatic systems in the early teenage years permits the adolescent to review formal operations, find flaws with them, and create new operations (Allison, 1992).

Because of their developmental level, young children cannot draw relationships; therefore their communication uses concrete, literal interpretations. No richness and fullness to the communication is present. The communication of an individual unable to form and use concepts resembles the communication of a young child and requires persons trying to communicate with the individual to use concrete, literal language as well.

Older persons appear to form language concepts and to use abstract concepts as readily as younger persons. However, older persons form visual-spatial concepts and abstract less readily.

SPEECH

Speech is a highly coordinated, sequential pattern of muscular contractions of the respiratory, larynx, pharynx, palate, tongue, and lip musculature (Adams et al., 1997). This results in verbal output. Speech development is considered part of language development and was discussed in the Linguistics section. Speech does not decline with normal aging.

Dysarthria

Dysarthria has been defined as a defect in articulation. *Anarthria* has been defined as the complete loss of articulation. However, speech problems that arise in dysarthrias are not exclusively articulatory but include respiratory deficits, phonation problems, and resonation difficulties. Loss of control of the vocal tract muscles produces phonation deficits that distort consonant and vowel sound production, which distorts the language.

Dysarthrias are caused by central or peripheral nervous system motor disorders that produce weakness or paralysis, incoordination, or alteration in the muscle tone of the speech musculature (Kirscher, 1995). Different forms of dysarthria have specific characteristics. Adams et al. (1997) described five types of dysarthria: lower motor neuron (flaccid), spastic and rigid, ataxic, hypokinetic, and hyperkinetic. Darley, Aronson, and Brown (1969) described a sixth type of dysarthria, mixed.

Flaccid Dysarthria

Flaccid dysarthria, the most common type of dysarthria, is caused by paresis or paralysis of the muscles used for articulation. The neurological damage is located in the motor nuclei of the lower brainstem or in cranial nerves VII (the facial nerve), IX (the glossopharyngeal nerve), X (the vagus nerve), and XII (the hypoglossal nerve). With this dysarthria, there is a marked hypernasality (nasal speech) due to palatal immobility. Speech sounds are thick and slurred but feeble. Indistinctness of speech results from paresis or paralysis of the tongue musculature. Consonant production is imprecise, especially with vibratory consonants such as *r.* With severe paresis or complete paralysis of all three cranial nerves, no lingual or labial consonants can be pronounced. Inspiration is audible. The voice is breathy. Persons with myasthenia gravis have flaccid dysarthria.

Hypokinetic Dysarthria

With hypokinetic dysarthria there is a slowness of articulatory movements. The range, direction, and force of muscle contraction are limited, making speech muffled and indistinct. Speech is monopitch and monoloudness. Clusters of prosodic insufficiencies are present. Persons with extrapyramidal system disorders (e.g., parkinsonism or Wilson's disease) may have this dysarthria.

Hyperkinetic Dysarthria

Hyperkinetic dysarthria is also caused by extrapyramidal system dysfunction. Hyperkinetic dysarthria is characterized by movements that are irregular, random, unpatterned, and rapid. Patterns of articulation are highly varied. Sudden variations in loudness are present. Rhythmic hypernasality is present. Speech is described by Adams et al. (1997) as "hiccup speech," a speech pattern with abrupt breaks in flow due to the superimposed abnormal movements of the muscles used to speak. Persons with Huntington's chorea have this type of dysarthria.

Spastic Dysarthria

Spastic dysarthria is caused by the loss of inhibitory cortical influxes on the brainstem reflexes due to damage within the corticobulbar system. This is called a *spastic bulbar palsy* or *pseudobulbar palsy.* In spastic dysarthria diffuse reduction, weakening, or loss of motor speech movement activity is present. Speech usually is slow with short utterances. Articulation is imprecise, and pitch is low. The voice is harsh. An acute brainstem trauma or stroke producing bilateral injury may initially produce complete flaccid anarthria. If there is some improvement with time, the person may exhibit the slow, thick, and indistinct speech of spastic dysarthria.

Ataxic Dysarthria

Ataxic dysarthria results from a cerebellar dysfunction. Ataxic dysarthria is characterized by errors in timing, speed, range, and force of vocal tract muscles. These errors result in dysrhythmia of speech manifested by explosive and intermittent speech. Some words and syllables are spoken with too great a force, and other words and syllables are not audible because the person's breath is gone. Syllable repetition may be present. Phoneme and interval prolongation produce an unnatural separation of the syllables of words called *scanning speech.* Imprecision in enunciation is present, speech is monotonous, and the rate of speech is slow. Respiratory and speech patterns are not coordinated. Persons with multiple sclerosis may have ataxic dysarthria, as may an intoxicated person.

Mixed Dysarthria

In mixed dysarthria, two or more of the previously described types of dysarthria are present in the same person. Two or more different neurological systems have sustained injury. Persons with amyotrophic lateral sclerosis (ALS) may have combined flaccid and spastic mixed dysarthria.

Dysfluency in Children

In children, speech impairment may be classified as a dysfluency (rhythm disorders), an articulation deficiency, or a voice disorder (Klein, 1996). Dysfluencies are usually characterized by repetition of sound, words, or phrases. The disturbance in the normal fluency and time pattern of speech is inappropriate for the child's age. Frequent occurrences of sound and syllable repetitions, sound prolongations, interjections, broken words, audible or silent blocking, circumlocutions, words produced with excess physical tension, and monosyllabic whole-word repetitions are present (Wong et al., 1999). Stuttering is the most common dysfluency. Articulation errors are sounds that the child makes incorrectly or inappropriately. Clinical signs of an articulation problem include unintelligible conversational speech after age 3 years, omission of consonants at beginnings of words after age 3 years and at the end of words after age 4 years, persisting articulation errors after age 7 years, omission of a sound where one should be, distortion of a sound, and substitution of an incorrect sound for a correct one (Wong et al., 1999).

Voice disorders involve deviations in pitch (too high or too low, especially for age and sex), monotone speech, deviations in loudness, and deviations in quality (hypernasal or hyponasal speech) (Wong et al., 1999).

Stuttering

As with dyslexia, in stuttering multiple areas of disruption are found. Stuttering has been demonstrated to produce widespread activity in motor areas throughout the brain, particularly the right hemisphere (Fox et al., 1996). The cerebellum has also been shown to be particularly active during stuttering (Bower, 1996). On the other hand, stuttering is correlated with nearly a complete absence of neural activity in parts of the cortex that regulate conscious monitoring of one's own speech and in areas that are thought to provide the ability to string words together fluently.

PATTERNS OF RECOVERY AND FACTORS INFLUENCING RECOVERY

Brain imaging technology is now allowing researchers to examine the brain as it recovers from an aphasia. Using imaging, training-induced improvement in verbal comprehension is correlated with activity in the posterior part of the right supertemporal gyrus and the precuneus (Musso et al., 1999). Left activation on imaging has also been found in persons recovering from aphasia. Often this activity is localized in perilesional areas (Samsom et al., 1999)

A strong tendency for some degree of spontaneous recovery from aphasia exists. At times, recovery is early, rapid, and extensive. Early recovery (i.e., in 1 to 2 weeks) is due to improvement in anoxia, edema, cellular infiltration, and intracranial pressure. The most dramatic language recovery is seen in the first 2 or 3 weeks after a cerebrovascular accident. Striking language recovery may still be found in the first 3 months, but there is a considerable decrease in language recovery after 6 months. Spontaneous recovery follows the path of a return of old knowledge and in no way resembles relearning of a child. Comprehension recovers more quickly and more completely than expression. Oral language improves more than written language. Language training centered on oral remediation also improves written language.

Recovery from Aphasia

Handedness, Etiology, and Severity

Consistent data across studies have emerged related to the influence of handedness, etiology, and severity on recovery from aphasia. Left-handed and right-handed persons with a family history of left-handedness recover language more often than right-handed persons, but Basso, Farabola, Grassi, Laiacona, and Zanobio (1990) challenge this belief.

Persons with posttraumatic aphasia improve more often than do persons with dysphasia after a stroke. Persons with focal damage are more likely to demonstrate overt speech and language disturbances. Anomic aphasia is the most commonly occurring disturbance. Persons with severe aphasias recover less language than persons with milder aphasias. Samson et al. (1999) have found that the size of the lesion is not a predictor of initial severity or recovery from aphasia. These researchers have also found that the site of the lesion in nonfluent aphasias, where language production is the problem, is not a predictor of recovery, but site in recovery of comprehension is predictive. The more severe the injury to the superior temporal gyrus, the less comprehension is recovered.

Age and Type of Deficit

The empirical data are contradictory regarding the influence of age and type of deficit on recovery. Influence of age on recovery is debated. Culton (1971) and Sarno (1980) found age to have no effect on recovery. Marshall, Tompkins, and Phillips (1982) found older adults recovered less language than did young adults. Recently, growing evidence has led pediatric experts to assert that cognitive skills, including language undergoing rapid development, usually are more impaired with neurological insult. Children aged 4 months to 5 years with injury are more prone to have overall language impairment. Children aged 6 to 9 years after head injury have been found to show much more impairment of written language skills. Injury in teenagers threatens their ability to extrapolate from concrete to basic abstraction, leaving them with only literal meaning.

Basso, Faglioni, and Vignolo (1975) found no difference in recovery between fluent and nonfluent aphasias. Burfield and Zangwell (1946); Messerli, Tissot, and Rodriguez (1976); and Kertesz and McCabe (1977) found the prognosis better for persons with Broca's aphasias. Vignolo (1964) found the prognosis to be better in persons with Wernicke's aphasias, and comprehension recovers more quickly and to a greater extent than expression in aphasic persons (Prins, Snow, & Wagenaar, 1978).

Intelligence and Sex

Inconsistent data have been found regarding the prognostic value of intelligence and sex. Intelligence was found to be a factor in recovery from aphasia by Darley (1975), but Basso (1987) could demonstrate no correlation between intelligence and recovery of verbal comprehension.

Basso, Capitani, and Vignolo (1979) found no difference between men and women on 6-month recovery of comprehension, but 6-month recovery of oral expression was significantly better in women. Pizzamiglio, Mammucari, and Razzano (1985) found that at 6 months or less, no difference existed between men and women on naming, but comprehension was better recovered on three of four tasks by women. Kertesz and Benke (1989) argue their data dispute sex differences in intrahemispheric cerebral organization.

Speech Therapy

The effects of therapy on recovery are highly debated. Vignolo (1964); Sarno, Silverman, and Sands (1970); and Levita (1978) found no difference with or without speech therapy, whereas Hagen (1973) and Basso et al. (1975, 1979) found the treatment group had greater improvement. Meikle et al. (1979) found no difference in recovery using a therapist versus volunteers. Wertz et al. (1981) in a multicenter study found greater improvement with individual versus group therapy sessions. Lincoln, Pickersgill, Hankey, and Hilton (1982) and David, Enderby, and Bainton (1982) found all clients improved regardless of treatment. Basso et al. (1979) found that the time lapse between onset of dysphasia and client evaluation correlated with degree of improvement. Generally the findings could be summarized as inconclusive, although Johnson and Pring (1990) argued that the benefit of speech therapy is documented by more recent experimental studies.

Other Factors

Little research has been conducted on the influence of education, social milieu, general health, and occupational status on recovery from aphasia, although these factors generally are considered prognostic.

Recovery from Pragmatic Deficits

Patterns of recovery from pragmatic deficits are not well described. Persons are believed to recover more gestural ability than verbal prosody. In global prosody clinical experts believe that affective-prosodic comprehension and gesturing improve over time. Spontaneous affective prosody usually remains severely compromised.

Recovery from Dysarthria

Patterns of recovery from dysarthria are somewhat unclear. Some dysarthrias progressively worsen because of the progressive nature of the disease producing the dysarthria (e.g., ALS). If essential functions such as respiration are compromised by the disease process, prognosis is said to be poor. Recovery from dysarthria is not good. Enderby and Crow (1990) found that persons with severe dysarthria remain severely dysarthric, but improvement was seen at 18 months, 24 months, and 30 months in three of four persons. Small gains continued until 48 months after speech therapy initiation.

Related to pragmatics, cognitive systems, and speech, empiric evidence of the factors influencing recovery is lacking.

NURSING PROCESS

Assessment of Communication

Nurses and other health-related professionals, as well as families and significant others, ignore or dismiss language and speech errors. It would be rude to focus on the deficit. Nurses mistakenly may view this deficit as solely within the arena of the speech-language pathologist and beyond the assessment skills of the nurse. Unfortunately such attitudes may mean that the deficit is never carefully and thoroughly evaluated, and appropriate therapeutic interventions are not instituted. The informality possible with the nurse and the continuous intimate contact with the nurse make nursing contribution to the assessment valuable. The best assessment takes place by observing clients in natural communication situations conversing with a partner, who may be the nurse.

A comprehensive nursing assessment concerning communication includes information on health history, developmental level of the client, previous cognitive and communication abilities, and present communication abilities. A comprehensive evaluation of communication function would include assessment of language, cognition, pragmatics, and speech. An aphasia battery in particular is not sufficient for the diagnosis and description of language impairments associated with diffuse brain injury such as in closed head injury because it does not address cognitive factors and pragmatic skills. This comprehensive nursing assessment also is used to identify areas of competence that may help the person cope with the communication deficits.

Before the assessment is begun, its purpose needs to be explained to the client. Describe what is to be done and why. Acknowledge the difficulty for the client. During the assessment, observe for fatigue, pain, and undue frustration. Stagger the assessment as needed.

Aphasia Assessment

An aphasia assessment includes evaluation of spontaneous speech, comprehension of verbal language, comprehension of written language, ability to name, ability to repeat, and ability to write. The nurse observes the following:

Spontaneous speech
- Is the client fluent or nonfluent?
- Is the speech hesitant and slow?
- Are there misused words, grammatical errors, word substitutions, or neologisms?
- What is the client's response to his or her own speech?

Comprehension of the spoken word
- Ask the client to follow simple midline (truncal) commands (e.g., "Stand up" or "Sit down").
- Ask the client to follow simple extremity commands (e.g., "Point to the floor" or "Point to the door").
- Increase the complexity of the commands by joining two or more requests together (e.g., "Stand up and walk to the bed"). Be careful not to give nonverbal cues.

Comprehension of written language
- Ask the client to read aloud.
- Ask the client to follow a written command (e.g., write out "Point to the chair").
- If reading is impaired, determine the client's ability to recognize letters and words.

Ability to name objects
- Ask the client to name objects in the room.

Ability to repeat
- Ask the client to repeat what is said (e.g., "It is a cloudy day").

TABLE 25-5 Outline of the Long Form for the Examination of an Aphasic Client

Background information	Handedness, level of education, language history (e.g., native language, delayed speech, stuttering)
Spontaneous speech	Listen to client during a conversation and note the following: fluency, rhythm and melody, articulation, phrase length, paraphasia, and word content
Comprehension	Test client's comprehension by the following: Commands: although client may comprehend, he or she may be apraxic; therefore also test with questions that can be answered with yes/no responses Pointing (pointing to ceiling)
Repetition	Ask client to repeat grammatical phrases (e.g., "no ifs, and, or buts"), numbers, and words
Naming	Test client's ability to name an article presented visually; test with objects, pictures of objects, colors, hospital-related items, and actions If client has difficulty with visual naming, try alternate afferent pathways (i.e., tactile, auditory, olfactory, taste) If client fails in naming, see if he or she will correct with the following tests: phonetic cueing (e.g., if one holds up a pencil and client cannot name it, give a "p" sound); multiple choice questions (e.g., give client a list of names that includes the correct name and see if he or she can choose it); sentence completion (e.g., "Summer is hot and winter is ——")
Series speech	Ask client to name the days of the week in order or to count sequentially
Reading skills	Listen to client read aloud; assess reading comprehension by asking client to respond to the following: commands, matching words to pictures, yes/no, multiple choice questions To test spelling, say a word and have client spell it; spell a word aloud and have client say it or point to object
Writing skills	Test writing in response to command (i.e., "Write a sentence about the weather today"), to dictation (i.e., "Write this"), or as an exercise in copying

From Boss, B.J. (1984). Dysphasia, dyspraxia, and dysarthria: Distinguishing features, part 2. *Journal of Neurosurgical Nursing, 16,* 212. Copyright by AANN. Reprinted by permission.

Ability to write

- Ask the client to write a spontaneous thought in a sentence (e.g., "Write in a sentence what you are thinking"). If this does not work, be more structured (e.g., "Write a sentence about your breakfast this morning").
- Ask the client to write what is dictated (e.g., "It is a sunny, warm day") (Boss, 1984b).

Table 25-5 represents a detailed bedside aphasia testing outline.

Language Disorders in Children

Related to assessing for language disorders in a child, the nurse asks the following questions of the parents:

- How old was your child when he or she began to speak his or her first words?
- How old was your child when he or she began to put words into sentences?
- Does your child have difficulty learning new vocabulary words?
- Does your child omit words from sentences or use short or incomplete sentences?
- Does your child have trouble with grammar, such as the verbs "is," "am," "are," "was," and "were"?
- Can your child follow two or three directions given at once?
- Do you have to repeat directions or questions?
- Does your child respond appropriately to questions?
- Does your child ask questions beginning with "who," "what," "where," and "why"?
- Does it seem that your child has made little or no progress in speech and language in the last 6 to 12 months? (Wong et al., 1999, p. 1108)

Pragmatic Assessment

Pragmatic assessment is not well established (Sohlberg & Mateer, 1989). A screening assessment includes evaluation of prosody, gestures, pantomime, facial recognition, and facial expression. The nurse observes the following:

Spontaneous use of affective prosody and gesturing during conversation

- Is there affective prosodia in client's voice, especially to emotionally loaded questions? (e.g., "How do you feel?").
- Does client convey emotional or attitudinal information appropriate to the situation?

Ability to repeat through imitation or linguistically neutral sentences with affective prosodia

- Select a declarative sentence with no emotional words (e.g., "It is cloudy").
- Ask client to repeat the sentence with same affective tone used by the examiner: happy, sad, tearful, angry, surprised, or disinterested voice.

Ability to auditorily comprehend affective prosodia

- Select a declarative sentence with no emotional words in it (e.g., "It is cold").
- Standing behind client so he or she cannot see gestures and facial expression, ask client to identify the affect voiced by the examiner in saying the sentence.

Ability to visually comprehend gestures

- The examiner conveys an affected state by using gestures of face and limbs (e.g., "It is hot") said neutrally but with facial expression indicating happiness, sadness, or anger.
- Ask client to identify emotion or describe emotion.

In addition, the nurse asks about the client's internal emotional state (e.g., "How does this news make you feel?" or "Tell me how you feel inside"). It is important to remember that clients with motor aprosodia will not display depression but remain able to experience depression.

Cognitive Assessment

Cognitive networks assessment that must accompany language, pragmatic, and speech assessment includes evaluation of arousal, selective attention, recent memory, remote memory, concept formation, and executive attention networks. The nurse observes the following:

Arousal

- Is the client awake?

Selective attention

- Is the client able to focus his or her attention?
- Does the client focus on external stimuli? If so, to what does the client respond?
- What overt orienting behaviors are evidenced?

Recent memory

- Is the client oriented? If not, to what is the client disoriented: self, person, place, time, situation? Is the client confused? What confuses the client?
- Is the client able to learn new information? Language-related memory? Nonlanguage-related memory? If so, to what degree? Is emotional memory affected?

Remote memory (pattern recognition)

- Is the client able to recall (retrieve) previously learned information? Language-related memory? Nonlanguage-related memory? If so, to what degree?

Concept formation (semantic processing)

- Does the client misinterpret information (illusion)?
- Is the client able to categorize? Sort? Identify similarities and differences?
- Is the client able to interpret the current situation? Does the client exhibit concrete thinking?
- Can the client abstract?

Vigilance

- Does the client search his or her environment?
- Does the client scan his or her environment?

Detection

- Does the client lack motivation? Initiative? Does the client initiate communication?
- Does the client exhibit a flat affect? Appear emotionless?
- Is the client able to self-monitor communication? Is the client able to appreciate his or her communication deficits? Does the client recognize communication omissions and errors in communication? Does the client recognize mistakes in speech?
- Does the client exhibit careless speech?
- Does the client overestimate his communication ability?
- Does the client lack social graces in conversation?
- Is the client able to use communication cues?

Working memory

- Is the client distractible or inattentive?
- Is the client's communication impulsive?
- Is the client able to attend to and respond to questions?
- Does the client require redirection?
- Can the client maintain attention with the presence of competing stimuli?
- Is the client able to form or set communication goals?
- Is the client able to make decisions about communication?
- Does the client think through his or her communications?
- Is the client able to initiate, maintain, and/or terminate communication activities? Does the client know where to begin? Is the client able to carry out a communication sequence?
- Is the client slow to shift or alter his or her communication responses?
- Is speech preservation present?

High-level language tests reflecting sensitivity to abstract language such as thematic pictures, synonyms, antonyms, metaphors, verbal power, and speed (e.g., word fluency) exist. The neuropsychologist is the resource person to consult for further information on such tests. However, Johnstone and Frank (1995) caution that clinical utility in rehabilitation populations of most neuropsychological measures have not been demonstrated.

Dysarthria Assessment

A dysarthria assessment includes evaluation of articulation, respiration, phonation, resonation, and prosody. The nurse:

1. Listens to the client during normal conversation or while the client reads aloud and notes the speech pattern. With a dysarthria, the same speech sounds are equally affected consistently; self-correction is minimal and articulation errors are consistent throughout repeated testing.
2. Asks the client to repeat test phrases or to rapidly repeat lingual (la-la-la-la), labial (me-me-me-me), or guttural (k-k-k-k) sounds.
3. Assesses movement of pharynx, tongue, face, and lips. The motor function of facial, vagus, and hypoglossal nerves is tested (Box 25-1).
4. Notes muscle tone of facial, palatal, and tongue muscles. Are there signs of spasticity, rigidity, or flaccidity?

Box 25-1 Assessment of Lower Cranial Nerves

Facial Nerve

- Observe client's face for symmetry and form. Are nasolabial folds equal? Is expression mobile, stiff, or excessive? Have client puff out his or her cheeks or whistle. Have client smile to differentiate emotional from voluntary facial weakness.
- Inspect for adventitious movements, fatigability, or automatic associated movements.
- Test deep tendon reflexes by gently tapping with reflex hammer.

Glossopharyngeal and Vagus Nerves

- Test palatal movement. Does palate elevate in midline? Do pharyngeal walls approximate on saying "ah"?
- Test swallowing (also refer to Chapter 17). Is there nasal regurgitation or choking on swallowing? Does larynx elevate on swallowing?
- Is client's voice hoarse? Can client say "a, e, i, o, u"?
- Test reflexes (cough, gag). When there is obvious deficit, testing gag is foolish and perhaps dangerous.

Hypoglossal Nerve

- Inspect client's tongue at rest for symmetry, size, shape, and presence of fasciculations.
- Is client able to protrude tongue in midline as well as against the cheeks? If there is paresis, tongue will protrude toward the weak side.
- Test rhythmic movement and coordination by repetitive protrusion as well as by test phrases (e.g., "Round the rugged rock the ragged rascal ran").

From Boss, B.J. (1984). Dysphasia, dyspraxia, and dysarthria: Distinguishing features, part 2. *Journal of Neurosurgical Nursing, 16,* 213.

5. Identifies any other factors that may contribute to a speech problem (e.g., drooling, ill-fitting dentures) (Boss, 1984b).

To assess for speech impairment in a child, the nurse asks the parents the following questions:

1. Does your child ever stammer or repeat sound or whole words?
2. Does your child seem anxious or frustrated when trying to express an idea?
3. When your child stammers, have you noticed certain behaviors, such as blinking the eyes, jerking the head, or attempting to rephrase thoughts with different words?
4. What do you do when any of the above occurs?
5. Does your child omit sounds from the words?
6. Does it seem like your child uses *t, d, k,* or *g* in place of most other consonants when speaking?
7. Does your child omit sounds for words or substitute the correct consonant with another one (such as "wabbit" for "rabbit")?
8. Do you have any difficulty in understanding your child's speech? How much of it is intelligible?
9. Has anyone else ever remarked about having difficulty in understanding your child?
10. Has there been any recent change in the sound or your child's voice? (Wong et al., 1999, p. 1108).

When a speech disorder is present, the rehabilitation nurse additionally assesses the client for other health problems often associated with a speech problem, including eating difficulties (Chapter 17), inability to cough (Chapter 18), and skin integrity problems (Chapter 16) due to drooling (Boss, 1984b).

The nurse documents the findings of these assessments in the client record. Serial assessments are performed to evaluate and document changes over time so that the treatment plan may be modified appropriately.

Magazines and books are excellent resources for pictures that can be used in assessing language, speech, pragmatics, and cognition. Standardized tests for aphasias, pragmatics deficits, and dysarthria are available.

Nursing Diagnosis

The accepted diagnostic category is impaired verbal communication (Gordon, 2000). Other relevant nursing diagnoses are impaired written, emotional, and/or gestural communication; anxiety; and impaired societal interaction (Table 25-6).

Therapeutic Goals

Comprehensive assessment provides a method for translating information gleaned through observation into treatment goals and establishing objectives such as the following:

- Assist the client in achieving optimum communication
- Establish a functional means of communication
- Establish an environment conducive to communication
- Prevent injury
- Preserve the client's self-esteem
- Promote social interaction
- Assist the client in returning to social roles
- Provide communication opportunities
- Educate the client and family regarding the communication deficit or deficits
- Assist the client and family in establishing effective support systems

Specific therapeutic goals for dysarthria are (1) to improve articulation and (2) to improve respiration, phonation, and resonance, which will make speech more intelligible. These goals and related nursing interventions are appropriate to inpatient, outpatient, and home care situations. They are applicable to acute, subacute, long-term care, and rehabilitation settings.

Likewise these goals fall under the broad goals of *Healthy People 2000* and *Healthy People 2010* to increase the span of healthy life for Americans, to reduce health dis-

TABLE 25-6 Nursing Diagnoses, Nursing Outcomes Classification (NOC), and Nursing Interventions Classification (NIC)

Nursing Diagnosis	Suggested Nursing Outcomes Classification	Suggested Nursing Interventions Classification
Impaired verbal communication	Communication ability Communication: expressive ability Communication: receptive ability	Communication enhancement: speech deficit Environment management Presence Energy management Support system enhancement
Impaired written, emotional and/or gestural communication	Communication ability Communication: expressive ability Communication: receptive ability	Support system enhancement Energy management Presence Environment management
Impaired social interaction	Social interaction skills Social involvement Social isolation Role performance	Socialization enhancement Support group Support system enhancement
Anxiety	Anxiety control Coping Rest	Anxiety reduction Coping enhancement Presence Anticipatory guidance
Knowledge deficit	Knowledge: disease process Knowledge: treatment regimen Family participation in professional care	Teaching: disease process Teaching procedure/treatment Teaching: prescribed activity/exercise Teaching: individual Anxiety reduction

Data from Johnson, M., Maas, M.L., & Moorhead, S. (2000). *Nursing outcomes classification (NOC)* (2nd ed.). St. Louis: Mosby; McCloskey, J.C., & Bulechek, G.M. (2000). *Nursing interventions classification (NIC)* (3rd ed.). St. Louis: Mosby; and North American Nursing Diagnosis Association. (2001). *Nursing diagnosis: Definitions and classification 2001-2002* (4th ed.). Philadelphia: Author.

parities among Americans, to harness technology, and to heighten demands for quality in health care services. The more specific *Healthy People 2010* indicators are survival disability free and health system access.

Interventions

Rehabilitation nursing interventions for the client with a communication deficit depend on the client's unique needs. The members of the rehabilitation team, in addition to the nurse, who most commonly work with the client with a communication deficit are the speech-language pathologist, physical therapist, occupational therapist, audiologist, dentist, social worker, psychologist, nutritionist, clergy member, and primary physician or psychiatrist. A primary nursing role in this team is communicating to all members of the team information about the whole client so that they all know the client's underlying diseases, the client's physical/cognitive/psychological/social communicative limitations, the client's coping and adaptation styles, and any current changes in the client. Nursing interventions are designed to provide a therapeutic, supportive environment for the client to facilitate actual communication and to educate the client and family. The Nursing Intervention Classification (NIC) is communication enhancement: speech deficit. Other nursing interventions are given in Table 25-6.

Therapeutic Environment

The rehabilitation nurse plays a primary role in creating an environment that makes attempts at communication easier and less stressful. Specific interventions to promote the existence of a therapeutic environment are given in Box 25-2.

In the acute rehabilitation setting, when a room is shared, the client with a problem in communication output (e.g., Broca's aphasia, motor aprosody, or dysarthria) benefits most from having a roommate who can understand the client's communication problem. The environment most supportive of the client with a comprehension problem is one that does not cause excessive auditory or visual stimulation. The roommate of a client with Wernicke's aphasia who is talkative should not be troubled by frequent spontaneous, meaningless verbalizations.

Impaired communication may seriously compromise the client's safety. Careful assessment of each client with a communication deficit for any needed safety precautions is appropriate. Ways to call for help either in the acute rehabilitation setting or at home need to be established, and the client should be taught how to use them. The client needs to be in-

Box 25-2 Creating a Therapeutic Environment

With Any Communication Deficit

- Maintain a calm, relaxed, and unhurried environment
- Maintain an uncluttered environment with equipment placed in least distracting areas
- Maintain a routine in the schedule of activities
- Avoid isolation
- Recognize anxiety-provoking stimuli and eliminate stressors
- Institute anxiety-reducing measures as appropriate

When Output of Communication Is Impaired While Comprehension Is Relatively Preserved

- Help client to communicate; create an environment where communicating is a pleasant experience, and praise client for trying to communicate even when the results are far from perfect
- Stimulate communication during routine nursing care activities
- Provide client with frequent opportunities to experience communication: hear speech; practice listening to family and social conversation; read; and practice interpretation of emotion, gestures, and pantomime as appropriate; radio and television may be used to some degree
- Encourage client to participate in group activities for social value and communication stimulation

When a Comprehension Deficit Is Present

- Avoid continuous noise and interaction
- Avoid fatigue
- Set limits on amount of praise given
- Limit frequency and length of time that communication is stimulated
- Limit frequency and length of group activities
- If activity or interaction is confusing or stressful, discontinue the activity or interaction (Boss, 1984b)

formed about environmental hazards despite the communication deficit by pictures, pantomime, or whatever means necessary. Two examples to illustrate the safety hazards are given in Box 25-3.

Box 25-3 Examples of Safety Hazards Experienced with Clients with Communication Deficits

Example 1

Mr. Jones, a 65-year-old man with a history of a myocardial infarction, had Broca's aphasia as a result of a stroke that occurred 6 weeks earlier. While ambulating in the hospital corridor, he experienced a severe episode of left-sided chest pain that radiated down his left arm. He became weak, fell to the floor, and remained there rubbing his arm. Initially the staff thought he had injured his arm in the fall. No one understood why he looked so apprehensive and pale. On taking his vital signs, the nurse discovered he was hypotensive and experiencing significant cardiac dysrhythmia. Fortunately, because the vital signs were taken, early treatment for the cardiac condition was initiated.

Example 2

Mrs. Brown experienced Broca's aphasia as a result of an automobile accident. She continually rubbed her right eye but never verbally complained (she could not). She frequently was restless and often appeared uncomfortable, but no one could determine the cause. Sometimes when the eye became red, a wrist restraint was applied to stop her from irritating the eye by rubbing. The eye became severely inflamed, so an ophthalmologist was consulted. Examination revealed that a piece of glass had become embedded in the eye at the time of the accident. Unfortunately the prolonged irritation left Mrs. Brown's cornea scarred.

Support Behaviors

All rehabilitation team members who interact with the client need to monitor themselves for postures, behaviors, tone of voice, and facial expressions. All of these types of communications need to be positive and supportive. Team members need to behave as if communications are understood when in the presence of the client and need to assume that misunderstanding because of the communication deficit may readily occur. Misunderstanding is assessed continuously, and corrective actions are taken immediately.

Embarrassment about the inability to communicate in a meaningful way can discourage the client from interacting with others and participating in treatment. The nurse, other rehabilitation team members, and family can help reduce embarrassment by demonstrating acceptance and interest. Supportive behaviors are listed in Box 25-4.

As the client physically recovers from the nervous system injury that produced the communication deficit, social interactions are encouraged. Initially interactions involve rehabilitation team members with whom the client regularly interacts, family, and close friends. Interaction involving one or two persons usually is best because this makes it easier for the client to focus. Visitors or other clients need to be instructed regarding appropriate communication techniques. The nurse monitors visits to ensure that the encounters are pleasant and not too long.

When a client returns home, resumption of a "normal" social life often is difficult. Frustration and embarrassment about communication may result in a loss of interest in socializing: the stress itself is fatiguing.

Old friends often feel uncomfortable in initiating interactions because the interests once shared can no longer be pursued. Friends also may be frustrated by their inability to communicate effectively or to help the client communicate more effectively. They may be frightened by the changes seen in their friend (Broida, 1979). The nurse and the family can teach the client's friends ways to communicate. Friends, like family, need to be encouraged to visit and should receive recognition for the support offered. They also need a chance to verbalize their fears and frustrations.

Box 25-4 Supportive Behaviors

- Show genuine concern for client
- Recognize frustration and difficulty client is experiencing; be patient and accepting of his or her anger and depression
- Treat client as an adult even during times when his or her behavior may regress; involve client in decision making regarding his or her care and activities
- Attempt to anticipate client's needs and validate specific needs with client; be observant and sensitive
- Encourage client in all of his or her communication efforts
- Praise even the smallest gain
- Help client develop constructive and positive outlook: emphasize things that client can do, build his or her confidence, reassure client that everyone has difficulty at times with self-expression
- Do not be overly helpful; allow client to take pride in being able to provide self-care as much as possible
- Encourage client to be as independent as he or she wishes regardless of the communication deficit
- Be honest with client regarding prognosis and difficulties in regaining communication abilities
- Limit communication goals to those that can be accomplished; emphasize short-term goals
- Avoid placing demands that cannot be met on client
- Do not force client to communicate or to see persons when he or she does not wish
- Do not remind client that once the client communicated well
- If client laughs or cries uncontrollably, attempt to change subject or activity; if crying or laughing continues, remove client from situation
- Begin speech-language therapy when client is interested and psychologically ready

When Comprehension and Cognition Are Intact

- Do not behave or permit other persons to behave as if client does not understand or has lost some of his or her cognitive abilities

When Comprehension Is Impaired

- Do not discuss client in the client's presence without direct attempts to communicate information to client as well
- Accept paraphasia, "jargon speech," cursing, and other such output nonjudgmentally, but attempt to inform client that you do not understand his or her communication
- Use touch, tone of voice, and other nonverbal behaviors to communicate calmness, reassurance, and trustworthiness when language comprehension is impaired; when prosodic comprehension is impaired, put all emotions and gestural intentions into verbal language and say what you mean
- Carry out all activities in an unhurried manner (Boss, 1984b)

Self-help organizations such as the American Heart Association stroke clubs, the National Head Injury Association chapters, and the National Alzheimer's and Related Disorders Association chapters help fulfill social, support, and education needs. These organizations are helpful not only to the client experiencing the communication deficit but also to spouses and family members. These organizations may be particularly valuable when the client and/or family have few support systems. These organizations can serve as a source of new friends who understand, share good ideas regarding mutual problems, and are seeking new friends themselves.

Facilitation Techniques to Improve Communication

All members of the rehabilitation team need to be knowledgeable about communication processes and facilitation techniques used to promote effective communication in clients with communication deficits. Often experimentation with various techniques is necessary to determine what works best for a particular client. Behaviors the rehabilitation nurse can use to facilitate communication are shown in Box 25-5.

Rehabilitation Approaches

The many widely different language interventions may be categorized into four main approaches. These approaches have sometimes arisen in different countries under the influence of different psychological theories, but they are not necessarily mutually exclusive. Specific treatment applications depend on what theories are accepted by the therapist. Some treatments have a clear research base. Others are derived more from the theory but are without empiric evidence of efficacy.

Classic Approach. The classic (or stimulation) approach encompasses many different intervention techniques, but all techniques are based on two assumptions. The first assumption is that aphasia is a central language deficit. An overall language pattern pervades all different language modalities; thus types of aphasia reflect only different levels of language dissolution. Aphasias are quantitatively different. The breakdown is in the one single central language mechanism. This assumption heavily influences rehabilitation because under this assumption improvement is simultaneous across all modalities. No need to focus on each modality using different techniques exists. Most therapists focus on oral language. The same exercises for comprehension and expression are sometimes used.

The second assumption is that "aphasia is characterized by reduced efficiency in gaining access to language knowledge" (Basso, 1987). Aphasia is a restriction of language availability; therefore therapy addresses levels of language availability (e.g., informative content versus automatic language) and focuses on improving accessing strategies.

Soviet Approach. The Soviet approach is built on Luria's theory that "any functional system may be deranged by lesions in diverse parts of the cortex, but the quality of the impediment is dependent on the localization of the lesion" (Luria, 1970). Recovery occurs through reorganization of the functional system under treatment in such a way that transfers affected function to a new structure. The defective link is replaced with a new one so that the function can reestablish

Box 25-5 Behaviors to Facilitate Communication

- Use spontaneous communication topics that are of interest to client or of immediate importance to him or her
- Recognize that frequent but short communications are more beneficial
- Postpone communication if client is fatigued or upset
- Encourage use of gestures and other forms of communication when client's verbalizations are misunderstood

When Communication Output Is Disturbed but Comprehension Is Intact

- Allow client to communicate for himself or herself; provide opportunity for client to speak first and provide the necessary time to communicate
- Encourage all attempts to verbalize by acknowledging attempts and efforts; encourage automatic speech or imitation (e.g., prayers, social responses such as hello); encourage singing if client enjoys singing
- Use self-talk (i.e., speaking about the activity as nurse performs it)
- Use parallel talk (i.e., describing aloud the activity client is carrying out with nurse)
- Use expansion, which adds substance to the statement (e.g., adding to statement "drink of water," "You want a drink of water")
- Attend very carefully to communications
- With dysarthria, encourage client to say one word at a time with all sounds in each word produced and consonants emphasized; encourage client to increase volume of voice
- React with physical actions or verbalizations to convey your understanding of verbalizations
- Assume some responsibility for misunderstanding communications
- Do not interrupt while client is trying to communicate unless client becomes frustrated; only then interpret or supply words
- Encourage use of shorter phrases, single words, or slower verbalization if client is distressed or fatigued or if verbalizations are misunderstood
- Allow mistakes; only occasionally correct client, if clearly appropriate; do not insist that each word be pronounced perfectly
- If client is having trouble with a word, use cueing (i.e., pronouncing the initial syllable of word), have client repeat the word after you, give an open-ended sentence to fill in the blank, or try writing down word for client to read
- Request statements be repeated or rephrased if not understood
- Serve as a good communication model to imitate when client is having difficulty

When Even a Slight Comprehension Deficit Is Present (as with Any Aphasia or Aprosodia)

- Provide a quiet environment for communication on a one-to-one basis at least initially
- Turn off televisions and radios; remove unnecessary items and equipment from client's visual field
- Gain client's attention first, get client to look at communication partner, and redirect client to communication partner if client becomes distracted
- Speak slowly and distinctly, using natural pauses; use short, simple instructions and/or explanations, and use gestures and pantomime along with verbalizations
- Use simple, direct questions that are answerable with one word or short phrases; use gestures and pantomime with verbal questions
- Reinforce appropriate responses
- Tell client when you do not understand him or her; ask simple questions and systematically point and gesture until the point is uncovered
- Do not raise your voice if client fails to understand or misunderstands; signal client that there was a miscommunication and reword the communication; try to use strong gestures and facial expressions; do not become annoyed (Boss, 1984b).

When Helping a Child Learn Language

- Select a small group of words connected to a specific activity (e.g., say "close" each time a door is closed); repeat the word with the activity several times and then repeat the word but wait for the child to initiate the activity
- Choose vocabulary that is useful, easy to pronounce, and understandable to the child
- Encourage vocabulary development by having the child say the word rather than gesture the word before fulfilling a request
- Speak at a level slightly above the child's level
- Expand the statement, preserving the child's intent
  - *Expand the statement using the same noun*
    - Child: Dog runs
    - Adult: The dog is running into the house
  - *Replace the noun with a pronoun*
    - Child: Dog runs
    - Adult: He is running
  - *Expand the statement adding new information*
    - Child: Dog runs
    - Adult: The cat is running, too
- Respond by indicating the meaning of the child's utterance, rather than its linguistic accuracy (or inaccuracy)
- Substitute questions with statements about an observed activity (Wong et al., 1999, p. 1109)

itself. Intrasystem reorganization may take place at a more primitive (low) level or at a more intentional level. Therapy is directed at helping the person understand the nature of the impediment and to learn to do things intentionally that were previously automatic. There is conscious analysis of speech and thought processes, a step-by-step reconstruction of a functional language operation that is exemplified in the substitute skills model therapies. External operations for each of the different links composing the function must then be progressively internalized. There are two fundamental rehabilitation rules: (1) the deficit must be rigorously differentiated, so there must be an accurate qualitative analysis of the deficit; and (2) each deficit calls for its own rehabilitation program.

Operant Conditioning Approach. The operant conditioning approach is based in Skinner's principles of operant conditioning. The consequences (reinforcement) are manipulated. Baseline data are collected, and criteria for success are defined. Then the steps within the treatment program are implemented. Basso (1987) argued that this approach is a methodological, not a content, approach, but it is useful at systematically implementing any rehabilitation program.

Psycholinguistic Approach. In the psycholinguistic approach, linguistic criteria are the focus. Although the approach is not well established, examples are the substitute symbols systems, including the deblocking technique, melodic intonation therapy (MIT) and its variant melodic rhythm therapy (TMR), the visual communication program, and visual action therapy (VAT). American Sign Language also has been used with some reported success, especially with severe Broca's aphasia. This approach has had a major impact on the diagnosis and classification.

Regardless of the approach used, therapeutic efforts generally are tailored on an individual basis. Generally therapies concentrate on improving spoken language. Impaired auditory language comprehension often is directly approached by exercises in listening to words and sentences. In severe cases lipreading or reliance on writing may be used. Alexia and agraphia commonly are treated with traditional classroom work and then homework assignments. Children usually are taught language by traditional educational methods. The communication problems most resistant to direct therapeutic approaches and substitute skills models are profound anomia, severe agrammatism, severe alexia, profound impairment of word retrieval and language comprehension via both speech and writing, and severe impairment initiating or formulating an utterance (e.g., transcortical motor aphasia) (Goodglass, 1987).

General Therapeutic Considerations

Some general principles that may help guide rehabilitation nurses as they attempt to facilitate the client's communication include:

1. It is common to distinguish between comprehension of communication and production of communication and reeducate each separately.
2. Because comprehension is believed to be easier than production, target it first.
3. Language in context is easier to deal with than words or phrases isolated from immediate experience. Nurses have ample opportunity to provide language exchange in context.
4. Improvement brought about by retraining in one modality may be accompanied by corresponding improvement in untrained skills.
5. With sufficient repeated practice, it is possible either to restore functional efficiency to a defective capacity or to bring an alternative route to a level of voluntary and eventual automatic skill. Interact with the client while giving care and during activities as well as in practice sessions. Use facilitation techniques given in Box 25-5.

Pragmatic Treatment Protocols

With regard to pragmatics, treatment protocols are in the very early stages of development. There are some trial remediation programs mostly with head-injured clients. Some therapists have used a group approach. Solhberg and Mateer (1989) use a modular format to address four behaviors: nonverbal communication, communication in context, message repair, and cohesiveness of the narrative. The module is introduced by describing and demonstrating target behaviors to be learned. Then role-play is videotaped, followed by review by the group. Participants are helped to look at specific behaviors that increase success or failure and identify ways to modify the communication behavior. Other therapists use an individual approach targeting particular communication behaviors that are deficient in individual clients. The therapist attempts to address the communication behaviors in a broad range of naturalistic communication environments. Family members receive descriptions of communication goals and suggestions for providing appropriate feedback. Opportunity is provided to practice appropriate behaviors and to modify existing problem areas as well as to establish new, effective modes of communication.

Dysarthria Therapy. With regard to dysarthria, rehabilitation nurses need to understand the specific treatments prescribed and the methods for applying the treatments during nurse-client interactions. Dysarthria therapy has three approaches:

1. Medical care of the underlying neurological disorder to prevent further deterioration
2. Prosthetic and/or surgical management
3. Therapeutic approach of a speech pathologist, which is usually behavioral in nature with some instrumental aids when available

The speech therapy approach is basically symptomatic and supportive or compensatory (McNeil, 1997). To improve articulation, the speech pathologist determines the reason for the articulatory errors and designs and implements a hierarchy of exercises starting with sounds that sometimes are correct and ending with those sounds impaired most seriously. To improve resonance, which will reduce hypernasality, the palatal muscles (palatine vault) are strengthened using exercises such as sucking and blowing and by producing oral and nasal sounds alternately (e.g., "pa, ma, pa, ma"). To improve phonation, laryngeal valve exercises may be used (e.g., production of "i-i-i" or rapid pitch changes). To strengthen the respiratory muscles, clients may use incentive spirometry, count aloud during expiration, and increase loudness rapidly and dramatically. Exercises to help prevent air waste may be prescribed (e.g., "pa-pa-pa" to improve bilabial air control and "ta-ta-ta" for linguoalveolar air control).

The nurse needs knowledge about the use of prosthetic devices and alternate forms of communication used by the client. Some common strategies used when interacting with the person who is dysarthric are given in Box 25-5.

Clients with aphasia, pragmatic deficits, and cognitive impairments need time to process incoming information. If the nurse has trouble eliciting a response from the client, the nurse's own communication needs to be examined.

Alternate Forms of Communication

Some persons with only speech problems, such as dysarthria involving only speech, can communicate in writing. Other persons, because of speech and arm motor problems, cannot put out verbal or written language but can use communication boards, a spelling board, or cards that use printed words or require spelling out words, sentences, and so on. Typewriters, computers, and voice simulators address the same communication problems.

When aphasia is present, the communication boards, notebooks, or cards must use pictures of objects, persons, needs, actions, faces expressing moods, and so on. A computer-aided visual communication system (Figure 25-6) has been developed for clients with aphasia.

Client and Family Education

Both the client and family need to understand the cause of the communication deficit, understand the purpose of speech-language therapy, and have a realistic view of the potential for recovery. All rehabilitation team members need to have knowledge of what the client and family have been told and by whom. Information on prognosis for recovery initially may be presented by the primary physician, physiatrist, or speech-language pathologist. Realistic hope for recovery of communication ability by the client and family is supported, but the client and family are informed that full recovery is not common.

The family is taught the importance of creating an environment that is physically and emotionally supportive and how to create that environment. Facilitation techniques found to promote more effective communication are taught to all persons who interact with the client. A team approach for education of clients, family, and friends begins with their learning about the communication deficit. Clients learn self-help techniques, including ways to assist others to use supportive behaviors that enhance communication. In turn, family and friends can use supportive behaviors to facilitate communication. They need reassurance about the client's behavioral changes resulting from language and prosodia comprehension deficits, and they need to understand why these changes occur. Clients also learn how to participate in daily home activities and to manage their environment. Family and friends learn ways to help clients such as offering them encouragement to participate in appro-

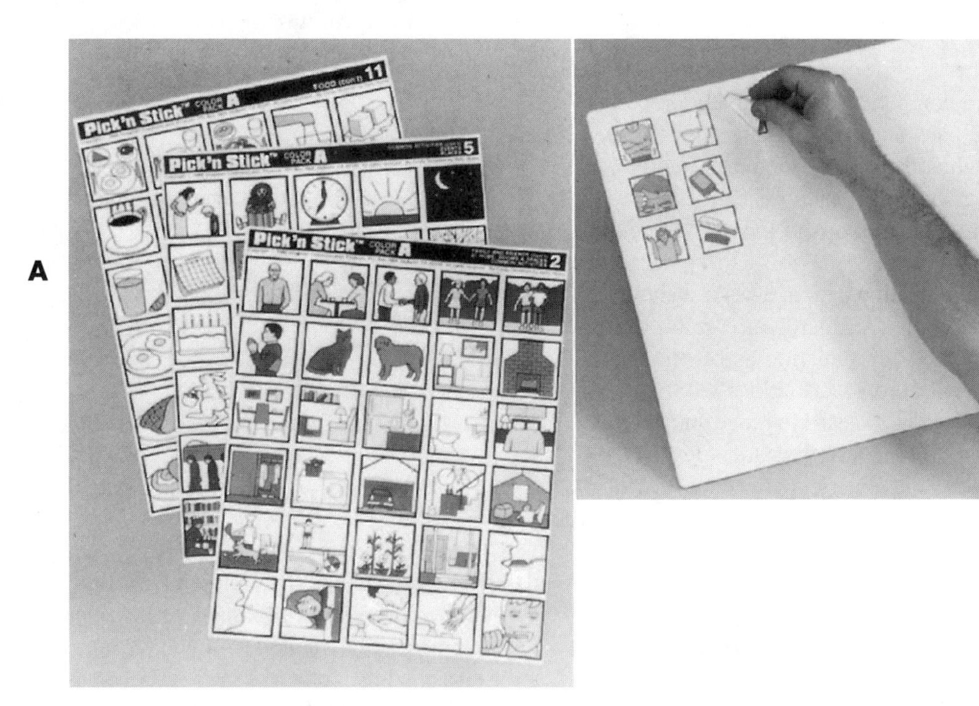

Figure 25-6 Many assistive devices for improving communication with clients who have aphasia can be made at home. Some clients may have computers and software packages available. Easy-to-use and excellent commercial products include identification stickers **(A)** and picture boards **(B).** (Reprinted by permission of Sammons Preston, Bolingbrook, IL.)

priate activities and including them in making mutually satisfying decisions, without allowing insignificant daily hassles to be burdensome or becoming overly protective (Boss, 1984a).

Referrals

The nurse assumes a key role in the referral of clients to various health disciplines within rehabilitation institutions and the community. Close and often long-term interactions with the client provide the opportunity for identifying obvious and subtle problems. The nurse's findings need to be carefully and completely documented in the client's record.

Nurses can assume a major role in seeing that information regarding communication techniques used with the client is communicated to other health care professionals. Nurses need to ensure that techniques health care providers have found useful are noted and shared both in the acute care facility and in the community setting.

Growing numbers of clients are receiving speech-language therapy on an outpatient basis in clinics and private practice settings. Likewise, more and more community health agencies and home health organizations are beginning to offer speech-language therapy services. Because of prohibitive costs for continued therapy, some speech-language pathologists have designed programs that the family can use with the client. They see the client only for reevaluation and adjustment of the therapy program. The nurse may need to be involved in finding such resources for clients and encouraging the development of such programs.

Evaluation

Evaluation is an essential component of the nursing process to document quality of care and cost-effectiveness. Both process and outcome evaluations are appropriate when providing health care to a person with a communication deficit.

Process evaluation provides a means to judge and document the caring giving process and behaviors carried out for a person who has a communication deficit. The Association of Rehabilitation Nurses' (ARN) standards of care provide one means to conduct a process evaluation and document nurses' as well as other health providers' actions.

Outcome evaluation provides a means to judge and document the effects of the care provided at the patient level. Although outcome criteria for the client experiencing a communication deficit are determined individually based on the client and situation, three nursing-sensitive patient outcomes with specific indicators and measurement scales have been developed in the Iowa Outcomes Project (Table 25-6). Other potential outcome criteria are presented in Box 25-6. The nursing-sensitive outcomes can be used for initially documenting the patient's performance, for monitoring changes over time, and for documenting outcomes at specific points in time (e.g., at inpatient discharge, at outpatient discharge, or on home visits). Outcome criteria shown in Box 25-6 can also be used at specific points, such as discharge to home or discharge from outpatient therapy.

Box 25-6 Outcome Criteria for Communication Deficits

- Client participates in all activities planned to improve communication:
  - Participates in speech therapy sessions and periodic evaluation
  - Interacts and communicates with health team members, family, and friends
  - Explains, demonstrates, or recognizes speech therapy methods and communication techniques designed to improve communication
  - Explains and appropriately uses alternate forms of communication
- Client is in control of anxiety and frustration permitting client to:
  - Participate in speech therapies
  - Effectively express anxieties and frustrations via verbalizations or gestures
  - Communicate needs to others
- Client functions safely and independently including searching for and accepting assistance of others as needed
- Client establishes a defined method of communication
- Client demonstrates ways to maximize communication
- Client demonstrates attitude of self-worth as evidenced by:
  - Spontaneous communication to others
  - Awareness and interest in other persons and environment
  - Expression of interest in appearance
- Client enjoys social interactions as evidenced by:
  - Identification of opportunities for social interaction
  - Participation in chosen activities
- Family provides effective support for client by:
  - Identifying safety needs of client
  - Explaining cause of communication deficit
  - Explaining expected prognosis for recovery of communication
  - Providing realistic and honest support for client
  - Identifying importance of psychological support for themselves as well as client
  - Explaining and using facilitation techniques, methods for maximizing communication, and alternative methods of communication
  - Explaining importance of promoting maximum independence
  - Identifying methods for promoting maximum recovery

IMPLICATIONS

New technologies have opened the way to study communication networks in healthy children and adults and in adults and children who have sustained neurological insult. With these studies comes a better understanding how complex and overlapped the networks involved in communication really are. These networks involve many different specialized areas and require remarkable coordination and synchronization. Additionally genes are being linked to language and speech as well as to cognition (Bower, 1998a; Glausiusz, 1999; Travis, 1999). These advances also open the way to examine the effectiveness of language, speech, and pragmatic therapies in both children and adults. Genetic interventions may become feasible in the future for some communication deficits.

Rehabilitation nurses traditionally remain on the sidelines in the area of communication rehabilitation, but the ever-increasing demand for cost containment, cross-trained rehabilitation specialists, early return to the community, and home-based health care services mandate that nurses play a larger role in communication interventions. Evidence-based nursing practices with established efficiency and effectiveness grow out of process and outcome evaluations related to communication enhancement. Payers and, more recently, the public are increasingly demanding these data-based interventions from all health providers, including nurses.

Resource allocation and distribution of services remain issues for patients, families, nurses, and other health care providers.

CRITICAL THINKING

Mr. T.J. is a 62-year-old divorced man with a dense Wernicke's aphasia from a thrombotic stroke involving only the left inferior branch of the middle cerebral artery. He has no motor primary sensory deficits and will be returning to live alone at home. During the course of his stroke workup, he was diagnosed with diabetes mellitus. He has been prescribed an 1800-calorie American Dietetic Association diet, a walking regimen, and 70/30 insulin daily with frequent glucose checks while his diabetes is regulated. He understands no verbal or written language. Develop a teaching plan so that he can learn about the disease, its signs and symptoms, complications, his diet, glucose testing, insulin injection, foot care, and other related information.

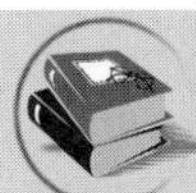

Case Study

T.R., a 29-year-old woman, experienced an ischemic stroke involving the left superior trunk of the middle cerebral artery 2 weeks after oral anticoagulation therapy was discontinued. She had been receiving anticoagulation drugs for 6 months because of deep vein thrombosis (DVT). She initially presented with a right hemiparesis, arm>face>leg, and a Broca's (motor, expressive) aphasia.

Her relevant medical history related to this cerebrovascular accident included the following: (1) a history of DVT immediately after resection of a right ovarian cyst at the age of 24 years, and (2) an iliofemoral DVT (confirmed by echo Doppler imaging and phlebography) at the age of 28 years that developed in her right leg a few days after hospital admission for a fractured left tibia that required casting. At this time her coagulation screening tests were abnormal, affirming her hypercoagulable state. For 6 months after anticoagulation with heparin, warfarin therapy was initiated. When T.R. had completely recovered from the DVT, the warfarin was discontinued. She had no history of nicotine use, hyperlipidemia, vascular abnormalities, or vasculitis.

Relevant family history obtained during hospitalization was that two of her female cousins had had episodes of DVT while taking oral contraceptives.

Relevant physical examination findings included vital signs within normal limits, regular rate and rhythm of heart without murmurs or extra sounds, absence of carotid and abdominal bruit, good peripheral pulses, and awake and alert neurologically but with an apprehensive and frustrated mood. Memory networks and executive attention networks appeared to be intact. On cranial nerve testing, T.R. was weak, related to the motor component of central nerves V, VII, IX, X, XI, and XII. The sensory components of V, VII, and IX were intact. Central nerves II, III, IV, and VIII were intact. Motor testing demonstrated movement against gravity in the right face and arm, but weakness was present with hypotonia and mild weakness in the lower right extremity. Sensation was intact. Deep tendon reflexes on the right side were diminished. Specifically related to communication, T.R. attempted little spontaneous speech (nonfluent). T.R.'s comprehension of both verbal and written language was generally intact; comprehension of pragmatics was intact. Language output both verbally and in writing was minimal with slow speech and much hesitation. Mostly the output was one or two words. Repeating was more fluent, and she could swear and sing. Use of pictures, drawing, and gestures was intact. T.R. could not name objects but understood their purpose and use. There was a fairly dense nonfluent aphasia.

Diagnostic Testing

Computed tomography (CT) initially showed no mass lesion or bleeding. Transcranial Doppler imaging suggested an occlusion of the left middle cerebral artery. Carotid Doppler study results were normal. Transthoracic echocardiogram findings were normal. A transesophageal echocardiogram showed no embolic source and no patent foramen ovale or shunt. There was no reoccurrence of DVT by compression ultrasound. The second CT a few days later showed a large hypodense area consistent with ischemia in the left inferior-posterior frontal area. Clotting studies confirmed an abnormal tendency to clot. Her lipid profile was within normal limits, and there was no laboratory evidence of an autoimmune process.

Medical Diagnosis

The medical diagnosis included left inferior-posterior frontal CVA with hemiparesis, Broca's aphasia, dysarthria (presence or absence of an apraxia was not able to be determined in view of the weakness), and a primary hypercoagulable state.

Nursing Diagnosis

The nursing diagnosis included impaired verbal communication (written language was also impaired).

The remainder of this case study addresses only communication issues. The therapeutic goals listed on page 587 are all appropriate for T.R.

T.R. began receiving heparin therapy and was discharged to the rehabilitation center on 7500 units of subcutaneous heparin twice daily for 1 month. At that time warfarin therapy in conjunc-

Continued

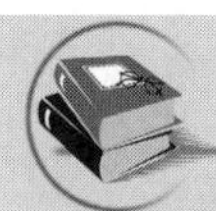

Case Study—cont'd

tion with a lower dose of subcutaneous heparin was planned, and intermittent International Numeric Ratios (INRs) were to be maintained after discharge to home.

During the acute care hospitalization T.R. was provided with a calm, relaxed, and unhurried environment and as routine a schedule of activities as possible in light of the numerous diagnostic studies undertaken in a short period of time. Staff demonstrated concern, patience, acceptance, and recognition of her frustration. She was treated as a capable adult and was encouraged to carry out as much self-care as feasible with the right hemiparesis. She was encouraged to socialize with staff, her family, and other patients. Generally, effective communication was achieved by her using gestures, pictures, and drawings. Education of the patient and family focused on the nature of the communication problem, its cause, and ways to enhance communication using environmental manipulation, supportive behaviors, and facilitation techniques. The speech therapy department was consulted and worked predominantly to provide alternate means of communication and help the family communicate effectively with the patient.

On completion of the stroke workup and confirmation of the hypercoagulable state, T.R. was transferred to an inpatient rehabilitation center. Speech therapy addressing both the aphasia and dysarthria was started along with other physical and occupational therapies. Rehabilitation staff continued to provide a therapeutic environment, to exhibit supportive behaviors, and to facilitate verbal language output. Family support and education continued as well. The patient was discharged to home with ongoing outpatient therapy in 2 weeks. The hemiparesis and Broca's aphasia persisted to a large degree, but T.R. learned compensatory techniques readily and showed little disability at the end of her rehabilitation period. Her anticoagulation regimen continues.

The outcome criteria listed in Box 25-6 can be used to document the progression and effectiveness of communication enhancement across inpatient acute care, inpatient rehabilitation, and outpatient rehabilitation. Likewise the nursing-sensitive patient outcome titled "Communication: Expressive Ability" is an appropriate tool to document progression and effectiveness of language rehabilitation over time for T.R.

REFERENCES

Acredolo, L., & Goodwyn, S. (1996). *Baby signs: How to talk with your baby before your baby can talk.* New York: NTC Publishing Group.

Adams, R., Victor, M., & Ropper, A.H. (1997). *Principles of Neurology* (5th ed.). New York: McGraw-Hill.

Allison, M. (1992). The effects of neurologic injury on the maturing brain. *Headlines, 3,* 2-6, 9-10.

Basso, A. (1987). Approaches to neuropsychological rehabilitation: Language disorders. In M. Meier, A.L. Benton, & L. Diller (Eds.), *Neuropsychological rehabilitation* (pp. 294-314). New York: Guilford Press.

Basso, A., Capitani, E., & Vignolo, L.A. (1979). Influence of rehabilitation on language skills in aphasic patients: A controlled study. *Archives of Neurology, 36,* 190-196.

Basso, A., Faglioni, P., & Vignolo, L.A. (1975). Etude controlée de la rééducation du language dans l'aphasia: Comparaison entre aphasiques traités et non-traités. *Revue Neurolgique, 131,* 607-614.

Basso, A., Farabola, M., Grassi, M.P., Laiacona, M., & Zanobio, M.E. (1990). Aphasia in left handers. Comparison of aphasia profiles and language recovery in non-right-handed and matched right-handed patients. *Brain and Language, 38,* 233-252.

Bavelier, D., Corina, D.D., Jezzard, P., Clark, V., Karni, A., Lalwani, A., Rauschecker, J.P., Brown, A., Turner, P., & Neville, H.J. (1998). Hemispheric specialization for English and ALS. Left invariance-right variability. *Neuroreport, 9*(7), 1537-1542.

Benson, D.G., & Ardila, A. (1996). *Aphasia: A clinical perspective.* New York: Oxford University Press.

Boss, B.J. (1984a). Dysphasia, dyspraxia, and dysarthria: Distinguishing features, part 1. *Journal of Neurosurgical Nursing, 16,* 151-160.

Boss, B.J. (1984b). Dysphasia, dyspraxia, and dysarthria: Distinguishing features, part 2. *Journal of Neurosurgical Nursing, 16,* 211-216.

Boss, B.J. (2000). Concepts of neurologic dysfunction. In S.E. Huether & K.L. McCance (Eds.), *Understanding pathophysiology.* St. Louis: Mosby.

Bower, B. (1996). Cerebellum. *Science News, 150, 23.*

Bower, B. (1998a). Family gives genetic clue to language. *Science News, 153, 71.*

Bower, B. (1998b). The name game. *Science News, 153,* 268-269.

Broida, H. (1979). *Coping with stroke: Communication breakdown with brain injured adults.* San Diego: College Hill Press.

Burfield, E., & Zangwell, O.L. (1946). Re-education in aphasia: A review of 70 cases. *Journal of Neurology, Neurosurgery and Psychiatry, 9,* 75-79.

Courtney, S.M., Petit, L., Maisog, J.M., Ungerleider, L.G., & Haxby, J.V. (1998). An area specialized for spatial working memory in human frontal cortex. *Science, 179*(5355), 1347-1351.

Culton, G.L. (1971). Reaction to age as a factor in chronic aphasia in stroke patients. *Journal of Speech and Hearing Disorders, 36,* 563-564.

Darley, F.L. (1975). Treatment of acquired aphasia. In W.J. Friedlander (Ed.), *Advances in neurology* (Vol. 7) (pp. 111-145). New York: Raven Press.

Darley, F.L., Aronson, A.E., & Brown, J.R. (1969). Clusters of deviant speech dimensions in the dysarthrias. *Journal of Speech and Hearing Research, 12,* 462-496.

David, R., Enderby, P., & Bainton, D. (1982). Treatment of acquired aphasia: Speech therapists and volunteers compared. *Journal of Neurology, Neurosurgery and Psychiatry, 45,* 957-961.

Enderby, R, & Crow, E. (1990). Long-term recovery patterns of severe dysarthria following head injury. *British Journal of Disorders of Communication,* 25, 341-354.

Fox, P.T., Ingham, R.J., Ingham, J.C., Hirsch, T.B., Downs, J. H., Martin, C., Jerabek, P., Glass, T., & Lancaster, J.L. (1996). A PET study of the neural systems of stuttering. *Nature, 382*(6587), 158-161.

Glausiusz, J. (1999). The genes of 1998. *Discover, 20*(1), 33.

Goodglass, H. (1987). Neurolinguistic principles and aphasia therapy. In M. Meier, A. Benton, & L. Diller (Eds.), *Neuropsychological rehabilitation* (pp. 315-326). New York: Guilford Press.

Gordon, M. (2000). *Manual of nursing diagnosis.* (9th ed.) St. Louis: Mosby.

Groher, M. (1977). Language and memory disorders following closed head trauma. *Journal of Speech and Hearing Research, 20,* 212-223.

Grossi, D., Trojano, L., Chiacchio, L., Soricelli, A., Mansi, L., Postighone, A., & Salvatore, M. (1991). Mixed transcortical aphasia: Clinical features and neuroanatomical correlates: A possible role of right hemisphere. *European Neurology, 31,* 204-211.

Hagen, C. (1973). Communication abilities in hemiplegia: Effect of speech therapy. *Archives of Physical Medicine and Rehabilitation, 54,* 454-463.

Hartshorn, K., Rovee-Collier, C., Gerhardstein, P., Bhatt, R.S., Klein, P.J., Aaron, F., Wondoloski, T.L., & Wurtzel, N. (1998). Developmental changes in the specificity of memory over the first year of life. *Developmental Psychobiology, 33*(1), 61-78.

Haxby, J.V., Ungerleider, L.G., Horwitz, B., Maisog, J.M., Rapoport, S.L., & Grady, C.L. (1996). Face encoding and recognition in the human brain. *Proceedings of the National Academy of Sciences of the United States of America, 93*(2), 922-927.

Hill, B.P., & Singer, L.T. (1990). Speech and language development after infant *tracheostomy. Journal of Speech and Hearing Disorders, 55,* 1520.

Hirsch, J., & Kim, K. (1997). The bilingual brain. *Discovery, 18,* 16.

Horwitz B., Ramsey, J.M., & Donohue, B.C. (1998). Functional connectivity of the angular gyrus in normal reading and dyslexia. *Proceedings of the National Academy of Sciences of the United States of America, 95*(15), 9039-44.

Johnson, J.A., & Pring, T.R. (1990). Speech therapy and Parkinson's disease: A review and further data. *British Journal of Disorders of Communication, 25,* 183-194.

Johnstone, B., & Frank, R.G. (1995). Neuropsychological assessment in rehabilitation: Current limitations and applications. *NeuroRehabilitation, 5,* 75-86.

Kertesz, A., & Benke, T. (1989). Sex equality in intrahemispheric language organization. *Brain and Language, 37,* 401-408.

Kertesz, A., & McCabe, P. (1977). Recovery patterns and prognosis in aphasia. *Brain, 100,* 1-18.

Kirscher, H.S. (1995). *Handbook of neurological speech and language disorders.* New York: Marcel Dekker.

Klein, E. (1996). *Clinical phonology: Assessment and treatment of articulation disorders in children and adults.* San Diego: Singular Publishing Group.

Layton, M. (1999). *Sign and say baby's first words.* New York: Peek-A-Boo Publishing.

Levita, E. (1978). Effects of speech therapy on aphasics' responses to the functional communication profile. *Perceptual and Motor Skills, 47,* 151-154.

Lincoln, N.B., Pickersgill, M.J., Hankey, A.I., & Hilton, C.R. (1982). An evaluation of operant training and speech therapy in the language rehabilitation of moderate aphasics. *Behavioral Psychotherapy, 10,* 162-178.

Locke, J.L., & Pearson, D.M. (1990). Linguistic significance of babbling: Evidence from a tracheostomized infant. *Journal of Child Language, 17,* 1-16.

Luria, A.R. (1970). *Traumatic aphasia: Its syndromes, psychology and treatment.* La Hauge: Mouton.

Marshall, R.C., Tompkins, C.A., & Phillips, D.S. (1982). Improvement in treated aphasia: Examination of selected prognostic factors. *Folia Phoniatric, 34,* 305-315.

Masataka, N. (1998). Perception of motherese in Japanese sign language by 6-month-old hearing infants. *Developmental Psychology, 34*(2), 241-246.

McNeil, M.R. (1997). *Clinical management of sensorimotor speech disorders.* New York: Thieme.

Meikle, M., Wechsler, E., Tupper, A.M., Benenson, M., Butler, J., Mulhall, D., & Stem, G. (1979). Comparative trial of volunteer and professional treatments of dysphasia after stroke. *British Medical Journal, 2,* 87-89.

Messerli, P., Tissot, R., & Rodriguez, J. (1976). Recovery from aphasia: Some factors of prognosis. In Y. Lebrun & R. Hoops (Eds.), *Recovery in aphasia.* Amsterdam: Swets & Zeitlinger.

Mesulam, M.M. (1990). Large-scale neurocognitive networks and distributed processing for attention, language, and memory. *Annals of Neurology, 28,* 597-613.

Milton, S.B., Prutting, C.A., & Binder, G. (1984). Appraisal of communicative competence in head injured adults. In R.H. Brookshire (Ed.), *Proceedings from the clinical aphasiology conference.* Minneapolis: BRK Publishers.

Monrad-Krohn, G.H. (1947). Altered melody of language ("dysprosody") as an element of aphasia. *Acta Psychiatrica Neurolgica, 46*(Suppl.), 204-212.

Morris, J.S., Frith, C.D., Perrett, D.I., Rowland, D., Young, A.D., Calder, A.J., & Dolan, R.J. (1996). A differential neural response in the human amygdala to fearful and happy facial expressions. *Nature, 383*(6603), 812-815.

Musso, M., Weiller, C., Kiebel, S., Muller, S.P. Bulau, O., & Rijntjes, M. (1999). Training-induced brain plasticity in aphasia. *Brain, 122,* 1781-1790.

Nagarajan, S., Mahncke, H., Salz, T., Tallal, P., Roberts, T., & Merzenich, M.M. (1999). Cortical auditory signal processing in poor readers. *Proceedings of the National Academy of Sciences of the United States of America, 96*(11), 6483-6488.

Neville, H.J., & Bavelier, D. (1998). Neural organization and plasticity of language. *Current Opinion in Neurobiology, 8*(2), 254-258.

Neville, H.J., Bavelier, D., Corinia, D., Rauschecker, J., Karni, A., Lalwani, A., Braun, A., Clark, V., Jezzard, P., & Turner, R. (1998). Cerebral organization of language in deaf and hearing subjects: Biological constraints and effects of experience. *Proceedings of the National Academy of Sciences of the United States, 95*(3), 922-929.

Nishimura, H., Hashikawa, K., Doi, K., Iwaki, T., Watanabe, Y., Kusuoka, H., Nishimura, T., & Kubo, T. (1999). Sign language "heard" in the auditory cortex. *Nature, 397*(6715), 116.

Nyberg, L., McIntosh, A.R., Cabeza, R., Habib, R., Houle, S., & Tulving, E. (1996). General and specific brain regions involved in encoding and retrieval of events: What, where, and when. *Proceedings of the National Academy of Sciences of the United States of America, 93*(20), 11280-11285.

Paul, R. (1995). *Language disorders from infancy through adolescence: Assessment and treatment.* St. Louis: Mosby.

Peterson, S.E., Fox, P.T., Posner, M.I., Mintun, M. & Raichle, M.E. (1998). Positron emission tomographic studies of cortical anatomy of single word processing. *Journal of Cognitive Neuroscience, 1*(2), 153-170.

Pizzamiglio, L., Mammucari, A., & Razzano, C. (1985). Evidence of sex differences in brain organization from recovery in aphasia. *Brain and Language, 25,* 213-222.

Posner, M.I., & Raichle, M.E. (1994). *Images of mind.* New York: Scientific American Library.

Prins, R.S., Snow, C.E., & Wagenaar E. (1978). Recovery from aphasia: Spontaneous speech versus language comprehension, *Brain and Language, 6,* 192-211.

Richardson, S. (1996). Tarzan's little brain. *Discover, 17*(11), 100-102.

Ross, E.D. (1985). Modulation of affect and nonverbal communication by right hemisphere. In M-M. Mesulam (Ed.), *Principles of behavioral neurology* (pp. 239-257). Philadelphia: FA Davis.

Ross, E.D., Holzapfel, D., & Freemen, R. (1983). Assessment of affective behavior in brain damaged patients using quantitative acoustical phonetic and gestural measurements. *Neurology, 33*(Suppl. 2), 219-220.

Rovee-Collier, C. (1997). Dissociations in infant memory; Rethinking the development of implicit and explicit memory. *Psychological Review, 104*(3), 467-498.

Samson, Y., Belin, P., Zilbovicius, M., Remy, P., Van Eeckhout, O., & Rancurel, G. (1999). Mechanisms of aphasia recovery and brain imaging. *Revue Neurologique, 155*(9), 725-730.

Sarno, M.T. (1980). Language rehabilitation outcome in the elderly aphasic patient. In L.K. Obler & M.L. Albert (Eds.), *Language and communication in the elderly: Clinical therapeutic and experimental issues.* Lexington: DC Heath.

Sarno, M.T., Silverman, M., & Sands, E. (1970). Speech therapy and language recovery in severe aphasia. *Journal of Speech and Hearing Research, 13,* 607-623.

Schooler, C., Neumann, E., Caplan, L.J., & Roberts, B.R. (1997). Stroop theory, memory, and prefrontal cortical functioning: Reply to Cohen et al. (1997) [Comment]. *Journal of Experimental Psychology: General, 126*(1), 42-44.

Shaywitz, S.E., Shaywitz, B.A., Pugh, K.R., Fulbright, R.K., Constable, R.T., Mencl, W.E., Shankweiler, D.P., Liberman, A.M., Skudlarski, P., Fletcher, J.M., Katz, L., Marchione, K.E., Lacadie, C., Gatenby, C., & Gore, J.C. (1998). Functional disruption in the organization of the brain for reading in dyslexia. *Proceedings of the National Academy of Sciences of the United States of America, 95*(5), 2636-2641.

Schmahmann, J.D., & Sherman, J.C. (1998). The cerebellar cognitive affective syndrome. *Brain, 121,* 561-569.

Sohlberg, M.M., & Mateer, C.A. (1989). *Introduction to cognitive rehabilitation: Theory and practice.* New York: Guilford Press.

Travis, J. (1999). Gene tinkering makes memorable mice. *Science News, 156,* 149.

Vignolo, L.A. (1964). Evolution of aphasia and language rehabilitation: A retrospective exploratory study. *Cortex, 1,* 344-367.

Wertz, R.T., Collins, M.J., Weiss, D., Kurtzke, J.P., Friden, T., Brookshire, R.H., Pierce, J., Holtzapple, P., Hubbard, D.J., Porch, B.E., West, J.A., Davis, L., Matovitch, V., Morley, G.K., & Resurreccion, E. (1981). Veterans Administration cooperative study on aphasia: A comparison of individual and group treatment. *Journal of Speech and Hearing Research, 24,* 580-594.

Wong, D.L., Hockenberry-Eaton, M., Wilson, D., Winkelstein, M.L., Allman, E., & DiVito-Thomas, P.A. (1999). *Whaley and Wong's nursing care of infants and children* (6th ed.) St. Louis: Mosby.

26 Cognition and Behavior

Cindy Gatens, MN, RN, CRRN-A
A. René Hébert, MS, RN, CRRN-A

If rehabilitation nurses could follow their clients back in time and live inside their bodies and minds during the course of an illness such as Alzheimer's disease, the nurses might find the experience both enlightening and disturbing. For example:

- *I'm having trouble remembering simple things. I have a weekly hair appointment in town but I get to town and forget why I am there.*
- *A year later—I'm driving and I pull out in front of another car. I don't know what happened, so I drive home. My husband meets me at home and tells me that I left the scene of an accident. No one is hurt, I am glad, but I don't remember.*
- *Months later—The neurologist asks me questions and tells me that I have major memory problems. It could be Alzheimer's. I'm scared. What will happen to me?*
- *Two years later—I cannot remember how to cook or do laundry. They took my keys away. People come to visit, I don't know them. My husband tells me they are my children and grandchildren.*
- *One year later—My husband is so patient, but he gets upset when I cannot find the bathroom and I'm incontinent.*
- *Six months later—Someone is packing my clothes into a suitcase. She says she is my daughter. My husband is crying. They tell me that my husband is worn out taking care of me, and I will be going to an intermediate care facility. He will come to see me every day.*
- *Four years later—I am no longer talking or walking. The nurses in the ECF (extended care facility) toilet me, shower me, dress me, and feed me. I'm glad that I can still swallow. I don't recognize anyone, but my husband is still sure that I know who he is. He comes to see me every day. The nurses are so good to me and my husband. They talk to him every day about how I am doing and how much they like me. They encourage him to come in for Sunday dinner, bingo, and all the social activities. They are a good source of support for both of us.*
- *A week later—The flu is rampant in the ECF. My favorite nurse comes in on the night shift and tells me that I'm ill and must go to the hospital. I am taken to an acute medical unit. I hear the doctor talking to my husband about my poor quality of life. I have a different nurse every day. No one gets me out of bed or takes me to the bathroom. No one even talks to me here. My husband comes and sees me daily. He finds a pressure sore on my heel and skin breakdown from the incontinence. I had a swallowing test and I did fine, but no one takes the time to feed me. They told my husband that I refused to eat. He comes for dinner and feeds me. I eat well.*
- *The next day—I hear them say that I am OK now and will be going back to my ECF tomorrow. I am glad and so is my husband. My rehabilitation nurses there know me, respect me, and care about me and my husband.*
- *That night—I'm having chest pain, what is going on?? I cannot call for help. I'm having a heart attack but no one knows that.*
- *The next morning—I'm not doing well, but the doctors do not know why. My liver and kidneys are failing. The doctor tells my husband that I won't live much longer and there is nothing they can do. My husband is with me when I die.*
- *Looking back—What would my husband and I have done without the rehabilitation nurses? They facilitated quality for the final years of my life. They kept me healthy and independent as long as they could. They talked to me all the time even though I didn't understand. They were patient and treated me with respect. They kept my husband involved and informed, and made him feel that he had a purpose in watching over me and my care. We will always remember them for their expertise. Rehabilitation nurses—thank you for all you do!*

Rehabilitation nurses provide care for clients who have experienced cognitive alterations after illness or injury across the continuum of rehabilitation care and throughout the life span. Cognition plays a major role in the determination of a person's rehabilitation potential—including the ability to remember and the capacity to learn new information, relearning self care, returning to a previous lifestyle, and maintaining independence despite specific deficits in cognitive functioning. Concepts of growth and development, learning, and the cognitive changes of aging provide structure for rehabilitation nurses in designing care for patients with deficits in cognition.

Grzanikowski (1997) defines cognition as the abstract concept of thinking. Intact cognitive function reflects the highly integrated functions of many parts of the cerebral hemispheres, cortex, and subcortical structures. The functional components of cognition include attention, memory, orientation, judgment/reasoning, problem solving, and executive function. Causes of cognitive impairment or alterations in thinking vary with age, severity, geographic location, and even season of the year. The location and nature of the insult or disease bear a direct relationship to the physical or cognitive impairment incurred.

INCIDENCE AND PREVALENCE OF COGNITION DEFICITS

Brain Injury

An estimated 5.3 million Americans (approximately 2% of the U.S. population) currently live with disability from traumatic brain injuries (TBI) according to the latest report by the Centers for Disease Control and Prevention (CDC) (Marino, 1999). The leading causes of TBI are motor vehicle crashes, violence (mostly from firearms), and falls, especially among the elderly. The risk in men is twice the risk in women. The risk is higher in adolescents, young adults, and people older than 75 years of age.

Shaken Baby Syndrome

Children younger than 1 year of age sustain brain injuries commonly as a result of abuse. According to the Pediatric Trauma Registry, shaken baby syndrome (SBS) is the fastest growing incidence of traumatic brain injury in children younger than 1 year. Every year an estimated 3,000 children are diagnosed with SBS. Twenty-five percent of the children die, whereas 60% sustain permanent lifelong disabilities. The outcome for children with SBS is permanent brain damage or death (Brain Injury Association [BIA], 1998).

Falls in Children and Adolescents

Falls are a significant cause of TBI in children ages 1 through 4 years. Children 10 to 15 years old are at high risk for experiencing TBI in motor vehicle or bicycle incidents or while playing sports (BIA, 1998).

Hypoxia/Ischemia in Children

Hypoxia/ischemic brain injury occurs frequently in infancy and childhood. This may include near drowning, respiratory arrest, and near sudden infant death syndrome. Despite current critical care practices, the outcomes from these injuries are often lifelong neurological deficits (Biagas, 1999).

Sports Injuries

Sports and recreational activities are thought to be a significant source of brain injury. There has been a paucity of information in the literature evaluating sports activities and the incidence of brain injury. Kraus and McArthur (1999) found their review of available data difficult to interpret, but they concluded by suggesting that helmet use for many recreational activities should be explored, specifically horseback riding, skateboarding, in-line skating, sledding, and skiing.

With the growing popularity of soccer in the United States and worldwide, reports of adverse effects of "heading" on brain function have become a concern. Baroff (1998) reviewed the neurological and neuropsychological findings in the research literature. Abnormalities were reported in a significant minority of older former professional players in Norway. The findings showed cerebral atrophy and impairment on intelligence test abilities that are vulnerable to brain damage. Also noted were persistent complaints (physical, cognitive, and emotional) consistent with post-concussion syndrome. Younger amateur players were free of major abnormalities, but some reported continual problems with memory and concentration. The author concluded that these problems may be the result of soccer-related head injuries, but not necessarily specific to heading. Kelly and Rosenberg (1998) emphasized the importance of detection of mild forms of concussion through detailed observation and examination of athletes. They described the practice parameters adopted by the American Academy of Neurology for sports sideline evaluation and management strategies for injured athletes. These guidelines are meant to educate and provide a balance between maintaining a competitive edge (letting an athlete return to competition) and an objective assessment of injury (that may prevent an athlete from further participation in a sport).

Sosin, Sacks, and Webb (1996) analyzed data on pediatric death from bicycling in the United States from the National Center for Health Statistics from 1989 through 1992. They found an average of 247 TBI deaths and 140,000 head injuries among children and adolescents younger than 20 years of age were related to bicycle crashes each year in the United States. They found that as many 184 deaths and 116,000 head injuries might have been prevented annually if these riders had worn helmets.

Alcohol/Substance Abuse

The positive association between blood alcohol level and risk of injury is well established for almost every type of external cause of injury, including motor vehicle crashes, drowning, and violence. Studies have examined frequency of intoxication at time of injury in adolescents and adults, but excluding children because of lack of data. The TBI Model System Project reported that 39% of their subjects were intoxicated at time of injury (Harrison-Felix, 1996).

There has been little or no systematic study of intoxication caused by drugs other than alcohol. Better data regarding the presence of drugs other than alcohol could increase estimates of the incidence of intoxication at the time of injury. The high frequency with which alcohol is used in conjunction with other drugs results in an overlap between intoxication secondary to alcohol and that secondary to the drugs. Almost two thirds of adolescents and adults admitted for rehabilitation have histories of alcohol or other drug abuse (Corrigan, Bogner, & Lamb-Hart, 1999).

Falls in the Elderly

Falls are the leading cause of TBI for people age 65 and older. Eleven percent of fall-related TBIs were fatal (BIA, 1998). Pedestrian injuries and lower speed motor vehicle crashes are the next most common causes of brain injury in the elderly (Englander & Cifu, 1999).

Human Immunodeficiency Virus/Acquired Immunodeficiency Syndrome

It has now been established that the human immunodeficiency virus (HIV) can have a direct effect on the brain. Acquired immunodeficiency syndrome (AIDS) dementia complex is the term used to describe the dementia in people with AIDS caused by HIV. HIV is not the only cause of dementia in people experiencing AIDS. As a result of the body's weakened immune system, other viruses and organisms can attack the brain. This type of dementia is called "opportunistic infection of the brain" because it literally takes opportunity of the weakened body. It is important for professionals to recognize that this is a side effect of the presence of HIV in the body; opportunistic infections are often treatable (Alzheimer's Association, 2000).

The CDC semiannual HIV/AIDS surveillance report (2000) revealed that the number of newly reported AIDS cases continues to decrease in the United States as a result of highly active antiretroviral therapy. The overall numbers of AIDS cases remain significant. The cumulative number of AIDS cases reported to the CDC is 688,200. Adults and adolescent AIDS cases total 679,739, with 570,425 cases in males and 109,314 cases in females. The proportion of cases among women increased slightly in 1998. Through the same time period, 8,461 AIDS cases were reported in children younger than age 13 (National Center for HIV, STD, and TB Prevention, 1998). It is estimated that 8% to 16% of people with AIDS develop dementia (Alzheimer Europe, 2000). Those who do tend to develop it in the later stages of AIDS.

Stroke

Stroke is the leading cause of disability in older adults and the third leading cause of death in the UnitedStates. The risk of stroke increases with advancing age. In the over-75 age group, approximately 10% of this age group will experience a stroke. The factors precipitating this seem to be more age related progressive changes in blood vessels, whereas the factors associated with those younger than 75 years old seem to be more related to lifestyle choices.

More than half a million people will experience a new or recurrent stroke each year; about 500,000 of these are new strokes and 100,000 are recurrent strokes. About 150,000 people die each year from a stroke. Strokes account for half of all clients hospitalized for acute neurological disease. Twenty-eight percent of those who have strokes are younger than age 65. Generally, men are at greater risk of stroke than women; however, women have a higher mortality from stroke. The mortality rate from a stroke for African-American females is higher than for Caucasian females. Women are reported to survive longer than men. These ethnic differences are directly related to their risk factor of hypertension. Hypertension occurs more frequently in certain African and Hispanic cultures. Hypertension is considered a major contributory factor causing stroke. One in every five Americans has hypertension, putting them at considerable risk for a stroke. Today, at least 3 million stroke survivors live with some degree of disability (American Heart Association, 2000).

Alzheimer's Disease

Alzheimer's disease is an insidious, progressive disorder that alters memory, executive function, language, visual-spatial, and other cognitive abilities. In addition to cognitive decline, behavioral disturbances occur such as agitation, hallucinations, and a decline in executive and self-care functions. Alzheimer's disease affects approximately 4 million people in the United States. Age is one of the greatest risk factors for developing Alzheimer's disease. It is estimated that 14 million Americans will have Alzheimer's disease by the middle of the next century unless a cure is found. One in 10 people older than 65 years of age and nearly half of those older than 85 have Alzheimer's disease. An average life span is 8 to 20 years from the onset of symptoms. Half of all nursing home clients experience Alzheimer's disease, which costs an average per client of $42,000, up to $70,000 per year. The average lifetime cost per client is estimated to be $174,000 (Alzheimer's Association, 2000). The financial burden of Alzheimer's disease, including both direct costs and indirect costs, is estimated at $90 billion annually in the United States.

Multiple Sclerosis

Multiple sclerosis (MS) is a common neurological disease in northern climates. The prevalence of this disease is difficult to determine because in many instances the diagnosis is not made. Most people with MS are diagnosed between the ages of 20 and 40. The disease course can be progressive. There appear to be various causes, including viruses and environmental, genetic, and immune system factors. Studies of patterns of this disease reveal that MS occurs with much greater frequency in higher latitudes (above 40°) away from the equator. In the United States, MS occurs more frequently in states that are above the 37th parallel than in states below it. From east to west, the parallel extends from Newport News, Virginia, to Santa Cruz, California. The northern borders include North Carolina to the northern border of Arizona, including most of California. There are at least 250,000 people with MS in the United States. Women are affected twice as often as men. MS is more common among Caucasians than other races, and is almost unheard of in other races (i.e., Alaskan Native Americans). In certain populations a particular genetic trait has been identified that may be activated thus causing MS (Multiple Sclerosis Foundation, 2000).

It is estimated that approximately 50% of people with MS will develop some cognitive deficits. Typical areas of deficits include slower thinking, delayed responses, impaired judgment, poor concentration, and short-term memory problems. These deficits do not cause the client to be unable to function within his or her home. Usually the cognitive symptoms are subtle and gradual. During stressful times and exacerbations, cognitive function can be significantly impaired. A person may need constant care until this episodes pass. When assessing cognitive function in a person with MS, one must remember to incorporate age, education, learning style, communication patterns, stress, and disease management before diagnosing with Altered Thought Processes.

PATHOPHYSIOLOGY OF DEFICITS IN COGNITION

Traumatic Brain Injury

TBI, often referred to as *head injury* or *head trauma,* is an acquired injury to the brain tissue caused by an external force and ranges from very mild to severe. General physiological effects that commonly are seen in moderate to severe head injury include cerebral edema, increased intracranial pressure, sensorimotor deficits, and cognitive deficits (Graham, 1999).

Brain damage is categorized as focal or diffuse, depending on the mechanism of how the damage occurred. Focal damage is discrete damage localized on either hemisphere to produce a specific deficit pattern. Focal damage generally results from falls, gunshot wounds, intracranial hemorrhage (including stroke), MS, or brain tumors.

Closed head injury (a nonpenetrating injury with no break in the skull), anoxia, and Alzheimer's disease produce a more diffuse damage to the brain. The primary mechanism of injury in closed head injury is injury to brain tissue resulting from the movement of the brain against the skull (rapid acceleration, deceleration, and rotational forces). These are high-acceleration injuries, often secondary to motor vehicle accidents.

Concussion is a jarring or shaking of the brain without bruising that frequently is accompanied by a brief loss of consciousness and loss of memory. A contusion is a bruising of the brain and is generally a result of more severe damage than a concussion.

Primary traumatic damage to the brain is worsened by secondary damage occurring after injury. These may be intracranial or systemic and can occur during initial management or within the first few days after injury. Potential secondary injury can occur from cerebral edema, increased intracranial pressure, brain herniation, hematoma development, elevated temperature, hypoxia, and ischemia. Systemic factors that can lead to secondary brain damage include cardiac arrest, hemorrhage, hypertension, and emboli. Each of these can cause an increase in intracranial pressure, which increases brain damage.

Hydrocephalus is a late secondary complication resulting from obstruction in cerebrospinal fluid circulation or absorption. Often late complications include abscesses and seizures. Approximately 7% of those experiencing TBI will develop a seizure disorder after brain injury (Rocchio, 2000). A seizure occurs when a large group of cells misfire or short circuit. In brain injury, misfires occur as a result of damage in the brain that interrupts the normal flow of cell firings. Katz and Black (1999) classify seizure events as immediate, early, or late. Immediate seizures (within minutes after injury) are frequent among children, but do not necessarily mean that the child will have posttraumatic epilepsy. Early seizures (within the first week after injury) have an incidence of approximately 5% and present a 20% to 30% risk of late seizures. For those with late seizures (after the first week postinjury), the risk of late posttraumatic epilepsy may be as high as 70%. More than half of the clients with posttraumatic seizures experience onset within the first year and 75% to 80% by the second year. At 5 years, the risk is most likely back to preinjury levels, but seizures can still occur (Katz & Black, 1999). Posttraumatic seizures may be generalized onset (grand mal), petit mal, focal, or complex partial (Rocchio, 2000).

Mild Traumatic Brain Injury

The clinical and scientific communities have found no consensus regarding the etiology of symptom presentation and duration after mild head injury. Consensus is also lacking on a single definition of mild head injury (Barth, Macciocchi, & Diamond, 1999).

The American Congress of Rehabilitation Medicine Head Injury Interdisciplinary Special Interest Group proposed a common definition for mild traumatic brain injury (MTBI) as follows: An injury to the head or mechanical forces applied to the head producing physiological disruption of brain function, as manifested by at least one of the following.

- Any period of loss of consciousness
- Any loss of memory for events immediately before or after the incident
- Any alteration in mental status at the time of the incident (i.e., feeling dazed, disoriented, or confused)
- Focal neurological deficits which may or may not be transient; but when the severity of the injury does not exceed the following:
  - Loss of consciousness of approximately 30 minutes or less
  - After 30 minutes, a Glasgow Coma Scale of 13 to 15 (Table 26-1)
  - Posttraumatic amnesia (PTA) not greater than 24-hours (Evans, 1992, p. 430)

People with MTBI can exhibit persistent emotional, cognitive, behavioral, and physical symptoms, alone or in combination, which may produce a functional disability. The symptoms generally fall into one of the following three categories and provide additional evidence that a MTBI has occurred.

1. Physical symptoms of brain injury (e.g., nausea, vomiting, dizziness, headache, blurred vision, sleep disturbance, fatigue, lethargy, or other sensory loss) that cannot be accounted for by peripheral injury or other causes.
2. Cognitive deficits (e.g., involving attention, concentration, perception, memory, speech/language, or higher level executive functions) that cannot be accounted for by emotional state or other causes.
3. Behavioral changes or alterations in degree of emotional responsivity such as irritability, quickness to anger, disinhibition, or emotional lability that cannot be accounted for by a psychological reaction to physical or emotional stress or other causes (American Congress of Rehabilitation Medicine [ACRM], 1991).

It is estimated that the number of individuals experiencing MTBI is quite high, but underestimated. Gordon et al. (1998) described a group of individuals with "hidden" TBI. They were defined as those who sustained a blow to the head with altered mental status, and who experienced a substantial number of the cognitive, behavioral, and emotional sequelae typically associated with brain injury, but did not make the causal connection between the injury and its consequences. It is estimated that 20% to 40% of those who experience mild brain injury do not obtain medical attention. Children and adolescents with isolated prefrontal injury associated with MTBI may appear well and without obvious problems and be discharged after a short hospital stay (Christensen, 1997).

TABLE 26-1 Glasgow Coma Scale

Response	Points
Eye Opening	**E**
Spontaneous	4
To speech	3
To pain	2
None	1
Best Motor Response	**M**
Obeys commands	6
Localizes pain stimuli	5
Withdraws from pain stimuli	4
Abnormal flexion	3
Extension response	2
None	1
Verbal Response	**V**
Oriented	5
Confused conversation	4
Inappropriate words	3
Incomprehensible sounds	2
None	1

Coma score (E + M + V): 3 to 15 points.

Anoxia/Hypoxic Brain Injury

Anoxic brain injury (ABI) refers to injury to the brain caused by inadequate oxygen supply. The terms "anoxia" and "hypoxia" often are used interchangeably. Although the terms can be used to refer to the oxygen supply of the lungs or bloodstream, it is the lack of oxygen availability at the brain tissue level that causes ABI.

Frequently, ABI occurs secondary to cardiac arrest. Although cardiopulmonary resuscitation restores some circulation, it is difficult to estimate the duration and severity of compromise of oxygen supply to the brain. When the oxygen supply to the brain is interrupted for a period of time, brain cells die and serious ABI can occur. Other causes of ABI include trauma, lightning injuries, choking on food, near-drowning, drug overdose, and perioperative complications (Long, 1989).

Secondary hypoxic damage also can occur after the initial brain insult. Arterial hypoxemia is present in more than a third of severely head-injured people when they arrive at a major hospital after injury. When arterial partial pressure of oxygen falls, a desaturation of arterial blood begins to occur, with a consequent fall in the volume of oxygen carried per unit volume of blood. Under normal circumstances this fall in oxygen content would be compensated for by a brisk cerebral vasodilatation. In the damaged brain, however, a compensatory boost in blood flow does not occur or occurs to a lesser extent. Thus, there is a reduction in oxygen reaching the brain cells in the most severely injured parts of the brain. Causes can range from airway obstruction secondary to blood, foreign bodies, poor positioning, aspiration of gastric stomach contents, and chest injury resulting in pneumothorax, hemothorax, or pulmonary contusion (Rosenthal ,Griffith, Bond, & Miller, 1990).

Depending on the severity of the ABI, certain "generic" symptoms may be characteristic, as shown in Box 26-1.

Other symptoms secondary to anoxia/hypoxia are receptive or expressive aphasia, apraxia (difficulty performing requested tasks despite adequate comprehension, strength, and coordination), and visual agnosia (inability to recognize something despite seeing it adequately).

Certain parts of the brain are especially sensitive to a lack of oxygen. Symptoms specific to brain regions/lobes occur depending on the severity of the anoxia. For example, anoxia/hypoxia to certain cells in the temporal lobe produces memory difficulty, whereas anoxia/hypoxia to cells in the cerebellum produces balance difficulties. If the oxygen shortage is prolonged and severe, numerous brain cells are damaged and the effects can be severe.

The brain areas affected after ABI differ from those affected by TBI; thus symptoms and course of recovery differ. For instance, anoxia injuries occur posteriorly, whereas TBI frequently causes damage to frontal or temporal areas of the brain; ABI causes loss of brain cells, whereas TBI leads to hemorrhage or bruising and edema.

It is difficult to predict the course of recovery after an anoxic/hypoxic event because most people are comatose immediately after an anoxic event, but there are indicators for estimating severity or extent of impairment. One indicator for predicting outcome is papillary response to light reflex. The duration of time a client requires to follow commands or speak is predictive of the course of recovery. Clients with ABI almost always regain communication abilities within the first 1 or 2 months when continuous recovery is occurring. On the other hand, clients with TBI sometimes show dramatic improvement after several months of unresponsiveness. Others demonstrate initial rapid improvements followed by a decrease in responsiveness, usually between the second and tenth days after anoxia; the reason for this is unknown.

Youth is an asset for recovery in ABI. With mild ABI many older people become able to return to independent living. For all age groups difficulty in cognition indicates problems with attention, concentration, and memory that can severely limit a person's safety and ability to function independently in society (Long, 1989). More specifically, research indicates that memory processes are impaired after hypoxic brain injury. Implicit memory processes (cognitive skill learning that occurs without awareness) appears to be spared after ischemic hypoxic encephalopathy; whereas the process of consciously accessing memory stored information is impaired (Mecklinger, von Cramon, & Matthes-von Cramon, 1998). The development of new therapies for hypoxic-ischemic brain injury depends on findings from such studies.

Box 26-1 Characteristics of Anoxic Brain Injury

Mild Anoxic Brain Injury

Decreased attention/concentration
Memory impairment (amnesia)
Decreased balance
Agitation/restlessness

Severe Anoxic Brain Injury

Decreased attention/concentration
Memory impairment (amnesia)
Agitation (may be persistent)
Soft, mumbled speech
Dysphasia
Balance/coordination difficulty
Seizures
Spasticity (may be monoclonus—sudden muscle jerking caused by movement)

Most Severe Anoxic Brain Injury

Inability to communicate consistently
Not fully comatose
Able to open eyes
Inconsistent response to the environment

HIV/AIDS

It is not easy to make a definitive diagnosis of HIV/AIDS. A computerized tomography (CT) scan can identify certain opportunistic infections. Magnetic resonance imaging (MRI) can sometimes show white matter changes in the brain of people with AIDS who have dementia. Regular neuropsychological testing can draw attention to slight changes in cognition by testing memory, concentration, and quick thinking. AIDS dementia complex develops when HIV "unlocks" and enters T_4 cells in the body, which are responsible for the body's defense system against infection and disease. HIV can enter the spinal cord and brain because certain cells in the brain have the same "locking system" as T_4 cells. The cells that allow HIV in are in the white matter, and thus interfere with the high-speed transmission of messages between different parts of the brain. Thus, thinking processes are slowed. The HIV kills the cells and the body cannot replace them, so the damage is irreversible (Alzheimer Europe, 2000).

Stroke

Stroke's medical definition is cerebrovascular accident. Stroke is closely associated with certain risk factors. These risk factors are divided into three categories: nonreversible, partially reversible, and reversible. The nonreversible risk factors include sex, age, race, and heredity. The partially reversible risk factors are hypertension, diabetes mellitus, cardiac impairments, and blood lipid abnormalities. Any of these diseases will significantly increase a person's risk for stroke. The reversible risk factors include smoking, obesity, salt intake, cholesterol level, sedentary lifestyle, and the use of some oral contraceptives. Smoking increases the risk in both men and women. The risk increases directly with the number of cigarettes smoked. Also increased total serum cholesterol levels correlate with increased production of plaques in the arteries causing a narrowing of the lumen of blood vessels.

Strokes result from impaired blood flow to a particular area of the brain. The carotid and vertebrobasilar arteries are the main arterial blood systems to the brain. The vertebral arteries enter the brain to form the basilar arteries. The Circle of Willis is a ring of arteries formed by the major arteries and circulates the blood between the right and left hemispheres of the cerebrum (brain). This cerebrovascular system is very stable; it is able to maintain a constant blood flow to the brain despite changes in circulation. Factors that affect cerebral blood flow can be divided into extracranial and intracranial factors. Extracranial factors are related to the circulatory diseases such as hypertension. Intracranial factors are related to diseases causing an increase in intracranial pressure such as hemorrhage and tumors.

There are three classifications or types of strokes: thrombotic, embolic, and hemorrhagic. Thrombosis, the most common type of stroke, is the formation of a blood clot or coagulation that results in narrowing of the lumen of a blood vessel with eventual occlusion. Atherosclerosis promotes this type of stroke. Gradual occlusion of an artery allows time for development of collateral circulation and thus can cause a less serious neurological deficit. Collateral circulation can develop via the Circle of Willis and other cerebral blood vessels thus preventing ischemia if a relatively large vessel is occluded by a clot or complete occlusion resulting from atherosclerosis. Because thrombotic strokes follow a pattern of a gradual narrowing of a blood vessel, a person usually exhibits signs referred to as transient ischemic attack (TIA) warning symptoms. This occurs when a person experiences a neurological deficit lasting no more than 24 hours, and is usually caused by the atherosclerotic plaques impeding constant blood flow through the vessel, or spasm of blood vessels.

Another stroke classification is an embolic stroke, the second most common type of stroke. This type of stroke is usually as a result of heart disease. People with atrial fibrillation are most likely to experience this type of stroke. With atrial fibrillation tiny clots are allowed to form and travel to the brain. The clot or embolus lodges at the point where an artery becomes too narrow for it to pass and causes ischemic infarction. Rapid occlusion, as with an embolus, does not allow for collateral circulation development. Neurological dysfunction will be more sudden and often more serious.

Regardless of whether the stroke is thrombotic or embolic, edema forms in the area of the infarction and contributes to the neuronal dysfunction. Edema can cause compression of brain structures or herniation of the brain. Brain edema develops within a few minutes of artery occlusion and peaks 3 to 4 days after the stroke. The location, extent of infarction, and severity of edema determine the neurological manifestations.

The third type of stroke is a hemorrhagic stroke. This occurs when a blood vessel in the brain leaks or bursts. The blood extravasates into the brain or subarachnoid space. This compresses and displaces the brain tissue. In a large hemorrhage, herniation of the brain tissue may occur. The signs and symptoms will be drastic and sudden when a large vessel is involved. Death may be immediate.

Signs and symptoms of a TIA or stroke are as follows: speech difficulties, numbness or tingling, blurred vision, dizziness, loss of consciousness, loss of balance, lack of comprehension, amnesia, loss of muscle control, or sensory disturbances. The problem with stroke identification is that many of these symptoms are vague and similar to other problems, especially if they resolve in less than 24 hours (TIA sign), and people do not seek medical attention. However, when a person experiences an abrupt onset of any of these neurological deficits, he or she is more apt to seek medical attention urgently, but irreversible damage may have already taken place.

Medical treatment is aimed at reducing neurological deficits and complications associated with the stroke, and improving functional outcome. The initial concern with a stroke is assessing the damage, cause, and onset. This will require thorough assessment and use of a CT scan or MRI study to determine location and cause of stroke. Other diagnostic tests might include cerebral arteriography, electrocardiogram, Doppler flowmeter studies, and laboratory studies. After the cause of a stroke is identified (i.e., clot verses hemorrhagic), treatment is determined.

Several drugs are used to prevent thrombotic stroke by reducing blood coagulability. These include aspirin, Coumadin, and other drugs that require regular blood level checks to ensure optimal range. Clients with acute nonhemorrhagic strokes are given a drug such as tissue plasminogen activator (TPA) in the emergency setting because it must be given within 3 hours of onset of symptoms. The problem occurs when a client waits to seek medical attention, hoping symptoms will resolve. If a person seeks care after 3 hours from onset of symptoms, drugs like TPA are no longer effective. Treatment at this point usually consists of heparin therapy or warfarin sodium (Coumadin) therapy, which have not proven to be as effective in halting the stroke, but do prevent additional clots. Steroids and osmotic diuretics are commonly used to reduce increased intracranial pressure. Carotid endarterectomy is the treatment of choice in 70% to 90% carotid stenosis. However, stroke is a possible complication to this procedure.

The neurological manifestations of stroke depend on brain site, rate of onset, size of lesion, presence of collateral circulation, and timeliness of seeking medical treatment. Neuromuscular deficits are the obvious manifestations of stroke. The left hemisphere is dominant for 93% of the population who are right-handed. When a stroke, regardless of type, occurs in the dominant hemisphere, the person usually experiences communication difficulties or aphasia because the speech center is located in the left hemisphere. When the stroke involves Wernicke's area of the brain (found in the lobe in the dominant hemisphere) a person will experience what is commonly called receptive aphasia. This person is not able to understand the sounds of speech or read written language. A stroke affecting Broca's area of the brain (found in the lobe in the dominant hemisphere) will cause expressive aphasia. This insult will cause the person to have problems in both speaking and writing. When both areas are damaged from a stroke (commonly referred to as global aphasia), a person will not be able to understand what he or she hears or reads and cannot communicate thoughts in speech or writing.

Other manifestations associated with left hemisphere damage are paralysis or paresis in the right side, cautious behavioral manner, language impairment, and cognitive deficits. Manifestations of a right hemisphere stroke include paralysis or paresis on the left side, spatial-perceptual deficits, impulsive behavior, and cognitive deficits. Regardless of location or type of stroke, many people experience some form of cognitive impairment and behavior change.

Recovery after a stroke has predominantly been focused on independent mobility and self-care activities. However, learning to perform old skills or new skills requires the person's ability to think and process information. Studies are beginning to identify neuropsychological consequences of stroke and their role in a person's recovery after a stroke. Hochstenbach and Mulder (1999), found the most relevant cognitive dysfunction after a stroke to include: "disorders in attention; memory; executive functions; perception, selection, and evaluation; communication; emotion, and behaviors" (p. 12).

This study found people with problems in attention had a decline in their flexibility, difficulties in concentrating on a task for a longer time, difficulties performing tasks in a stimulating, noisy environment, and difficulty performing more than one task at a time. It has been found that many stroke victims, if not all, have problems with processing information, causing a delay in thinking and response.

In addition to attention deficits, memory processes may be affected by a stroke. Without memory, a person cannot care for self or others. The seriousness of memory loss after a stroke depends on the location and type of stroke and the recovery of the person. Quantifying the extent of memory impairment after a stroke is done by tests such as the Salford Objective Recognition Test (SORT). The SORT has proven to be an acceptable tool in measuring memory in clients with stroke and could be used as a screening test to detect memory problems (Lincoln & Rother, 1998). In trying to determine the extent of memory impairment after a stroke, a study used the Mini-Mental State Exam (MMSE) (see Table 30-5) to compare the cognitive performance of 74 subjects matched for age and sex. This study found there was a significant decline in cognitive performance/memory processes when nonstroke and poststroke measurements were compared. Furthermore, this study found that depression was not a direct cause of the cognitive decline (Kase et al., 1998).

Another common finding found poststroke were problems in executive function. This leads to problems in planning and carrying out activities, thus forcing the person to be dependent on others. Neglect is another common disorder poststroke that impedes cognitive performance. Neglect occurs when a person has difficulty in reporting or responding to stimuli on the contralateral side of the stroke. Neglect is commonly referred to as a perceptual dysfunction. It significantly impedes a person's understanding of self and environment, thus hindering his or her cognitive abilities.

In addition to cognitive decline poststroke, many people experience emotional and behavioral problems. Compulsive laughing or crying, often referred to as emotional lability, is a classic behavior seen poststroke. The person's reaction or emotion is not appropriate. Depression is also another common reaction after stroke. Before managing depression, it is important to determine if the depression is the result of brain damage from the stroke or is a normal reaction to the stroke. Regardless of cause, depression should be addressed because it can impede recovery. Other behavioral problems identified poststroke are impulsivity, impatience, or being overly cautious. All of these neuropsychological factors need to be assessed carefully so that a plan of treatment can be activated to minimize the consequences (Hochstenbach & Mulder, 1999).

When designing a rehabilitation plan for a person with a stroke, attention needs to be on physical, functional, emotional, and cognitive changes. Cognitive decline can affect a person's rehabilitation outcome. Galshi, Bruno, Zorowitz, and Walker (1993) found that cognitive deficits poststroke have a direct correlation in predicting functional status. Clients who had a stroke with cognitive changes in the areas of abstract thinking, judgment, short-term memory, comprehension, and orientation, performed poorly in self-care activities at discharge from rehabilitation.

Incorporating cognitive rehabilitation into the traditional physical/language rehabilitation will make a person's recovery poststroke more meaningful. Sisson (1998) found that stroke survivors with mental changes in mood, judgment, memory, and personality during rehabilitation continued with problems such as depression, memory loss, nervousness, irritability, frustration, lack of energy, and decreased initiative 6 months after rehabilitation. In another study, Pound, Gompertz, and Ebrahim (1998) found that stroke survivors reported that in addition to the common physical limitations (in mobility and self-care), confusion and deteriorating memory were also issues.

As a result of the consequences of stroke, many people are placed in long-term care facilities. Those that are fortunate enough to return home usually report a wide range of differences in household responsibilities and socialization. Enterlante and Kern (1995) looked at changes in the roles of wives when their spouses became disabled because of a stroke. They found that wives' responsibilities increased significantly after a husband's stroke; wives' satisfaction with household responsibilities decreased significantly; and wives' degree of marital unhappiness increased significantly after the husband's stroke. The role responsibilities that the wives absorbed as part of their role change include managing household financial matters, fixing things around the house, and making decisions about family matters. It was not providing for the spouse's physical care, but rather the cognitive aspect of care that led to the wives' dissatisfaction.

It is well known that rehabilitation after a stroke provides most stroke survivors with functional improvement. However, very few rehabilitation programs assess, intervene, or evaluate for cognition deficits. A comprehensive rehabilitation program tailored to a client's physical and cognitive impairments can better facilitate a client's return to a worthwhile life.

Dementia/Alzheimer's Disease

Cognitive imperfections occur at all ages. Complaints of failing memory are a frequent issue in the elderly. Everyday events like forgetting the name of a person, misplacing objects, and forgetting events are common events that most attribute to the stigma of aging. However, not all cognitive problems are part of normal aging. Sometimes cognitive failure is a symptom of a disease. Problems with attention, memory, and learning in older adults can be the result of illness, drug therapy, deafness, and impaired vision. Therefore, when an older person complains of problems with their "thinking skills or memory" it is imperative to do further assessment. One test, the Fuld Objective Memory Evaluation, is useful in assessing memory impairments in older adults. This assessment tool uses multiple sensory modalities to test encoding of information, and was found to be valid compared to logical memory from the Wechsler Memory Scale—Revised and the memory scale of the Mattis Dementia Rating Scale (Wall, Deshpande, MacNeill, & Lichtenberg, 1998). Many researchers use a variety of cognitive/memory tools to determine if cognitive outcome is improved, status quo, or deteriorated. Most use observational measures or clinical scales, and fewer use specific neuropsychological tests for memory or cognition. Simard and Reekum (1999) reviewed specific neuropsychological tests used for cognitive testing in older adults (Table 26-2).

Whether in clinical practice or in a research setting, there is a need to establish if an elderly person's cognitive complaints are age-related and benign or early symptoms of dementia. Regardless of tool or assessment used, the expert administering the test must be sensitive to a person's cultural and educational biases. It is not uncommon for highly educated people to get high scores even when experiencing dementia, whereas lower educated people get low scores when there is no indication of dementia (Gauther, Panisset, Nalbantoghe, & Poirer, 1997).

TABLE 26-2 Neuropsychological Testing for Cognition in Older Adults

Type of Memory Test	Common Tests
Working Memory Testing	Complex visual search test
	Various cancellation tasks test
	Trial Maluny Test
	Barbizet–Cany's; 7 day/24 hour immediate recall test
	Short memory test for figures
	Sequential visual memory test
	*WAIS–Wechsler Adult Intelligence Scale
Episodic Memory Testing	Logic Memory subtests of the Wechsler Memory Scale (WMS)*
	Buschke Selective Reminding Test
	Paired Associates Learning subtest of the WMS
	Key Auditory Verbal Learning Test
	5-item Test
	Names Learning Test
	Various tests of verbal and visual recall and recognition
Semantic Memory	Boston Naming Test
	Vocabulary subtest of the WAIS
	Verbal Fluency Tasks*
Clinical and Cognitive Scales	Mini-Mental State Examination
	Alzheimer's Disease Assessment Scale
	Sandoz Clinical Assessment Geriatric
	Self-Assessment Scale–Geriatric
	Blessed Dementia Scale
	Gottfried-Brane-Steele Scale
	Global Deterioration Scale
	WAIS
	WMS
	Clinical Global Impression of Change (CGIC)*
	Clinical Interview Based Impression of Change*

*Most commonly used.

In addition to testing for dementia, a careful history must be obtained before a diagnosis can be made. Dementia is a condition in which global impairment of higher cortical functions occur. This includes memory, capacity to solve day-to-day living problems, performance of learned skills, correct use of social skills, and control of emotional reactions (Uren, 1984). Dementia is a descriptive term based on the presence of symptoms and signs. Dementia is the combination of progressive loss of cognitive skills and of functional abilities (in the absence of delirium) (Bayer, 1998).

After a diagnosis of dementia has been established, the next step is to identify the underlying clinical condition. The differential diagnosis of dementia includes common diagnoses such as Alzheimer's disease (AD), vascular dementia, and Lewy Body disease. Many of these conditions are combined with other diseases, such as Parkinson's disease.

AD is the most common cause of progressive deterioration of cognitive functioning in the aged. Because a brain biopsy is the only true assessment measure to determine AD, clinical history, neuropsychological testing, and serial observation are the primary means to diagnose AD. Increased evidence suggests that early intervention can delay the progression of AD and improve the symptoms and function of those affected. Thus, research to identify a means to diagnose AD early is of great importance. Serial imaging of the hippocampal fissure of the brain by MRI is being studied as a possible assessment tool in identifying AD in the early phase.

The etiology of AD is unclear. Pathological changes associated with this disease include neurofibrillary tangles and B-amyloid plaques in the cerebral cortex and hippocampus. The neuritis plaque is a cluster of degenerating axonal and dendritic nerve terminals that contain an abnormal protein, B-amyloid. Neurofibrillary tangles are abnormal neurons within which the cytoplasm is filled with bundles of abnormal protein. There is also an excessive loss of cholinergic neurons, particularly in the regions essential for memory and cognition. Research is looking into the possible genetic component of AD. We already know that some chromosomes are involved in familial AD. Additional research is supporting the idea that estrogen protects against the development of AD. Another focus in AD research is the relationship between nonsteroidal antiinflammatory drugs (NSAIDs), vitamins, and overall good nutrition in reducing the risk of AD.

All older people have plaques and tangles in their brains, but people with AD have a much higher number of them. Gross atrophy occurs as neurons die. Loss of neurons occurs primarily in the neocortex and hippocampus, which are essential structures for cognition. Neurons provide the cholinergic innervation of the hippocampus and neocortex. Loss of cholinergic innervation is one of the major biochemical changes that occurs in AD. The definitive diagnosis of AD can be made only at autopsy when the presence of neurofibrillary tangles are observed.

Progressive impairment of memory and other cognitive skills have been outlined in three stages (Box 26-2).

Box 26-2 Outline of Progressive Impairment of Memory and Other Cognitive Skills

Stage I (1 to 3 Years)

Mild memory impairment
Some naming errors
Indifference, occasional irritability

Stage II (2 to 10 Years)

Moderate memory impairment
Spatial disorientation
Fluent aphasia
Ideomotor apraxia (difficulty dressing and difficulty using utensils of daily living)
Indifference or irritability
Delusions in some
Restlessness, pacing

Stage III (11 Years and Older)

Severely impaired cognitive function
Limb rigidity, flexion posture
Urinary and fecal incontinence

From Luckman, J. (1997). *Manual of nursing care* (p. 714). Philadelphia: WB Saunders.

These three stages are only a guide of function and capacity and help in monitoring or anticipating the progression of the disease. Symptoms and behaviors often overlap stages. Many factors beyond the disease can contribute to the loss of functional capacity or cognition changes, such as illnesses, changes in the environment, drug therapy, and sensory changes. When a deficit occurs, the attention must be toward identifying the potential cause.

The idea of treatment for people with AD is relatively new and a growing area of research. For a long time there was no cure or treatment to manage AD. Knowledge of the neurobiological and environmental factors contributing to the pathogenesis of AD has substantially increased. Despite research, treatments to reverse the dementing process have yet to emerge. Most pharmacological agents in development target a specific symptom (i.e., memory loss, agitation).

Pharmacological approaches to AD were used to improve cerebral blood flow and oxygen use because the belief was that cerebral arteriosclerosis was the primary cause of senile dementia. The most widely used drug, first-generation compound, was Hydergine. The positive clinical outcomes are believed to be from the mild activating or mood elevating effects. Other first generation compounds used were drugs such as Germinal (engoloid mesylates), Niloric, chelation therapy, *N*-acetylcarnitive, lecithin, methylphenidate, and piracetam. Most failed to show clinical improvements over time.

The most important recent advance in treatment is the development of second-generation cholinesterase inhibitors. The loss of presynaptic neurons in the cortex and hippocampus is a significant aspect of AD. Studies have found a strong correlation between the extent of damage to the cholinergic system and the degree of dementia. Acetylcholinesterase inhibitors (AchE1s) prevent the breakdown of acetylcholine, thereby increasing the level of acetylcholine available to postsynaptic neurons. They do not alter the accumulation of senile plaques and neurofibrillary tangles in the brain. Tacrine, acridine, was the first drug to be approved for the treatment of AD in 1993. This was followed by the approval of donepezil in 1996. In clinical studies donepezil has been shown to improve cognitive and global functions in mild and moderate severe cases (Rogers & Friedloft, 1996). Treatment effects decline a few weeks after discontinuation of therapy. Tacrine therapy was associated with a high discontinuation rate because of side effects. The recommended starting dose of donepezil, a piperidine-based cholinesterase inhibitor, is 5 mg daily, and can be increased to 10 mg. Higher dose has a greater tendency to cause cholinergic side effects such as nausea, diarrhea, and insomnia.

Other cholinesterase (ChE) inhibitors have been, or will shortly be, approved for treating AD. These drugs target the cholinergic system, but with different modes of action. These drugs are physostigmine, rivastigmine, quilostigmine, metrifonate, galanthamine, and huperzine-A. Most of these drug studies determine the efficacy of AChEls as measured by improvements in cognition in the drug treated clients verses placebo-treated clients in controlled clinical trials. Thus far, AchEl therapy in AD can be used to treat cognitive losses or delay the progression of the disease, but provides no cure or reverse effect for the disease. Although providing only transient benefit, cholinesterase inhibitor therapy is the best option available to people with AD. It does improve quality of life by delaying a loss of activities of daily living.

Alternative approaches to the treatment of AD that appear promising include the development of cholinergic muscarinic and nicotinic receptor agonists, particularly selective muscarinic-m, agonists. Xanomeline tartrate, a muscarinic cholinergic receptor agonist, was studied and found to effectively reduce treatment of emergent noncognitive behavioral problems, including vocal outbursts, delusions, agitation, suspiciousness, and hallucinations; but it had many side effects (Bodick, Offen, & Levey, 1997).

Early studies suggested that smoking and nicotine enhanced delayed recall and attention performance in people without AD. Therefore, it was part of a trial in people with AD. Most studies evaluating the effects of nicotine are supporting memory improvement. White and Levin (1999) found that nicotine administered through a dermal patch produced a statistical significant improvement in attention, but no improvement in memory among AD subjects as measured by the Conners' continuous performance test. However, further studies are needed to determine the efficacy of nicotine in the treatment of AD.

Reports of women receiving estrogen therapy having lower rates of AD has sparked much interest in the possible correlation. Estrogen improves cerebral blood flow through direct effects on the endothelium and may play an important role in both the preservation and the repair of neurons. In addition, estrogen modulates antiinflammatory processes. Thus far clinical trials have shown a benefit from estrogen therapy in the delay and prevention of AD. However, estrogen may also have negative effects such as an increase in breast and uterine cancers. Currently, large studies are in process looking at the use of estrogen in the treatment and prevention of AD.

Inflammation has been considered in the etiology of AD. Chronic use of NSAIDs is being considered as a way to lowering the risk of AD. Rogers, Kirby, and Hempelman (1993) found that symptoms of AD were reversed. However, there was a high dropout rate because of the side effects.

Other studies in progress that are looking at halting the disease progression of AD include antioxidants such as vitamins C, E, and beta carotene. In recent years, there has been an interest in the role of reactive oxygen species (ROS) in the normal process of aging and the pathophysiology of diseases, such as AD. An antioxidant is any substance that is able to protect against the damages of oxidative stress caused by ROS. Antioxidant therapies are being promoted to the community at large as a drug therapy to enhance mental functions and delay cognitive losses with aging. Physicians are recommending antioxidant therapies such as high doses of vitamin E, gingko biloba, and selegiline. Limited research has been done using antioxidants and looking at their role in slowing the progression of AD.

High doses of vitamin E can be potentially dangerous, and prothrombin time in clients receiving oral anticoagulants should be monitored and adjusted frequently. In March 1999, the National Institute on Aging launched a prospective, randomized clinical study to compare the effects of vitamin E and a placebo.

In Oken, Storzbach, and Kaze's (1998) study on the efficacy of gingko biloba on cognitive function in Alzheimer's disease, they found a small but significant positive effect with a 3- to 6-month treatment of 120 to 240 mg of gingko biloba extract. Studies have shown no absolute improvement with gingko biloba, but it does merit further investigation.

Currently, with the exception of the modest effects of tacrine, there are no clinically effective drug treatments for the cognitive dysfunction associated with AD. However, third- and fourth-generation compounds are being developed, aimed at providing symptomatic relief or delaying deterioration in AD. Some of the newer investigations are looking at drugs to stimulate nerve growth factors and act as plaque busters. Many age-dementia brain changes are associated with the loss of neurons and plaque formation. Medications that target these areas may prevent or retard further cell loss, which could dramatically affect preservation of memory and other cognitive functions. In Florida, The National Institute of Aging is conducting a trial on an "Alzheimer's vaccine," which supposedly provokes the body's immune system into recognizing the brain plaque as an enemy and attacking it. If it is found to be effective, it could eliminate AD.

Multiple Sclerosis

MS is a disease of the central nervous system. The course of this disease involves unpredictable exacerbations and remissions that last throughout the person's life. The primary symptoms of MS are the result of multiple demyelinating lesions throughout the central nervous system. There are four major classifications of MS:

1. Relapsing-remitting MS
2. Secondary progressive MS
3. Primary progressive MS
4. Progressive-relapsing MS

In managing MS the focus is on altering the course of the disease and improving the quality of life. In treating MS exacerbations, a common drug of choice is methylprednisolone. In altering the course of MS or preventing exacerbation of MS, interferon, a protein that interferes with a virus' ability to attack a cell, has been found to significantly decrease the number of acute exacerbations over time. There are various interferon products available and not one is found to be better than another. The difference in these interferon products has to do with the way the drug is manufactured. Interferon potential side effects include fever, weakness, aches, and flulike symptoms.

Other drugs being used to alter the course of MS are glatiramer acetate (copolymer-1) and immunosuppressive and immunomodulating agents. Many new drugs are being investigated to impede the disease process. However, the ultimate goal is to eliminate the disease.

In addition to treatment of exacerbations and slowing the disease, focus needs to be on treatment to relieve specific symptoms with which a client presents at a particular point in the progression of the disease. Various studies have identified cognitive impairments as a symptom of MS. Cognitive impairments may include deficits in memory, attention span, speech, comprehension, information processing, planning, and problem solving. Stuifbergen's study (1995) explored the relationship between the nature and severity of cognitive impairment, perception of impairment, and physical, psychological, and social functioning as well as quality of life. This study found that only 51% of the subjects passed a cognitive test, with subjects scoring lowest on the measures of sustained attention and speed of information processing. Also found was the number of tests failed was significantly associated with age, education, time since diagnosis, employment, physical functioning, and regular use of medication. Cognitive impairment is not always an obvious symptom, but usually is a gradual change over time. It is important that a cognitive assessment be done on a routine basis so a plan of action can be implemented early before a client sustained injury from it.

NEUROBEHAVIORAL PROCESSES AND DEFICITS

Neurobehavioral Processes

No one area of the brain is the primary section for cognition. The brain functions as a whole with lesions of specific areas of the hemispheres producing characteristic dysfunctions (Table 26-3).

Cognitive function is made of many components. The

TABLE 26-3 Cognitive Functions Affected by Brain Injury

Area of Brain	Function	Results of Injury
Reticular activating system	For arousal, alertness, basic orientation. Alerts cerebral hemisphere of incoming stimuli	Loss of arousal, coma, confusion, decreased attention
Frontal lobe	Controls higher intellectual and social processing (judgment, attention span, sequencing thoughts, abstraction)	Loss of intellect, inappropriate social behaviors, poor judgment, decreased attention
Temporal lobe	Controls new memory and learning. Holds information for short-term memory	Impaired learning, impaired short-term memory
Temporal lobe (hippocampus)	New learning	Temporary memory loss, lack of contralateral orientation, distractibility, hyperactivity, attention deficits, perseveration
Right hemisphere	Controls recognition of faces, forms of artistic intelligence such as painting, music, 3-dimensional objects, sense of direction, and memory for pictures	Learning impairments, memory impairments
Left hemisphere	Controls memory for language, letters, words, verbal memory (i.e., reading, writing, speech), math and analytical skills	Deficits with math and communication
Limbic lobe of both hemispheres	Controls attention that affects socialization (affect, emotions, self-preservation)	Deficits with socialization, motivation, and sexual behavior

Adapted from Brillhart, B. (2000). Psychosocial healthcare patterns and nursing interventions. In P. Edwards (Ed.), *The specialty practice of rehabilitation nursing: A core curriculum.* (4th ed., p. 144). Glenview, IL: Association of Rehabilitation Nurses; and Grzanikowski, J.A. (1997). Altered thought processes related to traumatic brain injury and their nursing implications. *Rehabilitation Nursing, 22*(1), 24–28.

most crucial processes involved in carrying out daily living activities are as follows:

- Orientation
- Memory
- Attention
- Judgment/reasoning
- Problem solving
- Intellectual functioning skills
- Organization
- Initiation
- Sequencing
- Motivation

Orientation refers to the ability to understand self and the relationship of self to the environment: person, place, and time. Those individuals who experience disorientation lack the very basic skills needed to participate in society (Rosenthal et al., 1990).

The ability to remember, or *memory,* is crucial to all other aspects of cognitive function. Memory is a complex process of placing information in memory banks, keeping it there, and producing it when needed. Memory is divided into immediate recall, short-term memory, and long-term memory. Immediate recall, or incidental recall, is the memory ability to recall information from the moment of reception and up to 1 minute after its reception. Short-term memory is the ability to reproduce or recall information from 1 minute to 1 hour after its reception. Long-term memory is the ability to store and retrieve information for more than 1 hour. Long-term memory is practically limitless. Short-term memory appears to be a necessary step in the storage of long-term memories. No specific brain location is associated with long-term memory; it appears that storage of such memory involves the brain as a whole (Mitchell et al., 1984).

Attention refers to the ability to respond to relevant information and to screen out information that is not important (DeBoskey et al., 1991). The three components of attention include alertness, effort or maintenance, and selection. Alertness is the degree of generalized readiness of the central nervous system to receive information. Effort or maintenance is the amount of attention needed for a task. Concentration, persistence, and the ability to maintain focus over long periods are examples of effort. Selection is the ability to choose the information while suppressing irrelevant stimuli. Attention is required for information to be coded and stored (Rosenthal et al., 1990).

Judgment/reasoning is the ability to determine what the consequences of a given action may be, and the ability to act in a safe and appropriate manner.

Problem solving is the ability to define and analyze a problem, choose and execute a strategy, and evaluate the results.

Intellectual functioning/thinking comprises remembering, planning, foresight, judgment, abstraction, and the ability to transfer information from one situation to another. Problem solving is one form of thinking ability. Scholastic achievement is another.

Organization is the ability to establish a consistent relationship between objects, events, or features.

Initiation is the ability to start actions independently, continue, and carry them through to completion.

Sequencing is the ability to perform the steps of a task from start to finish.

Motivation refers to inner forces that regulate behavior to satisfy needs and achieve goals. Multiple factors influence a person's motivation to participate in self-care and rehabilitation.

To function as a fully functioning person, the quality and quantity of cognition must be intact. Being independent requires consciousness, mentation, and the ability to integrate cognitive and motor functioning.

Neurobehavioral Deficits

The effects of altered cognition can range from minor annoyances to profound disruption of every aspect of living. Most people with cognition impairments from any source may exhibit a broad range of behaviors. These behaviors are apt to be most evident in situations in which the brain is being asked to process multiple stimuli or to respond to new situations. The source or cause of the behavior may be different depending on the type of insult, injury, or disease that the individual has experienced, but the techniques of management often are similar. The following are behaviors that often accompany altered cognition:

- Disorientation/confusion
- Apathy
- Lack of initiation
- Attention-span deficits
- Impaired judgment
- Poor problem-solving skills
- Impulsivity
- Depression
- Perseveration
- Confabulation
- Emotional lability
- Disinhibition
- Agitation
- Lack of insight

Disorientation/confusion can be a result of attentional problems, fluctuating states of alertness, and memory problems. An individual often appears incoherent. As a result of the loss in sense of direction, getting lost may be a real problem. The disoriented or confused individual most often will not know where he or she is, what time it is, or be unable to recall minute-to-minute, hour-to-hour, or day-to-day events. As a result the individual is unable to understand his or her current situation in light of what has happened or will occur.

Apathy presents a bland affect, general lethargy, and low motivation. This behavior may be a result of an individual's frustration over what seems to be an impossible task or confusion. In response to this behavior, the individual may refuse to participate in daily self-care tasks, lose interest, and refuse to get out of bed or participate in rehabilitation.

Lack of initiation is when an individual is motivated to perform an activity but cannot determine how to carry it out. Lack of initiative may be evident when an individual does not experience self-starting and self-directed behavior. This often is mistaken as apathy, but it is important to differentiate the two behaviors.

Those exhibiting *attention-span deficits* may be highly distractible by either internal or external events, go off on tangents when a single thought occurs to them, move quickly from one idea to another, and fail to attend for any period.

Individuals with *impaired judgment* may misinterpret the actions and intentions of others, may be unable to handle multiple pieces of information simultaneously, and may have an inaccurate perception of strengths and weaknesses. These poor self-monitoring skills can lead to problems with safety and ultimately functional independence.

Those individuals who have difficulty with the high-level skill of *problem solving* generally have difficulty planning and organizing their thoughts and behaviors, formulating alternative solutions, and comprehending the potential consequences of their choices.

Impulsivity is the tendency to act without thought of consequences. Impulsive individuals may appear to act quickly, make continuous and unrelenting demands, and grab and reach for everyone and everything.

Depression is sadness that may be evident in social withdrawal, crying, self-degrading comments, anxiety, and irritability.

Perseveration is an individual's reflexive repetition of certain behaviors, either verbalizations or actions. There often is a consistent theme to perseverance, such as "I want to go home" or washing one extremity repeatedly during a bath.

Some individuals demonstrate episodes of *confabulation* where they compensate for memory loss and other deficits by inventing details to meet their needs. Although it is not done purposefully, it often reflects a person's inability to find other explanations for what is occurring to them. It may serve a purpose for the person, such as to reduce anxiety.

Emotional lability is the inability to control emotions. It generally is evidenced in easily triggered bouts of crying or laughing even though the individual is not sad or happy. An exaggerated emotion may occur suddenly and then disappear suddenly.

For individuals to function within the social and cultural norms of society, they must be aware of behavioral norms and the feelings and needs of others. Lack of inhibition, or *disinhibition,* is the inability to control verbalizations or behaviors in a socially appropriate way.

Agitation can be generally defined as excesses of behavior. It often is characterized by restlessness, inability to focus or maintain attention, and irritability, and may escalate to combativeness.

Lack of insight results in denial. These individuals may lack motivation for rehabilitation because they do not have internal feedback about their capabilities. They may blame others for their frustrations.

The cumulative effects of these emotional and behavioral changes often cause problems with personal and social relationships that can lead to increasing isolation for individuals and their families. Because the primary goal of rehabilitation is a return to family and community, simple containment or toleration of inappropriate behaviors within rehabilitation is not enough. The community will not tolerate such behavior. The plan for management should include elimination of socially unacceptable behaviors and restoration of self-regulated and socially acceptable responses to environmental demands. The basic premise is to acknowledge an individual's limitation, but assume that with structure and guidance a person can gain control over behavior. It is essential that we teach family members about an individual's cognitive impairment and resulting behavior changes so they can deal with the behaviors appropriately.

LIFE SPAN ISSUES AND COGNITION

Children and Adolescents

Brain injury at different developmental stages produces different challenges for the child as well as family and rehabilitation professionals. Because children are "in development," brain injury has the potential to not only take away knowledge and skills already learned and create obstacles to success at the current developmental stage; but also to jeopardize the child's ability to master new skills, acquire new knowledge, and successfully negotiate progressively more difficult developmental challenges over the years after injury (Ylvisaker, Chorazy, Feeney, & Russell, 1999).

Piaget emphasized the importance of early physical experience and motor activity in cognitive and intellectual development. Piaget's theory centers around the concept that motor actions, manipulation of objects, and physical exploration of the environment are the sources from which mental operations and intelligence emerge. According to Piaget's stages of description of intellectual development (Box 26-3), one stage must be attained before transition to the

Box 26-3 Piaget's Stages of Intellectual Development

Sensorimotor stage: birth to 2 years
Preoperational stage: 2 to 7 years
Preconceptual thought: 2 to 4 years
Intuitive thought: 4 to 7 years
Concrete operational thought: 11 to 15 years

From Luckman, J. (1997). *Manual of nursing care* (p. 472). Philadelphia: WB Saunders.

next stage can occur. A child in elementary school may perform adequately and without obvious problems during the first few years of life after a mild brain injury because the developmental stage is the same post injury as it was before the injury. When this same child transitions from elementary to middle school and thus moves from a highly structured setting to a more flexible setting requiring organization and independent functioning in a number of classes, this adolescent may begin to have difficulty (Christensen, 1997). After children with cognitive deficits reach adolescence there is a tendency for development of personality and behavior problems secondary to the cognitive deficits and difficulty adjusting to the residual disabilities. Professionals from pediatric rehabilitation and special education need to work closely with the family in providing services to meet the long-term needs for school age children with brain injuries (Blosser & Pearson, 1997; Janus, Mishkin, & Pearson, 1997; Savage, 1997;).

Shurtleff, Massagli, Hays, Ross, and Sprenk-Greenfield (1995) described the need for children to have a continuum of carefully planned services from emergency care to acute care, to rehabilitation services, to initial school reentry, to grade-to-grade transitions, and to school-to-community transitions. Neuropsychologists should be intimately involved along the continuum to diagnose subtle changes in cognitive behavior, and to revise the plan for services as the changes occur.

Changes in health care as a result of managed care (i.e., delivery of services efficiently with less cost) are requiring many professionals to make early referrals to existing educational services once funding for rehabilitation has run out. Under public law, schools are responsible (Savage, 1997). This makes the need for model programs combining rehabilitation and special education services even more essential.

Commonly used tests for screening in children include the following:

- Denver II Developmental Screening Test
- Pediatric Evaluation of Disability Inventory
- Bailey Scales of Infant Development
- Vineland Adaptive Behavior Scales
- Children's coma scale
- Neuropsychological testing

Rehabilitation goals for the child with altered cognition promote age-appropriate growth and maturation. A child's altered cognition affects the entire family (Gill & Wells, 2000; Kreutzer et al., 1997; Rocchio, 2000). Rocchio (2000) supports the need for increased and more productive dialogue between service providers and parents, and better access to community support systems over the life span of individuals with brain injuries. Gill and Wells (2000) qualitative exploratory study examined the experiences of siblings living with a brother or sister who had experienced a TBI. They discussed the presence of one overwhelming theme: The well sibling's life was forever different. There were four primary supporting themes: Change in the sibling with a brain injury (the reason for the difference in the well sibling's life), mixed emotions (well sibling's reactions to the experience), different life rhythm (changes in the way the well sibling went about day to day life), and change in self (ways that the well sibling became a different person). Education and appropriate support services are essential in empowering and enabling family members to become advocates—not only for their child with a brain injury, but for the entire family.

Aging and Cognition

Older adults may experience alterations or impairments in cognition as a result of falls, motor vehicle accidents, strokes, or secondary to illness or drugs. Falls are serious, often preventable problems for older adults

Research findings vary in regard to cognitive changes associated with normal aging. Katzman and Terry (1983) describes a decline in some aspects of fluid intelligence with aging—such as intellectual performance as measured by timed cognitive performance tasks, associative memory, logical reasoning, and abstract thinking; whereas crystal intelligence—such as intellectual performance as measured by tests of verbal abilities in vocabulary, information, and comprehension is preserved. The ability to learn is preserved but often at a slower rate.

The decline in fluid intelligence may be related to a decrease in the rate of central information processing. Performance on timed motor or cognition tasks or reaction time tasks or other tests requiring speed in processing of new information, deteriorates progressively after 20 years of age. Age-related impairments have also been shown consistently in tasks involving episodic short-term memory and incidental learning. This is not likely the result of slowed central processing (Katzman & Terry, 1983). Overall, the more complex the mental task, the greater the effects of aging. Because much of rehabilitation requires learning, these findings have major implications for rehabilitation professionals.

After an older adult is transferred into rehabilitation, the intensity of the daily therapies is tailored to meet the individual's tolerance. Before coming to acute rehabilitation, almost all clients have been on bed rest for several days. Reconditioning presents greater risks for older adults. Long-term outcomes for the elderly with altered cognition are related to cognitive status, behavioral status, and social situation.

FAMILY ISSUES

Rocchio (2000) describes the emotions that families experience from the moment of injury to various levels of client recovery. No family is ever prepared to comprehend the full magnitude of the life changes that brain injury or chronic disease affecting cognition creates. Most manage from day to day—learning as they go and drawing on resources to get through what they hope will be a short-term situation that comes to a satisfactory conclusion. Family friends share relief at the first signs of awakening after a brain injury, get excited at the first attempts to communicate and walk, and feel confidence that rehabilitation can restore functional abilities. But the physical recovery may be misleading, and families are often not prepared for the cognitive and behavioral changes that may persist.

Brzuzy and Speziale (1997) describe life after TBI this way: "The demands of TBI on a young adult seeking independence from the family, in siblings who are in a similar stage, and in parents moving toward a new stage of coupling, threaten normal developmental tasks and aspirations of all persons involved" (p. 86). Because of the consequences of TBI, young adults often lose recently attained independence and regress to a stage of dependency on family members. Many move back to their parents' home. Typically, family members rely on themselves to care for an adult member with a severe disability. This forced self-reliance creates, over time, a burden, more stresses than family members can handle, and one that generally decreases life satisfaction.

Practice interventions that help to reestablish normal individual and family life cycles also help in the facilitation of reintegration with other social systems. The use of larger social support systems and settings other than the home to meet needs that are currently being met by family can lower family stress.

For those whose family members sustain severe brain damage to the frontal and temporal lobes of the brain from trauma or disease, life may never be the same. The public seems to accept physical limitations but few understand and or tolerate cognitive deficits and the accompanying behaviors.

The manner in which the family deals with the residual deficits in cognition will determine the quality of life for the person with the injury, as well as for the remaining family. The amount of time that health care professionals spend gathering data and planning interventions to help the family deal with these issues, the more positive results can be expected.

Most individuals are very happy to return home after inpatient rehabilitation. Not only is home a safe place, but it is often perceived as a place where life will return to normal. Friends and family are happy, but after a period of welcoming, friends usually return to their own routines, leaving the person with brain injury isolated. Brain damage, especially from trauma, but also from stroke, MS, AD, and AIDS can change the individual dramatically, and it is difficult for others to understand the changes.

It does not take long for the individual with brain injury to realize that life is not the same. Friends quit coming around, driving privileges are gone, and life can become boring. This may begin a vicious cycle of behavioral deterioration. The goal of treatment should be to circumvent this cycle by advance planning.

Several tools are being tested for use in helping families cope. Weeks and O'Conner (1997) describe rehabilitation nurses as the change agents, educators, and encouragers working with families faced with the unexpected uncertainty of living with disabilities and caregiving responsibilities after brain injury or chronic illness. By including the family health system in the initial assessment of clients entering the rehabilitation system, nurses can help families identify their needs, highlight their strengths, and start the process of normalizing their family life. They designed and validated the FAMTOOL (Table 26-4), an assessment tool that can be used by nurses and family members to identify and reinforce the positive aspects of family health with families in any health care settings. It is a quick, positive approach for helping family members recognize the strengths in their family, compare their responses, and see possibilities they might not have considered otherwise.

Burges (1999) designed the Family Burden of Injury In-

TABLE 26-4 FAMTOOL: A Family Health Assessment Tool

Statement	False	Mostly False	Mostly True	True
As a Family,				
We work well together	0	1	2	3
We communicate effectively	0	1	2	3
We share beliefs	0	1	2	3
We play together	0	1	2	3
We put energy into the family	0	1	2	3
We value connectedness	0	1	2	3
We work toward physical health	0	1	2	3
We work toward emotional health	0	1	2	3
We work toward social health	0	1	2	3
We work toward spiritual health	0	1	2	3
We value one another	0	1	2	3
We have hope for the future	0	1	2	3

Please circle the number that best describes your family. Thank you for completing this family health analysis.

From Weeks, S.K., & O'Connor, P.C. (1994). Concept analysis of family + health = A new definition of family health. *Rehabilitation Nursing, 19,* 207–210.

terview to assess the impact of childhood brain injury and its effect on family. Their study interviewed the mothers of 99 children with moderate to severe TBI to assess family burden. The authors concluded that this is a first step in development of a promising tool for measuring the impact of a broad range of injury-related stress on the family. They anticipate that this tool will be useful in identifying families that experience high levels of stress after a child's head injury, and thus likely will be helpful in designing family interventions with anticipatory guidance in managing the impact of injury-related stressors.

There is an increasing focus in the clinical and research literature on family input and feedback on what works and what does not in helping families achieve success in dealing with individual and family issues after traumatic injury and chronic disease (Delehanty & Kieren, 1998; Gill & Wells, 2000; Kreutzer, Sunder, & Fernandez, 1997; Rocchio, 2000). Delehanty and Kieren's (1998) study of family perceptions of health professionals in family problem solving after brain injury provides data on the roles that health professionals can play in facilitating and promoting problem solving. Data include the need for professionals to:

- Provide sensitive direction, not authoritative, demands
- Respect families for who they are and have been while they are making decisions on changes in family
- Provide professional knowledge and emotional support as families work through the initial trauma and long-term adaptation they are dealing with
- Be a professional advocate (dealing with schools, government, agencies, and employers)

Kreutzer, Sunder, and Fernandez (1997) presented examples of case analyses and their suggestions for interventions to help clinicians working with family members to recognize and avoid common errors in evaluation and interventions. Rocchio (1997) described parental experiences in managing children and adolescents after brain injury. She identified the need for professionals to be better communicators by doing the following:

- Recognize that people respond differently in crises
- Communicate clearly with nonjargon
- Identify one family member as a contact
- Tape record important information and conferences for other family members
- Involve client and family as team members
- Place family on equal footing with professionals throughout recovery and school reentry
- Link client and family with existing community agencies for services (i.e., a brain injury association)
- Keep a list of potential peer support and advisors
- Facilitate support groups for families of children younger than 18 years of age
- Suggest an attorney for potential consultation for families (e.g., benefits, educational rights, advocacy)
- Be sensitive to special needs of family members struggling with guilt for not preventing the injury
- Help families plan and initiate a simple informational in-service they can use to inform others about the child's injury and the effects on daily living

The caregiving experience for those with cognitive deficits from brain injury and stroke are different from those who care for those with HIV dementia or AD. With HIV, the caregivers experience the difficulties related to specific HIV medical problems and problems with service shortfalls. The caregiver is more likely to be a parent or partner because of early age onset of HIV. HIV and AIDS are still often surrounded by prejudice and stigma. The burden may also be worse because of worries about confidentiality of diagnosis and the wish to guard privacy. With HIV-associated dementia, caregivers witness the loss of personality, vitality, and potential of the loved one they have cared for. Meadows, LeMarechal, and Catalan's (1999) observational study of caregivers of those with HIV-associated dementia identified potential needs of these individuals and their caregivers:

- Need for clear communications between caregiver, client, and medical profession, especially related to disease progression and prognosis
- Need for services to be flexible and provide continuity and reliability in support of the client and caregiver (i.e., respite care)
- Need for information about entitlements, how to claim benefits
- Need for immediate access to services/medical advice if needed
- Need for services after the death of the person they were caring for (i.e., counselors, support, drop-in centers)

In AD, because of the older age of the individual affected, primary caregivers often are the children or spouses who are elderly. The issues identified above by HIV-associated dementia caregivers are similar to those of AD, but the cognitive deficits associated with AD progress over time; and the life expectancy of those with AD is generally longer because HIV-associated dementia generally occurs in late stages of the disease. Because many caregivers experience loneliness and may be burdened by their responsibilities, counseling on problem solving is thought to help caregivers cope, but few studies have proven the effectiveness of counseling for those caregivers (Roberts et al., 1999).

Rehabilitation nurses who provide care at all points along the continuum are in an essential position to educate, support, and advocate for clients and caregivers for those with cognition deficits and dementia.

NURSING PROCESSES

Assessment

Because cognition has a major impact on a client's rehabilitation potential, nursing has a major role in determining baseline cognition, participating with the interdisciplinary team in formulating a plan of care to treat the deficits, monitoring for changes in cognition, carrying out the treatment plan, and evaluating outcomes. To begin the assessment, the nurse will need to talk with family members and significant others to determine the client's preinjury cognitive abilities. This will assist in defining the baseline normal cognitive strengths and weaknesses. The neuropsychologist's assessment provides a description of the client's mental status, covering both cognitive processes and affective status. Among the major cognitive processes that are assessed are attention, executive function, perception, memory, motor performance, language, and intelligence. It is equally important that the presence of depression, agitation, and emotional lability be evaluated because these affective disturbances are prime determinants of a client's ability to participate in rehabilitation.

Preinjury Nursing Assessment

Obtain data before disease, injury, or alteration in thought processes, including medical history in regard to thought processes and cognitive and behavioral functioning. Ask family and friends to describe an individual's preinjury behaviors and intellectual functioning. Ask family and friends about the individual's preinjury recreation, socialization, and occupation. Assess a pediatric client's level of development preinjury by talking with parents and the pediatrician. Obtain history of medications, alcohol, or substance abuse. Obtain history of activities of daily living and sleep-wake patterns.

Postinjury Nursing Assessment

Obtain data immediately after injury or onset of disease or alteration in thought process. Assess level of consciousness, cognition, or behavior with the Glasgow Coma Scale (see Table 26-1) or the Children's Coma Scale (Table 26-5). Assess short-term memory (1 minute to 1 hour) and long-term memory (greater than 1 hour). Assess attention span and concentration deficits. Monitor judgment and intellectual functioning and thought content. Assess cognitive function with Rancho Los Amigos Levels of Cognitive Function Scale (Table 26-6). Obtain sequence of recovery from coma and tracking of behaviors.

Assess body systems. Identify onset of symptoms, gradual onset versus sudden onset, and the etiology of impairment. Review medications and identify those that could alter thought processes.

Monitor for seizures. Observe physical status and motor functioning. Assess level of communication and determine if it is verbal or nonverbal. Assess sensory and perceptual function.

Apply tactile stimulation to skin and monitor response. Assess level of responsiveness. Assess visual-spatial alterations.

TABLE 26-5 Children's Coma Scale (Modified Glasgow Coma Scale, Recommended for Children 3 Years and Younger)

Response		Score
Eye Opening		
Spontaneous		4
Reaction to speech		3
Reaction to pain		2
No response		1
Best Motor Response		
Spontaneous (obeys verbal command)		6
Localizes pain		5
Withdraws in response to pain		4
Abnormal flexion in response to pain (decorticate posture)		3
Abnormal extension in response to pain (decerebrate posture)		2
No response		1
Best Verbal Response		
Smiles, oriented to sound, follows objects, interacts		5
Crying	*Interacts*	
Consolable	Inappropriate	5
Inconsistently consolable	Moaning	3
Inconsolable	Irritable, restless	2
No response	No response	1

Courtesy of Yoon Hahn, MD, with the help of pediatricians and a neonatologist at Children's Memorial Hospital, Chicago, IL.

Assessment Concurrent with Rehabilitation

Assessment concurrent with rehabilitation consists of data collected throughout the rehabilitation process by nurses and members of the rehabilitation team. It includes general orientation to person, place, and time. A common bedside assessment for memory is the following:

1. Recall for immediate memory (0–60 seconds)
2. Short-term memory (1 minute–1 hour)
3. Long-term memory (longer than 1 hour)

Examine the client's ability to follow a sequence of commands. Assess the client's ability to problem solve and follow simple assignments and instructions. Assess the client's ability to solve problems and choose alternatives. Assess the client's ability to use self-monitoring skills and remain safe.

Monitor for phobias, perseveration of thought, or delusions. Assess for changes in behavior. Note any changes in medications and observe patterns of seizures. Monitor vital signs and test values.

Observe progression of physical status and motor control. Note patterns of communication/language skills. Monitor changes in sensory and perceptual functioning. Assess the client's ability to perform activities of daily living.

Observe the client's motivation and cooperation with the rehabilitation program. Note sleep-wake cycles. Assess community and social support systems available to the

TABLE 26-6 Levels of Cognitive Function Scale

Level	Description
I—No response	No response to pain, touch, sound, or sight
II—Generalized reflex response	To stimulation or pain
III—Localized response	Blinks to strong light, turns toward or away from sound, responds to physical discomfort, gives inconsistent response to commands
IV—Confused-agitated	Alert, very active, aggressive, or bizarre behaviors; performs motor activities but behavior is nonpurposeful; extremely short attention span
V—Confused-nonagitated	Gross attention to environment, highly distractible, requires continual redirection, difficulty learning new tasks, agitated by too much stimulation
VI—Confused-appropriate	Inconsistent orientation to time and place, retention span/recent memory impaired, begins to recall past, consistently follows simple directions, goal-directed behavior with assistance
VII—Automatic-appropriate	Performs daily routine in highly familiar environment in nonconfused but automatic robotlike manner, skills noticeably deteriorate in unfamiliar surroundings, lack of realistic planning for own future
VIII—Purposeful-appropriate	

Adapted from C.A. Downey. (1979). *Levels of cognitive function* scale. Rancho Los Amigos Medical Center, Adult Brain Injury Service.

client. Assess tests of orientation, mental clarity, and memory.

Assessment Tools

Assessment tools examine orientation, mental clarity, and memory. A common bedside examination is the MMSE, which is a brief screening tool to measure orientation, attention, short-term memory, ability to register new information, and recall (see Chapter 30). It was developed to benchmark mental status, including several questions to determine orientation (Alverzo & Galski, 1999).

Common neuropsychological tests include the Galveston Orientation and Amnesia Test, which measures cognition serially during recovery from closed head injury. It gives a total score on orientation and amnesia (Alverzo & Galski, 1999). The Halstead Reitan Battery measures problem solving, attention, vigilance, abstraction, motor speed, and incidental memory (Putnam & Fichtenberg, 1999). The Wechsler Memory Scale–Revised measures verbal and nonverbal memory functioning. It measures the level of cognitive functioning and allows a quantitative discrimination between verbal and performance abilities (Putnam & Fichtenberg, 1999). The Luria-Nebraska Neuropsychological Battery measures simple and complex abilities in each sensory area under varying conditions (Bondy, 1994).

Cognitive impairments can affect how well an individual will function in rehabilitation and in society. Neuropsychological assessment tests have been developed to quantitate the severity of cognitive deficits by identifying brain-behavior relationships. For many the deficits are transient, and for some the cognitive deficits are permanent. In either situation a neuropsychological assessment test is used to clarify the nature and type of cognitive deficits. Vast numbers of neuropsychological tests are available. They derive from many scientific and clinical traditions. As a result of the diversity in tests, a single index or measure cannot capture the pattern of cognitive strengths and weaknesses. Comprehensive neuropsychological assessment should be done with overlapping tests to survey cognitive functions. Comprehensive sampling permits the analysis of patterns of cognitive performance within an individual client. After specific deficits are identified and quantified, a plan of individual care can be established and implemented.

Nursing Diagnoses

It is a frightening experience for a person experiencing cognitive deficits as well as for his or her family. Clients respond differently to problems with cognition depending on many factors including etiology, age, prior health status, education about and understanding of injury or disease, support systems, and available treatments. When a rehabilitation nurse identifies that a person is having cognitive problems, an essential management strategy is consistency. A number of nursing diagnoses can be formulated for the person with an impairment in cognition. The major diagnoses are included in Table 26-7.

Goals

Many goals are appropriate for people with cognitive deficits. Goals are formulated based on the etiology of the problem. Goals need to target interventions that focus on assisting the person in using effective communication, improving memory, increasing sensory awareness, and promoting safety.

Identifying the numerous settings in which rehabilitation nurses practice while caring for people with cognitive deficits, will serve as a guide in planning quality care. If the

Table 26-7 Nursing Diagnoses: Defining Characteristics

Nursing Diagnosis	Functional Health Pattern*	Definition	Defining Characteristics	Common Medical Diagnoses/Concerns
Disturbed thought processes	Cognitive-perceptual pattern	Disruption in cognitive operations or activities relative to chronological age expectation	Cognitive dissonance Memory deficit/loss Impaired perception/judgment/decision making Distractibility Inappropriate behavior Impaired attention span	Dementia Alzheimer's disease Neurological diseases, such as brain tumors, seizures, stroke, multiple sclerosis Head injuries Anoxia/hypoxia injuries Mental disorders Drug and alcohol abuse Fluid and/or electrolyte imbalance Infections (older adults)
Chronic confusion	Cognitive-perceptual pattern	Irreversible long-standing or progressive deterioration of intellect and personality, characterized by decreased ability to interpret environmental stimuli and decreased capacity for intellectual thought processes, and manifested by disturbances of memory, orientation, and behavior	Disoriented to person, place, or time Clinical evidence of organic impairment Altered interpretation or response to stimuli Progressive or long-standing cognitive impairment No change in level of consciousness Impaired memory Altered personality Impaired socialization	Alzheimer's disease Multi-infarct dementia Stroke Head injury Anoxia/hypoxia injuries Multiple sclerosis
Impaired memory	Cognitive-perceptual pattern	Inability to remember or recall bits of information or behavioral skills	Memory problems only Forgetfulness Difficulty learning new skills or information Inability to perform a previously learned skill Inability to recall recent or past events Forgetting to perform a behavior at a scheduled time	Hypoxia/anoxia injuries Anemia Congestive heart failure Neurological disturbances, such as multiple sclerosis, mild-moderate Alzheimer's disease, brain injury, dementia, stroke, etc. Fluid and electrolyte imbalance Excessive environmental disturbances Stress/fatigue

*Functional Health Pattern data from Gordon M. (2000). *Manual of nursing diagnosis* (9th ed.). St. Louis: Mosby.
Other potential nursing diagnoses are uncompensated memory loss, risk for cognitive impairment, acute confusion, and knowledge deficit.

Continued

TABLE 26-7 Nursing Diagnoses: Defining Characteristics—cont'd

Nursing Diagnosis	Functional Health Pattern*	Definition	Defining Characteristics	Common Medical Diagnoses/Concerns
Attention-concentration deficit	Cognitive-perceptual pattern	Inability to sustain a focal awareness	Distractibility Lack of focus Unable to attend to a task for any prolonged period (e.g., more than 5 minutes)	Head injury Hypoxia/anoxia injuries During agitation/outbursts Fatigue/stress syndromes Neurological disturbances
Impaired environmental interpretation syndrome	Cognitive-perceptual pattern	Consistent lack of orientation to person, place, time or circumstances over more than 3-6 months that necessitates a protective environment	Consistent disorientation in known and unknown environments for more than 3-6 months Chronic confusional states Loss of occupation or social functioning from memory decline Inability to follow simple directions Inability to reason Inability to concentrate Slow in responding to questions	Alzheimer's disease AIDS dementia Parkinson's disease Huntington's disease Depression Alcoholism Head injury

*Functional Health Pattern data from Gordon M. (2000). *Manual of nursing diagnosis* (9th ed.). St. Louis: Mosby.

Other potential nursing diagnoses are uncompensated memory loss, risk for cognitive impairment, acute confusion, and knowledge deficit.

etiology of a cognitive deficit is abrupt and sudden, such as a stroke or brain injury, the person usually enters into the health care system through the emergency department. Depending on the seriousness of the injury, a person may enter a critical care life supportive environment, where the goal is survival. For a person with cognitive deficits or behavioral problems, other primary goals are safety and effective communication. The cognitive problem may be temporary or permanent. Once stabilized, the person most likely will be admitted to an acute care unit.

After entering the acute care unit, the goals for the client are prevention of complications and return to medical stability. Many times people are admitted to acute care medical units because of acute confusional states, change in level of consciousness, altered personality, new onset of dementia, or behavioral disturbances. It is through examination, testing, and assessments that the etiology of cognitive dysfunctions is identified—such as AIDS, AD, stroke, or head injury. If the person needs therapy to regain strength, practice activities of daily living, speech enrichment, or memory strategies, it may be initiated in acute care. Because of shortened length of stay in acute care, there is not much time for improvement. If acute care treatment does not promote the person's ability to return to his or her premorbid living situation, other options may be needed.

Rehabilitation Nursing Interventions and Outcomes

Postacute Levels of Care

Postacute care units vary in several ways. Each level of care has a unique purpose and criterion for admission. The major options of postacute care include subacute care units, inpatient rehabilitation, outpatient rehabilitation therapies, day rehabilitation care centers, home health services, transitional living homes, memory special care homes, and long-term convalescent homes. People may enter and leave many levels of postacute care. The goals of each postacute level of care usually involves a team effort between nurses, physicians, physical therapists, occupational therapists, speech therapists, recreation therapists, social workers, dietitians, psychologists, vocational counselors, and the client and family. Reimbursement can range from 100% coverage by health insurance providers to 100% private pay. Because of the cost of various postacute care levels and the nonreimbursement issues, many do not enter into the appropriate level of care.

Subacute Care Units

Subacute care units are considered to be less acute than a medical unit, yet they provide interdisciplinary therapies, as does a traditional inpatient rehabilitation unit, but on a smaller scale. Table 26-8 shows rehabilitation nursing interventions and outcomes for cognitive disturbances in a subacute care unit.

Inpatient Rehabilitation Units

Inpatient rehabilitation units are considered short-term units in which the client may receive physical therapy, occupational therapy, speech therapy, social services, nursing care, psychology, and ancillary services to promote his or her return to home or the next level of care (Table 26-9).

Outpatient Rehabilitation Units

Outpatient rehabilitation units are day rehabilitation care centers or home health services provided while the client resides at home but receives support and therapy (Table 26-10).

Postacute Levels of Care

Postacute levels of care include transitional living centers, special memory care homes, assisted living homes, and long-term convalescent homes. These are considered a client's home in which he or she receives specialized care services (Table 26-11).

Evaluation

To evaluate the effectiveness of nursing interventions, compare actual client and family behaviors with the expected client and family outcomes.

HEALTH PROMOTION AND PREVENTION

Both primary and secondary prevention should be integrated into programs facilitated and managed by rehabilitation nurses across the continuum of care. As people live longer lives, health care providers should encourage consumers to pursue healthy lifestyles. Prevention is often described in two forms: Primary prevention, aimed at the general population, and secondary prevention, designed to reduce the chance of future injury to an already injured individual (Sege, Schneps, Licenziato, & Lash, 1997).

Healthy People 2010 identified priorities and opportunities to improve health in both the public and private sector (Box 26-4).

Box 26-4 *Healthy People 2010* Areas of Focus

Healthy People 2010, the Nation's Prevention Agenda, has 28 focus areas; a number of them relate to injuries and illnesses that cause deficits in cognition, including:

1. Disability and secondary conditions
2. Access to quality health services
3. Education and community-based programs
4. Stroke and heart disease
5. Injury and violence prevention
6. Substance abuse

U.S. Department of Health and Human Services. (1999). *Healthy people 2000* [on-line]. Available http://www.health.gov/healthypeople/prevagenda/whatishp.htm.

TABLE 26-8 Rehabilitation Nursing Outcomes/Interventions for Cognitive Disturbances in a Subacute Care Unit

Potential Rehabilitation Nursing Outcomes	Potential Rehabilitation Nursing Interventions
Cognitive orientation intact as evidence by identifying person, place, and time	Promote comfort, safety, and reality orientation by the following activities: • Maintain safe environment • Provide appropriate level of supervision • Decrease environmental stimuli • Maintain daily, consistent routine • Assign consistent caregiver • Educate family and significant others about orientation strategies, • Post calendars, clocks for visual aids • Encourage clients to participate in orientation, reality groups (if available) • Maintain daily log • Keep schedule with client at all times
Concentration intact as evidence by the ability to focus on a specific task or stimulus appropriately	Promote attention span and the ability to focus, which allows the client to participate in an activity: • Minimize environmental stimuli • Keep distractions to a minimum • Promote adequate rest and sleep • Individualize schedule of activities and therapies • Gradually increase complexity of schedule as ability to focus improves
Neurological status: consciousness as evidenced by the individual's ability to arouse, orient, and attend to the environment	Promote recovery of consciousness by coma-stimulation activities such as: • Familiar strong odors (coffee, chocolate) • Familiar sounds (family member's voice, music) • Tactile stimulation with different fabric textures • Visual pictures or large colored codes
Activity tolerance increased to the point the client can participate in daily activities	Promote frequency and duration of individual's activity: • Establish baseline activity tolerance and gradually increase • Assist to choose appropriate activities consistent with cognitive capabilities (focus on what can be and not deficits) • Provide activities to increase attention span and concentration in therapies • Provide positive reinforcement for engaging in activities • Assist the client and family to monitor own progress toward goal achievement
Family participates in professional care as evidenced by their involvement in making decisions, delivering, and evaluating care provided by health care professionals	Promote family participation: • Educate family about disease, situation, and their role responsibilities • Facilitate coping and problem-solving skills • Assist family to maintain positive relationships • Facilitate open communication between health care workers and family • Encourage families to participate in support groups • Encourage family participation in care as appropriate • Schedule and facilitate family conferences to discuss and evaluate care
Family has the knowledge to understand the illness or injury causing deficits in cognition	Promote family understanding for reasons of deficits in cognition: • Assess family's education level (learning style and ability to learn new information) • Use resources from appropriate agencies such as American Heart Association, Multiple Sclerosis Society, Brain Injury Association, or Alzheimer's Association • Encourage interdisciplinary team strategies to provide information about deficits • Provide education one-on-one or in small groups as appropriate • Facilitate family participation in managing the cognitive deficits
Client and family participate in health care decisions regarding next level of care	Promote client and family to make appropriate decisions regarding next of level of care: • Keep family informed • Encourage participation in rehabilitation program • Use discharge planning resources (i.e., case manager, social worker, patient advocates) • Provide them with information about options and resources based on situation and benefits

TABLE 26-9 Rehabilitation Nursing Outcomes and Interventions for Cognitive Deficits in an Inpatient Rehabilitation Unit

Potential Rehabilitation Nursing Outcomes	Potential Rehabilitation Nursing Interventions
Cognitive ability intact as evidenced by ability to execute complex mental processes	Promote cognitive function: • Identify/assess current cognitive status via Mini-Mental State Exam/Rancho's Los Amigo's Scale • Facilitate reality orientation • Label items in environment to promote recognition • Provide access to current news events • Encourage participation in decision making • Encourage use of aids (e.g., eye glasses, hearing aids, and dentures) • Dress patient in personal clothing • Speak in concrete terms, avoid abstract terms
Decision making intact as evidenced by the ability to choose between two or more alternatives	Promote appropriate decision making: • Identify potential choices such as allowing the client to pick daily clothing • Allow the client to make choices in daily care • Help client identify the advantages and disadvantages of each alternative • Encourage the client to make decisions about self and care • Provide positive reinforcement when appropriate choices are made • Provide simple problems that can be controlled (e.g., card games, meal selection) • Gradually increase complexity of tasks (e.g., computer games, planning daily activities) • Develop a problem-solving training program that allows client to practice responses to common problem situations • Gradually introduce common problems the client may face in the community • Encourage client to participate in community outings to test decision making skills • Use computer programs to practice decision making
Thought control as evidenced by appropriate perception, thought processes, and thought content	Promote appropriate control of thoughts: • Monitor client's statements of self • Provide experiences that increase client's autonomy • Assist client to identify positive responses from others (discourage negative criticizing and teasing) • Identify client's inappropriate behavior when it occurs: provide feedback in behavior; if client cannot identify inappropriate behavior, nurse must identify it for client and provide counsel (videotape client when acting inappropriately and show to client for educational purposes), role-playing • Establish consistent interdisciplinary plan to deal with inappropriate behaviors • Establish a behavior modification plan • Provide positive reinforcement for appropriate behavior
Information processing will be consistently demonstrated as evidenced by acquiring, organizing, and using information	Promote accurate information processing: • Assess level of comprehension • Encourage the client to ask for clarification • Assess for nonverbal and verbal behaviors that would indicate the degree of understanding • Converse with client in one-on-one conversation • Provide discussion about events, current news, items found in print (reading is the highest level of comprehensive skills)
Memory intact as evidenced by ability to retrieve and report previously stored information	Promote memory function: • Assess memory problems • Stimulate memory by repeating client's last expressed thought • Implement appropriate memory techniques (i.e., memory cues, making lists, memory games, mnemonic devices, computers, rehearsing information) • Assist in associated learning tasks (such as practical learning and recalling information) • Provide for orientation training (i.e., client rehearsing personal information and dates) • Provide opportunities to use memory for recent events (i.e., questioning client about recent event) • Encourage client to participate in group memory training program • Provide repetition of information and make verbal or visual association that will promote remembering • Teach clients to organize information in a logical way (i.e., when dressing teach person to plan events in sequence of bathing, hygiene, underclothes, and clothes) • Model calm and friendly behavior to reduce fear and anxiety

Continued

TABLE 26-9 Rehabilitation Nursing Outcomes and Interventions for Cognitive Deficits in an Inpatient Rehabilitation Unit—cont'd

Potential Rehabilitation Nursing Outcomes	Potential Rehabilitation Nursing Interventions
Safety behavior as evidenced by fall prevention	Promote safety: • Assess client for potential for injury/risk for fall • Educate client and family about potential hazards in current environment and home • Assess environment for potential or actual risks and eliminate problem area • Use less restrictive devices to prevent falls from bed, wheelchair, commode, etc., such as a bed alarm, chair alarm, and constant supervision; restraint options include locking bed belt, side rails, and wheelchair belt • Identify risk factors and design plan of care to lessen the risk (i.e., call light within reach, toileting program, frequent observation checks, consistent caregivers and routine, adhering to schedule, visual cues in environment, anticipate client's needs, wear shoes or nonskid slippers) • Use wheelchair tippers to prevent wheelchair from tipping over • Consult physical therapist for wheelchair and ambulation safety • Use safety ambulation device (i.e., merry walker), if needed • Use specialty beds that are low or set up on the floor if frequent falls out of bed • Limit access to windows that can be opened by client • Avoid stairways, but if stairs are used make sure handrail is available • Manipulate lighting for therapeutic viewing of environment
Aggression control as evidenced by self-restraint of assaultive, combative, destructive, or agitation behaviors	Promote control of aggression: • Assess level of cognition in relation to potential for agitation and behavior control • Identify situations that precipitate aggression or agitation • Set up behavior management plan: communicate expectations to client and family the need to maintain control; set limits; refrain from arguing; establish routines; employ consistent caregivers; use soft, low speaking voice; redirect agitation away from source; ignore inappropriate behavior; praise efforts of self-control; provide consistent consequences for desired and undesired behaviors; break multiple-step instructions into simple steps; provide aids that will increase environmental structure, concentration, and task (i.e., watches, calendars, signs, step-by-step instructions, schedules); monitor and regulate level of activity and stimulation in environment; limit choices as necessary; use external controls as needed to control client (i.e., time out, physical restraint, chemical restraint); limit caffeinated foods and fluids; and teach/reinforce appropriate social skills • Teach behavior management plan to family and significant others • Facilitate family coping through support groups, respite care, and family counseling as needed

Much can be done in terms of prevention of those injuries and illnesses that affect cognition. Strategies include:

- Identification of and reduction of reversible risk factors for stroke
- Early detection and intervention with AD to delay disease progression and improve function
- Safe sex, safe needle use, and other prevention measures to prevent HIV/AIDS
- Use of seat belts, air bags in automobiles, and helmets when riding motorcycles, snowmobiles, and bicycles to prevent head injuries and fatalities
- Practice of gun control and firearm safety to reduce incidence of brain injury
- Reduction of substance abuse to lower incidence of motor vehicle accidents and violent activities
- Improve home environment safety features to reduce falls and injuries
- Prevention education for SBS and other forms of child abuse
- Prevention education and equipment for playground safety, school bus safety, sports and concussion safety to prevent brain injury

Violence is one of the most important and preventable causes of severe childhood neurological injury. For this reason, it is important for the rehabilitation clinician to understand the opportunities for violence prevention in any professional setting (Sege, Schneps, Licenziato, & Lash, 1997). The American Academy of Pediatrics further defines SBS as an act of "shaking/slamming that is so violent that any competent individual observing the shaking would recognize it was dangerous" (Kang, 2000). The trigger is typically a cry-

Text continued on p. 626

TABLE 26-10 Rehabilitation Nursing Expected Outcomes and Interventions for Cognitive Deficits in an Outpatient Rehabilitation Unit

Possible Rehabilitation Nursing Outcomes	Potential Rehabilitation Nursing Interventions
Home physical environment: safety as evidenced by no physical harm or injury in the home	Promote home safety: • Assess home by interdisciplinary team to assess for potential hazards • Provide good lighting • Place hand railings, ramps, and grab bars • Arrange furniture to reduce risk • Notify community safety personnel about cognitively impaired client at home in community (i.e., local police, neighborhood watch patrol) • Place telephone or communication device in an accessible location with phone numbers posted nearby • Ensure smoke detectors are in working condition in the home • Remove environmental hazards (i.e., rugs, cords, sharp objects) • Provide adaptive equipment for cooking (i.e., mirrors over stove so client can see, large knobs, key and lock use) • Secure rooms to keep client in to avoid elopement
Caregiver home care readiness as evidenced by being prepared to assume responsibility for the health care of family member with cognitive deficit	Promote caregiver readiness: • Assess caregiver potential to assume the role/responsibilities (emotional, knowledge, stress/coping) • Participate in home care decisions • Return demonstration and information about home care management/care plan: treatments, activity plan, schedule, emergency care, follow-up care/appointments, when to seek medical attention, identification of plans for home care backup, management of equipment/supplies • Establish a respite plan if needed
Caregiver performance, direct care, and indirect care given as evidenced by provision and oversight of appropriate care by family member or significant other	Promote caregiver performance, direct and indirect care: • Implement a care plan identified in acute or rehabilitation level of care • Monitor behavior of care recipient and anticipation of care recipient needs • Demonstrate confidence in monitoring caregiver skills • Demonstrate positive regard for care of recipient, confidence in performing needed tasks, and confidence in problem solving • Recognize changes in behavior and health status of recipient and care • Obtain and oversee needed services for care recipient
Caregiver physical and emotional health as evidenced by physical and emotional well-being of family care provider while caring for family member or significant other over extended period	Promote caregiver's physical and emotional health by continually assessing energy level, sleep pattern, physical function, perceived general health, mobility level, resistance to infection, medication use, use of health care providers, and physical comfort Promote wellness behaviors: • Encourage social support system • Identify stressors • Identify limitations in caregiving • Identify role performance • Use health care services • Encourage involvement in activities • Identify satisfaction/dissatisfaction with caregiver's role • Identify other potential needs for caregiver support • Identify potential support groups • Monitor factors promoting endurance • Observe satisfaction of care recipient/caregiver relationship • Master indirect/direct care activities • Identify services/social support needs for caregiver • Provide health care system support, resources, and respite for caregiver

Continued

TABLE 26-10 Rehabilitation Nursing Expected Outcomes and Interventions for Cognitive Deficits in an Outpatient Rehabilitation Unit—cont'd

Possible Rehabilitation Nursing Outcomes	Potential Rehabilitation Nursing Interventions
Family normalization as evidenced by the ability of the family to develop and maintain routines and management strategies that contribute to optimal functioning when a member has a cognitive impairment	Promote family normalization and integrity: • Assess family roles and structure preinjury/disease and current status • Identify family's ability to maintain usual routines • Monitor family's ability to accommodate the needs/care of recipient • Identify potential resources to support family integrity (counseling, psychology, social work, support groups) • Facilitate participation in the role changes required by cognition deficit of care recipient (i.e., breadwinner, parent, spouse no longer able to fulfill previous role responsibilities) • Promote communication between family members • Encourage problem solving and conflict resolution • Encourage participation in family events (i.e., meals, leisure activities, family traditions, rituals) • Identify potential support/resources in times of crisis
Health seeking and promoting behaviors as evidenced by actions promoting and sustaining optimal wellness, recovery, and rehabilitation	Promote health-seeking and health-promoting behaviors: • Assess family and client's ability to implement healthy behaviors: asking questions appropriately, completing health-related tasks, performing daily activities with energy tolerance • Describe strategies to eliminate unhealthy behaviors • Describe strategies to maximize health • Encourage health promoting behaviors • Monitor personal behaviors for risk • Seek balance among exercise, work, leisure, rest, and nutrition • Use effective stress reduction behaviors • Maintain satisfactory social relationships • Use financial, physical, and social support resources to promote health • Facilitate the reentry into school and work by monitoring current and ongoing cognition needs and potential services to improve cognitive recovery • Facilitate work site assessment and visit to determine appropriateness and potential resources for return • Promote work-simulated opportunities • Monitor performance and make changes based upon individual client's needs • Identify the child's or adolescent's ability to participate in formal schooling • Provide cognitive appropriate resources or sites for ongoing education • Promote long-term monitoring for changes in educational support based on changes in cognition/problems that may occur with developmental levels • Provide educational support based on developmental needs
Social interaction skills/involvement as evidenced by a client's ability and frequency of social interactions	Promote social interaction skills and involvement: • Encourage involvement within already established relationships • Encourage relationships with people who have common interests/goals • Encourage honesty in presenting oneself to others • Encourage respect for the rights of others • Refer client to a program that teaches appropriate social skills • Help client increase awareness of strengths and limitations in communicating with others • Use role-play to practice communication and social skills • Confront client about impaired judgment when appropriate • Give positive feedback when client reaches out to others • Encourage client to participate in leisure activities

TABLE 26-11 Rehabilitation Nursing Expected Outcomes and Interventions for Cognitive Disturbances in Postacute Levels of Care

Potential Rehabilitation Nursing Outcomes	Potential Rehabilitation Nursing Interventions
Safety behavior as evidenced by caregiver's ability to control client's behaviors that might cause physical injury	Promote personal safety: • Assess client's risk for injury/falls assessment tool • Create a safe environment for the client • Remove potentially harmful objects from the environment • Provide low-height beds or floor mats as appropriate • Provide adaptive devices (e.g., hand rails) • Place frequently used objects within reach (e.g., urinal) • Monitor environmental stimuli (e.g., noise, lighting, contact stimulation) • Individualize daily routine • Maintain consistency of staff assignment • Provide frequent or ongoing monitoring • Ensure client has access to nursing call light at all times (mark it with bright color such as orange) • Educate client and family about safety plan • Monitor client for inappropriate behaviors, attempt to identify trigger stimuli • Redirect client's attention away from agitation source • Ignore inappropriate behavior • Praise efforts at self control • Use chemical restraints as a last option • Use restraints or immobilization devices, if appropriate and according to facility's policy (may no longer allow them)
Aggression control as evidenced by self-restraint of assaultive, combative, or destructive behavior toward others	Promote control of aggressive behavior: • When aggressive outbursts occur, assess situation for patterns such as time of day, circumstances before event, environmental factors (lighting, noise, over- or understimulation), caregiver's approach, food/drinks (e.g., caffeinated products, high-sugar foods) eaten before episode, and visitors/people surrounding client before or during event • Refrain from arguing with client • Ensure client does not strike out at staff or other clients by removing them from scene • Secure environment so client doesn't have access to sharp objects • When client's anger escalates, assist client in identifying behavior (e.g., voice gets louder, makes threatening comments, strikes out), and provide client with alternative solution (e.g., throw pillow, hug stuffed animal, ambulate [if able to safely] or propel self in wheelchair, push in wheelchair [motion can have a calming effect], try rocking chair, put on calming music, dim lights, remove people [avoid gathering staff; this feels like an attack], or avoid conversation) • After outburst, discuss the situation to educate client on aggressive behaviors • Educate family about aggression and plan of care
Caregiver adaptation to client institutionalization as evidenced by family caregivers adaptation role when the care recipient is transferred outside the home	Promote caregiver's adaptation to client's institutionalization: • Assess caregiver's understanding/belief of institutional care • Promote a trusting relationship between family and staff • Encourage family to be involved in decision-making regarding care • Offer to let family participate in care • Establish a means of communication • Encourage family and client to express feelings about change or being in institution • When conflicts arise, promote family to be part of resolution • Allow client to be as independent as possible • Encourage family to bring in client's personal items/clothes to make the environment feel more familiar

Continued

TABLE 26-11 Rehabilitation Nursing Expected Outcomes and Interventions for Cognitive Disturbances in Postacute Levels of Care—cont'd

Potential Rehabilitation Nursing Outcomes	Potential Rehabilitation Nursing Interventions
Quality of life as evidenced by an individual's or family's expressed satisfaction with current life circumstances	Promote quality of life: • Assess client's code status and living will status • Promote client's productivity or usefulness by having client participate in self-care activities and mobility, as appropriate • Encourage client to express thoughts about past, present and future • Assist client in recognizing strengths • Encourage client to engage in social support system, leisure activities, and daily routine • Seek psychological support, if appropriate • Administer medications, if appropriate • Promote comfort and prevention of complications • Provide a balance between rest and activity • If not a group activity person, provide one-on-one activities • Maintain consistency in schedule; dress client in street clothes during the day and pajamas for bedtime • Provide meals at a table/dining room experience • Promote toileting in a bathroom environment • Provide hygiene and baths appropriately • Use pastoral and social services when indicated

ing, inconsolable child. It is important that caregivers of small children be provided with information on positive coping skills when dealing with a crying baby:

- Make sure all of the baby's basic needs are met (food, diapering, etc.)
- Offer baby a pacifier
- Take the baby for a walk in a stroller or ride in the car
- Call a friend, relative, or neighbor to come over for support or take care of the baby while you take a break
- Call the national help lines provided by Child Help USA (800-4-A-Child) or National Committee to Prevent Child Abuse (800-Children)
- If you are a child care provider and cannot handle a crying baby, let the parent know, and do not be afraid to tell the parent(s) you cannot care for the baby

Parents with children in child care should be mandated reporters of child abuse. In many instances, previous "unexplained injuries" of other children in a child care setting were never reported, with the end result being the next "unfortunate" child with serious abuse such as SBS (Kang, 2000).

The two main goals of primary prevention of youth violence are instilling the following in minds of youth:

- Methods of conflict resolution and
- Outlets for anger which are productive, yet not violent (Sege et al., 1997)

Emergency Medical Services for Children, through their national efforts have proposed several secondary prevention initiatives and recommendations regarding the development of a coordinated system of care for children with special needs that includes children with TBI. These initiatives include:

- Injury prevention
- Early referral to physical medicine and rehabilitation (PM&R) services
- Coordination of care for children with special needs that are admitted to the hospital
- Information and education for families of children with brain injury
- Linkages with public health programs
- Establishment of written emergency care plans for children at risk of a medical emergency
- Training for emergency medical technicians and paramedics on how to provide emergency for children with special needs (Savage, 1997)

After one brain injury, the risk for a second is 3 times greater; after the second injury, the risk for a third injury is 8 times greater (Brain Injury Association, 1998). In July 1996, Congress enacted Public Law 104-166 "to provide for the conduct of expanded studies and the establishment of innovative programs with respect to TBI." The TBI State Demonstration Grant Program is administered by the Health Resources and Services Administration, Maternal and Child Health Bureau. TBI demonstration grants emphasize activities by states to implement statewide systems that ensure access to comprehensive and coordinated TBI Services (Berube, 1998). A model was developed at The Ohio State University through the Ohio Valley Center for Brain Injury

Prevention and Rehabilitation programs for patients with brain injury. Considering shorter lengths of stay and fewer resources, but substance abuse risks of individuals with brain injury staying the same, this model serves as a practical source of secondary prevention for rehabilitation health professionals along the continuum of care (Corrigan et al., 1999). Every rehabilitation program serving people with brain injuries should screen for risk of substance abuse, provide client and family education related to alcohol and drugs, and provide appropriate referrals for those identified at risk. The Ohio Valley Center for Brain Injury Prevention and Rehabilitation (1997) also developed a guide for professionals to intervene with those clients who have substance abuse problems.

The Division of Research Sciences of the National Institute on Disability and Rehabilitation Research (NIDRR) also awards grants for TBI model systems. These grants are competitively awarded to rehabilitation hospitals, centers, and universities to carry out research, demonstrate and evaluate a comprehensive, multidisciplinary service delivery system to improve the care, rehabilitation, and community reintegration of individuals who have experienced TBI (1997). The network of these centers has established a national database (Traumatic Brain Injury [TBI] Model Systems, 2000).

Potential legislation is currently being proposed that allows law enforcement officers to stop motorists for seat belt violations as well as helmet violations for those states mandating helmets. "Campaign Safe and Sober" is a national traffic campaign that seeks to unite national, state, and local efforts to reduce alcohol-related crashes and increase safety belt and child safety belt use (Campaign Safe and Sober, 2000).

Hendrickson (1996) presented a school-based helmet intervention program to educate about bike safety and increased bicycle helmet use with fourth graders. This community experience increased children's recognition of the potential critical nature of brain injury and their personal susceptibility to injury. The author encourages rehabilitation nurses throughout the country to participate in similar prevention endeavors.

Prevention fact sheets are available from the Violence and Brain Injury Institute. The set of nine fact sheets contains information about the prevention of violence, accidents, and brain injury. Topics include bicycle safety, SBS, motorcycle safety, motor vehicle safety, playground safety, school bus safety, firearm safety, sports and concussions, and pedestrian safety (Violence and Brain Injury Institute, 2000).

Prevention is also important with older persons because they sustain a majority of TBIs in domestic falls. Tinetti and Speechley (1989) categorized fall risk factors for the elderly into groups:

- Chronic (i.e., neurological disease, sensory impairment, or musculoskeletal disease that especially affect the lower extremities)
- Short term (i.e., periodic postural hypotension, acute illness, alcohol use, or medication side effects)
- Activity related (i.e., tripping while walking, descending stairs, or climbing ladders)
- Environmental (i.e., throw rugs, poor lighting, poorly fitting shoes or pants) (p. 454) (see Chapter 14)

These same risk factors predispose the elderly to motor vehicle, pedestrian, and recreational accidents, all of which can result in TBI. Rehabilitation programs providing services for the elderly should address these risk factors and provide education related to prevention in each of these areas.

The National Safety Council, in cooperation with the National Retired Teachers Association and the American Association of Retired Persons, developed a home safety checklist to identify fall hazards in the home. It is a useful tool for rehabilitation professionals to use in identifying hazards that should be reduced or eliminated in homes of the elderly (Home Safety Checklist, 1982).

CRITICAL THINKING

Mrs. B is 37 years old and was diagnosed 6 years ago with Multiple Sclerosis (MS). She is a mother of three school-age children and works full-time as an occupational therapist. She is admitted to acute inpatient rehabilitation for a recent exacerbation of her disease causing her to be "weaker." During the assessment Mrs. B could not appropriately state her children's names, city where she lived, current president, or name of their pet. During her first few days in rehabilitation, it was assessed that Mrs. B had trouble staying focused on therapies, following her schedule, and remembering strategies to complete activities of daily living. The rehabilitation team met her with her and her significant other to address her cognitive disturbances. During this meeting, Mrs. B's spouse reported on many situations in which Mrs. B had forgotten important things and had trouble finding items. Mrs. B became very upset and threatened to leave the rehabilitation unit.

As the rehabilitation nurse on the unit, you will be managing the plan of care with Mrs. B and her family. Include the team in thinking critically about the following questions:

1. What are potential cognitive disturbances that may be causing Mrs. B's behavior?
2. How would you approach Mrs. B and her family about available and appropriate treatments?
3. What can you tell them about innovations, alternative or complementary therapies, or advances in conventional medicine?
4. Where will you look for resources and referral information?
5. Identify strategies (e.g., effective coping, memory enhancement, energy conservation, or compensatory actions) that may improve outcomes for Mrs. B.

Case Study ∽∽∽ *Traumatic Brain Injury Care Plan*

Mike is 24 years old and sustained a traumatic head injury from an assault. After completing an acute inpatient rehabilitation unit, he was discharged to his parents' home. He was evaluated as Rancho Level VI. Before his injury he lived with his girlfriend and worked full-time as a house painter. His girlfriend has remained supportive and active in his recovery. She worked full-time as a beautician and was unable to provide Mike's care. After returning home, Mike was scheduled to attend outpatient therapies (occupational and speech) for ongoing cognitive rehabilitation. Fortunately he was left with no physical disability from the incident. He was scheduled to attend therapies Monday, Wednesday, and Thursday. The rest of the time, he would be home under the supervision of his parents. His father worked outside the home, approximately 50 hours a week, and his mother worked out of their home office and was the primary caregiver.

At first Mike was excited and glad to be out of the rehabilitation center; however, by the second week he was restless. His mother found him several blocks away, walking aimlessly through the neighborhood. She started to lock all doors; however, a couple days later Mike was gone and could not be found. He was found by the police who suspected he was under the influence of drugs because of his cognitive deficits, confusion, and odd behavior. He spent several frightening hours in a local police station, while his family spent hours in panic searching for him. After being reunited, therapists decided that a rehabilitation home health nurse would be beneficial in helping prevent Mike from future elopements.

After assessing the situation, the rehabilitation home health registered nurse (RN) developed a care plan to address problems.

Nursing diagnosis: Altered thought processes: Rancho level VI related to traumatic brain injury

Nursing outcome: Caregiver performance: Direct care as evidenced by family able to provide appropriate care for client in their home; client will not leave home without supervision

Nursing Goal

Nursing goals include actions that will promote family providing appropriate care for Mike. Nursing interventions include:

- The pattern of elopement and potential causes were assessed.
- The parents' understanding of Mike's cognitive status and measures implemented to secure Mike's safety were assessed. After assessment, the RN discovered that Mike had no set routine and no responsibilities other than attending therapies. His mother spends most of her time in the office working, while Mike spends his time watching television. Mike reported that he gets the urge to leave because he is trying to get to his apartment.
- In mutual decision making, it was decided that Mike needed a planned routine and more activities. Thus Mike would attend a rehabilitation day care center from 8:00 AM to 4:30 PM, where he would receive daily therapies, social activities, leisure activities, home management activities, and work-simulated activities.
- His girlfriend participated in the plan. After day care, she would pick him up for dinner.
- Mike's father would bring him home.
- A planned schedule was established Monday through Friday, as well as the weekends.
- The family agreed that supervision would include close monitoring at all times.
- Bells were added to all doors to alert family when doors were opened.
- Bright red STOP signs would be placed on the inside of all doors to remind Mike not to leave.
- Mike agreed to wear an alert bracelet stating "Memory Problems" with a home phone number until his memory improved.
- Local community emergency medical services (police, fire department) were notified of Mike's condition and risk for elopement.
- The family and Mike were encouraged to participate in a local TBI support group. Within a few weeks, Mike's cognitive status had improved significantly and he was ready to return to his apartment and begin a return-to-work program.

REFERENCES

Alverzo, J.P., & Galski, T. (1999). Nurses' assessment of patient's cognitive orientation in a rehabilitation setting. *Rehabilitation Nursing, 24,* 7-12, 23.

Alzheimer Europe. (2000). *AIDS dementia complex* [On-line]. Available: http://www.alzheimer-europe.org/aids.html.

Alzheimer's Association. (2000). *Alzheimer's statistics* [On-line]. Available: http://www.alz.org/facts/left.htm.

American Congress of Rehabilitation Medicine. (1991). *Definition of mild traumatic brain injury.* Chicago. Author.

American Heart Association. (2000). *Stroke statistics* [On-line]. Available: http://americanheart.org/heartandstroke_ a-z_guide/strokes.html; http://americanheart.org/statistics/biostats/biowo.htm.

Baroff, G. II. (1998). Is heading a soccer ball injurious to brain functions? *Journal of Head Trauma Rehabilitation, 13,* 45-52.

Barth, J.T., Macciocchi, S.N., & Diamond, P.T. (1999). Mild head injury: current research and clinical issues. In M. Rosenthal, E.R. Griffith, J.S. Kreutzer, & B. Pentland (Eds.), *Rehabilitation of the adult and child with traumatic brain injury* (3rd ed., pp. 471-478). Philadelphia: FA Davis.

Berube, J.E. (1998). A good first step toward nationwide aid to persons with brain injury: The Traumatic Brain Injury Act of 1996. *Journal of Head Trauma Rehabilitation, 13,* 80-85.

Biagas, K. (1999). Hypoxic-ischemia brain injury: advancements in the understanding of mechanisms and potential avenues for therapy. *Current Opinions in Pediatrics, 1,* 223-228.

Blosser, J., & Pearson, S. (1997). Transition coordination for students with brain injury: A challenge schools can meet. *Journal of Head Trauma Rehabilitation, 12,* 21-31.

Bodick, N.C., Offen, W.W., & Levey, A.L. (1997). Effects of xanomeline, a selective muscarinic receptor agonist, on cognitive function and behavioral symptoms in Alzheimer's disease. *Archives of Neurology, 54,* 465-473.

Bondy, K.N. (1994). Assessing cognitive function: A guide to neuropsychological testing. *Rehabilitation Nursing, 19,* 24-30.

Brain Injury Association. (1998). *Brain injury prevention information* [On-line]. Available: http://www.biausa.org.

Brillhart, B. (2000). Psychosocial healthcare patterns and nursing interventions. In P. Edwards (Ed.), *The specialty practice of rehabilitation nursing care curriculum: A core curriculum* (4th ed., pp. 139-165). Glenview, IL: Association of Rehabilitation Nurses.

Brzuzy, S., & Speziale, B.A. (1997). Persons with traumatic brain injuries and their families: Living arrangements and well-being post injury. *Social Work in Health Care, 26,* 77-88.

Burges, E.S., Drotar, D., Taylor, H.G., Wade, S., Stanins, T., & Yeates, K.O. (1999). The family burden of injury interview: Reliability and validity studies. *Journal of Head Trauma Rehabilitation, 14,* 394-405.

Centers of Disease Control and Prevention. (2000). *HIV/AIDS surveillance report* [On-line]. Available: http://www.cdc.gov/.

Christensen, J.R. (1997). Pediatric traumatic brain injury rehabilitation: challenges in care delivery. *Neuro Rehabilitation, 9,* 105-112.

Corrigan, J.D., Bogner, J.A. Lamb-Hart, G.C. (1999). Substance abuse and brain injury. In M. Rosenthal, E.R. Griffith, J.S. Kreutzer, & B. Pentland (Eds.), *Rehabilitation of the adult and child with traumatic brain injury* (3rd ed., pp. 556-571). Philadelphia: FA Davis.

DeBoskey, D.S., Hecht, J., & Calub, C. (1991). *Educating families of the head injured: A guide to medical, cognitive, and social issues.* Gaithersburg, MD: Aspen.

Delehanty, R., & Kieran, D. (1998). Family perceptions of health professionals in family problem solving after brain injury. *The Journal of Cognitive Rehabilitation,* May/June, 14-23.

Englander, J., & Cifu, D. (1999). The older adult with TBI. In M. Rosenthal, E.R. Griffith, J.S. Kreutzer, & B. Pentland (Eds.), *Rehabilitation of the adult and child with traumatic brain injury* (3rd ed., pp. 453-470). Philadelphia: FA Davis.

Enterlante, T., & Kern, J. (1995). Wives' reported role changes following a husband's stroke: A pilot study. *Rehabilitation Nursing, 20,* 155-160.

Evans, R.W. (1992). Mild traumatic brain injury. *Physical Medicine and Rehabilitation Clinics of North America, 3,* 427-439.

Galshi, T., Bruno, R.L., Zorowitz, R., & Walker, J. (1993). Predicting length of stay, functional outcome and after care in the rehabilitation of stroke patients. *Stroke, 24,* 1794-1800.

Gauther, S., Panisset, M., & Nalbantoglu, J. (1997). Alzheimer's disease: Current knowledge, management and research. *Canada Medical Association Journal, 157,* 1047-1052.

Gill, D.J., & Wells, D.L. (2000). Forever different: Experiences of living with a sibling who has a traumatic brain injury. *Rehabilitation Nursing, 25,* 48-53.

Gordon, W.A., Brown, M., Sliwmski, M., Hibbard, M.R., Patti, N., Weiss, M.J., Kalinsky, R., & Sheever, M. (1998). The enigma of "hidden" traumatic brain injury. *Journal Head Trauma Rehabilitation, 13,* 39-56.

Graham, D.I. (1999). Pathophysiological aspects of injury and mechanisms of recovery. In M. Rosenthal, E.R. Griffith, J.S. Kreutzer, & B. Pentland (Eds.), *Rehabilitation of the adult and child with traumatic brain injury* (3rd ed., pp. 19-41). Philadelphia: FA Davis.

Grzanikowski, J.A. (1997. Altered thought processes related to traumatic brain injury and their nursing implications. *Rehabilitation Nursing, 22,* 24-28.

Harrison-Felix, C. (1996). Disruptive findings from the traumatic brain injury model systems national data base. *Journal of Head Trauma Rehabilitation, 11:*1.

Hendrickson, S.L. (1996). A bruise on the brain: Conveying the meaning of head injury to children. *Rehabilitation Nursing Research, 5,* 35-42.

Hochstenbach, J., & Mulder, T. (1999). Neuropsychology and the relearning of motor skills following stroke. *International Journal of Rehabilitation Research, 22,* 11-19.

Home safety checklist. (1982). *Falling—The unexpected trip. A safety program for older adults, program leader's guide.* National Safety Council.

Janus, P.L., Mishkin, L.W., & Pearson, S. (1997). Beyond school re-entry: addressing the long-term needs of students with brain injuries. *Neuro Rehabilitation 9,* 133-148.

Kang, K. (2000). *Shaken baby syndrome: The facts and hard realities. prevention matters newsletter* [On-line]. Available: http://www.biausa.org/pmatters.htm.

Kase, C.S., Wolf, P.A., Kelly-Hayes, M., Kannel, W.B., Beiser, A., & D'Agostino, R.B. (1998). Intellectual decline after stroke: the Framingham study. *Stroke, 29,* 805-812.

Katz, D., & Black, S.E. (1999). Neurological and neuroradiological evaluation. In M. Rosenthal, E.R. Griffith, J.S. Kreutzer, & B. Pentland (Eds.), *Rehabilitation of the adult and child with traumatic brain injury* (3rd ed., pp. 89-116). Philadelphia: FA Davis.

Katzman, R., & Terry, R. (1983). Normal aging of the nervous system in rehabilitation medicine. In J. DeLisa, B. Gans, W. Bockeneck, D. Currie, S. Geiringer, L. Gerber, J. Leonard, M. McPhee, W. Pease, William, & N. Walsh (Eds.). Rehabilitation Medicine: *Principles and practice* (3rd ed.) Philadelphia: Lippincott-Raven, pp. 15-50.

Kelly, J.P., & Rosenberg, J.N. (1998). The development of guidelines for the management of concussions in sports. *Journal of Head Trauma Rehabilitation, 13,* 53-65.

Kraus, J.F., & McArthur, D.L. (1999). Incidence and prevalence of, and costs associated with traumatic brain injury. In M. Rosenthal, E.R. Griffith, J.S. Kreutzer, & B. Pentland (Eds.), *Rehabilitation of the adult and child with traumatic brain injury* (3rd ed., pp. 3-18). Philadelphia: FA Davis.

Kreutzer, J.S., Sunder A.M., & Fernandez, C. (1997). Misperceptions, mishaps, and pitfalls in working with families after traumatic brain injury. *Journal of Head Trauma Rehabilitation, 12,* 63-73.

Lincoln, N.B., & Rother, L (1998). A further validation of the Salford objective recognition test in stroke patients. *British Journal of Occupational Therapy, 61,* 545-546.

Long, D.F. (1989). *What is anoxic brain injury?* Washington, DC: National Head Injury Foundation.

Marino, M.J. (1999). Centers for Disease Prevention and Control report shows prevalence of brain injury. brain Injury Challenge, 3(3), 12-13.

Meadows, J., LeMarechal, K., & Catalan, J. (1999). The burden of care: The impact of HIV-associated dementia on caregivers. *AIDS Patient Care and STDS, 13,* 7-56.

Mecklinger, A., von Cramon, Y., & Matthes-von Cramon, G. (1998). Event-related potential evidence for a specific cognition memory deficit in adult survivors of cerebral hypoxia. *Brain, 121,* 1917-1935.

Mitchell, P.W., Cammermeyer, M., O'Luna, J., & Woods, N.F. (1984). *Neurological assessment for nursing practice.* Reston, VA: Reston Publishing, Prentice Hall.

Multiple Sclerosis Foundation. (2000). *Multiple sclerosis statistics* [On-line]. Available: http://www.msfact.org/stats.htm.

National Center for HIV, STD and TB Prevention. (1998). *Division of HIV/AIDS prevention* [On-line]. Available: http://www.cdc.gov/nchstp/hiv_aids/stats/cumulati.htm.

Ohio Valley Center for BI Prevention and Rehabilitation. (1997). *Substance use and abuse BI: A programmer's guide.* Ohio Valley Center for BI Prevention and Rehabilitation. Columbus, OH.

Oken, B.S., Storzbach, D.M., & Kaze, J.A. (1998). The efficacy of ginkgo biloba on cognitive function. *Archives of Neurology, 55,* 1409-1415.

Pound, P., Gompertz, P., & Ebrahim, S. (1998). A patient-centered study of the consequences of stroke. *Clinical Rehabilitation, 12,* 338-347.

Putnam, S.H., & Fichtenberg, N.L. (1999). Neuropsychological examination of the patient with traumatic brain injury. In M. Rosenthal, E.R. Griffith, J.S. Kreutzer, & B. Pentland (Eds.), *Rehabilitation of the adult and child with traumatic brain injury* (3rd ed., pp. 147-166). Philadelphia: FA Davis.

Roberts, J., Browne, G., Milne, C., Spooner, L., Gatni, A., Drummond-Young, M., LeGois, J., Watt, S., LeClair, K., Beaumont, L., & Roberts, J. (1999). Problem-solving counseling for caregivers of the cognitively impaired: Effective for whom? *Nursing Research, 48,* 162-172.

Rocchio, C. (1997). Families of youngsters speak out: What works/what doesn't. *NeuroRehabilitation, 9,* 159-166.

Rocchio, C. (2000). *Family news and views—impaired cognition and behavior problems: double trouble!* [On-line]. Available: http://www.biausa.org/famviewnws/impairedcog_behaveprob.htm.

Rogers, J., Kirby, L.C., & Hempelman, S.C. (1993). Clinical trial of indomethacin in Alzheimer's disease. *Neurology, 43,* 1609-1611.

Rosenthal, M., Griffith, E., Bond, M., & Miller, J.D. (1990). *Rehabilitation of the adult and child with traumatic brain injury.* Philadelphia: FA Davis.

Savage, R.C. (1997). Integrating rehabilitation and education services for school-age children with brain injuries. *Journal of Head Trauma Rehabilitation, 12,* 11-20.

Sege, R.D., Schneps, S.E., Licenziato, V.G., & Lash, M. (1997). Violence: A preventable cause of head injury in children. *Neuro Rehabilitation, 9,* 167-176.

Shurtleff, H.A., Massagli T.L., Hays, R.M., Ross, B., & Sprenk-Greenfield, H. (1995). Screening children and adolescents with mild or moderate brain injury to assist school re-entry. *Journal of Head Trauma Rehabilitation, 10,* 64-79.

Simard, M., & Reekum, R. (1999). Memory assessment in studies of cognitive-enhancing drugs for Alzheimer's disease. *Neurology, 14,* 197-230.

Sisson, R. (1998). Life after a stroke: Coping with change. *Rehabilitation Nursing, 23,* 198-203.

Sosin, D.M., Sacks, J.J., & Webb, K.W. (1996). Pediatric head injuries and death from bicycling in the United States. *Pediatrics, 98,* 868-870.

Stuifbergen, A. (1995). Cognitive impairment and perceptions of quality of life among individuals with multiple sclerosis. *Rehabilitation Nursing Research, 2,* 11-18.

Tinetti, M.D., & Speechley M. (1989). Prevention of falls in the elderly. *New England Journal of Medicine, 320:*1055-1058.

Traumatic brain injury (TBI) model systems [on-line]. (2000). Available: http://www.ed.gov/offices/OSERS/NIDRR/tbims.htm.

Uren, R. (1984) Organic disorders. In C.K. Cassell, & J.R. Walsh. *Geriatric medicine* (2nd ed., p. 553). New York, Springer-Verlag.

Violence and Brain Injury Institute. (2000). *Violence and brain injury.* Available through electronic mail: btremblay@biausa.org.

Wall, J.R., Deshpande, S.A., MacNeill, S.E., & Lichtenberg, P.A. (1998). The Fuld object memory evaluation, a useful tool in the assessment of urban geriatric patients. *Clinical Gerontologists, 19,* 39-49.

Weeks, S.K., & O'Connor, P.C. (1997). The FAMTOOL family health assessment tool. *Rehabilitation Nursing, 22,* 188-191.

White, H., & Levin, E. (1999). Four-week nicotine skin patch treatment effects on cognitive performance in Alzheimer' disease. *Psychopharmacology, 143,* 158-165.

Ylvisaker, M., Chorazy, A.J.L., Feeney, T.J., & Russell, M.L. (1999). Children and adolescents: Assessment and rehabilitation. In M. Rosenthal, E.R. Griffith, J.S. Kreutzer, & B. Pentland (Eds.), *Rehabilitation of the adult and child with traumatic brain injury* (3rd ed., pp. 353-392). Philadelphia: FA Davis.

Sleep and Recreation 27

Pamela M. Duchene, DNSc, RN, CRRN

It is Sunday morning, and you worked the evening shift on Saturday. It was incredibly busy at work, with three admissions and one acute care transfer. As a result, you worked 2 hours of overtime, and did not get home until close to 2 AM. By the time you were able to unwind, roll into bed, and finally close your eyes it was almost 2:45. Now it is 10 AM, and you are doing your best to listen to the sermon at church. You had a 16-ounce cup of coffee on your way to church, but no matter how hard you try, your eyelids are so heavy that it has become impossible to keep them open. The minister is talking in a low voice, everyone is quiet, the room is warm, and the coffee has become ineffective in keeping you alert. You seem to sink deeper into the pew and relax against the side of the pew. Your eyes burn, and your eyelids feel so heavy that you allow them to close for the briefest of seconds. As your eyelids close, your head nods forward, and you feel complete relaxation for a few minutes, then your head jerks up, and you are awake once again. This cycle of eyelid closing, head nodding, and jerking awake continues throughout the 20-minute sermon. The minister closes his sermon, and everyone rises to sing. At once you feel a jolt of energy, rise, and begin singing. As you leave the sanctuary, you try not to meet the eyes of the minister, who probably noticed the nodding-off episodes. As you head for home, you vow to spend the next 2 hours catching up on sleep before starting the Sunday evening shift.

SLEEP

According to Shakespeare, sleep is "nature's soft nurse." In the United States, however, most adults sleep less than the recommended 8 hours a night (National Sleep Foundation, 1999a). The National Sleep Foundation, in their omnibus "Sleep in America Poll," conducted a telephone poll of 1014 adults living within the continental United States. They questioned sleep habits, problems, and disorders and found that most Americans sleep an average of 6 hours, 58 minutes during work nights, and an average of 7 hours, 38 minutes on weekends. Results of the poll indicate that during the past year, 62% of American adults experienced sleep problems a few nights a week. Unfortunately Americans consider sleep a waste of time, robbing the sleep hours for daytime activities. During the past century, average sleep time decreased by 20%, whereas work and commute times increased by a month. Although culture has changed, the physiology of the body and the need for sleep have not, resulting in the problems indicated in Box 27-1.

OVERVIEW OF SLEEP

Purpose of Sleep

Sleep is necessary for restoring energy and other anabolic processes. The actual homeostatic contribution of sleep is unknown (Beers & Berkow, 1999). Although sleep serves the purpose of providing rest and maximizing wakefulness, the functions of sleep are not well understood. Studying the effects of sleep loss, or deprivation, provides clues to the purpose of sleep. Sleep deprivation leads to problems with simple, short activities. An absence of sleep causes irritability, fatigue, decreased motivation, a shortened attention span, and reduced problem-solving capacity. Sleeplessness is a predictor of absenteeism and is estimated to be linked to more than 200,000 motor vehicle accidents annually. Such information indicates that sleep plays a major role in physical and emotional health and promotes healing from illness and injury.

Box 27-1 Qualities of Sleep in America

Results of the 1999 Omnibus Sleep in America Poll indicate that of U.S. adults:

- 65% receive less than the recommended 8 hours of sleep a night
- 62% experience sleep problems a few nights of the week
- 65% report problems with insomnia a few nights of the week
- 12% have symptoms of sleep apnea a few nights of the week
- 30% state that stress affects their ability to sleep
- 40% report that daytime sleepiness interferes with daily activities
- 62% state they have driven while feeling drowsy during the past year
- 30% do not keep regular sleep schedules

Adapted from National Sleep Foundation. (1999). *National Sleep Foundation's 1999 Omnibus "Sleep in America poll"* [On-line]. Available: http://www.sleepfoundation.org/publications/1999poll.html.

TABLE 27-1 Stages of Sleep

Stage	Description
Stage 1:	The onset of sleep, identified by muscle relaxation, slow side-to-side eye movements and reduction in eye blinking. Slow eye movement (non–rapid eye movement (REM).
Stage 2:	Slightly deeper sleep with muscle relaxation and little eye movement. Slow eye movement (non-REM).
Stage 3:	Deep sleep, with slow waves noted on electroencephalography, and some side-to-side eye rolling. Slow eye movement (non-REM).
Stage 4:	Deep sleep, similar to stage 3, with high-voltage and slow-frequency electroencephalographic activity. Slow eye movement (non-REM).
Stage 5:	Rapid eye movement (REM) sleep, characterized by dreams with vivid visual content.

Jackson, WJ. (1999). Brain function: Sleep. In T. Nosek (Ed). *Essentials of human physiology.* Atlanta: Gold Standard Multimedia Inc. and Medical College of Georgia.

Process of Sleep

Through polysomnography, a process involving electroencephalogram, electro-oculogram, and electromyogram studies, sleep may be classified into two major categories: slow eye movement or non–rapid eye movement (REM) sleep, and REM sleep. Slow eye movement sleep can be subdivided into four stages, with REM composing a fifth stage (Table 27-1).

In REM sleep, there are rapid oscillations of the eyes, with muscle atonia (linked with deep sleep), whereas with wakefulness, the electroencephalographic activity is low volume and high frequency (Jackson, 1999). Bursts of electroencephalographic activity in conjunction with decreased muscle activity occur during REM sleep.

During sleep, a person shifts through stages, initially proceeding through stages 1, 2, 3, and 4, and then re-versing through stages 3 and 2, followed by an REM episode. A sleeping individual will pass through the stages several times during the night, with five or six cycles during the night. Age, medication, and other differences will have an impact on sleep cycles, as discussed later in this chapter.

Physiology of Sleep

The midline raphe system, located in the midbrain, is considered a center for sleep activity. Serotoninergic mechanisms originating in the midline raphe affect the noradrenergic and cholinergic systems. During non-REM sleep, there is increased secretion of growth hormone (70% of secretion occurs during sleep), luteinizing hormone, and prolactin, and decreased secretion of adrenocorticotropic and thyroid-stimulating hormones. During deep sleep (stages 3 and 4), blood pressure and respiratory function decrease, whereas vagal tone in the cardiovascular system increases.

The systems work in a balance to prevent an immediate change from a wakeful state to REM sleep. One hypothesis on the cause of narcolepsy is an imbalance in the systems, with immediate change to REM sleep becoming possible. In such a situation (REM intrusion), an individual would be wide awake one minute and in a state of atonia with active hallucinations, or visual dreams, the next.

Circadian rhythm is linked with sleep/wake cycles. Stemming from the 24-hour Earth rotation, the term *circadian* means "around a day." During a 24-hour period, many changes occur within physiological parameters, including changes in temperature, respiratory rate, heart rate, and wakefulness. Minimum body temperature and maximum sleepiness coincide in time during the nighttime hours. A second low-temperature/sleepiness point typically occurs at 3 PM, a common time for naps and siestas. The suprachiasmatic hypothalamic nucleus is an important anatomical structure in the wakefulness/sleep cycle. The retina provides stimulation to the suprachiasmatic hypothalamic nucleus, cueing the body to the light/dark cycle and influencing wakefulness/sleep. Lesions of this area result in an impairment of circadian rhythm.

FACTORS AFFECTING SLEEP

Healthy Sleep Habits

Obtaining a good night's sleep is an elusive goal to many individuals. To ensure the optimal chances of getting enough sleep and of obtaining enough rest through sleep, the following strategies may be of assistance:

- Go to bed at a regular time

TABLE 27-2 Sleep Stealers

Psychological factors	The most common cause of sleep problems are stress, pressure, illness, or marital problems.
Shift work	Around 20% of workers in the United States are shift workers. For shift workers, sleep must occur while others are awake, resulting in a need to compete with usual biological rhythms developed over decades of life. Shift workers are as much as 5 times more likely to fall asleep at work as nonshift work employees.
Environmental interferences	Issues such as the room temperature, noise level, or lighting will influence the ability to sleep soundly. Likewise, the size of the bed, comfort of the mattress, and habits of the individual's sleep partner will influence sleep.
Physical factors	Pain, hormonal shifts, breathing issues, and pregnancy are just a few of the physical factors that can interfere with sleep.
Jet lag	Biological rhythms can be disturbed by traveling across time zones.
Lifestyle stressors	Intake of alcohol or caffeinated beverages before sleeping can interfere with sound sleep or the ability to fall asleep. Exercise or heavy mental activity completed immediately before sleep may interfere with the ability to sleep.
Medications	Steroids, antihypertensives, and antidepressants may interfere with sleeping.

National Sleep Foundation (1999b). *ABC's of ZZZ's* [On-line]. Available: http://www.sleepfoundation.org/.

- Establish a consistent waking time and do not vary the time during weekends and holidays
- Develop and maintain bedtime rituals, such as a warm bath or relaxation exercise
- Exercise during the daytime and avoid strenuous activity immediately before sleeping
- Reduce fluid intake close to bedtime
- Avoid eating a heavy meal right before going to bed
- Avoid alcohol, caffeine, and nicotine
- Use the bed only for sleeping and sex
- If unable to fall asleep within 15 minutes, get out of bed

The most common thieves of sleep are listed in Table 27-2.

Alcohol Use

Alcohol acts as a central nervous system depressant, inducing sleep; however, alcohol is linked with delay and disruption of REM sleep. Minimal alcohol intake results in fragmentation of sleep, with prolonged stages 1 and 2 and delayed stages 3 and 4 and REM sleep. As the alcohol is metabolized, a rebound may occur with REM sleep late in the sleep cycle (Brown, 1999).

Medications

Many medications have an impact on sleeping cycles—in particular, those known to influence mood (Table 27-3). Monoamine oxidase–inhibiting drugs suppress REM sleep more than any other drug class.

Natural Sleep Factors and Dietary Supplements Inducing Sleep

With the trend to look to natural and herbal remedies for relief of common problems, there is research on natural sleep factors. Factor S is one such natural sleep aid. Found in intestinal bacteria, factor S is linked with sleep induction and may be one cause of the fatigue and tendency to sleep associated with bacterial infection (Jackson, 1999).

Cholecystokinin (CCK), a neuropeptide released through the digestive system after ingestion of a large meal, is linked with sleepiness. The compound is under consideration for use as an appetite suppressant. Individuals who consumed CCK during European clinical trials experienced a decreased appetite but an increased feeling of sleepiness (Jackson, 1999). A side effect of CCK is panic attacks (Akiyoshi, 1999), so the usefulness of the drug for sleep induction or appetite reduction is limited.

Naturally occurring substances such as tryptophan (found in turkey and milk), melatonin, and valerian root may induce sleep. Synthetic tryptophan is not available, but natural tryptophan is easily accessible. A bedtime snack of milk or potatoes will provide sufficient tryptophan to induce sleep. Synthetic melatonin is available, but long-term studies on its safety are not available. Although synthetic valerian root is available, the extract (400 to 450 mg) is most effective. As with melatonin, long-term safety has not been documented (Brown, 1999). Other herbs and natural agents that may induce sleep include chamomile, catnip, hops, kava, lavender, and St. John's Wort (Cauffield & Forbes, 1999; Tyler, 1999) (Table 27-4). Because of the accessibility of such natural agents and their purported claims, many individuals with sleep disturbances are using them. In one study of 937 individuals with arthritis, 32.8% reported sleep disturbances. The most common reason for use of complementary relief strategies cited was sleep disturbance (Jordan et al., 2000).

Relaxation and Music

Although relaxation and sleep are not synonymous, they are related states. Without relaxation, one will find it difficult to sleep. Without sufficient sleep, a person may find it difficult to relax without sleeping. Relaxation exercises will aid in as-

TABLE 27-3 Impact of Medications on Sleep

Medication		Effect on Sleep		
Generic Name	**Classification**	**Heavy Sedation**	**Moderate Sedation**	**Low Sedation**
Amitriptyline	Tricyclic antidepressant	X		
Amoxapine	Tricyclic antidepressant	X		
Bupropion	Dopamine uptake inhibitor		X	
Desipramine	Tricyclic antidepressant			X
Doxepin	Tricyclic antidepressant	X		
Fluoxetine	Selective serotonin reuptake inhibitors			X
Fluvoxamine	Selective serotonin reuptake inhibitors	X		
Imipramine	Tricyclic antidepressant		X	
Mirtazapine	α^2-adrenergic blocker antidepressant	X		
Nefazodone	Postsynaptic serotonin 5-HT_{2A} antagonist and presynaptic serotonin reuptake inhibitor	X		
Nortriptyline	Tricyclic antidepressant	X		
Paroxetine	Selective serotonin reuptake inhibitors	X		
Phenelzine	Monoamine oxidase inhibitor		X	
Sertraline	Selective serotonin reuptake inhibitors		X	
Venlafaxine	Serotonin and norepinephrine reuptake inhibitor			X

From Brown, D. (1999). Managing sleep disorders. *Clinician Reviews, 9,* 69; Burnham, T. (Ed.) (2000). *Drug facts and comparisons.* St. Louis: Facts and Comparisons.

sisting a person to fall asleep. One manner of achieving a state of relaxation is through the use of music. In a study of 500 individuals undergoing surgery, one researcher found that pain scores decreased and relaxation was enhanced through the use of music (Stephenson, 1999). Johannes Brahms is best known for his lullabies, which many find sleep inducing. There is some evidence to show that Brahms himself may have suffered from sleep apnea (Margolis, 2000). Brahms had difficulty with heavy snoring, an obese neck, irritability, and was frequently seen sleeping at unusual times and places (most often in Viennese cafes). Each of these symptoms is associated with sleeping issues. Whether such problems with sleep led Brahms to compose beautiful lullabies is unknown; however, his music continues to lull people to sleep today.

Stimulants

The use of caffeine, nicotine, and other stimulants may significantly affect sleep. Coffee, tea, chocolate, and colas taken within 6 hours of bedtime may interfere with sleep. For some individuals, even a small amount of caffeine taken as much as 10 to 12 hours before sleep may prove problematic.

Psychological Stressors

Of the most common factors that interfere with sleep is psychological stress, including depression and anxiety. Sleeplessness or sleep disturbance is reported by 90% of individuals experiencing psychological stress, depression, and anxiety (Chokroverty, 1995).

Health Care Issues

Pain

Many of the issues that coincide with health care problems affect sleep. Health care problems associated with pain will interrupt sleep. Although analgesics may be necessary to decrease pain levels to allow sleep, the medications themselves will affect the architecture of sleep. Narcotics will facilitate relaxation and pain relief; however, they interfere with both deep and REM sleep. An individual using narcotics for pain relief may experience daytime sleepiness and nighttime restlessness, with reduced dreaming and deep sleep. One study of pain, fatigue, and sleep with individuals undergoing oncology radiation concluded that participants had a sleep efficiency of 71% compared with 90% for healthy control volunteers (Lamberg, 1999). This indicates that participants took longer to fall asleep and awakened frequently. Recommendations included daytime exercise, activity, better analgesic management, and planned naps.

Cardiopulmonary Problems

Individuals with cardiopulmonary problems may experience shortness of breath and orthopnea. These issues often result in sleep hypoxemia, which causes alterations in pulmonary, cardiac, and hematological functions (Brown, 1998). Persons with orthopnea frequently sleep with multiple pillows to ease the breathing difficulty they experience. Clinicians should inquire about multiple pillow use by clients because it may be a key indicator of cardiac failure or significant obstructive pulmonary disease. The elevated position is helpful for lung fluid clearance but is problematic for sleep, resulting in daytime drowsiness (Smith, 1996).

TABLE 27-4 Dietary Supplements Used to Impact Quality and Quantity of Sleep

Herb/Dietary Supplement	Description	Comments
Chamaemelum nobile [L] (Chamomile)	• Antispasmodic • Diaphoretic • **Sedative and sleep inducement** • Folk remedies have used the plant for asthma, fevers, colic, inflammation, and cancer	• Herbal plant, creeping perennial • Native to western Europe and North Africa
Garcinia mangostana L.	• Used to treat diarrhea, dysentery, cystitis • **Acts as a central nervous system depressant** • May cause elevation of blood pressure	• Derived from the fruit, mangosteen • Grown in Malaysia, Thailand, and Burma
Humulus lupulus L. (Hops)	• **Sedative** • Primary use is as a flavor for beer	• Perennial vine • Native to Europe
Hypericum perforatum L. (St. John's Wort)	• Relieve or reduce depression • Antibacterial • Spasmolytic • Antiseptic • **Increases latency to rapid eye movement sleep** • **Increases amount of deep sleep in total sleeping period**	• Native to Russia • Wild, flowering plant • Used in teas • Most popular drug (herbal or otherwise) in Germany for treatment of depression
Lavandula sp. (Lavender)	• **Used to induce sleep** • Used to reduce depression • Gives sense of happiness and relaxation • Antispasmodic • Diuretic • Tonic • Used for treatment of colic and headaches	• Aromatic shrub • Native to Europe • Fragrant blue and purple flowers
Melissa officinalis L. (Balm or lemon balm)	• **Sedative, central nervous system depressant** • Used for fever, flatulence, diaphoretic • Used to treat influenza, headaches, and toothaches	• Perennial herb • Native to southern Europe and North America
Nepeta cataria L. (Catnip)	• Used as an antispasmodic, diaphoretic, stimulant • **Mild sedative** • Used to treat diarrhea, colic, colds, and cancer	• Perennial herb • Native to Eurasia • Grown in North America • Smoking catnip causes euphoria and hallucinations
Papever somniferum L. (Opium poppy)	• Habit-forming narcotic used for manufacture of morphine, papaverine, codeine, and heroin • **Used as a hypnotic, sedative,** antitussive, and analgesic • Seeds contain no opium and are a source of energy	• Annual or biennial herb • Native to Mediterranean areas east of Iran
Tagetes minuta (Asteraceae)	• Remedy for colds • Diarrhea • Stomach upset • Liver ailments • **Oil of the plant has tranquilizing properties,** and may promote hypotension, brochodilation, anti-inflammation	• Erect annual herb • Native to South America • Has a slightly sweet taste and is similar to the taste of licorice
Valerian officinalis (Valerian)	• **Used to shorten sleep latency and to increase length of sleep** • Used as a flavor for tobacco • Antispasmodic, calmative • Used for fever, fatigue, headaches • Used to relieve stress and hysteria	• Tall, perennial herb • Native to western Asia and Europe • Linked with liver disease
Ziziphus sp. (Jujube)	• Used for memory enhancement • Anti-inflammatory • Analgesic • **Sedative, used for insomnia** • Antispastic	• Native to China • Medium-sized tree with deciduous foliage • Fruit is similar to figs • Used in candies and cooking

From Tyler, V.E. (1999). Herbs affecting the central nervous system. In J. Janick (ed.), *Perspectives on new crops and new uses* (pp. 442-449). Alexandria, VA: ASHS Press.

Urinary Problems

Urinary problems, including frequency and urgency, whether the result of diuretic use, urinary tract infection, or benign prostatic hypertrophy, may result in sleep disruption. Individuals waking multiple times during the night may have difficulty falling back asleep and will not cycle through deep and REM sleep in the manner necessary. Individuals with incontinence will, likewise, experience sleep disturbance, whether because of becoming wet or because of the disruption of nursing and hygiene care.

Sleep Apnea

Sleep apnea occurs as a result of relaxation and collapse of the upper airway during sleep, resulting in snoring and lowered oxygen saturation. As the individual continues to sleep, relaxation increases and oxygen saturation decreases until the point at which the individual wakes, gasps for breath, and falls back asleep. The individual's sleeping partner may be aware of this cycle, but often the affected person is oblivious to the problem. The indicators of this problem may be daytime sleepiness and excessive fatigue (Marrone, Bonsignore, Insalaco, & Bonsignore, 1998). Although polysomnography is useful in diagnosing sleep apnea, a self-administered questionnaire may be a good first effort at problem identification. The Berlin questionnaire (Netzer, 1999) is a low-cost, valid tool for early identification of individuals suspected to have sleep apnea. The tool was pilot tested in five primary care practices in Cleveland, Ohio.

Musculoskeletal Problems

Spasticity and limited mobility may affect sleep architecture. Individuals with spasticity may find the spontaneous movement of limbs and muscles awakens them. Although with neurological diseases such as Parkinson's, tremors may cease during sleep, they may reoccur during times of body movement and sleep arousal. In able-bodied individuals, position changes occur about every half hour during sleep. For those with weakness or impaired mobility, it may be difficult or impossible to obtain positions of comfort. Requesting and waiting for the assistance of others in order to move to a comfortable position may be difficult and result in an additional loss of sleep.

Cognitive Changes

Disorders that affect cognition, including Alzheimer's disease, may lead to impairment of normal circadian control of sleep and alertness, which may result in sundowning (increased confusion and behavioral changes during the late afternoon and early evening), nighttime insomnia, and wandering.

Aging

Although individuals of all ages sleep, the amount of time spent in stages of sleep varies with age. The amount of REM sleep is highest in neonates and decreases steadily until 20 years of age. REM sleep continues to decrease after 20 years of age but at a slower rate of reduction. Older persons spend little time in REM or stage 4 sleep and awaken during the night. As a result of these changes, as an individual ages, it may take longer to gain the needed amount of sleep in REM and stage 4.

SLEEP ASSESSMENT

Subjective

Few individuals will seek health care for sleep issues, although many people are affected. Because problems with sleep do not trigger a visit to a health care practitioner, it may be overlooked in the assessment process. With an estimated 30% of individuals getting less than sufficient sleep (Brown, 1999), a critical question to ask any client is, "Do you have difficulty getting enough sleep and do you have problems staying awake during the day?"

One of the most common tools for sleep assessment is the Epworth Sleepiness Scale (SleepQuest, 2000), which is available on the Internet. Individuals completing the questionnaire by Internet send the results to the SleepQuest site, where the results are interpreted and correspondence is returned to the individual. The website is managed through Stanford University and is linked with Dr. William Dement, a founder of the study of sleep.

The following questions should be included in an assessment of sleep hygiene and quality:

- Do you have difficulty sleeping?
- Do you feel rested upon rising?
- Do you keep a regular sleep schedule (go to bed and rise at consistent times)?
- Do you have any difficulty falling asleep?
- Do you use any routines to assist you in falling asleep?
- Do you use any medications to assist you in falling asleep?
- Do you drink alcohol? How often? Do you use alcohol to assist with sleep?
- Do you drink coffee, tea, or colas? Do you drink caffeinated beverages before bedtime?
- Do you smoke?
- Do you experience drowsiness during the daytime?
- Do you nap during the daytime? If so, for how long and how often?
- Do you rise during sleep time for any reason, for example, to urinate?
- Approximately how many times during an episode of sleep do you rise?
- Are you able to return to sleep after an interruption?

Objective

Observation of sleep patterns should include an hour-by-hour assessment of the time the client spends sleeping, the number of times the client is awakened because of pain, voiding, in-

continence, and interruptions. According to Winslow (1996), nurses' observations of sleep patterns match polysomnographic recordings with a correlation of 82%. In addition to assessing the pattern of sleep, nurses should review the environment, including lighting, noise level, and temperature. If lighting and noise levels are elevated, the individual attempting to sleep may be unable to achieve a deep sleep or REM sleep. Temperature is significant in that individuals who are too cold or too warm may not be able to achieve a sense of comfort and may not be able to sleep uninterrupted. Another factor that should be assessed is the perceived comfort of the bed, pillows, and linens. The need for comfort during sleep is critical in attaining deep and REM sleep. In one study (Wirz-Justice, 1999), investigators linked warm feet with inducing sleep and cold feet with a delay in falling asleep.

NURSING DIAGNOSIS: SLEEP PATTERN DISTURBANCE (SPECIFY TYPE)

Disturbance of sleep patterns may occur because of a variety of factors. Nursing assessment information appropriate to the nursing diagnosis of sleep pattern disturbance is included in this section. Nursing diagnosis, outcomes, and interventions are included with nursing diagnoses in Table 27-5.

Sleep pattern disturbances may present in different ways, including parasomnias, dyssomnias (insomnia and hypersomnia), and medical/psychiatric sleep disorders (discussed in the Health Care Issues section). Each pattern will be discussed in the following section.

Parasomnias

Disorders that disrupt sleep events and processes are known as parasomnias. Arousal disorders and sleep-wake transition disorders are considered parasomnias. Abnormal arousal disorders include sleepwalking (somnambulism), confusional arousals, and sleep terrors. In these disorders, individuals are sufficiently awake to act, but not aware of their actions. Somnambulism results in walking during sleep and most often starts before puberty. Complex behaviors are initiated during slow-wave sleep, usually during the first third of sleeping time. Individuals are difficult to arouse during such episodes and do not recall the event on waking. Intervention revolves around making the environment safe and preventing injury to the affected person. Benzodiazepines (diazepam and alprazolam) may be of assistance in preventing somnambulism activity. Relaxation before sleeping and prevention of overexertion may also be of help (Beers & Berkow, 1999).

Nightmares

Frightening dreams occurring during REM sleep are nightmares. Alcohol, excess fatigue, and fever may lead to the occurrence of a nightmare. Night terrors are nightmares with screaming and flailing. As with nightmares, the development of night terrors in adults is linked with alcohol use and psychological stress.

Nocturnal Leg Cramps

Muscle cramps of the lower calf or foot may occur in middle-aged and older individuals who are otherwise healthy. The cramps are severe and make cause an individual to awaken suddenly. Relief may be obtained through stretching the muscles after the spasm has subsided.

Restless Legs Syndrome

Uncomfortable sensations such as a crawling sensation, paresthesia, and dysesthesia occurring in the legs associated with motor restlessness may be restless legs syndrome. The

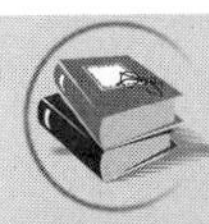

Case Study I ~ *Sleep*

Mr. Kessler had recently survived a triple coronary artery bypass, new diagnosis as an insulin-dependent diabetic, and, after 6 weeks in intensive care, 2 weeks on an acute telemetry and surgical unit, and a left below-the-knee amputation, he found himself on the physical rehabilitation unit. He and the therapists were disappointed with his progress. The evening nurse, Charlene, commented to the physiatrist that no matter what she did, Mr. Kessler did not seem to sleep at night. The physiatrist prescribed 400 mg of Skelaxin as needed at bedtime. Charlene administered the medication.

When she entered Mr. Kessler's room at 11 PM, he had the television on, was sitting up in bed, and requested a cup of hot tea. Although Mr. Kessler was adamant about his desires, Charlene questioned the wisdom of his choices. She made him a cup of hot herbal tea, and requested his permission to talk with him about his sleeping habits. After completing a sleeping history, she learned that ever since his time in ICU, whenever he drifted to sleep, he experienced severe nightmares. His attempt to stay up was in an effort to avoid them.

Charlene learned that Mr. Kessler enjoyed classical music and that a prior bedtime routine was a warm bath just before bed. She offered him a back rub with lavender lotion, located and played a classical radio station on the radio, and ensured he was in a position of comfort for the initial part of the night. She explained that she would have Elaine, the night shift nurse, not waken him for vital signs or assessment, unless he requested that she do so, or a change was noted in his status.

Charlene repeated the process each night she was working. She updated his care plan to assure continuity of care. Mr. Kessler began to sleep soundly at night. He no longer needed the bedtime medication and he began to make progress in therapy.

TABLE 27-5 Nursing Diagnosis/Nursing Outcome Classifications (NOC)/Nursing Intervention Classifications (NIC) for Sleep

Nursing Diagnosis	Suggested Nursing Outcome Classifications (NOC)	Suggested Nursing Intervention Classifications (NIC)
Sleep pattern Disturbance: sleep disruption	Anxiety control Rest Sleep Well-being Comfort level Leisure participation Medication response Mood equilibrium Pain level Psychosocial adjustment: life change Respiratory status: ventilation	Dementia management Environmental management Environmental management: comfort Medication administration Medication management Medication prescribing Security enhancement Simple relaxation therapy Touch Anxiety reduction Autogenic training Bathing Calming technique Coping enhancement Energy management Exercise promotion Exercise therapy: ambulation Meditation facilitation Music therapy Nutrition management Pain management Positioning Progressive muscle relaxation Self-care assistance: toileting Simple massage Urinary incontinence care: enuresis
Sleep pattern Disturbance: sleep deprivation	Sleep Anxiety control Cognitive ability Concentration Distorted thought control Endurance Energy conservation Information processing Memory Mood equilibrium Pain control Rest	Anxiety reduction Coping enhancement Dementia management Energy management Environmental management: comfort Medication management Meditation facilitation Pain management Progressive muscle relaxation Simple guided imagery Surveillance safety Music therapy Simple massage

Data from Johnson, M., Maas, M.L., & Moorhead, S. (2000). *Nursing outcomes classification (NOC)* (2nd ed.). St. Louis: Mosby; McCloskey, J.C., & Bulechek, G.M. (2000). *Nursing interventions classification (NIC)* (3rd ed.). St. Louis: Mosby; and North American Nursing Diagnosis Association. (2001). *Nursing diagnosis: definitions and classification 2001-2002* (4th ed.). Philadelphia: Author.

problem may affect the arms also and is typically worse during times of rest. This problem may result in sleep loss and distress because the legs may move every 20 seconds with bursts of movement. Individuals are unable to find a position of comfort because of the sensations, thereby delaying sleep. The individual affected with restless legs syndrome suffers sleeplessness, as does his or her sleeping partner. The problem is associated with peripheral neuropathy, uremia, anemia, and rheumatoid arthritis (Lamberg, 1999).

Dyssomnias (Insomnia and Hypersomnia)

Interruption of sleep may be linked with alcohol use, psychological stress, or pain. Initial insomnia may be caused by pain, emotional stress, respiratory problems, and problems with sleep hygiene. Early morning awakening is common with aging and with individuals experiencing depression. Sleep rhythm reversals are associated with disturbance of circadian rhythms and tend to affect nightshift workers and those with brain injury or damage to the hypothalamus. Lesions of the hypothalamus may cause hypersomnia, as may encephalitis, depression, and increased intercranial pressure. Additionally hypersomnia may be seen with hyperglycemia, hypoglycemia, hypothyroidism, uremia, anemia, hypercalcemia, liver failure, hypercapnia, multiple sclerosis, and epilepsy. Narcolepsy is an infrequent form of hypersomnia in which there is a sudden change from wakefulness to deep sleep with cataplexy (momentary paralysis with no loss of consciousness), hypnagogic phenomena (vivid visual and auditory hallucinations), and sleep paralysis (loss of voluntary movement as falling asleep or awakening). The majority of individuals with narcolepsy do not experience all of the symptoms of narcolepsy. Although longevity is not affected, there are clinical accounts of individuals who have experienced an episode of narcolepsy while driving, resulting in a collision or fatality.

RECREATIONAL, LEISURE, AND DIVERSIONAL ACTIVITY

Introduction

It is 2 weeks before you are scheduled to take a much-needed vacation to visit California. You have worked no less than 56 hours a week each week for the past 2 months. When you are not working, you are attending graduate school classes in an effort to complete the course work for a nurse practitioner certificate. At home, the situation is grim. The laundry has accumulated, and although a source of embarrassment, you have resorted to purchasing additional pairs of underwear in an effort to stay the need for laundry a few more days. It has been at least 2 weeks since you made a trip to the grocery store. The milk in the refrigerator soured about 3 days ago, and you have been using ice cream for your morning and evening coffee.

The day for the start of vacation finally arrives. You finish last-minute packing, slip in a few articles to read during the flight, and board the plane for California. You spend the first 2 days of vacation worrying about work, graduate school, mounting laundry, and other tasks left undone. By day 3, you are able to sleep without setting an alarm clock, and you are able to leave the unfinished articles for review in your carryon bag for the return trip home. It has taken 3 full days for you to remember how to rest and enjoy leisure time and activities.

OVERVIEW OF RECREATIONAL, LEISURE, AND DIVERSIONAL ACTIVITY

The question of a link between the "joyless striving" of the type A personality and cardiac disease has existed since the mid-nineteenth century (Januzzi, Stern, Pasternak, & DeSanctis, 2000). In 1910, Sir William Osler noted that the individual with angina pectoris is frequently a worrier and "a man whose engine is always set full speed ahead" (Larkins, 2000). The type A personality is characterized by hostility, aggressiveness, and a perpetual sense of urgency, and is linked with an increased risk of cardiovascular disease (Barefoot et al., 1989). Studies to reduce cardiovascular risks through stress reduction indicate that including stress reduction programs may positively affect morbidity and mortality (Blumenthal et al., 1997).

Stress and reduced physical activity and exercise are associated with other significant health care problems, including symptomatic cholelithiasis and diabetes. Recreational physical activity, including jogging, running, and bicycling, is inversely related to the incidence of symptomatic cholelithiasis (Leitzmann et al., 1999). In those at risk for cholelithiasis, recreational physical activity in conjunction with other risk factor modifications, such as maintaining ideal body weight, may be beneficial to decrease the risk (Vega, 1999). Although there is some debate on the correlation between risk of symptomatic cholelithiasis and recreational physical exercise (Lawlor & Hanratty, 2000), there is wide acceptance of the correlation between recreational physical exercise and blood sugar control for individuals with type 2 diabetes mellitus (Baron, Steinbuerg, Brechtel, & Johnson, 1994).

For those unable to participate in recreational physical exercise, alternative methods of simulating the exercise experience have been noted to positively affect risk factors. In one unusual study, the author correlated the use of hot tub therapy with stabilization of blood sugars and weight reduction for type 2 diabetics (Hooper, 1999).

In addition to the research findings identified above, recreational activities have a significant impact on the well-being of individuals with physical impairment and disability. Therapeutic recreation activities are linked with the outcomes indicated in Box 27-2. Through therapeutic interventions including recreational, leisure, and diversional activities, the physical, emotional, cognitive, and social functioning of individuals may be enhanced. Such therapeutic interventions

Box 27-2 Outcomes of Recreational Therapy

- Improvement in physical, social, cognitive, and emotional function
- Enhanced functional independence and improved quality of life
- Prevention of physical, cognitive, and psychosocial functional declines
- Reduction of secondary disability and prevention of increased health care costs

Adapted from Coyle, C., Kinney, W., Riley, B., Shank, J. (Eds.) (1991). *Benefits of therapeutic recreation: A consensus view.* Ravensdale, WA: Idyll Arbor, Inc.

include the environment and support systems of individuals and focus on maximizing physical and psychosocial well-being. Activities are structured around specific goals targeting improved independence, function, and symptom reduction (Coyle, Kinney, Riley, & Shank, 1991).

Participation in recreational physical activities result in enhanced cardiovascular and respiratory function, in addition to improved coordination, strength, and endurance (Rowland, Kline, Goff, Martel, & Ferrone, 1999). These improvements affect those who are able bodied, as well as those with physical disabilities and chronic illness (Karason, Lindroos, Stenlöf, & Sjöström, 2000). Related to the improvements in cardiopulmonary status, secondary medical complications that are associated with spinal cord injury and chronic illnesses are reduced through recreational physical activities (Wannamethee, Shaper, & Alberti, 2000). Specifically, complications such as pressure ulcers and urinary tract infections are less common in those participating in recreational physical activities. Health risk factors including cholesterol and blood sugar levels are improved through recreational physical activities (Pratt, 1999). Memory, attention, organizational skills, and perception may be enhanced through participation in recreational activities. Additionally, depression may be decreased and body image enhanced through recreational exercise and lifestyle activity (Blumenthal et al., 1999).

FACTORS AFFECTING RECREATION, LEISURE, AND DIVERSIONAL ACTIVITY

Although aspects of physical disability and chronic illness may impact *how* one participates in recreation and leisure activities, *whether or not* one participates is the result of inclusion and accessibility more than a restriction imposed by physical limitations.

Inclusion

The philosophy of inclusion holds that individuals with and without physical disabilities and chronic illnesses should participate in activities together. The perception of limitation should not interfere with an invitation to participate in an event. Rehabilitation professionals must understand that it is better to make the error of assuming an individual will want to participate in an event than to fail to invite the individual. Many individuals have painful memories of being the last individual selected for a team. The failure to include an individual in an event is far worse than simply being selected late.

Accessibility

Therapeutic recreational specialists work to design "ways around physical limitations" to enable individuals with physical disabilities and chronic illness to participate in recreation and leisure activities. In Jackson, Mississippi, one therapeutic recreational specialist, Ginny Boydston, has devoted her career to creating opportunities for individuals with significant physical disabilities to participate in sports activities (Boydston, personal communication, March 24, 2000). She offers a scuba program for individuals with quadriplegia. After participants have passed an initial training program at the local pool, she takes the participants to the Gulf of Mexico for actual diving experiences. Ginny has developed a program known as "Victory Sports" for racing, basketball, and other team types of activities for individuals with spinal cord injury. Additionally, she offers sports clinics throughout the state of Mississippi for individuals with significant physical limitations. The clinics include water skiing and bowling. Ginny's efforts provide proof that the extent of physical limitation need not interfere with participation in recreation and leisure activities (Figure 27-1). She has noted clients have increased self-esteem, body image, and social interaction as results of the unique sports clinics.

NURSING DIAGNOSIS: DIVERSIONAL ACTIVITY DEFICIT

Deficits in diversional activities may occur as a result of variety of factors. Nursing assessment information appropriate to the nursing diagnosis of diversional activity deficit is included in this section. Nursing diagnosis, nursing outcome

Case Study 2 ⌒ *Recreation*

Joe, 42, was diagnosed with amyotrophic lateral sclerosis in 1997. He is able to reside at home through home health nursing care, personal attendants, and a dedicated, caring, and supportive extended family. Joe's physical limitations have progressed to the point that he has a tracheostomy and respiratory assistance and uses a power chair for mobility. His voluntary muscle control is limited to flexion and extension of the index finger of his right hand. Joe's quality of life is linked with his involvement with his family and with his ability to remain current in news events and reading.

Through extensive modification of the living environment, and the installation of an environmental control unit, Joe is able to use the limited range of his index finger to control the world around him. Of most significance to Joe, however, through the use of his single digit, Joe is able to access a control switch to run the computer system for leisure and recreation. Although the computer system does not provide Joe with physical exercise and recreation, it allows his mind to continue to stretch and grow.

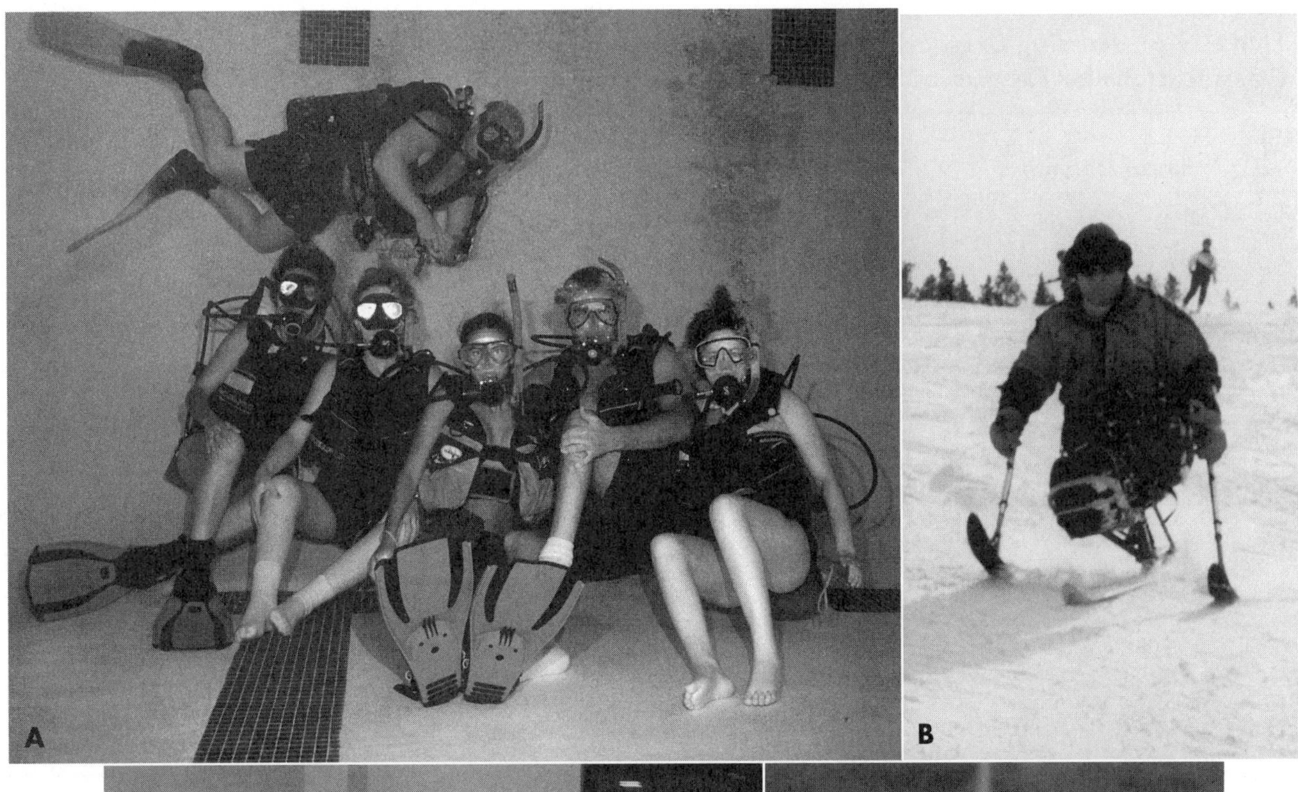

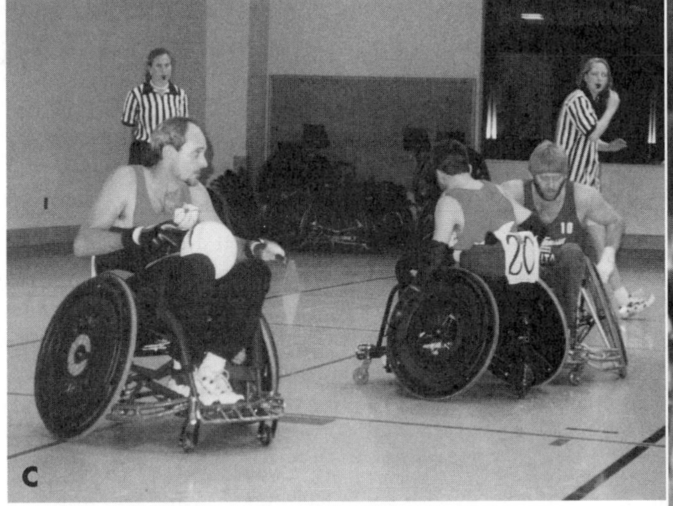

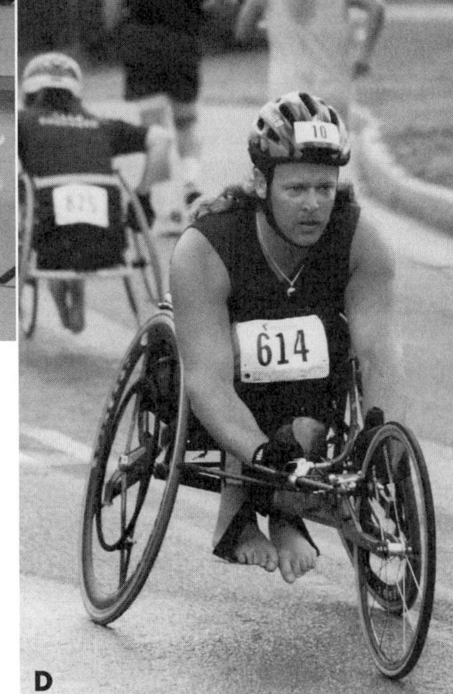

Figure 27-1 **A** to **D,** Clients with chronic illnesses and physical impairments can still participate in a wide range of recreational activities. (**A,** Reproduced with permission of Ginny Boydston, Jackson, MS. **D,** © Greg Campbell Photography, Jackson, MS.)

TABLE 27-6 Nursing Diagnosis/Nursing Outcome Classifications/Nursing Intervention Classifications for Recreation/Leisure Deficit

Nursing Diagnosis	Suggested Nursing Outcome Classifications (NOC)	Suggested Nursing Intervention Classifications (NIC)
Diversional activity deficit	Leisure participation Play participation Social involvement	Activity therapy Animal-assisted therapy Art therapy Milieu therapy Music therapy Mutual goal setting Reminiscence therapy Self-esteem enhancement Therapeutic play Visitation facilitation Energy management Environmental management Exercise promotion Pain management Pass facilitation Patient contracting Support group Surveillance: safety Teaching: individual

Data from Johnson, M., Maas, M.L., & Moorhead, S. (2000). *Nursing outcomes classification (NOC)* (2nd ed.). St. Louis: Mosby; McCloskey, J.C., & Bulechek, G.M. (2000). *Nursing interventions classification (NIC)* (3rd ed.). St. Louis: Mosby; and North American Nursing Diagnosis Association. (2001). *Nursing diagnosis: definitions and classification 2001-2002* (4th ed.). Philadelphia: Author.

classifications, and nursing intervention classifications are included in Table 27-6.

Assessment should include a review of the individual's likes and dislikes with respect to activities and leisure interests. An individual who routinely refuses to join the afternoon bingo game may simply not enjoy bingo. Not all individuals enjoy arts, crafts, or movies. In the rehabilitation setting, the more diverse the activities and leisure opportunities, the more likely that some activity will appeal to most individuals. Arts, crafts, and cooking are popular activities because they convey a sense of accomplishment, and many individuals find the activities relaxing with easy opportunities for socialization, fine motor exercise, and hobby development (Dixon, 2000).

In addition to assessing likes and dislikes, the nurse designing a therapeutic recreational program should assess energy and endurance levels. Individuals who are tired from a full day of therapy may not have an interest in an evening movie or game. Assessing the individual's exercise tolerance and the impact on cardiopulmonary function will be helpful. The therapeutic recreation program should be designed to accommodate changes in exercise tolerance, muscular fitness and range of motion limitations (Petajan & White, 2000).

SUMMARY

Sleep and recreation are activities essential for life satisfaction, yet both tend to be overlooked as "nonessential" or not critical to an individual's outcome. Rehabilitation nurses must recognize the key element that sleep and recreation play in recovery and rehabilitation from illness and disability. Through attention to sleep, individuals are able to make the gains necessary at the rate possible in therapy. Through attention to recreation and leisure activities, individuals may have the drive to regain function and to return to lives filled with adventure, excitement, and fun.

CRITICAL THINKING

Although, as nurses, we recognize the significance of sleep and recreation on the quality of life, we often fail to apply the principles to our own lifestyles. Identify some examples of how you can improve the quality of sleep and recreational activities with which you are involved.

REFERENCES

Akiyoshi, J. (1999). Neuropharmacological and genetic study of panic disorder. *Nihon Shinkei Seishin Yakurigaku Zasshi, 19,* 93-99.

Barefoot, J., Peterson, B., Harrell, F., Hlatky, M., Pryor, D., Haney, T., Blumenthal, J., Siegler, I., & Williams, R. (1989). Type A behavior and survival: A follow up study of 1,467 patients with coronary artery disease. *American Journal of Cardiology, 64,* 427-432.

Baron, A., Steinberg, H., Brechtel, G., & Johnson, A. (1994). Skeletal muscle blood flow independently modulates insulin-mediated glucose uptake. *American Journal of Physiology, 266,* (2 Pt 1), E248-253.

Beers, M.H., & Berkow, R. (Eds.). (1999). *The Merck manual of diagnosis and therapy* (17th ed.). Whitehouse Station, NJ: Merck Research Laboratories.

Blumenthal, J., Babyak, M., Moore, K., Craighead, E., Herman, S., Khatri, P., Waugh, R., Napolitano, M., Forman, L., Appelbaum, M., Doraiswamy, M.J., & Krishnan, R. (1999). Effects of exercise training on older patients with major depression. *Archives of Internal Medicine, 159,* 2349-2356.

Blumenthal, J.A., Jiang, W., Babyak, M.A., Krantz, D.S., Frid, D.J., Coleman, R.E., Waugh R., Hanson, M., Appelbaum, M., O'Connor, C., & Morris, J. (1997). Stress management and exercise training in cardiac patients with myocardial ischemia: Effects on prognosis and evaluation of mechanisms. *Archives of Internal Medicine, 157,* 2213-2223.

Brown, D. (1999). Managing sleep disorders. *Clinician Reviews, 9,* 51-54, 57-58, 60, 63-64, 69.

Brown, L. (1998). Sleep-related disorders and chronic obstructive pulmonary disease. *Respiratory Care Clinics of North America, 4,* 493-512.

Cauffield, J., & Forbes, H. (1999). Dietary supplements used in the treatment of depression, anxiety, and sleep disorders. *Primary Care Practice: A Peer-Reviewed Series, 3,* 290-304.

Chokroverty, S. (Ed.). (1995). *Sleep disorders medicine: Basic science, technical considerations, and clinical aspects.* Oxford, UK: Butterworth-Heinemann Medical.

Coyle, C., Kinney, W., Riley, B., & Shank, J. (Eds.). (1991). *Benefits of therapeutic recreation: A consensus view.* Ravensdale, Washington: Idyll Arbor.

Dixon, C. (2000). *Therapeutic recreation activities and treatment ideas: Arts and crafts* [On-line]. Available: http://www.recreationtherapy.com.

Hooper, P. (1999). Hot-tub therapy for type 2 diabetes mellitus. *New England Journal of Medicine, 341,* 924-925.

Jackson, W.J. (1999). Brain function: Sleep. In T. Nosek (Ed.), *Essentials of human physiology.* Atlanta: Gold Standard Multimedia Inc. and Medical College of Georgia.

Januzzi, J., Stern, T., Patsternak, R., & DeSanctis, R. (2000). The influence of anxiety and depression on outcomes of patients with coronary artery disease. *Archives of Internal Medicine, 160,* 1913-1921.

Jordan, J., Bernard, S., Callahan, L., Kincade, J., Konrad, T., & DeFriese, G. (2000). Self-reported arthritis-related disruptions in sleep and daily life and the use of medical, complementary, and self-care strategies for arthritis. *Archives of Family Medicine, 9,* 143-149.

Karason, K., Lindroos, A., Stenlöf, K., & Sjöström, L. (2000). Relief of cardiorespiratory symptoms and increased physical activity after surgically induced weight loss. *Archives of Internal Medicine, 160,* 1979-1802.

Lamberg, L. (1999). Patients in pain need round-the-clock care. *Journal of the American Medical Association, 281,* 689-690.

Larkins, R. (2000). A great life in medicine. *Lancet, 9206,* 852-856.

Lawlor, D., & Hanratty, B. (2000). Recreational physical activity and the risk of cholecystectomy in women. *New England Journal of Medicine, 342,* 212-214.

Leitzmann, M., Rimm, E., Willett, W., Spiegelman, D., Grodstein, F., Stampfer, M., Colditz, G., & Giovannucci, E. (1999). Recreational physical activity and the risk of cholecystectomy in women. *New England Journal of Medicine, 341,* 777-784.

Margolis, M. (2000). Brahms' lullaby revisited: Did the composer have obstructive sleep apnea? *Chest, 118,* 210-213.

Marrone, O., Bonsignore, M., Insalaco, G., & Bonsignore, G. (1998). What is the evidence that obstructive sleep apnoea is an important illness? *Monaldi Archives of Chest Disease, 53,* 630-639.

National Sleep Foundation. (1999a). *The National Sleep Foundation's 1999 Omnibus "Sleep in America Poll"* [On-line]. Available: http://www.sleepfoundation.org/publications/1999poll.html.

National Sleep Foundation (1999b). *ABC's of ZZZ's* [On-line]. Available: http://www.sleepfoundation.org/ publications/ZZZs.html.

Netzer, N. (1999). Self-administered survey helps identify patients with sleep apnea syndrome. *Annals of Internal Medicine, 131,* 485-491, 535-536.

Petajan, J., & White, A. (2000). Tailored physical activity programmes beneficial for patients with multiple sclerosis. *Drug and Therapeutic Perspectives, 15,* 7-9.

Pratt, M. (1999). Benefits of lifestyle activity vs structured exercise. *Journal of the American Medical Association, 281,* 375-376.

Rowland, T., Kline, G., Goff, D., Martel, L., & Ferrone, L. (1999). One-mile run performance and cardiovascular fitness in children. *Archives of Pediatrics and Adolescent Medicine, 153,* 845-849.

SleepQuest. (2000). *The Epworth Sleepiness scale* [On-line]. Available: http://sleepquest.com/s_sleepquestionnaire2.html.

Smith, T. (1996). Heart failure. In R. Cecil, F. Plum, & J. Bennett, J. (Eds.). *Cecil textbook of medicine* (20th ed., p. 217). Philadelphia: WB Saunders.

Stephenson, J. (1999). Tuneful tonic. *Journal of the American Medical Association, 281*(23), 2175.

Tyler, V.E. (1999). Herbs affecting the central nervous system. In J. Janick (Ed.), *Perspectives on new crops and new uses* (pp. 442-449). Alexandria, VA: ASHS Press.

Vega, K. (1999). Exercise and the gallbladder. *New England Journal of Medicine, 341,* 836-837.

Wannamethee, S., Shaper, A., Alberti, K. (2000). Physical activity, metabolic factors, and the incidence of coronary heart disease and type 2 diabetes. *Archives of Internal Medicine, 160,* 2108-2116.

Winslow, E. (1996). Testing nurses' skill in sleep assessment. *American Journal of Nursing, 96,* 51.

Wirz-Justice, A. (1999). Warm feet may encourage sleep. *Nature, 401,* 36-37.

28 Spirituality

Mary Ann Solimine, MLS, RN

She has chronic problems with arthritis and a heart condition. When asked to evaluate her health, she says, "Very good." How can she say this when she has arthritic pain, angina, shortness of breath, and other problems? "Well, that's my body," she answers, and smiles. "I just don't live there all the time. You can ask me questions about my thoughts and my soul—I spend time with the Lord, and that is more healing than anything else could ever be. This body is temporary, you know; it just depends on whether He wants me to hang around this planet for awhile, or not." Furthermore, she offers, "For there is hope of a tree if it be cut down, that it will sprout again, and that the tender shoot thereof will not cease" (Job 14:7). Now where and how does the rehabilitation nurse document this assessment data or evaluate outcome?

With knowledge of all that is natural in the biological, psychological, and sexual nature of humanity, rehabilitation nurses observe, assess, plan, and intervene to solve problems involving the "whole person." Long before the paradigm of holism officially reentered professional nursing, the tradition of a spiritual context extended beyond the biopsychosocial approach, adding dimension to nurses' personal lives and professional practice. "Seek and you shall find" (Matthew 7:7); coping with a spiritual crisis, recognizing and gauging the need for the spiritual aspects of daily care, as well as feeling comfortable with interventions of spiritual support, is not only ethical, but in keeping with rehabilitation principles (Davis, 1994).

Spiritual Distress *is a designated nursing diagnosis (Gordon, 2000),* Spiritual Well-Being *is a nursing outcome classification (NOC) (McCloskey & Bulechek, 2000), and* Spiritual Growth Facilitation and Spiritual Support *are nursing intervention classifications (NIC) (Johnson, Maas, & Moorhead, 2000). Many nurses remain uncertain of their spiritual role and give higher priority and prominence to the safer, physical aspects of care; more at home in a milieu of action and immediate realities, rather than reflection. They ask clients about religious preferences and practices that are substantive and deliverable, but often ignore important aspects of their spirituality. As an agreed on definition, "spiritual" eludes experts, they may have a valid point. Affecting their clients' lives longer than do nurses in acute care, and concerned with care and wholeness of being, rather than cure alone, rehabilitation nurses may make an enviable holistic contribution to clients' spiritual quality of life.*

CARING OVER TIME

The universal function of humanity even in prehistoric times was wellness as survival of the fittest, adapting and obtaining resources, and caring for the sick. In primitive societies, care for the sick was according to religious rituals and difficult to distinguish from medical or nursing measures. The Oracle at Delphi proclaimed a regimen of physical therapies, baths, and medications, and in the sixth century BC Aesculapius was the first to promote the idea of health other than in the absence of illness or in the context of scientific study. Men and women served the sick in the temples, acquiring basic nursing skills beyond fundamental family caregiving.

In diverse populations, traditional healers (Druids, spiritists, witches, shamans, and more) melded religion with magic, herbs, fertility, and healing. Throughout ancient and preindustrial cultures, people able to enter into visionary states, ranging from ecstatic trances to revelations, became sources of artistic inspiration, religious enthusiasm, predictions, and remarkable healing.

In Old Testament times, Jewish priests and others—such as physician and philosopher Moses Maimonides—were custodians of public health. He was convinced that a healthy soul required a healthy body that enabled one's moral and intellectual capabilities to develop toward greater knowledge of God and an ethical life. Healing was the art of repairing both the defects of the body and the turmoil of the mind (Feldman, 1986).

Later, the ideals of charity, piety, service, self-sacrifice and brotherhood, espoused by the early Christian church inspired workers to tend the ill and needy in everyday life. With few cures, healing consisted of rest and cleanliness, dressed wounds, herbal pain remedies empowered by clients' beliefs in the placebo effect, or "remembered wellness" (Benson, 1996, p. 109). The caregivers tried to reconcile the sick to the inevitabilities of fate in this world while preparing their souls for the next; comfort for a peaceful death much as in today's hospices. Religious orders provided nursing care; Knights Templar built hospitals along Crusade routes, the Alexian Brotherhood emerged when the Black Death struck Europe, and the Imams in Indian mosques were often physicians. Cloisters sheltered the disabled, a hospice housed the blind in ancient Turkey, and pious foundations proliferated to support health institutions throughout Islam as they assimilated Greek, Persian, and Indian medical traditions while providing a spiritual home (Rahman, 1989).

After the Protestant Reformation, hospitals in many parts of Europe drifted from their religious moorings and secular administrators began to work alongside motivated religious directors of daily operations (Marty & Vaux, 1982); some religious order hospitals remained. Individuals connected science to the spiritual, such as Puritan Cotton Mather (1663-1728), who championed inoculations against small pox and practiced spiritual and physical healing as an "angelical conjunction"; or Charles Boyle (Boyle's Law) (1627-1691), chemist and physicist, who wrote theological treatises.

Although Bacon, Copernicus, Galileo, Newton, and Descartes theorized science as separate from theology, not until the industrial and scientific revolutions would rationality become the watchword; this mechanistic paradigm was seized on as the total explanation, rather than a tool, for certain situations. It totally replaced spiritual and religious beliefs (Grof & Grof, 1989). Everything remotely connected to mysticism was relegated to disbelief and mistrust; nothing sacred stood. Modern medicine, neither art nor science, became the new religion. Rather than faith and trust, the new church had doctors as high priests performing their rituals, leading Dr. Benjamin Rush to state the physician's abilities were superior to the powers of nature in 1769 (Mendelsohn, 1979).

Florence Nightingale originated the scientific, professional perspective in nursing as a practical art. Her action philosophy aligned organized nursing with allopathic medicine as a way for women to engage in meaningful work. Yet, her spiritual beliefs were that all creativity, insight, and sense of purpose were evidences of divine intelligence and a potent resource for healing; that physical laws were evidence of the divine; that carrying out the natural laws and taking responsibility for them brought healing. She did not seek miracles, but thought prayer could bring a person in tune with universal law and the spiritual energy of the divine. While emphasizing her abilities as theorist, administrator, and statistician, she entrusted nurses to smooth away any hindrances that hindered the healing nature from within the client to operate (holism) (Macrae, 1995).

Social forms and values have changed with sanitation and new technologies as medicine became more mechanistic; that is, specialized, institutionalized, technical, and fragmented with bureaucracy. Religious beliefs, remembered wellness, and natural imbalance receded; unity, balance and harmony were abandoned. Man was a mere biopsychosocial animal; the spirit subsumed. Clients viewed nuclear medicine, genetic engineering, and organ replacement as rights. Specialists made critical decisions and clients and relinquished control in hope of "cure," but distrusted their own bodies. Nurses lost sight of their clients and, "as faith in scientific medicine grew, faith in a caring capacity . . . diminished" (Benson, 1996, p. 109). Technology was the new medical religion and nurses were out of the "spirit-game."

Weaknesses and limitations of the new biomedical paradigm began to manifest themselves in mainstream medicine: contradictory advice, errors, costs, dilemmas, and failures. Other observations, patterns, behaviors, and ethics refused to fit the scientific paradigm. Clients' power diminished under paternalism; they felt dehumanized and viewed medicine as less reliable. A spiritual crisis was in the air. The 1960s brought a wave of interest in spirituality and consciousness exploration and changes in attitudes and beliefs toward medicine. Postmodern thought fostered acceptance of diverse medical systems and client empowerment. More than 150 years later, medicine and nursing began the return to the mind/body/spirit perception of health and care. The new challenge is to establish evidence of its effectiveness, as discussed in Chapter 13.

PARADIGMS AND HOLISM

The holistic theory originated in physics (von Bertalanffy's general system theory) in 1937, with parallel developments in the biological, behavioral, and social sciences, opening a previously mechanistic world to sets of integrated systems. "The mechanistic world view, . . .which glorifies physical technology, has led eventually to the catastrophes of our times. Possibly, the model of the world as a great organization can help us to reinforce the sense of reverence for the living which we have almost lost in the last sanguinary decades of human history" (von Bertalanffy, 1955, p. 49). Then came the therapeutic revolution, the stage for new paradigms of "wholeness," healing, "holiness," and "holism" coined by Jan Smuts (1926, p. 98), a South African historian, explorer, and military leader. He declared holism to be the "source of all values; Love, Beauty, Goodness, Truth are all of the whole; they are the Holistic Ideals . . . which lay the foundations of a new order in the universe. . . . Conception of wholes covers a much wider field than that of biological life; it applies in a sense to human associations like the state, and to the creations of the human spirit" (Smuts, 1926, p. 144).

Laszlo (1972) identified humans as self-contained living systems, functioning in continual interaction with, acting on, and being acted on by their environments, challenging Descartes' notion of the body as "nothing but" a machine, isolated from the mind/soul. Pastoral counselor and psychotherapist Roberto Assagioli (1974) had clients repeat phrases, "I have a body, but I am more than my body; I have a mind, but I am more than my mind . . .; I have emotions, but . . .," and so forth. The holistic model encourages viewing a person as composed of multidimensional and interrelated parts that combine to create something larger than the parts suggest. It inspires looking at larger relationships, underlying connections and systems, and considering family, social, political, cultural, and spiritual implications when observing an individual.

What holism is *not:* It is not "New Age," not mechanistic reductionism, and does not equal alternative or complementary medicine. It does invite an open mind to unconventional approaches or treatments. It is not a collection of therapies, but an approach to and honor of clients (Robinson, 1999) that is not restricted to one health environment. Holistic medical science has providers understand the whole person in the context of their total environment and the impact of multiple sources of causality. The term "holotropic" emphasizes movement toward wholeness as the objective of therapeutic interventions (Vash, 1994).

However, nursing's assertions of holistic caring form a way to define the profession's "linked-yet-subordinate relationship to medicine, as much as they are a statement about clinical aims and bedside practices. Nursing is, by definition, not medicine" (Rosenberg, 1998, p. 345). Nurses can embrace conventional medicine while employing methods to enhance health, emphasize prevention, and encourage clients' participation in decision-making and self-care. They can assess, diagnose, and intervene to help the client create healing based on interaction with their environments and a higher being, realizing it is impossible to separate parts that are intimately interconnected (Figure 28-1).

The perception of the mind as a tool for healing brought imagery, biofeedback, and self-hypnosis. Nursing theorists advanced disparate views of holism and attempted to incorporate the concept of soul into theory. Longway's (1970) "Circuit of Wholeness" was the first theory based on spirituality, with God as a power source. Newman's (1986) theory viewed health as expanding consciousness, with humans' inner selves interacting with plants and animals, on to spiritual beings. Illness or injury is a shock; a client must organize for harmony. Watson (1988) focused on a mental-spiritual-nursing role, with the body as access; disease is, or gives, disharmony. Dossey, Keegan, Guzzetta, and Kolkmeier (1988) combined the doing therapies of conventional medicine with being therapies, using states of consciousness as techniques to affect the body.

In the American Holistic Nurses' Association's Standards of Holistic Nursing Practice, one of the core values is Holistic Communication. It serves "to ensure that each person experiences the presence of the nurse as authentic and sincere; there is an atmosphere of shared humanness that includes a sense of connectedness and attention reflecting the individual's uniqueness" (American Holistic Nurses Association, 1998, p. 1). Nurses carry technical knowledge into the holism paradigm. Although not all nurses practice holism in the spiritual context, nursing is holistic; and practice holds many interventions to accomplish holistic-spiritual care of self and clients.

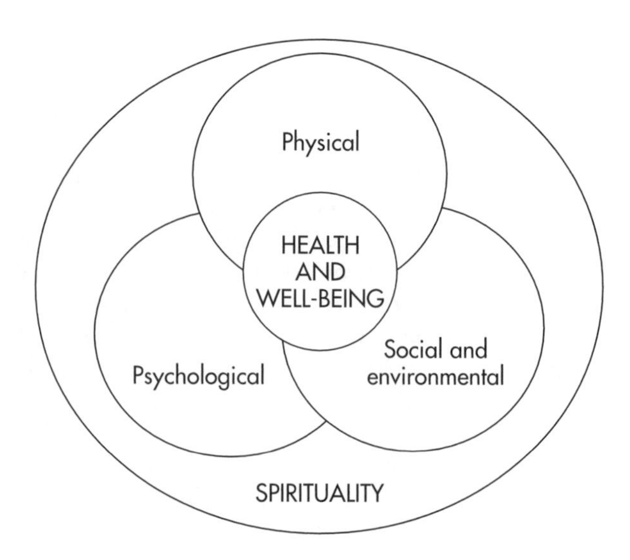

Figure 28-1 A model for incorporating spirituality into holistic biopsychosocial health.

RELATED CONCEPTS

Soul/Spirit/Spirituality

Often the soul is distinguished from the spirit. *Soul* is the depth and inner self-helper gazing at life's relationships, pleasure, pain, emotions, and sentiments, and enters inward. The sense of the soul is the power of life to worship God. "It immerses itself within the world through intimacy, relationships, pleasure and pain and aspires to attachment and engagement. It views human suffering and illness with reverence by honoring symptoms with its voice" (Karasu, 1999, p. 145).

Karasu separates the soul from the spirit; although used interchangeably and related, they differ. "The inner man, the place or voice of God within, a conscience; we are dealing with a symbol which we take to refer to that unknown human factor which makes meaning possible, turns events into experiences, is communicated in love, and has religious concern. It has the same ambiguity as have 'life,' 'health,' 'nature,' and 'energy'" (Hillman, 1972, p. 23). It is dependent on human relationships, yet clings to God. The three powers of the soul are memory, understanding, and will.

Soulfulness needs to be cultivated; the way to it requires love (Karasu, 1999).

Spirit is essence of being and is to the soul what blood is to the body (Karasu, 1999). Spirit breathes, pervading and integrating the system, is a repository of morality, energy, force, and life-giving power. The spirit synthesizes the total personality; it provides integration, energizing force, and balance and mediates between the heart and the mind. The spirit's power is available and experienced through others in times of joy, in crises, and suffering (Dreyer, 1994), but it needs to be fed as fear, anxiety, and pain hinder its expression. Finding faith and science in some degree of tension, the spirit seeks to repair the fracture between medicine and tradition, it wills to wellness (not health).

Spirituality or a *spiritual life* reflects the force of spirit giving wholeness of selves meaning and purpose, a unity of "innerness," "connectedness," or "interconnectedness." (Dreyer, 1994, p. 76). Communication with God through prayer, and the belief that prayer influences life, would be intrinsic spirituality; extrinsic spirituality addresses extraneous religious behavior, which may or may not be an expression of a client's interior spirituality. Basic to well-being, this internal guidance system influences life, behavior, and health, regardless of religion or philosophical beliefs or practices. A path of quiet contemplation to find the divine in the world and selves, harmony among mind, body, and soul—the spirit is the life of that interior self. A part of daily life, it embodies our thoughts and emotions and records them, from the mundane to the visionary; it is faith in everyday attitudes and behavior (Dreyer, 1994). Yet, according to Hardy, it is a biological phenomenon natural to the human species and has evolved because of biological survival value (Hardy, 1979). There is potential for exploitation and self-deception in spirituality.

The world of the spirit grows with human development as significant others and life events play major roles in spiritual growth. A vibrant spirituality is one that is in tune with, and therefore able to speak to, the culture in which it finds itself. One can look at spirituality from three perspectives: 1) falling in love with God; 2) a variety of religious expressions; and 3) scholarly reflection, analysis, interpretation, and organization. "The way to spirituality requires belief. . ." (Karasu, 1999, p. 145).

The greater the degree of spirituality, the more it influences life and health. The inherent vital force of spirit does not weaken of itself; a person's reflection of spirituality may be affected by physical, emotional, or personal environmental factors, obscuring spirituality. In a physical analogy, the body may suffer respiratory distress when a ventilatory problem causes misery and affects the mind, as with hypoxia. Multiple causes may contribute to impaired ventilation, including pneumonia, chronic obstructive pulmonary disease, asthma, emphysema, neoplasms, genetic predisposition, or occupational environment. The etiology of "dis-spiriting" is similarly multiple and diverse, but impaired spiritual needs are manifested through physical or psychosocial disquietude.

Nurses may assist clients to enact or persevere in an affirmative relationship with their higher power whether belief is in established religions, in their own power to succeed, in science, or in life itself. An individual's concept of "God" may be less sacred and more mundane; that which is valued—self, family, work, activity, or money among others. It is difficult to assist someone who is without inner resources (Vaillot, 1970).

The quality of spirituality is so elusive that without a universal definition it cannot be brought into research through the science-technology paradigm. "Theoretically, it is defined as the experiences and expressions of one's spirit in a unique and dynamic process reflecting faith in God (however defined by the person); connectedness with oneself, other, nature or God, and integration of the dimensions of mind, body and spirit" (Meraviglia, 1999, p. 19). Is it possible that practicing spirituality is akin to scientific thinking in that an enthusiastic seeker moves from intuition through a process of revision and comprehension of expanded discoveries.

In Longway's "Circuit of Wholeness," God is the power source. She postulated that a person is ill when he or she has nothing to give another, so he or she then has no power, and health problems become evident. The nurse's challenge is to define the agent responsible, be it physical, spiritual, social, or mental-emotional; serve in a giving and receiving relationship; and identify client's strengths and use them to enable him to give to others, thereby receiving energy for health (Longway, 1970). A client bound up in impaired mobility or loss of a limb has no available energy to give, but depression and despair are plentiful. When he or she receives care and identifies strengths, he or she can choose to move on and be a giving entity. Every attitude, every judgment is a source of positive or negative power for which we are accountable.

Spiritual Crisis

Being "holy" is no guarantee of good health—illness and injury do not imply spiritual shortcomings—and our physical bodies show imperfections through physical, emotional, and mental pain. Crisis or breakdowns occur when problems extend beyond a client's capacity. Rehabilitation nurses who understand and are receptive to spiritual concerns are comfortable knowing that clients and families need to make sense of their circumstances and to find meaning in daily events, relationships, and life. Mild concerns or anxiety, discouragement, or anticipatory grief can escalate to distress: crying, silence, expressions of guilt, sleep pattern disturbances, anger, and increasing anxiety. Without intervention, the situation may lead to despair and a client might exhibit psychotic behavior or depression, refuse to communicate or participate in therapy, and even state a death wish. Enhanced, inclusive spiritual support is a client's right; care that considers his or her personal dignity and respects his or her values as the client works toward spiritual well-being, is therapeutic (Sumner, 1998).

FACTORS INFLUENCING SPIRITUALITY

Religion and Health Care

Religion and spirituality are *not* the same. Religion, an organized social institution has doctrine, morality, and often a physical environment; beliefs are held in common. Worship through formal ritual and observances may be a framework to express spirituality, but not its core. Many in rehabilitation will seek some religious solace.

Religion can be extrinsic, used for security or status in the social structure or intrinsic wherein internalized beliefs empower a person to live accordingly regardless of social pressures. A spiritual person need not be religious, nor must a seemingly religious person be inwardly spiritual. Some rely on religion to lessen self-blame and improve psychological outcome (Dein, 1997). In contrast, clients may express anger with God because they believe impairment or disease is evidence of God's abandonment. However, nurses cannot rely solely on studies that find religion gives or fosters hope, meaning, optimism, security, peacefulness, or a sense of purpose. Religion, especially when coupled with guilt or anger can heighten self-doubt, guilt, depression, or codependency and lead to paranoia (Hill & Butter, 1995; Mayer, 1992). Certain sects and cults have exploited members for power or material gain.

Surveys and in-depth studies report greater impact and intensity of spiritual experience when a person is under stress related to illness or trauma. Whether consciously, or unconsciously, many only acknowledge their spiritual relationship with or dependency on God when faced with illness or incapacity. Gathering data about a client's religious affiliation is not sufficient to understand how beliefs, practices, and attitudes may influence responses to illness or disability, but it is a starting place. In the nursing literature many short guides or larger tables specifying cultural and specific religious beliefs are available; several sources are referenced at the end of this chapter as suggested resources.

Religion and Disability

Many clients with impairments receive no spiritual services or are unable to gain access to participate fully within their faith communities. Apart from religious organizations having inadequate knowledge concerning the disabled community, a gap remains between the ideals and practices. Religion might reclaim its prominent role in healing by halting even a trace of sanctions or negative perceptions concerning people with disabilities, and concentrating on their gifts to congregations and talents in leadership roles. The biblical Old Testament viewed illness and disability as punishment for transgression that could be continued throughout generations. Job eventually understood that God has a purpose for the whole person that overrules any misfortune, including disability. In the New Testament, Jesus rejected the punitive stance, but many Christians continue to hold that view. Islam maintains beliefs about Allah's will and punishment, whereas Hindus hold that one life is part of a journey of lives. Many other religions have their own world views.

Culture

Clients from differing cultures or religious preferences will have their own explanations for suffering, loss, or disability. They may require certain individuals to perform specific interventions and behaviors to alleviate pain and ward off suffering. People of many faiths consider suffering a product of wrongdoing or failure to perform some action. For others an event or person outside of their control caused their suffering. The extensive array of beliefs that individual clients may have about the universal experience cannot be listed, but a well thought out and careful assessment will help a nurse to determine the unique nature underlying a particular client's suffering.

Spiritual interventions will vary according to the culture of both client and nurse. Recognizing typical patterns of behavior without relying on stereotypes increases a nurse's cultural sensitivity and relevance. Clients may respond more openly to a nurse who offers opportunities for discussions about beliefs and practices and who asks perceptive questions indicating an awareness and respect for diversity. Local or traditional helpers who are involved in healing, spirituality, holistic health, or related activities may be available to provide practical information that would prevent unintended errors or forestall awkward situations arising from assumptions.

It is not difficult to find specific information about a culture or ethnic group, many nursing texts list tables of cultural or religious comparisons; however, resources and clients do not always agree. For instance, a source may state that African-Americans view health as harmony with nature and that they occasionally visit healers or that elderly Hispanics believe that illness is the result of imbalance, as punishment for wrongdoing, the "evil eye," or because of fright or envy. Do all Hispanics and Asians revere elders and expect and respect privacy? Do elderly people of all cultures value their faith and tend to feel fatalistic about the burdens God has given them to bear? Is it unlikely they will be convinced otherwise; what are their thoughts about the story of Job (Ebersole, 1997)?

However, nurses will agree that people do not adhere uniformly to the beliefs and practices of their culture or ethnic group; in fact, few practice all commonly known rituals, and most practice variations. Those who have become acculturated into Western medical practices may not employ any culturally specific practices apart from personal idiosyncrasies or choices. Education, economic status, length of time in the dominant culture, English language ability, and goals influence health behaviors and beliefs. Clearly, the cultural charts are useful as reminders and starting points, but not as protocols. Sensitive inquiry on the part of the nurse will provide enlightenment and clarification. Refer to Chapter 13 for more information about health systems and cultural influences.

Health Services and Parish Nursing

Religious communities and organizations can do more charitable work through changing attitudes, as well as by providing health-related services, operating church sponsored adult day-care centers and nursing homes, and providing community-based education and health-testing programs for elderly people who are disabled and disadvantaged (Hill & Butter, 1995). Clergy can encourage illness prevention by ministering to the "whole" person and by influencing the community—healing services, laying on of hands, home visitation, sharing needs with serious or chronic illness involves congregations, and encouraging personal roles.

Parish nursing is a concept of working with faith communities to deliver holistic health care nursing. More than 4,000 strong since the revival of congregation-based health ministry in the 1980s, parish nurses are most active where the church is a meeting place (Wishmant, 1999). Nurses may work with one or a group of parishes or may volunteer, collaborate with community nursing agencies, or share employment with a local hospital. In addition to preventive care, parish nurses use many rehabilitation principles in practice. Their functions are important in cultural groups, such as African-Americans, because they link health care with an institution, which is seen as a useful and agreeable idea (Barnum, 1996). Likewise, many Hispanics associate spirituality with healing through prayer and rituals. The parish nurse is in excellent position to work as a culture broker.

The Health Ministries Association developed standards for parish nursing as it evolves into an advanced practice professional role. The nurses serve by advocating, outreaching, teaching (clients and volunteers), listening, counseling, referring, and empathizing and praying; they can spearhead services, such as home visitation, respite programs, and peer counseling. Most community health services understand their differing roles. Parish nurses do not provide home health care services or perform invasive nursing procedures, but work collegiality with agencies; all their functions need not be spiritual work. In many situations they link the purpose of the church and nursing, rather than attempting to make nursing more of a spiritual base (Barnum, 1996). They collaborate with clergy to establish programs for health promotion, education about chronic health problems, and information about impairment and healing from a more spiritual viewpoint (Easton & Andrews, 2000). Those nurses decide for more spiritual roles may train in pastoral care.

Some rehabilitation facilities have initiated ecumenical prayer groups intending for clients who already share goals and therapies in rehabilitation, to foster self-esteem, mutual support, and prayer, and "deepen their hopes and make use of the present moment" (Durkin, 1992, p. 53). Groups may be regularly planned events or contacts with clergy and other religious leaders who will serve as professional resources after a client's discharge to the community. A pastoral care provider or a spiritual leader can lend insight to rehabilitation team members and help them form therapeutic liaisons for clients with the religious community. Some team members may volunteer at retreats or camps or train for specialization in spirituality therapy. However, at no time are professionals required to abdicate their own beliefs, make statements, or practice behaviors that are inconsistent with, or in opposition to, their faith or spiritual beliefs, nor are they allowed proselytizing.

Pain and Suffering

Pain is physical; suffering is mental; both are part of human life and caring. Pain signals that the body is in danger; suffering warns us that the entire structure of memories and habits that we consider a person is threatened (Vash, 1994). Suffering includes the way we experience pain and how we understand that experience to be affective in our lives (Lindholm & Eriksson, 1993).

Suffering is not a feeling or a pain. It is the state of severe distress associated with events that threaten the intactness of a person: the strain of trying to endure, the alienation of forced exclusion from everyday life, the shock of institutionalization, and the uncertainty of anticipating the ramifications of disability (Hinds, 1993). Spirituality encourages the reevaluation and reinterpretation of pain and suffering in the light of our relation to the beneficial force of God. Although suffering has no meaning, the client can give meaning to the experience.

Foley (1988) reviewed the various meanings for suffering found in our society, and categorized them into 11 "interpretations of suffering":

- Punishment (such as for sins)
- Testing (such as loyalty to God)
- Bad luck (negative odds)
- Submission to the laws of nature (nature taking its course)
- Resignation to the will of God (accepting what happened without knowing why)
- Acceptance of the human condition (including suffering and pain)
- Personal growth (becoming a better person as a result of suffering)
- Defensiveness and denial (not thinking about it)
- Minimalization (downplaying the severity or significance of suffering)
- Divine perspective (transcending personal perspective)
- Redemption (finding joy in suffering)

Physical pain often engenders spiritual pain as clients, families, and providers struggle to find meaning and hope in the suffering they experience and witness. Spirituality can be threatened, as well as strengthened, by pain. A Christian athlete, disabled in an accident, Tada (1999) views suffering as, ". . .nothing more than hell's splashover, warning us of coming judgment. The disabling condition can be an advantage to an individual's soul. God has a message for that person, and he is sitting right on it." Many Hindu believers envision pain as a divinely ordained punishment, or resulting from personal actions (Desai, 1989). In Islam, it can be punitive or fatalistically, Allah's will (Haddad & Hoeman, 2000). A popular Buddhist belief is that suffering is the cost of attachment. Pelka (1994) discussed purposes served by the attitude that disabilities are caused by sin, bad karma or negative emotions held by the media and even by religious healers. Chapter 12 discusses suffering and effective coping in detail.

Intuition and perception may alert a nurse that clients are suffering; understanding what pain means to clients gives insight into interventions. A client's most profound response to suffering is frequently a shift to, and an emphasis on, spirituality. The outcome is to create a healing environment for client and family to relieve suffering; avoiding ready answers, listening, and accepting. Through true compassion and love, clients, family, and nurses encounter the domain of spirituality; suffering and spirituality become the soul of clinical work with the family (Wright, 1997).

Viktor Frankl's concentration camp experiences led him to logotherapy, a model for overpowering suffering by finding meaning in it. His version of modern existentialism proposes:

- Life has meaning under all circumstances, even the most miserable
- Humans have a will to meaning, which is their main motivation for living
- Persons have freedom to find meaning in what they do, what they experience, or at least in the stand they take in the face of a situation of unchangeable suffering (Frankl, 1984).

The object and challenge of logotherapy is to weave the slender threads of a broken life into a firm pattern of meaning and responsibility. It focuses on the future.

Loss and Change

Any deficit or impairment is a loss that forces confrontation with limitations in life, recognition of events, and reevaluation of goals and hopes. Although everyone must let go of various things during life, each loss is a big step, and each person experiences the reality of loss uniquely. Losses of any kind may be easier to manage when the person:

- Takes time to say goodbye (to whatever has been lost and to how life was lived)
- Reaches out to others
- Accepts change
- Learns to trust in God
- Makes happiness a habit
- Lives a life well (Idowu, 1993).

To these add:

- Prays constantly.

Early on, clients must be allowed time to grieve throughout whatever stages for whatever they had, now lack, and what "might have been." Mourning affirms the life, but the pace and pathway differ for each one. Increased demanding and faultfinding, withdrawal, and low ability to control frustration may occur, perplexing both client and family with anger and revolt against religion or labile emotions.

It requires time for clients to become accustomed to their altered body image and to regain a sense of purpose, priorities, goals, moral choices, a philosophy of life, and spiritual orientation. Clients must learn to take self-responsibility without fostering self-blame. Whatever people value gives them meaning and purpose and inherently influences behavioral response and adjustment to the event, even a traumatic one. (The better terms for "find meaning" might be "make sense of" in the context of a life.) Gaynor (1995) writes that clients can turn an adversity or negativity into a capacity—fear into the capacity for experiencing faith and trust; anger into experiencing infinite forgiveness. An independent person, with a positive and stable sense of self, can come to accept personal limitations and hold onto the person he or she is. (But, beware the "too cheerful" client; at what energy cost is this denial maintained?) Acceptance can stimulate deeper religious conviction, but the too cheerful client may expend great in denial. Ideally, clients will be uplifted spiritually where they can regard whatever occurs, including their struggle against frustration, as opportunity for spiritual growth. "We all tend to look upward when the ground beneath our feet shifts out of control" (Myss, 1996, p. 48).

- Is the problem a lesson? What will it teach?
- Is it a divinely ordained detour? From what are you being saved?
- Is it an invitation to grow in a new direction? What direction would that be?

Spiritual maturity results in capacity to let go of a need to be perfect and think of the loss as a challenge to exceed previous goals, to choose better over bitter. Clients may resist rehabilitation or using a prosthesis or an assistive device, but a rehabilitation nurse who creates a safe atmosphere for emotional and spiritual expression enables the client to know it is acceptable to experience and communicate feelings. Time for reflection, meditation, and contemplation can be planned, as much a part of routine as food, drink, and human contact.

Loss begins internally and moves out until it affects relationships. After personal emotional shock, client concerns shift to the effects of the loss on others, their love and acceptance or understanding and comfort. Family roles, relationships, and coping are addressed in Chapter 12. Sharing a loss is the gentlest way of living it. Nurses may arrange opportunities for sharing among consenting people or groups who have similar impairments or special interests. For instance, in many rehabilitation facilities, self-help groups for people with amputations meet monthly and hold social events, invite professionals for education programs, and help conduct summer camps for adolescents and young children who have amputations. Although the physical aspects of disability are of concern, the spiritual and psychosocial aspects are more challenging for rehabilitation nurses. "God, why are people physically handicapped?" (Michaux, 1970, p. 61) may not have a ready answer. Clients who desire healing do not have to become "spiritual dropouts"; beyond scientific explanations, at the depth of all understanding there is God.

Chronicity

Chronic illness poses continuing unpredictable and multidimensional demands; social resources are shifting toward their care and management. As early as 1951, chronic illness was described as "all impairments or deviations from normal which have one or more of the following characteristics: permanence, residual disability, caused by nonreversible pathological alteration, require social training for rehabilitation, and may need supervision, observation, or care over time" (Young, 1993, p. 298). Chronic conditions last longer than 3 months and lead to "a health condition that results in permanent and usually progressive limitations of activity, frequently precipitating undesirable changes in the level of independence and lifestyle" (p. 298). The Chronic Illness Trajectory (Corbin & Strauss, 1988) is explained further in Chapter 2 and contains concepts that are foundational to this book.

Corbin & Strauss (1988) classified the seven salient features of chronic illness as

- Long-term nature
- Uncertainty of prognosis and that caused by episodic nature
- Requires great efforts for palliation
- Requires a variety of ancillary services
- Overwhelming financial burden
- Intrusive

Goal of which is to maintain a stable phase of the trajectory. Trajectory framework is based on the notion that chronic illnesses vary over time, and have a course that may be shaped or managed, extended, or stabilized.

INDIVIDUAL EXPERIENCE AND SPIRITUALITY

The rehabilitation nurse in the community finds clients with chronic conditions at any stage of the trajectory as they attempt to cope with a multitude of impairments and adjust to altered situations. Individuals experience serious chronic illness in three ways. As an interruption of life, they look for recovery. As an intrusive illness, they seek to accommodate as the effects continue. And when immersed in illness or disability, these occupy the foreground, ever present and ever vexing. Receiving a diagnosis is both good and bad news: good in that it ends the question "What is this?" and bad in that it opens the door of uncertainty to "What now?" Loss, or fear of loss, invades the world soon after a person learns of a chronic illness and loss becomes part of the lived experience of being in that world (Schaefer, 1995).

How a loss is experienced depends on the client's definition of the illness experience because its meaning derives from the client's bodily feelings, thought, and sentiments (Charmaz, 1991). His or her illness or pain permeates his or her mind, body and spirit, as well as relationships, roles, and lifestyle (Narayanasamy, 1996). When asked if he ever felt sorry for himself, acute lateral sclerosis (ALS) sufferer Morrie Schwartz answered: "Sometimes in the mornings. That's when I mourn. I feel around my body. I move my fingers and my hands—whatever I can still move—and I mourn what I've lost. I mourn the slow, insidious way in which I'm dying. But then I stop mourning. I give myself a good cry if I need it. But then I concentrate on all the good things in my life . . . I don't allow myself any more self-pity than that. A little each morning, a few tears, and that's all. It's only horrible if you see it that way. It's horrible to watch the body wilt, but wonderful because there is time to say good-by. Not everyone is so lucky" (Albom, 1997, p. 49).

The client must honor every ability or capacity as it remains present. "To meet one day with defeat, the next with hope, the great adversity of chronic illness, with its many losses and threats, surely is a moral lesson that can keep most of us from despair" (Kleinman, 1988, p. 145). If the body is playing out the symphony of life, it now "includes a long movement of pure chaos, somber and discordant, but one that would lead somewhere worth going if I learned to listen" (Doyle, 1994, p. 32).

Many problems, as previously discussed, fit the holistic picture of the client with chronic illness. The crisis of loss with chronicity requires letting go in a myriad of small stages spread out over time, often being healthy between times. This "health in illness" is understood as coping in the best way with inevitable changes; the honest assessment of the situation; the marshaling and use of resources to make experiences not overwhelming. It consists of willful courage—functioning in spite of fear. The themes of such health participation are honoring the self, seeking and connecting with others, creating opportunities, celebrating life, transcending the self, and acquiring the "state of grace" that is wholeness and connectedness (Lindsey, 1996).

Transcendence is a fragile state; a self is more than its body and much more than an illness or disability; it is self-acceptance. Spiritual courage can grow through the client's willingness to keep remembering the moments of grace, when he or she experiences love, gratitude, awe, joy, security, and compassion, with no fear, and to keep on searching for the sacred behind all the mundane and terrible facets of life (Borysenko, 1987). Support groups, family, and friendship networks are of prime importance to someone with chronic illness (Hale, 1996).

REHABILITATION NURSING ROLES

The role for nurses with clients who are chronically ill are comforter, counselor, and challenger; necessary skills include self-awareness and the ability to communicate, build trust, and encourage hope (Narayanasamy, 1996). A client whose condition is potentially threatening or terminal may need time to express his or her rage, terror, depression, and sadness before he or she is receptive to prayer or a relevant spiritual message.

Importantly, spiritual well-being has been associated with improved quality of life for people who have sustained illness or injury. Those who experience changes in body image may benefit when they are able to focus on values of spiritual growth apart from their outward appearance. A client who centered personal worth on physical appearance or abilities may be at risk for psychosocial breakdown when body image is altered. Former levels of self-confidence, self-esteem, assertiveness, trust, and hope, as well as interpersonal relationships, often are threatened or destroyed. Clients want a sense of being in control after the invasive procedures associated with many medical treatments, leaving feelings of powerlessness. Nurses can target interventions that improve a client's comfort, strength, well-being, and attitude by establishing a spiritual presence.

The team is challenged to assist the client to find a meaning and purpose according to the person's belief system. Many people believe that God will impart direction amidst crisis and within the limitations imposed by the client's condition. Some clients may desire a traditional healer or spiritual leader to intervene against the perceived causes or may seek to "make right" or "undo" events that they believe led to the present situation. Others may wear a talisman or keep objects of spiritual importance to them, abstain from certain foods or activities, or any number of rituals that have meaning to the person.

Rehabilitation nurses help clients set goals that are mutually agreed on, feasible, attainable, realistic, and appropriate. A client who has a chronic illness or disability tends to set goals that are general rather than specific, open-ended rather than finite, and focused on adapting to altered functional status, reflecting expectations and avoiding disappointment. Promoting optimism, this type of goal setting helps integrate hope into the client's existence, kept alive by hope in God. Librarians in university and medical libraries can help providers identify and locate information about organizations, education programs, support groups, and treatments relevant to any particular illness or disability. Researchers suggest that future studies will reveal more about possible relationships among spirituality, quality of life, health, and life satisfaction for populations served by rehabilitation nurses. Also open to study is whether correlations exist among diagnoses, treatment interventions, and type of spiritual well-being (Riley et al., 1998).

In a study of clients with ALS who showed strengths and positive aspects in the face of the crippling neurological malady, Young & McNicoll (1998) discussed adaptive strategies of wisdom, human relationships, and leisure activities. Clients saw intellectual stimulation and relationships as extremely important. They would silence their sadness and despair in the interest of maintaining friendships, such as with pastors and church members. They all believed that something positive resulted from their experiencing ALS; and that taking life 1 day at a time was a strategy for managing the progressive disease. Challenges were often reframed as adventures, and all 13 clients in the study described finding new meaning to their lives.

A severe disability or terminal chronic illness initially brings disorientation and depression. over the long term a crisis ultimately affects the world view, and the client may cry "Enough!" Wanting to maintain control, yet unable to carry out the act of putting himself to death, either type of client may cry for help for the soul to overcome the bondage of the body. The battle rages on, in and out of our courts, over the benefits and dangers of allowing physician-assisted suicide. Many books (Maxson, 1987; Thobaben, 1996) and articles (Miller, 1993) often written by people with impairments, have been published on the subject, as have statements made by leaders and organizations in health care and various faith and interfaith communities.

The National Council on Disability (1997) published a lengthy position paper opposing the legalization of assisted suicide. The American Nurses Association's (ANA) position is that a nurse must uphold the ethical mandate of the profession and not participate in assisted suicide, defining it as "making a means of suicide (e.g., providing pills or a weapon) available to a client with knowledge of a client's intention. Assisted suicide is distinguished from active euthanasia; in assisted suicide, someone makes the means of death available, but does not act as the direct agent of death . . . The nurse's caring approach assists patients and families in finding meaning and purpose in their living and dying and furthers the attainment of a meaningful death" (American Nurses Association, 1985). Refer to Chapter 4 for more discussion regarding ethical issues.

FAITH STAGES

Children in rehabilitation may be slow to enter into a relationship with nurses who are responsible for painful procedures and the invasion of their privacy; however, they do value the times when a nurse is willing to listen when they question pain and suffering. A nurse's central task is not to talk to children, but to have children talk to them; nurses should feel free to express anger and bewilderment over what they may consider injustice, punishment, or betrayal. When a child expresses an intimate concern, a nurse can convey authentic hope, beginning with a willingness to share their concerns. Talking baby talk, smothering, offering platitudes, or threatening divine retribution do little to increase trust and rapport with a child. Although it is difficult to confess a lack of understanding about why and to whom accidents and illness happen, nurses should understand that children recognize honesty.

Children have a fine-tuned relationship with God; a trusted nurse can reassure them that He looks beyond their imperfections and sees them as special, not punishing them with disability. With this knowledge they can gain strength to survive, come to terms with their condition, or move forward with the power of prayer and relationships. A visit from the family's spiritual leader or hospital chaplain early in the hospital stay can be particularly beneficial to open the door of communication and lay groundwork for future support.

A six-item self-report index, the Children's Hope Scale, is used with children 8 to 16 years of age (Snyder et al., 1997) to identify support for less hopeful children. Taking each day as it comes within their stage of faith development, children are able to respond to parables, shared stories, and experiences of others that affirm their perceptions and offer hope. They are in close touch with their spirits through vivid imaginations, making relaxation, imaging, and centering techniques possible, as do imagination games in support groups (Hendricks & Wills, 1975). Telling their own life stories, stories about who they are and whose they are, hold importance for children (Webb-Mitchell, 1993). Spiritual-based stories on tape followed with instructions on how to "create your own TV show in your head about the story" help reinforce the message, especially when centered on the child's abilities. Therapeutic play with puppets, equipment models, storytelling, and drawing materials allow children to work through feelings and gain a different perspective on the situation. Parents are involved in these sessions and given prayer homework as part of their inclusion.

Children need a nurse who will honor their truth and understanding of life. Faith rituals such as bedtime prayers appropriate to their heritage and beliefs can be important and comforting at all ages. Preschoolers enjoy picture books or puzzles with Bible characters or other religious people, small items, and religious objects. Some cultures do not use objects, pictures, or other materials, so be clear before introducing this type of content. Different religions and belief systems will have their own ways of making contact with key people, relating the stories and performing the ceremonies important to their children and families. Rituals can be ways of letting children know that they have a remembered place in their families and that their God will always be with them (Sommer, 1989). New ceremonies can be created with the families; ideally, a quiet, private area is provided to meet clients' religious needs.

Hopefulness contributes to the psychosocial development of adolescents. They are inclined to look to God as they move toward independence from authority, questioning family values and ideals. Given to emotion and introspection, they need support while sorting out conflicts; peer influence is valued highly and may create conflict with values gained during formative years. Adolescents may reject formal worship services, then worship in the privacy of their rooms or reveal deep spiritual concerns and then get silly and deny the feelings. A spiritual and religious concerns questionnaire for hospitalized adolescents, ages 11 to 19 years, showed that spirituality and religious experiences become more important in direct relationship to the severity of the adolescent's condition, a finding usually attributed to the elderly (Silber & Reilly, 1985).

For various reasons, sects and evangelical types of worship are attractive to older adolescents; possibly they serve as rites of passage to enter adulthood. Adolescents are searching for values and may welcome discussion about interventions such as meditation, visualization, and relaxation. Nurses must anticipate clients will have spiritual or religious questions and be prepared for responses and appropriate referrals. To discern what any child's questions really mean, the nurse must listen to the child within.

NURSING PROCESS

"Many writers assume that spiritual needs can be assessed by the same methods as other human needs, and the literature attests to the attempts made to develop measurement tools that could be incorporated into a care plan. . . . It is pertinent to keep questioning the assumption that spirituality can be classified and controlled, quantified and written up in nursing notes, and processed in such a way that questions about ultimate values and intimate areas of relationship can be asked, answered, and recorded in the same way as questions about fluid balance, bowel function and body chemistry. And if is deemed possible, then further questions need to be asked about whether it should be. . . . But the determination to formulate care plans and schemes of intervention to achieve meaning for patients may reflect the nurse's need for order and meaning rather than the patient's" (Mayer, 1992, p. 51).

Taking Mayer's beliefs into account, the rehabilitation nurse builds clients' spiritual resources, needs, or distress into an individualized care plan. Observations, such as religious books or objects, facial expressions and gestures, or references to God or religion must be validated to eliminate false assumptions. Religious items or practices from some cultures may not be recognized, especially when a client and nurse have different cultures or heritage.

Spiritual Assessment

The ANA Code of Ethics specifies, "The nurse, in providing care, promotes an environment in which the values, customs, and beliefs of individuals are respected" (American Nurses Association, 1985). The International Code of Nursing Ethics makes the same statement, with specific reference to "religious beliefs" (International Council of Nurses,

2000, p. 3). Helping clients maintain their individuality without conflicting with the dominant culture demonstrates personal respect and conforms to Joint Commission on Accreditation of Healthcare Organizations standards. Interpreting the meaning of spirituality from the client's perspective and keeping aware that spirituality is a global concept may create responses more therapeutic to clients' immediate needs and certainly is in line with professional standards (Sumner, 1998). Whether formal or ongoing, assessment elicits information about how clients' spiritual beliefs affect their needs.

The initial spiritual assessment is conducted toward the end of admission history, when there has been opportunity to assess psychosocial background and gain trust and rapport with the client. Clients need reassurance that someone will attend to basic religious needs, such as dietary requirements, receiving sacraments, access to water for washing, or the means to perform other rituals (Mayer, 1992). A number of multidimensional tools measure religious parameters based on clients' responses in an attempt to identify and define true needs over vague or elusive concepts. However, the data alone do not offer insight into spiritual recesses. Clients may not discuss their spiritual coping strategies in rehabilitation because the kind of information collected for planning care was limited to religious data.

When a nurse remains open and respectful of privacy, a client may be relieved to share spirituality; conversely, a client may express offense, feel threatened, or appear to be puzzled by spiritual assessment. The nurse explains the holistic approach of understanding individual sources of strength. A client may not associate the need to belong or have meaning in life as spiritual. The ways a client responds and content of responses, not the degree or absence of expressed concern, form the assessment. A client has a right to object and not to answer questions about beliefs and religious preferences. Others may manifest spiritual needs, recall spiritual events, spontaneously acknowledge problems, and confide in the nurse. Spiritual needs may be expressed subjectively in conversation during daily care, giving opportunity to interject questions about a client's spiritual integrity and intervene to strengthen the responses to disability or participate in therapy.

Rehabilitation nurses may advocate for incorporating a spiritual component into the history. Assessment questions must be validated as relevant, sensitive, and reflective of the fundamental values of respect, understanding, caring, and fairness—both for client and interviewer. Offer a continuing education program before instituting any change, and conduct a broader assessment to determine the various patterns of culture and beliefs held by clients in the community. This will help nurses anticipate client needs and learn specific information about common beliefs and practices. Stoll's (1995) spiritual history guide can be incorporated into any general nursing history. Based on four areas of concern, the questions in Box 28-1 may be arranged in any order to elicit data about spirituality from client.

Box 28-1 Spiritual History Guide

Sources of Hope and Strength (Support System)

Who is the most important person to you?
To whom do you turn when you need help? Are they available?
In what ways do they help?
What is your source of strength and hope?
What helps you most when you feel afraid or need special help?

Concept of God/Deity

Is religion or God significant to you? If yes, can you describe how?
Is prayer helpful to you? What happens when you pray?
Does God/deity function in your personal life? If yes, can you describe how?
How would you describe your God or what you worship? (Draper, 1965)

Relation Between Spiritual Beliefs and Health

What has bothered you most about being sick (or in what is happening to you)?
What do you think is going to happen to you?
Has being sick (or what has happened to you) made any difference in your feelings about God or the practice of your faith?
Is there anything that is especially frightening or meaningful to you now?

Religious Practices

Do you feel your faith (or religion) is helpful to you? If yes, would you tell me how?
Are there any religious practices that are important to you?
Has being sick made any difference in your practice of praying? Your religious practices?
What religious books or symbols are helpful to you?
To this might be added:
Is there anything I can do to help you in your practice of faith?

Additional Modes of Spiritual Assessment

The Spiritual Well-Being Scale (SWBS) is a 20-item Likert scale that measures the individual's relationship with God and his or her satisfaction with life (Ellison, 1982). Forbes (1994) developed a 10-question structured interview as a companion to the SWBS. Although in use for many years, the SWBS has been criticized for its limitations: it may not address several key components of spirituality, has a potentially narrow focus within the Judeo-Christian religious perspective, and focuses on assessing spiritual beliefs rather than actions.

Other scales are the Religious Orientation Scale; the Index of Religiousness, which is a three-item measure asking about the frequency of attendance at services, perceived religiousness, and the degree to which religion is a comfort (Passman, 1990); and the Royal Free Interview for Religion

Spiritual Involvement and Beliefs Scale

How strongly do you agree with the following statements? Please circle your response.

	Strongly agree	Agree	Mildly agree	Neutral	Mildly disagree	Disagree	Strongly disagree
1. I set aside time for meditation and/or self-reflection.	7	6	5	4	3	2	1
2. I can find meaning in times of hardship.	7	6	5	4	3	2	1
3. A person can be fulfilled without pursuing an active spiritual life.	7	6	5	4	3	2	1
4. I find serenity by accepting things as they are.	7	6	5	4	3	2	1
5. Some experiences can be understood only through one's spiritual beliefs.	7	6	5	4	3	2	1
6. I do not believe in an afterlife.	7	6	5	4	3	2	1
7. A spiritual force influences the events in my life.	7	6	5	4	3	2	1
8. I have a relationship with someone I can turn to for spiritual guidance.	7	6	5	4	3	2	1
9. Prayer does not really change what happens.	7	6	5	4	3	2	1
10. Participating in spiritual activities helps me forgive other people.	7	6	5	4	3	2	1
11. I find inner peace when I am in harmony with nature.	7	6	5	4	3	2	1
12. Everything happens for a greater purpose.	7	6	5	4	3	2	1
13. I use contemplation to get in touch with my true self.	7	6	5	4	3	2	1
14. My spiritual life fulfills me in ways that material possessions do not.	7	6	5	4	3	2	1

Figure 28-2 Spiritual involvement and beliefs scale. (From Hatch, R.L., Burg, M.A., Naberhaus, D.S., & Hellmich, L.K. [1998]. The spiritual involvement and beliefs scale: Development and testing of a new instrument. *Journal of Family Practice, 46,* 485–486.) *Continued*

and Spiritual Beliefs. Most scales are generally based on North American Christian precepts.

The Spiritual Involvement and Beliefs Scale (SIBS) (Hatch, 1998) offers a broader scope than SWBS, uses terms that avoid cultural bias, and assesses both beliefs and actions. The SIBS was modified after publication, administered to 154 people of widely varied spiritual backgrounds, and revised. Feedback on the modified version (Figure 28-2) will be solicited when the scale is next administered (Hatch, 1998). The Jarel Spiritual Well-Being Scale is a brief, reliable, and valid scale to assess spiritual well-being in older adults (Hungleman, Kendel-Rossi, Klassen, & Stollenwerk, 1989), and the Correlates of Spiritual Well-Being Scale measures spiritual well-being, loneliness, health hardiness, social support, functional status and pain (Pace & Stables, 1997). The Index of Core Spiritual Experience is a sample of an instrument that measures intrinsic spirituality (McBride, Arthur, Brooks, & Pilkington, 1998).

Oncology nursing often generates spiritual needs assessment tools; Taylor, Amenta, and Highfield (1995) developed

	Strongly agree	Agree	Mildly agree	Neutral	Mildly disagree	Disagree	Strongly disagree
15. I rarely feel connected to something greater than myself.	7	6	5	4	3	2	1
16. In times of despair, I can find little reason to hope.	7	6	5	4	3	2	1
17. When I am sick, I would like others to pray for me.	7	6	5	4	3	2	1
18. I have a personal relationship with a power greater than myself.	7	6	5	4	3	2	1
19. I have had a spiritual experience that greatly changed my life.	7	6	5	4	3	2	1
20. When I help others, I expect nothing in return.	7	6	5	4	3	2	1
21. I don't take time to appreciate nature.	7	6	5	4	3	2	1
22. I depend on a higher power.	7	6	5	4	3	2	1
23. I have joy in my life because of my spirituality.	7	6	5	4	3	2	1
24. My relationship with a higher power helps me love others more completely.	7	6	5	4	3	2	1
25. Spiritual writings enrich my life.	7	6	5	4	3	2	1
26. I have experienced healing after prayer.	7	6	5	4	3	2	1
27. My spiritual understanding continues to grow.	7	6	5	4	3	2	1
28. I am right more often than most people.	7	6	5	4	3	2	1
29. Many spiritual approaches have little value.	7	6	5	4	3	2	1

Figure 28-2, cont'd For legend see previous page.

spiritual assessment questions for clients with cancer pain, which could be adapted for a person with chronic pain. Highfield and Cason (1983) give descriptors of four spiritual needs that are comparable to the nursing diagnosis of Spiritual Distress and four signs of spiritual "more-being," or achievement." Adapted for rehabilitation, the information in the tables could serve as an assessment checklist.

Nursing Diagnosis and Interventions

Whatever form assessments take, spirituality fits within the value-belief pattern (Gordon, 2000). The value-belief pattern is used to identify clients' actual or at-risk health problems or wellness regarding their spiritual well-being (Gordon, 2000; Kim, McFarland, & McLane, 1997). Clients may have clinical manifestations of discouragement, alienation, resentment, or become unable to conduct their usual religious practices. These, and related diagnoses of fear or anxiety, anger, grief, hopelessness, powerlessness, or ineffective coping may be the first clues to an overall spiritual deficit. With the advent of the NIC (McCloskey & Bulechek, 2000), the choices of interventions, once targeted become broader and easier to implement.

Nurses are challenged to manage religious needs of clients to the best of their ability, either directly or through referral. Also they contribute to client's mentally restorative experiences, including environmental control, using interventions from spirituality. The next section details a number

	Strongly agree	Agree	Mildly agree	Neutral	Mildly disagree	Disagree	Strongly disagree
30. Spiritual health contributes to physical health.	7	6	5	4	3	2	1
31. I regularly interact with others for spiritual purposes.	7	6	5	4	3	2	1
32. I focus on what needs to be changed in me, not on what needs to be changed in others.	7	6	5	4	3	2	1
33. In difficult times I am still grateful.	7	6	5	4	3	2	1
34. I have been through a time of great suffering that led to spiritual growth.	7	6	5	4	3	2	1

Please indicate how often you do the following:

	Always	Almost always	Usually	Some-times	Not usually	Almost never	Never
35. When I wrong someone, I make an effort to apologize.	7	6	5	4	3	2	1
36. I accept others as they are.	7	6	5	4	3	2	1
37. I solve my problems without using spiritual resources.	7	6	5	4	3	2	1
38. I examine my actions to see if they reflect my values.	7	6	5	4	3	2	1

39. How spiritual a person do you consider yourself? (With "7" being the most spiritual.)

1 2 3 4 5 6 7

Scoring instructions:
Reverse score all **negatively** worded items (3, 6, 9, 15, 16, 21, 28, 29, 37) (i.e., Strongly Agree, 1; Agree, 2; ..... Strongly Disagree, 7; or Always, 1; Almost Always, 2; ..... Never, 7). For all other items, the score is the number circled by the subject.

Figure 28-2, cont'd For legend see p. 655.

of spiritual health interventions recognized for nursing practice.

Spiritual Listening through Presencing or Centering

"I was afraid and the procedure was going to be quite uncomfortable. The nurse leaned over to help me into position, but also gave me an extended hug; I couldn't see her after that, but I could feel her hand on my shoulder and I knew she was there with me. It still was painful, but I knew wasn't alone amidst all the medical technology; I am not sure I learned her name, but I knew her presence" (S.P. Hoeman, personal communication, December 5, 2000).

In an age where communication tends to be swift, short, and superficial, many clients acknowledge that "presencing" or "accompanying" has proven important. They simply want someone to be present to listen, acknowledge, touch, empathize, show concern, quietly reassure, patiently explain, allow their crying or crying out, or exercise nonjudgmental understanding (Ellis, 1980). Rehabilitation nurses will recall times of "being there" at the invitation of the client to listen with respect and support, and being emotionally, spiritually, and intellectually present in the moment with a client. The voice of the spirit heard in this silence is intuition; listening develops wisdom, and the nurse is able to honor the spirituality of others through intuition (Keating, 1996).

Presencing is a sense of meaningful self-giving when the

client needs it most. Offered and never forced, it is revealed in a glance and through a touch or tone of voice. It implies closeness, openness, receptivity, readiness and availability, willingness to hear, and involvement; it is "skilled companionship." There is healing and being healed without "saying or doing the right thing." Risks are exposure to feelings of awkwardness and discomfort, possibly to fear and pain, and vulnerability in safe silence. A nurse can practice spiritual listening to establish a caring rapport and sense of being with a client. Avoid lectures or advice and appeals to religious dogma; encourage clients to examine their ethical or spiritual conflicts and support their beliefs about ways to live and resolve conflicts.

In Western culture, people have an impulse to fill silence with speech that intensifies when nervous or tense. Holding still the impulse to speak may allow a person to experience a subtle quieting of the mind and a magnified awareness of inner wisdom, a centering.

Centering requires excluding extraneous, distracting thoughts and feelings and focusing on the client, without intrusion of conflicts or personal concerns. Once established in a relationship, presencing does not require time; it is known by real attentive being there as well as physical presence. The spiritual nature of presencing is "kything," the nonverbal communication that brings about a loving spirit-to-spirit connection, union, or communion between two or more people or living things; the remembered face that continues to inspirit long afterward (Pettigrew, 1990).

The Relaxation Response

Training to achieve the relaxation response that decreases anxiety and fatigue helps clients dissociate from pain and gain periods of rest. The response may be accomplished through autogenic training (self-hypnosis), deep-breathing exercises, progressive muscle relaxation, prayer repetition, or other techniques such as the relaxation exercises in Box 28-2. A client may be individually guided in relaxation by a nurse or be provided with earphones and specific relaxation audiotapes. Biofeedback may serve as a complementary intervention when weaning a client from a ventilator.

Meditation

Meditation is an age old means of achieving relaxation and is used in many cultures. Rather than searching for quiet, meditation is finding the quiet within. It is listening long and deeply with calmness and deep concentration for the subtleties and sensibilities of the spirit that evoke intuition, nurturing one's spiritual voice with open-mindedness and without judgment. Meditation techniques include yoga, Zen, transcendental meditation, and hypnosis. Classically, meditation was conducted in a comfortable position within a quiet environment (the spirit loves silence), with some object, mantra, or thought to dwell on in a passive attitude. More recent introductions are walking, running, dancing, and laughing meditations. Those who practice regular meditation twice a day have shown themselves to be in better health, have sharper minds, and live longer than their contemporaries (Di Meo, 1991).

Eastern religions, Judeo-Christian literature, and Native American religions, among others, describe and advocate meditation. Thoughts and words chosen from one's religion or belief system are repeated and meditated upon. Although some meditation prescriptions suggest "emptying the mind," others suggest a person may prepare specific acts or petitions, consider basic truths, or come to conclusions; some may be resolutions for change, such for service to God.

Box 28-2 Relaxation Exercises

Exercise 1

Slow, rhythmic breathing for relaxation requires a comfortable position and the ability to put aside distractions. Instruct clients to breathe in and out slowly and deeply. Guide them to concentrate on releasing tension, relaxing, and breathing regularly; try abdominal breathing. On inspiration they silently count 1-2-3 and, maintaining a slow rhythm, count 1-2-3 while exhaling, or they concentrate on a word or thought. Perform relaxed breathing for 5 to 10 minutes initially, working up to 15 to 20 minutes. Clients end the exercise with a slow, deep breath, saying, "I feel alert and relaxed."

Exercise 2

The examples of simple touch, massage, or warmth for relaxation can be integrated with other nursing interventions and activities of daily living. Touch is useful contact for infants and older persons. Massage can be whole body or a 3- to 10-minute massage of the back, hands, and feet. Use a warm lubricant, and as clients prefer and are permitted, vary massage techniques or add aromatics. Place the person in an appropriate position and use rhythmic stokes (60/minute) with continuous hand contact during a back rub. Begin at the crown of the head and move to the lower back, avoiding the spine.

Exercise 3

Drawing on memories of peaceful past experiences helps some persons to gain present calm and comfort. However, avoid this technique for persons who may draw on sad or uncomfortable memories. Clients may recall special times with family or events or religious experiences and try to regain those happy feelings. Music, poetry, daydreams, photographs, or memorabilia may help clients recall. Clients may choose to write or tape record their memories and review them later.

Exercise 4

For clients who are able, active listening to recorded books, old radio or comedy programs, music, or religious messages is a popular and inexpensive form of relaxation. Materials are available from a variety of public and private sources. A comfortable position, appropriate volume, and pleasurable content aid relaxation. Clients may choose their level of participation, such as keeping time with a musical selection or focusing steadily, to bypass discomfort.

At any time in the exercise of meditation, the client can engage in thoughts of the topic or in conversation with God, returning to the simple breathing formula from time to time. When other thoughts intrude during meditation, they are only acknowledged, not engaged, and then deliberately set aside for later consideration. Throughout the day, recall of meditation reinforces the technique until the person is able to create an atmosphere of prayer. Thus, someone who began meditation after breakfast and continued it into therapy sessions could make the work of therapy a prayer or offering.

Meditation advocates believe that practicing the technique of breathing and gazing downward while mentally saying the chosen word or prayer ensures a client is never far away from immediate personal contact with the infinite and intimate spiritual presence within. This breath of spirit can then flow out, carrying the holy words, prayer lines, Bible phrase, Hebrew word, mantra, or whatever the client has chosen. Some clients use a technique in which they focus on an image that embodies their sense of the divine.

Centering, mentioned previously and performed by nurses who practice the principles of therapeutic touch (TT), has been likened to the sensations attained through meditation. Although TT is not associated directly with meditation techniques or mental effort, it depends on the universal healing power being channeled through the nurse as a conduit to provide comfort or healing. One who desires that a time be set aside for a meditation period may need assistance from a nurse to find a secluded place in a rehabilitation facility, a "sacred space" within daily routines to attend to spiritual practices, alone, or with others.

Visualization and Imagery

Visualization may help clients to live in alignment with their purpose. Nurses can guide a client in asking questions about envisioning life—for example, "How does life look?," "How do you feel inside?," "What am I doing?," "How do I interact, and with whom?," and "What is a typical day?" Clients adjust their personal visions until an inner voice says yes, then they adjust their actions until the vision becomes the reality. Journal writing is a complementary method for keeping track of goals and helping to make decisions or to take actions in alignment with the goals.

Imagery is related closely to visualization. It is the internal experience of memories, dreams, and fantasies that requires focused concentration. Imagery uses imagination and all the senses in attempts to dismiss anxiety and reach inner spiritual resources. Imagery techniques may influence the peripheral and autonomic nervous systems by reducing stressful symptoms and speeding recovery from illness, as well as produce change in a client's perceptions about disability and treatment. Many clients choose symbolic images related to God or an inner guide because these hold personal healing significance. A nurse who is interested in helping clients access their inner healing resources first becomes familiar with types of imagery (receptive, active, concrete, symbolic process end-of-state, and general healing) and studies ways to guide clients on their healing journey. A commercial audiotape or one made from a personalized script can facilitate visualization. The power of the process increases with the time invested. Drawing after relaxation and imaging, without thought to artwork complements these therapies and may reveal areas of negative images.

Prayer

Prayer is back! And it is slowly being given the blessing of the medical profession because numerous studies show results prayer is moving toward center stage in modern medicine (Dossey, 1996). Although petitionary prayer does not always produce the precise desired benefit from the human point of view, the results given time may be welcomed. Science has been forced to concede that some prayer generally is preferable to no prayer, although faith need not be validated by science. Although prayer and the relaxation process operate on the same biochemical pathways, and neurologists may have located a place in the brain activated during prayer, it is not necessary to understand how prayer works to use it. What is necessary for prayer is to think and live in the presence of one's God. When a client in spiritual distress feels unable to pray, then prayer becomes an outcome rather than an intervention.

Among various forms of prayer, Dossey (1993) suggests prayers for petition (asking something for self), intercession (asking something for others), confession (repentance of wrongdoing), adoration (giving honor and praise), invocation (summoning the Almighty), lamentation (crying in distress), and thanksgiving (offering gratitude). Levin (1996) describes four independent dimensions of prayer: ritual or recitational, conversational or colloquial, petitionary or intercessory, and meditative.

Other types of prayer include centering (contemplative), soaking (in-depth directed outpouring), the laying on of hands, and dream prayer. Soaking prayer is like radiation therapy without the side effects, using a gentle touch over time to let power and love seep through to a dry spiritual core in need of revival. Although prayer forms used most for health problems are petitionary and intercessory, clients often request God to fulfill spiritual or material needs, so the best prayer petition is open-ended and not specific.

Conversational and meditative prayer relate closer to spiritual well-being than do petitionary or intercessory prayers; prayers of confession and for thanksgiving are interrelated. Meditative prayer may be part of the relaxation response intervention; thus, prayer may be an attribute of being spiritual or characterized as an outcome of spirituality.

Regardless of a provider's beliefs, all a client has to do is start a conversation with God, who can reach down and touch the soul to prayer, then God will keep it going. Many an ill or disabled person has recognized that an ailment eventually can be a gift after they "let go and let God, be God." Many people report trading their weakness for God's strength and then beginning to "do" for others. Although physically challenged or impaired, they find they are doing without doing; that is, they cooperate with the natural order in thoughts and prayers (Soeken & Carson, 1987).

Prayer has cultural roots, but remains highly personal. With that in mind, a Jewish client might believe that sympathetic prayer by others is a value in itself and part of a larger sympathetic act. Native American clients may pray for dreams, spirited insight, or wisdom. Some clients of Hispanic heritage might ask penance or divine intervention from patron saints; Islamic clients may invoke Allah's blessing for their fate; or those in touch with nature may invoke those channels or resources. It is impossible to have a bad prayer day.

Not offering a client the opportunity to pray is tantamount to withholding medication. If clients evince any interest in prayer, a nurse first tells them to pray, then offers presence during prayers, and finally may choose to offer to pray with them. Prayer is the sense of being aligned with something higher, thus prayers are not directed out into the universe, but inwardly to the spirit. An outward demonstration does not indicate quality or level of prayer, but some may desire a leader or spiritual person to assist them in meditation or to perform ceremonial acts as a part of prayer. As with other techniques, prayer may be expressed while meditating, keeping a journal, or creating art. In a prayerful state, a client may have "a sense in which a 'cure' can occur—the realization that physical problems, no matter how painful or severe, are at some level of secondary importance in the total scheme of existence. One's authentic higher self is completely impervious to the ravages of any ailment whatsoever—utterly beyond the ravages of disease and death" (Dossey, 1993, p. 36).

Humor

Norman Cousins and Patch Adams, MD, brought popular medical humor to the forefront, but it has been known throughout medical history to be health promoting. Dr. Thomas Sydenham (1624–1648), the founder of clinical medicine and epidemiology, said that a clown arriving in town was worth 20 donkeys laden with drugs. Humor has physiological and psychological effects to ease tension in situations, act as a great distraction, play up the eustress (positive, motivating energy) in situations, and can be shared to enhance interpersonal relationships. People with impairments or disfigurements have borne the brunt of humor over time, frequently being endowed with negative traits associated with ill-willed humor. Recently, people with disabilities have launched their own forms of humor, self-initiated and self-directed. "The shortest distance between two points . . . is usually not accessible," is an example of so-called disability humor. Providers are cautioned not to develop or spread this specific humor—it belongs to the group, not society at large.

As a spiritual intervention, humor helps clients to think creatively and contend with mortality. It may give a feeling of belonging and social cohesion, facilitate coping, and counteract feelings of alienation and giving a sense of control in life. The benefits of comedy have been likened to the functions of religion: to raise self-awareness and one's spirits; to accept reality and its contradictions; to reveal harmony by increasing connections to each other and to life. Humor is a God's-eye view of the universe. (Why do ghosts ride on elevators? To raise their spirits.)

Smiling and laughing are contagious and can occur for no reason. Laughter is likened to jogging on the inside. It is an inexpensive and nonfattening way to relieve stress. Laughter provides a perspective for suffering, acknowledging it while momentarily relieving the tension and grief. One should laugh only lovingly at oneself. Compassionate laughter means finding something to laugh about in the face of tragedy because life's drama can be both extremely serious and exquisitely funny. (The doctor fell on his funny bone, and the nurse charted it as a humerus incident.)

As with any intervention, it is wise to assess the client's sense and use of humor to learn if and what type is appropriate. The concept of humor lies in each client's mind and each has a personal, favorite brand. Humor does not travel well across cultures; in fact, intended humor may be interpreted as insulting, ridicule, or even threatening to clients of other cultures. Likewise, humor differs among age groups, religious believers, and even persons from different regions of the United States. Laughing with a client can be therapeutic, when appropriate. The various types of humor that can act as stimulus for healing are word play, satire, jokes, stories, cartoons, witticisms, clowning, games, videos, books, and pictures. Ridicule, sarcasm, and racist jokes have no place and are strictly taboo, and wit can be hurtful. ("Soap is to the body as laughter is to the soul"—Yiddish proverb.)

Humor has found a home in children's hospital or residential units. In another example, a retired nurse educator, also trained as a clown, gives examples of a retired clergyman acting as staff clown in an Iowa regional health center, a clown working out of pastoral care in a South Dakota hospital, and a hospital clown newsletter (Gustafson, 1996). Some facilities have collections of small toys, games, comedy tapes, and joke books available in a humor basket; a recreation department can host a humor cart. Nurses' continuing education venue often includes humorists who impart wise humor skills for clients, but also attend to teaching stressed-out nurses how to laugh and replenish their own cheer. "A joyful heart is good medicine, but a crushed spirit dries up the bones" (Proverbs 17:22).

Arts Therapy

The symbolism inherent in dance, painting, poetry, music, quilting, gardening, and other arts communicates a language of the soul. Art has great power to uplift, communicate, enhance understanding, educate, and impart beauty. Typically the arts refer to the creative and interpretive works that express perceptions, feelings, and intuitions. Recently the martial arts, such as T'ai Chi, and some sports have been recognized as fostering psychospiritual development. All levels and aspects of art can be used to aid in recovery from suffering, and transforming it into something valuable (Vash, 1994).

Music has a long history in the art of medicine, as an antidote for many ills. It washes away the everyday dust from the soul, and can promote inner silence. The client's individual choice of music can enhance the relaxation response and imagery states. Individual tastes dictate the kind of music for various situations, but research and clinical studies show "designer music" produces significant effects in listening and physiological and psychological status, as reflected in relaxation, mental clarity, vigor, fatigue, sadness, and tension. Also, caring increases and hostility decreases.

Bibliotherapy

In bibliotherapy, medical librarians join the team by identifying appropriate readings in the literature that can guide clients to cost-effective, low-technology, and high-quality tools so they can learn about their disabilities or conditions, as well as about the spiritual and emotional aspects. At first, clients may do better with "escape" literature and progress to material that aids nurse-client discussions. Because many clients identify with others having similar problems, uplifting narratives and book reading groups, spiritual readings, or poetry may be interesting. When reading is not possible, a family member or volunteer may assist, or the nurse can read short passages when appropriate or possible. Audiotapes with inspiriting and informational messages are available. Individual interests vary greatly. Librarians are aware of and know how to obtain a variety of materials and specialized resources (Solimine, 1995).

Reminiscence Therapy

Reminiscence therapy is characterized by conscious and progressive calling of positive experiences from the past into current memory. A type of bibliotherapy, it involves listening, being present, and caring for the distinct purpose of encouraging a client in recalling memories. This process evokes questions that lead clients to review their life by focusing on successful victories over challenges. Only at the client's request would other memories be retrieved, and then only when the client wished to explore what actually happened to cause them distress to achieve closure. Rehashing of past wounds or failures is not part of the therapy.

Looking over old photographs and memorabilia can enhance memory in reminiscence. These times often create an atmosphere for family involvement and storytelling. Through stories, clients can make sense of life, connect with listeners, and even leave a legacy when they are recorded on video or audiotape. The images etched in a person's imagination, as well as the parts of the life story, are bits of individual soul carried within. When people tell their tales, they give away part of their soul, and this should be honored (Hillman, 1972). Other strategies are to create a time line, a collage, or a journal for reflection. Writing about stressful experiences to reduce symptoms also has gained some medical research attention (Smyth, Stone, Hurewitz, & Kaell, 1999).

OUTCOMES

Forgiveness

One of the most powerful things a person can accomplish in a lifetime is to decide to make peace with oneself and others, letting go of grudges and the pain of hurtful relationships—forgiving oneself and others—and say yes to life. It is the necessary first step in the passage to spiritual quality of life that entails a struggle with feelings of denial, anger, bargaining, and depression, much as the dying client makes.

Although anger is an appropriate initial response to hurt, clients may become victims of their own mistaken judgment. The error of the self as right and powerful prevails and clients damage themselves, for anger weakens rather than empowers (Borysenko, 1993). When a person cannot find it in his or her heart to forgive someone, the other party may or may not experience grief, but the person will continue to anguish and mourn not being a loving, peace-filled person. Remaining unforgiving holds back and limits spiritual growth. The process of forgiving is a dynamic energy force—an act of will consciously undertaken to heal self and memories, to restore self-determination and strengthen spirituality. Children can learn about forgiveness, as well as self-esteem, and moral principles enjoyably, through animated videos, such as the series called "Veggie Tales."

It takes grace to forgive and ask God's forgiveness; forgiving others follows. Asking for another's forgiveness for any conscious or unconscious sorrow one has inflicted means learning about responsibility, sensitivity, empathy, and kindness—and internalizing them. When a person forgives self, loses any attachment to the deed, and considers the consequences of not forgiving; then a person can celebrate becoming a new being. However, telling someone they have been forgiven may not be necessary or even wise; forgiveness is an internalized process. As amputee, Andre Dubus (1991), says: "After the physical pain of grief has become, with time, a permanent wound in the soul, . . . then comes the transcendent and common bond of suffering, and with that comes forgiveness, and with forgiveness comes love . . ." (p. 138).

This love can guide both nurse and client on the spiritual path to wholeness, but resources help. Mariposa Ministry online holds workshops on "Healing our Disabilities through Forgiveness," sharing a confession litany with able-bodied Christians. Dr. Carol Gill (Chicago Center for Disability Research, University of Illinois at Chicago) received a grant to study the role of forgiveness in positive adjustment to disability. Her research explores the role of forgiveness in making someone who has become physically disabled to have a positive adjustment. Ideally, findings will help health providers understand more about the role of forgiveness and how to plan effective support for clients.

Hope and Coping

Recent developments toward understanding disease etiology, improving treatment methods, validating research findings, and instituting interdisciplinary teamwork with rehabilitation have stimulated social services and programs for clients and their families. More choices of effective interventions and treatments that can be blended with rehabilitation techniques give optimism, and team members are able to help clients generate hope. Hope is future-oriented and changes across the illness trajectory. It is essential to achieving goals and strong interpersonal relationships—hope is the force between a client and perception of the Almighty. Hope has power and energy—wishes might happen, hope must happen, but is more likely when grounded in reality.

Particularized hope begins with achieving a desired goal and dissipating a stressful experience. This success contributes to an immediate sense of peace and well-being and creates an overall generalized hope about future success. Hope is a positive phenomenon to activate effective coping; it is activity, not passivity. However, the process and meaning of hope across cultures requires further investigation.

The opposite of hope is not pure hopelessness because a remnant of hope remains. Pain and suffering, depleted energy, and impaired cognition impede hope. Hopelessness often accompanied by helplessness and is preceded by loss of control of one's own life and independence. Thus the same life situation can be an occasion for either hope or hopelessness, or for both. Clients who feel hopeless are not demanding or noisy; rather, they appear passive and depressed, wreaking further adversity on their quality of life. Acknowledging a client's seeming hopelessness, offering to discuss problems, and assisting in constructive ways may begin a supportive nurse-client relationship from which to foster hope. Acknowledging grief and despair may be more important than converting a client to a premature goal; assessment for potential self-injury may be appropriate. Helping people realize that developing hope is an evolving process allows them to identify outcomes and resources that have little meaning now, but may be pursued later.

Hope is important in the lives of clients with spinal cord injury, regardless of how long it has been since the injury (Nelson, 1990). Strategies to build hope include teaching effective coping, setting mutual goals, reframing health problems as opportunities for adaptation and physical growth, and fostering improved self-esteem and social supports. Although hope is directive and willful, spiritual hope is most likely to emerge when a client lets go of will and opens self to trust in God.

Serenity

Trauma, major illness, and increasing age give way to a search for inner peace, or serenity, to be sustained regardless of life events. Serenity, an awakened state, "gives one a healthy mastery of emotions, decreases stress, and leads to improved relationships with others and especially with God, through prayer, zest for living, acceptance of one's self as worthy, increased compassion and self-possession during trying times, and trust in a higher power" (Dossey, 1993). A serene person is caring, active, involved and responsible, not passive or detached. Serenity is not always being happy, rather it is being able to have a quiet inner-directed action and calm despite negative circumstances.

Nurses themselves need to acquire serenity to reach their own inner haven where they find detachment, belonging, giving, trust in a higher power, acceptance, problem solving, presentness, forgiveness, and a view of the future. Conversely, anxiety, anger, lack of faith, impatience, and unhealthy lifestyle behaviors are samples found in the nonserene.

An individual who is able to achieve serenity may have a strategy for coping with chronic illness, other comorbid conditions, or addictive behaviors that may accompany disabilities. One addicted to food, gambling, drugs, alcohol, nicotine, and the like may be longing for wholeness. Consider the language references to "drinking spirits" and "using drugs to get high." Alcoholics Anonymous (AA) and similar organizations ground their recovery programs in a relationship to a higher power. Clients may suffer a spiritual emergency that reflects a crisis in learning about their spiritual self and eventually experience a spiritual transformation. Many gain insights when they break through addiction and learn to substitute a drug routine with a spiritual focus. The AA prayer has become famous in the quest for serenity, "God grant me the serenity to accept the things I cannot change, courage to change the things I can, and wisdom to know the difference" (Niebuhr, 1943).

Healing/Wholeness/Spiritual Quality of Life

Disability and chronic illness interrupt the fabric of life; clients adjust by weaving their lives together in whatever ways make sense to them. This is healing, but does not cure the physical problem. Authentic healing is an expression of spiritual maturity that leads to integrity and wholeness and psychospiritual growth may be nearly equivalent to healing. Self-healing can bring clients to meaningfulness in life through separation from daily routine, transition to the inner self, and finally a return with an inner peace. "Healing is an active and internal process that includes investigating one's attitude, memories and beliefs with the desire to release all negative patterns that prevent one's full emotional and spiritual recovery. This internal review inevitably leads one to review one's external circumstances in an effort to recreate one's life in a way that serves activation of will—the will to see and accept truths about one's life and how one has used one's energies, and the will to begin to use energy for the creation of love, self-esteem and health" (Myss, 1996, p. 48).

Although healing is a goal, it is a means to serve a purpose in life regardless of impairment, and not the purpose itself. The process of curing is passive; the client authorizes physicians, healers, and treatments that do not necessarily alleviate psychological and emotional stresses that accompany the illness, and that may trigger its return. Healing involves emotional, psychological, physical, and spiritual recovery. The nurse and client are mutually involved as healers. "The nurse-healer uses the art of guiding to help others discover and recognize new health behaviors, make choices and discover insights about how to cope effectively. . . . The nurse acts as a facilitator to evoke the patient's process of inner healing" (Dossey, Guzzetta, & Keener, 1992, p. 8).

Nursing Education and Research

Spiritual care is an inseparable part of client care and has an intrinsic value and importance, beginning with basic professional education it is not extra or optional content. Every nurse can feel confident to give as a caring and integrated person having been educated to set personal development and relationships with others—that is to say, that the spiritual care of the nurse and client are priorities (Mayer, 1992).

Research in the field of spirituality is sparse. Questions for investigation include nurses' perceptions of spirituality, techniques that facilitate spiritual healing and clients' responses, values, and other spiritual factors that influence outcomes with disability or chronic illness, complications from spiritual interventions, or the roles of lay and religious communities in rehabilitation. Although conceptual frameworks and definitions are challenging, a definition of spirituality that will accommodate the uniqueness of all clients and nurses is a need. Few reliable tools measure the effects of interventions used with disabled clients and control groups or validate changes. Interest in spirituality is growing in many areas of health and it is a responsible area of research for rehabilitation nurses.

Interdisciplinary Focus

Spirituality is a sought-after topic in professional conferences, continuing education courses, publications, media, and Web sites. Often spiritual and ethical issues are discussed along with alternative or complementary therapies. The Internet promotes spiritual resources and support groups; Pope John Paul II's computer activities, such as his letters to the elderly (1999), have earned him the title "Cyber Pope." Many journals that publish spiritual articles still are not indexed on MEDLINE, such as *The Journal of Religion in Disability and Rehabilitation,* the *Journal of Christian Healing,* the *Journal for the Scientific Study of Religion,* and the *International Journal for the Psychology of Religion.* However, Dossey (1996) notes that major medical journals are beginning to publish findings from research about the effects of prayer and faith on healing, as well as reports of physicians' activities in the spiritual areas. Certainly the media has opened the topics of prayer, healing, and spirituality in print and on the airwaves.

However, a great deal of confusion and disagreement exists about whether spiritual interventions are to be performed, by whom, and under what circumstances. Meanwhile, prestigious health professionals are praying with clients, courses in medical schools emphasize spiritual issues, and researchers are examining spiritual phenomena and healing. The Panel of Mind/Body Interventions also has examined evidence surrounding the effectiveness of prayer and spiritual healing (National Center for Alternative and Complementary Medicine at the National Institutes of Health, http://nccam.nih.gov/nccam).

Some believe that science is the enemy of spirituality and that research will replace its beauty with cold, hard data, whereas others hope to open a window and watch God work, expanding spiritual healing. Physicians as a group do not lack faith, but their profession demands precision, not unsubstantiated claims. "Testing prayer can actually be a form of worship, a ritual through which we express our gratitude for this remarkable phenomenon" (Dossey, 1996, p. 10). Wilber (1991) states that genuine mysticism, as opposed to dogmatic religion, is very scientific, because it relies on the direct experiential evidence of meditation in the laboratory of the mind.

Psychoneuroimmunologists (PNI), or psychoneuroendoimmunologists, study connections and relationships among meaning, attitude, hope, and prayer—expressions of the invisible spiritual power within—and the transformation of disease. Thus, the spirit, mind, and body are seen again as integrated components of a common system, with considerable biodirectional activity. It is not simply mind over matter, but that the mind matters. All an individual's experiences affect health, or as Myss (1996, p. 34) states: "Your biography becomes your biology." For instance, expectancy is one of the variables linked to placebo outcome. High expectancy in both nurse and client predict and facilitate the healing process in a spiritual healing encounter (Wirth, 1995). Combining the PNI principles with nursing practice may add value to the profession.

Many psychiatrists throughout history, Jung among them, maintained belief in the spiritual nature of man, and added the diagnosis of Religious or Spiritual Problems to the *Diagnostic and Statistical Manual of Mental Disorders* (American Psychiatric Association, 1994). The diagnosis includes the loss or questioning of faith or spiritual values and is considered a problem, not a mental disorder. Training in religious and spiritual issues is now required in psychiatric residency programs, and a model curriculum has been published. Holotropic breathwork, developed by a psychiatrist, is a powerful technique for self-exploration and healing, activating nonordinary states of consciousness (Grof & Grof, 1989).

Psychologists have identified changes in clients' lives based on spirituality and are among those arguing for holism in their practice. The transpersonal perspective (i.e., having experiences in which the sense of identity of self extends beyond [trans] the individual [personal] to encompass wider aspects of life or psyche) has gained many adherents among psychologists. The transpersonal is a revolutionary aspect in astronomy, physics, and biology as well. Genetics scientist Lerner believes that we have spent 100 years of reductionism trying to understand biological processes by looking at the pieces. Now we're going to try to understand complexity, how the pieces work together.

Although modern physics does not itself prove Eastern mysticism, many pioneering physicists were mystics. They desired to go beyond the intrinsic limitations of physics to higher and more enduring realities, wanting neither physics nor mysticism cheapened (Wilber, 1991). A movement among some middle-class people seeking enlightenment, emotion, and personal relationship with a higher power not found in traditional worship has intermingled mainline religion with Eastern meditative practices and New Age beliefs. Called "designer faith," its precepts are under study by the New Religious Group panel of the American Academy of Religion.

One can but guess at the future of spirituality if materialists such as Kurzweil (1999) prevail. Believing that spiritualism is possible, materialists would resolve the mind-body issue with the premise that machines are the answer. Because machines can outstrip human capacities, human beings need to be transcended by scanning their brains into computers to be immortal; the next great step in the evolution of intelligence. The spirituality of any machine could only be an impoverished one, compared with that of a human being who communes with God.

Collaboration of health care with religious professionals may yield an inclusive and universal spirituality. "Scientific data and spiritual perspective can be quite compatible when one's convictions about the 'highest' and 'deepest' human potentials and values are based on both reason and intuition, both intellect and feeling, both personal observation and the accumulated wisdom of one's medical, nursing, or therapeutic discipline" (Krippner & Welch, 1992, p. 196). In the long run, scholars in the field will rely on many health disciplines, as well as those from anthropology, history, sociology, literary analysis, ecology, and economics.

SPIRITUALITY AND THE REHABILITATION NURSE

Rehabilitation nurses can, and should, provide for their clients; but what about the plight of the overworked, underspiritualized nurses within the profession? Previously, basic nursing educational content was reduced to lists and reviews of major religions and their tenets, with no attempts to infuse a nurse with spiritual purpose or belief. So, some nurses have no idea of their role in what is now a new and spiritual component of nursing. "Spiritual development, or religious affiliation has seldom been a criterion for nursing . . . practice. As there are different levels of maturity, even in religion, different nurses bring different limitations and talents in providing patient care . . . she/he can't be what she/he isn't" (Barnum, 1996, p. 142).

Self-care or self-respect is not even discussed—although nurses are caring people, ethically, the first object of their care should be themselves—take the time to love and care for selves to be able to care and minister to others; refresh and revitalize the body, mind, and spirit. The nurses who choose to become a spiritual resource to clients cannot allow themselves to become personally depleted, either physically or spiritually. Regardless of spiritual background or personal beliefs, nurses who fortify others' personal spiritual perspectives must find the time to renew their spirits, for they can help clients grow only as much as they have grown. Are you caring for your whole self as conscientiously as you do for others? Taking responsibility for your own spiritual health is one way to focus creatively on your own needs, and to achieve a better balance in caring for yourself. If you list the things that you do for yourself that are physical, then emotional, intellectual, social, and spiritual, you can see which category you may need to enhance, where you need more "re-creation."

To strengthen wellness and self-esteem, list these same categories with what you like best about yourself in each of them, what others have said they like about you, and for what you would like to be remembered. If you are critical of yourself in any area, this is where you need to cultivate something positive. As a personal prescription for your wellness, do the following. Focus on your positive aspects, set realistic goals and reward yourself for progress, be gentle, practice centering, learn to ask for what you need, learn to say no, and think and say positive things to yourself. Develop intuitive skills, take time for fun and laughter, walk a labyrinth, learn to take mental health breaks and minivacations, identify your stressors and find coping mechanisms for them, and mentally inventory the good things that happen to you daily and give thanks. We are all eligible for small pleasures (Uustal, 1992). In your practice, trust your intuition; trust that there will be change from day to day. Walk the path of humility, let go of control outcomes, hold your highest healing intention in your thoughts and actions; be open (Towey, 1997). To all of these add, pray for guidance and seek counsel when needed. Sharing and demonstrating the benefits of personal renewal with a client may result in mutual reinforcement.

Inspiriting Colleagues

The caring ethic, when shared among nurses, is collegiality in their practice area; it inspirits. Nurse managers are challenged to foster spiritual growth in themselves as leaders and human beings and fuel and brighten the spirituality of ones they work for and with, and those they serve (Kerfoot, 1995). Spirituality shapes the quality of the working atmosphere by building morale and increasing nursing satisfaction, providing a "holding environment" that is balanced, where nurses can feel sustained, and where they feel safe and can reach their potential (Karl, 1993). The need is great for a network of support that surrounds an individual nurse and makes it possible to focus energies beyond self.

Practical ideas, which can make significant difference in the sharing of support and love, include an important ground rule of no "put downs"! A team can state expectations, such as expect the best and hold safe gripe sessions, identify areas of expertise, collaboration, and standards of excellence, and be patient. They can celebrate behavior that adds value, encourages intuitive skills, and activates team support to keep morale high.

One team put envelopes (with individuals' names) on the bulletin board to hold one-line notes of praise and encouragement from others. Another team designated a time to share what needs healing during weekly informal sessions and requested education on spiritual topics. Some teams meditate or perform yoga together during lunch or after work. Logotherapy can be applied to nursing through Frankl's summary: "Get to work! Work is not merely being productive in the hospital or clinic, but rather to re-establish a moral and spiritual dimension to the profession that brings you the satisfaction of lasting value" (Scully, 1995, p. 43). Although he was not speaking directly to nurses, all health care professionals may heed this. However, one must want to do this more than anything else, for those who bear a God in them bring genius to their work. The spirituality of work demands reverential focus on what is now; in the present moment, not wishing you were somewhere else. If you so choose to work at spiritually enhancing your profession and your clients by becoming a spiritual resource, you would do well to execute a self-contract, stating things you would like to see changed in your life; a plan and its steps; indicators of progress; ways you might impede the progress and how to overcome them; by what deadline; and share it and have it witnessed by a friend (Uustal, 1992). This is a means of preventing procrastination and reaching your goals.

Beliefs and Rehabilitation Nursing Practice

Nurses who agree spirituality is important, but respond negatively to its use in their practice, may hold one or more of the following beliefs.

- Clients are uncomfortable discussing spiritual matters with a nurse (social restraint).
- Matters of spirituality do not concern nurses, but rather psychologists or pastoral caregivers.
- A person lacks time to devote to what is perceived as an arduous task.
- Nurses are so technologically oriented that they are not comfortable with spirituality.
- A person lacks maturity/education/experience necessary to have anything to do with spiritual issues (own shortcomings).
- A nurse's own beliefs/culture, differing from that of the client, would contradict the client's perspective or would demand self-expression.
- A person's own spiritual wellspring is depleted and not equal to the task (vulnerability; emotional risk).
- After clients' spiritual fears surfaced, a nurse would not be able to deal with the issues presented (counseling skills).

Many nurses fear they are meddling in a client's spiritual life, and correctly so. However, clients interviewed concerning spiritual needs have chosen nurses second to clergy as those with whom they wish to discuss spiritual matters. A nurse educates a client about the condition and rehabilitation techniques that may seem strange or frightening, addresses most physical needs without calling on a physician, and intervenes with many psychosocial or emotional responses without relying on a psychologist.

A nurse advocates for a client and understands when a referral is needed, then selects the appropriate professional. When a client believes illness or impairment appears as a punishment for wrongdoing (especially perceived sexual transgressions), clerical intervention is needed. For example, those who value the ministry of confession are taught through grace to view God as a present friend rather than perceiving a punishing enemy. Other spiritual leaders have specific views for followers of their religion. Some clients, who continue to have serious adjustment problems of conscience, may benefit from referral for psychological help.

The foundation for religious belief is formed during the same developmental stage as the ability to trust. Thus, a nurse may work with clients to create a healing environment and foster an atmosphere of trust wherein a client is encouraged to relax and be able to confide religious and spiritual needs. The professional must be as comfortable with the subject and setting as the client.

The pattern of how sexuality was treated is a comparison. For many years, sexuality was a topic seldom mentioned in rehabilitation and less often with the client. When the subject was introduced, professionals felt unqualified and that it was out of bounds, whereas clients wondered if their questions were inappropriate and experienced frustration because they were left without answers. Today, sexuality is discussed freely, whereas spirituality remains a less approachable topic. In a nurse-client relationship bound by trust, confidentiality, and respect, spirituality becomes an acceptable topic. The rehabilitation nurse needs to be aware of the essential role of spirituality in clients' lives.

SUMMARY

If life is a trip all people are taking and health is the vehicle that carries them, then impairment is the spiritual flat tire that happens on some vehicles. Seemingly disastrous when it occurs, repairs are made with the spiritual resources at hand and their adventure continues, hopefully in a redirected, meaningful manner. The rehabilitation nurse can play a part as a professional who guides the repair and assists them on their way, stronger in spirit for having had the experience. It is through the spiritual life in each client that rehabilitation nurses can nourish the spirit to fruition and flourish in their own spirituality.

"I reserve the name 'caregiver' for the people who are willing to listen to ill persons and to respond to their individual experiences. Caring has nothing to do with categories of illness; it shows the person that his life is valued because it recognizes what makes his experiences particular. When the caregiver communicates to the ill person that she cares about this uniqueness, she makes the person's life meaningful. And as that person's narrative becomes part of her own, the caregiver's life is made meaningful as well. Listening to another, we hear ourselves. Caring for another, we care for ourselves as well" (Frank, 1995, p. 48).

CRITICAL THINKING

Respond to the following quote in an open debate or discussion with peers. Use a real (confidential and anonymous) client or situation, if possible.

"My concern is that these issues (i.e., of assisted suicide) be confronted in such a way as to create a social climate in which people with disabilities perceive life to be an honorable choice. And that means sending the social message that disabled people are valued and valuable, precious even, by investing, financially and emotionally, in institutions and practices that help them out. Everybody, well or ill, disabled or not, imagines a boundary of suffering and loss beyond which, she or he is certain, life will no longer be worth living" (Mairs, 1996, p. 114).

REFERENCES

Albom, M. (1997). *Tuesdays with Morrie: An old man, a young man, and life's greatest lesson.* (Large print edition). Rockland, MA: Wheeler Publishing.

American Holistic Nurses Association. (1998). *Standards of holistic nursing practice.* Flagstaff, AZ: Author.

American Nurses Association. (1985). *Code of ethics for nurses.* Washington, DC: Author.

American Psychiatric Association. *DSM–IV: Diagnostic and Statistical Manual of Mental Disorders.* (4th ed.). Washington, DC: Author, 1994.

Assagioli, R. (1973). *The act of will.* New York: Viking Press.

Barnum, B.S. (1996). *Spirituality in nursing: From traditional to new age.* New York: Springer.

Benson, H. (1996). *Timeless healing: The power and biology of belief* (p. 109). New York: Scribner.

Borysenko, J. (1987). *Minding the body, mending the mind.* Reading, MA: Addison-Wesley.

Bryant, M.D. (1993). Religion and disability: Some notes on religious attitudes and views. In M. Nagler (Ed.), *Perspectives on disability* (pp. 91-95). Palo Alto, CA: Health Markets Research

Charmaz, K. (1991). *Good days, bad days: The self in chronic illness and time.* New Brunswick, NJ: Rutgers University Press.

Corbin, J.M., & Strauss, A. (1988). *Unending work and care: Managing chronic illness at home.* San Francisco: Jossey-Bass.

Davis, M.C. (1994). The rehabilitation nurse's role in spiritual care. *Rehabilitation Nursing, 19,* 298-301.

Dein, S. (1997). Does being religious help or hinder coping with chronic illness? A critical literature review. *Palliative Medicine, 11,* 291-298.

Desai, P.N. (1989). *Health and medicine in the Hindu tradition* (p. 20). New York: Crossroads.

Di Meo, E. (1991). Rx for spiritual distress. *RN, 54,* 22-24.

Dossey, B., Keegan, L., Guzzetta C., & Kolkmeier, L. (1988). *Holistic nursing practice: A handbook for practice.* Rockville, MD: Aspen.

Dossey, B., Guzzetta, C.E., & Kenner, C.V. (1992). Body-mind-spirit. In B. Dossey, C.E. Guzzetta, & C.V. Kenner (Eds.), *Critical care nursing: Body-mind-spirit* (3rd ed., pp. 3-16). Philadelphia: JB Lippincott.

Dossey, L. (1993). *Healing words: The power of prayer and the practice of medicine.* San Francisco: Harper & Row.

Dossey, L. (1996). *Prayer is good medicine: How to reap the healing benefits of prayer.* San Francisco: Harper San Francisco.

Doyle, B. (1994). Graceful falls: How physical injuries can lead to spiritual growth. *U.S. Catholic, 60,* 27-34.

Dreyer, E.A. (1994). *Earth crammed with heaven: A spirituality of everyday life.* New York: Paulist Press.

Dubus, A. (1991). *Broken vessels.* Boston: D.R. Godine.

Durkin, M.B. (1992). A community of caring patients in a rehabilitation unit experience holistic healing through a spiritual support group. *Health Progress, 73,* 48-53, 70.

Easton, K.L., & Andrews, J.C. (2000). The roles of the pastor in the interdisciplinary rehabilitation team. *Rehabilitation Nursing, 25,* 10-12.

Ellis, D. (1980). Whatever happened to the spiritual dimension? *Canadian Nurse, 76,* 48-53, 70.

Ellison, C.W. (1982). Spiritual well-being: Conceptualization and measurement. *Journal of Psychology and Theology, 11,* 330-340.

Feldman, D.M. (1986). *Health and medicine in the Jewish tradition.* New York: Crossroads.

Foley, D.P. (1988). 11 interpretations of personal suffering. *Journal of Religion & Health, 27,* 321-328.

Forbes, E.J. (1994). Spirituality, aging, and the community-dwelling caregiver and care recipient. *Geriatric Nursing, 15,* 297-302.

Frank, A.W. (1995). *At the will of the body: Reflections on illness* (p. 48). Boston: Houghton Mifflin.

Frankl, V. (1984). *Man's search for meaning: An introduction to logotherapy.* (Reprint). New York: Simon & Schuster.

Gaynor, M.L. (1995). *Healing essence: A cancer doctor's practical program for hope and recovery.* New York: Kodansha International.

Gordon, M. (2000). *Manual of nursing diagnosis* (pp. 542-547). St. Louis: Mosby.

Grof, S., & Grof, C. (1989). *Spiritual emergency: When personal transformation becomes a crisis.* Los Angeles: Tarcher.

Gustafson, M.B. (1996). The newest member on the healthcare team: Clowns. *Creative Nursing: 2,* 14.

Haddad, L.G., & Hoeman, S.P. (2000). Home healthcare and the Arab-American client. *Home Healthcare Nurse 18*(3), 189-197.

Hale, T.W. (1996). Spiritual response to traumatic illness. *Polio Network News, 12,* 6-7.

Hardy, A. (1979). *The spiritual nature of man.* Oxford: Clarendon Press.

Hatch, R.L., Burg, M.A., Naberhaus, D.S., & Hellmich, L.K. (1998). The spiritual involvement and beliefs scale: Development and testing of a new instrument. *Journal of Family Practice, 46,* 476-486.

Hendricks, G., & Wills, R. (1975). *The centering book: Awareness activities for children, parents and teachers.* Englewood Cliffs, NJ: Prentice Hall.

Highfield, M.F., & Cason, C. (1983). Spiritual needs of the patient: Are they recognized? *Cancer Nursing, 6,* 187-192.

Hill, P.C., & Butter, E.M. (1995). The role of religion in promoting physical health. *Journal of Psychology & Christianity, 4,* 141-155.

Hillman, J. (1972). *The myth of analysis.* New York: Harper & Row.

Hinds, C. (1993). Suffering: A relatively unexplored phenomenon among family caregivers of non-institutionalized patients with cancer. *Journal of Advanced Nursing, 17,* 718-725.

Hunglemann, J., Kendel-Rossi, E., Klassen, L., & Stollenwerk, R. (1996). Focus on spiritual well-being: Harmonious interconnectedness of mind-body-spirit—including the use of the Jarel spiritual well-being scale. *Geriatric Nursing, 17,* 262-266.

Idowu, F. (1993). Let go and let live. *America, 169,* 20-21.

International Council of Nurses (ICN). (2000). Code of ethics. Geneva: ICN. Available on-line at: http://www.icn.ch/icncode.pdf.

Johnson, M., Maas, M., & Moorhead, S. (2000). *Nursing outcomes classification (NOC)* (2nd ed.). St. Louis: Mosby.

Karasu, T.B. (1999). Spiritual psychotherapy. *American Journal of Psychotherapy, 53,* 143-145.

Karl, J.C. (1993). Being there. Who do you bring to practice? In D. Gault (Ed.), *The presence of caring in nursing.* New York: National League of Nursing.

Keating, T. (1996). *Intimacy with God.* New York: Crossroads.

Kerfoot, K. (1995). Today's patient care unit manager: Keeping spirituality in managed care: the nurse manager's challenge. *Nursing Economics, 13,* 449-451.

Kim, M.J., McFarland, G.K., & McLane, A.M. (1997). *Pocket guide to nursing diagnoses* (7th ed., pp. 81-83, 423-427). St. Louis: Mosby.

Kleinman, A. (1988). *The illness narratives: Suffering, healing, and the human condition.* New York: Basic Books.

Krippner, S., & Welch, P. (1992). *Spiritual dimension of healing:* From Native shamanism to contemporary health care. New York: Irvington.

Kurzweil, R. (1999). *The age of spiritual machines: When computers exceed human intelligence.* New York: Viking.

Laszlo, E. (1972). *The systems view of the world: The natural philosophy of the new developments in the sciences.* New York: George Braziller.

Levin, J.S. (1996). How prayer heals: A theoretical model. *Alternative Therapy in Health & Medicine, 2,* 66-73.

Lindholm, L., & Eriksson, K. (1993). To understand and alleviate suffering in a caring culture. *Journal of Advanced Nursing, 18,* 1354-1361.

Lindsey, E. (1996). Health within illness: Experiences of chronically ill/disabled people. *Journal of Advanced Nursing, 24,* 465-472.

Longway, I. (1970). Toward a philosophy of nursing. *Journal of Adventist Education, 32,* 20-23, 27.

Macrae, J. (1995). Nightingale's spiritual philosophy and its significance for modern nursing. *Image—The Journal of Nursing Scholarship, 27,* 8-10.

Mairs, N. (1996). *Waist-high in the world: A life among the non-disabled.* Boston: Beacon Press.

Maxson, G. (1987). 'Whose life is it, anyway?' Ours, that's whose! In *On moral medicine: Theological perspectives in medical ethics* (pp. 591-594). Grand Rapids, MI: Eerdmans.

Mayer, J. (1992). Wholly responsible for a part, or partly responsible for a whole? *Second Opinion, 17,* 26-56.

McBride, J.L., Arthur, G., Brooks, R.E., & Pilkington, L. (1998). The relationship between a patient's spirituality and health experience. *Family Medicine, 30,* 122-126.

McCloskey, J.C., & Bulechek, G.M. (Eds.) (2000). *Nursing Interventions Classifications (NIC).* (3rd Ed.) St. Louis: Mosby.

Mendelsohn, R.S. (1979). *Confessions of a medical heretic.* Chicago: Contemporary Books.

Meraviglia, M.G. (1999). Critical analysis of spirituality and its empirical indications: Prayer and the meaning of life. *Journal of Holistic Nursing, 17,* 18-33.

Michaux, A. (1970). *The physically handicapped and the community: Some challenging breakthroughs.* Springfield, IL: C Thomas.

Miller, P.S. (1993). The impact of assisted suicide on persons with disabilities—Is it a right without a freedom? *Issues in Law & Medicine, 9,* 47, 58.

Myss, C. (1996). *Anatomy of the spirit: Seven stages of power and healing.* New York: Harmony.

Narayanasamy, A. (1996). Spiritual care of chronically ill patients. *British Journal of Nursing, 5,* 41-46.

National Council on Disability. (1997). *Assisted suicide: A disability perspective.* Washington, DC: Author.

Nelson, P.B. (1990). Intrinsic/extrinsic religious orientation of the elderly: relationship to depression and self-esteem. *Journal of Gerontological Nursing, 15,* 29-35.

Newman, M. (1986). *Health as expanding consciousness.* St. Louis: Mosby.

Niebuhr, R. (1943). *Serenity prayer.* Heath, MA: Written for service in the Congregational Church.

Pace, J.C., & Stables, J.L. (1997). Correlation of spiritual well-being in terminally ill patients with AIDS and terminally ill patients with cancer. *Journal of the Association of Nurses in AIDS Care, 8,* 31-42.

Pelka, F. (1994). Hating the sick. *Humanist, 54,* 17-20.

Pettigrew, J. (1990). Intensive nursing care: The ministry of presence. *Critical Care Nursing Clinics of North America, 2,* 503-508.

Pope John Paul II (1999, October 1). *Letter of His Holiness Pope John Paul II to the elderly.* Vatican City: Author.

Rahman, F. (1989). *Health and medicine in the Islamic tradition.* New York: Crossroads.

Riley, B.B., Perna, R., Tate, D.G., Forchheimer, M., Anderson, C., & Luera, G. (1998). Types of spiritual well-being among persons with chronic illness: Their relation to various forms of quality of life. *Archives of Physical Medicine and Rehabilitation, 79,* 258-264.

Robinson, J. (1999). Holistic care is an exercise in open-mindedness. *Cincinnati Business Courier, 16,* 31.

Rosenberg, C.E. (1998). Holism in 20th century medicine. In Lawrence, G., Weisz, G. (Eds.), *Greater than the parts: Holism in biomedicine, 1920-1950* (pp. 335-355). New York: Oxford Press.

Schaefer, K.M. (1995). Women living in paradox: Loss and discovery in chronic illness. *Holistic Nursing Practice, 9,* 11-14.

Scully, M. (1995). Viktor Frankl at ninety: An interview. *First Things, 52,* 39-43.

Silber, T.J., & Reilly, M. (1985). Spiritual and religious concerns of the hospitalize adolescent. *Adolescence, 20,* 217-223.

Smuts, J. (1926). *Holism and evolution.* New York: Macmillan.

Smyth, J.M., Stone, A.A., Hurewitz, A., & Kaell A. (1999). Effects of writing about stressful experiences on symptom reduction in patients with asthma or rheumatoid arthritis: A randomized trial. *Journal of the American Medical Association, 281,* 1304-1309.

Snyder, C.R., Hoza, B., Pelham, W.E., Rapoff, M., Ware, L., Danovsky, M., Highbeerger, L., Rubinstein, H., & Stahl, K.J. (1997). The development and validation of the Children's Hope Scale. *Journal of Pediatric Psychology, 22,* 399-421.

Soeken, K., & Carson, V. (1987). Responding to the spiritual needs of the chronically ill. *Nursing Clinics of North America, 22,* 603-611.

Solimine, M.A.E. (1993). Seek and you will find: The librarian and the team. *Holistic Nursing Practice, 7,* 82-90.

Sommer, D.R. (1989). The spiritual needs of dying children. *Issues in Comprehensive Pediatric Nursing, 12,* 225-233.

Stoll, R. (1995). Personal communicatior. Messiah College, PA.

Sumner, C.H. (1998). Recognizing and responding to spiritual distress. *American Journal of Nursing, 98,* 26-30.

Tada, J.E. (1999). How to minister to the disabled: Q and A with Joni Eareckson Tada. [On-line]. Available: http://www.rts.edu/quarterly/spring99/qa.html.

Taylor, E.J., Amenta, M., & Highfield, M. (1995). Spiritual care practices of oncology nurses. *Oncology Nursing Forum, 22,* 31-39.

Thobaben, J.R. (1996). Long-term care. In J.R. Thobaben (Ed.), *Dignity and dying: a Christian appraisal* (pp. 191-207). Grand Rapids, MI: Eerdmans.

Towey, S. (1997). Spiritual self-care: The healer's journey. *Creative Nursing, 3,* 12.

Uustal, D.B. (1992). Rx: Holistic caring in the caregiver. In B.M. Dossey, C.E. Guzzetta, & C.V. Kenner (Eds.), *Critical care nursing: Body-mind-spirit.* (3rd ed., pp. 41-50). Philadelphia: JB Lippincott Co.

Vaillot, S.M. (1970). Hope: the restoration of being. *American Journal of Nursing, 70,* 268.

Vash, C.L. (1994). *Personality and adversity: Psychospiritual aspects of rehabilitation.* New York: Springer.

von Bertalanffy, L. (1955). *General system theory: Foundations, developments, applications.* New York: George Braziller.

Watson, J. (1988). *Theory of nursing: Human science and human care.* New York: National League for Nurses.

Webb-Mitchell, B. (1993). *God plays piano, too: The spiritual lives of disabled children.* New York: Crossroads.

Wilber, K. (1991). *Grace and grit: spirituality and healing in the life and death of Treya Killam Wilber.* Boston: Shambhala.

Wilke, H. (1984). "Get me to the church on time! But can I get in?" *Journal of Rehabilitation, 50,* 55.

Wirth, D.P. (1995). The significance of belief and expectation within the spiritual healing encounter. *Social Science in Medicine, 41,* 249-260.

Wishmant, S. (1999). The parish nurse: Tending to the spiritual side of health. *Holistic Nursing Practice, 14,* 84-86.

Wright, L.M. (1997). Suffering and spirituality: The soul of clinical work with families. *Journal of Family Nursing, 3,* 3-14.

Young, C. (1993). Spirituality and the chronically ill Christian elderly. *Geriatric Nursing, 14,* 298-303.

Young, J.M., & McNicoll, P. (1998). Against all odds: Positive life experiences of people with advanced amyotrophic lateral sclerosis. *Health & Social Work, 23,* 35-43.

SUGGESTED RESOURCES

Kuhn, T.S. (1962). *The structure of scientific revolutions.* Chicago: University of Chicago Press.

L'Arche, a community founded in 1964, with emphasis on the dignity of all persons within. "The rejected, isolated, oppressed, abandoned . . . are welcomed, loved and liberated, as well as are those who care for them; for all there have been wounded. Healing their wounds requires a faithful and tender relationship, a 'being with' the other" (Bryant, 1993). www.larche.org.uk

Healing Community, founded in 1973 by Harold Wilke, a minister who is disabled, was created to help congregations throughout the world become accessible in attitude, architecture and communication in behalf of persons with all types of disabilities and handicaps, not only with regard to mobility-impaired. It was to provide models for the creating of caring congregations, act as consultant to denominations and agencies, and guide theological educators in teaching this concern (Wilke, 1984).

Joni and Friends, an organization helping people with disabilities use evangelical Christian precepts in psychological recovery and adjustment, was founded by a young woman athlete who became quadriplegic. It wants to communicate the Gospel and disciple disabled people—to integrate them into church fellowship as indispensable believers. To this end, it offers practical ways to address their needs (Tada, 1999).

Pediatric Rehabilitation Nursing 29

Deirdre F. Jackson, MSN, APRN, CRRN

Marcus and Patricia had tried to become pregnant for years and finally were successful. Patricia had excellent prenatal care and there were no pregnancy complications until Patricia went into labor at 32 weeks. When Amanda was born 36 hours later, she was taken immediately to the neonatal intensive care unit. Amanda was weaned from oxygen and was breathing well on her own; however, she continued to need tube feedings because of poor oral feeding skills. By the day of discharge, all test results were normal. But doctors were concerned about some abnormal motor signs and her continued irritability and poor feeding. Amanda was referred to the developmental follow-up clinic for further assessment in 3 months.

I met Marcus, Patricia, and Amanda on their first visit to the developmental follow-up clinic. During this first visit, Patricia reported that Amanda was still very irritable and hard to console. She was gaining weight slowly but Patricia was frustrated that she often took more than 60 minutes to feed. Marcus and Patricia knew that "something was wrong" with their daughter but we could not give them a definitive diagnosis. After that first visit, I spoke with Patricia by telephone on an almost daily basis to provide support and encouragement.

By the 6-month visit, Amanda still could not hold her head up. She slept poorly, was difficult to calm, and still had very poor feeding skills. When she cried her legs were so stiff that Patricia could not undress her. There was no question that Amanda had cerebral palsy.

I remember Marcus' and Patricia's faces when we explained Amanda's diagnosis and what they could expect. They were upset by the news but also relieved to finally have an answer to many of their questions. They were also encouraged that there were early intervention services close to their home to help them. At the early intervention program (EIP), Patricia learned feeding and calming strategies and therapy exercises to help Amanda. Patricia also established a support network with other mothers who were experiencing the same sense of loss and frustration. Several months later, they were transferred out of state to another army base. The Christmas after they moved I received a card that read,

Well we're here in Texas but I think of you every day. I miss our daily talks more than you know. I have found a new EIP and the staff there is great, too. Amanda is making small gains. Thank you for listening, supporting, and encouraging but never lying to us about how challenging and yet rewarding it would be to raise Amanda. Every day I remember to think of her as my daughter (first) who just happens to have cerebral palsy (second).

Pediatric rehabilitation nursing is a specialty practice area that continues to grow within the field of rehabilitation. This chapter traces the evolution and the expanding scope of this specialty. The unique role of the pediatric rehabilitation nurse is described. A developmental framework is suggested as a conceptual model for practice, and applied to discussion of the impact of disabilities across pediatric age groups. Medical and societal trends that affect the field are examined. Public laws protecting the educational rights of children with disabilities are identified. Strategies for assessment are presented along with interventions and outcomes based on nursing diagnoses commonly associated with selected chronic illnesses and disabilities. The chapter concludes with several case histories that highlight the complexity of care needs—a common finding in children receiving pediatric rehabilitation services.

EVOLUTION OF PEDIATRIC REHABILITATION

The field of pediatric rehabilitation has experienced marked development over the past century. In the late nineteenth century, "homes" and training schools were established for individuals with specific problems such as blindness and crippling conditions (Edwards, 1992). Near the turn of the century, the concept of a multidisciplinary approach emerged as restorative and reconstructive procedures were incorporated into the care of people with disabilities. During the 1940s many new rehabilitation facilities were established, some of which specialized in the care of children (Allan, 1958). Congenital neurological and orthopedic problems commonly were seen.

Through the end of the twentieth century, the scope of the field has continued to broaden. Many pediatric rehabilitation facilities now provide care for children with chronic conditions, acquired disabilities, and developmental disabilities. Some of these children are also dependent on technology for their survival. The Centers for Disease Control and Prevention (CDC) introduced the new National Center for Birth Defects and Developmental Disabilities (NCBDDD) in April 2001. Goals of the new center are prevention of birth defects and developmental disabilities, promotion of optimal development for children, and wellness for persons with disabilities. The Children's Health Act of 2000 provided for the NCBDDD (CDC, 2001).

UNIQUENESS OF THE PEDIATRIC REHABILITATION NURSE

Although rehabilitation services have been provided for children for quite some time, the field of pediatric rehabilitation nursing is relatively new (Selekman, 1991). In the mid-1980s the Pediatric Special-Interest Group was formed within the Association of Rehabilitation Nurses. The membership described the role of the pediatric rehabilitation nurse in the publication *Pediatric rehabilitation nursing-role description* (Pediatric Special Interest Group, 1992). Pediatric rehabilitation nurses are both specialists and generalists: specialists by virtue of age of their clients and generalists as a result of the broad diagnostic categories they serve.

Inherent in the specialized approach is the nurse's acceptance of a child with disability as a valued member of society who is first and foremost a child, and secondly a child with special needs. This approach requires the nurse to be able to accept and celebrate small accomplishments and establish outcomes that focus on optimal levels of performance for that child.

Advanced Practice Pediatric Rehabilitation Nurse

Advanced practice pediatric rehabilitation nurses can assume a wide variety of roles across the health care continuum, including expert clinician, care coordinator, primary care provider, early intervention nurse, school nurse, educator, consultant, researcher, political activist, administrator, or manager (Neal, 1997). Regardless of the role assumed or the practice setting, advanced practice pediatric rehabilitation nurses must have in-depth knowledge of the theories, issues, and legislation affecting the pediatric rehabilitation population. They must also have a strong knowledge of client management strategies across pediatric rehabilitation settings and be able to effect positive outcomes through teams of professionals (Jackson & Wallingford, 1997).

PEDIATRIC REHABILITATION POPULATION

In 1994, 18% of children in the United States had a special health care need. The Maternal Child Health Bureau defines this population as follows:

Children with special health care needs are those who have or are at increased risk for a chronic physical, developmental, behavioral, or emotional condition and who require health and related services of a type or amount beyond that required by children generally (McPherson et al., 1998, p. 138).

These are the children cared for in pediatric rehabilitation settings. Children with special health care needs may have congenital or acquired disorders. Many of these disorders are also rare. The increased numbers of survivors of childhood illness, prematurity and serious injuries contribute to this population. This variety in disorders is a defining characteristic of pediatric rehabilitation (Table 29-1). Several specific groups of children that are relatively new to pediatric rehabilitation settings are discussed below.

Human Immunodeficiency Virus/Acquired Immunodeficiency Syndrome

The first case of acquired immunodeficiency syndrome (AIDS) in the pediatric population was reported in 1982. From that time through December 1999, there were 8,718 cases in children younger than 13 years of age reported to the CDC. Perinatal transmission accounts for 90% of pediatric AIDS cases and almost all new human immunodeficiency virus (HIV) infections in children (CDC, 1999a). Multiple studies have shown that HIV testing during pregnancy and drug therapies for HIV-infected mothers have decreased perinatal transmission rates over the past 5 years to as low as 5% (Lindegren, Steinberg, & Byers, 2000).

Diagnostic advances and combination drug therapies have increased life expectancy for many children who are HIV positive. As a result of these advances, rehabilitation specialists may need to treat clients who have a variety AIDS-related conditions, including severe failure to thrive, developmental delays, learning disabilities, and encephalopathy (Dwyer, 2000). Modifications in typical treatment approaches may be necessary to accommodate the deconditioned state of the acutely ill child. In addition to the medical aspects of this disease, many psychosocial issues must be considered.

TABLE 29-1 Common Pediatric Rehabilitation Conditions/Situations

Acquired Disabilities	Problems of Premature and Low Birth Weight	Developmental Disabilities	Congenital Disorders	Chronic Illnesses	Miscellaneous Disorders	Technology-Dependent
Burns	Bronchopulmonary dysplasia	Cerebral palsy	Congenital heart disease	Asthma	Neuromuscular diseases	Ventilator
Traumatic brain injury	Short gut	Spina bifida	Down syndrome	Human immunodeficiency virus	No diagnosis	Oxygen
Spinal cord injury	Infants of drug and alcohol addicted mothers	Limb deficiencies	Miscellaneous syndromes	Juvenile diabetes	Encephalitis	Total parenteral nutrition
Near drowning	Feeding disorders	Muscular dystrophy		Juvenile rheumatoid arthritis	Meningitis	Tracheostomy
Cerebral vascular accident				Seizure disorders	Anoxia (suicide attempts, drug overdose, birth asphyxia)	Enteral feeding tube
				Renal failure	Orthopedic conditions	
				Hematology/oncology disorders		

Hematology/Oncology Disorders

The sequelae of hematology/oncology problems are being seen more frequently in rehabilitation settings. In the recent past, limited survival rates precluded the need for such services. However, Philip, Ayyanger, Vanderbilt, and Gaebler-Spira (1994) described the positive effects of rehabilitation on functional outcome after treatment for primary brain tumors. Goals in the rehabilitation setting are generally focused on managing complications from surgeries, radiation and chemotherapy, and reintegrating the child into the community. Complications include cardiomyopathies, pulmonary fibrosis, orthopedic problems, and neurological deficits.

Technology-Dependent Children

Another population that is increasing is that of children who are dependent on or assisted by technology for survival (e.g., total parenteral nutrition, oxygen, or ventilators). These children may be cared for in intensive care units, long-term care facilities, pediatric rehabilitation centers, or in the home. Each setting has its own limitations. Intensive care units are extremely costly. Technology-dependent children take up beds that may be more appropriately used for children with acute care needs. These units are generally not able to meet the long-term developmental needs of these children and their families. There are a very limited number of long-term care facilities that accept children on ventilators. Often a long-term care facility's staffing ratios do not provide for developmental interventions, intensity of care, or the vigilance that some children on ventilators require. Pediatric rehabilitation units are better able to meet the ongoing developmental needs of clients, but again bed space may be limited. In each of these hospital-based settings the child has limited exposure to the real world (e.g., sunshine, breezes, rain, and snow) and too much exposure to hospital routines and infections.

The home setting provides another care alternative. Discharge to the home setting requires an extensive and comprehensive multidisciplinary plan. Community resources such as a primary care pediatrician, a case manager, home nursing services, and durable medical equipment must be available. School systems must be able to accommodate and provide a safe environment for the child who is dependent on technology. Common issues for families in the home setting are fear of technological failure, exhaustion from constant care needs, inadequate respite, loss of personal freedom and employment opportunities, lack of full-time nurses, and transportation challenges. Although home care presents a more cost-effective alternative to long hospital stays, there are many "hidden" expenses that are not covered by insurance—such as utility bills, electrical renovations, and lost income (Capen & Dedlow, 1998).

DEVELOPMENTAL FRAMEWORK

Developmental theory is fundamental to pediatric rehabilitation nursing because children are continuing to grow and mature throughout the rehabilitation process. The pediatric rehabilitation nurse must continuously revise goals and tailor interventions to the child's currently expected level of development rather than the level of development that was expected at the time of admission to the care setting. Age-specific communication skills, knowledge of developmentally appropriate play, and creative problem solving are necessary skills for promoting developmental milestones (Selekman, 1991). In addition, emphasis should always be placed on the child's abilities rather than limitations. Clearly, special skills are needed to optimally care for children with disabilities, as "children are not small adults" (Figure 29-1).

Children grow and develop in several realms: physical, cognitive, social, and emotional. Growth and development proceed in a predictable, sequential fashion for all children. It is the individual rate and level of achievement that vary.

Physical Growth, Gross Motor, and Fine Motor

In the physical realm, growth occurs in a cephalocaudal manner. Height, weight, and head circumference are important indicators of health and disease. These growth parameters should be tracked serially and plotted on standardized charts. Children must also acquire mobility to negotiate their environment and fine motor skills to eat, dress, toilet, and groom themselves.

Cognitive, Social, and Emotional Development

Cognitive development progresses from concrete to abstract thinking, which ultimately provides for learning and problem solving (Piaget, 1952). In the social realm children develop a trusting relationship first with their parents or primary caregivers, then their siblings, and ultimately with strangers (Erickson, 1963). They also learn socially appropriate behavior and culturally acceptable norms. A positive body image and self-esteem are essential building blocks of healthy emotional development.

Play, Sports, and Recreation

Play is the life work of children, occupying the majority of the day. It is the child's vehicle for exploration and learning. Play also helps children to master anxiety-provoking situations—for instance, catheterizing a doll during medical play. Involvement in sports provides fun and exercise, while allowing for development of peer relationships and self-esteem. There is a wide range of adapted equipment and organized programs available to enable children with special health care needs to participate in sports and recreational activities (e.g., Special Olympics, National Wheelchair Athletic Associations, U.S. Cerebral Palsy Athletic Association) (Kaitz & Miller, 1999).

Camps provide another recreational outlet for children with disabilities and chronic illnesses. Camps may be organized around a particular disability or chronic illness or they may provide the opportunity for children to be mainstreamed into programs for children without disabilities. Some camping programs operate year-round to provide recreation during school vacations or ongoing respite for families.

IMPACT OF DISABILITY

The meaning and impact of chronic illness and disability varies for each child. However, the effects of disability are similar in that they create "differentness" in performance or achievement, services required, participation in life events or sequences, and connectedness. Physical growth and development may be below expected age or qualitatively unusual. Special services or assistive technology and devices may be necessary for success and participation in school and recreation. Relationships with family, peers, and significant

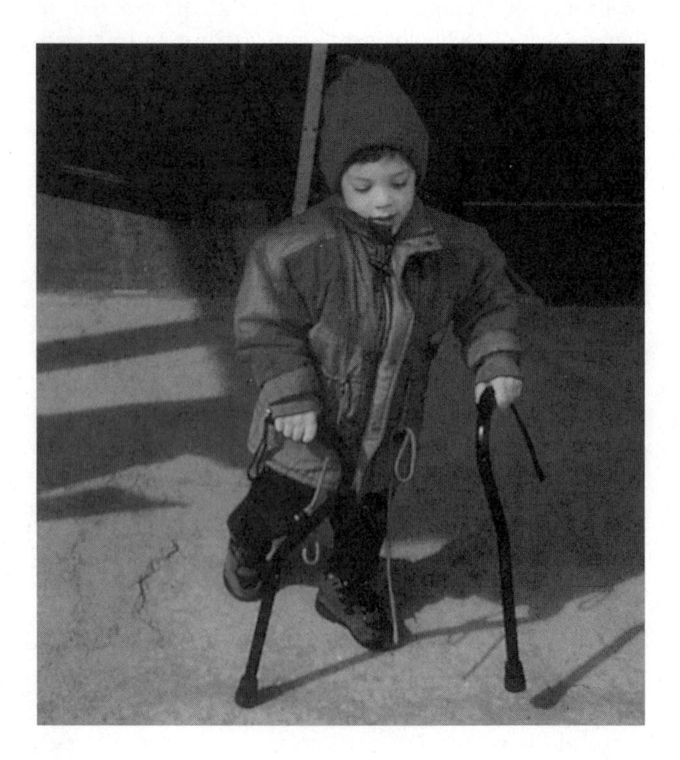

Figure 29-1 Children are not miniature adults. They require care and equipment designed especially for their growth, development, and disabling disorders. (From Wong, D.L., Hockenberry-Eaton, M., Wilson, D., Winkelstein, M.L., & Schwartz, P. [2000]. *Wong's essentials of pediatric nursing* [6th ed.]. St. Louis: Mosby.)

others may be altered (Crocker, 1996). These psychosocial factors may be greater determinants of overall success in life that the severity of the child's disability (Easton, Rens, & Alexander, 1999). The following sections discuss the impact of disability across pediatric age specific populations. Developmental tasks, effects of disability, and intervention strategies are summarized in Table 29-2.

Infancy (Birth to 1 Year of Age)

When a child is born with or acquires a chronic or disabling condition during infancy, the implications are far reaching. Parents often experience guilt and may grieve the loss of the child of their dreams (Solnit & Stark, 1962). Parent-infant bonding may be interrupted or impaired because of the physical or behavioral characteristics of the infant. Infants with disabilities are often difficult to calm and they may have impaired ability to communicate their basic needs (Easton et al., 1999). Separation anxiety may be exacerbated by multiple hospitalizations.

Toddlerhood (1 to 4 Years of Age)

The toddler is a concrete thinker who affords life and function to all objects. Reasoning is transductive; therefore, illness may be viewed by the child as a consequence of "bad" behavior (Pontious, 1982). Disability and hospitalization may separate parents and children for extended periods of time. Equipment and physical environments may limit mobility. Toddlers are often forced to be dependent (e.g., spica cast prevents getting to toilet independently or safety dictates that child sleep in crib). At times parents may be reluctant to set appropriate limits for children with special health care needs; however, failure to do so may interfere with development of impulse control (Perrin & Gerrity, 1984).

Early Childhood/Preschool (4 to 6 Years of Age)

The preoperational phase of cognitive development (Piaget, 1952) provides the preschool child with a basic understanding of rules of social behavior and a basic sense of right and wrong (Kohlberg, 1969). Disability and chronic illness can limit mobility and disrupt established routines. Body invasion and mutilation are key fears; thus, treatments including burn dressings, bladder catheterization, and injections may be perceived as punishment for bad behavior. Time constraints and overprotection may prevent parents from expecting children to perform activities of daily living (ADLs) independently.

Middle Childhood/School Age (6 to 12 Years of Age)

The school-aged child has a greater understanding of the body, causation of illness, and treatment processes than does the younger child. There is a shift in emphasis from home to peers and school. School-aged children with special health care needs may need help with personal care and often take more time to move through the environment. Learning disabilities may also become evident during early elementary school years. In addition to academic learning, the structure of the classroom and interactions with classmates provide an opportunity for learning social skills and making friends. But having the "opportunity" does not guarantee these children will accepted. School-aged children with disabilities need to develop the social skills to overcome the fears and prejudice they may face (Easton et al., 1999). Isolation, withdrawal, depression, and social dysfunction can result if the child is not well integrated into family, school, and community life. Whenever possible, therapies and other health-related activities should be scheduled so that they do not interfere with critical academic subjects and peer relationships.

Adolescence (12 to 18 Years of Age)

Adolescence is a period marked by rapid growth, profound physiological changes, development of higher order reasoning abilities, an emerging personal identify, and a budding interest in the opposite sex (Molnar, 1988). The peer group is highly influential, and there is a strong need to be a part of the crowd. It is a tumultuous time for adolescents as they strive to attain independence from their parents.

Whether the disability is congenital, as with limb deficiency, or acquired, such as traumatic amputation, the impact on psychosocial functioning can be great. The adolescent may have to adapt to separation from school and peers, changes in body image, discomfort, limitations in mobility, and involvement with the health care system.

During adolescence there is a preoccupation with physical characteristics, and "different" automatically implies "imperfect" (Perrin & Gerrity, 1984). A person whose physical appearance is altered or who may require assistive devices for mobility may be perceived as less attractive to members of the opposite sex (Thompson, 1990). Because body image is so important and control over one's body increases self-esteem and confidence, every attempt should be made to get adolescents out of diapers through intermittent catheterization programs or external devices as appropriate.

Socialization is another problem area for adolescents with special health care needs. They may find themselves with limited friends and minimal opportunities for social interactions. Getting to social functions may be logistically difficult. Limited ability to perform the "3Ds"—dating, driving, and dressing—may create social isolation (Thompson, 1990).

Sexuality is a concept that should be addressed throughout the life span of an individual. However, specific issues may surface at this stage related to sexual functioning and fertility. Any teen that is capable of communicating should be allowed time alone with the physician or nurse to ask questions and voice their concerns. Their goals and issues may be very different from those of their parents. However, it is not uncommon for adolescents to be hesitant about sharing thoughts and feelings, particularly with adults. Therefore

TABLE 29-2 Summary of Developmental Tasks, Effects of Disability, and Coping Skills and Intervention Strategies

Stage	Developmental Profile	Effects of Disability	Coping Skills	Intervention Strategies
Infancy	Trust versus mistrust Sitting, crawling, walking Sensorimotor exploration and discrimination Visual tracking Pincer grasp Recognizes bottle Eats solid foods Differentiate self from environment Cause and effect Separation anxiety Object permanence (beginning)	Unpredictable caretakers Delays in having needs met Pain Limited exploration of environment Inappropriate sensory stimulation	Crying Motor activity (e.g., kicking legs, thumb sucking, pacifier sucking)	Give information about child's condition and trajectory of condition Provide consistent nurturing and caregiving Support breast-feeding, if desired Respond to needs in a timely fashion Give appropriate sensory stimulation Permit freedom to move and explore Provide verbal and vestibular soothing Provide toys and activities adapted to disability (e.g., switch-activated)
Toddlerhood	Autonomy versus shame and doubt Walks alone Climbing Hand dominance Drinks from cup Language acquisition and development Says "no" Begins toilet training Object permanence (established) Asserts independence Separation from parents Imitation, fantasy, and play Concrete thinking Egocentricity (limited ability to see another viewpoint)	Separation difficulties Limited mobility and exploration Forced dependence Overprotection No limit setting Lack of ability to control elimination functions	Crying Protest Temper tantrums Demanding attention Repetitive activity Play and fantasy Behavioral regression Time-out	Allow parents and siblings to be involved in care Provide independent mobility Promote independence in activities of daily living (ADLs) Provide safe outlets for tension reduction Set limits Break instructions down into small parts Teach basic sign language to communicate needs Teach parents caregiving and limit-setting skills
Early childhood (preschool)	Initiative versus guilt Exploration and mastery of environment Running Rides tricycle Toilet trained Independence in self care activities Fantasy and magical thinking Fears (e.g., dark, body mutilation) Asks why, when, how Identifies self as boy or girl	Lack of stamina Difficulty establishing body image Overprotection No limit setting Limited mobility Impaired communication Lack of normal routine Lack of choice	Routines and ritualized activities Imaginative play Physical or verbal aggression	Use pictures to help communication Integrate play and fantasy into therapies and treatments Support established routines Allow parents to be present to decrease anxiety Provide independent mobility Offer realistic choices Encourage and assist with independence in ADLs Teach parents caregiving and limit settings skills

Data from Jackson, D., & Wallingford, P. (1997). Nursing care across the age continuum: Children and adolescents. In K.M.M. Johnson (Ed.), *Advanced practice nursing in rehabilitation: A core curriculum* (pp. 87-108). Glenview, IL: Association of Rehabilitation Nurses.

TABLE 29-2 Summary of Developmental Tasks, Effects of Disability, and Coping Skills and Intervention Strategies—cont'd

Stage	Developmental Profile	Effects of Disability	Coping Skills	Intervention Strategies
Middle childhood (school-aged)	Industry versus inferiority Rides bicycle Roller skates Increased independence Starts school Competition and cooperation Starts to read Same-sex peer relationships Consideration of other points of view Logical thought Develops academic skills (conservation, reversibility, and time concepts)	Lack of stamina Inability to participate in social/ recreational activities Inaccessible schools Missed school Feelings of inferiority Forced dependence Incontinence (when should be continent)	Humor Withdrawal Verbal aggression Physical aggression Depression Hides disability or chronic illness from peers and others	Allow participation in or direction of self care and procedures Use models and diagrams to teach self care Correct disability-related misconceptions Maintain peer and sibling relationships when hospitalized Assign household responsibilities and chores Set up situations where child can be successful Educate school personnel and classmates about child's disability Obtain assistive devices and adaptations to make schools and playgrounds accessible Foster friendships with sleepovers and outings Enhance opportunities to relate to others with similar difficulties Facilitate participation in organized sports and recreation expectations
Adolescence	Identity versus role confusion Rapid growth Puberty Establishes identity Sexuality development Increased emotional independence Need for privacy Conflicts with parents Peer relationships with larger groups Dating Driving Set future career and personal goals Abstract thinking Transition to adult roles	Altered body image Separation from peers Missed school Forced dependence Delayed puberty Limited behavioral and style experimentation (hair color, tattoos, piercings) Limited risk taking Vocational and social limitation	Denial Intellectualization Despair Resentment Conformity Withdrawal Noncompliance Risk-taking behavior	Give independence in self care and decision making as much as possible Allow to fail Respect need for privacy Listen to perceptions of illness and clarify misconceptions Give honest, accurate sexuality information Dress in developmentally appropriate clothing Assist in giving attention to overall appearance and cleanliness Teach how to deal with unwanted sexual advances and emergency situations Provide electric wheelchairs for independent mobility Facilitate peer interactions through clubs, dances, and sports and recreation

clinicians must be alert to cues that may indicate a desire to talk and be willing to listen. The nurse and other members of the rehabilitation team are highly influential in the development and adjustment of children with chronic illness and disability as they mature into productive adults.

TRANSITION TO ADULTHOOD

The majority of children born today with a chronic illness or disability will survive into adulthood (Scal, Evans, Blozis, Okinow, & Blum, 1999). Unemployment, reliance on public assistance and social security, and poverty are realities for many adults with disabilities. Few people with disabilities achieve a college education and the majority do not live independently (Betz, 1998). According to Betz (1998), "the goal of transition care is to foster the achievement of responsible self-care and linkages to adult health care services, thereby enabling the most optimal prospects for educational options, employment, social relationships and networks, and community living" (p. 23). Thus it is crucial that preparations for the fully functioning adult lifestyle begin at the person's point of entry into the rehabilitation system.

Barriers to Success

The transition from childhood through adolescence to adulthood is challenging for all children, but often it is more difficult for the child with a special health care need. These adolescents are often not well prepared for the transition to adulthood. People without disabilities often feel the need to protect and make decisions for them; thus, an adolescent may not have had the opportunity to develop decision-making skills. Parents often continue to speak for their adolescents, (i.e., during visits with nurse practitioners or physicians), further limiting opportunities for the adolescent to express feelings and concerns. The adolescent with a special health care need may have been protected from family responsibilities and therefore may be lacking in basic skills such as performing household chores.

Health Transition

The passage into adulthood brings with it some unique concerns related to health maintenance. One issue is that of transitioning from the pediatric to the adult rehabilitation team. Ideally the stage is set for this transition in the mid-to-late teenage years. Both adolescents and parents must be prepared to leave the team of health professionals with whom they have a long-standing relationship. Many adolescents and young adults continue to be followed by their pediatrician, but this typically occurs because of difficulty finding an adult general physician willing and capable of providing care rather than unwillingness to transition on the part of the family (Scal et al., 1999). Insurance coverage is another consideration. It may be difficult to impossible for young adults to obtain insurance coverage if they are no longer considered a dependent (Betz, 1998).

Comprehensive transitional health care models are lacking. Demonstration models are currently being funded. These models need to include provision of comprehensive services for health maintenance as well as vocational and social counseling (Betz, 1998; Scal et al., 1999).

Vocational Transition

At this point in life, most young adults without disabilities have solidified their self-identity and career plans and have established or are working toward personal and financial independence. Individual transition plans (ITPs) are the tools used to assist adolescents with disabilities in moving toward the same level of independence. ITPs, which are mandated by Public Law 101-476, the Individuals with Disabilities Education Act, are developed in the educational setting between the ages of 14 and 16. Rehabilitation professionals, educators, parents, and the student conduct an assessment of student's abilities and skills. The plan that is developed includes details of the services and supports needed for successful postsecondary education, job training, employment, and community living (Betz, 1998).

Community Mobility

Community mobility is important for employment, as is participation in social and recreational activities. Driver's evaluation and training programs are available through some vocational rehabilitation centers or departments. Assessments can be made of the cognitive and physical abilities required for safe driving skills. If driving is not feasible, educating the adolescent or young adult in how to use public transportation of all types can increase locus of control. Feeling in control of one's life is essential in establishing the independence and self-determination needed to function as an adult in society.

The pediatric rehabilitation nurse can play a key role in supporting adolescents through the transition process. Health professionals can assist families in accessing appropriate health care services, encourage parents to allow teens to make informed decisions about their health care, and educate adolescents about their rights. Teaching self-care management strategies and connecting teens with peer or adult mentors with similar disabilities are other ways that nurses can support transition.

FAMILY ISSUES

Coping and Adjustment

Disability and chronic illness have a far-reaching impact on the entire family system. A variety of events that may be directly or indirectly related to child's illness produce stress. Travel to distant trauma or rehabilitation centers, high care needs, lost time from work, problems with school systems, fatigue, trouble finding baby-sitters, and lost leisure time are just a few of the challenges families face (Sterling, Jones,

Johnson, & Bowen, 1996). And these are in addition to major and daily life stresses we all experience. Siblings experience altered family routines, competition for parents' time and attention, and increased responsibility.

But in spite of these issues, most parents and siblings make a positive adjustment. Having appropriate resources can help them cope with stress and manage the child effectively. For adults, professionals and family are the primary support system (Easton et al., 1999). Involvement in support groups, time alone with parents, the ability to continue their own activities, and participation in family decision-making can support sibling adjustment (Crocker, 1996). Additional family supports that have been identified as important include:

- Nurses and other health professionals
- Support from spouses, extended families, and friends
- Formal parent networks
- Training on the child's health needs
- Adequate transportation
- Education on rights and entitlements
- Available financial resources and insurance coverage
- Religious beliefs and prayer
- Legal services (Crocker, 1996; Sterling et al., 1996)

Identifying resources for respite care and day care has been identified as crucial for successful management in the community (Cernoch & Newhouse, 1996; Sterling et al., 1996).

Respite Care

All parents need an occasional break from parenting and this is also true for parents of children with special health care needs. In addition to providing direct relief, respite has added benefits for families (Box 29-1).

Box 29-1 Benefits of Respite Care

*R*elaxation. Respite gives families peace of mind, helps them relax, and renews their humor and energy
*E*njoyment. Respite allows families to enjoy favorite pastimes and pursue new activities
*S*tability. Respite improves the family's ability to cope with daily responsibilities and maintain stability during crisis
*P*reservation. Respite helps preserve the family unit and lessens the pressures that might lead to institutionalization, divorce, neglect, and child abuse
*I*nvolvement. Respite allows families to become involved in community activities and to feel less isolated
*T*ime off. Respite allows families to take that needed vacation, spend time together and time alone
*E*nrichment. Respite makes it possible for family members to establish individual identities and enrich their own growth and development

Data from National Information Center for Children and Youth with Disabilities. (1996, June). Respite care. *NICHCY News Digest* (No. ND12). Available: http://www.nichcy.org/pubs/newsdig/nd12txt.htm.

Federal legislation authorizes funding to states for respite care, but access and affordability are still issues in many communities. Connecting with groups and professionals in the community who work with children of similar ages to the child with the disability can assist in locating these critical services (National Information Center for Children and Youth with Disabilities, 1996). Assisting parents in locating respite services, either within the extended family network or community, can be an extremely valuable role for nurses and social services.

Day Care

Despite the increasing number of laws and incentives, parents of young children with disability or chronic illness still are struggling with limited programs and waiting lists. More than 1 million children with special needs younger than 6 years of age have mothers who could be in the workforce. Fewer than 10% of mothers of children with special health care needs can locate adequate child care (Fewell, 1993). Crowley (1990) found that some privately owned centers and all publicly funded centers *could* accept children with disabilities. However, most mainstream day care centers lack staff who are adequately trained or experienced in the management of children with disabilities. Space, support services, and staffing ratios are also barriers; therefore, they are reluctant to undertake this responsibility.

By providing day care personnel with the appropriate resources and training, there is hope that a greater comfort level will be achieved in caring for this population, thus increasing enrollment. Increased enrollment provides opportunities for nurses to become involved in health education of child care providers and legislative activities, to serve as liaisons to the community, and to advocate with parents for increased services.

Family-Centered Care

Disability and chronic illness bring families and health care workers together over the continuum of pediatric rehab settings. The family is responsible for advocating for the child's rights to the best care, education, and resources available. Role conflicts, differing opinions, and limiting hospital policies were part of the driving force behind a major philosophical change in care delivery. In 1997, the Rehabilitation Accreditation Commission (CARF) endorsed pediatric family-centered rehabilitation programs for comprehensive inpatient rehabilitation. This philosophy involves the client and family at all phases of care with full membership on the interdisciplinary team. Within family-centered care the child must be viewed as an integral part of a family system, with the family and home as the central focus of the child's world. Key elements of family-centered care include:

1. The family is the constant, but health care systems and personnel change
2. Recognition of family diversity, strengths, and individuality

3. Complete unbiased information exchange
4. Family-to-family support is encouraged and facilitated (Hostler, 1999)

Rehabilitation nurses and other personnel who have contact with children with special health care needs share an important role and responsibility with the families in shaping each child's future.

CARE SETTINGS

Infants, children, and adolescents with special health care needs are major users of health care services in a wide variety of settings.

Acute Inpatient Rehabilitation

Pediatric rehabilitation services were traditionally provided on acute inpatient pediatric rehabilitation units. These units may have been part of a larger acute care hospital, a larger rehabilitation facility, or a freestanding pediatric rehabilitation center. Like many other types of hospitals, changes in reimbursement have had a profound effect on pediatric rehabilitation service delivery during the past decade. Many facilities that have been freestanding for more than 100 years have merged, affiliated, reduced the number of inpatient beds, or closed altogether. Inpatient stays, once long and intensive, have been streamlined significantly. For example, hospitalizations for spinal cord injury, which once spanned 6 to 12 months, have now been reduced to 60 days in some cases.

Day Hospital and Medical Day Care

Today the trend is clearly toward outpatient and community-based services. Children can attend comprehensive outpatient day hospital or medical day care programs during the day Monday through Friday. Nursing care, cognitive retraining, therapies, and educational services are provided by the multidisciplinary team. The children return home each evening. This trend supports the philosophy of keeping children in their most natural environment: family and community. In addition, it provides a more cost-effective alternative to the inpatient approach to rehabilitative care. Unfortunately these types of programs are not available in all communities and may not be covered by all insurance carriers.

Home Care

Home care is a rapidly growing segment of the health care continuum. This growth has been driven by consumer desire, technological improvements such as portable ventilators, and health care financing issues. To meet the needs of the varied pediatric rehabilitation population, home care agencies must be able to provide or access a full range of services including skilled nursing care, home health aides, professional therapies, infusion services, and durable medical equipment services (Madigan, 1997). They must also have staff with the same level of expertise as hospital- and clinic-based pediatric rehabilitation nurses with the added skill of dealing with situations that happen only in the community environment.

Reimbursement for home care services varies widely among insurers. State medicaid programs are the major payment source for the majority of pediatric cases (Clemens, Davis, Novak, & Connell, 1997). Federal medicaid waiver programs provide coverage for many technology-dependent children cared for in the home setting. Waiver programs allow families to bypass the usual income requirements for medicaid eligibility. Other sources of payment include funds from state and community organizations for children with special health care needs (Madigan, 1997).

The role of the pediatric rehabilitation nurse in a home care setting is to teach the family about the chronic illness or disability so that they can provide care, administer medication, identify problems, and intervene appropriately (Madigan, 1997). Insurers may discharge children home with 16 hours of nursing care reimbursed, only to decrease that reimbursement to 8 hours within weeks. As reimbursement from insurers continues to change, parental training and identification of alternate care providers is critical for the health and safety of the child in the home care setting.

Outpatient Services

Outpatient services include clinics and therapy services. The increased demand for outpatient pediatric rehabilitation services has given rise to private, for-profit outpatient therapy practices. These practices often are appealing because of more convenient locations, flexible service hours, and minimal waiting lists.

School

Pediatric rehabilitation services may also be provided in school settings as an adjunct to facility-based services. Public laws mandating these services in early intervention, preschool, and school settings will be discussed later in this chapter.

ACCESS TO CARE

Access to health care includes having insurance to pay for care and having identified providers for regular and specialty care. In 1998, 15% of all children less than 18 years of age in the United States had no health insurance coverage. Poor children represented 30.6% of the total uninsured child population. Of those children with coverage 19.8% were covered by public health insurance (U.S. Census Bureau. United States Department of Commerce, 1999).

In an effort to control health care costs, state medicaid

and other insurance providers have changed from traditional fee-for-service to managed care plans. Most managed care plans require a primary care pediatrician who serves as the gatekeeper to the health system. These plans could benefit children with special health care needs by improving access to primary health care and case management services.

On the other hand, managed care plans may increase the difficulty in accessing rehabilitation services. Families may be required to leave physicians with whom they have an established relationship. They may be "forced" to receive care from physicians who have no interest or time to coordinate and provide care for children with special health care needs. Most pediatricians have little experience and have received limited training in skills needed to manage these children effectively (Sneed, May, & Stencel, 2000). Access to pediatric specialists and other rehabilitation services may also be affected if these providers are not part of the managed care plan (Committee on Children with Special Needs, 1998). As more children with chronic illness and disability survive and return to the community, these issues become more critical. Continued work is needed to educate primary care providers and develop community-based networks to meet the complex needs of these client populations (Hoeman, 1997).

Case Management

The shift to community-based services and managed care has contributed to the growth in need for case management services. Case management includes "direct and indirect service provision, service coordination across programs and over time, and assurance of achieving planned goals" (Biehl, 1997, p. 260). Implicit in this definition is the requirement of helping families meet both current and future goals in a timely and cost-effective manner. High care-coordination needs occur when children with disabilities and chronic illness are discharged from the hospital, enter school or the special education setting, transition to adulthood, or when their health status changes (Ziring et al., 1999).

Parents, an agency, a health professional, or a combination of these people may assume the role of case manager. Qualifications for a case manager include knowledge of the issues of infants, children, and adolescents with chronic illness and disabilities; knowledge of the requirements of relevant disability legislation; knowledge of the nature and scope of services available in the state; and knowledge of insurance benefits and other available funding. Case managers also must have expert documentation skills and ability to effectively communicate information to the rehabilitation team and family. Pediatric rehabilitation nurses have traditionally cared for children and families from a holistic perspective, thereby uniquely qualifying them to function in the role of case manager. With greater numbers of children and families requiring these services, it is likely that pediatric rehab nurses will increasingly assume case management responsibilities.

FACTORS ASSOCIATED WITH PEDIATRIC REHABILITATION

Poverty

Poverty is a societal problem that influences chronic illness and disability in children and adolescents. The poverty rate for children was 18% in 1998. The typical profile of a child living in poverty is a child younger than the age of 6 years, living in a household led by a single woman, who is black or Hispanic. Children who are living below the poverty level or who are homeless are more likely to have to no usual source of health care. Health problems among these children include poor general health, underimmunization, malnutrition, high infant morbidity and mortality rates, lead poisoning, illicit drug use, HIV infection, and child abuse (Federal Interagency Forum on Child and Family Statistics, 1999).

Foster Care

Many children in foster care come from homes where parents have HIV or AIDS or problems with drugs and alcohol abuse. Some have suffered child abuse as well. Young children with chronic illness and disability are the fastest growing population of children in foster care. Although there are some families willing to assume the added responsibility of caring for children with complex medical and behavioral problems, more families are needed. Foster parents need adequate financial support, education and training regarding the child's care, and support and respect from health care professionals for their knowledge and love of these special children (Barton, 1999).

Unintentional and Intentional Injury

Unintentional injury is the leading cause of death and disability in children ages 14 and under. Motor vehicle–related events (includes children injured as automobile occupants or pedestrians, riding on bicycles, motorcycles or other recreational vehicles) are the leading cause of injuries in children. Falls are the second leading cause of injuries. Injury profiles are determined by the child's developmental level; the child's gender, race, and socioeconomic level; the prevalence of the threat in the child's community; and prevention strategies in use (CDC, 1999b). For example, burn injuries in young children are generally caused by scalds from hot liquid spills or hot tap water whereas burns in older children are often the result of playing with fire (e.g., matches, fireworks). Urban African-American children have higher overall injury rates than do other children in the United States. Near drownings are more prevalent in areas where there are outdoor swimming pools. Children with attention deficit hyperactivity disorder are at greater risk for severe injury from motor vehicle-pedestrian and bicycle accidents (DiScala, Lescohier, Barthel, & Li, 1998).

Violence

The United States ranks first among industrialized nations in violent deaths, with homicide and suicide claiming more than 50,000 lives each year. Youth are increasingly involved both as perpetrators and victims. In addition to the deaths, significant numbers of adolescents and children sustain long-term disability as a result of violence. Immediate access to handguns is a major contributing factor. Public awareness, education, primary prevention programs, offering alternative school and community-based activities, and increasing effort of mental health and substance abuse programs are among the intervention strategies necessary to reduce violence-related deaths and injuries among our youth (U.S. Department of Health and Human Services, 2000).

Child Abuse

Child abuse is another significant contributor to childhood injury, disability, and mortality. In 1997, professionals reported approximately 1 million children under the age of 18 were victims of child abuse or neglect. Neglect is the largest component with additional contributions by physical abuse, emotional abuse, and sexual abuse (U.S. Department of Health and Human Services, 1999). Children who are victims of abuse are usually very young and have a history of prematurity or medical problems. Their abuse often results in fatality or severe neurological compromise (DiScala, Sege, Li, & Reece, 2000). Burns, head injuries, and other injuries that result from child abuse are all too often witnessed in the pediatric rehabilitation setting. By increasing public awareness regarding child abuse and neglect as well as providing such services as hot lines, parenting classes, and mentor programs, health professionals are attempting to decrease the incidence of abused children. The increasing number of people with substance abuse problems, however, is adversely affecting such efforts.

Special Education and the Laws

Education is a critical aspect of all children's lives. Involvement in a stable school setting can help provide normalcy. Changes are being made in our federal and state laws as the public becomes more aware of the needs of children with chronic illness and disabilities, and as parents become more verbal regarding the challenges of caring for these children. The focus is now on access and full inclusion. Special education includes services provided for children in early intervention, preschool, elementary, and secondary school settings. Table 29-3 outlines federal legislation with implications for special education.

In 1990 then-President George Bush signed the amendment to the Education for All Handicapped Children Act, Public Law 101-476, naming it the Individuals with Disability Education Act (IDEA). This amendment changed the term *handicapped* to *disabled* and placed more emphasis on the cultural needs of children served. It also expanded the populations of children covered by the legislation.

IDEA currently mandates that education be provided to all eligible children through 21 years of age in the least restrictive appropriate placement at no cost to parents. Additional mandates include the development of an annual Individualized Education Plan and protection of parents' rights.

Part B of IDEA provides separate allotments for preschool (ages 3 to 5 years) education and related services. Part H of IDEA provides grants for coordination of early intervention services for children from birth to 3 years of age. Each state has the responsibility to set up systems to serve their children; however, the following components are requirements for all early intervention programs.

- Child find—Identifies infants and toddler who have or are at risk for developmental delays
- Diagnostic evaluation—Multidisciplinary assessment of the child to determine if they qualify for services; family assessment is also included
- Individualized family services plan—Plan for needed services that is developed jointly between family and health care team
- Early intervention service delivery—Full range of services provided by multidisciplinary team in the child's home or at a center-based facility (Berger, Holt-Turner, Cupoli, Mass, & Hageman, 1998)

Despite public laws, parents still face many challenges within the educational system. The "appropriate" placement is not always the best placement in the parents' eyes. There is also wide variability in services between states and different communities within those states. School nurses, teachers, and administrators have unmet needs for health information about individual students; education and training about specific disabilities; and effective, timely communication with the multidisciplinary team. School systems need to continue to develop the structure and personnel to support the child with special health care needs in the school setting (Esperat, Moss, Roberts, Kerr, & Green, 1999). Parents, professionals, and children with disabilities need to have a full awareness of the laws related to special education so they can advocate effectively and work toward making full inclusion a reality.

NURSING PROCESS

Assessment

Strategies for Assessment

Children with chronic illness or disability are assessed at regular intervals and at all points along the health care continuum: from preadmission through postdischarge follow-up. Assessment is a critical element in the nursing process. It is the basis from which planning and evaluation of therapeutic interventions emerge.

Holistic assessments encompass the physical, cognitive, social, emotional, cultural, and spiritual aspects of a child's life. The child also is assessed within the context of the family system. An additional consideration for some children

TABLE 29-3 Special Education Legislation

Date Enacted	Legislation	Practice Implications
1973	Rehabilitation Act of 1973, Public Law 93-112 Section 504	Prohibited discrimination based on disability in any program or activity receiving financial assistance from the federal government, including schools
1974	The Family Education Rights and Privacy Act (FERPA), Public Law 93-380	Addressed issues of confidentiality and access to student records in school
1975	Education for All Handicapped Children Act, Public Law 99-142	Mandated free and appropriate public education to all eligible handicapped children and provided federal funding States had to: • Identify and locate all handicapped children between 6 and 18 years of age in need of special education • Evaluate them to determine eligibility for special education and related services • Provide education in the least restrictive environment • Implement systems to protect parents' rights • Provide an Individualized Educational Program (IEP).
1986	The Education of the Handicapped Act Amendment, Public Law 99-457	Lowered the age of eligibility for special education services to 3 years of age Added comprehensive Early Intervention services for children 0 to 3 with or at risk for developmental delay (Part H) Required the development of an Individualized Family Service Plan (IFSP) Mandated case management services
1990	Individuals with Disabilities Education Act (IDEA), Public Law 101-476	Amended and renamed the Education for All Handicapped Children Act, Public Law 99-142 Expanded definition of disability to include children with autism and traumatic brain injury among others Added transition services and assistive technology to services that must be included in IEP Added rehabilitation counseling and social services to related services
1991	The Individuals with Disabilities Education Act Amendments, Public Law 102-119	Reauthorized the Education of the Handicapped Act Amendment, Public Law 99-457 Changed language of case management to service coordination Authorized additional services (vision, assistive devices and technology, and transportation) and additional qualified personnel (family therapists, orientation and mobility specialists, pediatricians, and other physicians)

Data from Gittler, J. (1996). Legal rights of children with disabilities. In H.M. Wallace, R.F. Biehl, J.C. MacQueen, & J.A. Blackman (Eds.), *Mosby's resource guide to children with disabilities and chronic illness* (pp. 97-105). St. Louis: Mosby; Lynch, E.W., & Fisher, D.B. (1996). Special education. In H.M. Wallace, R.F. Biehl, J.C. MacQueen, & J.A. Blackman (Eds.), *Mosby's resource guide to children with disabilities and chronic illness* (pp. 360-369). St. Louis: Mosby.

with disabilities is the application of chronological versus developmental age. Neurological deficits and limited or abnormal experiences can delay the child's development. This must be considered during the assessment.

Privacy and dignity must be provided for the child or adolescent during the assessment process. Fear and anxiety can be allayed or minimized by providing honest, concise, and age-appropriate information to the child. Toys for younger children and other age-appropriate items such as puppets, anatomically correct dolls, diagrams, and books may also help to calm and elicit information from the child. Although parents or guardians usually are the primary historians, older children and adolescents should never be overlooked or excluded from conversations regarding themselves. The nurse's behavior must convey the fact that the child is the central focus of the interaction and a valuable source of information. Figure 29-2 is a sample data collection tool that can be used to guide nursing assessment of the child with rehabilitative needs across the continuum of health care settings.

Tools for Developmental Assessment

Nurses can use screening tools to detect delays in development. The Denver II (the revised Denver Developmental Screening Test) is a standardized basic screening tool that can assist the practitioner in evaluating young children in the following areas: gross motor, fine motor-adaptive, language, and personal-social. The administration of the Denver II is relatively simple, requiring minimal and easily accessible equipment and can be done in any pediatric rehabilitation setting (Frankenburg, Dodds, Archer, Shapiro, & Bresnick, 1990). Parent-completed screening tools, such as

Text continued on p. 690.

PEDIATRIC ASSESSMENT GUIDE

Date ____________________

Client name ____________________ Date of birth ____________________

Historian ____________________ Sex ____________________

Client/parent/guardian goals ____________________

____

____

T ________ P ________ R ________ B/P ________ WT ________ HT ________

Head circumference (cm) ____________ (clients ≤ 5 yrs)

Arm span ____________ (Spina Bifida clients and SCI clients ≤ 5 yrs)

1. Medical diagnosis (include date of onset, course, and other significant information)

____

____

____

2. Significant medical history

A. Diabetes no/yes ____________________

B. Recent infection no/yes ____________________

C. Past surgeries no/yes ____________________

D. Allergies no/yes (describe) ____________________

E. Latex allergy no/yes (describe) ____________________

F. Medications no/yes ____________________

____

____

G. Immunizations

DTaP: (date) 1st ________ 2nd ________ 3rd ________ 4th ________

Hepatitis B (date) 1st ________ 2nd ________ 3rd ________

IPV: (date) 1st ________ 2nd ________ 3rd ________ 4th ________

MMR (date) 1st ________ 2nd ________

Hib (date) 1st ________ 2nd ________ 3rd ________ 4th ________

Figure 29-2 Pediatric assessment guide. (Adapted from the inpatient nursing admission form and pediatric nursing admission form supplement from the Division of Nursing, Rehabilitation Institute of Chicago, Chicago, IL.)

Tetanus booster (date) ______

Tuberculosis (date) ______ Result ______

Pneumovax (date) ______

Varicella (date) ______

Other ______

H. Childhood disease history

Has your child had any of the following?

If yes, when?

Chicken pox no/yes ______

Measles no/yes ______

Mumps no/yes ______

Rubella no/yes ______

Tetanus no/yes ______

Pertussis (whooping cough) no/yes ______

Rheumatic fever no/yes ______

Tuberculosis no/yes ______

CMV no/yes ______

Rotavirus no/yes ______

Hepatitis no/yes ______

Has your child been in contact with any of these illnesses in the past 4 weeks? no/yes ______

3. Cognitive/communicative

A. Mental status

Alert yes/no ______

Orientation (circle) person place time

Memory intact: short term yes/no ______

long term yes/no ______

Loss of consciousness no/yes ______

Client responds to (circle) voice pain neither ______

Client is "yes/no" reliable (circle) yes/no ______

Figure 29-2, cont'd See legend on opposite page.

B. Safety issues no/yes ____________________

History of restraint use no/yes ____________________

Seizures no/yes ____________________

Shunt no/yes ____________________

C. Communication: language spoken ____________________

Spontaneous speech yes/no ____________________

Speech intelligible yes/no ____________________

Alternative communication system used no/yes ____________________

Was child speaking before onset of illness/disability no/yes ____________________

D. Visual problems no/yes Glasses no/yes ____________________

Hearing problems no/yes ____________________

Assistive device no/yes ____________________

4. Cardiovascular

H/O cardiac problems no/yes ____________________

H/O hypertension no/yes ____________________

Chest pain no/yes ____________________

Pulses palpable: brachial __________ radial __________ pedal __________

5. Respiratory

H/O respiratory problem (asthma) ____________________

Current status (breath sounds) ____________________

Tracheostomy no/yes ____________________

(size, type, date last changed, plugging schedule) ____________________

Respiratory management (include oxygen, assistive cough, suctioning, incentive spirometer) ____________________

____

Respiratory support (including BiPap, CPAP, ventilator type and settings, weaning schedule and history) ____________________

____

____

6. Nutrition

Type and texture of diet ____________________

Route ____________________

Enteral feedings no/yes (type; amount of feeding) ____________________

____

Figure 29-2, cont'd See legend on p. 682.

Type/size tube Date last changed ______

Problems sucking, chewing, pocketing food, swallowing no/yes ______

______

Dentition ______

Likes ______

Dislikes ______

Appetite: good ______ poor ______ fussy eater ______

Uses: cup ______ bottle ______ straw ______ pacifier ______

fork ______ spoon ______

Special feeding techniques/adapted equipment ______

______

Indicate means of communicating: drink ______ water ______ milk ______

hunger ______ other ______

7. Elimination

A. Bowel: continent yes/no ______

Last bowel movement ______

Premorbid pattern ______

Current status (include bowel sounds) ______

______

Indicate means of communicating need for toileting/BM ______

______

Stoma: yes/no ______

B. Urinary: continent yes/no ______

Last void ______

Management program ______

Indwelling catheter no/yes (type, size, date last changed) ______

______

Intermittent catheterization program (include size, type of catheter; clean or sterile technique; level of independence) ______

______

______

Indicate child's means of communicating need to void ______

______

______

Figure 29-2, cont'd See legend on p. 682.

8. Gynecologic

A. Age at menarche ______________ Date LMP ______________

B. Date last PAP smear ______________

C. Performs breast self-examination no/yes ______________

Frequency ______________ Date last done ______________

Level of independence ______________

Genitourinary

Performs self-testicular examination yes/no ______________

____

Frequency ______________ Date last done ______________

Level of independence ______________

9. Integument

A. Sensation (circle) intact impaired absent

B. Skin intact yes/no ______________

(describe type lesion, location, grade/stage, measurements, treatment) ______________

____

Photo optional

C. Prevention program (describe turning, sitting tolerance) ______________

____

Special mattress/cushions used ______________

____

Method and frequency of pressure relief ______________

____

Method and frequency of skin checks ______________

____

10. Activity/mobility

A. Motor function (i.e., describe paraplegia; left-sided hemiparesis) ______________

____

B. Ambulatory yes/no ______________

Assistive device(s) no/yes ______________

C. Decrease in ROM no/yes ______________

D. Spasticity no/yes ______________

Figure 29-2, cont'd See legend on p. 682.

E. Contractures no/yes ____

E. Edema no/yes ____

F. Pain no/yes rating scale used ____

Relief measures ____

G. Recent fracture no/yes ____

H. Mobility equipment used ____

____

Has child outgrown equipment no/yes ____

11. Rest/sleep

A. Naps no/yes ____

B. Normal AM waking time ____

C. Normal bedtime ____

D. Does child sleep through the night yes/no ____

E. Child sleeps in (circle) bed crib

F. Does child sleep alone yes/no (if shares bed/room, with whom) ____

____

12. Psychosocial

A. Family unit (with whom does child live; list names and ages of siblings) ____

____

____

B. Primary caretaker ____

C. Others that care for child (grandparents; neighbors; baby sitters) ____

____

D. Pets ____

E. Religious affiliation ____

F. Any religious/cultural/traditional beliefs of which staff should be aware ____

____

G. Leisure/play activities enjoyed by child ____

____

H. Does child have special toy or comfort item no/yes ____

Was it brought with child today no/yes ____

I. Does child play well with other children yes/no ____

Figure 29-2, cont'd See legend on p. 682.

J. Does child attend school yes/no ________________ Grade ________________

K. Does child have any problems in school yes/no ________________

____

L. Parent/guardian-child interaction ________________

____

M. Home assessment ________________

13. Developmental ________________

A. Milestones: before illness/disability--was child

Walking no/yes ________________ (age) ________________

Talking no/yes ________________ (age) ________________

Feeding self no/yes ________________ (age) ________________

Toilet training no/yes ________________ (age) ________________

B. Fears

Does child have any fears about which staff should be aware (dark; strangers; needles; animals; other) ________________

____

____

What behavior does child exhibit when frightened ________________

____

How is your child comforted ________________

14. Safety

A. Birth to 4 years

Do you have a car safety seat for your child yes/no ________________

Do you consistently use safety seat yes/no ________________

B. Four years and older

Does your child use an approved child restraint and ride in the back seat? yes/no ________________

C. Does your child wear a helmet for bike riding; skating yes/no ________________

D. History of tobacco use no/yes ________________

E. History of alcohol use no/yes ________________

F. History of drug use no/yes ________________

15. Discharge planning (for inpatient)

Where will child be going at discharge ________________

Figure 29-2, cont'd See legend on p. 682.

Is residence accessible yes/no ____________________

Pediatrician

____

School to which child will be returning

____

16. Functional levels: activities of daily living

[Scale: 5 = Independent; 4 = Minimal physical assistance (client does 75% or more); 3 = Moderate assistance (50% or more); 2 = Maximal assistance (25% to 50% or may direct); 1 = Dependent]

Oral/facial ____________ Eating ____________

Hygiene/bathing ____________ Turning ____________

Dressing UE ____________ Transfers ____________

Dressing LE ____________ Toileting ____________

17. Nursing diagnoses

____

____

____

____

____

18. Mutual goals

____

____

____

19. Educational needs (include assessment of learning style)

____

____

____

____

____

RN ____________ Signature

Adapted from Inpatient Nursing Admission Form (1991) and Pediatric Nursing Admission Form Supplement, Division of Nursing, Rehabilitation Institute of Chicago, Chicago, Illinois.

Figure 29-2, cont'd See legend on p. 682.

the Revised Denner Prescreening Developmental Questionnaire (R-PDQ), are also available. They require very little professional time and are a cost-effective alternative for basic developmental screening. More focused assessments should be performed by the appropriate interdisciplinary team member if delays are identified during the basic screening. There are numerous tools available for these diagnostic assessments.

Nursing Diagnoses and Interventions and Outcomes for Common Chronic Conditions and Disabilities in Children and Adolescents

It is beyond the scope of this chapter to provide a comprehensive review of all the diagnoses encountered in the field of pediatric rehabilitation; however, this section addresses four of the more common conditions with respect to nursing diagnoses, outcomes, and interventions.

Cerebral Palsy

Children with cerebral palsy (CP) are the largest population requiring pediatric (re)habilitative services (Matthews & Wilson, 1999). Bax & Molnar (as cited in Matthews & Wilson, 1999) define cerebral palsy as "a disorder of movement and posture that results from a nonprogressive lesion or injury to an immature brain" (p. 193). The injury may occur in utero, near the time of delivery, or during early childhood. The incidence of CP is 2 per 1,000 live births, but more children acquire the disability in early childhood, resulting in 10,000 per year in the United States (CDC, 2000). Among the multiple causes of CP (i.e., intrauterine infections, toxins, and delivery complications), prematurity is the most significant contributing factor (Matthews & Wilson, 1999). Lifetime costs for each newly diagnosed child (using 1992 dollar values) are $503,000. Families pay at least half of this amount and still remain short on access and availability of the multiple disciplines and services they require (CDC, 2000).

CP is classified as spastic, dyskinetic, ataxic, or mixed. These types are further divided according to the number of extremities or parts of the body involved. The majority of children with CP have the spastic form. CP is usually diagnosed in the second half of the first year of life. Suspicious signs are reflex abnormalities, abnormal muscle tone and posture, delayed development, and poor feeding.

The broad span of causes accounts in part for the number of associated problems seen in children with this condition: hearing, vision, and speech impairments; feeding problems and malnutrition; seizures; and mental retardation; in addition to various motor impairments (Matthews & Wilson, 1999).

Spasticity is a particularly difficult to manage complication. Figure 29-3 illustrates two children who have spasticity producing "scissoring." The goal of spasticity management is functional mobility. Daily passive/active range of motion (ROM) exercises, warm baths, and other relaxation techniques can be used to facilitate movements. Follow-through of physical and occupational therapy exercises in the rehabilitation, home, and school settings is essential. Roughly half of those with CP use assistive devices that are prescribed for individual needs; furthermore the prescriptions are reevaluated frequently and change rapidly as children grow and develop. Strollers, wheelchairs, walkers, standers, splints and orthotics, and positioning devices must be evaluated frequently to ensure proper fit as the child grows. Other strategies to manage spasticity and promote mobility include medications (baclofen), phenol injections, Botox injections, surgeries, and rhizotomy. Surgical procedures should be scheduled for summertime or vacation to minimize time lost from school.

The ability to communicate opens doors. Children with CP need adequate time and a supportive environment for communication. Communication skills can be increased with augmentative (enhance existing speech) or alternative (replace written or spoken word) communication devices that are recommended by a speech language pathologist. If an augmentative or alternative device is recommended the child, family, school, and health care personnel need education to ensure consistency in use.

Feeding is a very time-consuming task in caring for many children with CP. Collaboration with the physician and speech language pathologist is necessary to establish a safe feeding regimen. Swallowing studies may be recommended to rule out aspiration and ensure safe oral feeding. Consistency of food and fluid may need to be adjusted to ensure safe consumption. Occupational therapists can provide adaptive feeding utensils and techniques; physical therapists can ensure proper seating and positioning for feeding. Families and school personnel require education regarding feeding regimen and techniques to ensure community follow through. If adequate nutrition cannot be taken orally in a reasonable time, education in the care and use of an enteral feeding tube may be necessary.

Safe transport is another consideration for children with CP. Convertible car seats approved for the forward-facing semireclining position are useful for children with poor head control. Other modifications to maintain appropriate posture and alignment can be made using rolled towels, diapers, or blankets. Parents must be trained in proper techniques so that modifications do not interfere with proper function of safety features of the car seat. Wheelchairs should be secured with proper tie downs with trays and adaptive equipment removed. Community resources to provide specialized restraint systems and training in proper car restraint use should be identified. Transportation should also be incorporated into the individualized education plan at school (Bull et al., 1999).

Constipation in children with CP is related to decreased fluid and bulk intake and decreased mobility. Bowel programs should focus on the least invasive, most cost-effective

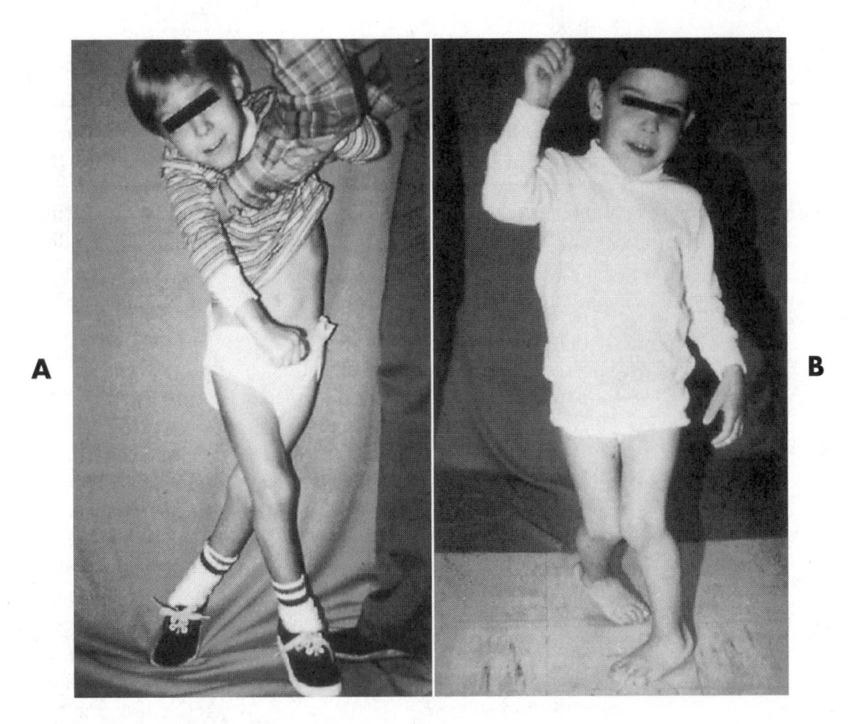

Figure 29-3 Two children with adductor spasticity producing scissoring. **A,** Severe spasticity in nonambulatory child who has adduction deformity and severe scissoring. **B,** Ambulatory child with spastic diplegia whose legs scissor during walking. (From Canale, S.T., & Beaty, J.H. [1991]. *Operative pediatric orthopaedics.* St. Louis: Mosby.)

measures first (i.e., dietary and fluid measures, regular exercise/increased mobility, and scheduled toileting). Stool softeners and laxatives are added as adjuncts to dietary measures and exercise as necessary. The physical therapist can provide supported seating (commode chair) for relaxation of tone and facilitation of elimination. The child's ability to communicate the need to use toilet is also a consideration. Support of family and school personnel is necessary for a successful program.

Many children with CP have specialized dental care needs. Consultation with a pediatric dentist who specializes in care of children with special health care needs can provide solutions for problems such as gingival hyperplasia, malocclusion, and caries and periodontal disease (Matthews & Wilson, 1999). Case managers can collaborate with a child's dentist to identify funding for dental care. Routine oral hygiene consisting of toothbrushing and flossing is essential for dental health. Drooling is an additional problem with significant social implications. Medications and oral stimulation and behavior modification can be effective in reducing this problem. Refer to Table 29-4 for specific nursing diagnoses, outcomes, and interventions for children with CP.

Spina Bifida

Spina bifida is a term used to describe a group of neural tube defects that include spina bifida occulta, meningocele, and myelomeningocele (see Figure 15-1). Neuromuscular function is affected below the level of lesion, resulting in lower extremity paralysis, impaired bowel bladder and sexual function, sensory deficits, respiratory problems, and hydrocephalus. Over the past 3 decades, use of antibiotics and surgical advances have increased survival and life expectancy for children with spina bifida. Spina bifida occurs in about 1 in 1,000 live births in the United States (Hays & Michaud, 1994). It is the second most common developmental disability (Molnar & Murphy, 1999). Although the exact cause of spina bifida is unknown, a contributing factor has been identified—inadequate folic acid intake. The U.S. Public Health Service and Academy of Pediatrics currently recommend that all women of child-bearing age consume 400 μg folic acid daily before conception and during pregnancy to prevent neural tube defects (Committee on Genetics, 1999).

Controlling incontinence, preventing infections, and preserving kidney function are common rehabilitation goals for the child with spina bifida. Routine urological evaluation by a physician is recommended every 6 to 12 months to monitor these goals. Families are educated regarding urinary tract health maintenance; adequate fluid intake; signs, symptoms, and steps to take for urinary tract infection; prevention of bladder overdistention; and performing clean intermittent catheterization. They must also learn about medications to increase bladder volumes (oxybutynin) and treat infection (nitrofurantoin or trimethoprim). By 4 to 8 years of age, children have the manual dexterity, psychological readiness, and postural balance to learn and perform self-care for clean intermittent catheterization (Hoeman, 1997). Appropriate direct care providers should be educated regarding bladder

TABLE 29-4 Nursing Diagnosis, Outcomes, and Interventions for Cerebral Palsy

Nursing Diagnosis	Suggested Nursing Outcome Classification (NOC)	Suggested Nursing Intervention Classification (NIC)
Impaired swallowing (uncompensated)	Swallowing status	Aspiration precautions Enteral tube feeding Feeding Nutrition therapy Surveillance Positioning Self-care assistance: feeding Swallowing therapy
Impaired physical mobility	Mobility level	Exercise promotion: stretching Exercise therapy: ambulation Exercise therapy: balance Exercise therapy: joint mobility Exercise therapy: muscle control Medication management Positioning: wheelchair Self-care assistance Teaching prescribed activity/exercise
Impaired verbal communication	Communication ability	Active listening Communication enhancement: hearing deficit Communication enhancement: speech deficit
Risk for constipation	Bowel elimination	Bowel training Constipation/impaction management Fluid management Exercise promotion Medication management Self-care assistance: toileting
Impaired urinary elimination	Urinary continence	Urinary habit training Urinary continence care
Risk for impaired skin integrity	Immobility consequences: physiological	Skin surveillance
Total self-care deficit	Self-care: activities of daily living	Self-care assistance
Impaired dentition	Oral health	Oral health maintenance
Delayed growth and development	Child development: 2 months through adolescence	Developmental enhancement: child Developmental enhancement: adolescent
Social isolation or social rejection	Social involvement: play participation	Socialization enhancement
Risk for caregiver role strain	Family coping or role performance	Caregiver support Respite care

Data from Johnson, M., Maas, M.L., & Moorhead, S. (2000). *Nursing outcomes classification (NOC)* (2nd ed.). St. Louis: Mosby; McCloskey, J.C., & Bulechek, G.M. (2000). *Nursing interventions classification (NIC)* (3rd ed.). St. Louis: Mosby; and North American Nursing Diagnosis Association. (2001). *Nursing diagnosis: definitions and classification 2001-2002* (4th ed.). Philadelphia: Author.

program so they can provide support, encouragement, and privacy needed. Families, school personnel, and health professionals must encourage the child's progression toward maximal independence with bladder program because continence gives self-esteem. The need for intermittent catheterization puts the child at personal risk for child sexual abuse. Children should be taught from an early age that they are in charge of their own bodies and that they have the right to say no to anyone who tries to touch them in a private place.

Obesity is a another common problem among children with spina bifida that only adds to their musculoskeletal, mobility, and skin problems (Hoeman, 1997). Children and families need early education regarding healthful nutrition patterns. Even young children can participate in selection and preparation of healthy meals and snacks. Dietitians can assist by calculating appropriate calories for weight control. Regular exercise and involvement in adapted sports and recreational activities should also be encouraged.

Unique safety issues are present for the child with spina bifida. Some children have ventriculoperitoneal (VP) shunts in place to manage hydrocephalus. Parents must be able to identify signs of increased intracranial pressure and shunt failure and perform shunt care. Neurosurgical evaluations are necessary as children grow to ensure they do not out-

TABLE 29-5 Nursing Diagnosis, Outcomes, and Interventions for Spina Bifida

Nursing Diagnosis	Suggested Nursing Outcome Classification (NOC)	Suggested Nursing Intervention Classifications (NIC)
Impaired urinary elimination	Urinary continence Urinary elimination	Urinary catheterization: intermittent Urinary elimination management
Imbalanced nutrition: risk for more than body requirements	Weight control	Exercise promotion Nutrition management
Risk for injury (trauma) or risk for latex allergy response	Risk control	Latex precautions Surveillance: safety Sports injury prevention: youth Teaching: disease process
Bowel incontinence	Bowel elimination Bowel continence	Bowel training Self-care assistance: toileting
Risk for impaired skin integrity	Immobility consequences: physiological	Skin surveillance
Impaired physical mobility	Ambulation: walking Ambulation: wheelchair	Exercise promotion: strength training Exercise therapy: ambulation Positioning: wheelchair
Body image disturbance or low self-esteem	Body image Self-esteem	Body image enhancement Self-esteem enhancement
Delayed growth and development	Child development: 2 months through adolescence	Developmental enhancement: child Developmental enhancement: adolescent
Risk for caregiver role strain	Family coping Role performance	Caregiver support Respite care

Data from Johnson, M., Maas, M.L., & Moorhead, S. (2000). *Nursing outcomes classification (NOC)* (2nd ed.). St. Louis: Mosby; McCloskey, J.C., & Bulechek, G.M. (2000). *Nursing interventions classification (NIC)* (3rd ed.). St. Louis: Mosby; and North American Nursing Diagnosis Association. (2001). *Nursing diagnosis: definitions and classification 2001-2002* (4th ed.). Philadelphia: Author.

grow their shunts, which would inhibit function. Families can expect that children will need three or more shunt revisions by age 12 (Hoeman, 1997).

Sensory alterations place these children at risk for pressure ulcers, burns, frostbite, and trauma. Skin checks should be performed at least twice daily to prevent development of impaired skin integrity. A long-handled mirror can increase the child's involvement and promote independence. Special attention should be given to areas under braces and other orthoses. Frequent hygiene care is necessary in children who are incontinent or adolescents who are menstruating.

The child with spina bifida needs adaptive equipment for exploratory play. Adapted seats, carts, standers, and wheelchairs are available to support involvement in play and activities. When children move to the school setting, wheelchairs should be motorized so children can keep up with peers. School-aged and adolescent children should be able to instruct others in use of their adaptive equipment and wheelchairs. Refer to Table 29-5 for specific nursing diagnoses, outcomes, and interventions for children with spina bifida.

Traumatic Brain Injury

Traumatic brain injury (TBI) is a major and costly cause of disability in children. The annual incidence of pediatric TBI is estimated to be 185 per 100,000 per year (Krach & Kriel, 1999). The highest incidence is in the adolescent and young adult population (15-24 years of age) with a smaller peak in children younger than 5 years of age. Motor vehicle, pedestrian, and bicycle accidents are responsible for the majority of brain injuries. Falls, sports and recreation, violence, and assault are other major contributors (Kraus, Rock, & Hemyari, 1990). Child abuse is the cause in most children under 3 years of age (Reece & Sege, 2000).

A wide spectrum of problems is seen as a result of TBI. The severity and type of disability varies with the amount, type, and location of brain damage. Common motor consequences in children are balance problems, ataxia, hemiparesis, and spasticity. Hearing and vision may also be impaired. But it is the cognitive deficits that have the largest impact on the child and family. Impaired attention, agitation, altered memory, behavior problems, and emotional lability are all common cognitive consequences of TBI in children (Krach & Kriel, 1999).

Nursing and rehabilitative intervention to manage these consequences and other associated medical disorders must focus on the child's current level of cognitive functioning. The Rancho Los Amigos Scale of Cognitive Functioning is one scale that is used to facilitate use of common language between rehabilitation team members (see Chapter 26). Throughout the rehabilitation process, the three most important strategies are structure, repetition, and consistency.

Stimulation activities are the focus of care before the child is able to follow simple commands (levels I-III). ROM exercises and positioning to prevent pressure ulcers and contractures are also important at this stage. Bowel and bladder programs, tracheostomy care, gastrostomy feedings, and seizure management are common aspects of nursing care during this phase.

When the child is agitated (levels IV-V), safety and limit setting are key. Using simple commands, providing concrete explanations, and providing orientation help the child to cooperate and participate in ADLs. Decreased environmental stimulation (i.e., decrease light, noise, and schedule medical and nursing procedures so that sleep is not disturbed), relaxation techniques (i.e., warm bath or shower, deep breathing, guided imagery, soft music, comfort items within reach), and prescribed medications help promote adequate rest during these stages.

By level VI, the child is often ready to return to the community and school. Neuropsychological testing should be performed to ensure proper school placement. More complex commands can generally be understood and followed. Memory books and daily schedules will help children with TBI gain independence. A low-stimulation environment will increase their ability to attend to tasks. Increased emotional support is often needed as they begin to realize the magnitude of their disabilities. They often lose friends and need to adjust life goals because of their disabilities. Schools are often not prepared to deal with the learning disabilities, attention deficits, poor impulse control, lack of motivation, and impaired social judgment that are common behavioral consequences of TBI. Behavior management programs must be communicated, understood, and implemented consistently by the interdisciplinary team, family, and school personnel.

Families need support during community reentry. Structured counseling sessions and spontaneous interactions through the course of daily activities help family members verbalize feelings related to their situation. Referrals to head injury support groups and identifying appropriate community resources (i.e., day care programs, respite services, and attendant care) also help families cope with ongoing care needs in the home setting. Refer to Table 29-6 for specific nursing diagnoses, outcomes, and interventions for children with traumatic brain injury.

TABLE 29-6 Nursing Diagnosis, Outcomes, and Interventions for Traumatic Brain Injury

Nursing Diagnosis	Suggested Nursing Outcome Classification (NOC)	Suggested Nursing Intervention Classification (NIC)
Disturbed thought process	Cognitive ability or information processing	Behavior management: overactivity/inattention Elopement precautions Environmental management: safety Medication management Memory training
Disturbed sensory perception (auditory, olfactory, visual)	Risk control Hearing compensation behavior Vision compensation behavior	Communication enhancement: hearing deficit Environmental management
Impaired verbal communication	Communication ability	Communication enhancement: speech deficit
Sleep-pattern disturbance	Sleep	Environmental management Sleep enhancement
Risk for injury (trauma)	Neurological status	Seizure precautions Surveillance: safety Physical restraint
Impaired physical mobility	Ambulation: walking Ambulation: wheelchair	Exercise therapy: ambulation Exercise therapy: balance Exercise therapy: joint mobility Positioning: wheelchair
Impaired swallowing (uncompensated)	Swallowing status	Swallowing therapy
Bowel incontinence	Bowel continence	Bowel training Self-care assistance: toileting
Impaired urinary elimination	Urinary continence	Urinary incontinence care Self-care assistance: toileting
Delayed growth and development	Child development: 2 months through adolescence	Developmental enhancement: child Developmental enhancement: adolescent
Risk for caregiver role strain	Family coping or role performance	Caregiver support Respite care

Data from Johnson, M., Maas, M.L., & Moorhead, S. (2000). *Nursing outcomes classification (NOC)* (2nd ed.). St. Louis: Mosby; McCloskey, J.C., & Bulechek, G.M. (2000). *Nursing interventions classification (NIC)* (3rd ed.). St. Louis: Mosby; and North American Nursing Diagnosis Association. (2001). *Nursing diagnosis: definitions and classification 2001-2002* (4th ed.). Philadelphia: Author.

Bronchopulmonary Dysplasia

Bronchopulmonary dysplasia (BPD) is a chronic lung disease that occurs primarily in premature infants. Excessive intravenous fluid, exposure to high concentrations of oxygen, and mechanical ventilation all contribute to lung injury. Surfactant replacement therapy has improved survival of preterm infants but has not had a conclusive effect on reducing the number of children with BPD (McColley, 1998). Many infants with BPD have additional developmental disadvantages such as extreme prematurity, intraventricular hemorrhage, and prolonged hospitalization.

Early rehabilitation goals for children with BPD are often focused on stabilizing respiratory status. These children may receive supplemental oxygen through nasal cannula, tracheostomy, or mechanical ventilators. A common long-term goal is to wean them from respiratory support. Supportive care is needed from both nursing and respiratory staff. Portable oxygen and ventilators enable these children to have mobility despite their need for continuous respiratory support. Activity intolerance is an obstacle to full involvement in the rehabilitation program. Clustering care and paying attention to early signs of distress can help prevent acute deterioration and clinical setbacks.

Oral hypersensitivity, prolonged periods without food or drink, increased caloric demands, and poor feeding skills combine to place many infants at increased nutritional risk. Collaboration with the registered dietitian is important for nutritional planning and growth monitoring. Growth is the key to improving respiratory status. Speech-language pathologists can help enhance these children's oral feeding skills.

Parents of children with BPD require extensive training and support for success in the home environment. Care regimens should be simplified whenever possible to enable parents to get several hours of uninterrupted sleep at night (e.g., eliminate feedings and medications in the middle of the night). Parents should be educated on illness warning signs, respiratory care, feeding, positioning, calming strategies, and cardiopulmonary resuscitation. Health emergency plans must be established before discharge.

Parents often need training in well child care, as many of these infants have never been home. Positioning devices, age-appropriate toys, and calming strategies promote development in the hospital, home, and early intervention settings. Considerations for safe transportation should also be included in the training plan. Strollers can be adapted to accommodate suction equipment, portable oxygen, and ventilators. Infant-only car seats that can be reclined are helpful for children with difficulty breathing in the sitting position. To prevent injury to the neck and face or blockage of the tracheostomy during impact, premature and small infants and infants and children with tracheostomies should not be placed in car seats with a harness-tray/shield combination or an armrest. According to the American Academy of Pediatrics' Committee on Injury Prevention and Poison Prevention, a rear-facing car safety seat with a three-point harness or a car safety seat with a five-point harness is the best option for children with a tracheostomy. Oxygen tanks and monitors should be secured on the floor of the vehicle (Bull et al., 1999). Refer to Table 29-7 for specific nursing diagnoses, outcomes, and interventions for children with BPD.

TABLE 29-7 Nursing Diagnosis, Outcomes, and Interventions for Bronchopulmonary Dysplasia

Nursing Diagnosis	Suggested Nursing Outcome Classification (NOC)	Suggested Nursing Intervention Classification (NIC)
Ineffective airway clearance and impaired gas exchange	Respiratory status: gas exchange Respiratory status: ventilation	Airway management Respiratory monitoring Mechanical ventilation Mechanical ventilation weaning
Activity intolerance	Activity tolerance	Oxygen therapy
Ineffective infant feeding pattern	Swallowing status	Enteral tube feeding Nonnutritive sucking Swallowing therapy
Imbalanced nutrition: less than body requirements	Nutritional status: food and fluid intake nutritional status: body mass	Nutrition management Environmental management: attachment process
Ineffective protection	Immunization behavior	Immunization/vaccination management
Delayed growth and development and disorganized infant behavior	Child development: 2 months through 3 years	Developmental care
Risk for impaired parent-infant/child attachment	Parent-infant attachment; parenting Caregiver performance: direct care	Environmental management: attachment process

Data from Johnson, M., Maas, M.L., & Moorhead, S. (2000). *Nursing outcomes classification (NOC)* (2nd ed.). St. Louis: Mosby; McCloskey, J.C., & Bulechek, G.M. (2000). *Nursing interventions classification (NIC)* (3rd ed.). St. Louis: Mosby; and North American Nursing Diagnosis Association. (2001). *Nursing diagnosis: definitions and classification 2001-2002* (4th ed.). Philadelphia: Author.

EVALUATION

Outcomes

Outcomes have always been important to professionals, patients, and families, but measurement of outcomes has become increasingly important in all pediatric rehabilitation settings. In the current health care environment, insurance carriers use outcomes to justify spending of limited health care dollars. Accrediting bodies also integrate outcome data into organizational accreditation processes. Outcomes in pediatric rehabilitation are related to age at initiation of services severity, extent and location of injury, overall health and nutrition, comorbidities, psychosocial issues, and quality and quantity of interventions. As length of stay decreases, traditional measure of outcomes need to be adjusted to include measures of quality of life and school and community reintegration.

Program Evaluation

Rehabilitation facilities, like most organizations, use outcome measurement as a method of evaluating the effectiveness of their programs. Outcome measurement tools are used to identify the level at which a client is functioning on admission and discharge, thus enabling detection of improvement in functional categories or ADLs. These measures are being evaluated for use in home and community settings as well. Some examples of areas that are rated include transferring, toileting, bathing, and cognitive functioning (i.e., communication, problem solving, and memory). Rehabilitation programs use the information to assess their effectiveness and make necessary adjustments to improve client outcomes.

Individual programs or facilities traditionally developed outcome measurement tools; however, it became apparent that there was a nationwide need for documenting the severity of disability and the outcomes of medical rehabilitation in a uniform language. The uniform data system (UDS) for medical rehabilitation was established to ensure uniformity in definitions and measures of disabilities and outcomes in rehabilitation.

The functional independence measure (FIM) tool was developed to assess 18 items relative to self-care, sphincter management, mobility, locomotion, communication, and social cognition on a seven-level scale. The UDS serves as a central repository for client data and provides reports of comparable data for quality management to subscribing facilities. The process is dependent on reliable data collection and reporting by facilities and quality control of data received by the UDS. Raters are credentialed to ensure knowledge of FIM definitions and levels (Uniform Data System, 1991). Chapters 7 and 8 provide additional information on these topics.

A FIM for children (WeeFIM) was developed to reflect functional and criteria differences seen in children as a result of developmental age. The tool is used with children from 6 months to 16 years of age. Although very young children may score with a higher dependency factor at both admission and discharge because of developmental age, scores for older children can reflect gains in any or all areas measured. The WeeFIM can be used in both inpatient and outpatient settings, as well as in schools and community-based agencies.

The pediatric evaluation of disability inventory (PEDI) is another functional evaluation measurement tool (Table 29-8). The PEDI provides a comprehensive clinical assessment of key functional capabilities and performance in children between the ages of 6 months and 7 years. Older children, whose functional abilities are not equivalent to

TABLE 29-8 Functional Skills Content of the Pediatric Evaluation of Disability Inventory

Self-Care Domain	Mobility Domain	Social Function Domain
Types of food textures	Floor locomotion	Comprehension of word meanings
Use of utensils	Chair/wheelchair transfers	Comprehension of sentence complexity
Use of drinking containers	Opening and closing doors	Functional use of expressive communication
Toothbrushing	In and out of car	Complexity of expressive communication
Hair brushing	Bed mobility	Problem resolution
Nose care	Stand/sit in tub or shower	Social interactive play
Hand washing	Method of indoor locomotion	Peer interactions
Washing body and face	Distance/speed indoors	Self-information
Pullover/front-opening garments	Pulls/carries objects	Time orientation
Fasteners	Method of outdoor locomotion	Household chores
Pants	Distance/speed outdoors	Self-protection
Shoes/socks	Locomotion on outdoor surfaces	Community function
Toileting tasks	Scooting up and down stairs	
Control of bladder function	Walking up and down stairs	
Control of bowel function		

From PEDI Research Group, New England Medical Center Hospitals, Boston, MA.

chronological norms, may also be evaluated. The unique feature of the PEDI is the attempt to include social outcome measures, as well as those for ADLs. The three domains attempt to measure what a child "does do" rather than what cannot be accomplished and the level of caregiver assistance required. A separate scale, the modifications scale, documents environmental modifications or adaptive equipment a child uses to perform ADLs. The PEDI has been standardized on a sample of children without disabilities in the targeted age range (Feldman, Haley, & Coryell, 1990). Rehabilitation professionals administer the PEDI in a clinical setting or by structured interview of parents, requiring approximately 45 minutes. Individual record booklets for maintaining a long-term profile are available. Software for data entry, scoring, and individual profile summaries is also available.

IMPLICATIONS FOR PEDIATRIC REHABILITATION NURSING PRACTICE

Prevention Summary

Prenatal intervention is one of the major defenses against children with congenital disabilities resulting from prematurity, low birth weight, and associated medical problems. A good prenatal diet with adequate folic acid intake; absence of smoking, alcohol, and recreational drugs; and appropriate medical monitoring increase the chances of having a healthy infant. Women, particularly those in high-risk areas, should be tested for HIV and treated during pregnancy if found to be positive. Teenage pregnancies, which often result in premature deliveries, contribute to the numbers of infants born at risk for special health care needs. Ongoing well-child care, including immunizations, can prevent disabling illnesses such as measles encephalopathy, influenza, meningitis, and polio.

Unintentional injury is the leading cause of death and acquired disabilities in children older than 1 year of age. Prevention strategies must focus on the specific type of injury and population at greatest risk for that injury. For example, manufacturers' changes in infant walkers and shopping carts have decreased head injuries from falls in young children. Ongoing use of infant and child car seats, car safety belts, and helmets and other protective gear while bicycling or skating can continue to decrease disability related to traumatic brain injury and other physical injuries (Consensus Conference, 1999). Educating children and adults in all areas of safety and injury prevention is key to decreasing the incidence of injuries. It is clearly less costly from a financial and societal perspective to prevent rather than treat injuries. Combined efforts from many professionals and organizations such as National Safe Kids Campaign and National Pediatric Trauma Registry are necessary to identify and implement further prevention strategies.

Unmet Needs

The field of pediatric rehabilitation continues to grow and evolve. Federal and state legislation has helped to ensure the rights of children and adults with disabilities. A fully integrated system of health care to meet the needs of children with special health care needs is not yet a reality. This system has been described as the "medical home" by the American Academy of Pediatrics (1992). It includes:

1. Provision of preventive care
2. Assurance of ambulatory and inpatient care 24 hours a day
3. Strategies and mechanisms to ensure continuity of care (from infancy through adolescence)
4. Identification of and medically appropriate use of subspecialty consultation and referrals
5. Interaction with school and community agencies
6. Maintenance of a central record and database containing all pertinent medical information including hospitalizations (p. 774)

Forsman (1999) adds to this list the importance of a family-centered approach to care and geographical and financial accessibility. She further stresses the need for commitment to this concept by the entire team of professionals that may be involved in the care of the child with special health care needs. Nurses at all levels will clearly play an important role in quality, efficiency, and cost-effectiveness in this system. Development of standards for care of special populations in different settings will help in outcome and quality measurements of this system of care.

Other National Resources

National associations, such as for CP and spina bifida, are resources for consumers and professional providers—The American Academy of Pediatrics, the Academy of Cerebral Palsy and Developmental Medicine, and Nurses of Developmental Disabilities are examples. The National Center for Environmental Health at the Centers for Disease Control and Prevention has four branches, one of which is devoted to developmental disabilities. This resource is important to pediatric rehabilitation nurses because 2% of school-aged children in the United States have serious developmental disabilities and learning impairments. Additionally, the National Center for Environmental Health's Web site contains links to other national institutes and centers concerned with pediatric rehabilitation as well as to sites with Spanish or other non-English language information (CDC, 2000).

CRITICAL THINKING

How do you work with parents who are suspected of having caused their child's injuries?

Should a child be admitted to a rehabilitation center far away from home because it is a center of excellence?

Should insurance companies be required to pay for rehabilitation services for children across all care settings (inpatient, day hospital, and outpatient)?

Is it ethical to spend scarce health care resources on maintaining severely neurologically compromised children on ventilators in any rehabilitation setting?

Where do medically complex children go if their parents cannot or refuse to learn their children's care?

Should schools be required to provide special services for one child when the money could be spent on programs to benefit many children?

What responsibility do we have as a society for supporting families of children with disabilities in the community?

Could you do what we often ask families to do? (Capen & Dedlow, 1998; Deaton, 1996).

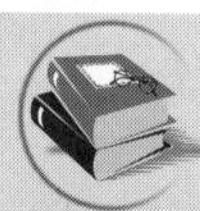

Case Study 1 ⌒ *Spina Bifida*

Ryan is a 6-year-old child with myelomeningocele who began first grade a few weeks before coming in for an outpatient evaluation. During this evaluation with the rehabilitation team, his mother reported to the nurse that Ryan recently had expressed embarrassment about wearing diapers and had been teased by his classmates. She was concerned that Ryan was becoming more withdrawn and irritable. After completing the assessment, the following nursing diagnoses were identified:

1. Altered urinary elimination pattern
2. Bowel incontinence
3. Ineffective coping (individual)
4. Family coping: potential for growth

Short-term goals were to establish urinary continence through intermittent catheterization or external collecting device, to establish bowel continence through a regulated bowel program, and to promote effective coping for Ryan and his family. Long-term goals included independence in bladder and bowel program and continued individual family coping.

In developing an educational plan, it is important to consider both the developmental age and any associated learning disabilities common in children with myelomeningocele. Ryan was encouraged to express his feelings about being different and being teased by peers. His desire to get out of diapers was established and his participation in the plan was elicited. Because school-aged children are industrious and eager to master skills, Ryan was given clear and concrete information regarding his urinary and gastrointestinal systems. Pictures and anatomically correct dolls were used to facilitate understanding of the body systems and the relationship between dietary measures and elimination.

Both Ryan and his mother were taught how to perform the bladder and bowel programs. Ryan was allowed to practice catheterization skills first on the doll and then on himself. Because he could not yet tell time, the catheterization schedule was linked to familiar events (when he awakened, after lunch and school, and before bedtime). A watch with an alarm helped to remind Ryan of his schedule. The teacher and school nurse were also involved to facilitate success of the program. Ryan was given the responsibility of recording his catheterization volumes on a chart by coloring in the appropriate amount on a predrawn graduated cup. Ryan's mother was responsible for supervising, coaching, and praising her son's efforts and achievements. She also maintained contact with the teacher, school nurse, and rehabilitation nurse. Both Ryan and his mother were referred to the local Spina Bifida Association for support groups and family activities.

Over time, Ryan gained more control over his body by participating in self-catheterization and bowel regulation. He achieved continence, which increased his self-esteem and allowed him to get out of diapers. Ryan's mother and teacher reported that he seemed happier and more confident and that the teasing had stopped.

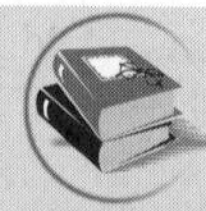

Case Study 2 ⌒ *Spinal Cord Injury*

Juan, a 10-year-old Hispanic boy, was admitted to the inpatient rehabilitation unit 6 weeks after sustaining a C2-3 spinal cord injury. He had been hit by a car while playing in the street near his apartment house. Juan was ventilator-dependent with no movement below his shoulders. A gastrostomy tube was in place. Along with his physical disabilities, Juan had a history of attention deficit hyperactivity disorder. Juan lived in a third-floor apartment with his mother and older brother. His father was incarcerated. Juan's mother spoke very little English.

For the first few days after admission, Juan was impossible. He cried, spit at his nurses and therapists, and refused to eat by mouth. His mother did not discipline him but rather sat at his bedside and cried. The following nursing diagnoses were the focus of care:

1. Altered nutrition: less than body requirements
2. Risk for fluid volume deficit
3. Impaired physical mobility: level III
4. Ineffective coping (individual)
5. Altered parenting

Short-term goals were to improve nutrition intake by mouth, maintain adequate fluid intake, establish independent wheelchair mobility, and promote effective parenting. Long-term goals included discharge to home and return to school.

The primary nurse worked with the dietitian to set minimal re-

Case Study 2 ~ *Spinal Cord Injury—cont'd*

quirements for fluid and nutrition intake. The team agreed that the gastrostomy tube should only be used for medication administration and critical fluid supplements. Juan was allowed to select preferred foods from the menu. Physical therapy worked to teach Juan to operate his power wheelchair. Mouth controls were provided so he could operate the wheelchair independently and move around the unit.

Psychology and nursing developed a behavior management plan. Reinforcers were given in the form of time tokens to play the switch-adapted video game. Tantrums were handled by placing him behind a curtain for a set period in bed or with the wheelchair controls turned off. A core group of experienced nurses and therapists were assigned to his care to provide consistency and establish a daily routine. Psychology provided supportive counseling sessions to help him express his feelings and deal more appropriately with his disability. Social services worked with the mother to develop her skills in limit setting and to help her cope with the stress of the situation.

Nursing, respiratory, and therapy staff trained Juan's mother in all aspects of his care. Teaching materials were provided in Spanish and a translator was used to overcome the language barrier. Within 2 months all training was complete, but discharge to home was delayed while the mother continued to try to find affordable, accessible housing.

Juan is currently attending school accompanied by a nurse who is funded through his school system. His mother and primary nurse have set clear academic and behavioral expectations. He returns to the inpatient unit in the afternoon to do his homework. He manipulates a computer and turns pages with a mouthstick. Juan takes a full regular diet by mouth and has independent mobility in his power wheelchair. He directs staff in performing his ADLs and selects his school clothes in the morning. He has regained his sense of humor and is more pleasant and polite to staff. Juan is looking forward to going home.

REFERENCES

Allan, W.S. (1958). *Rehabilitation: A community challenge.* New York: John Wiley & Sons.

American Academy of Pediatrics Ad Hoc Task Force on the definition of the medical home: The medical home. (1992). *Pediatrics, 90,* 774.

Barton, S.J. (1999). Promoting family-centered care with foster families. *Pediatric Nursing, 25,* 57-59.

Berger, S.P., Holt-Turner, I., Cupoli, J.M., Mass, M., & Hageman, J.R. (1998). Caring for the graduate from the neonatal intensive care unit: At home, in the office, and in the community. *Pediatric Clinics of North America, 45,* 701-712.

Betz, C.L. (1998). Adolescent transitions: A nursing concern. *Pediatric Nursing, 24,* 23-28.

Biehl, R.F. (1997). Case management and service coordination. In H.M. Wallace, R.F. Biehl, J.C. MacQueen, & J.A. Blackman (Eds.), *Mosby's resource guide to children with disabilities and chronic illness* (pp. 259-267). St. Louis: Mosby.

Bull, M., Agran, P., Laraque, D., Pollack, S.H., Smith, G.A., Spivak, H.R., Tenenbein, M., Tully, S.B., Brenner, R.A., Bryn, S., Neverman, C., Schieber, R.A., Stanwick, R., Tinsworth, D., Tully, W.P., Garcia, V., & Katcher, M.L. (1999). American Academy of Pediatrics. Committee on Injury and Poison Prevention. Transporting children with special health care needs. *Pediatrics, 104,* 988-992.

Capen, C.L., & Dedlow, E.R. (1998). Discharging ventilator-dependent children: A continuing challenge. *Journal of Pediatric Nursing, 13,* 175-184.

Centers for Disease Control and Prevention. National Center for HIV, STD, & TB Prevention. (1999a, December). *HIV/AIDS surveillance report: U.S. HIV and AIDS cases reported through December 1999* [On-line] (Vol. 11 No. 2). Atlanta: Author. Available: http://www.cdc.gov/hiv/stats/hasr1102.htm.

Centers for Disease Control and Prevention. National Center for Injury Prevention and Control. (1999b, July 2). *Childhood injury fact sheet* [Online]. Atlanta: Author. Available: http://www.cdc.gov/ncipc/factsheets/childh.htm.

Centers for Disease Control and Prevention. National Center for Injury Prevention and Control. National Center for Environmental Health. (2000). Developmental Disabilities Branch. Atlanta: Author. Available: http://www.cdc.gov/nceh/cddh/ddhome.htm.

Centers for Disease Control and Prevention (2001) National Center for Birth Defects and Developmental Disabilities. Available: http://www.cdc.gov/NCBDDD/.

Cernoch, J.M., & Newhouse, E.E. (1996). Respite care: Support for families in the community. In H.M. Wallace, R.F. Biehl, J.C. MacQueen, & J.A. Blackman (Eds.), *Mosby's resource guide to children with disabilities and chronic illness* (pp. 402-410). St. Louis: Mosby.

Clemens, C.J., Davis, R.L., Novak, A.H., & Connell, F.A. (1997). Pediatric home health care in King County, Washington. *Pediatrics, 99,* 581-584.

Committee on Children with Special Needs. (1998). Managed care and children with special health care needs: A subject review. American Academy of Pediatrics. *Pediatrics, 102,* 657-660.

Committee on Genetics. (1999). Folic acid for the prevention of neural tube defects. American Academy of Pediatrics. *Pediatrics, 104,* 325-327.

Consensus conference. NIH Consensus Development Panel on Rehabilitation of Persons with Traumatic Brain Injury. (1999). Rehabilitation of persons with traumatic brain injury. *Journal of the American Medical Association, 282,* 974-983.

Crocker, A.C. (1996). The impact of disabling conditions. In H.M. Wallace, R.F. Biehl, J.C. MacQueen, & J.A. Blackman (Eds.), *Mosby's resource guide to children with disabilities and chronic illness* (pp. 22-29). St. Louis: Mosby.

Crowley, A. (1990). Integrating handicapped and chronically ill children into day care centers. *Journal of Pediatric Nursing, 16,* 39-44.

Deaton, A.V. (1996). Ethical issues in pediatric rehabilitation: Exploring an uneven terrain. *Rehabilitation Psychology, 41,* 33-52.

DiScala, C., Lescohier, I., Barthel, M., & Li, G. (1998). Injuries to children with attention deficit hyperactivity disorder. *Pediatrics, 102,* 1415-1421.

DiScala, C., Sege, R., Li, G., & Reece, R.M. (2000). Child abuse and unintentional injuries: A 10-year retrospective. *Archives of Pediatrics and Adolescent Medicine, 154,* 16-22.

Dwyer, M.L. (2000). Advanced practice nursing for children with HIV infection. *Nursing Clinics of North America, 35,* 115-124.

Easton, J.K., Rens, B., & Alexander, M.A. (1999). Psychosocial aspects of childhood disabilities. In G.E. Molnar & M.A. Alexander (Eds.), *Pediatric Rehabilitation* (3rd ed., pp. 111-124). Philadelphia: Hanley & Belfus.

Edwards, P. (1992). The evolution of rehabilitation facilities for children. *Rehabilitation Nursing, 17,* 191-195.

Erickson, E.H. (1963). *Childhood and society* (2nd ed.). New York: Norton.

Esperat, M.C.R., Moss, P.J., Roberts, K.A., Kerr, L., & Green A.E. (1999). Special needs of children in the public schools. *Issues in Comprehensive Pediatric Nursing, 22,* 167-182.

Federal Interagency Forum on Child and Family Statistics. (1999). *America's children: Key national indicators of well-being 1999* [On-line]. Washington, DC: Author. Available: http://childstats.gov/ac2000/econtxt.asp.

Feldman, A.B., Haley, S.M., & Coryell, J. (1990). Concurrent and construct validity of the pediatric evaluation of disability inventory. *Physical Therapy, 70,* 602-610.

Fewell, R.R. (1993). Child care for children with special needs. *Pediatrics, 91,* 193-197.

Forsman, I. (1999). Children with special health-care needs: Access to care. *Journal of Pediatric Nursing, 14,* 336-338.

Gittler, J. (1996). Legal rights of children with disabilities. In H.M. Wallace, R.F. Biehl, J.C. MacQueen, & J.A. Blackman (Eds.), *Mosby's resource guide to children with disabilities and chronic illness* (pp. 97-105). St. Louis: Mosby.

Hays, R.M., & Michaud, L.I. (1994). Principles of pediatric rehabilitation. In R.M. Hays, G.H. Kraft, & W.C. Stolov (Eds.), *Chronic disease and disability: A contemporary rehabilitation approach to medical practice* (pp. 215-229). New York: Demos.

Hoeman, S.P. (1997). Primary care for children with spina bifida. *The Nurse Practitioner, 22,* 60-72.

Hostler, S.L. (1999). Pediatric family-centered rehabilitation. *Journal of Head Trauma Rehabilitation, 14,* 384-393.

Jackson, D. & Wallingford, P. (1997). Nursing care across the age continuum: Children and adolescents. In K.M.M. Johnson (Ed.), *Advanced practice nursing in rehabilitation: A core curriculum* (pp. 87-108). Glenview, IL: Association of Rehabilitation Nurses.

Kaitz, E.S. & Miller, M.A. (1999). Adapted sports and recreation. In G.E. Molnar & M.A. Alexander (Eds.), *Pediatric rehabilitation* (3rd ed., pp. 139-155). Philadelphia: Hanley & Belfus.

Kohlberg, L. (1969). Stage and sequence: The cognitive-developmental approach to socialization. In D.A. Goslin (Ed.), *Handbook of socialization theory and research.* Chicago: Rand McNally.

Krach, L.E. & Kriel, R.L. (1999). Traumatic brain injury. In G.E. Molnar & M.A. Alexander (Eds.), *Pediatric Rehabilitation* (3rd ed., pp. 245-268). Philadelphia: Hanley & Belfus.

Kraus, J.F., Rock, A., & Hemyari, P. (1990). Brain injuries among infants, children, adolescents, and young adults. *American Journal of Diseases of Children, 144,* 684-691.

Lindegren, M.L., Steinberg, S., & Byers, R.H. (2000). Epidemiology of HIV/AIDS in children. *Pediatric Clinics of North America, 47,* 1-21.

Madigan, E.A. (1997). An introduction to pediatric home health care. *Journal of the Society of Pediatric Nurses, 2,* 172-178.

Matthews, D. J. & Wilson, P. (1999). Cerebral palsy. In G.E. Molnar & M.A. Alexander (Eds.), *Pediatric rehabilitation* (3rd ed., pp. 193-218). Philadelphia: Hanley & Belfus.

McColley, S.A. (1998). Bronchopulmonary dysplasia: Impact of surfactant replacement therapy. *Pediatrics Clinics of North America, 45,* 573-586.

McPherson, M., Arango, P., Fox, H., Lauver, C., McManus, M., Newacheck, P.W., Perrin, J.M., Shonkoff, J.P., & Strickland, B. (1998). A new definition of children with special health care needs. *Pediatrics,* 102, 137-140.

Molnar, G.E. (1988). A developmental perspective for the rehabilitation of children with physical disability. *Pediatric Annals, 17,* 766, 768-771, 773-776.

Molnar, G.E., & Murphy, K.P. (1999). Spina bifida. In G.E. Molnar & M.A. Alexander (Eds.), *Pediatric rehabilitation* (3rd ed., pp. 219-244). Philadelphia: Hanley & Belfus.

National Information Center for Children and Youth with Disabilities. (1996, June). Respite care [On-line]. *NICHCY News Digest* (No. ND12). Available: http://www.nichcy.org/pubs/newsdig/nd12txt.htm.

Neal, L.J. (1997). Characteristics of the advanced practice nurse in rehabilitation. In K.M.M. Johnson (Ed.), *Advanced practice nursing in rehabilitation: A core curriculum* (pp. 18-22). Glenview, IL: Association of Rehabilitation Nurses.

Pediatric Special Interest Group. (1992). *Pediatric rehabilitation nursing—role description.* Skokie, IL: Association of Rehabilitation Nurses.

Perrin, E.C., & Gerrity, P.S. (1984). Development of children with a chronic illness. *Pediatric Clinics of North America, 31,* 19-31.

Philip, P., Ayyanger, R., Vanderbilt, J., & Gaebler-Spira, D. (1994). Rehabilitation outcome in children after treatment of primary brain tumor. *Archives of Physical Medicine and Rehabilitation, 75,* 36-39.

Piaget, J. (1952). *The origins of intelligence in children.* New York: International Universities Press.

Pontious, S. (1982). Practical Piaget: Helping children understand. *American Journal of Nursing, 82,* 114-117.

Reece, R.M. & Sege, R. (2000). Childhood head injuries: Accidental or inflicted?. *Archives of Pediatrics and Adolescent Medicine, 154,* 11-15.

Scal, P., Evans, T., Blozis, S. Okinow, N., & Blum, R. (1999). Trends in transition from pediatric to adult health care services for young adults with chronic conditions. *Journal of Adolescent Health, 24,* 259-264.

Selekman, J. (1991). Pediatric rehabilitation: From concepts to practice. *Pediatric Nursing, 17,* 11-14, 33.

Sneed, R.C., May, W.L., & Stencel, C.S. (2000). Training of pediatricians in care of physical disabilities in children with special health needs: Results of a two-state survey of practicing pediatricians and national resident training programs. *Pediatrics, 105,* 554-561.

Solnit, A., & Stark, M. (1962). Mourning and the birth of a defective child. *Psychoanalytical Study of Children, 17,* 523-536.

Sterling, Y.M., Jones, L.C., Johnson, D.H., & Bowen, M.R. (1996). Parents' resources and home management of the care of chronically ill infants. *Journal of the Society of Pediatric Nurses, 1,* 103-109.

Thompson, C.E. (1990). Transition of the disabled adolescent to adulthood. *Pediatrician, 17,* 308-313.

Uniform Data System (UDS). (1991). *Uniform data system for medical rehabilitation.* Buffalo: State University of New York at Buffalo.

U.S. Census Bureau. United States Department of Commerce. (1999, October). *Health insurance coverage: 1998* [On-line] (P60-208). Available: http://www.census.gov/prod/99pubs/p60-208.pdf.

U.S. Department of Health and Human Services. (1999). *Child maltreatment 1997: Reports from the states to the national child abuse and neglect data system.* Washington, DC: U.S. Government Printing Office.

U.S. Department of Health and Human Services. (2000, January). *Healthy People 2010, Conference Edition* [On-line] (Vol. 1). Available: http://www.health.gov/healthypeople/Document/HTML/Volume1/15Injury.htm

Ziring, P.R., Brazdziunas, D., Cooley, W.C., Kastner, T.A., Kummer, M.E., Gonzalez de Pijem, L., Quint, R.D., Ruppert, E.S., Sandler, A.D., Anderson, W.C., Arango, P., Burgan, P., Garner, C., McPherson, M., Michaud, L., Yeargin-Allsopp, M., Johnson, C.P., Wheeler, L.S., Nackashi, J., & Perrin, J.M. (1999). American Academy of Pediatrics. Committee on Children with Disabilities. Care coordination: integrating health and related systems of care for children with special health care needs. *Pediatrics, 104,* 978-981.

Gerontological Rehabilitation Nursing 30

Maria B. Radwanski, MSN, RN, CS, CRRN

Mr. Leisawitz was an 85-year-old man who was confused, agitated, and paranoid. He had Parkinson's disease and chronic renal failure. Before coming to the acute rehabilitation hospital, he fell repeatedly while "trying to get away from the nurse." He was admitted to the rehabilitation facility from an assisted living facility. The rehabilitation team used a very traditional approach and questioned, "Our clients must come from the hospital to qualify for rehabilitation, right?" "What is he doing in rehabilitation?" "What are his goals?" "After all, he has Parkinson's disease."

The rehabilitation nurse's assessment found that Mr. Leisawitz had orthostatic hypotension as a side effect of his levodopa/carbidopa medications. She intervened with a medication holiday, better nutrition, and better hydration; his blood pressure stabilized. Then his levodopa/carbidopa was resumed. In therapy, he began to walk safely using a rolling walker, eventually with only supervision. His cognition cleared after the changes in his medication and fluid management. Indeed—what was he doing in rehabilitation?

Tithonus was a mortal in Greek mythology; he won the heart of the goddess Aurora. Aurora asked Zeus to grant Tithonus eternal life as a mortal. What he got was eternal life, but not eternal youth. Tithonus grew increasingly frail and old, cursed with the infirmities of old age (Tennyson, 1952). Modern medicine also grants longevity. The struggle for many older adults today is to answer the question of Tithonus, how to live long while maintaining health and quality of life. This is one goal of Healthy People 2010; *however, for quality of life to keep pace with the quantity of life has proven difficult.*

DEMOGRAPHICS

The number of people age 65 and older will more than double by 2030 in comparison to 1989 (Haber, 1994), and the population 85 years and older will grow from 4 million in 1998 to 8.5 million in 2030 (Administration of Aging, 1999). The challenges of aging are compounded by the onset of chronic illnesses and disabling conditions and use of health resources, including costly acute services (Fowler & Machisko, 1997). However, physiological old age occurs much later in life when compared with half a century ago. Vaccines, antibiotics, surgical advances, new treatments for cancer, heart disease, and other potentially fatal chronic diseases deserve much of the credit. Work, housing, and sanitary conditions are better. Some speculate that the amount of time spent being old is short, which is a paradigm shift. As people live longer, vibrant lives into their 60s, 70s, and 80s, changes in social construction of older adults move to positive, popular images. John Glenn stated, "Old folks have dreams and ambitions, too; don't sit on the couch," after his 1999 space mission. Thirteen million older adults volunteer in some capacity, accounting for 3 billion volunteer hours (National Council on Aging, 1999). Obviously, many older adults have found productivity is one part of maintaining health. Today's "baby boomers" anticipate working for economic reasons beyond traditional retirement age.

The "golden years" have three separate categories: the young old (60-74), the middle old (75-84), and the very old (85+). Although the young old group of seniors face fewer health problems than in years past, the very old are the frailest, least educated, and have the lowest functional levels (Ansello, 1988). Advanced age is related to the high incidence and prevalence of chronic and disabling conditions. For example, national figures show people between 18 and 44 years report arthritis in 50.1 per 1,000 population. By ages 44 to 64 years, arthritis is reported by 240.1 per 1,000 population; between ages 65 and 74 years, 453 per 1,000, and older than 75 years, 523.6 per 1,000 (1994-1995 National Health Interview Survey on Disability, 1999). Perception of health is the number one indicator of quality of life for older adults. In one study, clients who were home bound with health problems and functional impairments had their quality of life affected by one additional symptom, such as urinary incontinence (McDowell, Engberg, Rodriguez, Engberg, & Sereika, 1996). In another study of older adults with hypertension, quality of life also was correlated with their physical symptoms. Quality of life is also an issue for family caregivers. For a disabled family member to be cared for in a community-based setting, establishing a care support network is essential for the family's health and quality of life (Canam & Acorn, 1999). Well-being and self-perception of health can improve for those who are able to participate in an exercise program over time (Bravo et al., 1996).

HEALTH CARE FINANCES

Finances affect the general health of older adults; they rely heavily on medicare. Medicare coverage is not comprehensive—there is substantial cost sharing and many services are not covered, including health promotion and prevention. Medicare beneficiaries spent an average of $2330 (19% of income) for out-of-pocket health care in 1999 (American Association of Retired Persons, 1999) for medicare cost sharing, coinsurance premiums, prescriptions, and balance billing for physicians.

The highly publicized discussions on health care reform did not produce the promised outcomes that providers or consumers envisioned. Everyone bears a piece of the burden for health care but disagreements continue about to whom services are provided and at what point in the system or at what level of preventive intervention. The Balanced Budget Act of 1997 intended $115 billion in medicare savings through 2002 by limiting payments to health care providers through prospective payment systems and by establishing incentives for medicare beneficiaries to embrace lower cost health care alternatives, such as health maintenance organizations (HMOs) (Turnball, 2000). These provisions affected the practice of gerontology rehabilitation nurses and interventions for older clients in all treatment settings. For older people to receive needed and appropriate services, rehabilitation nurses must acquire a working knowledge of the reimbursement system and practice according to nationally accepted clinical guidelines while treating clients' problems quickly and aggressively. They must document thoroughly and communicate effectively with a multidisciplinary team (Turnball, 2000).

Social security and medicare benefits continue to be the sole income and support for many older adults; improvements for health promotion and disease prevention services are inadequate. Rehabilitation nurses have a responsibility in every setting to provide consumer education to promote health and welfare of today's seniors. Assumptions that consumer education is provided by primary care physicians are idealistic and erroneous. Older adults need nurses' time. Experienced rehabilitation nurses listen to their symptoms, use communication skills to understand what underlies the vague symptoms that they report, to answer their questions, to clear up confusion or unwarranted concerns, avoid unnecessary health-related expenses, and to provide necessary information to maximize health and wellness. Opportunities for rehabilitation nurses to interact with older adults occur across the service continuum, especially in community settings they can target services to meet precise needs of the elderly population.

DEFINITION OF GERONTOLOGICAL REHABILITATION NURSING

Gerontological rehabilitation nursing is a subspecialty of rehabilitation nursing, practitioners hold the CRRN credential and practice in multiple settings. The gerontological rehabilitation nurse "provides care and expertise to promote health, maintain and restore function, and provides education and counseling to older clients and their families. Gerontological rehabilitation nurses combine rehabilitation knowledge and skills with gerontological principles to focus on individuals who are 65 years of age and older" (Association of Rehabilitation Nurses, 1994, p. 1). In the care of the older adult, the rehabilitation nurse uses assessment skills and tailors interventions that recognize the effect of chronic disease and age-related changes. Chronic disease and disabilities that occur in the aging process make it difficult to discern whether a client's impaired function is the result of a preexisting limitation, a sequela, or from an acquired condition or disability. Early, rapid intervention and long-term management and protection of health ultimately improves outcomes (Brummel-Smith, 1990). Gerontological nurses consider the age-related changes that are anticipated and functional limitations brought on by an acute illness or injury in older adults. Specific disabling conditions and their concomitant medical issues dictate specific consideration of nursing interventions and techniques (Association of Rehabilitation Nurses, 1994). Equally, and perhaps more importantly, gerontological rehabilitation nurses give effort to assist older adults in preventing disability and chronic illness.

THEORIES AND SOCIETAL ATTITUDES OF AGING

A number of theories have been advanced to explain the aging process. Some theories set forth stereotypes, not only of the elderly, but for cultural bias against the process of aging socially, behaviorally, and physiologically (Table 30-1). This bias is called ageism, prejudice against older adults expressed through beliefs, practices, and attitudes. Society provides many myths and cruel humor about aging that un-

TABLE 30-1 Theories of Aging

Aging Theory	Description
Biological theories	Describe cause-and-effect relationship between body system function and effect on individual over time.
Cross-link theory	Explains that chemical reactions within the body's DNA block cell division and affect normal function of the cell.
Immune theory	Implies that immune responses create an internal war within the aging body, which essentially destroys itself from an autoimmune response.
Free-radical theory	States lipofuscin occurs from fat-protein metabolism. In the aging body this chemical increases in amount and interferes with diffusion and intracellular transport.
Stress theory	Accounts for aging due to "wear and tear" of physiological parts over time and load on psychosocial responses.
Programmed theory	States that aging occurs as a result of a genetically predetermined time clock that runs out, causing aging to occur in every individual.
Psychosocial theories	Indicate there are some interactions between aging adult and society that result in changes in relationships.
Disengagement theory	Suggests a norm for society and aging person to withdraw from one another to allow society to continue its function without interference with youth.
Activity theory	Suggests society and aging adult continue to have an interdependent relationship, and although roles change for aging persons, they have continued importance. New roles and activities are expected to fulfill needs of the community.
Developmental theory (or continuity theory)	Implies that there are a wide variety of relationships between aging individual and society, which is influenced by individual's previous life roles and behaviors. Erickson's last developmental stage of integrity versus despair states that developmentally certain tasks are necessary for aging person to successfully adjust to the last years. Failure to achieve integrity results in despair, even death. These tasks include retirement, adjusting to loss and relocation, as well as maintaining generational ties. Other developmental tasks are to find new interests and hobbies while trying to find meaning to life and prepare for death.

fortunately mold older adults' beliefs about themselves and their worth, however inaccurate. An older person who has impairments or chronic conditions that prevent independent function bears a double burden. The rehabilitation nurse recognizes the role society plays in shaping beliefs and attitudes and assists older adults and their families to transform their beliefs into a more accurate vision of who older adults are and what they can expect from themselves (see case study). They advocate and support goals of *Healthy People 2010* to reduce disparities in access to health care.

ANATOMY AND PHYSIOLOGY

Few changes occur as a result of the aging process; however, the majority of problems previously attributed to aging now are recognized as consequences of chronic disease, social adversity, and behavior. It is difficult to discern whether aging or disease produces certain changes. For example, cardiopulmonary disease may cause some symptoms that also occur with aging (Table 30-2). Aging does produce changes in muscles and joints, particularly atrophy and in the back and legs. Changes in flexibility and strength, posture and gait, and pain make older adults more vulnerable. Osteoporosis, for instance, leads to postural instability, further exacerbated by medications. Medications used in Parkinson's disease or hypertension increase susceptibility to falls as a result of orthostatic hypotension. Strength and flexibility are decreased, endurance to a lesser extent.

NURSING PROCESS: ASSESSMENT

Functional Assessment

Developing rapport with the older adult is an important initial step in obtaining a thorough assessment. Ask questions about lifestyle to understand the client's current function and well-being. For example, how does the person spend the day; what leisure, social, or other activities take place outside the home? Do family members, neighbors, or friends assist with any activities of daily living (ADLs)? Instrumental activities of daily living (IADLs), such as grocery shopping, transportation, financial management, laundry, or cleaning are the first activities that older adults call on others for assistance with when function becomes impaired. Successful long-term or discharge planning takes into account the person's lifestyle, health beliefs, and practices. When older adults are seemingly resistant to answer assessment questions, ask for details about their premorbid self-care practices, management of health and chronic disease, self-perception of the impairment, and ways altered function effects their health. A number of functional evaluation tools can provide objective, reliable, and valid data to help the rehabilitation team fully appreciate the person's functional

TABLE 30-2 Changes from the Aging Process Versus Chronic Illness or Disease

System	Expected Aging Changes	Changes from Disease or Chronic Illness
Cardiopulmonary	Increased risk for arteriovenous blocks or other arrhythmia Decreased pumping force of heart Reduced work capacity Higher resting systolic blood pressure Decreased vital capacity Increased risk of pulmonary infection Increased significance for risk factors of cardiopulmonary disease Reduced chest wall compliance Reduced cough reflex Reduced ciliary activity	Orthostatic hypotension Reduced reflex tachycardia
Musculoskeletal	Decreased height Decreased mobility Decreased stature and posture Redistribution of bone minerals Redistribution of body mass and fat	Muscle atrophy from disuse Slowed movement to accommodate for decreased range of motion Diminished strength Stiffening of joints
Skin changes	Thinner, paler skin Less vascularity to skin and subcutaneous tissue Fewer sweat and sebaceous glands Dryer Less thermoregulatory control Nails more brittle Increased incidence of corns and calluses	Delayed healing time
Neurological	Decreased short-term memory Decreased brain weight Slowed reflexes Increased response time Decreased sensory receptors for temperature, pain, and tactile discrimination	Decreased cerebral blood flow Decreased balance and coordination
Sleep patterns	Longer to fall asleep Less rapid eye movement sleep More nighttime awakenings Quicker transition between sleep cycles	Frequent daytime and early evening "catnaps"
Bowel function	Less saliva Decreased gastric juices Decreased peristalsis Slower absorption	Gastroparesis Dysphagia
Genitourinary function	Vaginal atrophy resulting in urethral changes Prostatic enlargement	Hypertrophy of bladder wall Diverticula formation Decreased size and capacity Elevation of postvoid residual Change in sensation
Liver function	Decreased size Decreased drug metabolism Decreased protein synthesis	Elevated liver enzymes
Renal	Decreased vascularity of nephrons Decreased glomerular filtration rate Decreased creatinine clearance Decreased sodium conservation Slower adjustment to acid-base balance	Increased serum blood urea nitrogen and creatinine
Endocrine	Reduced insulin secretion Decreased glucose tolerance Decline, then plateau of estrogen production Gradual decline in testosterone production	Hypoglycemia

Adapted from Rossman, I. (1986). *Clinical geriatrics* (3rd ed.). Philadelphia: JB Lippincott.

status. When the nurse's assessment data are integrated with other observations, the nurse can work with the older adult and the family to determine the meaning of impairments in their lives and develop a plan that improves the likelihood for a safe and effective discharge plan.

Environmental assessment is a crucial assessment for the safety and well-being of the older adult with disabilities (see Box 14-1). Extrinsic risk factors for falling include living alone and being socially isolated. Other extrinsic factors that can be assessed by the rehabilitation nurse to increase the safety of elders within their environment. Intrinsic risk factors for falls include the number of comorbid conditions, medications, cognition including awareness and insight, attention, judgment, depression, and slow walking speed. Most falls occur from a combination of extrinsic and intrinsic factors (Tiderksaar, 1992).

Medication History

Conduct a thorough medication history with the client and the family. Determine any beliefs or expectations, concerns, or problems the person is experiencing with medications. Ask specifically about each step of the medication regimen. Assess the older adult's technical skills including ability to read the labels, open the container, and take the medication properly. Cognitively, assess whether the person understands why the medication is taken, how many and how often it is taken, and any special instructions, such as take with milk or store out of direct sunlight. Over-the-counter preparations may not be viewed as a medication, nor may home remedies, such as herbal teas, or folk and cultural treatments. Take time to justify the number of pills in each container with the date of the last refill to obtain a sense of compliance. Inspect all medications. Too often people continue to take medications after they are no longer needed, when the drugs are old or outdated, or in undesirable food medication or multiple medication combinations. Older clients have been known to frugally share their medications with others or hoard medications obtained by prescriptions from several providers. Excellent problem-solving and communication skills are needed to determine whether medications are being taken accurately.

Physical Assessment

Other assessment parameters specific to the older adult are outlined in Table 30-3. The sections that follow this outline present content critical to nursing management of the older adult, but not in ranked order. Although concepts are discussed separately, multiple variables and complex factors interact in a given situation. Only through an assessment can the rehabilitation nurse identify how one factor affecting an older adult's health may exacerbate or aggravate another problem, and then reconvene to complicate the first. For example, an older adult who is depressed develops urinary incontinence; the incontinence exacerbates the underlying depression, and eventually malaise leads to poor hygiene and skin breakdown.

Fall Risk Assessment

Decreased mobility is one of the most frequent complaints of older adults. A sensitive, but quick, test to assess the ambulatory older adult's transfer, balance, and walking ability is the "Get up and Go Test." In this test, the adult is asked to sit in a chair, rise from the chair, stand still, walk 10 feet and 9 inches, turn without touching anything, and return to the chair. Deviations in the ability to complete the test warrants further exploration of balance and strength (Mathias & Nayak, 1986). Another screening is the client's ability to stand on one foot without losing balance, repeated with the other foot. Being able to stand on one foot for more than 6 seconds means low risk for falls. A client's ability to reach forward without taking a step also predicts risk for falling. The person stands parallel to a wall, raises the outside arm to a 90-degree angle from the body, and then leans forward as far as possible without taking a step. The distance the person can lean forward is measured from neutral position. Risk for falling is low if the person is able to lean at least 10 inches. Later in this chapter are interventions to decrease the risk for falling.

PLAN OF CARE: NURSING DIAGNOSES

The plan of care for the older adult includes secondary and tertiary care strategies necessary to prevent further disabilities. Co-morbid conditions resulting from chronic illnesses often complicate the rehabilitation process and need attention in the rehabilitation plan to halt complications and prevent sequela.

Health Perception-Health Management Pattern

Risk for Injury Related to Falls

Falls are the second leading cause of traumatic death in older adults (Corrigan et al., 1999), and more than 172,000 older adults fall each year with a cost of more than $7 billion (Gibson, 1990). Of all age groups, elderly people have the highest mortality and experience the greatest degree of disability and dysfunction from falls. Many people live a compromised lifestyle, avoiding any exercise or outings for fear of falling. Older adults who fall have characteristics that differentiate them from their healthy age mates who do not fall. Factors responsible for falls can be intrinsic or extrinsic. Intrinsic factors include age-related physiological changes in balance and gait, cognitive impairment, medical conditions, nutritional status, and the use of certain medications. The chance of falling increases with age when a sedentary lifestyle alters body weight, fat, and muscle distribution, and

TABLE 30-3 Physical Assessment of the Geriatric Rehabilitation Client

Parameters	Assessment	Comments
General appearance	Height	Weight is considered the fifth vital sign of the older adult
	Weight	
	Appropriateness of facial expression	
	Verbal and nonverbal communication	
	Grooming	
	Appropriateness of clothing to the season	
	Grooming of hair, nails	
	Odors	
Head, eyes, ears, nose, and throat	Extraocular muscle coordination and movement	
	Cranial nerve testing	
	Visual acuity	
	Pupillary reflexes	
	Hearing acuity	
	Patency of ear canals	
	Intactness of tympanic membranes	
	Moisture of tongue	
	Color of lips, tongue, and gingival tissue	
	Condition of teeth/fit of dentures	
	Quality of voice	
	Swallowing ability	
Cardiac	Vital signs	
	Blood pressure and pulse lying, sitting, and standing	
	Carotid pulsations, presence of bruits	Assessment of orthostatic hypotension
	Jugular venous pressure	
	Hepatojugular reflux	
	Arterial pulses	
	Peripheral edema	
Respiratory	Rate and rhythm of breathing	
	Chest expansion	
	Presence of adventitious lung sounds	
	Presence of shortness of breath at rest or with activity	
Abdomen	Presence of bowel sounds in all four quadrants	
	Firmness of abdomen	
	Presence of abdominal pain or tenderness	
	Abdominal circulation	
	Liver tenderness, size	
Rectal and pelvic examination	Rectal sphincter tone	Pelvic floor examination necessary in incontinence evaluation. Older adult should otherwise be counseled to have yearly pelvic examination with primary care physician or gynecologist
	Presence of rectal nodules	
	Presence of occult blood	
	Firmness/nodularity of prostate	
	Presence of hemorrhoids	
	Pelvic floor muscle strength	
	Vaginal discharge	
	Presence of rectocele, cystocele	

Adapted from Lueckenotte, A. (1998). *Pocket guide to gerontologic assessment* (3rd ed.). St. Louis: Mosby.

changes the center of gravity. Loss of strength, flexibility, and decreased mobility are risk factors (Allison, 1997).

Diminished stamina and strength attributed to aging may be preceded by reduced physical activity. Remaining physically active is necessary to maintain heart and lung health, muscle and bone mass, flexibility, and independence and to keep a quality of life that the older adult so richly deserves. However, only 39% of older adults exercise on a regular basis (Barry & Eathorne, 1994); pain may impede mobility for elders. Falls are attributed to alcohol and prescription drug use, fear of falling, dizziness, orthostatic hypotension, neuropathic changes, balance problems, urinary urgency, hearing or vision loss, lack of exercise, environmental hazards, and poorly designed or ill fitting shoes. Use of mechanical restraints has been found to increase risk of falling for the hospitalized elder (Arbesman & Wright, 1999). Table 30-4

TABLE 30-3 Physical Assessment of the Geriatric Rehabilitation Client—cont'd

Parameters	Assessment	Comments
Mobility/neurological	Arm and leg strength Range of motion of all joints Gross deformities Atrophy Localized joint or soft tissue inflammation, nodules Joint swelling, tenderness, crepitations Dynamic and static sitting and standing balance; single leg standing balance Quality of gait Speed and coordination of movement Walking posture Range of motion of joints Presence of ataxia Romberg test Sensory testing of extremities: position-sense, temperature-testing, sharp and dull testing Presence of arm drift Rigidity and cogwheeling Position-change induced dizziness and/or vertigo Deep tendon reflexes, including (−, +) presence of Babinski reflex Presence of kyphosis/scoliosis of spine Deviation of leg lengths	The get-up-and-go-test is useful as screening of balance and gait function Ataxia can be assessed by finger-to-nose-to-finger testing and the heel-to-shin test
Skin	Condition of feet and toenails, deformities of toes, feet, and ankles or fingernails Condition of hair Pigmentation Intactness of skin Bruising	
Cognitive	Attention Calculation Short-term memory Long-term memory Orientation Verbal comprehension Nonverbal comprehension Judgment Insight Affect	The Mini-Mental State Exam is useful to use as a screening of cognitive function The Geriatric Depression Scale is useful as a screen of affect

identifies chronic illnesses that may increase susceptibility of older adults to falls and injury.

Alcohol Abuse

Misuse of alcohol is often overlooked as a possible culprit. Zulkowski and Kindsfater's study (2000) of wellness behaviors among independent living older adults found 71% had at least one alcoholic beverage a day.

Fifteen percent of older adults consume four or more alcoholic beverages daily. Women, in particular, drink alone and may conceal it; late-onset alcohol abuse is more common among women (Gomberg, 1994). Signs of abuse or misuse include history of falls, self-neglect, confusion, and family problems (Ruth, Sedlak, Doheney, & Martsoff, 2000). Alcohol is often overlooked as the culprit, causing cognitive changes, confusion, depression, elevated blood pressure,

TABLE 30-4 Chronic Illnesses That Make Older Adults More Susceptible to Falls and Injuries

Type	Illness
Neurological	Transient ischemic attacks, vertigo, syncope, stroke, cerebellar disorders, spinal stenosis, cervical spondylosis, delirium, dementia, myelopathy, normal pressure hydrocephalus, Parkinson's disease, peripheral neuropathy, seizure disorder
Musculoskeletal	Muscle weakness, arthritis, inflammatory joint disorders, myopathy, podiatric problems
Sensory	Vision loss: cataracts, glaucoma, macular degeneration; vestibular disorders: acute labyrinthitis, Meniere's disease, benign positional vertigo, vertebrobasilar disease, drug toxicity
Genitourinary	Incontinence, micturition syncope, nocturia, frequency, urgency leading to unsafe maneuvering to toilet
Cardiovascular	Aortic stenosis, arrhythmia, carotid sinus sensitivity, conduction disorders, myocardial infarction, postural hypotension, syncope, vertebrobasilar insufficiency, volume depletion
Respiratory	Pneumonia, hypoxemia
Environmental/ functional	Improper clothing such as long nightclothes or robes, improper use of wheelchairs and walkers, especially on transfers
Psychological	Anxiety, confusion, depression, stress, fear of falling, impaired judgment, impulsiveness
Drugs	Polypharmacy (4+ medications), new medication, increased dosage, type of drug, (alcohol, antihypertensive, barbiturate, diuretics, narcotics, nonmiotic eye medications, phenothiazines, tricyclic antidepressants, oral hypoglycemics, cardiac medications)

weight loss, self-neglect, neuropathy, gait or balance abnormalities, tremors, jaundice, and ascites. It is essential to address the effects of alcohol on existing conditions, interactions with medications, and increased risk for injuries.

Alcohol is a depressant and affects judgment, coordination, alertness, and reaction time. Research has shown that older adults are negatively affected by smaller quantities of alcohol than their younger cohorts. Older adults are also more likely to be taking prescription and over-the-counter medications. When taken with alcohol, drugs effects are potentiated (National Institute on Aging, 1999). During assessment, the rehabilitation nurse must ask rather than avoid questions regarding alcohol use. Several useful screening tools, such as the Geriatric Michigan Alcohol Screening Test, CAGE (see Chapter 33), and the Alcohol Use Disorders Test are not diagnostic.

Driving

The aging process frequently leads to medical conditions that impair the older adult's ability to operate a car safely. It is essential to identify driving safety hazards resulting from functional impairments that occur from specific medical conditions. Older adults with decreased functional ability drive at reduced skill, putting themselves and others at risk for serious injury. Definite changes in mobility occur when older adults stop driving because they must depend on others for trips outside of the home. A few are fortunate to have spouses or significant others who drive will and will not experience the same consequences, at least until those people are unable to drive. Otherwise, activities and expectations narrow to meet the current circumstances (Burkhardt, Berger, Creedon, & McGavock, 1998).

Elder Abuse

Most elders who are abused have dementia and are women. The characteristics of their abusers help in detection and in assisting potential victims. Caregivers who have extreme stress, anxiety, lack of knowledge as caregivers, and a maladaptive personality may conduct abuse (Buckwalter, Campbell, Gerdner, & Garand, 1996). The person who has been abused may not be able or may not wish to disclose the abuse for fear of retribution. Although many symptoms may be part of changes in the aging process, it is keen assessment of clusters or specific types of symptoms that may detect abuse. For example, numerous bruises that are in various stages of healing and in different colors clustered together in the same area on arms, trunk, or legs may indicate repeated squeezes, grabbing, or blows. Other common indicators are outlined in Box 30-1.

Self-Care Deficit

Adult Failure to Thrive

It is difficult to estimate the number of older adults with functional impairments. Estimates vary. Many needs for assistance are unmet. The core components of self-satisfaction and quality of life are ADLs and IADLs. A growing number of elderly are presenting with deterioration in functional abilities that cannot be directly attributable to an active disease process. Drugs, alcohol, dysphagia, sensory deficits, and depression may trigger adult failure to thrive that may occur rapidly or over several months.

Older adults with chronic functional abilities primarily reside at home. Frail older adults are vulnerable and at highest risk for adverse health outcomes. These definitions com-

Box 30-1 Indications of Possible Elder Abuse

Poor hygiene
Unexplained bruises in different stages of healing
Broken bones
Malnutrition
Dehydration
Depressed mood
Withdrawn, fearful
Cowering
History of treatment in a variety of facilities and by different physicians
Person left alone in the home
Person brought for treatment by someone other than the caregiver
Elder expresses feelings of hopelessness, helplessness
Elder expresses ambivalent feelings toward family

Adapted from Easton, K. (1999). *Gerontological rehabilitation nursing.* Philadelphia: WB Saunders.

monly equate frailty with functional dependence in performing ADLs; common geriatric syndromes of confusions, falls, immobility, incontinence; and extreme old age. Decreased ADLs result in a downward spiral and cause increased frailty, more caregiver services, frequent hospitalizations, and nursing home placements. Using Folstein's Mini-Mental State Exam (Table 30-5), Gill, Williams, Richardson, Berkman, & Tinetti (1997) found domains of cognition measuring most closely associated with ADL dependence were orientation and short-term memory impairments. Furthermore, when older adults lose the ability to manage money or make a telephone call accurately and simultaneously experience decline in their lower body function, they have higher morbidity rates.

Sleep-Rest Pattern

Interrupted Sleep Pattern

Although one third of all Americans report sleep problems, the elderly are the most deprived. In 1990, the National Institutes of Health reported that half of all adults older than 65 years of age living at home had sleep disturbances. Sleep-related complaints are the second most common reason for elderly visits to physicians. Age-related changes are related to diminished blood flow, structural changes, and neuron loss that occurs as the brain ages resulting in a decline of stages 3 and 4 of the non–rapid eye movement stage of sleep; stage 5 is less prominent. These may be associated with age-related changes in core body temperature increases in the elderly, usually occurring between 2:00 and 8:00 AM, the same pattern as in poor sleepers. Psychosocial changes as well as chronic illness are factors. For example, sleep disturbances among those with Parkinson's disease as well as for their spouses' were best predicted by their depression rating. Caregivers reported awakening to assist their loved ones as secondary (Smith, Ellgring, & Oertel, 1997). Sleep pathologies including sleep apnea, neurological diseases affecting the respiratory center and cardiac-respiratory loops, restless leg syndrome in kidney disease, diabetes, and circulatory diseases account for many sleep disturbances. Other conditions attributing to insomnia among the elderly include chronic pain from arthritis and other disorders, esophageal reflux, hiatal hernia, Alzheimer's disease, and Parkinson's disease.

Insomnia

Insomnia, the most frequently encountered sleep problem among older adults is described as a perceived disturbance of the usual sleep pattern that has troublesome consequences. Insomnia is more prevalent in women and increases with age and socioeconomic class. Taking longer than 40 minutes to fall asleep with an average sleep time of less than 6 hours in 24 hours, or feeling of distress, tenseness, or upset resulting from the lack of sleep, are diagnostic. It is characterized by the inability to fall asleep, fragmented sleep because of increased arousal, decreased total time asleep, decrease in sleep efficacy, and early awakenings.

Although there may be a specific reason for insomnia, it is often the result of multiple factors, representing many different underlying causes. Insomnia may begin in response to a crisis situation, such as illness or death and progress into a chain of ineffective behaviors. Assessment of all the underlying factors is necessary to resolve the problem of insomnia.

Cognitive Perceptual Pattern

Chronic Pain

Pain is not always considered relevant in the care of elders, and their perceptions of pain may be devalued or considered inaccurate. Physical signs vary and may be confused with distress or anxiety, experiences of pain are influenced by culture and social norms, and may be altered because of communication and cognitive deficits. Many older adults are reluctant to report pain because they continue to believe that analgesia is addicting and they will become dependent on the medication, regardless of past experiences. They are fearful that use of any analgesia will cause confusion.

Frequent, intense pain is associated with depression and affects independence and self-care abilities that are quality of life issues (Luggen, 1998). Assessment of depression is essential. The Geriatric Depression Scale (see Table 30-8) has dual use in that it can help evaluate the effects of pain on the person's quality of life. Nearly three quarters of community-dwelling older adults acknowledge pain, the greatest prevalence being degenerative joint diseases, rheumatoid arthritis, cancer, and vascular diseases. Impaired or al-

TABLE 30-5 Mini-Mental State Exam

Maximum Score	Score	
		Orientation
5	( )	What is the (year) (season) (date) (month)?
5	( )	Where are we: (state) (country) (town) (hospital) (floor)?
		Registration
3	( )	Name 3 objects: 1 second to say each. Then ask the client to repeat all 3 after you have said them. Give 1 point for each correct answer. Then repeat them until the client learns all 3 Count trials and record. Trials
		Attention and calculation
5	( )	Serial 7's; 1 point for each correct. Stop after 5 answers. Alternatively, spell "world" backwards.
		Recall
5	( )	Ask for the 3 objects repeated above. Give 1 point for each correct.
		Language
5	( )	Name a pencil, and watch (2 points) Repeat the following "No ifs, ands, or buts" (1 point) Follow a three stage command: *"Take a paper in your right hand, fold it in half, and put it on the floor"* (3 points) Read and obey the following: CLOSE YOUR EYES (1 point) Write a sentence (1 point) Copy design (1 point)
______		Total score
		ASSESS level of consciousness along a continuum______________ Alert Drowsy Stupor Coma

Instructions for Administration of Mini-Mental State Examination

Orientation

(1) Ask for the date. Then ask specifically for parts omitted, e.g., "Can you also tell me what season it is?". One point for each correct.
(2) Ask in turn "Can you tell me the name of this hospital?" (town, country, etc.). One point for each correct.

Registration

Ask the client if you may test his or her memory. Then say the names of 3 unrelated objects, clearly and slowly, about 1 second for each. After you have said all 3, ask the client to repeat them. This first repetition determines the score (0–3), but keep saying them until the client can repeat all 3, up to 6 trials. If the client does not eventually learn all 3, recall cannot be meaningfully tested.

Attention and calculation

Ask the client to begin with 100 and count backwards by 7. Stop after 5 subtractions (93, 86, 79, 72, 65).
Score the total number of the correct answers.
If the client cannot or will not perform this task, ask him or her to spell the word "world" backwards. The score is the number of letters in correct order (e.g., dlrow = 5, dlorw = 3).

Recall

Ask the client if he or she can recall the 3 words, you previously asked him to remember. Score 0–3.

Language

Naming: Show the client a wristwatch and ask what it is. Repeat for pencil. Score 0–2
Repetition: Ask the client to repeat the sentence after you. Allow only one trial. Score 0–1
3-Stage command: Give the client a piece of plain blank paper and repeat the command. Score 1 point for each part correctly executed.
Reading: On a blank piece of paper print the sentence "Close your eyes," in letters large enough for the client to see clearly. Ask the client to read it and what it says. Score 1 point only if the client actually closes his or her eyes.
Writing: Give the client a blank piece of paper and ask him or her to write a sentence for you. Do not dictate a sentence; it is to be written spontaneously. It must contain a subject and verb and be sensible. Correct grammar and punctuation are not necessary.
Copying: On a clean piece of paper, draw intersecting pentagons, each side about 1 inch, and ask the client to copy it exactly as it is. All 10 angles must be present, and 2 must intersect to score 1 point. Tremor and rotation are ignored.
Estimate the client's level of sensorium along a continuum, from alert on the left to coma on the right.

From Mini-Mental State: a practical method for grading the cognitive state of patients for the clinician. 1975, *Journal of Psychiatric Research, 12,* 189-198.

tered sensory function, such as vision or hearing and reduced sensation and perception, alter the pain experience. An older adult may guard movement or positioning, change patterns of walking, pace level of activity, or "work around" painful activities without reporting pain. Those with cognitive or communication impairments may become frustrated, angry, or contentious because they cannot express or explain their pain. Careful interviews are important because older adults may experience chronic transient pain, but describe the experience as discomfort, ache, or other names that avoid the name or nature of pain (Flahery, 2000).

Acute Confusion

Acute confusion is defined as an abrupt onset of global, transient changes and disturbances in attention, cognition, psychomotor activity, level of consciousness, and the sleep/wake cycle. Acute confusion or delirium is present at hospital admission for at least 18% of older adults, increasing to 24% after admission. Those with delirium are likely to have chronic cognitive impairment, severe acute illness, multiple comorbid conditions, and functional disability. Acute confusion is characterized by fluctuations in mental function and may be accompanied by hallucinations. Delirium is usually caused by sudden changes in environment (sometimes referred to as transfer trauma). Acute confusion may precipitate an acute illness, but more often it develops as a result of iatrogenic factors: infections, polypharmacy use, or other hospital-acquired complications (O'Keeffe & Lavan, 1997). Acute confusion is treatable, but left undiagnosed can continue indefinitely and progress to a more chronic confusional state.

Chronic Confusion

Chronic confusion or dementia may be caused by a number of conditions (Table 30-6). Dementia is a progressive decline in several dimensions of cognition that severely interfere with a person's everyday living and ability to perform ADLs, but without a decreased level of consciousness. Dimensions of cognition that may be affected include memory, verbal and nonverbal learning, visual-spatial perception, aphasia, apraxia, and agnosia. Changes in personality and motor and gait disturbances may occur. Table 30-7 compares characteristics of chronic and acute confusion. Chapter 26 discusses cognition in detail.

Confusion in older adults remains an enigma for most health providers. Although acute and chronic cognitive impairment are problems for the elderly, providers have inadequate understanding and poor detection and offer inadequate treatment and care (Neelon & Champagne, 1992). Confusion has become known as a normal part of the aging process. This is inaccurate. As a result, health providers fail to attend to this significant cause of acute illness. Confusion in the form of delirium and dementia is prevalent in up to 80% of older adults in acute care hospitals (Evans, Kenny, & Rizzuti, 1993). Confusion also inhibits functional ability that is a direct affect on the outcome of rehabilitation. For example, complications from failure to thrive may occur in older adults who develop chronic confusion. Their weight loss occurs before cognitive changes are apparent but this is subtle because the cognitively impaired person is unwilling or unable to eat (Barrett-Connor, Edelstein, Corey-Bloom, & Wiederholt, 1996).

Self-Perception Self-Concept

Reactive Depression

Ten percent of the general population will experience a major depressive episode in their lifetime. Depression is the most frequent and most treatable disorder in older adults, after delirium and dementia. Depression can be difficult to distinguish from dementia because some symptoms of depression (disorientation, memory loss, and easy distraction) are

TABLE 30-6 Diseases or Conditions and the Relationship of Dementia to the Cause

Disease or Condition	Relationship of Dementia to Cause
Alzheimer's disease	Degeneration of the cells and neurons of the basal forebrain, cerebral cortex and other areas of the brain
Multiinfarct dementia	Small and large cerebral infarcts often associated with hypertension
Normal pressure hydrocephalus	Caused by impeded cerebrospinal fluid and absorption
Metabolic disorders	Chronic anoxia, nutritional deficits, hepatic or uremic encephalopathy, hypercalcemia. Hypothyroidism, hypoglycemia, B_{12} deficiency
Intracranial mass lesions	Caused by benign as well as malignant masses
Medication toxicity	Benzodiazepines, methyldopa, neuroleptics, cimetidine, anti-Parkinson drugs, and others
Wernicke's dementia	Alcoholism
Dementia pugilistica	Repeated head injuries leading to frontal lobe dementia syndrome
Infections	Tertiary syphilis, human immunodeficiency virus
Other degenerative diseases	Anterior lateral sclerosis, Parkinson's disease, multiple sclerosis, Pick's disease, Huntington's chorea, Wilson's disease, epilepsy

TABLE 30-7 Characteristics of Confusion States

Acute Confusion (Delirium)	Chronic Confusion (Dementia)
Acute onset, short duration	Long duration
Fluctuation in symptoms	Progressive symptoms
Short attention span	Short attention span
Reduced ability to shift attention	Personality changes and progressive behavioral problems
Impaired orientation (severity fluctuates)	Severe disorientation with confusion and mood fluctuation
Impaired short-term memory	Impaired short- and long-term memory
Distorted thinking	Impaired thinking and judgment
Distorted perception (delusions, hallucinations, or illusions)	Confabulates, no insight into memory deficits; impaired abstract reasoning
Variable psychomotor behavior	Impairments interfere with social and functional abilities
Reversal of sleep-wake cycles	Chronic confused sleep-wake cycles

Box 30-2 Medications That Can Cause Reactive Depression

Analgesics and antiinflammatory agents
Hormones
Antihypertensives
Anticonvulsants
Digoxin
Estrogen
Anti-Parkinson drugs
Antibiotics
Cardiac drugs
Chemotherapy agents
Immunosuppressives
Sedatives and tranquilizers

similar; it coexists with early to mid dementia in nearly one third of cases. Unrecognized and untreated, it is life threatening. Biological, social, and psychological changes make older adults at higher risk for developing or recurring depression. Examples might be central nervous system changes, adjustments in lifestyle, reduced income, or decline in physical health that negatively affect the older adult (Small et al., 1996). Medications that may cause depression are listed in Box 30-2.

Symptoms of depression in older adults are more difficult to identify because older adults preoccupied with a problem are less likely to express their feelings. They may present with masked depression, denying that they are depressed by covering up symptoms such as crying spells, apathy, and diminished appetite. Others who are more anxious and somatic may display vague, nonspecific complaints that cannot be confirmed during physical assessment. The 30-item Geriatric Depression Scale (Table 30-8) is useful in evaluating depression in older adults. A score of 8 or higher suggests depression and indicates a referral to a psychologist for further evaluation.

PLAN OF CARE: NURSING INTERVENTIONS

Health Perception-Health Management Pattern

Health Promotion and Prevention Strategies

Some aging studies have demonstrated longitudinally that there is a loss of mobility and function among older adults over time; one such study examined 21 functional activities over 2 years. By the end of the second year, functional abilities such as sitting, standing, walking distances, and climbing stairs declined steadily among the participants. However, when looking at individual results, function of specific tasks improved. Getting worse was associated with a decline in health. Getting better was more likely when losses were more recent. Early intervention and therapy were essential variables to prevent further decline in function and improvement in specific tasks (Resnick, 2000; United States Department of Health and Human Services, 1996). Daily activities need to be adapted to medical conditions, but at the same time, exercise and therapy are necessary to increase muscle mass and maintain balance. Good balance is one of the prerequisites of mobility and performing ADLs without difficulty; good balance in turn may enable a physically active life (Era et al., 1997).

Prevention, screening, and wellness programs positively affect elders. Screening for osteoporosis and risk of falls are a few of the many prevention strategies that rehabilitation nurses can implement within the community for clients and for primary care providers. T'ai Chi, strength training, and seated "sit and fit" classes have been well shown not only to improve cardiovascular health, but also physical function including muscle strength, balance, and bone density measures.

Self-efficacy and outcome expectations were variables influencing exercise behaviors in older adults; exercise in turn helps maintain functional performance. In a study of older adults, the only significant factors affecting functional

TABLE 30-8 Geriatric Depression Scale

Question	Score	Question	Score
Are you basically satisfied with your life?	Score 1 if no	Do you think it is wonderful to be alive now?	Score 1 if no
Have you dropped many of your activities and interests?	Score 1 if yes	Do you often feel downhearted and blue?	Score 1 if yes
Do you feel that your life is empty?	Score 1 if yes	Do you feel worthless the way you are right now?	Score 1 if yes
Do you often get bored?	Score 1 if yes	Do you worry a lot about the past?	Score 1 if yes
Are you hopeful about the future?	Score 1 if no	Do you find life very exciting?	Score 1 if no
Are you bothered by thoughts that you cannot get out of your head?	Score 1 if yes	Is it hard to get started on new projects?	Score 1 if yes
Are you in good spirits most of the time?	Score 1 if no	Do you feel full of energy?	Score 1 if no
Are you afraid that something bad is going to happen to you?	Score 1 if yes	Do you feel that your situation is hopeless?	Score 1 if yes
Do you feel happy most of the time?	Score 1 if no	Do you think most people are better off than you are?	Score 1 if yes
Do you often feel helpless?	Score 1 if yes	Do you frequently get upset over little things?	Score 1 if yes
Do you often get restless and fidgety?	Score 1 if yes	Do you frequently feel like crying?	Score 1 if yes
Do you prefer to stay at home rather than go out and try new things?	Score 1 if yes	Do you have trouble concentrating?	Score 1 if yes
Do you frequently worry about the future?	Score 1 if yes	Do you enjoy getting up in the morning?	Score 1 if no
Do you feel you have more problems with your memory than most?	Score 1 if yes	Do you prefer to avoid social gatherings?	Score 1 if yes
		Is it easy for you to make a decision?	Score 1 if no
		Is your mind as clear as it used to be?	Score 1 if no

From Yesavage, J.A., Brink, T.L., Rose, T.L., Huang, V., Adey, M., et al. (1983). Development and validation of a geriatric depression screening scale: A preliminary report. *Journal of Psychiatric Research, 17,* 37-49. Reprinted with permission.

performance were people developing contractures or cognitive impairments (Resnick, 2000). Six activities affect adherence to an exercise program: beliefs about exercise, benefits of exercise, experiences with exercise, goals, personality, or unpleasant sensations associated with exercise (Resnick & Spellbring, 2000). T'ai Chi improves balance through exercise movements consisting of turning, shifting weight from one leg to the other, bending and unbending the legs, and conducting various arm movements. T'ai Chi increases muscular strength and helps prevent physical deterioration (Liu, 1990). Although postural sway increases with age, T'ai Chi incorporates single-stance postures that aid in balance and thus reduce risks of falling (Ross & Presswalla, 1998).

Fall Prevention Strategies

Multifactorial interventions such as medication adjustments, behavioral changes, and balance training exercises used in combination were most significant in reducing falls (Tiderksaar, 1992). Strategies aimed at preventing falls among the very old focus on modification of intrinsic factors. Modification of environmental hazards has the greatest potential for prevention among the young old and those living in private homes (Norton, Campbell, Lee-Joe, Robinson, & Butler, 1997). A careful history as outlined previously is important in identifying the cause of falls for each individual, including possible causes and whether intrinsic, extrinsic, or iatrogenic factors are involved. Fall-related consultation services may involve a physical and occupational therapist, physiatrist, and rehabilitation nurse. A home environment assessment is beneficial to identify and correct potential causes that can prevent further falls. Fall prevention programs offered by community health nurses are geared toward eliminating risks. Table 30-9 lists nursing interventions targeting reduced risk for falls.

Interventions to Decrease Alcohol Use

Misuse of alcohol contributes to falls. Education and counseling increase awareness of the effects of alcohol. Counseling interventions include socialization for older adults who are socially isolated. They may be encouraged to join a senior center or garden club to meet people and participate in activities. Many counties, services for the aging, senior centers, or churches offer transportation at no cost or for a small fee. Referral to a drug and alcohol rehabilitation program is indicated for those with severe alcohol dependency. Older adults usually fare well in treatment programs that address the physiological struggles encountered in withdrawal, as well as the psychosocial roots of alcohol dependence.

Driver Evaluations

Assessment of potential for mobility and functional skills is important before taking the step of revoking an older adult's license to drive because he or she has reduced function and is at risk for injury. Driver evaluation programs, available in most communities, employ occupational and physical therapists to evaluate whether the older adult's function can be enhanced and deficits corrected or adjusted to retain independence. When restricted mobility follows the loss of a dri-

TABLE 30-9 Nursing Interventions to Reduce the Risk of Falls

Risk Factors	Nursing Interventions
New admission or relocation	Orient thoroughly to environment including use of call bell and bedside items
	Introduce to staff and roommates
	Instruct client to call for assistance with movement
	Provide agreed-on place to store belongings and personal care items, dentures, prostheses, or assistive devices
	Place articles within easy reach of the client
	Encourage family involvement and visits
	Provide visible clock, calendar, familiar objects, family pictures, favorite pillow
	Use night light at bedside at night; keep surroundings well-lit during the day
	Provide frequent observations by nursing staff, especially at night
History of fall or physical weakness	Assess thoroughly for risk factors and causes
	Explore associated events (before, during, after falls)
	Use wheelchair, chair, bed alarm devices
	Provide antiskid mat at bedside
	Ensure easy access to bathroom and assure call bell is answered promptly; observe frequently
	Encourage timed voiding every 2 hours during the daytime, every 4 hours at nighttime
	Use bedside commode during hours of sleep for patients experiencing severe urgency, frequency, nighttime confusion, dizziness, unsteadiness at night
	Use comfortable chairs of proper height, with backrests and armrests for easy transfer
	Use comfortable chairs such as rockers, recliners, instead of wheelchair when client is in bedroom or lounge
	Encourage mobility and activity
	Monitor gait, balance, and fatigue level when ambulating
	Provide close supervision
	Encourage reconditioning exercises
	Encourage frequent, short rest intervals
	Provide nonrestrictive reminders to stay seated
	Use appropriate assistive devices
	Avoid clutter on floor surface
Altered mental status	Provide visual cues to client to remind him to call for help
	Eliminate unnecessary noise
	Reduce visual stimulation
	Assign a room near nurses' station
	Provide adequate lighting
	Provide family education and encourage involvement

From Strumf, N., Evans, L., & Patterson, J. (1992). *Reducing restraints: Individual approaches to behavior: A teaching guide.* Huntington Valley, PA: Geriatric Research and Training Center. Copyright 1992 by University of Pennsylvania, School of Nursing. Adapted with permission.

ver's license, the rehabilitation nurse must facilitate communication about options with the client and family. This involves a significant amount of planning to ensure the client has optimal mobility especially when the older adult does not live in close proximity to shopping, recreation, or appropriate accessible transportation. Rehabilitation nurses have a responsibility for educating clients, families, community agencies, and other providers about mobility needs of older adults, and unique needs of individual elders. The nurse can facilitate education and counseling by elder peers and the multidisciplinary team to help people plan ahead to retire from driving, just as they retired from work (Burkhardt et al., 1998).

Improving Functional Skills

Health problems and complications are the most frequent contributors to the loss of functional abilities. If impairments in ADLs, visual-spatial skills, or perception are apparent, refer to occupational therapy for evaluation and treatment. The rehabilitation nurse monitors clients who use adaptive devices to ensure they are able to attend to personal hygiene, grooming, toileting, and eating. The older adult performs as much self-care as possible; those who are confused need additional cues, simple commands, and directions for a step at a time. People who develop receptive aphasia after a stroke or other cognitive impairment benefit from nonverbal gestures to assist them. Encouragement and

TABLE 30-9 Nursing Interventions to Reduce the Risk of Falls—cont'd

Risk Factors	Nursing Interventions
Altered mental status—cont'd	Use companion or closer supervision Implement orientation exercises Consider medication, dehydration, or nutritional or electrolyte imbalances as potential causes
Altered psychosocial or emotional status	Encourage decision making Involve in establishing short-term goals or plan of action Perform psychosocial or psychiatric assessment and treatment as indicated Ask client and family to identify measures to aid in relaxation for inducing sleep (back rub, tea, music) When appropriate, gradually expand psychosocial environment
Visual impairment	Assess vision Ensure eyeglasses are cleaned regularly Assess eyeglasses Encourage use of visual aids Provide adequate lighting Remove unnecessary furniture Avoid highly polished floors that produce glare Have unobstructed and nonskid floor surfaces Use colors to increase visibility (avoid blue-green combinations, use contrasting colors)
Actual or potential incontinence	Ensure easy access to bathroom and assure call bell is answered promptly Assess cause of incontinence Encourage time voiding every 2 hours during daytime, every 4 hours during hours of sleep Use bedside commode during hours of sleep for patients experiencing severe urgency, frequency, night-time confusion, dizziness, unsteadiness at night Encourage using easily manipulated clothing such as elastic waistbands
Postural hypotension	Perform initial assessment of blood pressure lying, sitting, and standing Ensure adequate hydration (1500–2000 ml/24 hours unless restricted) Use elastic stockings Provide education regarding slow, gradual position changes
Medications	Assess drug actions, interactions, side effects; include self-medication and over-the-counter products Assess drug substitutions or elimination Consider changing medications that produce adverse side effects or discomfort Consider drug holidays with physician's order
Comfort	Use relaxation measures identified as helpful by client and family Provide pain medication on a schedule if client is experiencing pain (or when suspected in client who is unable to communicate)

a consistent repetitive routine help most elders establish patterns for incorporating personal health practices into ADLs. Other strategies to assist the older adult with cognitive impairment are in Box 30-3.

Nutritional Considerations

Nutritional deficits often contribute to adult failure to thrive. Oral health is a major problem for all ages, but older people often develop difficulty with dentition. Tooth decay and breakage, receding gums that cause dentures to fit poorly, changing food preferences some brought on by altered glucose tolerance, and chronic diseases such as hypoglycemia and diabetes increase risk. In one study, two thirds of institutionalized or hospitalized older adults had serum albumin levels below normal; only 27% ever received prescriptions for nutritional supplements (Zulkowski & Kindsfater, 2000). Poor nutrition is a known risk for skin breakdown, delayed wound healing, and increased mortality when older adults become ill.

Other inaccurate assumptions are about older adults who are overweight and believed to be getting adequate protein and nutrients. Again, alcohol use affects nutrition and self-care abilities as do food preferences, cultural and dietary habits, financial resources, and transportation to obtain food. Remembering to eat is a subtle culprit. When telephoned by family members, older adults with mild to mod-

Box 30-3 Key Points in Treatment of Chronically Confused Older Adults

Keep requests and demands relatively simple
Keep explanations simple, with one concept or idea stated at a time
Avoid complex tasks that might lead to frustration
Avoid confrontation; defer requests if the client becomes angered or upset
Remain calm, firm, and supportive if the client becomes upset
Allow the client brief periods of quiet time if he or she becomes upset
Be consistent and avoid unnecessary changes in routine
Provide a structured routine
Provide simple explanations and reminders
Provide orientation clues such as clocks, calendars, name outside of room, personal items in surroundings
Recognize decline in function and adjust explanations accordingly
Bring sudden changes or decline in function to the physician's attention; evaluate for medical causes of decline
Review physical activity limitations, such as no driving, need for supervision at all times, assistance for medication management

Adapted from McCloskey, J.C., & Bulechek, G.M. (2000). *Iowa Intervention Project: Nursing classification.* St. Louis: Mosby.

erate cognitive impairment may confabulate sufficiently to affirm that they have eaten. When queried further to identify what time or what they ate, their answers are vague. It is imperative to identify the underlying cause of the nutritional problem and employ nursing interventions. For example, the family of an older adult who experienced chronic confusion believed a microwave would be easier than a gas stove for the person and avoid risk of creating a fire. However, an older adult with chronic confusion is not likely to be capable of new learning; the microwave would most likely be useless.

Interrupted Sleep Patterns

Behavioral Strategies to Treat Insomnia

Transient and intermittent insomnia of short duration does not require treatment Longer episodes of insomnia accompanied by recurrent daytime sleepiness and impaired performance may improve with behavioral interventions and medications may reverse the insomnia. Sleeping pills remain controversial because of the potential side effects, particularly among the elderly. When used, low doses for the shortest duration are recommended. Behavioral techniques to improve sleep include eliminating evening fluids to avoid nocturia and eliminating foods and fluids containing caffeine. Caffeine is found in coffee and tea; in carbonated drinks such as Mountain Dew, Pepsi, Coca-Cola, and Dr. Pepper; and in chocolate.

Relaxation therapy helps reduce or eliminate anxiety and body tension, inducing muscle relaxation and restful sleep. With practice elders can learn these techniques to achieve effective relaxation. Sleep-deprived older adults spend too much time in bed trying to get to sleep. If sleep does not occur within a half an hour after retiring, the person is to get up and leave the room for some type of activity and return to bed a half hour later. Other recommendations are to restrict the hours of sleep during the night, gradually reintroducing time until a normal night's sleep. Another treatment is to recondition elders to associate the bed only with sleep and sexual activity. Activity in bed, such as reading or watching television, are halted because these activities may stimulate the brain and derail sedation and drowsiness in preparation for sleep. Sleep disorders associated with medical problems, such as sleep apnea and depression, require referral for medical evaluation and testing.

Cognitive Perceptual Pattern

Chronic Pain Management

Back pain is associated with impaired function. X-rays and bone density tests of older adults with vertebral fractures reveal that many also have osteoporosis. Pain is an important issue, and activity worsens back pain and pain promotes dependency in ADLs. Pain associated with fractured vertebra leads to lack of sleep, social isolation, and increased dependence; maintaining function prevents debilitation. Active and active-assistive exercises to stretch and exercised to reduce stiffness and pain intensity may be interventions (Bravo et al., 1996).

Nurses know to take report of pain at the person's word (McCaffery & Pasero, 1999). Older adults with chronic confusion may describe their immediate experience with pain accurately, but experiences and pain relief methods may be clouded by their memory deficits. Of 80% of older adults in a nursing home, the majority have chronic confusion, and were able to complete the Visual Analogue Scale (Chapter 24) that continues to be highly effective for assessing pain. The American Geriatrics Society (1998) contributed to guidelines for management of pain in older persons.

Analgesic management of acute, chronic, and neuropathic pain in older adults becomes somewhat cumbersome because of age-related changes in drug metabolism. To offer clients maximum pain relief, it helps to have a menu of at least two prescribed analgesics to administer according to the client's report of pain severity. For example, a pain report of 8 requires a stronger analgesic than a level 4 report. Acetaminophen and Coxx-3 inhibitors (Luggen, 1998) are considered the safest analgesic agents for long-term chronic pain. They may be used concomitantly with neuroleptics or antidepressants depending on the nature and source of the pain. The selective serotonin reuptake inhibitors do not have the anticholinergic, antihistaminic, or α-adrenergic receptor blocking activities of tricyclic antidepressants, and thus have low risk for adverse reactions when used for chronic pain in the elderly.

TABLE 30-10 Medications That May Cause Delirium/Acute Confusion

Drug Class	Generic Names
Anticholinergic agents	Scopolamine, orphenadrine, atropine, trihexyphenidyl, benztropine, meclizine, homatropine
Tricyclic antidepressants	Amitriptyline, desipramine, doxepin, trazodone, fluoxetine,
Antimanic agents	Lithium
Antipsychotics	Thioridazine, chlorpromazine, fluphenazine, prochlorperazine, trifluoperazine, haloperidol
Antiarrhythmics	Quinidine, disopyramide, tocainide
Antifungals	Amphotericin B, ketoconazole
Sedative/hypnotic agents	Diazepam, chlordiazepoxide, lorazepam, oxazepam, flurazepam, triazolam, alprazolam
Barbiturate acid derivative	Phenobarbital, butabarbital, butalbital, pentobarbital
Chloral and carbonate derivatives	Chloral hydrate, meprobamate
Beta-adrenergic antagonists	Propranolol, metoprolol, atenolol, timolol
Alpha-2 antagonists	Methyldopa, clonidine
Alpha-1 antagonists	Prazosin
Calcium channel blockers	Verapamil, nifedipine, diltiazem
Inotropic agents	Digoxin
Corticosteroids	Hydrocortisone, prednisone, methylprednisolone, dexamethasone
Nonsteroidal antiinflammatory agents	Ibuprofen, naproxen, indomethacin, sulindac, diflunisal, choline magnesium trisalicylate, aspirin
Narcotic analgesics	Codeine, hydrocodone, oxycodone, meperidine, propoxyphene
Antibiotics	Metronidazole, ciprofloxacin, norfloxacin, ofloxacin, cefuroxime, cephalexin, cephalothin
Radiocontrast media	Metrizamide, iothalamate, diatrizoate, iohexol
H_2 receptor antagonists	Cimetidine, ranitidine, famotidine, nizatidine
Immunosuppressives agents	Chlorambucil, cytarabine, interleukin-2, spirohydantoin mustard
Anticonvulsants	Phenytoin, valproic acid, carbamazepine
Anti-Parkinson agents	Levodopa, levodopa/carbidopa, bromocriptine, pergolide
Antiemetics	Prochlorperazine, methocarbamol, carisoprodol, baclofen, chlorzoxazone
Antihistamines/decongestants	Diphenhydramine, chlorpheniramine, brompheniramine, pseudoephedrine, phenylpropanolamine

Chronic pain also requires a holistic approach, using behavioral strategies along with medications. The impact the pain has on function is one indicator for implementing aggressive pain management strategies and appropriate modalities. Nonpharmacological techniques are helpful before, during, and after painful activities; before pain occurs or increases; and along with other pain relief measures. Alternative methods for pain relief may be effective, especially when used to complement conventional modalities. Older adults who are engaged actively in making decisions about which modalities to use and are willing to participate in planning a program of pain management have a significant impact on the outcome. Examples of alternative methods include biofeedback, hypnosis, music and activity therapies, guided imagery and distraction, applied heat or cold, massage, acupressure, and transcutaneous electrical nerve stimulation (TENS), as well as the relaxation exercises described in Chapter 28.

Eliminating Acute Confusion

A safe and therapeutic environment is essential for the older adult who is acutely confused. The cause or source of delirium is important to the type of treatment. Assessment includes review of medications, over-the counter drugs, and any supplements. Review the medical history for possible precursors of delirium including head injury, hypertension, cerebral vascular disease, B_{12} deficiency, and emotional or psychiatric disease. Ask family members about past and present drug and alcohol use and dietary habits.

The rehabilitation nurse works with the physician to review drugs that may cause acute delirium in light of the assessment and the individual's history (Table 30-10). When it is not possible to eliminate a drug causing acute delirium because it is the only option for treating a chronic illness, a short medication holiday may be effective to clear the body of the drug. A drug holiday must be supervised. The medication is reintroduced at a lower dose; "start low and go slow" because the goal of therapeutic dosing is to optimize function with chronic disease. Avoid medications that aggravate acute confusion in this age group, namely hypnotics, sedatives, antianxiety agents, tricyclic antidepressants, and others that have anticholinergic side effects.

People experiencing acute confusion have difficulty with abstract concepts; give information in concrete terms. Short-term memory is usually impaired, but may cycle as the delirium clears and many experience delusions and hallucinations. Specific interventions improve the person's outcome and reduce their anxieties. Recognize and accept the client's perceptions, stating your perception of the situation in a calm, reassured and nonargumentative manner. It is important to respond to the client's theme or feelings and not on the content of hallucinations. Quizzing clients with orientation questions they cannot answer only adds frustration. Remove anything in the environment that appears to trigger misperceptions. For example, flower pollen that has fallen onto a tabletop may appear as insects to a person who is acutely confused. Nursing interventions to maintain the client's safety and well-being are outlined in Table 30-9; those for treatment of chronically confused older adults are in Box 30-3. These interventions are appropriate for the acutely confused client until the delirium clears.

Chronic Confusion

Treatment for chronic confusion is targeted to the specific medical or neurological disorder. Some dementia is reversible with treatment. Clients may be able to participate in some decision making, but their degree of insight, reasoning ability, and judgment will vary depending on the diagnosis and the progression of the disease. Use specific examples with families when defining a client's abilities to participate because it is not unusual for families to reflect what they have been taught to only to ask the client who is chronically confused to understand the information. By diagnosis, older adults with chronic confusion is not able to remember complex conversation or understand abstract concepts. They need a supportive, structured, and supervised environment. Family education must extend beyond treatments and medications to incorporate their awareness of these more insidious manifestations of chronic confusion. Interventions are outlined in Box 30-3.

Rehabilitation is appropriate for older adults with chronic confusion, with some caveats. Chronically confused older adults often experience acute illnesses that alter their function and mobility; however, those with early to middle stages of chronic confusion can perform most ADLs when guided by simple verbal and visual cues. The rehabilitation nursing principle of offering guidance to older adults to function within their capabilities applies to family education as well. Emphasize that although it is more time consuming, clients will maintain a higher level of function and general health with fewer complications if they remain engaged and practice self-care as fully as possible.

Self-Perception Self-Concept

Treating Depression

Older adults experience reactive depression as a result of loss, chronic illness, impaired cognitive function, disability, stress, social isolation, and underlying medical illnesses, such as a thyroid disorder. Elderly women experience depression twice as often as men (Phoenix, Irvine, & Kohr, 1997). Interventions for older adults with depressed mood focus on providing safety, stabilization, recovery, and maintenance.

Because older adults are less likely to report feelings associated with depression, the rehabilitation team must weigh the merits of implementing psychotherapy as part of the treatment plan. Psychotherapy has been found to be effective in reducing symptoms of short-term depression in the older adult who is physically ill. Depression is a biochemical illness; antidepressant medications benefit older adults in the same way they do in younger cohorts. Chronic physical illness does not alter responses to antidepressant drugs (Small et al., 1996), but they may take longer to become effective, in some cases as long as 6 weeks from the time of implementation. It is imperative that clients take their medication as prescribed; clients are inclined to discontinue the antidepressant when they begin to feel better. Many clinicians become frustrated with the high incidence of reported side effects to the antidepressant, often symptoms are inherent in reactive depression and are not responses to the medication. Encourage continuing the antidepressant. As with chronic pain, older adults respond best to selective serotonin reuptake inhibitors for the treatment of depression and experience fewer side effects when compared with more traditional tricyclic antidepressants.

Complementary interventions are therapeutic to the older adult include regular exercise and involvement in self-care, both of which improve quality of life (Ellingson & Conn, 2000). Social support, loneliness, and conflict affect depression; the most significant factor is a sense of belonging (Hagerty & Williams, 1999). Increasing socialization may eliminate a cause of depression, particularly in those who have been socially isolated. This intervention is most successful if a companion, perhaps a family member or friend accompanies the older adult for initial at socialization, such as at a senior neighborhood center or other community program. A self-report questionnaire like the Geriatric Depression Scale is useful to use periodically to evaluate outcomes and need for ongoing follow-up.

Health Promotion and Prevention Interventions

Geriatric rehabilitation nurses cannot prevent the aging process; however, they can promote a healthy lifestyle to maximize quality of life and actively engage older adults in the community and in rehabilitation settings. In some settings, inpatient and outpatient rehabilitation ends when the person becomes independent with a set of home maintenance exercises regardless of their preferred style for activity. Many older adults maintain a higher level of function and mobility when given the opportunity to interact socially with their peers. Wellness-maintenance classes targeted at providing recreational activities; structured but safe standing and modified seated exercises classes; and informal social time needed in most communities. For example, The Arthritis Foundation rents the heated swimming pool in the acute rehabilitation hospital every day during lunch although it is not being used for inpatient and outpatient therapy; the pool is then used by the hospital's community-based wellness program in the evening for water aerobics classes. These programs are well attended and worth the effort. The reha-

TABLE 30-11 ***Healthy People 2010:* Health Promotion and Prevention Topics for the Older Adult**

Topic	Key Points
Diet and exercise	Fat, cholesterol, complex carbohydrates, fiber, sodium, calcium Caloric balance Selection of exercise programs
Substance use	Tobacco cessation Alcohol and other drugs: limiting alcohol consumption, driving /other dangerous activities while under the influence, treatment for abuse
Injury prevention	Prevention of falls Medications/abuse practices that increase the risk for falls Safety belts Smoke detectors Smoking near bedding or upholstery Hot water heater temperature Safety helmets Home safety awareness Abuse and neglect awareness Burn prevention
Dental health	Regular dental visits, toothbrushing, flossing
Myths of aging	Dispel myths that urinary incontinence, falls, confusion are normal results of aging
Cardiovascular disease in women	Effects of estrogen as a natural protector, changes after menopause, prevention and treatment
Vaccinations	Flu clinics Pneumonia vaccines
Senior consumer awareness	Scam prevention

Data from U.S. Department of Health and Human Services. (2000). *Healthy people 2010.* Available: http://web.health.gov/healthypeople/document.

bilitation team can refer clients and reduce reliance on expensive inpatient and outpatient resources.

Each encounter with an older adult in a rehabilitation setting is an opportunity for rehabilitation nurses to address goals for health promotion and prevention that will affect quality of life positively. A speaker's bureau with lists of topics sent to women's clubs, nonprofit groups, church groups, senior centers, senior clubs, and similar groups offers opportunity for reaching older adults and the family members involved in their care. Suggestions for health promotion and health prevention topics for the older adult are outlined in Table 30-11.

OUTCOMES

Age-related variables related to actual age, including cognitive skills, socialization status, physical ability, and presence of depression and comorbid conditions are thought to influence functional outcomes. Age is a relevant variable for functional outcomes; those in the young old age group (65-74 years) demonstrated better physical recovery in rehabilitation than the very old (older than 85 years) (Hanks & Lichtenburg, 1996). The very old group demonstrated poorer cognitive skills and more dependent social status at the time of discharge. Although results from the study cannot be generalized because specific comorbid conditions were not defined, other research has shown depression results in poorer health outcomes at discharge and later (Covinsky, Fortinsky, & Palmer, 1996). The outcomes listed in Table 30-12 are measurable in evaluating the effectiveness of nursing interventions.

CRITICAL THINKING

Elderly persons who have experienced chronic illness and functional deficits are at risk for developing other deficits and comorbid conditions. One factor affecting health may exacerbate or aggravate another, then reconfigure and complicate the first situation, and so forth until the seeming "snowball" effect or "cascade" of problems overwhelms clients and their families. Consider this dilemma with clients you encounter in your workplace, clinical site, community programs for the elderly, or your own circle of family and friends.

- Identify obstacles to and resources for preventing or ameliorating the "snowball" or "cascade" of problems; examine individual, family, and community levels.
- Identify gaps, barriers, and resources in the health system, including those occurring at different levels of nursing assessments and interventions, such as primary, acute, or tertiary care, that affect outcomes for elderly persons. Are some nursing processes interfering with rather than improving outcomes?
- Determine whether there are there particular changes associated with aging that are contributing factors.

TABLE 30-12 Nursing Diagnoses and Related Outcomes for Gerontological Rehabilitation

Suggested Nursing Diagnosis	Suggested Nursing Outcomes Classification
Risk for injury	Knowledge: personal safety
	Safety behavior: fall prevention
	Safety behavior: home physical environment
	Safety status: physical injury
	Risk control: alcohol use
	Safety behavior: driving
Adult failure to thrive	Cognitive ability
	Decision making
	Depression control
	Endurance
	Hydration
	Information processing
	Neglect recovery
	Nutritional status
	Self-care: activities of daily living
	Social involvement
	Weight control
Disturbed sleep pattern	Anxiety control
	Cognitive ability
	Memory
	Rest
	Sleep
	Well-being
	Comfort level
	Leisure participation
	Medication response
	Psychosocial adjustment
	Respiratory status: ventilation
Chronic pain	Comfort level
	Depression control
	Depression level
	Pain control
	Quality of life
	Sleep
	Symptom control
	Well-being
	Will to live
Acute confusion	Cognitive ability
	Distorted thought control
	Information processing
	Memory
	Neurological status: consciousness
	Sleep
	Blood glucose control
	Cognitive orientation
	Electrolyte and acid-base balance
	Fluid balance
	Respiratory status: gas exchange
	Risk control: alcohol use
	Risk control: drug use
	Safety behavior: fall prevention
	Safety behavior: personal
	Thermoregulation
Chronic confusion	Cognitive ability
	Cognitive orientation
	Concentration
	Decision making
	Distorted thought control
	Identity
	Information processing
	Memory
	Neurological status: consciousness
	Communication ability
	Safety status: fall prevention
	Safety behavior: home physical environment
	Safety behavior: personal
	Social interaction skills
Depression	Cognitive ability
	Decision making
	Depression control
	Endurance
	Hydration
	Information processing
	Neglect recovery
	Nutritional status
	Self-care: activities of daily living
	Social involvement

Data from Johnson, M., Maas, M.L., & Moorhead, S. (2000). *Nursing outcomes classification (NOC)* (2nd ed.). St. Louis: Mosby.

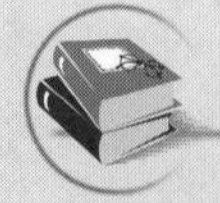

Case Study

Ellen W, 89 years old, was admitted to the acute rehabilitation unit after a brief hospitalization. She had been independent in all personal ADLs; her daughter assisted her with IADLs of transportation and grocery shopping. She fell down the basement steps of her two-story home and remained on the cellar floor for several hours before her daughter arrived on a regular visit to her home. She was admitted with a fractured pelvis to an acute rehabilitation unit where goals were mobilization and strengthening before she returned home. Medical history revealed a bowel resection 5 years prior for cancer, which was considered resolved. She has well-controlled hypertension, noninsulin-dependent diabetes mellitus, and osteoporosis. The physiatrist prescribed Vasotec 5 mg daily, docusate sodium 100 mg daily, psyllium 1 tablespoon daily, Glyburide 5 mg daily, Levsin 10 mg twice daily, and Miacalcin nasal spray two sprays alternating nostrils daily. She received oxycodone 30 mg every 4 to 6 hours for pain.

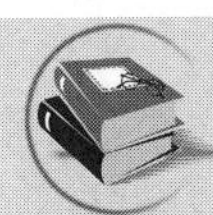

Case Study—cont'd

Although her blood sugar had been very stable, since hospitalization Ellen W experienced some elevations every morning and occasionally in the evening before her bedtime snack. The rehabilitation nurse consulted with the dietitian and the physician. As a team they adjusted her medication and changed her diet from an 1800 calorie American Diabetes Association (ADA) low-residue diet to a 1500-calorie ADA low-residue diet. Ellen also had loose stools and a poor appetite; her abdomen was tender to touch and bowel sounds were hypoactive. Reviewing Ellen's medical record, the rehabilitation nurse noted loose stools documented during the 3 days before her transfer to the rehabilitation unit. Frequent analgesia use prompted the rehabilitation nurse to assess Ellen for fecal impaction. The physiatrist ordered an abdominal x-ray series to rule out obstruction; none was found. The diarrhea disappeared after 2 days, when Ellen began to complain of constipation.

The physiatrist reviewed the medical record from the acute care unit and found a consult with a gastroenterologist that indicated Ellen had "Berks County Bowel Syndrome." Berks County is heavily populated by older adults who were perceived by the medical establishment as being "fixated" on their bowels. The rehabilitation nurse decided to take another look at the problem beginning with reviewing the medical history and medication with Ellen. Ellen knew she was taking Levsin but not *why.* The rehabilitation nurse and physiatrist had assumed the medication was for chronic bladder incontinence, but Ellen denied any history of incontinence. The daughter told the rehabilitation nurse that Ellen began the medication after bowel surgery. Apparently, because of her managed care-medicare HMO, her primary care physician resumed Ellen's care shortly after surgery and continued to prescribe Levsin, which is indicated for use only for several weeks after surgery. Telephoning the surgeon and primary care physician, the rehabilitation nurse obtained agreement, and the physiatrist discontinued the Levsin. Ellen's constipation resolved, but she experienced loose stools again for 2 days. One afternoon after therapy, the nurse walked in to find Ellen putting away her "treat"—sugar-free (sorbitol) gummy bears! She knew that sorbitol can cause bowel hyperirritability; Ellen soon returned to a normal bowel elimination pattern. She continued with her rehabilitation program and returned home after an 8-day inpatient stay. She continued strengthening and gait training as an outpatient.

REFERENCES

Administration of Aging. (1999). A profile of older Americans. Publication. Available on-line http://aoa.gov/stats/profile/profil99.html.

Allison, L. (1997). Identifying and managing elderly fallers. NeuroCon International.

American Association of Retired Persons. (1999). A profile of older Americans. Washington, DC: Department of Health and Human Services.

American Geriatrics Society. (1998). The management of chronic pain in older persons: New guidelines from the American Geriatrics Society. *Journal of the American Geriatrics Society, 46,* 128-150.

Ansello, E. (1988). A view of aging America and some implications. *Caring, 4*(8), 62-63.

Arbesman, M., & Wright, C. (1999). Mechanical restraints, rehabilitation therapies, and staffing adequacy as risk factors for falls in an elderly hospitalized population. *Rehabilitation Nursing, 24*(3), 122-128.

Association of Rehabilitation Nurses. (1994). *Rehabilitation nurses make the difference.* Skokie, IL; Author.

Barrett-Connor, E., Edelstein, S., Corey-Bloom, J., & Wiederholt, W. (1996). Weight loss precedes dementia in community-dwelling older adults. *Journal of the American Geriatrics Society, 44,* 1147-1152.

Barry, H., & Eathorne, S. (1994). Exercise and aging: Issues for the practitioner. *Medical Clinics of North America, 78,* 357-376.

Bravo, G., Gauthier, P., Payette, H., Gaulin, P., Harvey, M., Peloquin, L., & Dubois, M. (1996). Impact of a 12-month exercise program on the physical and psychological health of osteopenic Women. *Journal of American Geriatrics Society, 44*(7), 756-762.

Buckwalter, S., Campbell, J., Gerdner, L., & Garand, L. (1996). Elder mistreatment among rural family caregivers of persons with Alzheimer's disease and related disorders. *Journal of Family Nursing, 2,* 249-265.

Burkhardt, J., Berger, A., Creedon, M., & McGavock, A. (1998). *Mobility and independence: Changes and challenges for older drivers.* U.S. Department of Health and Human Services, Administration on Aging.

Canam, C., & Acorn, S. (1999). Quality of life for family caregivers of people with chronic health problems. *Rehabilitation Nursing, 24,* 5.

Corrigan, B., Allen, K., Moore, J., Samra, P., Stetler, C., & Thielen, J. (1999). Preventing falls in acute care in geriatric nursing protocols for best practice. In I. Abraham, M. Bottrell, T. Fulmer, & M. Mezey (Eds.), *Geriatric nursing protocols for best practice.* New York: Springer.

Covinsky, K.E., Fortinsky, R.H., & Palmer, R. (1996). Relation between symptoms of depression and health status outcomes in acutely ill hospitalized older persons. *Annals of Internal Medicine, 126,* 417-425.

Ellingson, T., & Conn, V. (2000). Exercise and quality of life in elderly individuals. *Journal of Gerontological Nursing, 26,* 17-25.

Era, P., Avlund, K., Jokela, J., Gause-Nilsson, I., Heikkinen, E., Steen, B., & Schroll, M. (1997). Postural balance and self-reported functional ability in 75-year-old men and women: A cross-national comparative study. *Journal of the American Geriatrics Society, 45,* 21-29.

Evans, C.A., Kenny, P.T., & Rizzuti, C. (1993). Caring for the confused geriatric surgical patient. *Geriatric Nursing, 12,* 237-241.

Flahery, E. (2000). Assessing pain in older adults. *Journal of Gerontological Nursing, 26*(3), 5-6.

Fowler, F., & Machisko, F. (1997). The geriatric continuum. *Continuing Care, 1,* 20-23.

Gibson, M. (1990). Falls in later life. In R. Kane, G. Evans, & D. MacFayden (Eds.), *Improving the Health of Older People.* New York: Oxford University Press.

Gill, T., Williams, C., Richardson, E., Berkman., L., & Tinetti, M. (1997). A predictive model for ADL dependence in a community living older adults based on a reduced set of cognitive status items. *Journal of the American Geriatrics Society, 45,* 441-445.

Gomberg, E. (1994). Risk factors for drinking over a woman's life span. *Alcohol Health and Research World, 19,* 220-227.

Haber, D. (1994). *Health promotion and aging.* New York: Springer.

Hagerty, B., & Williams, R. (1999). The effects of sense of belonging, social support, conflict, and loneliness on depression. *Nursing Research, 48,* 215-219.

Hanks, R., & Lichtenberg, P. (1996). Physical, psychological and social outcomes in geriatric rehabilitation patients. *Archives of Physical Medicine and Rehabilitation, 77,* 783-792.

Liu, D. (1990). *The Tao of health and longevity.* New York: Prager.

Luggen, A. (1998). Chronic pain in older adults. *Journal of Gerontological Nursing, 24*(2), 48-53.

Mathias, S., & Nayak, I. (1986). Balance in elderly patients: The "get-up and go" test. *Archives of Physical Medicine and Rehabilitation, 67*(6), 387-9.

McCaffery, M., & Pasero, C. (1999). *Pain clinical manual* (2nd ed.). St. Louis: Mosby.

McDowell, J.B., Engberg, S., Rodriguez, E., Engberg, R., & Sereika, S. (1996). Characteristics of urinary incontinence in homebound older adults. *Journal of American Geriatrics Society, 44,* 963-968.

National Council on Aging. (1999). A new world of longevity: 12 ideas on vital aging [On-line]. Available: http://www.ncoa.org.

National Institute on Aging. (1999). Bethesda, MD: National Institute on Alcohol Abuse and Alcoholism. Available: http://www.nih.gov/nia.

Neelon, V., & Champagne, M. (1992). Managing cognitive impairment: The current basis for practice. In S. Funk, E. Tornquist, M. Champagne, & R. Wise (Eds.). *Key aspects of elder care: Managing falls, incontinence and cognitive impairment.* New York: Springer.

Norton, R., Campbell, J., Lee-Joe, T., Robinson, E., & Butler, M. (1997). Circumstances of falls resulting in hip fractures among older people. *Journal of the American Geriatrics Society, 45,* 1108-1112.

O'Keeffe, S., & Lavan, J. (1997). The prognostic significance of delirium in older hospital patients. *Journal of the American Geriatric Society, 45,* 174-178.

Phoenix, E., Irvine, Y., & Kohr, R. (1997). Sharing stories: Group therapy with elderly depressed women. *Journal of Gerontological Nursing, 23,* 10-15.

Resnick, B., & Spellbring, A. (2000). Understanding what motivates older adults to exercise. *Journal of Gerontological Nursing, 26,* 34-41.

Resnick, P. (2000). Functional performance and exercise of older adults in long term care settings. *Journal of Gerontological Nursing, 26,* 7-16.

Ross, W., & Presswalla, J. (1998). The therapeutic effects of tai chi for the elderly. *Journal of Gerontological Nursing, 42,* 45-47.

Ruth, T., Sedlak, C., Doheney, M., & Martsoff, D. (2000). Alcohol use in elderly women. *Journal of Gerontological Nursing, 26,* 44-49.

Small, G., Birkett, M., Meyers, B., Koran, L., Bystritsky, A., Nemeroff, C., & the Fluoxetine Collaborative Study Group. (1996). Impact of physical illness on quality of life and antidepressant response in geriatric major depression. *Journal of the American Geriatric Society, 44,* 1220-1225.

Smith, M., Ellgring, H., & Oertel, W. (1997). Sleep disturbances in Parkinson's disease patients and spouses. *Journal of the American Geriatrics Society, 45,* 194-199.

Tennyson, Alfred Lord. (1952). Tithonus. *British literature: Blake to the present day.* Boston: DC Heath.

Tiderksaar, R. (1992). Falls among the elderly: A community prevention program. *American Journal of Public Health 82,* 892-893.

Turnball, G. (2000). Understanding the Balanced Budget Act of 1997. *Ostomy Wound Management, 46*(1), 3-4.

U.S. Department of Health and Human Services. (1996). *Physical activity and health: A report of the Surgeon General*. Atlanta, GA: United States Department of Health and Human Services, Centers for Disease Control and Prevention, National Center for Chronic Disease Prevention and Health Promotion.

Yesavage, J.A., Brink, T.L., Rose, T.L., Huang, V., Adey, M., et al. (1983). Development and validation of a geriatric depression screening scale: A preliminary report. *Journal of Psychiatric Research, 17,* 37-49.

Zulkowski, K., & Kindsfater, D. (2000). Examination of care-planning needs for elderly newly admitted to an acute care setting. *Ostomy Wound Management, 46*(1), 32-36, 38.

31 Cardiac and Cardiovascular Rehabilitation

Linda Brewer, MSN, RN, CFNP, CACNP
Billie R. Phillips, PhD, RN, CDFS
Barbara J. Boss, PhD, RN, CFNP, CANP

Mr. B.J. was a 51-year-old man who retired from engineering at age 40 years after suffering a large myocardial infarction (MI) with complications. His risk factor profile included: (1) history of tobacco use/significant exposure to tobacco smoke, (2) dyslipidemia, (3) positive family history, and (4) sedentary lifestyle. He was 1 year postoperative from his second quadruple coronary artery bypass graft (CABG) surgery. His first CABG surgery was 10 years earlier. Mr. B.J.'s deconditioned state and ventricular dysrhythmias made him an excellent candidate for outpatient cardiac rehabilitation. He was started in a Phase 2 program that provided close supervision and cardiac monitoring. Initially his exercises were at low metabolic equivalent units (METs). Mr. B.J. successfully completed phases 2, 3, and 4 of the cardiac rehabilitation program with significant improvement in MET work tolerated. Shortly after completing the program, Mr. and Mrs. B. J. safely traveled in their motor home to Nova Scotia for an extended trip. Later they traveled in an recreational vehicle caravan with friends to Alaska for an extended summer trip. Today, some 15 years after entering the outpatient cardiac rehabilitation program, he travels cross-country with his energetic golden retriever to participate in national target shooting competitions. Needless to say the authors feel his cardiac rehabilitation was "right on target."

Cardiac rehabilitation nursing is an essential professional nursing area within an interdisciplinary specialty—a specialty that is growing in response to needs of an aging population and an increased awareness of the benefits available from cardiac care programs for people of all ages. Technological advances, treatment options, early intervention procedures, and medications have rescued many lives.

Cardiac rehabilitation is defined by the World Health Organization as "the sum of activities required to ensure clients the best possible physical, mental and social conditions so that they may resume and maintain as normal a place as possible in the community" (Wenger et al., 1995). The U.S. Public Health Service definition states that cardiac rehabilitation services are comprehensive, long-term programs involving medical evaluation, prescribed exercise, cardiac risk factor modification, education, and counseling (Wenger et al., 1995).

PREVALENCE OF HEART DISEASE

In the United States, heart disease remains a major threat health. Coronary heart disease (CHD) affects 12.4 million Americans. Sixty percent of the 1.1 million persons survive their myocardial infarctions (MIs) (45% are younger than age 65 years) each year; 6.4 million persons have stable angina; 553,000 persons have coronary artery bypass graft (CABG) surgery (45% younger than age 65 years), and 539,000 have percutaneous transluminal coronary angioplasty (PTCA) (54% younger than age 65 years) each year. In addition, 4.7 million persons have congestive heart failure (CHF) (American Heart Association, 2001). The cost of health care services, institutional care, medications, and lost productivity for clients who have cardiovascular disease exceeded $117 billion in 1993, $56 billion of which was in revascularization procedures in 1994 (American Heart Association, 1994). Cardiovascular diseases and stroke costs exceeded $298.2 billion in 2000 (American Heart Association, 2001). At the same time the pattern of coronary care has changed, as have treatment philosophies; early hospital discharge is a major force. Supervised programs of exercise, education, and lifestyle changes have improved outcome for clients who have coronary artery disease, MI, and other severe cardiovascular conditions.

CANDIDATES FOR CARDIAC REHABILITATION

The Agency for Health Care Policy and Research (AHCPR) clinical practice guidelines list candidates for cardiac rehabilitation to include the million survivors of MI, the million persons with stable angina, and the 671,000 persons who undergo CABG surgery and PTCA. In addition persons with CHF benefit from rehabilitation. But Thomas et al. (1996) found on a national survey of cardiac rehabilitation programs that only a minority of those who are eligible, particularly women, nonwhites, and elders, participate in cardiac rehabilitation programs. Likewise Evenson, Rosamond, and Luepker (1998) found a disparity in cardiac rehabilitation utilization with lower usage among women, persons with less education, and unemployed persons.

Some participants in supervised programs would have been rejected as candidates for cardiac rehabilitation programs in the past. Twenty years ago clients were restricted to bed rest with limited activities over several months after an MI. By the early 1970s eligible applicants to participate in hospital-based cardiac rehabilitation programs exceeded the number of programs and trained staff available. In 10 more years community-based cardiac rehabilitation programs and supervised outpatient clinic programs began to serve low-risk clients. Researchers continue to investigate client risk factors, client self-help, and program methods. Researchers seek the optimal amount and type of exercise that is safe. For example, DeGroot, Quinn, Kertzer, Vroman, and Olney (1998) found weight training of varied intensity is safe, whereas Barnard, Adams, Swank, Mann, and Denny (1999) found one repetition maximum (RM) did not result in injury or soreness and a high-intensity strength training program with an aerobic-based program increased strength with no rate, rhythm, or blood pressure changes (Adams et al., 1999; Beniamini, Rubenstein, Faigenbaum, Lichtenstein, & Crim, 1999).

ADHERENCE CHARACTERISTICS

The characteristics of clients who will adhere to and benefit from programs have been examined. The studies of cardiovascular disease, treatment for cardiovascular disease, and cardiac rehabilitation for many years used predominantly men in the samples. Only recently has this area of research been broadened to study women, minorities, and elders. Eligibility rates compared to referral rates continue to show higher male referral (Halm, Penque, Doll, & Beahrs, 1999) whereas elders are still not admitted to cardiac rehabilitation programs (Heldal, Steine, & Dale, 1996). But Willoughby, Roozen, and Barnes (1997) demonstrated that post-CABG surgery elders had increased functional capacity and cardiovascular efficiency with either a low- or high-intensity aerobic exercise program, whereas Fragnoli-Munn, Savage, and Ades (1998) found elders increased body strength with a combined resistive-aerobic exercise program.

Interestingly compliance rates are higher in men (e.g., Halm et al., 1999). Moore, Ruland, Pashkow, and Blackburn (1998) studied women's exercise patterns and adherence to recommendations for exercise and found that women exercise well below recommendations, which has led to studies addressing why fewer women complete phase 2 programs (Halm et al., 1999); what are the obstacles to participation for women (e.g., Johnson & Heller, 1998); and preferences/perceptions related to aspects of cardiac rehabilitation programs (e.g., Missik, 1999; Moore & Kramer, 1996; Wallwork, 1996). Women tend not to push to peak exercise oxygen consumption maximum with testing. American women have tended to be less athletic in general. This may change now that young women are being encouraged in more athletic careers, including professional sports. Women are now being studied in relation to psychosocial factors in recovery (e.g., Brezinski, Dusseldorp, & Maes, 1998; Con, Linden, Thompson, & Ignaszewski, 1999). Social networks and support as they related to recovery in women are also being examined (e.g., Fridlund, 1997). Researchers around the world are pursuing this line of study.

MENTAL HEALTH EFFECTS OF CARDIAC REHABILITATION

The hostility component of the type A personality is currently viewed as the predominant feature associated with CHD and adverse health outcomes (Wenger et al., 1995). More studies are under way to examine this relationship.

Moser and associates (1999) have examined neuropsychological functioning to determine how this might affect cardiac rehabilitation clients. Recently clients with moderate to severe depression have been found to be twice as likely to die in the 2 years after a severe cardiac event (Shaw, 2000), apparently because depressed clients have an increased tendency to clot (Shaw, 2000). Lavie, Milanni, Cassidy, and Gilliland (1999) have found dramatic improvement in depression, energy level, and exercise capacity when clients enroll in cardiac rehabilitation programs. Social isolation has been found to have a negative impact on prognosis (Wenger et al., 1995). Cardiac rehabilitation improves social adjustment and functioning (Wenger et al., 1995). Training in behavior modification, stress management, and relaxation techniques is effective in lowering levels of self-reported emotional distress and modifying negative affective behaviors (Wenger et al., 1995).

Many clients who enter cardiac rehabilitation programs already have comorbid or disabling conditions. Some develop complications involving additional body systems such as neuromusculoskeletal problems or obstructive vascular impairments in a lower extremity, which must be considered in a plan to improve cardiac function. The interdisciplinary approach and follow-up offered by rehabilitation is an understandable choice for dealing with the complex array of clinical and psychosocial variables associated with these clients and their families.

PROGRAM SERVICES

A cardiac rehabilitation program may be located in a community health setting, major medical center, local hospital, or self-directed home programs. The scope, size, goals, and variety of services can be expected to vary among programs. Although clients enter a cardiac rehabilitation program after a cardiac event, prevention is a program cornerstone. Exercise training is a generic ingredient in all programs; however, for clients with severe cardiac disease and who are high risk, programs offering a broad range of services and a full interdisciplinary team is recommended. This chapter provides information that applies to any cardiac rehabilitation program.

Several professional and governmental organizations have developed standard competencies for professionals in cardiac rehabilitation (e.g., Southard et al., 1994) (Box 31-1), which include qualifications specific to each discipline, as well as additional preferred qualifications. A number of leading organizations that have set program standards is listed at the end of this chapter.

Box 31-1 Core Competence for Cardiac Rehabilitation Professionals

Needs Assessment

Pathophysiology and comorbidity
Professional communication
Standards of practice
Restoration of functional capacity
Biopsychosocial
Risk factors management
Emergency procedures

Goal Setting

Pathophysiology and comorbidity
Professional communication
Standards of practice
Restoration of functional capacity
Biopsychosocial
Risk factors management
Emergency procedures

Intervention

Pathophysiology and comorbidity
Professional communication
Standards of practice
Restoration of functional capacity

Outcome Evaluation

Pathophysiology and comorbidity
Professional communication
Standards of practice
Restoration of functional capacity
Biopsychosocial
Risk factors management
Emergency procedures

From Southard, D.R., Certo, C., Comoss, P.M., Gordon, N.F., Herbert, W.G., Protas, E.J., Ribisl, P., & Swails S.H. (1994). *Core competencies for cardiac rehabilitation professionals.* Position Statement of the American Association of Cardiovascular and Pulmonary Rehabilitation *Journal of Cardiopulmonary Rehabilitation, 14,* 87-92. Copyright 1994 by American Association of Cardiovascular & Pulmonary Rehabilitation. Reprinted by permission.

INTERDISCIPLINARY TEAM APPROACH

The minimum cardiac rehabilitation team is composed of a medical director or supervising physician, a program director or coordinator, and a registered professional nurse in instances when the coordinator is an allied health professional other than a nurse. Although the nurse's role may vary from program to program, the most consistent role functions are (1) coordination and (2) client and family education, essential activities in all programs. Nursing is viewed as vital to all phases of cardiac rehabilitation in all settings, largely because of the holistically oriented goals inherent in nursing. Ideally professionals will include a cardiologist and a physiatrist with training in cardiac rehabilitation as regular or consulting members, an exercise physiologist, and a specialty trained cardiac rehabilitation nurse. A cardiac rehabilitation team may consist of professionals from, but not limited to, those listed in Box 31-2.

Although team members have specialized cardiac knowledge appropriate to their discipline, each professional must understand the role and contribution of the other disciplines. Roles and responsibilities vary across programs. The concept of cross training is valued among members of cardiac rehabilitation teams who regularly share specialty knowledge during team meetings. As a result, the team members participate in developing one another's expertise within the specialty and improve outcome for clients. Regardless of program size, individualized services are one hallmark of quality in a cardiac rehabilitation program, which means the client and family are always active members of the interdisciplinary team.

The success of a cardiac rehabilitation program has been attributed in part to the professional quality of the team members. Composition of the team reflects the program philosophy, available resources, client population demand, and administrative policies of the institution or agency. Taken together, members of a team of cardiac rehabilitation professionals have advanced practice knowledge about (1) cardiovascular disease; (2) current intervention strategies; (3) educational goals, methods, and tools, (4) health psychology; (5) nutrition;, (6) exercise physiology; (7) emergency procedures; (8) rehabilitation principles and care for clients with comorbid conditions; and (9) common over-the-counter (OTC) supplements used by clients, especially those with potential risk when used in conjunction with exercise (eg., Ma Huang) and with thrombolytics (eg., ginseng and ginkgo).

Box 31-2 Cardiac Rehabilitation Team Members

Client
Physician
Social worker
Exercise physiologist
Physical therapist
Clergy member
Occupational therapist
Respiratory therapist
Family
Professional registered nurse
Dietitian/nutritionist
Mental health professional
Health educator
Pharmacist
Vocational rehabilitation counselor
Case manager and others, as needed

An ideally functioning team is characterized by collaborative relationships and collective decision-making that includes client and family members. The obvious advantage is full integration of professional expertise and an informed and involved client. However, many teams tend to function as multidisciplinary, rather than interdisciplinary, teams. As a result each member contributes uniquely to a client's cardiac program but all members do not have equal status in decision-making processes. Decisions may not be arrived at jointly and may exclude clients' preferences or ignore their lifestyles. The nurse coordinator who is able to work effectively with each team member to assure continuity and integrated planning is a key to success. (Chapter 2 provides additional discussion of team models for practice.)

CHANGING REHABILITATION SCENE

As changes in the health system reduce hospital length of stay, rehabilitation nurses in facilities and community settings are working with clients who are more acutely ill and who have more complex health problems than in the past. Similarly these same clients have fewer days to accomplish rehabilitation goals in a facility before they move on to community settings. Rehabilitation nurses are called on to function as case managers and consultants to community programs and to assist with preventing clients from reentering hospitals.

In this reperfusion era, early triage and treatment of persons with acute coronary syndromes changes the immediate course of an acute MI and alters long-term prognosis (Cummins, 1997). Early reperfusion via thrombolytic agents or PTCA decreases the size of infarction and improves regional and global left ventricular function (Cummins, 1997). Secondary prevention through cardiac rehabilitation has an increasingly important role.

Cardiac rehabilitation is one of several emerging rehabilitation nursing specialties that deals with clients and settings where increased acuity raises the potential for cardiac and other life-threatening emergencies. Preparation in rehabilitation facilities requires written procedures and equipment to respond to clients' needs and for nurses to be knowledgeable about managing cardiopulmonary emergencies for clients and how to implement any advanced directives. As a result nurses may decide to review critical care and medical-surgical content with current clinical guidelines for practice and to learn how to operate equipment or perform procedures associated with these specialty practices.

DEEP VENOUS THROMBOSIS

Because deep venous thrombosis (DVT) is such a serious risk and is not covered elsewhere in this text, DVT is covered here during the inpatient discussion. Many rehabilitation clients carry a high-risk score for DVT during the course of hospitalization and rehabilitation. There is a relatively high incidence of DVT in persons with acute MI and CHF. A large number of clients, even with preventive measures, still suffer DVT and its complications.

Thrombophlebitis refers to an inflamed vein as a result of thrombus formation. Phlebothrombosis is probably the same entity, but it does not exhibit a marked inflammatory component. DVT refers to either thrombophlebitis or phlebothrombosis in the deep venous system of the legs (Bullock, 1996; Rubin & Farber, 1994). The most important consequences of DVT are pulmonary embolism and the syndrome of chronic venous insufficiency (Launius & Graham, 1998). DVT accounts for 600,000 hospitalized clients in North America per year (Collins, 1998) and results in 100,000 deaths each year. To minimize client morbidity and mortality, prevention, early diagnosis, and treatment of DVT is paramount (Launius & Graham, 1998).

Factors Associated with DVT

The triad associated with DVT was described in 1846 by Virchow as (1) stasis of blood, (2) increased blood coagulability, and (3) vessel wall injury. One or a combination of these factors may produce the formation of a thrombus (Bullock, 1996). Bed rest and immobilization are associated with decreased blood flow and venous pooling in the lower extremities, increasing the risk of DVT. Persons immobilized by hip fracture, joint replacement, or spinal cord injury are especially vulnerable to DVT. The risk of DVT is increased in situations of impaired cardiac function. Older persons have a higher incidence compared to younger persons, probably because disorders that produce venous stasis occur more frequently in older persons. The homeostatic mecha-

TABLE 31-1 DVT Risk Assessment Scoring Tool

Underlying Conditions	Points
Obesity (>20% Metropolitan Life Table)	2
Malignancy	2
Abnormal coagulation factors at admission	2
Pregnancy (including 8 weeks postpartum)	2
History of thromboembolism	2
Injury-Related Factors	
AIS ≥ 3 for chest	2
AIS ≥ 3 for abdomen	2
Spinal fracture	2
Coma (Glasgow Coma Scale score < 8 for > 24 hours)	3
Immobility (excluding pelvic fractures)	3
Required bedrest > 5 days	3
Complex leg fracture	3
Pelvic fracture requiring bedrest > 5 days or operative fixation	4
SCI (complete or incomplete with paraplegia or quadriplegia)	4
Iatrogence Factors	
Central femoral line > 24 hours	2
Four or more transfusions during past 24 hours	2
Surgical procedure > 2 hours	2
Repair or ligation of vessels	3
Age	
≥ 40 but < 60	2
≥ 60 but < 75	3
≥ 75	4

From Lehigh Valley Hospitals and Networks (1997).
AIS, Abbreviated Injury Scale (an anatomically based system that classifies individual injuries by body region on a 6-point ordinal severity scale [a score of ≥ 3 is considered serious]); *DVT,* Deep vein thrombosis; *SCI,* Spinal cord injury.

nism hypercoagulability is designed to increase clot formation and any conditions that increase the concentration or activation of clotting factors increase the risk of DVT. The loss of body fluids associated with hemoconcentration cause the clotting factors to become more concentrated. Deficiencies in certain plasma proteins that normally inhibit thrombus formation, such as antithrombin III, protein C, and protein S, predispose to DVT. Any conditions that increase the levels of fibrinogen, prothrombin, and other coagulation factors increase the risk of DVT. Women in the postpartum state are at increased risk. The use of oral contraceptives appears to increase coagulability and predispose to DVT. DVT has been associated with certain cancers. Although the reason for this is largely unknown, it is thought that substances that promote blood coagulation may be released from tissues because of the cancerous growth. Introduction of catheters traumatizes vessels and increases the risk of DVT (Porth, 1994) (Table 31-1).

Anatomy and Pathophysiology

A thrombus develops as a result of slowed flow in the venous bloodstream and is associated with platelet aggregation. The thrombus organizes from its outer margins centrally. In some veins, the entire thrombus becomes organized with complete and permanent occlusion of the lumen. If the thrombus is large, involution usually occurs by a process of partial fibrosis and partial lysis, which is probably the result of the action of naturally occurring fibrinolysins in the blood. The center may disappear but the periphery organizes into a fibrous ring or in other instances, bands of fibrous tissue extend across the old lumen of the vein and divide it into many small lumina. The result is some restoration of function of the vein but there is partial obstruction of the lumen by the remaining fibrous tissue and a decrease in circular diameter (Bullock, 1996; Spittell & Spittell, 1994).

There are varying degrees of inflammatory reaction, depending on the different layers of the vein involved. The accumulation of inflammatory cells, leukocytes, lymphocytes, and fibroblasts cause congestion of the capillaries in and around the venous walls. The amount of obstruction to venous blood flow is directly related to the size and location of the involved vein. Collateral circulation compensates through superficial veins, and this may also be true in obstruction of the saphenous vein of the leg. Because of the numerous anastomoses that exist, collateral channels may become evident even after obstruction of the superior or inferior vena cava (Bullock, 1996; Joyce, 1994). When thrombosis occurs in the iliofemoral or axillary veins, there is only partial collateral circulation causing, increased venous pressure in the veins. The result is distension of all veins, venules, and capillaries, which causes intense congestion and impedes normal reabsorption of fluids and electrolytes. Progressive edema in the affected limb results (Bullock, 1996).

Assessment

Signs and symptoms of DVT develop acutely and usually persist for 1 to 3 weeks. Acute thrombophlebitis in small or medium veins rarely produces systemic reaction, whereas involvement of the larger vessels may cause the temperature to rise as high as 102° F (39° C) (Bullock, 1996). The most common signs of DVT are related to the inflammatory process and include pain, swelling, and deep muscle tenderness. Accompanying signs may be fever, malaise, and an elevated white blood count as well as sedimentation rate. The site of the thrombus formation is somewhat determined by the location of the physical findings (Figure 31-1). The most common sites are in the venous sinuses in the soleus muscle, the posterior tibial veins, and the peroneal veins. Swelling of the foot and ankle is usually present, although it may be slight or absent. Calf pain and tenderness are common complaints. Femoral vein thrombosis will produce pain and tenderness in the distal thigh and popliteal area. The most profound signs are produced when there are thrombi in

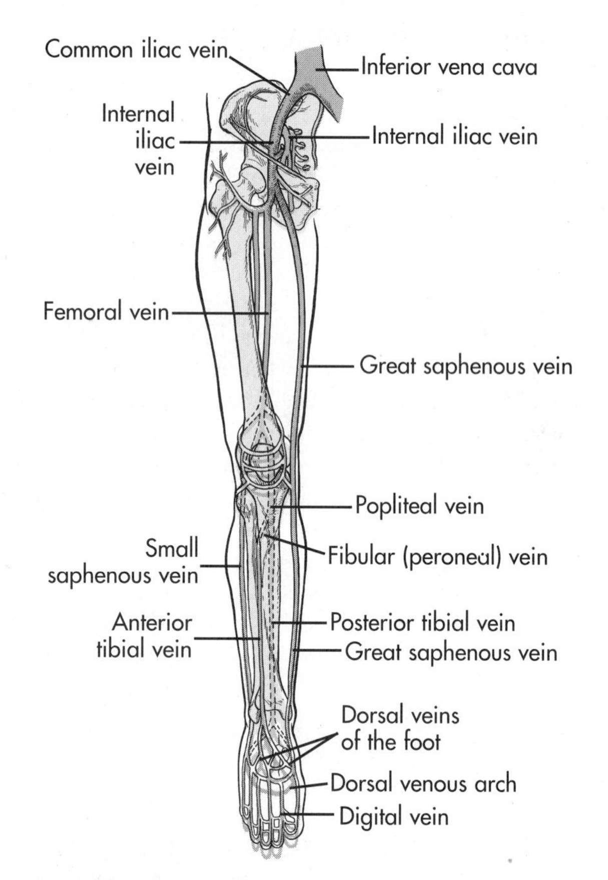

Figure 31-1 Major veins of the lower extremity (anterior view). (From Thibodeau, G.A., & Patton, K.T. [1999]. *Anatomy & physiology* [4th ed.]. St. Louis: Mosby.)

ileofemoral veins. There is swelling, pain, and tenderness of the entire extremity. DVT in the calf veins produces pain with active dorsiflexion of the foot (Homans' sign) (Porth, 1994).

Because of the risk of pulmonary embolism, the need for early detection and treatment of DVT is paramount. Diagnostic aids that assist with the diagnosis of DVT include contrast DVT scans, Doppler ultrasonic flowmeter studies, impedance plethysmography, and ascending venography. Radioactive fibrinogen is intravenously injected. Any developing thrombus incorporates the radioactive fibrinogen. This allows detection and recording of the location of the thrombus. These diagnostic measures assess venous flow and fibrinogen accumulation. They are also useful in monitoring persons at risk for developing DVT.

Nursing Diagnosis

Nursing diagnoses appropriate when DVT exists include (1) altered tissue perfusion: peripheral, (2) risk for anxiety or anxiety, and (3) ineffective management of the therapeutic regimen.

Therapeutic goals in the presence of DVT are to arrest the thrombosis, dissolve existing clots, prevent clot migration, and provide supportive care. With DVT in large veins another goal may be to remove the thrombus (Figure 31-2).

Intervention

The nursing intervention classification related to DVT is embolus precautions, anxiety, and possibly pain in affected extremity. Elevation, antiembolism stockings, passive and active range of motion, position change, and pain medication are the appropriate nursing interventions.

CORONARY ARTERY CIRCULATION

Coronary Artery Perfusion

The following anatomic and physiological review describes coronary artery perfusion— impairments are common factors in many cardiac disorders—and contains information that influences nursing assessment and rehabilitation interventions.

The epicardial section of the coronary arteries lies on the surface of the heart. Perforator vessels enter the myocardium, delivering blood to the endocardial and subendocardial areas of the myocardium during diastole. The subendocardial area is the last area of the heart muscles fed by the coronary arteries. This explains why, in an MI, the damage spreads from the endocardial area outward to the epicardial area. The resting coronary blood flow is 5% of the total cardiac output (Guyton & Hall, 1996).

Three special factors affecting coronary artery perfusion are (1) cardiac cycle, (2) heart rate, and (3) diastolic intraventricular pressure. These factors must be considered while making all nursing assessments related to the cardiac cycle. In systole the ventricular wall tension greatly limits blood flow through the coronary perforator arteries. Most coronary circulation occurs during ventricular diastole, while the ventricular walls are "relaxing," which allows a significant reduction in ventricular muscle tension (Guyton & Hall, 1996). The significant anatomic parts of the heart are illustrated in Figure 31-3; distribution of the coronary arteries throughout the heart and great vessels via the coronary arteries is illustrated in Figure 31-4.

The left anterior descending (LAD) artery of the left coronary artery supplies the septum and the anterior portion of the heart, the major portion of the left ventricle. The circumflex artery supplies the lateral portion of the heart, the lesser portion of the left ventricle. The right coronary artery (RCA) supplies the inferior portion of the heart which includes parts of the right atrium and right ventricle, the sinoatrial node in 55% of persons, and the atrioventricular (AV) node in 90% of persons. The left atrium is supplied by branches arising from the LAD.

Altered Coronary Artery Perfusion

Since 1994, the term acute coronary syndromes (ACS) has been used to refer to clients with ischemic chest pain. ACS

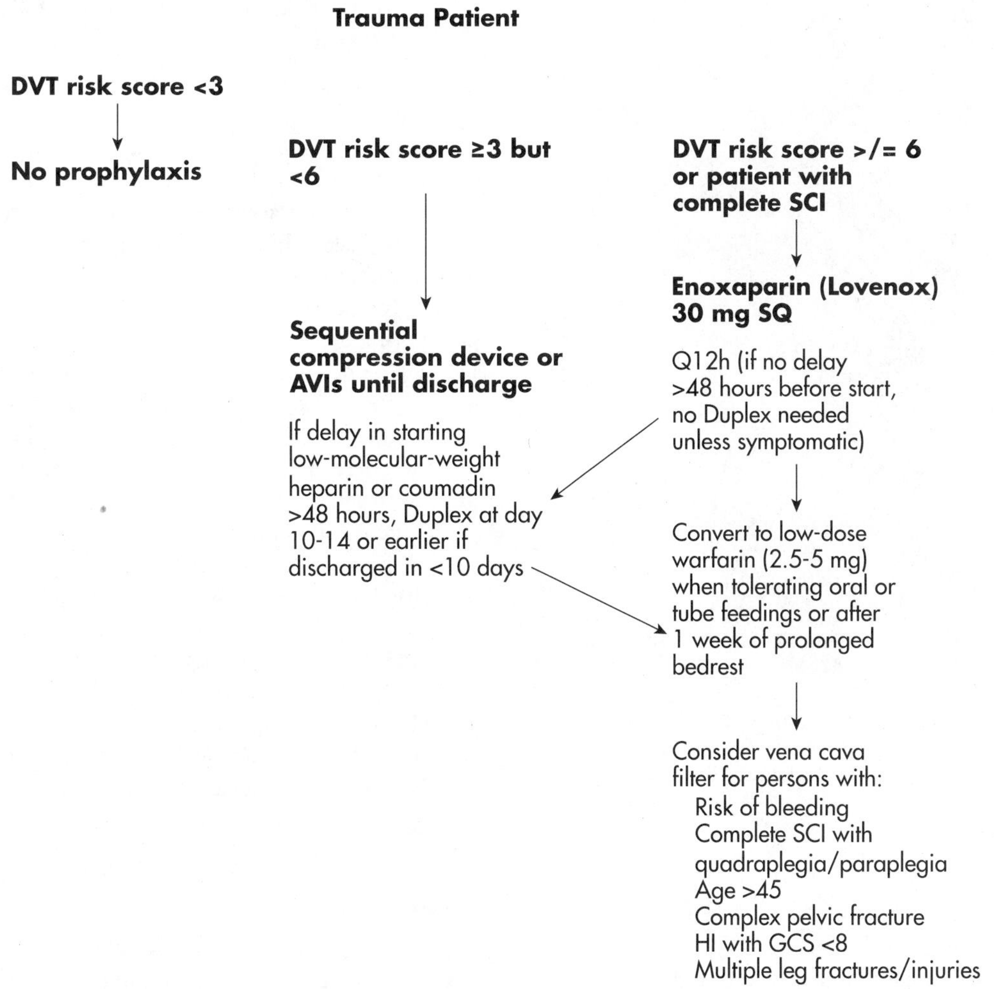

Trauma Patient

DVT risk score <3

↓

No prophylaxis

DVT risk score ≥3 but <6

↓

Sequential compression device or AVIs until discharge

If delay in starting low-molecular-weight heparin or coumadin >48 hours, Duplex at day 10-14 or earlier if discharged in <10 days

DVT risk score >/= 6 or patient with complete SCI

↓

Enoxaparin (Lovenox) 30 mg SQ

Q12h (if no delay >48 hours before start, no Duplex needed unless symptomatic)

↓

Convert to low-dose warfarin (2.5-5 mg) when tolerating oral or tube feedings or after 1 week of prolonged bedrest

↓

Consider vena cava filter for persons with:
- Risk of bleeding
- Complete SCI with quadraplegia/paraplegia
- Age >45
- Complex pelvic fracture
- HI with GCS <8
- Multiple leg fractures/injuries

Figure 31-2 Deep vein thrombosis prophylaxis algorithm for trauma client. (From Lehigh Valley Hospitals and Networks, Allentown, PA, 1997.)

represents a continuum of a similar disease process. The continuum is stable angina, unstable angina, non-Q-wave infarction and Q-wave infarction (Cummins, 1997).

Heart rate is a crucial factor in clients with a coronary syndrome. *Heart rate dictates the length of diastolic perfusion time for coronary arteries.* As the heart rate increases, the diastolic filling time shortens. A client with stable angina has a threshold heart rate in which diastolic filling time shortens to a point where adequate coronary artery perfusion cannot perfuse stenotic arteries. Rest thwarts anginal episodes. Rest enables the heart rate to slow, and slowed heart rate lengthens the diastolic filling time of the coronary arteries, thereby increasing perfusion. Beta-blockers may also be an important adjunctive therapy to control heart rate.

Conditions associated with higher circulating blood volume, such as CHF, may cause myocardial ischemia and anginal symptoms when blood flow to subendocardial areas is reduced. Diastolic intraventricular pressure alters perfusion of blood through the perforator arteries. A high diastolic interventricular pressure reduces the blood flow to the subendocardial area. Sublingual nitroglycerine or other nitrates relieve anginal symptoms by causing blood to pool in tile extremities, which in turn decreases blood return to the heart (preload) and reduces intraventricular diastolic pressure, thereby increasing perfusion.

Stable angina indicates an unchanging atherosclerotic process in the coronary perfusion. Precipitation and relief of anginal symptoms are predictable. In contrast, unstable angina or preinfarction angina suggests an active, dynamic atherosclerotic progression. Symptoms of unstable angina become unpredictable, appear with less exertion, occur more frequently, and tend not to be relieved as readily as with stable angina.

Various symptoms, including angina, are associated with myocardial ischemia. With atherosclerosis, fixed stenotic lesions develop in the coronary arteries. A lesion that occludes 60% or more of an artery can produce myocardial ischemia and anginal symptoms, which often are precipitated by exertion or emotional (dis)stress, accompanied by increased heart rate. Thus rest is a key intervention once again. At

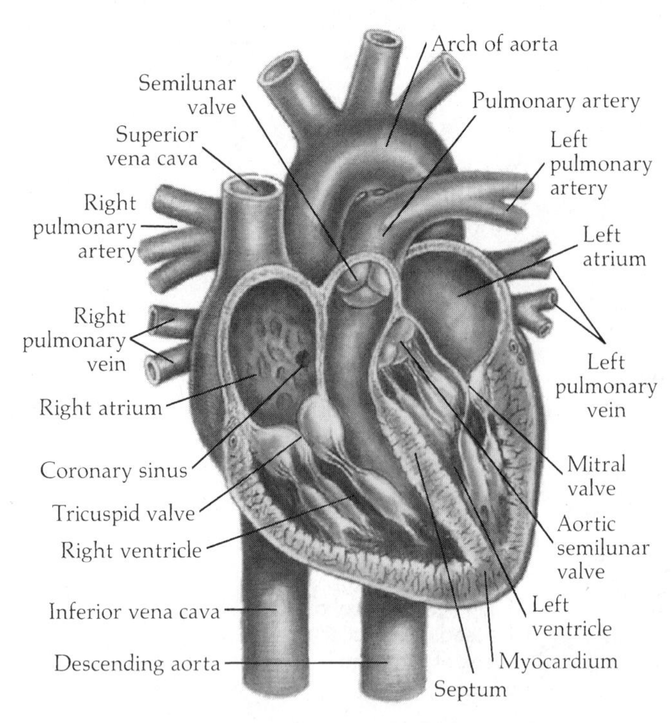

Figure 31-3 Frontal schematic view of the heart. (From Thompson, J.M., McFarland, G.K., Hirsch, J.E., & Tucker, S.M. [1997]. *Mosby's clinical nursing* [4th ed.]. St. Louis: Mosby.)

times ischemia of the left ventricle may precipitate transient congestive heart disease. Symptoms of CHF include dyspnea and paroxysmal nocturnal dyspnea. Elderly clients who develop congestive heart disease classically become fatigued, gain weight resulting from edema, and develop cough with dyspnea . A rise in heart rate also occurs in CHF, also decreasing coronary perfusion and further aggravating the situation.

Occlusion of the LAD causes an acute anterior wall infarction. These infarctions have a variety of more specific labels depending on the site of occlusion. The higher the occlusion is in the LAD, the more extensive the anterior wall damage and the more extensive is the left ventricular pump problem. These persons will always be at risk for CHF. Conduction problems (e.g., third-degree heart block) have a poor prognosis because of the extent of muscle loss. Occlusion of the circumflex artery is associated with less risk for pump problems.

Occlusion of the RCA produces an acute inferior wall infarction. Inferior MIs are often associated with conduction disorders (frequently temporary) because of disruption of blood supply to the AV node. Right ventricular cardiogenic shock occurs in massive right ventricular infarctions and is often associated with complete heart block. Cardiogenic shock from a right ventricular failure requires definite diagnosis because the therapeutic management is quite different from left ventricular failure.

A CARDIAC REHABILITATION PROGRAM

A cardiac rehabilitation program begins within a few days after an MI; coronary angioplasty, CABG surgery, heart transplant, or other cardiovascular surgery when a client participates in a predischarge assessment based on a protocol involving exercise testing. Testing provides one basis for assigning risk to clients to determine their need for further medical treatment, their exercise tolerance and abilities, potential for exercise training, and level of safe exercise with an appropriate level of supervision in a rehabilitation program. Client risk, cardiac drugs and other medications, types of exercise, parts of the body exercised, and specific therapeutic exercises are all factors in initial prescriptions for exercise training. The following principles apply to cardiac rehabilitation:

- Client and family are active participants in the team
- Early assessment using exercise testing is repeated and used to decide activities and medical treatment or medication needs
- Individual prescriptions for exercise training are designed to reach optimal level of function
- Interdisciplinary assessment, intervention, and evaluation of risk factors; and psychosocial and occupational status are completed and communicated (Miller, 1991)

Phases of Cardiac Rehabilitation Management

Cardiac rehabilitation is a continuous process that commonly is categorized according to phases. Although phases have been numbered 1 through 4 traditionally, many programs use the terms *inpatient* and *outpatient* to designate phases. AHCPR guidelines identify three phases—beginning during hospitalization, followed by a supervised ambulatory outpatient program lasting 3 to 6 months, and continuing in a lifetime maintenance stage (Wenger et al., 1995). Each component or phase of a program needs to be defined and the specific functions described clearly to avoid confusion due to variations among programs.

Inpatient Cardiac Rehabilitation (Phase 1)

Phase 1 is usually a program to limit physical and psychological consequences of the acute cardiac illness for the client who is still hospitalized. This phase lasts between a few days for persons with percutaneous transluminal angioplasty or uncomplicated MI to 2 weeks with persons who have complicated MI and other CHD pathology. The major components are risk assessment, early ambulation and physical activity, and education of clients and families.

Assessment

Identifying a client's level of risk not only assures lifesaving measures are available for those with serious conditions but

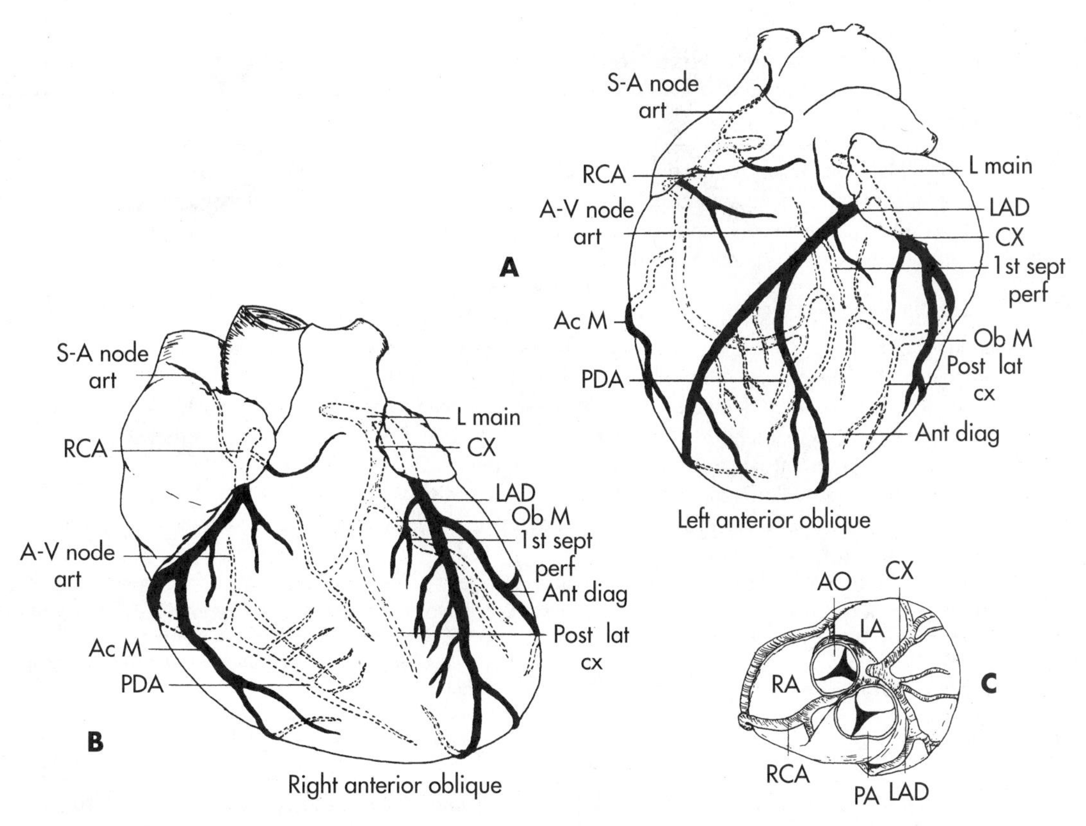

Figure 31-4 **A** and **B,** Left and right anterior oblique views of coronary arteries and their distribution. **C,** Cephalad view of coronary artery distribution in relation to the great vessels. (From Gravanis, M.S. [1993]. *Cardiovascular disorders: Pathogenesis and pathology.* St. Louis: Mosby.) *S-A,* Sinoatrial; *Art,* artery; *RCA,* right coronary artery; *A-V,* atrioventricular; *Ac M,* acute marginal; *PDA,* posterior descending artery; *Ant,* anterior; *Post,* posterior; *Lat,* lateral; *Cx,* circumflex; *Ob M,* obtuse marginal; *Sept,* septal; *Perf,* perforator; *LAD,* left anterior descending; *L,* Left; *AO,* Aorta; *LA,* Left atrium; *RA,* Right atrium; *PA,* Pulmonary artery.

prevents unnecessary restrictions for clients with low risk levels. A treadmill test is a means of evaluating risk and usually is conducted before hospital discharge.

Treadmill Exercise Test

Most people have become familiar with or performed a "stress test." Exercise tolerance test using a treadmill to categorize their cardiac risk. Risk stratification is based on clinical assessment of functional capacity, myocardial ischemia, ventricular dysfunction, and arrhythmias (Wenger et al., 1995) (Table 31-2). After acute MI, clients perform a supervised and monitored treadmill exercise test. Test results are correlated with other factors to form an individualized risk stratification—high, low, or moderate—that is used in the exercise prescription and long-term treatment plan.

The test uses treadmill equipment with recording monitors and with controls to vary the speed and raise the elevation of the exercise surface as the client "walks" to evaluate the level of fitness. The test is conducted at an intensity that is appropriate for the client's physical activity at the time. Predischarge testing is important to determine a home program and activity or work capacity, as well as to minimize a client's anxiety about activity. Repeated testing at certain intervals helps in determining whether the exercise prescription needs to be altered. For instance, a client's health status, medications, or symptoms may change. Repeated exercise testing at intervals may occur as necessary but is recommended at 6 months and 1 year after the initial testing.

Other modalities for exercise tests include the graded exercise test, stationary cycling, or arm crank ergometry. The arm crank enables clients with lower body paralysis or paresis, such as with paraplegia, to be tested provided they have sufficient upper body strength and function. A variety of modified or adapted equipment and devices have been used in exercise testing of persons with disabilities. Generally these consist of modified bicycles to suit clients' abilities such as a supine model or arm- and leg-powered model, or equipment attached to existing wheelchairs that connects the equipment to cycles or similar circular modifications. With modifications that rely on the parts of the body with functional abilities to supply crank or cycle power, the exercise workload should not overtax some parts of the body while

TABLE 31-2 Minimal Guidelines for Risk Stratification

Risk Level	Characteristics
Low	No significant left ventricular dysfunction (i.e., ejection fraction $>$ 50%)
	No resting or exercise-induced myocardial ischemia manifested as angina or ST-segment displacement
	No resting or exercise-induced complex arrhythmias
	Uncomplicated myocardial infarction, coronary artery bypass surgery, angioplasty, or atherectomy
	Functional capacity $>$ 6 METs on graded exercise test 3 or more weeks after clinical event
Intermediate	Mild to moderately depressed left ventricular function (ejection fraction 31%-49%)
	Functional capacity $<$5-6 METs on graded exercise test 3 or more weeks after clinical event
	Failure to comply with exercise intensity prescription
	Exercise-induced myocardial ischemia (1–2 mm ST-segment depression) or reversible ischemic defects (echocardiographic or nuclear radiography)
High	Severely depressed left ventricular function (ejection fraction, 30%)
	Complex ventricular arrhythmias at rest or appearing or increasing with exercise
	Decrease in systolic blood pressure of $>$15 mm Hg during exercise or failure to rise with increasing exercise workloads
	Survivor of sudden cardiac death
	Myocardial infarction complicated by congestive heart failure, cardiogenic shock, or complex ventricular arrhythmias
	Severe coronary artery disease and marked exercise-induced myocardial ischemia ($>$2 mm ST-segment depression)

From American Association of Cardiovascular and Pulmonary Rehabilitation. (1995). *Guidelines for rehabilitation programs* (p.14). Champaign, IL: Human Kinetics Books. Copyright 1995 by American Association of Cardiovascular and Pulmonary Rehabilitation.
MET, Metabolic equivalent units.

achieving necessary cardiovascular levels (Wenger et al., 1995; ACSM, 1998).

Client and Family Assessment

Clients and families are enabled to participate as members of the team when they receive information, individualized to their needs, as soon as possible after hospitalization and throughout the program. A nursing assessment of stressors and coping ability is initiated for both client and family, with referral for mental health counseling as needed. Clients and family members may have misconceptions or misunderstandings about the disease trajectory or the benefits from participating in a cardiac rehabilitation program (Moranville-Hunziker, Sagehorn, Conn, Feutz, & Hagenhoff, 1994). For instance, some may believe that bypass surgery is a curative procedure that expunges cardiac risk. Health beliefs have been found to be important factors influencing a client's decision and ultimate participation in a cardiac rehabilitation program. Assessment questions related to pertinent learner characteristics are presented in Table 31-3.

Nursing Diagnoses and Therapeutic Goals during Inpatient Cardiac Rehabilitation

For clients who have uncomplicated cardiac disease, MI, or who have received angioplasty, the relevant North American Nursing Diagnosis Association (NANDA) diagnostic category are risk for activity intolerance under the typology of exercise-activity pattern, anxiety, and knowledge deficit (Gordon, 2000). Inpatient goals for these clients are early risk assessment and early ambulation so they can be discharged promptly to outpatient rehabilitation care and reenter the community.

Some clients who survived sudden cardiac death or who have severe cardiac conditions, CHF, serious ventricular arrhythmias or complex dysrhythmias, left ventricular dysfunction, myocardial ischemia, or certain specific electrocardiogram (ECG) changes with exercise. Diagnostic categories for these persons also may include activity intolerance, decreased cardiac output, and altered tissue perfusion. Inpatient goals are risk reduction via intensive monitoring and early diagnosis and treatment of problems and complications, conditioning or reconditioning through mobilization (physical activity and exercise), and reentry into the community.

Therapeutic Plan and Interventions

When clients have uncomplicated disease, some Nursing Intervention Classifications are Cardiac Care and Cardiac Care: Rehabilitation, Teaching: Disease Process, Teaching: Diet, Teaching: Activity/Exercise, Teaching: Individual, and Teaching: Prescription Management. Clients with more severe cardiac problems may fall into several Nursing Intervention Classifications including Cardiac Precautions, Cardiac Care: Acute, Dysrhythmia Management, Shock Management: Cardiac, and Hemodynamic Regulation (Table 31-4). These clients receive intensive monitoring using electrocardiographic telemetry in order to detect problems immediately during activity and exercise. Referral to appropriate members of the cardiac rehabilitation team begins in phase 1.

The first and foremost goal in rehabilitation as well as in acute and chronic care is prevention of DVT. Risk assessment and implementation of a DVT prophylaxis plan accomplish this. A risk assessment tool is presented in Table 31-1. A DVT prophylaxis plan is shown in Figure 31-2.

TABLE 31-3 Education-Related Variables and Assessment Questions

Variable	Questions
Existing knowledge base	What do the client and family already know? What illness-related experiences have the client and family had?
Readiness to learn (motivation)	What priority does the client and family place on learning? What questions or comments are being raised? What factors may be impeding motivation (denial, anger, depression)?
Learning needs	Do the client and family state these needs specifically? Do nurse, client, and family agree on needs and on the resulting plan?
Client and family goals	What goals, if any, do the client and family have in relation to illness, lifestyle changes, or therapeutic regimens?
Client and family energy for learning	Are symptoms present that must be taken into account? Can teaching strategies be geared to the energy level?
Presence of support systems	Will others be learning with the client and family? Do learning needs of client and family coincide with those of other support persons?
Time for learning	How much time is available? Can a "time line" be designed with the client and family?
Potential for understanding	What factors will influence understanding of the content (educational level, language, presence of sensory dysfunction, amount of anesthetic, medications that depress central nervous system, anxiety level)? What resources are available that will promote understanding?

From Jillings, C. R. (1988). *Cardiac rehabilitation nursing.* Rockville, MD: Aspen. Copyright 1988 by Aspen. Reprinted by permission.

TABLE 31-4 Relevant Nursing Interventions during Inpatient Cardiac Rehabilitation

Monitor

Cardiac status—preload, afterload, perfusion (angina, ST changes), conduction (prolonged PT interval, frequent PVs, ectopy close to T)
Trends in blood pressure, hemodynamics parameters (CVP, PCWP, PAP, CO, cardiac index, left ventricular work load index as appropriate)
Intake and output, urine output, daily weights if appropriate
Electrolytes (K^+, Mg^{++}) as appropriate
Oxygen delivery deficit (PaO_2, Hgb, CO), if appropriate
Renal function (BUN, CR), if appropriate
Acid-base balance, if appropriate
Liver function, if appropriate
Coagulation studies (PT, PTT, platelets, fibrinogen, fibrin degradation/split products)
Medication effectiveness and side effects

Assess

Chest pain
Heart sounds, cardiac rhythm, heart rate, pulses, capillary refill, temperature and color of extremities
Neurological status
Jugular vein distention
Peripheral edema

Other

Maintain cardiac monitoring and intravenous (IV) access
Obtain serial ECGs
Relieve/prevent pain/ischemia
Correct oxygen deficits, acid-base balance, and electrolytes
Provide a calm/supportive environment. Decrease external stressors
Administer IV fluids and medications (vasodilators including nitrates, diuretics, vasoconstrictors, inotropics)
Promote optimal preload (e.g., nitrates, position)
Promote afterload reduction (vasodilators, pump devices)
Promote coronary artery perfusion (mean arterial pressure > 60 mm/Hg), control tachycardia
Prevent Valsalva maneuver (stool softeners, antiemetics, no rectal temperatures)
Prevent DVTs
Maintain nutrition (small frequent feedings, healthy diet, decreased caffeine, sodium, cholesterol, and fats)
Document dysrhythmias (frequency/duration, hemodynamics response, activities associated with inset, pain, or syncope)

Exercise Component

The exercise component is a foundational piece of cardiac rehabilitation. A major physiological effect of exercise training is improved functional capacity resulting from peripheral effects (Cottin et al., 1996; Fletcher et al., 1995) with reduced fatigue, dyspnea, angina, or related symptoms. Overall musculoskeletal condition improves, but the constriction of coronary arteries and collateral circulation is not known to be directly affected. Limited left ventricular function improvement has been found (Goodman et al., 1999). Exercise training has produced improvement in exercise tolerance in both men and women of every age group, including those older than 75 years (Balady, Jette, Scheer, & Downing, 1996). Exercise training also results in improvement of symptoms including decreased angina, decreased symptoms of heart failure, and improvement in clinical measures of ischemia (Wenger et al., 1995).

Recently, low to moderate intensity strength training soon after an infarction has been found to be effective and may actually have lower complication rates than aerobic exercise (Daub, Knapik, & Black, 1996; Maoirana, Briffa, Goodman, & Hung, 1997). Strength training did not increase peak oxygen consumption or reduce myocardial oxygen demand. Combined training improved aerobic and muscle fitness (Adams et al., 1999; Beniamini et al., 1999; Stewart et al., 1998;). The increased basal metabolic rate helps with obesity. Increased insulin sensitivity decreases blood glucose levels and cholesterol.

Regular physical activity is known to protect against the progression of many acquired chronic diseases or development of others and assists in maintaining functional abilities. Low-intensity exercises, 3 times a week for 30 minutes plus warm-up and cool-down time, have been found to be more effective in improving functional capacity and endurance than once believed (Pashkow & Dafoe, 1993; Wenger et al., 1995) during the maintenance phase. Initially more frequent exercise may be needed.

Progressive physical activity is supervised and performed in a gradual sequence of steps to increase a client's work demand as a means to counter deconditioning, as well as to prevent DVT or pulmonary emboli. Activities and exercise often improve a client's sense of well-being and control, reduce confusion and depression, and stimulate outlook. Thus within the first 1 to 2 days, clients without medical complications are encouraged to perform grooming and self-care activities, get out of bed for toileting when this requires walking short distances, and perform range-of-motion (ROM) exercises.

Throughout the day a client takes several short walks after which the nurse monitors blood pressure, heart rate, and ECG readings for signs of changes that would indicate a need for reduction of activities. Principles of energy conservation are important considerations as ROM exercises progress from passive to active; eventually 1- to 2-lb weights can be used as resistance. Soon thereafter, warm-up and stretching activities or mild calisthenics are added to ambulation or treadmill work; clients who will encounter stairs at home or work practice climbing and descending stairs.

Exercise Prescription. The exercise component of cardiac rehabilitation is individualized for each client as a means of reaching cardiovascular conditioning goals. This is in effect an exercise prescription. Data collection begins with the client's complete medical history, current health status, medication profile, lifestyle data, and level of fitness based on multiple results from exercise testing including workload, heart rate, and blood pressure, and any signs of dysrhythmia or ischemia. The prescription is a written program or "dosage" for exercise that describes the type or mode of exercise; how often it is to be performed; and the duration, intensity, and rate of progression of intensity.

Intensity describes the level of demand at which an activity is performed and is tailored to each client's status. Clients are monitored closely for signs or symptoms of myocardial ischemia or ventricular dysrhythmias, or various other criteria (Box 31-3) for termination of the exercise session. The mode of activity describes how the exercise will employ which large muscle groups in sustained and rhythmic activity, most commonly walking. Other appropriate modes include cycling, jogging, rowing, arm ergometry, and aquatic exercises. Duration of exercise refers simply to the length of time an activity is to be performed. When upper extremities are exercised, care is taken related to intensity so that blood pressure is not increased. Clients are taught not to use the Valsalva maneuver with upper extremity exercises and when lifting weights. Learning yoga breathing helps to prevent clients from holding their breath. Initially exercises are performed at low intensity and should not produce sore muscles or undue fatigue.

Related to weight training, the American Congress of Re-

Box 31-3 Criteria for Termination of Exercise Session

Fatigue
Dizziness
Dyspnea
Nausea
Change in cardiac rhythm
Anginal symptoms
Drop in heart rate > 10 beats/minute
Drop in systolic blood pressure > 10 mm Hg
Rise in heart rate > 20 beats/minute for myocardial infarction clients (or number determined with previous exercise testing)
Rise in blood pressure more than amount determined with previous exercise testing

From American College of Sports Medicine. (2000). *Guidelines for exercise testing and prescription* (6th ed.). Philadelphia: Lippincott, Williams & Wilkins.

habilitation Medicine and the American Academy of Physical Medicine and Rehabilitation published DeGroot et al.'s recommendation that stable cardiac clients on a circuit weight training program start with initial load between 40% and 60% 1-RM (one repetition maximum and at least 60 seconds of rest between exercise) (1998).

The exercise prescription ensures that the exercise session is both beneficial and safe; age related target heart rates are not used as guides for cardiac programs. Guidelines for the prescription are based on results from research, and it is written by a specialist such as an exercise physiologist, who understands the principles and physiology of exercise (ACSM, 1998). Each component of the exercise session is modified further by a client's prognosis of risk (risk stratification factor), which is used to identify clients who may be a higher risk for developing complications during an exercise session. Other guidelines contain information about client selection for exercise and contraindications for exercise. Remember that current guidelines are not predictive of complications during supervised activity (Paul-Labrador, Vongvanich, & Merz, 1999). Criteria for terminating an exercise session are listed in Box 31-3. The Borg rate of perceived exertion can be used by health care provider and clients to estimate heart rate. This scale, commonly used during exercise studies and in cardiac rehabilitation program, correlates symptoms with the heart rate to guide the client toward an optimal intensity of exercise. Perceived intensity is rated numerically, to give an estimated heart rate (see Chapter 18).

Metabolic Equivalent Unit (MET) Method. Exercise and activity requirements are described using the MET method. One MET is equivalent to the amount oxygen an individual requires while standing at rest or 3.5 ml of O_2/kg/minute (Woods, Froelicher, & Motzer, 2000). Increased expenditure of energy levels results in multiplication of MET values—that is, a 2-MET activity uses oxygen twice the rate of a 1-MET resting activity, or an 8-MET activity uses oxygen at 8 times the resting rate.

The MET method is easy to understand and can be related to both occupational and leisure activities (Tables 31-5 and 31-6). For example, a client may have ischemic ECG changes at a level of 6 METs on a graded exercise test. Therefore this client's instructions should direct him or her to perform activities that are at or below the level of 5 METs. Clients often do not estimate the actual energy requirements—METs—for daily activities or leisurely pursuits. Women routinely have been found to underestimate the energy requirements needed to complete household tasks

Table 31-5 Activities of Daily Living: Household Tasks (Energy Requirements in METs)

Very Light Activity		Light Activity		Moderate to Heavy Activity			
1	2	3	4	5	6	7	8
Eat	Dress						
Drive car	←	Grocery shop	→				
Sit to do hygiene	Stand to do hygiene						
Lie awake	Take tub bath	Shower					
Sit		Do general housework	Paint				
		←	Have sexual intercourse	→			
	Cook while standing	Mop	←	Move furniture	→		
Walk: 1 mph	Walk: 2 mph	Walk: 3 mph	Walk: 3.5 mph	Walk: 4 mph			
		Iron		Walk upstairs			
		Hang clothes					
		Dust					
		Make bed			Carry suitcase		
		Wash clothes by machine					
		Clean floors					
Sweep		Clean windows					
		Ride mower			Cut grass: hand mower		
		Cut grass: push mower			Shovel snow		
	Do light gardening	Do heavier gardening					
		Polish floor					
			Rake leaves				
		Vacuum	Trim hedges/trees				
	Wash dishes		Wash windows	Clean gutters	Wash car		

METs, Metabolic equivalent units.

Table 31-6 Activities of Recreation/Vocation (Energy Requirements in METs)

Very Light Activity		Light Activity		Moderate to Heavy Activity				Heavy Activity		
1	2	3	4	5	6	7	8	9	10	11
	Play billiards		Play volleyball							
		Bowl								
		Canoe: 2.5 mph			Ski				Ski (fast downhill)	
Play cards	Do wood work	Paint					Run cross-country			
Knit	Play musical instrument		Do masonry							
Read		Cycle: 5 mph	Cycle: 6 mph	Cycle: 8 mph	Cycle: 10 mph	Cycle: 11 mph	Cycle: 12 mph	Cycle: 13 mph		
Sew	Sew on machine		←	Aerobic dance	→					
Watch TV	Play shuffle board		Folk dance	In-line skate						
		Slow dance	Ballroom dance	Square dance		Play racquetball	Play soccer			
	Fish in boat		Climb ladder	Stream fish		Dig ditch	Wrestle			
		←	Play table tennis	→	Split wood					
		←	Throw Frisbee	→						
Ride in golf cart		Pull golf cart	Carry golf clubs							
Walk: 1 mph	Walk: 2 mph	Walk: 3.5 mph	Walk 4 mph			Run: 1 mi in 10 min	Run: 1 mi in 11 min	Run: 1 mi in 12 min		
Do desk work	Do computer repair		Swim slowly			Swim back stroke	Swim breast stroke		Crawl	
Type	Work auto assembly line									
	Bake		Do light carpentry							
	Bartend				Play tennis: singles					
	Operate hand tools		Play tennis: doubles							

METs, Metabolic equivalent units.

and thus often work at higher MET levels than recommended soon after an MI.

Special Client Populations. Several subgroups of clients require special considerations when planning exercise testing and formulating exercise prescriptions. Elderly persons have more frequent complications that involve deconditioning and may lead to functional limitations and responses that result in ineffective coping. These clients may require a longer time to achieve training goals; they may benefit from learning and practicing energy conservation measures, using low-impact exercises (especially walking or swimming), having longer warm-up periods, modifying or abstaining from exercise under undesirable climatic conditions, and attending to primary health needs.

Clients who have one or more chronic or disabling conditions in addition to cardiac disease require special exercise considerations that will take into account requirements of each specific condition and the combined requirements of all the conditions. For example, increased exercise most likely will alter the MET needs and carbohydrate metabolism for a client with diabetes, creating a change in insulin or caloric balance. Clients with lower body impairments will need to strengthen the upper body to achieve cardiovascular fitness. Likewise, adjustments are required for clients with respiratory disorders, arthritic conditions, chronic fatigue syndrome, or those who have had a stroke and clients who have been recipients of a pacemaker or a heart transplant.

Modified exercise routines or adapted equipment are needed for those who have altered or impaired function and sensation resulting from spinal cord injury or amputation or who have hemiplegia. However, cardiac rehabilitation teams must use care not to focus only on cardiac management of the disability for these latter clients without attention to the client's one or more chronic conditions and primary care needs.

Rehabilitation nurses examine program plans to meet cardiac goals to assure these do not interfere with other constraints or needs a client may have due to comorbidity. This entails a holistic assessment with provisions to prevent further complications or disabilities in facilities or community settings. (Chapter 9 provides for additional content on clients reentering the community.)

Pertinent issues include safety in the home, primary care and health maintenance, pain management, medication regimens that may become complex or costly, rest and energy conservation, recreation and activities, social network, nutritional requirements, religious or cultural dietary preferences, and use of health systems or products from sources other than the cardiac rehabilitation program.

Education Component

Education in phase 1 includes:

- Empowerment for client and family as team members such as answering questions and concerns, determining learning style and needs, and introducing them to the disease trajectory and anticipated interventions
- Disease- or condition-specific content such as anatomy and physiology, medical procedures and tests, purposes of monitoring equipment, cardiac precautions, wound care/precautions, self-care of chest pain, access to emergency services
- Specific guidelines or instructions such as activity types and levels including lifting/pushing and weight limitations for lifting, specific exercises, prescribed and OTC medication actions and side effects, diet, tobacco use, activities of daily living, and rest
- Preparatory information such as about return to work, stress reduction, sexual activity, risk factor and lifestyle modifications, and follow-up care
- Ongoing monitoring of client status

During inpatient cardiac rehabilitation, ongoing monitoring of client status includes vital signs, cardiovascular status, respiratory status, fluid balance, and pertinent laboratory values. The client is monitored for dysrhythmias, signs and symptoms of decreased cardiac output, and pacemaker function if appropriate.

Early Outpatient (Phase 2)

Clients require close supervision and monitoring during the first 2 to 3 months after discharge. Ideally clients will have access to a supervised cardiac rehabilitation program and then will enroll and attend. This is a phase when clients and families experience the greatest adjustment. They are vulnerable to experiencing a great deal of anxiety about the type and amounts of activities, developing fears and depressions, misinterpreting instructions about medications or regimens, and encountering problems with instituting lifestyle changes such as preparing diets, stopping smoking, or managing stressors.

Assessment

Many clients recover from a cardiovascular event only to succumb to depression, anxiety, and other behaviors that prevent them from resuming family and social relationships or returning to a satisfactory and productive life. As survival rates from MI improve, attention to issues surrounding a client's quality of life have become more common. For example, Engerbretson and associates (1999) have studied quality of life and anxiety during early output cardiac rehabilitation. Wenger et al. (1995) have concluded "education, counseling, and/or psychosocial interventions, either alone or as a component of multifactorial cardiac rehabilitation, result in improved psychological well-being and are recommended to complement the psychosocial benefits of exercise training" (p. 121).

Quality of Life. Quality of life and self-esteem, along with adherence to self-care, medication, and exercise regimens may be deciding factors in a client's continued participation in a cardiac rehabilitation program (Conn, Taylor, & Casey, 1992). Concepts such as quality of life are not easy to measure or evaluate. One group of rehabilitation nurse researchers has used the Perceived Quality of Life Scale

(Patrick, Danis, Southerland, & Hong, 1988), which has internal consistency reliability to predict participation and outcomes (Conn et al., 1992). Rukholm and McGirr (1994) tested the reliability and validity of a Quality of Life Index (QLI), which has been adapted to specifically measure quality of life for clients who have cardiac problems. The QLI also has been tested for use as an outcome measure after a cardiac rehabilitation program (Rukholm & McGirr, 1994).

Self-Esteem. Clients may have difficulty maintaining self-esteem as they face changes in their lifestyle and roles. Depression and anxiety are heightened when a client is unable to return to former activities, including work. In a downward spiral, the client assumes a sick role, learns helplessness, and becomes fearful of impending cardiac emergencies—even sudden death. Family members may respond by overly protecting the person or by labeling the client as being overly concerned or having a "cardiac psychosis."

Loss of Control. Some clients respond with rebellious behaviors to regain a sense of control or conversely with avoidance and denial by resorting to addictive behaviors, compulsions, and perhaps substance abuse. Clients may develop symptoms of illness secondary to depression such as vague discomfort or pains in the chest, headache, restlessness, insomnia, fatigue, feelings of panic, or altered concentration and memory. A comprehensive cardiac rehabilitation program provides for a client's psychosocial needs, as well as for physical training. Clients may feel as if they have "given up" control over many areas of their lives and find lifestyle preferences a solace. Change requires energy and commitment, which may be emotionally or psychologically overwhelming for them.

Client and Family Concerns. Each client and family needs to receive guidance and coaching to cope with the potential psychosocial problems that commonly occur after a cardiac event and often provoke stressful responses. As a group clients and families predictably ask questions about similar concerns (Box 31-4). Rehabilitation nurses who are aware of these commonly expressed concerns are able to provide anticipatory guidance about specific responses and work through coping responses that enable clients and families to resist or eliminate stressors.

Learning Needs. The nurse and other team members will be educating clients and families who are coping at different levels and using various coping behaviors. Educational materials are more effective when they meet individual needs. Readability of all educational materials can be tested in order to meet the needs of specific populations. When selecting educational materials, assess the client and family concerning the following:

- Diagnosis and health status
- Education and socioeconomic background
- Interest in material and mode of presentation
- Availability of videocassette recorder, tape players, or other devices
- Cultural or religious preferences
- Literacy level, primary language
- Visual, auditory, or other sensory impairments
- Functional abilities
- Age or developmental factors

Millions of persons in the United States are unable to comprehend materials written above the sixth-grade reading level; many are functionally illiterate or speak a primary language other than English. Elderly persons, who account for a large percent of the population, who have cardiovascular conditions, also have a 30% to 40% rate of illiteracy. Additionally many elderly persons require large print, which is visualized better against a contrasting color. For example, dark letters printed on yellow, light blue, or white paper are easier for them to read.

Educational resources are becoming more sophisticated and readily available. For example, educational materials may include anatomic views of coronary arteries showing blockages of the coronary arteries after the angiograms or pictures that illustrate surgical procedures or complementary product guides from companies that manufacture prosthetic valves and pacemakers. A number of major organizations, such as the American Heart Association, and private vendor or manufacturing companies, have available educational materials, charts, videocassette tapes, handout materials, interactive computer programs, and anatomic models. Many Web sites are available. Preview any prepackaged or "canned" educational materials to individualize the content to meet client goals, match program philosophy, and ensure information is current and accurate.

Although clients and family members clearly benefit from a variety of educational materials, materials are se-

Box 31-4 Commonly Expressed Concerns after a Cardiac Event

What Can Be Expected from a Client Regarding

Emotions
Symptoms
Medication side effects
Response to exercise or activity

When Can a Client Resume

Sexual activity
Driving a car
Recreational activities or sports
Work-related activities
Housework or laundry

How Does a Client

Manage stress effectively
Exercise safely
Know when to call a physician or emergency responder
Eat properly
Meet financial needs
Modify lifestyle to control risk factors

Data from Karem, C. (1989). *A practical guide to cardiac rehabilitation.* Philadelphia: Aspen.

lected based on the assessment of their learning needs and styles. As a rule families prefer simple and illustrated materials that provide complete and informative explanations over highly technical data, unless they request otherwise. The nurse controls the temptation to overload them with materials they will *never* use.

Nursing Diagnoses and Therapeutic Goals

Many of the relevant NANDA diagnostic categories for early outpatient cardiac rehabilitation continue to apply except shock management. Additional diagnostic categories may be impaired adjustment, health management deficit, depression, and sexual dysfunction.

The early outpatient goals are to improve functional abilities, to control weight, and to build cardiovascular levels. The key lifestyle changes recommended for clients in a cardiac rehabilitation program are the same as those proposed as preventive measures for others:

- Control obesity and make dietary changes, especially reducing calorie and fat intake
- Institute measures to reduce serum cholesterol levels and improve low-density lipoprotein/high-density lipoprotein (LDL/HDL) ratio; may include medications
- Stop cigarette smoking or other tobacco use and exposure
- Reduce or eliminate alcohol intake
- Incorporate stress management and measures for effective coping
- Develop or maintain a prescribed exercise program

Therapeutic Plan and Interventions

In addition to Cardiac Care, Cardiac Care: Rehabilitation and Teaching: Diet, Activity/exercise, Disease process, the Nursing Interventions Classifications in early outpatient cardiac rehabilitation include Risk Detection, Risk Control, Anticipatory Guidance, Role Enhancement, Coping Enhancement and Anxiety Reduction. Lifestyle education joins exercise as a foundational component.

Risk Detection and Control (Lifestyle Changes). Clients and families need to be informed and knowledgeable for effective decision making and problem solving about lifestyle choices, behaviors, and specific interventions. Clients are taught to understand their risk factors and learn about those lifestyle habits or preferences that may help modify or reduce their coronary risk level. Lifestyle changes are one of the few areas over which a client has direct control. Because lifestyle behaviors are embedded in everyday activities and patterns, as well as having cultural or emotional values, they are difficult to change in the short term and more difficult on a long-term basis.

Education is a key function in cardiac rehabilitation programs and a crucial factor in a client's long-term outcome, but the "window of opportunity" to provide education may be extremely short. The site and format for an educational program can be adapted to meet the available space and group size. For instance, one-on-one interactions, group classes, discussion groups, peer or support groups, and other configurations are conducted in person, via video, closed circuit television, and chat rooms via the Internet.

Many programs offer a series of educational sessions conducted by the members of the cardiac team. As far as possible, scheduling for educational sessions should be modified so both families and clients are able to attend all sessions. Many programs are offered in the evening or on Saturday mornings. The content of the program will provide information about the cardiac event, treatments and procedures, lifestyle activities, exercise prescriptions, and medical alerts. Time for participants to raise concerns and ask questions is exceedingly important. As a result clients and families often are able to provide assistance to one another by passing along information or sharing solutions to otherwise troublesome problems, which is an empowering activity.

Although an educational program necessarily contains standardized content and information, the nurse assesses each client and family to identify learner variables that will influence their perspective on learning, identify any barriers to learning, and determine the type and mode most appropriate to be used for this client's educational materials (Table 31-7).

Teaching Techniques

For clients and each family member, it is important to use educational techniques that educate both hemispheres of the brain. The left hemisphere is the analytic side of the brain, which deals with factual information when delivered in a language format. To illustrate, the left hemisphere of the brain is learning when a person makes statements such as, "Tell me about . . ." or "Explain to me . . ." or "I don't understand. . . ." Written materials are examples of tools for left-brain education programs.

In contrast, the right hemisphere is the visual-spatial side of the brain, which prefers to deal with models, drawings, figures, and pictures. The right hemisphere of the brain is learning when a person makes statements such as, "Show me . . ." or "Let me see it . . ." Diagrams and drawings are methods for educating persons with right brain learning. (Chapter 25 provides additional information in this area.)

Calendars and other data management tools are inexpensive, portable, and easy to use and interpret. They are useful for recording appointments, class times, reminders for follow-up such as with laboratory test results, and other scheduling matters. The same calendar functions as an activity log. Data records can be maintained to show a profile of a client's changes in weight, daily glucose levels, vital signs or blood pressure, as needed medication use, occurrence of symptoms, exercise levels, diet changes, or similar events. When these logs are analyzed to show patterns of behavior, the results become a powerful teaching tool created by the client.

Exercise Regimen

Prescribed exercise programs continue to be key interventions for improving functional abilities controlling weight

TABLE 31-7 Assessment of Learner Variables in Cardiac Rehabilitation

Variables	Assessment Area
Individual	Demographics Developmental stage Education Prior illness experience
Sociocultural	Culture/ethnicity Beliefs about condition Social construction or meaning
Illness related	Status of illness Stage of intervention Anticipated outcome Physical limitations Social limitations Diagnostic activities
Situational	Client/family system Extended family/significant others Social network or support system
Cardiac status	Specific symptoms and impact Diagnostics and treatment Therapeutic regimens: diet, exercise, medications Illness trajectory

From Jillings, C. R. (1988). *Cardiac rehabilitation nursing.* Rockville, MD: Aspen. Copyright 1988 by Aspen. Reprinted by permission.

and building cardiovascular levels. The exercise session or activity program consists of warm up, conditioning or activity, and cool down (Woods, Froelicher, & Motzer, 2000). The purpose of a warm up is to prepare muscles and joints for the pending activity, which is exercise. This requires between 5 and 15 minutes of stretching activities and ROM exercises, by which time the resting metabolic rate (1 MET) has increased to a level necessary for beginning the conditioning segment of the session.

The composition of the conditioning activity is guided by the individualized dosage written in the exercise prescription for frequency, intensity, mode, and duration of exercise, which are approximately 20 to 30 minutes. Although frequencies may be set at several times daily, exercises sessions for outpatient clients generally are set for 3 to 5 times a week because little benefit has been found to be derived from exercises more frequent than 5 times weekly (Wenger et al., 1995). Persons with diabetes mellitus may need to exercise daily related to maintaining their insulin sensitivity, however. The 5- to 10-minute cool-down segment of the session is important to prevent exercise-related complications and should not be overlooked.

Ideal climates for exercise are those with less than 65% humidity and temperatures between 40 and 75° F. Exercising under ideal conditions is not always feasible but certainly is preferable for clients who have cardiac conditions. Extremes of heat and humidity are major concerns to health; whenever the humidity exceeds 65%, the metabolic rate required for activities is increased. Excessive heat results in vasodilation, which reduces blood return to the heart, decreasing the blood pressure and elevating the heart rate. Heat stress may occur in hot air or hot water temperatures and may result in the vasodilatation cycle when a client is using alcohol or nitrates.

Clients may choose to modify the environment or alter their exercise time. For example, in hot, humid climates as found in the South, clients may exercise outdoors in the cooler morning or late evenings; during the day they would use an air-conditioned or environmentally controlled indoor space. On the other hand, cold temperatures also increase peripheral resistance and thus a raise the workload of the heart. Clients should consider the fabric and type of clothing worn for exercise so it is appropriate for the weather conditions. For example, covering the mouth and nose with a scarf is effective prevention of cold-induced bronchospasms. Polypropylene/cool max wicks away moisture (especially important for persons with diabetes mellitus).

Because this early outpatient phase is the period within which clients experience the highest cardiac mortality rates after hospitalization, frequent contact, monitoring, and support are essential to assist clients in judging their behaviors and activities and for determining when they have medical complications or emergencies. Many clients return home at low risk and can be monitored effectively by nurses from community-based cardiac rehabilitation programs. A number of models to serve low-risk clients who live in geographically distant areas or who do not have cardiac rehabilitation programs nearby exist (Wenger et al., 1995). Strategies for promoting success in early outpatient cardiac rehabilitation include:

- Provide referrals to community agencies or self-help groups for smoking cessation, weight loss or control, or spousal support meetings
- Provide referrals for professional assistance such as psychosocial or mental health professionals, nutrition counseling or computerized dietary analysis, or professional assistance with comorbid conditions such as diabetes
- Provide resources to assist with stress reduction and management when appropriate
- Encourage accessible activities and events within tolerance levels to promote socialization
- Generate written health contracts with assigned responsibilities for accomplishing mutually agreed-upon goals
- Use logs, checklists, calendars, and other record keeping aids to encourage clients to perform tasks and steps for meeting goals
- Assess and intervene with the entire family system and any significant others, not only the client
- Assure programs, groups, and referrals are culturally and religiously relevant and sensitive

Late Outpatient Cardiac Rehabilitation (Phase 3)

Assessment

Components of phases 2 and 3 tend to blend for clients who do not have complications; activities may intensify as they continue over a longer period. As a rule clients who were monitored with telemetry during phase 2, but who have achieved goals to this point, continue to be supervised but are no longer monitored with telemetry.

Nursing Diagnoses and Therapeutic Goals

The additional nursing diagnostic categories for late outpatient cardiac rehabilitation may include ineffective coping (individual), dysfunction grieving, noncompliance, and risk for noncompliance. The therapeutic goals are to integrate lifestyle changes and reconstruct one's life in context of health status. By 6 months after hospitalization, clients and families have begun to recognize that exercise, self-monitoring, and lifestyle changes are lifelong goals. At the same time they have been able to reconstruct their lives within the parameters of the client's condition and abilities. For some clients this will mean few changes beyond eliminating detrimental habits and adhering to exercises; others will encounter major adjustments and complications; some will have great difficulties or fail.

Therapeutic Plans and Interventions

In addition to Cardiac Care: Rehabilitation, the Nursing Interventions Classifications in late outpatient cardiac rehabilitation may include Support Group, Support System Enhancement, Emotional Support, Coping Enhancement, Counseling and Anxiety Reduction. All these interventions are addressed in the following paragraphs specific to cardiac rehabilitation.

Support Systems. Services that are enjoyable, accessible, and acceptable for a client are more likely to be used. Support groups and social activities for clients and families may promote attendance. Social networks and social support are two factors that have been found to be valid predictors of outcome after MI. Networking among clients and family members is one way to provide needed psychological support throughout all stages of illness and rehabilitation. Involvement of all family members is imperative because the numbers of family members grow alongside the numbers of clients. Family members benefit from networking and sharing experiences whether the client is in a critical care unit or any of the other stages of recovery. Psychosocial issues require the interdisciplinary team to function with awareness and coordinated intervention, with the coordinator ensuring communication among team members.

Support Groups. Support groups may be organized or informal; many become very creative, but they exist to meet the needs of the persons who participate in them. For example, separate groups may be organized for spouses, children and parents, or clients to present issues or address specific concerns of a group. Some programs organize groups according to diagnostic criteria such as clients with pacemakers, those with congestive heart disease, clients who receive medical treatment, or those who have surgical interventions.

To be successful, organized groups in a facility meet on a regular schedule that takes into account other activities or client needs that may interrupt or overrun their gathering time and place. For example, clients may need to meet in a location near a telemetry monitor or with access to emergency equipment. Others may choose a time when family members are not visiting, after physicians' rounds on the unit, or times that will avoid conflict with medication or meal times.

Suggestions for improving participation in late outpatient cardiac rehabilitation include the following.

- Involve client and family in plan
- Educate client to make realistic assessments of status; educate family to client's limitations and abilities
- Refer to counseling program where professionals are knowledgeable about concerns and issues for clients who have had cardiac events; include family counseling
- Reinforce exercise program
- Reinforce medication and dietary regimens
- Reinforce lifestyle modifications
- Promote activities and programs that enable return to usual lifestyle as much as possible for client
- Evaluate client and family psychosocial status regularly

Electronic support groups are flourishing among clients and families who have personal computers with modem, communications software and Internet access (Box 31-5). Personal computers offer a new form of networking that can extend locally, nationally, or even internationally (Kinney et al., 1998). Advantages of electronic support groups include:

1. Twenty-four-hour access is available
2. The system can be used from home or facility
3. Client chooses topics to read and respond to
4. Client and family are assured privacy, anonymity, and control
5. A hard copy of all transactions can be printed
6. Professional personnel are able to exchange information and obtain interactive consultations (Box 31-6)

Maintenance (Phase 4)

The maintenance phase of cardiac rehabilitation is lifelong. Because clients are more clinically stable and knowledgeable about their activity limits, professional supervision is tapered. Activities and exercises are more aggressive, and organized educational programs designed to maintain participation and accomplish lifestyle changes become more important.

Assessment

Many clients who have participated in cardiac rehabilitation programs eventually are able to return to work. Older persons are less likely to return to work than those who are in primary wage earning years unless there are preexisting

Box 31-5 Electronic Resources and Support Group Information

Heartlink
Heartlink House (support group)
351 Fishponds Road
Eastville, Bristol B556RI
England
http://www.pcug.co.uk/nrwall

Heartmates
PO Box 16202
Minneapolis, MN 55416
http://www.heartmates.com/cardiac.html

Heart Information Network (information resource)
Center for Cardiovascular Education, Inc.
New Providence, NJ
http://www.heartinfo.org

Krames Communication
800-333-3032 (6 AM to 5 PM Pacific time)
http://www.krames.com

National Heart, Lung and Blood (NHLBI) (information resource)
U.S. Department of Health and Human Services
Public Health Service
National Institutes of Health
NHLBI Information Center
PO Box 30105
Bethesda, MD 20824-0105
NHLBI Educational Materials Catalog (Publication No. 94-3085), April 1994
Phone 202-783-3238 or fax 202-512-2250
http://www.nhlbi.nih.gov/nhlbi/pubs.htm

Prichett and Hull Associates, Inc. (information resource)
Suite 110, 3440 Oak Cliff Road NE
Atlanta, GA 30340
http://www.p-h.com

Adapted from Kinney, M.R., Dunbar, S.B., Brooks-Brunn, J., Molten N. & Vitello-Cicciu, J.M. (1998). *AACN's clinical reference for critical care nursing* (4th ed.). St. Louis, Mosby.

medical reasons. Although work and working have high value in the United States, clients and employers may have a sense of fear or confusion about an employee's health status after a cardiovascular incident. As with other behavioral questions, sorting out the complex variables in determining whether a client actually returns to work is not an exact science. Assessment of an individual client's ability to return to work and the capacity for a safe expeditious return to the workforce is conducted by the full team.

Box 31-6 Cardiac Rehabilitation Reference Organizations

American Association of Cardiovascular and Pulmonary Rehabilitation
7611 Elmwood Avenue
Suite 201
Middleton, WI 53562
http://www.aacvpr.org

American College of Sports Medicine
401 W. Michigan Street
Indianapolis, IN 46202-3233
http://www.acsm.org

American Heart Association
7272 Greenville Avenue
Dallas, TX 75231-4596
http://www.amhrt.org//affili/mend.htm

American Nurses Credentialing Center
1101 14th Street, NW
Suite 700
Washington, D.C. 20005
http://www.nursingworld.org/acc

Return to Work

Physical, psychosocial, and medical factors as well as age, access to work, financial situation, and family support are all factors in a client's return to work. Examples of questions a client, family, and employer ask include:

- Is the person medically stable and able to return to work?
- How soon can work be resumed and at what level of function?
- Are other comparable, less strenuous positions available?
- Can the same job functions be performed?
- Are there any types of barriers?
- Are physical structure or equipment modifications necessary?
- How does the environment need to be altered?
- Does the person have disability coverage or other financial support?
- Do the client and company want the client to return to work?

The cardiac rehabilitation team is prepared to work with a client and family to assess the readiness to return to work and the conditions for doing so. Initially a client completes a treadmill test to identify and calculate the MET level at which she is able to function safely without encountering problems or warning sips (MET max). Table 31-6 supplies representative amounts of METs for certain vocational tasks. Some clients will be able to improve their MET score after exercise training for cardiovascular fitness.

Workplace Assessment

It is important for clients to have a realistic evaluation of the ability to perform work and other activities so they do not overextend themselves on the job or restrict themselves needlessly. The client's view of self in the sick role or with learned helplessness is an indicator for a psychosocial assessment, which may reveal a need for counseling before work is attempted.

In some work hardening programs, a client and team member conduct a detailed workplace assessment, documenting activities that would occur during a typical day. They note details of the work style, such as whether a client is sitting at a computer terminal versus climbing or lifting versus standing in an assembly line. The workplace environment and availability of services, such as food choices in the cafeteria and location and accessibility of lavatories are inspected; the client's commute to work and means of transportation are taken during regular commuting hours; and the number of stressful situations and the degree to which the client identifies stressors are noted. The workplace load is calculated in METs, which are compared with the client's exercise test METs level. The MET level, health status, and exercise prescription are important determinants of the client's ability to return to work.

Nursing Diagnoses and Therapeutic Goals

The additional nursing diagnostic category for phase 4 may be altered role performance and social isolation. The therapeutic goals are to accomplish lifelong lifestyle changes and reintegrate into the community.

Therapeutic Plans and Interventions

Cardiac Care: Rehabilitation, Support System Enhancement Role Performance and Family Support continue as nursing interventions in phase 4. These interventions are addressed below and specifically focus on return to work and a home-based exercise program.

Work Hardening Program. Work hardening is a general term as well as the title for a program that has specific characteristics and goals to determine whether a client realms to work, or under what auspices. The work hardening program may range from 2 to 8 hours per day. It consists of simulated work-related tasks that may become progressively difficult until the client is able (or unable) to perform the functional tasks as he or she would be required to do on the job. These tasks are performed under supervision of a trained therapist and in a structured environment.

Other common components of a work hardening program include functional activities; cardiovascular conditioning; education about proper use of body mechanics to prevent overtaxing, strain, or injury; and a variety of techniques for managing job-related and personal stressors.

Home-Based or Unsupervised Exercise Programs. Clients who are unable to attend or access medically supervised exercise classes may be candidates for home exercise training according to a specific exercise prescription. Under certain conditions clients may be eligible for partial reimbursement for intermittent community health nursing services, therapies, and medical supplies. A large number of community-based providers offer a wide array of health care services for clients with varying payment options. However, clients and families need to be educated to choose services that will assure a complete assessment followed by ongoing coordination, continuity, and communication with the cardiac rehabilitation program.

Modern technology has made home exercise programs more practical by improving communications between a client and the cardiac rehabilitation center. With the availability of telephone, fax, or electronic mail transmissions; transtelephonic ECG recordings; videocassette tape recordings, home educational video, and other electronic telecommunication devices, clients who would otherwise be without services can access a cardiac rehabilitation team. The nurse as coordinator, educator, advocate, and assessor-evaluator is a key link in communication.

Clients and family members need to be able to demonstrate their knowledge about the individualized exercise prescription, precautions including environmental conditions, signs and symptoms to be reported to the cardiac rehabilitation team, and criteria for terminating exercise. Emergency telephone numbers should be posted near the telephone where family members and other persons in the home can locate them quickly. Emergency response or electronic emergency systems are available in many communities. As additional precautions, clients may wear medical alert bracelets, carry diagnosis and treatment cards, and place a Vial of Life in the refrigerator. Those who have implanted cardiac pacemakers or cardioverter defibrillators should have special information regarding their status and care readily available.

Clients and families need to make arrangements with the primary physician and members of the cardiac rehabilitation team concerning content of any advanced directives or do-not-resuscitate orders. The client's situation, preferences, and special needs should be known to members of the local emergency response units, the pharmacist, vendors who supply equipment or goods such as oxygen and backup supplies for electricity or heat, and other similar services or personnel.

EVALUATION

Evaluation is a necessary component of a cardiac rehabilitation program to provide evidence of the quality of care and cost effectiveness. Likewise evaluation is part of the nursing process. Both process and outcome evaluations are appropriate for all phases of the cardiac rehabilitation program.

Process Evaluation

Process evaluation provides a means to judge and document the rehabilitation process, including the activities and behaviors of all team members. The cardiac rehabilitation program can be compared to the published program standards and the published standard competencies for professionals in cardiac rehabilitation. Appropriate standards of care also provide a means to conduct a process evaluation and document all team members actions.

Outcome Evaluation

Outcome evaluation provides a means to judge and document the effectiveness of the cardiac rehabilitation program. Several different outcomes have been studied related to cardiac rehabilitation programs. For example, Schairer et al. (1998) found that most clients (83%) in a maintenance cardiac rehabilitation program exercise below the 300 Kcal per session stated goal. Merz, Felando, and Klein (1996) found that participation in a long-term cardiac rehabilitation program improved cholesterol awareness, use of lipid lowering therapy and achievement of total serum cholesterol lower than 200 mg/dl. Verges, Patois-Verges, Cohen, and Casillas (1998) and Ades et al. (1999) found improved lipidemic status in cardiac rehabilitation clients. Suter, Suter, Perkins, Bona, and Kendrick (1996) studied maintenance of life style changes and perceptions of program value. Similarly Liddell and Fridlund (1996) studied cardiac events, physical and psychological condition, life habits and cardiac health knowledge in cardiac rehabilitation. Gulanick, Bliley, Perino, and Keough (1998) have examined recovery patterns and life style changes after PTCA.

Biological factors such as fat distribution (McConnell, Palm, Shearn, & Laubach, 1999), body mass index, and body shape are being studied to determine their impact on cardiac rehabilitation outcomes.

Many of the nursing-sensitive client outcomes with specific indicators and measurement scales have been developed in the Iowa Outcomes Project that may be appropriate to cardiac rehabilitation during one or more of the phases (Table 31-8).

TABLE 31-8 Potential Nursing Sensitive Outcomes (NOC) for Cardiac Rehabilitation

Phase 1	*Phase 2*	*Phase 3*	*Phase 4*
Activity tolerance	Adherence behavior →	→	Acceptance of health status
Ambulation: walking →	→		
	Anxiety control		
Cardiac pump effectiveness →	→	→	→
Circulation status →	→	→	→
Coagulation status →	→	→	→
		Compliance	
		Coping	
	Depression control →	→	
Endurance →	→	→	
Energy conservation			
Family participation in professional care			
Fluid balance →	→		
		Grief resolution →	→
Knowledge: disease process	Knowledge: diet		
Knowledge: energy conservation	Knowledge: medications		
Knowledge: illness care	Knowledge: prescribed activity		
Knowledge: treatment regime			
Medication response →	→	→	→
Rest →	→		
			Quality of life
		Risk control: Cardiac health →	→
			Role performance
Self care ADL	Self care: instrumental ADLs →	→	→
		Self-direction of care →	→
		Support group	
		Social support →	→
	Symptom control →	→	→
Tissue perfusion: cardiac →	→	→	→
Tissue perfusion: peripheral →	→	→	→
			Well-being

ADLs, Activities of daily living.

The most important outcome measurement related to DVT is to decrease the incidence of DVT and decrease the incidence of pulmonary emboli. Nursing-sensitive client outcomes with specific indicators and measurement scales in the Iowa Outcome project that are appropriate for DVT are Tissue Perfusion: Peripheral, and Knowledge: Treatment Regimen.

IMPLICATIONS

The future of cardiac rehabilitation programs includes offering more individualized services to a greater variety of clients and families regardless of their geographic location. The needs of an aging population in an era of shrinking hospital stays are accompanied by social changes in work patterns and lifestyles, electronic technology, and a growing body of research knowledge. Clients with chronic CHF need to be further incorporated into cardiac rehabilitation programs. Reconditioning strategies need to be explored; e.g., low-frequency electrical stimulation of quadriceps and calf muscles have been found to increase exercise capacity without increase in cardiac output (Maillefert et al., 1998). Besides weight training additional strategies such as T'ai Chi Chuan, yoga, stress management, and relaxation strategies need to be studied for their possible contribution to cardiac rehabilitation.

Findings from research of highly structured and uniform aspects of cardiac rehabilitation programs need to be translated into programs that are available to all clients who have experienced a cardiac event and their families, not only those who are geographically available. Sparks, Shaw, Jenning, and Quinn (1998) have examined the complications with use of transtelephonic exercise monitoring for home sites and satellite sites and found this to be safe. McConnell et al. (1998) have demonstrated that it is safe not to have an entry exercise test. Prevention, education for self-care, and lifestyle modification are key components for improved outcomes.

CRITICAL THINKING

1. Consider this dilemma. Persons with inflammatory arthritis—i.e., rheumatoid arthritis (RA) and systemic lupus erythematosus (SLE)—are at high risk for heart disease. Inflammation in rheumatic disease is a predictor of cardiovascular disease. With the evidence linking inflammation to diseased blood vessels, it is now thought that the inflammation in RA and SLE accelerates the process of atherosclerosis. But the new COX-2 inhibitors avoid altering COX-1 enzymes that also promote blood clots; therefore, the heart is not protected with these agents as with acetylsalicylic acid (ASA) and nonsteroidal antiinflammatory drugs. Likewise steroids promote high cholesterol and clogged arteries but the antimalarials have cholesterol-lowering capabilities. What aspects of cardiac rehabilitation may be helpful to RA and SLE clients?
2. Complete a risk assessment scale for DVT using the tool given in this chapter for the case study client presented in Chapter 25.

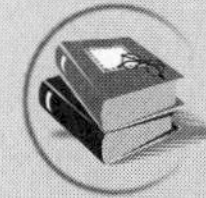

Case Study I

Mr. B.W. is a 79-year-old married gentleman with a long-standing history of atrial fibrillation treated with Digoxin 0.25 mg qd and ASA 325 mg qd. He and his wife are very reluctant to take Coumadin (warfarin sodium). In May Mr. B.W. had an episode of severe bilateral pneumonitis requiring ventilatory support for several days; weaning was difficult. His hospitalization lasted more than 3 weeks; the last 10 days were spent on an inpatient rehabilitation unit of the hospital. His risk score for DVT was 10 (immobility, required BR > 5 days and he was > 75 years of age). Embolism precautions per NIC were in place. Sequential compression devices were in place. On discharge to home he was able to transfer barely from bed to chair and walk to the bathroom. Home PT was arranged and assistive devices obtained. His discharge medications were Cardizem 240 mg and high dose steroids.

In mid June Mr. B.W. suffered a GI bleed from a stomach ulceration that had to be surgically closed since cautery failed to stop the bleeding. He was on the ventilator a few days postoperatively and was started on tube feedings as soon as possible postoperative. By now his weight had dropped from 140 before the May illness to 104 pounds. His risk score was now 13 (a surgical procedure of >2 hours was added). Embolism precautions per NIC were again in place. He was again sent to the inpatient rehabilitation unit for one week. This time on discharge he was able to walk a short distance and get in and out of bed with minimal assistance. Again PT was received at home after discharge.

In early September Mr. B.W.'s right leg began to swell and he was experiencing more fatigue and weakness than usual. The PT notified the physician and he was rehospitalized with a diagnosis of DVT. He was started on Coumadin which he was told he would have to continue at home for the foreseeable future.

The nursing diagnoses at the time of hospitalization related to the DVT problem were (1) tissue perfusion impaired: peripheral, (2) anxiety, (3) impaired mobility, (4) risk for ineffective management of therapeutic regimen (fearful of Coumadin), (5) role strain, caregiver (his wife was very stressed with the long illness and many complications). The neurogenic intermittent claudication (NIC) interventions for impaired tissue perfusion are circulatory care: venous insufficiency and embolism precautions.

After discharge Mr. B.W. was continued on physical therapy and his anticoagulation status was monitored weekly. His Cardizem was decreased to 120 mg qd and then discontinued. He remains on Prilosec and Coumadin. Since discharge he has gained weight, strength, and endurance. He is walking up and down stairs, driving his car short distances, and beginning to work outside in his yard.

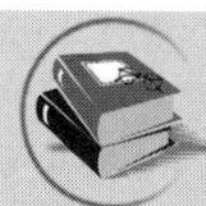

Case Study 2

Mrs. Doe, a 68-year-old widow, suffered an acute anterior MI complicated by CHF. She now has an ejection fraction of 30%, no signs or symptoms of CHF, no murmur or gallop, and no crackles. She lives 100 miles from the nearest "formal" cardiac rehabilitation program in a rural area with two pets. Her children live out of state. She describes her neighbors as "helpful whenever I call."

A treadmill test before hospital discharge documented her tolerance of 1 to 2 METs. Mrs. Doe had been very active with yard and garden work before her MI. Her risk factors for atherosclerosis include cholesterol 220 (high), HDL 40 (low). She does not use tobacco but has had heavy tobacco smoke exposure until 1.5 years ago, and has non-insulin-dependent diabetes. She has had a hysterectomy with oophorectomy 10 years ago and is not on estrogen replacement therapy.

Care Plan: Educational Component

First, what are the client's questions and concerns?

A few facts: 80% clients experiencing an acute MI return to preinfarction activity level; proper education, activities, and follow-up facilitate this return to "normal" lifestyle.

Home health referral is appropriate for continued education, continued assessment, and on-site follow-up. Consult a home health agency that has a formal program for post-MI and CHF clients using specialty nurses and additional disciplines such as physical therapy, dietary, and social worker. Jointly decide roles and responsibilities of "consultant and consultee" of client, who is to continue under the umbrella of formal cardiac rehabilitation. For example, the home health nurse may need to confer with appropriate cardiac rehabilitation personnel regarding an increase in exercise or activity plan.

Regarding MI: definition, cause, healing process, rationale for activity/exercise limitations and recommendations, signs and symptoms to report, awareness of preinfarctional anginal symptoms.

Regarding CHF: definition, cause, factors that lower/raise risk of reoccurrence, signs and symptoms to report, rationale of no-added salt diet, rationale regarding client continuing daily weights and reporting cumulative weight gain of 2 pounds to the home health nurse, physician, or cardiac rehabilitation personnel, daily weight rules (approximate same time, same amount of clothing, no weights on carpeted floor and use only on set scale (home health personnel should use client's scales also), importance of early symptom awareness and reporting.

What is to be expected? Emotions, symptoms, medication side effects, and response to exercise and activity: Which to report and to whom.

When can client resume work, sex, driving, recreation (e.g., gardening, club activities), housework (carefully review which MET activities are permitted and project when additional activities may be added to the established schedule).

How does the client exercise and eat properly and safely, manage stress, control risk factors—specifically for this client: lower cholesterol to below 200 and raise HDLs to above 65, investigate estrogen replacement therapy, which also will assist in the elevation of HDLs. Maintain NIDDM status under strict control.

Know when to call physician, home health nurse, or cardiac rehabilitation personnel. Be sure lines of communication are clearly in place among all parties involved.

Exercise and activity: specific information on which activities are allowed and which are not. What type of exercise is best for client's life and routines of daily living? What symptoms indicate client should terminate an activity or exercise? A good rule of thumb is that 30 minutes after an activity or exercise the client should feel good. If the client is tired after 30 minutes, he or she probably has overdone. Usually people push speed of an activity or exercise too fast. Gradually increasing the time of an exercise or activity is preferred before increasing the speed of work

REFERENCES

Adams, K.J., Barnard, K.L., Swank, A.M., Mann, E., Kushnick, M.R., & Denny, D.M. (1999). Combined high-intensity strength and aerobic training in diverse phase II cardiac rehabilitation patients. *Journal of Cardiopulmonary Rehabilitation, 19,* 209-215.

Ades, P.A., Savage, P.D., Phehlman, E.T., Brochu, M., Fragnoli-Munn, K., & Carhart, R.L. Jr. (1999). Lipid lowering in the cardiac rehabilitation setting. *Journal of Cardiopulmonary Rehabilitation, 19,* 255-260.

American College of Sports Medicine. (1998). *Guidelines for exercise testing and prescription* (5th ed.). Baltimore: Williams & Wilkins.

American Heart Association. (1994). Cardiac rehabilitation programs: A statement for health care professionals from the American Heart Association (position statement). *Circulation, 90,* 1602-1610.

American Heart Association. (2001). *Heart and stroke update.* Accessed June 9, 2001. Available: http://www.amhrt.org//affili/mend/htm.

Balady, G.J., Jette, D., Scheer, J., & Downing, J. (1996). Changes in exercise capacity following cardiac rehabilitation inpatients stratified according to age and gender: results of the Massachusetts Association of Cardiovascular and Pulmonary Rehabilitation Multicenter Database. *Journal of Cardiopulmonary Rehabilitation, 16,* 38-46.

Barnard, K.L., Adams, K.J., Swank, A.M., Mann, E., & Denny, D.M. (1999). Injuries and muscle soreness during the one repetition maximum assessment in a cardiac rehabilitation population. *Journal of Cardiopulmonary Rehabilitation, 19,* 52-58.

Beniamini, Y., Rubenstein, J.J., Faigenbaum, A.D., Lichtenstein, A.H., & Crim, M.C. (1999). High-intensity strength training of patients enrolled in an outpatient cardiac rehabilitation program. *Journal of Cardiopulmonary Rehabilitation, 19,* 8-17.

Brezinski, V., Dusseldorp, E., & Maes, S. (1998). Gender differences in psychological profile at entry into cardiac rehabilitation. *Journal of Cardiovascular Rehabilitation, 18,* 445-449.

Bullock, B.L. (1996). Alterations in systemic circulation. In B.L. Bullock (Ed.), *Pathophysiology: Adaptations and alterations in functions* (4th ed.). Philadelphia: JB Lippincott.

Collins, L.M. (1998). Deep venous thrombosis. *Nurse Practitioner Forum, 9,* 163-169.

Con, A.H., Linden, W., Thompson, J.M., & Ignaszewski, A. (1999). The psychology of men and women recovering from coronary artery bypass surgery. *Journal of Cardiopulmonary Rehabilitation, 19,* 152-161.

Conn, V.S., Taylor, S.G., & Casey, B. (1992). Cardiac rehabilitation program participation and outcomes after myocardial infarction. *Rehabilitation Nursing, 17,* 58-62.

Cottin, Y., Walker, P., Rouhier-Marcer, I., Cohen, M., Louis, P. Didier, J.P., Casillas, J.M., Wolf, J.E., & Brunotte, F. (1996). Relationship between increased peak oxygen uptake and modifications in skeletal muscle metabolism following rehabilitation after myocardial infarction. *Journal of Cardiopulmonary Rehabilitation, 16,* 169-174.

Cummins, R.O. (Ed.). (1997). Advanced cardiac life support. Dallas: American Heart Association.

Daub, W.D., Knapik, G.P., & Black, W.R. (1996). Strength training early after myocardial infarction. *Journal of Cardiopulmonary Rehabilitation, 16,* 100-108.

DeGroot, D.W., Quinn, T.J., Kertzer, R., Vroman, N.B., & Olney, W.B. (1998). Lactic acid accumulation in cardiac patients performing circuit weight training: implications for exercise prescription. *Archives of Physical Medicine & Rehabilitation, 79,* 838-841.

Engerbretson, T.O., Clark, M.M., Niaura, R.S., Phillips, T., Albrecht, A., & Tilkemeier, P. (1999). Quality of life and anxiety in a phase II cardiac rehabilitation program. *Medicine & Science in Sports & Exercise, 31,* 216-223.

Evenson, K.R., Rosamond, W.D., & Luepker, R.V. (1998). Predictors of outpatient cardiac rehabilitation utilization: the Minnesota Heart Survey. *Journal of Cardiopulmonary Rehabilitation, 18,* 192-198.

Fletcher, G.F., Balady, G., Froelicher, V.F., Hartley, L.H., Haskell, W.L., & Pollock, M.L. (1995). Exercise standards: A statement for health care professionals from the American Heart Association. *Circulation, 91,* 580-615.

Fragnoli-Munn, K., Savage, P.H., & Ades, P.A. (1998). Combined resistive-aerobic training in older patients with coronary artery disease early after myocardial infarction. Journal of *Cardiovascular Rehabilitation, 18,* 416-420.

Fridlund, B., (1997). Social network and support among MI-women during the three months following upon a first myocardial infarction. Vard i Norden. *Nursing Science & research in the Nordic Countries, 17,* 9-14.

Goodman, J.M., Pallandi, D.V., Reading, J.R., Plyley, M.J., Liu, P.P., & Kavanah. T. (1999). Central and peripheral adaptations after 12 weeks of exercise training in post-coronary artery surgery patients. *Journal of Cardiopulmonary Rehabilitation, 19,* 144-150.

Gordon, M. (2000). *Manual of nursing diagnosis* (9th ed.). St. Louis: Mosby.

Gulanick, M., Bliley, A., Perino, B., & Keough, V. (1998). Recovery patterns and lifestyle changes after coronary angioplasty: the patient's perspective. *Heart & Lung: Journal of Acute & Critical Care, 27,* 253-262.

Guyton, A.C. & Hall, J.E. (1996). *Textbook of medical physiology* (9th ed.). Philadelphia: WB Saunders.

Halm, M., Penque, S., Doll, N., & Beahrs, M. (1999). Women and cardiac rehabilitation: referral and compliance patterns. *Journal of Cardiovascular Nursing, 13,* 83-92.

Heldal, M., Steine, K., & Dale, J. (1996). Elderly patients are still deprived the benefits of cardiac rehabilitation. *Cardiology in the Elderly, 4,* 167-170.

Johnson, N.A., & Heller, R.F. (1998). Prediction of patient nonadherence with home-based exercise for cardiac rehabilitation: the role of perceived barriers and perceived benefits. *Preventive Medicine, 27,* 56-64.

Joyce, J.W. (1994). The diagnosis and management of diseases of the peripheral arteries and veins. In R.C. Schlant & R.W. Alexander (Eds.), *Hurst's The Heart* (8th ed.). New York: McGraw-Hill.

Kinney, M.R., Dunbar, S.B., Brooks-Brunn, J., Molter, N., & Vitello-Cicciu, J. M. (1998). *AACN's clinical reference for critical care nursing.* St. Louis: Mosby.

Launius, B. K., & Graham, B.D. (1998). Understanding and preventing deep vein thrombosis and pulmonary embolism. *AACN Clinical Issues: Advanced Practice in Acute & Critical Care, 9,* 91-99.

Lavie, C.J., Milanni R.V, Cassidy, M.M., & Gilliland, Y.E. (1999). Effects of cardiac rehabilitation and exercise training programs in women with depression. *American Journal of Cardiology, 83,* 1480-1483.

Lehigh Valley Hospital and Health Network. (1997). *Clinical management protocols for trauma and surgical critical care.* Allentown, PA: Author.

Liddell, E., & Fridlund, B. (1996). Long-term effects of a comprehensive rehabilitation program after myocardial infarction. *Scandinavian Journal of Caring Sciences,* 67-74.

Maillefert, J.F., Eicher, J.C., Walker, P., Dulieu, V., Rouhier-Narcer, I., Branly, F., Cohen, M., Brunotte, F., Wolf, J.E., Casillas, J.M., & Didier, J.P. (1998). *Journal of Cardiopulmonary Rehabilitation, 18,* 277-282.

Maoirana, A.J., Briffa, T.G., Goodman, C., & Hung, J. (1997). A controlled trial of circuit weight training on aerobic capacity and myocardial oxygen demand in men after coronary artery bypass surgery. *Journal of Cardiopulmonary Rehabilitation, 17,* 239-247.

McConnell, T.R., Klinger T.A., Gardner, J.K., Lauback, C.A., Jr., Herman, C.E., Hauck, C.A. (1998). Cardiac rehabilitation without exercise test for post-myocardial infarction and post-bypass surgery patients. *Journal of Cardiopulmonary Rehabilitation, 18,* 458-463.

McConnell, T.R., Palm, R.J., Shearn, W.M., & Laubach, C.A. Jr. (1999). Body fat distribution's impact on physiologic outcomes during cardiac rehabilitation. *Journal of Cardiopulmonary Rehabilitation,* 19, 162-169.

Merz, C.N.B., Felando, M.N., & Klein, J. (1996). Cholesterol awareness and treatment in patients with coronary artery disease participating in cardiac rehabilitation. *Journal of Cardiopulmonary Rehabilitation, 16,* 117-122.

Miller, N.H. (1991). Cardiac rehabilitation. In M.R. Kinney, D.R. Packa, K.G. Andreoli, & P.P. Zipes (Eds.), *Comprehensive cardiac care* (7th ed.). St. Louis: Mosby.

Missik, E. (1999). Personal perceptions and women's participation in cardiac rehabilitation including commentary by Easton KL. *Rehabilitation Nursing, 24,* 158-165.

Moore, S.M., & Kramer, F.M. (1996). Women's and men's preferences for cardiac rehabilitation program features. *Journal of Cardiopulmonary Rehabilitation, 16,* 163-168.

Moore, S.M., Ruland, C.M., Pashkow, F.J. & Blackburn, G.G. (1998). Women's patterns of exercise following cardiac rehabilitation. *Nursing Research, 47,* 318-324.

Moranville-Hunziker, M., Sagehorn, K.K., Conn, V., Feutz, C., & Hagenhoff, B. (1994). Patients' perceptions of learning needs during the first phase of cardiac rehabilitation following coronary artery bypass graft surgery. *Rehabilitation Nursing Research, 2,* 75-80.

Moser, D.J., Cohen, R.A., Clark, M.M., Aloia, M.S., Tate, B.A., Stefanik, S., Forman, D.E., & Tilkemeier, P.L. (1999). Neuropsychological functioning among cardiac rehabilitation patients. *Journal of Cardiopulmonary Rehabilitation, 19,* 91-97.

Pashkow, F.J., & Dafoe, W.A. (1993). *Clinical cardiac rehabilitation: A cardiologist's guide.* Baltimore: Williams & Wilkins.

Patrick, D., Danis, M., Southerland, L., & Hong, G. (1988). Quality of life following intensive care. *Journal of General Internal Medicine,* 3, 218-223.

Paul-Labrador, M., Vongvanich, P., & Merz, C.N.B. (1999). Risk stratification for exercise training in cardiac patients: Do the proposed guidelines work? *Journal of Cardiopulmonary Rehabilitation, 19,* 118-125.

Porth, C.M. (1994). Alteration in blood flow. *Pathophysiology: Concepts of altered health states* (pp. 355-377). Philadelphia: JB Lippincott.

Rubin, E., & Farber, J.L. (1994). *Pathology* (2nd ed). Philadelphia: JB Lippincott.

Rukholm, E., & McGirr, M. (1994). A quality-of-life index for clients with ischemic heart disease: Establishing reliability and validity. *Rehabilitation Nursing, 19,* 12-16.

Schairer, J.R., Kostelnik, T., Proffitt, S.M., Faitel, K.I., Windeler, S., Rickman, L.B., Brawner, C.A., & Keteyian, S.J. (1998). Caloric expenditure during cardiac rehabilitation. *Journal of Cardiopulmonary Rehabilitation, 18,* 290-294.

Shaw, G. (2000). *For depressed heart patients rehab can be a lifesaver* [Online]. Available: http://healthwatch.medscape.com/medscape/p/G_library/article.asp?RecID=2062527channel=11.

Southard, D.R., Certo, C., Comoss, P.M., Gordon, N.F., Herbert, W.G., Protas, E.J., Ribisl, P., & Swails, S. (1994). Core competencies for cardiac rehabilitation professionals: Position statement of the American Association of Cardiovascular and Pulmonary Rehabilitation. *Journal of Cardiopulmonary Rehabilitation, 14,* 87-92.

Sparks, K.E., Shaw, D.K., Jennings, H.S. III, & Quinn, L.M. (1998). Cardiovascular complications of outpatient cardiac rehabilitation programs utilizing transtelephonic exercise monitoring. *Cardiopulmonary Physical Therapy Journal, 9,* 3-6.

Spittell, P.C., & Spittell, J.A. (1994). Diseases of the peripheral arteries and veins. In J.H. Stein (ed.), *Internal medicine* (4th ed.). St. Louis: Mosby.

Stewart, K.J., McFarland, L.D., Weinhofer, J.J., Cottrell, E., Brown, C.S., Shapiro, E.P. (1998). Safety and efficacy of weight training soon after acute myocardial infarction. *Journal of Cardiopulmonary Rehabilitation, 18,* 37-44.

Suter, P.M., Suter, W.N., Perkins, M.K., Bona, S.L., & Kendrick, P.A. (1996). Cardiac rehabilitation survey: Maintenance of lifestyle changes and perception of program value. *Rehabilitation Nursing, 21,* 192-195.

Thomas, R.J., Miller, N.H., Lamendola, C., Berra, K., Hedback, B., Durstine, J.L., & Haskell, W. (1996). National survey on gender differences in cardiac rehabilitation programs: patient characteristics and enrollment patterns. *Journal of Cardiopulmonary Rehabilitation, 16,* 402-412.

Verges, B.L., Patois-Verges, B., Cohen, M., & Casillas, J.M. (1998). Comprehensive cardiac rehabilitation improves the control of dyslipidemia in secondary prevention. *Journal of Cardiopulmonary Rehabilitation, 18,* 408-415.

Wallwork, M. (1996). Targeting women for cardiac rehabilitation. *Health Visitor, 69,* 179-180.

Wenger, N.K., Froelicher E.S, Smith L.K., Ades, P.A., Berra, K., Blumenthal, J.A., Certo, C.M., Dattilo, A.N., Davis, D., & Debusk, R. (1995, October). Cardiac rehabilitation (Clinical Practice Guidelines No. 17, AHCPR Publication No. 96-0672). Rockville, MD: U.S. Department of Health and Human Services, Public Health Service, Agency for Health Care Policy and Research and the National Heart, Lung, and Blood Institute.

Willoughby, D.S., Roozen, M., & Barnes, R. (1997). Effects of aerobic exercise on the functional capacity and cardiovascular efficiency of elderly post-CABG patients. *Journal of Aging & Physical Activity, 5,* 87-97.

Woods, S. L., Froelicher, E.S.S., & Motzer, S.U. (2000). *Cardiac nursing* (4th ed.). Philadelphia: JB Lippincott.

SUGGESTED READINGS

Brannon, F.J., Foley, M.W., Starr, J.A., & Saul, L.M. (1998). *Cardiopulmonary rehabilitation: Basic theory and application* (3rd ed.). Philadelphia: FA Davis.

Messecar, D.C. (1998). The rehabilitation home health nurse and clients with cardiac or pulmonary conditions. In L. Neal (Ed.), *Home health and rehabilitation* (pp. 227-247). Glenville, IL, Association of Rehabilitation Nurses.

Restoration after Burn Injury

32

Patricia L. McCollom, MS, RN, CRRN, CDMS, CCM, CLCP

"I'm ready! I've been ready for a year!" With those words, Buck Simpson (not his real name) hopped up into the cab of a "14 wheeler," slammed the door, and started the ignition. The roar of the diesel engine almost drowned his words . . . "Thanks—I couldn't have made it without you!" Eighteen months before, I had met Buck in the burn intensive care unit of a large hospital in the Midwest. A semi driver, he had made a near fatal error during a cold January winter night. Diesel fuel "coagulates" in below-zero weather, requiring an additive to make the fuel liquid and move through the engine. After stalling along the Interstate, Buck added the material to the gas tank. He reached for a flashlight to check the tank and found it did not work. Quickly, in the frigid air, he grabbed a cigarette lighter and held it above the fuel tank. The next thing he remembers was his physician telling him he may not live. Buck was diagnosed with full thickness burns over 55% of his body surface area. His right arm was amputated below the elbow; his left arm was amputated above the elbow. Multiple surgeries were necessary, and long inpatient stays seemed they would never end.

This day, as I watch Buck with two specialized prostheses drive a semi truck down the highway, I was reminded about an old definition of rehabilitation nursing: "assisting clients to where they have the potential to be." Rehabilitation nursing practice has evolved beyond that simple definition, but Buck fits the definition well. He is back driving over the road, where he chooses to be, because a rehabilitation team believed in his potential.

OVERVIEW OF BURN INJURY

Epidemiology

It has been estimated that 2.5 million people experience a burn injury every year in the United States. Of these, 60,000 people are admitted to hospitals and more than 7,000 die as a direct result of the injury (Fritsch & Yurko, 1999). Half of those with burns will have injuries severe enough to restrict daily activities in the home, school, or workplace. Rehabilitation is a critical component of recovery and community reentry.

Though statistics are significant, review of data reveals declines in the national incidence of burn injury in the past two decades. This decline is in direct relation to prevention and a focus on burn injury treatment. Additionally, during this time, regional burn centers have been developed, smoke detectors are widely used, burn prevention education has expanded, occupational safety has increased, and consumer product information about burns has been emphasized. The decrease in burn incidence also reflects societal changes, such as decrease in smoking, changes in cooking practices, and reduced industrial employment (Brigham & McLoughlin, 1996).

This chapter provides information about burn injuries, treatment, and rehabilitation nursing interventions and outcomes. Although intensive care is necessary for acute burn injury care, it is the rehabilitation philosophy that facilitates return to function, coping with body image change and dealing with long-term health issues.

Incidence

Children ages 2 to 4 years old and young adults ages 15 to 25 years old are the age groups with greater numbers of injuries from burns. Burn injuries rank second only to motor vehicle accidents as a cause of death during childhood.

Elderly people experience high mortality and morbidity from burns (Covington, Wainwright, & Parks, 1996); they may not detect danger when preexisting problems such as altered or impaired judgment, decreased coordination and tactile sensation, or impaired vision or smell inhibit awareness.

Seventy percent of burns result from thermal injury. Thermal injury may be from dry heat (flame) or moist heat (hot liquid). Thermal injury results in marked changes in the vascular and metabolic responses of the body, resulting in increased risk for infection resulting from loss of skin integrity and postburn immunosuppression. Burns may also be caused by chemicals, electric current, or radiation. Scald injuries are the most frequent type of burn; however, flame injuries are more serious. Electrical and radiation burns may appear less severe on the skin surface, but may affect underlying organs with damage that may not be known for days after the injury. The direct cost of treating burn injuries is more than $1 billion per year. Indirect costs, including resulting disability, are several billion dollars annually (Fletchall & Hickerson, 1995).

PATHOPHYSIOLOGY

Burns are currently described in the clinical context as partial thickness and full thickness. This terminology more accurately describes the burn, indicating depth and severity of tissue injury (Figure 32-1).

Partial thickness burns result in destruction of varying depths of the epidermis (outer layer of skin) and the dermis (middle layer of skin). The depth of tissue injury is described as superficial (involving only the epidermis) or deep partial thickness (involving the entire epidermis into the dermis). Partial thickness burns are painful because nerve endings are injured and exposed. However, because epithelial cells are not destroyed, partial thickness burns will heal. Blistering indicates deep partial thickness burns. Blisters may increase in size, resulting from collection of tissue fluid. Dryness and itching are common during healing; itching is caused by increased vascularization, reduced secretions, and decreased perspiration.

Full thickness burns destroy the epidermis and the dermis and cause possible damage to the subcutaneous tissue, muscle, and bone. Nerve endings are destroyed. The wounds become covered by eschar, a dark, thickened substance composed of denatured protein. Surface dehydration causes the eschar to form. Full thickness burns require skin grafting because epithelial cells are destroyed.

Normal skin function is diminished as a result of burns. There is a loss of protective covering, escape of body fluids, lack of temperature control, loss of sweat and sebaceous glands, and loss of sensory receptors. The severity of these complex changes will determine local response or systemic response.

A major burn injury, despite the cause, is one of the most critical forms of trauma that an individual can endure (Brigham & McLoughlin, 1996). The initial physiological response to partial or full thickness burn injury is capillary vasoconstriction. Soon after, vasodilation occurs and plasma is released to the injury site. Within 24 hours, increased clot-

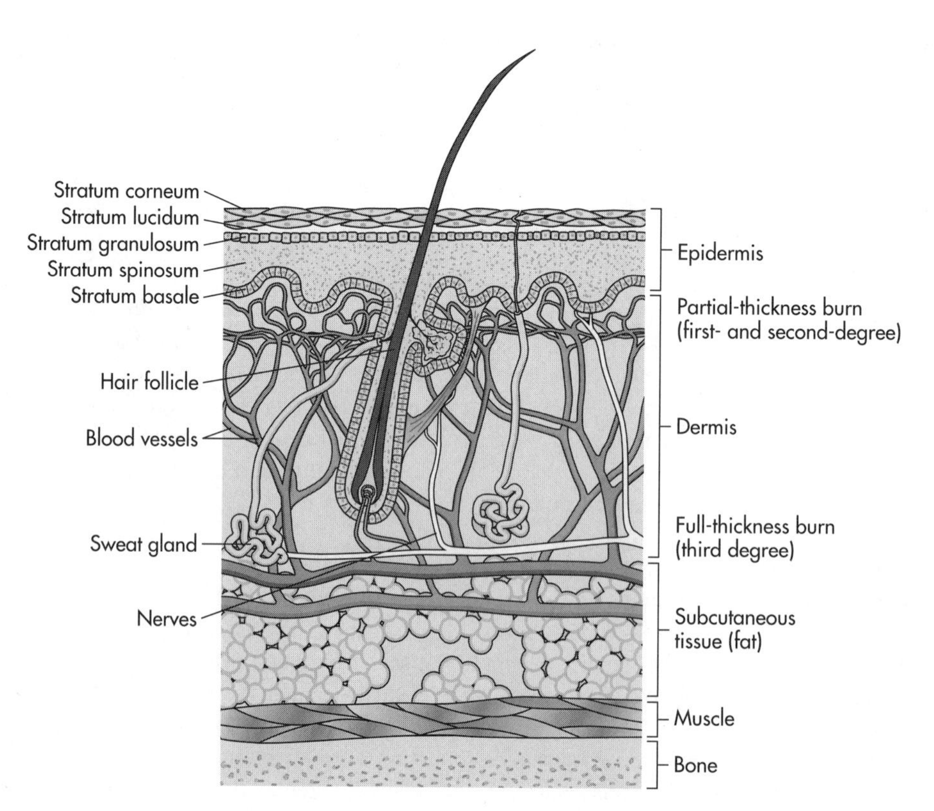

Figure 32-1 Levels of human skin involved in burns. (From Phipps, W.J., Sands, J.K., & Marek, J.F. [1999]. *Medical-surgical nursing: Concepts and clinical practice* [6th ed.]. St. Louis: Mosby.)

ting may occur, which will decrease or eliminate blood flow. Without proper blood supply, further cellular death will occur. Because of this dynamic process, the exact depth of a burn injury may not be apparent for 3 to 5 days. During this process, massive fluid loss from open wounds and evaporation will occur, resulting in heat loss and elevated metabolism. Furthermore, when skin integrity is compromised, the body is no longer protected from bacteria; local sepsis will occur rapidly as bacteria enter the wound. If the infection is not monitored closely and treated carefully, tissue will be destroyed. The depth of burn injury may deepen as a partial thickness burn coverts to full thickness. Life-threatening systemic involvement also may occur.

Burn shock may occur as a result of hypovolemia. As fluid escapes to surrounding tissue, edema progresses. Edema progresses until fluid impairs range of motion (ROM) and blood flow to other tissues. Cellular death, damage to peripheral nerves, and sensory or motor loss may occur. The respiratory system is affected either by facial and neck edema after burn injury or by hyperventilation and increased oxygen consumption from smoke inhalation, possibly requiring emergent intubation. Other systemic effects involve the gastrointestinal and renal systems. Because of the hemodynamic changes that occur with postburn crises, renal insufficiency as well as gastric dilation and gastrointestinal ileus are concerns. Additionally, a suppressed immune system creates an ongoing risk of infection.

Wound Healing

In partial thickness burns, the epidermal cells lining the hair follicles and sweat glands remain intact. Healing occurs as these cells migrate from the wound margin and join any small intact pieces of epithelium to form new epithelium, which will cover the burn wound in 14 to 21 days, depending on the depth of the injury. This newly formed epithelium is extremely delicate and must be shielded until it is capable of performing temperature regulation functions and protecting the body from infection.

Deeper full thickness burns heal with a different process, which begins with phagocytosis by white blood cells to clear the wound area of debris and bacteria. Fibroblasts secrete collagen at the same time as marginal epithelial cells migrate from the wound periphery and injured venule buds for capillary networks to restore circulation. This process creates granulation tissue that is reddened, highly vascular, warm to the touch, and hypersensitive.

Phases of Injury and Goals

The three phases of burn care are the emergent or resuscitative phase, the acute phase, and the rehabilitative phase.

The emergent stage involves critical care, often instituted in the emergency room or on-site at the place of the injury. Goals for this period are to maintain an airway, replace fluids, maintain client comfort, prevent infection, maintain body temperature, and provide emotional support.

The acute phase encompasses the period from burn injury until the client is considered stable and until all full thickness burns are covered with skin. The acute phase focuses on multisystem stabilization, wound care, infection control, mobility and function, and nutritional support (Box 32-1).

The rehabilitation period focuses on reentry into the life continuum. Restoration of function and emotional support are the goals of this phase of treatment. Although rehabilitation is an ongoing component of burn care, discharge planning and discharge require rehabilitation nursing interventions to deal with body image change, a societal response to the change in appearance resulting from burns and functional limitations that may affect activities of daily living (ADLs) and work potential. Initial goals set during acute care are directed toward preserving joint mobility strength, endurance, and controlling edema, with some attention to promoting independent self-care and educating clients and families about burn recovery (DeSanti, Lincoln, Egan, & Demling, 1998). Rehabilitation goals expand beyond acute care to prevent further disability and complications, such as disfigurement related to scar contracture (Staley, Richard, Warden, Miller, & Shuster, 1996). The goals of rehabilitation are directed toward minimizing scar contracture formation; increasing flexibility, strength, and endurance; and promoting independence in normal daily activities (Doctor, Patterson, & Mann, 1997). Long-term goals for clients are to improve physical skills for returning to work or school and for community reintegration.

Assessment

During initial assessment, information regarding the circumstances surrounding the burn injury must be obtained from the individual or witnesses. Data should include:

- How and when the injury occurred
- Duration of contact with the burning agent
- Location when burned
- Presence of explosion
- Age and general health
- Nature of thermal agent

Small children and the elderly have a higher mortality rate (Brigham & McLoughlin, 1996). Concurrent health conditions will affect the individual's ability to withstand the physiological stress of burns.

Objective data will identify the severity of the burn.

Box 32-1 Acute Phase Focus

Multisystem stabilization
Wound care
Infection control
Mobility and function
Nutritional support

Burns are classified as major, moderate, or minor, depending on the size of the burn, the depth, the location, and other complications (Box 32-2).

The "rule of nines" may be used clinically to describe the total body surface area (TBSA) that has been burned. A chart demonstrating anterior and posterior diagrams of the body is divided into areas equal to multiples of 9% (Figure 32-2). The burned areas are typically shaded on the diagrams, allowing the amount of area burned to be calculated. A pediatric chart for "rule of nines" exists; however, infants and children will have calculations modified because of their inherent size differences and the depth and location of burns.

Age

The severity of a burn also depends on the age of the individual. Infants younger than 2 years of age have a poor response to infection. Older people with preexisting health conditions may be unable to withstand the physiological stress of the burn injury.

Burn Site

The burn's location on the body is an important consideration in assessing the client with burns. A 5% burn to the abdomen of an obese adult female is far different from the same site on a 5-year-old child. Any burn that extends across a joint may cause mobility limitations and require extensive physical therapy. A circumferential burn may cause constrictive contracture, resulting in multiple complications. Any burn causing facial disfigurement results in severe emotional distress, as well as initial concerns about respiratory maintenance because of structural damage to respiratory anatomy.

Causative Agent

The cause of the burn must be identified because of the direct relationship to treatment and prognosis.

During the rehabilitation phase, ongoing assessment must include the individual's ROM, complaints of pain and pressure, and the individual's response to client teaching. Special attention must be given to the individual and family responses to body image change. Coping mechanisms must be specified.

Further, the rehabilitation nurse must be prepared to assess the individual's response to positioning, splinting, exercise, wound care, and ability to perform ADLs.

Box 32-2 Burn Classification by Total Body Surface Area (TBSA) Burn Estimate

Minor Burn Injuries

Less than 15% TBSA in adults (10% in children or elderly persons)
Less than 2% TBSA full thickness injury
Burns in patients with no preexisting disease

Moderate Burn Injuries

15-25% TBSA in adults, partial thickness (10-20% TBSA in children younger than 10 years and adults older than 40 years)
2-10% TBSA full thickness
Burns with no concurrent injury
Burns in patients with no preexisting disease

Major Burn Injuries

Partial thickness injury greater than 25% TBSA (greater than 20% in children younger than 10 years and adults older than 40 years)
Greater than 10% TBSA, full thickness (children and adults)
Involvement of face, eyes, ears, hands, feet, or perineum
Electrical burns
Burns complicated by inhalation injury or major trauma
Burns in patients with preexisting disease (diabetes, congestive heart failure, or chronic renal failure)

Source: Burn Unit Education Program, University of Iowa Hospitals and Clinics, Iowa City, Iowa.

NURSING DIAGNOSIS

Nursing diagnosis is defined as a clinical judgment about an individual, family, or community response to actual or potential health problems or life processes that provide the basis for definitive therapy toward achievement of outcomes for which the nurse is accountable (Gordon, 2000).

Determined from analyses of client data, nursing diagnoses for the person with burns during the rehabilitation period may include those found in Table 32-1.

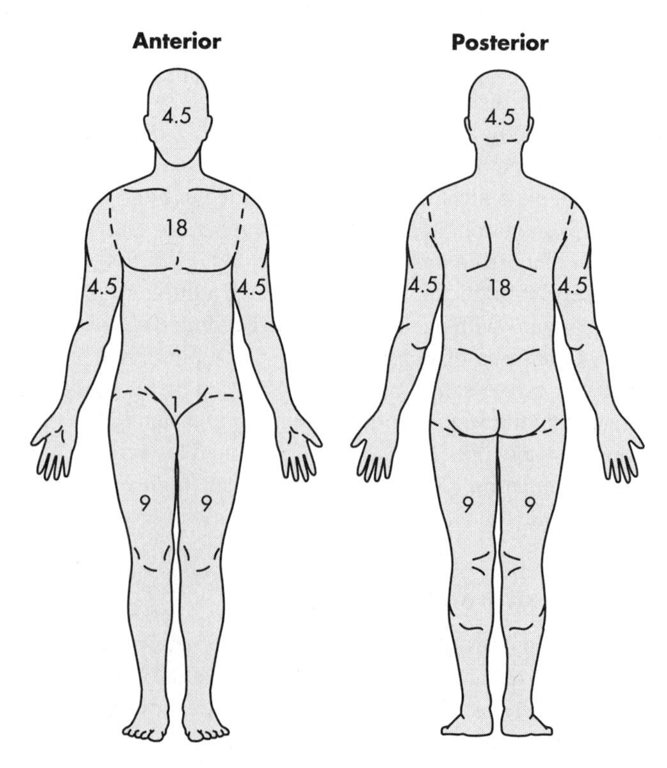

Figure 32-2 Rule of nines. (From Phipps, W.J., Sands, J.K., & Marek, J.F. [1999]. *Medical-surgical nursing: Concepts and clinical practice* [6th ed.]. St. Louis: Mosby.)

Expected Outcomes

Expected outcomes are defined as a client state, at a given point in time, reflecting improvement over a state at a prior assessment (Johnson, Maas, & Moorhead, 2000). Outcomes for the burn-injured individual during the rehabilitation phase include:

1. Endurance, increased mobility, and increased joint movement
2. Participating in health care decisions, self-direction of care, coping
3. Comfort level
4. Psychosocial adjustment: life changes
5. Social support
6. Family coping, family functioning
7. Coping, body image acceptance
8. Nutrition

INTERVENTIONS

Nursing interventions represent those activities that nurses do to assist the individual or family to move toward a desired outcome (McCloskey & Bulechek, 2000) (Table 32-2).

Interventions Related to Impaired Skin Integrity

Rehabilitation nursing assessment of the integumentary system goes beyond evaluation of injury sites. By the time the client has reached the rehabilitative phase, escharotomies, debridements, and grafting procedures have been completed; therefore, a client may enter rehabilitation with a wound that is covered with extremely fragile skin. The goals of wound care during rehabilitative recovery focus on attending to healed areas and donor sites, preventing infection, protecting new skin from further trauma, and preparing skin for compression. Understanding physiological alterations of skin resulting from burn injury, along with its impact on lifestyle, underlies all interventions and ongoing management of the individual with burn injury.

Topical agents may be used to prevent infection during the rehabilitation phase. No single topical agent has been demonstrated to be universally effective for burn care. Alternative agents may be used concurrently on different burn sites. The most popular topical agent in use is silver sulfadiazine 1% (Silvadene), a water-based cream effective against Gram-positive, Gram-negative and *Candida* organisms. Other agents commonly used include mafenide acetate (Sulfamylon), povidone-iodine, sliver nitrate 5%, and cerium nitrate 1.74%. Over-the-counter topical agents may include bacitracin with polymyxin B and neomycin sulfate.

People who have had a burn injury may experience impairments for an extended period after hospitalization. Many of these impairments are difficult to assess and document. For example, heat or cold intolerance, decreased strength and coordination, photosensitivity, or changes in sweating and psychosocial problems may complicate rehabilitation.

For example, a burn injury that extends to the dermis also will destroy hair follicles and sebaceous and sweat glands, which arise from this skin layer. Also lost are the abilities for these structures to regenerate. Scar tissue may take up to 2 years to mature; thus, the skin is continually changing, healing, and evolving during this posthospitalization phase. As a result the client must deal with skin that is thinner, less pliable, drier, more sensitive to temperature changes, and more prone to blistering and itching.

Dryness

Topical emollients supply external moisture and lubrication to the newly healed skin. Lotions that contain both water (for absorption) and lipid (to retard evaporation) are recommended. In general, it is best to avoid creams, lanolins, and cocoa butter with nonessential or poorly characterized ingredients such as fragrance, exotic plant oils, or extracts that only will mimic adequate lubrication. These nonessential ingredients can cause irritation or contact sensitization. As a supplement, a room humidifier may help to reduce epidermal dehydration.

Photosensitivity

Avoiding sunlight exposure for 6 months or longer after a burn injury is recommended to prevent sunburn and permanent hyperpigmentation. Return of melanin pigments to newly healed skin or grafts varies, depending on the extent of injury. Common sense measures include use of a hat and appropriate clothing, timing of outdoor activities for early morning or late afternoon, and application of sunscreen to newly formed skin. A product with a sun protection factor rating of at least 15 should be used when sunlight exposure cannot be avoided. Sunscreens labeled "water resistant" will retain their protective ability for 40 minutes of sweating or swimming, whereas those labeled "waterproof" will retain their effectiveness for up to 80 minutes of activ-

TABLE 32-1 Nursing Diagnoses for Clients with Burn Injury

Diagnostic Title	Etiological Factors
Impaired physical mobility	Joint stiffness or contractures; pain discomfort; musculoskeletal impairment
Ineffective health maintenance	Ineffective coping; impairment of support system
Risk for joint contractures	Imposed restrictions by scarring
Chronic pain	Physiological factors and knowledge deficit
Disturbed body image	Nonintegration of change in body characteristics
Social isolation	Alteration in physical appearance
Interrupted family processes	Situational transition
Posttrauma syndrome	Injury flashbacks
Imbalanced nutrition: less than body requirements	Loss of body fluid

TABLE 32-2 Suggested Nursing Outcomes Classification (NOC) and Nursing Interventions Classifications (NIC) for Burn Injury

Nursing Diagnosis	Nursing Outcome Classifications (NOC)	Nursing Intervention Classifications (NIC)
Risk for impaired skin integrity	Risk detention Risk control Tissue integrity: skin and mucous membranes Tissue perfusion: peripheral	Skin surveillance Pressure management Pressure ulcer prevention Foot care Positioning
Impaired skin integrity	Tissue integrity: skin and mucous membranes Wound healing: primary intention Wound healing: secondary intention Fluid balance Immobility consequences: physiological Treatment behavior: illness or injury Nutritional status	Skin surveillance Skin care: topical treatments Wound care Pressure ulcer care Nutrition management Fluid/electrolyte management Positioning Traction/immobilization care
Deficient knowledge of skin management	Knowledge: treatment regimen Knowledge: diet Knowledge: disease process	Teaching: procedure/treatment Teaching: prescribed diet Teaching: disease process Learning facilitation Learning readiness enhancement Health education
Imbalanced nutrition: less than body requirements	Nutritional status: nutrient intake	Nutrition management Fluid monitoring Fluid/electrolyte management Nutritional counseling Nutrition therapy Nutrition monitoring Weight management Weight gain assistance Teaching: prescribed diet

Data from Johnson, M., Maas, M.L., & Moorhead, S. (2000). *Nursing outcomes classification (NOC)* (2nd ed.). St. Louis: Mosby; McCloskey, J.C., & Bulechek, G.M. (2000). *Nursing interventions classification (NIC)* (3rd ed.). St. Louis: Mosby; and North American Nursing Diagnosis Association. (2001). *Nursing diagnosis: definitions and classification 2001-2002* (4th ed.). Philadelphia: Author.

ity. New sunscreen products are being developed each season.

Pruritus

Pruritus is a significant problem during the recovery period. If not treated and controlled, the scratching can destroy fragile grafts and healing donor sites. Strategies of daily hygiene, conscientious lubrication, appropriate thermal protection, alternatives to scratching, and antipruritic medications must be incorporated into the client's lifestyle if successful management is to be achieved. Itching of healing burn areas and new skin can be a severe discomfort. Using systemic antihistamines in conjunction with topical antipruritic agents may ease some symptoms. An emollient lotion containing menthol (¼%-½%) and camphor (½%-2%) feels cool to the skin and may provide temporary relief while countering dryness. Refrigerating lotions may be soothing for some people. Topical anesthetics (e.g., pramoxine hydrochloride 1%) are available in ointments, creams, and lotions. Topical benzocaine preparations are not recommended because of potential allergic sensitization.

Interventions Related to Pain Management

Pain

Severe pain often accompanies partial thickness burns because of damaged but not destroyed sensory nerve fibers. In contrast, little, if any, pain is associated with full thickness injury because nerve endings are in large part destroyed.

Nurses are aware that each client is the authority on the pain he or she is experiencing. Chapter 24 contains principles for nursing assessment and management of pain and pain relief that apply to clients who have burn injuries. The most valuable nursing intervention with clients who have pain is pain relief through prescribing medications (often narcotics), implementing comfort measures, and assisting clients to use alternative techniques. Relaxation techniques of imagery and distraction heighten the effects of analgesia for many clients. These are discussed in more detail in Chapter 28.

Coordinating therapy procedures, anticipating energy requirements for activities, planning for rest periods interspersed with therapies, and promoting time and guidance for self-help strategies contribute to minimizing pain; this in turn allows a client to participate in ADLs. A client who is involved in wound care and decision-making processes feels more empowered, thereby enhancing feelings of control related to pain management.

Interventions Related to Impaired Physical Mobility

Mobility

Assessment of the client's mobility status is an ongoing process because functional recovery may be a long and laborious process and usually involves interdisciplinary assessments and interventions. Positioning, exercise, compression, and splinting are basic burn rehabilitation treatment procedures. The purpose of these modalities is to prevent loss of function and promote functional independence.

With advances in splinting and other modalities, most clients can expect to approximate their preinjury level of function. Assistive devices or adapted equipment may be needed to ensure function. Reconstructive surgery may be necessary for a client to regain function when scar contractures have formed.

Positioning

Proper positioning begins at onset of injury and is evaluated regularly throughout rehabilitation. During the acute phase of injury, proper positioning minimizes edema, provides safe and proper joint alignment, and maintains tendon balance between overstretching and promoting contracture formation. During the rehabilitative phase of recovery, the goal is to continue effective positioning to prevent contractures (Fritsch & Yurko, 2000). Because clients are encouraged to become ambulatory as soon as possible, using an assistive device for proper positioning is part of learning upright sitting and standing posture. Whether a client's wound management dictates total body or partial positioning, various burn injury sites require special attention to prevent complications of pressure necrosis, dependent edema, or flexion contractures. Common factors that may affect positioning are edema, donor sites, graft areas, and respiratory function.

Figure 32-3 illustrates how cloth rolls, foam wedges, straps, foot boards, and slings may be used to assist with proper positioning. Burns involving the head, face, or neck require individualized positioning according to the area burned. Pillows are not recommended because their use may lead to secondary complications, such as neck flexion contractures and pressure on the ears. The supine position, using a small foam pad instead of a pillow, is recommended for severely burned clients. As a general rule, knees, hips, elbows, and interphalangeal joints are placed extended in neutral alignments. Ankles and feet are dorsiflexed at a 90-degree angle, wrists are dorsiflexed at 10 to 20 degrees, and a shoulder is placed in neutral alignment supported in a 90-degree abduction.

Splints are one way to immobilize an area of the body and place it in a position that will preserve or restore function. However, a client must adhere to a schedule for wearing a splint, practice routine cleaning, and inspect the skin before and on removal of the splint to achieve desired outcomes.

Exercise

Joint function may diminish as a result of bed rest, decreased protein, altered fluid and electrolytes, and poor circulation until ultimately contractures occur and heterotopic bone is formed. Full ROM joint exercises for all joints begin early in the wound management process and continue at regular daily intervals. Active and passive exercises may be combined, depending on a client's capabilities; however, joints are not moved beyond their free range unless prescribed by a physician and directed by a physical therapist.

Successful outcomes of burn injury cannot be achieved when a client relies solely on the benefits of scheduled therapies. In home and community settings, rehabilitation nurses can assist community health nurses and other community resources to intervene with exercise modalities for stretching and increasing ROM, which are both creative and cost-effective. In the home, assistive devices such as splints, wedges, pulley systems, slings, shoes or pillows may be effective in incorporating active or passive exercises into daily routines. As part of self-care, a client is expected to follow through with these mobility skills during nontherapy hours; family members are taught how to assist. A program or system established in the rehabilitation setting will be followed more consistently when it is appropriate and adaptable to the home environment. Ideally a client will understand, initiate, and incorporate these strategies into everyday routine.

Some clients may find it difficult to adhere to a prescribed exercise program because of pain, diminished endurance, low levels of motivation, other chronic or disabling conditions, or knowledge deficit. The rehabilitation nurse may be instrumental in educating a client and family about strategic ways to address issues such as anticipating and treating pain before exercise, developing and tolerating wearing schedules of compression garments and splints, coordinating wound management with other treatment regimens, and enduring effective positioning of extremities and trunk. Successful adaptations of these necessary lifestyle changes can be achieved better when clients have incentives for high levels of motivation.

Compression

A primary treatment for prevent and reduction of hypertrophic scarring is compression therapy. After wounds are

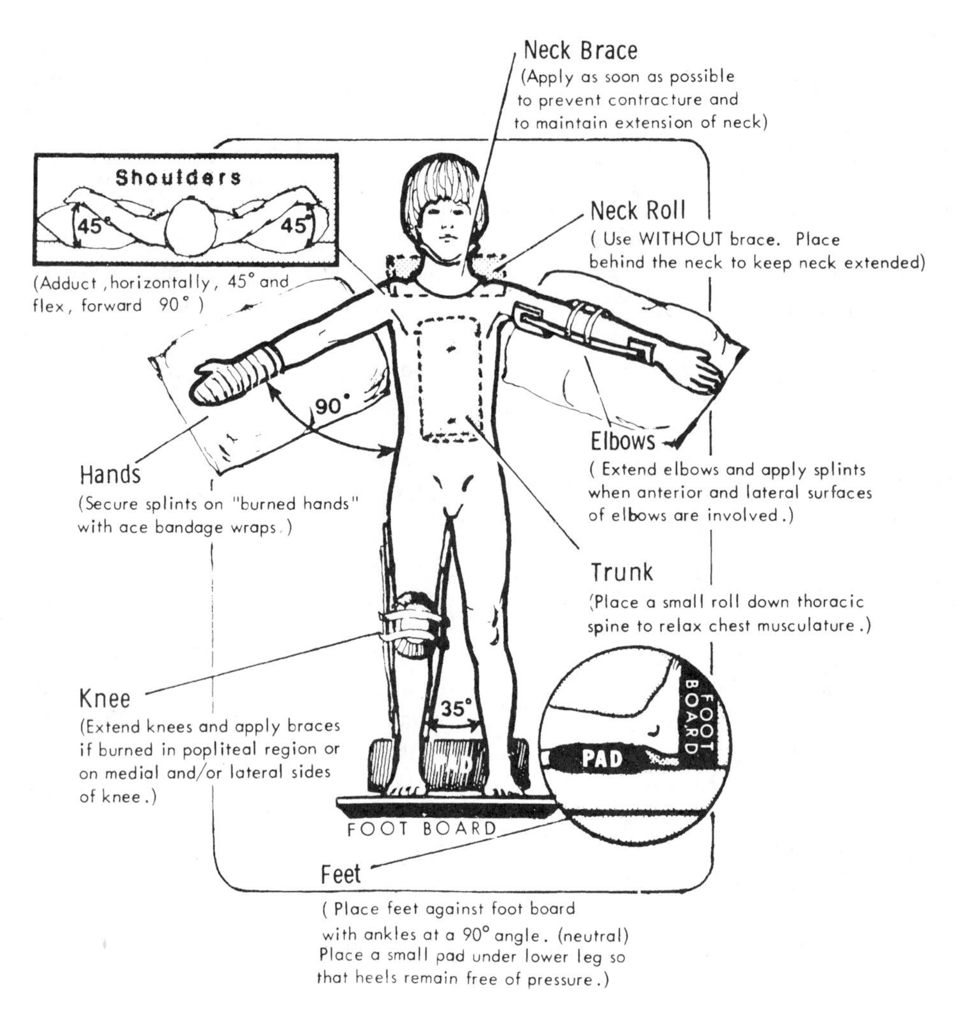

Figure 32-3 Supine positioning of the burn client to prevent contracture formation. (Courtesy Shriners Burns Institute, Galveston, TX.)

closed, custom-fitted garments are worn 24 hours every day and are removed only for hygiene and skin care. These garments are worn for as long as 1 to 2 years or until scar tissue matures. Clearly this long-term treatment relies on interdisciplinary teamwork with a fully participating client and family for successful outcome. Research has demonstrated in some burn centers that flexible dressings provide the same outcome.

Preparation and toughening of the skin to tolerate the custom-fitted garment for such long duration is a primary goal of the interdisciplinary team. Pressure may be applied to burn areas gradually and through various methods. Products such as elastic wraps (e.g., Ace bandages), premade tubular elastic garments (e.g., Tubigrip), or tailor-made burn garments (e.g., Jobst) are designed to apply varying degrees of pressure to the scar tissue. Inserts of foam or silicone may be applied underneath the pressure garment to increase direct pressure to a specific area. The length of time a client is scheduled to wear a particular pressure application is increased gradually and as tolerated.

Whenever the compression garment or other device is removed, the nurse conducts a complete head-to-toe skin assessment. The nurse pays specific attention to any pressure areas that may be developing and evaluates skin tolerance to compression treatment. With burn injuries, it is not uncommon for blisters to develop on healed areas; these differ from pressure areas. Blisters are evaluated and noted but left intact unless accompanied by signs of infection. Any sign of infection is reported to the physician immediately.

Splinting

Splints are fabricated by occupational therapist to prevent or correct contractures. As assistive devices they may be used on various parts of the body for support, to promote mobility and to enable a client to perform self-care activities. Splinting aids joint positioning and decreases scar contractures and hypertrophy. Splints are necessary to maintain the length of soft tissue joint structures; however, they are used cautiously to avoid prolonged immobilization and fibrosis of soft tissue. Static splints can be used over compression garments to maintain increases in motion that have been achieved with therapeutic exercise. Dynamic splints provide continuous gentle stretch when full motion is not achieved with exercise and activity. Some physicians prefer to use frequent exercise instead of splints (Fritsch & Yurko, 2000).

Nursing interventions with splint treatment include assisting client and team with initiating and adhering to a tolerable wearing schedule, monitoring skin status, and evaluating the effectiveness of the splint regimen on function and mobility in daily activities. Coordinated interventions with physical and occupational therapy regimens are critical in preventing contractures. Team members, the client, and the client's family must coordinate treatments and devote attention to each phase of the treatment to achieve desired outcomes, which are to preserve function and minimize complications associated with burn injury.

Interventions Related to Altered Health Maintenance

Lifestyle

Assessment of each client's lifestyle, preferences, and habits as they were lived before injury is essential in developing effective and realistic interventions. Clients who learn and practice new strategies to care for their "now-new body" will experience improved outcomes. Simple but regular strategies of daily hygiene, vigilant lubrication, avoidance of strong sun exposure and temperature changes, appropriate thermal protection, and antipruritic measures are incorporated as much as possible into lifestyle and preferences. Although these strategies may be intrusive for some, they are necessary for effective long-term skin care management.

Self-Care

Self-initiated programs give clients the psychological benefit of actively participating in their own rehabilitation and promote the habits of a daily routine, which must be conscientiously adhered to after discharge. Active participation in wound care, hygiene, and self-exercise programs are crucial to prevent complications and increase functional ability. The rehabilitation nurse educates client and family and reinforces modifications for the client's life-long lifestyle, not only for the duration of the rehabilitation wound management program.

PSYCHOSOCIAL ADJUSTMENT AND FAMILY INVOLVEMENT

The psychological implications for a client who has a burn injury are great. Nurses may encounter clients who exhibit a variety of responses and emotional reactions, depending on their phase of recovery. Initially, a client may be delirious as a result of burn shock and medications. Later, depression becomes a major factor as the realization of drastic changes in personal appearance, seemingly endless treatments, and functional implications for the future become more apparent. At some time fear of death is a major concern for many. Other fears commonly expressed by clients are fears of pain, suffering, disfigurement, and prolonged hospitalization, and concerns about disruption of lifestyle or survivor guilt.

The nursing goals during these early phases are to decrease pain, to ensure gentle physical care and handling, to answer questions as completely as possible, and to begin to elicit participation from both the client and the family. There is some evidence that children who have burn injuries ultimately may experience less psychological impact than their parents do; however, findings from this study certainly do not negate psychosocial adjustment problems for children.

The stress of lifestyle changes and the constant demands of active participation in various preventive procedures can be extremely difficult for many people. Coupled with body image concerns, functional limitations, and adapted lifestyle, and perhaps a changed vocation, the client reenters society essentially as a changed person with a "now-new body." Thus some type of grief response to changed body image usually occurs. These internal changes and adjustments are heightened by the multiple reminders of changes in appearance or ability that a client will encounter on reentering society. Assertiveness training may help many clients deal with social responses—ranging from avoidance, ridicule, stares, to excessive sympathy—that threaten a client's self-confidence.

The 1-year postinjury mark appears to be significant for people who survive burn injuries. For many, emotional issues are resolved as physical function is restored and most extensive treatment such as compression is completed and there has been time to adjust to social issues. These factors coincide with scar tissue maturation and improved sensation, which also may be occurring at approximately 1 year. Work and family roles may have been renegotiated by this time.

Family involvement is crucial during both initial and recovery periods. Tremendous sadness or guilt of being a survivor may accompany clients when a loved one was lost as a result of the burn injury event. The family is often the single most important continuing force in a client's life and the primary resource in redefining identify when the client reenters the community. Allowing and encouraging regular family visits during all phases of recovery may accomplish the following three goals:

1. Providing a client opportunity to express emotions and encouraging expression of frustrations and concerns
2. Allowing family members to observe wound healing and adjust to changes in client's physical appearance and functioning
3. Aiding family in understanding a client's day-to-day struggles and offering insight into physical and emotional challenges during rehabilitation

The absence of family or significant other in the ongoing recovery process impedes a client's motivation and creates further stressors in the discharge process. Depending on the extent of the burn injury and physical functioning, family involvement and support may be a deciding factor in whether a client returns to live at home or in a skilled-care facility.

Sexuality

Although the recovery period after a burn injury may require up to 5 years, a milestone is achieved when a client is able to look, touch, and care for affected areas. Many times clients have disassociated themselves from the burn areas, perhaps for as long as the first year. Rehabilitation nurses who conduct ongoing assessment will be attuned to a client's psychological readiness for redefining body image and self-esteem. Sexual functioning becomes a concern as other issues are resolved.

Unpleasant sensations may be the result of hypersensitivity of immature scar tissue, irritable feelings from itching, blisters, or changes in heat and cold sensation, which affect normal pleasure responses. Often, significant others do not know how to deal with sexuality issues. For instance, they may fear causing injury to fragile healing skin sites, may experience frustration with role changes, or in some circumstances may be dealing with their own discomforts resulting from burn injuries incurred during the same event.

If sexual and social adjustment is to be successful, preparation for privacy, time, and supporting client and family needs intimacy during all or any phases of recovery is planned. Information regarding sexual potential and emotional adjustment is provided along with specific sexual education on positioning, pleasuring, and alternative methods of sensuality in the reestablishment of intimacy. Questions of fertility may arise secondary to physical injury to genitalia or interruption of organ functioning (e.g., scrotal edema or amenorrhea). Chapter 23 presents a more complete discussion of sexuality and options for people with chronic or disabling disorders.

Vocational Implications

Research findings indicate that most people who are employed at the time of their burn injury will return to work (Vierling, 1999). The extent, etiology, and site of burn injury influence a person's return-to-work status. Functional limitations resulting from burn injuries may temporarily or permanently affect the ability to return to work. Related factors include stamina and endurance; tolerance to standing, walking, or sitting; and degree of hand grip and upper extremity strength. A comprehensive medical evaluation by a vocational specialist is required before a client is cleared to resume occupational roles. Personal fear of reinjury, concern about peer reaction, and an individual's confidence level about resuming a work role may hinder return to work (Vierling, 1999). Vocational issues are a major correlate of long-term psychosocial or emotional problems. When clients hold positive perceptions about how their roles in family, work, social network, and other activities will be resumed, these attitudes indicate strengths toward effective coping and adjustment.

Strength and Resources

All severe burn injuries, regardless of origin, can alter the function of many body systems. Although most systems will recover and resume normal functioning, some processes may be compromised and others will never regenerate. When a client is able to construct a realistic assessment of these functions, the nurse is able to assess the beginning of psychosocial and emotional recovery, just as wound healing marks the beginning of physical recovery.

Ongoing support from family members and the interdisciplinary team is critical during all phases of institutional care and on community reentry. The rehabilitation nurse functions as advocate, educator, and facilitator to assist clients in realistic appraisal of their status, emphasizing ability rather than limitations or disability. During follow-up appointments, clients need guidance, encouragement, empowerment, and reassurance about emotional adjustments; rehabilitation nurses may use these opportunities to promote effecting coping behaviors.

In the community clients and families benefit from association, awareness, and use of community-based services and resources. Examples include hospital- or center-based support groups, peer groups, volunteer or not-for-profit self-help groups established by people who have themselves survived burn injuries (e.g., Phoenix Foundation or the Knapp Foundation), and national organizations (e.g., American Burn Association).

OUTCOME AND RESTORATIVE NURSING PRACTICE

The transition from client with a burn injury to person who survived a burn injury and reentered the community is the ultimate outcome desired after a rehabilitation program. The client is educated, motivated, and empowered to become the director of his or her own care. The roles of rehabilitation are pivotal to achieving successful outcomes of burn rehabilitation. This is one practice area in the growing field of restorative nursing care. As medical advances continue and health care system changes occur, rehabilitation nurses can anticipate active practice roles in planning, implementing, and evaluating services for clients who require extensive, long-term restorative care for a variety of conditions, in addition to those people with burn injuries.

CRITICAL THINKING

These questions are based on the Case Study.

1. Considering general principles of psychological care, develop one nursing approach for each of the following issues associated with responses of Isabel D to the diagnosis of 10% TBSA deep partial thickness burns: fear, decreased control, inability to return to work.
2. Discuss the impact of limited mobility on the potential for rehabilitation in Isabel D's case.
3. List the differences in priorities of care for Isabel D during the emergent and rehabilitation phases of burn injury.

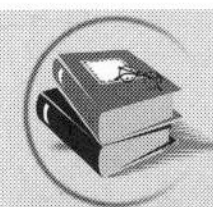

Case Study

Isabel D is a 61-year-old female who works as a certified nurse aide in a long-term care facility. She has a history of adult onset diabetes, obesity, and hypertension. Ms. D was in the process of preparing a meal and was carrying a pot of boiling potatoes to the sink to drain them, when she dropped the pot to the floor. Boiling liquid splashed over both feet and lower legs. She was wearing sport shoes and cotton socks. Emergency medical services transported her to the regional burn center for treatment.

On emergency evaluation, Ms. D was found to have a 10% TBSA, deep partial thickness burn, circumferential from the toes to midcalf, bilaterally. A wound culture was obtained, then wounds were cleansed with sterile water and mild soap. Nonadherent skin was removed. Nursing assessment identified the following:

- Ms. D has been prescribed an oral hypoglycemic and was directed to "avoid sweets." She does not monitor blood glucose.
- She lives with a significant other in a second-story apartment.
- She works more than 40 hours per week on the night shift.

Objectively, Ms. D was assessed as follows:

- Blood pressure 189/111; respirations 37 breaths per minute; heart rate 109 beats per minute
- Lower extremity pulses present per Doppler
- Burning, throbbing sensation described in lower extremities
- Blood glucose level of 210 mg/dl

Nursing diagnoses in this case are:

- Impaired skin integrity related to thermal injury
- Risk of infection related to loss of skin integrity and diabetes
- Pain related to tissue injury
- Impaired physical mobility
- Altered health maintenance related to burn injury, lack of knowledge of burn process, treatment, and complications

Relating to the nursing diagnoses, the plan of care may be developed as follows.

Nursing Diagnosis	Nursing Interventions	Client Outcomes
Impaired skin integrity	Wound care using strict asepsis Assess wound status with each dressing change Limit ambulation; maintain proper positioning of extremities Administer nutrients and supplements as prescribed Monitor blood glucose levels; to maintain control of diabetes	Burn sites healed; no complications
Risk of infection	Observe and monitor for signs and symptoms of infection Assess wound status for change in appearance, odor Obtain cultures as indicated Maintain asepsis	Infection control
Pain related to injury	Assess pain levels using rating scale Administer analgesics as prescribed Maintain positioning to decrease edema Implement nonpharmacological options for pain control Environmental management: comfort	Pain is managed
Impaired physical mobility	Assess joint mobility—active and passive Assess patterns of movement and ambulation Maintain positioning Teach regarding activity and exercise Energy management	Increased endurance and mobility
Altered health maintenance	Assess cognitive and physical abilities to perform wound care Teach client comfort measures Teach safety/surveillance procedures	Verbalizes understanding of wound care; performs wound care Identifies necessary care for burn sites Specifies actions to promote health

REFERENCES

Brigham, P.A., & McLoughlin, E. (1996). Burn incidence and medical care used in the United States: Estimates, trends and data sources. *Journal of Burn Care and Rehabilitation, 17,* 95-107.

Covington, D.S., Wainwright, D.J., & Parks, D.H. (1996). Prognostic indicators in the elderly patient with burns. *Journal of Burn Care and Rehabilitation, 17,* 222-230.

DeSanti, L., Lincoln, L., Egan, F., & Demling R. (1998). Development of a burn rehabilitation unit: Impact on burn center length of stay and functional outcome. *Journal of Burn Care and Rehabilitation, 19,* 414-419.

Doctor, J., Patterson, D.R., & Mann, R. (1997). Health outcome for burn survivors. *Journal of Burn Care and Rehabilitation, 18,* 490-495.

Fletchall, S., & Hickerson, W.L. (1995). Quality burn rehabilitation: Cost-effective approach. *Journal of Burn Care and Rehabilitation, 16,* 539-542.

Fritsch, D., & Yurko, L. (2000). Management of persons with burns. In W. Phipps, J.K. Sands, & J. Marek (Eds.), *Medical surgical nursing, concepts and clinical practice* (6th ed., pp. 2109-2145). St. Louis: Mosby.

Gordon, M. (2000). *Manual of nursing diagnosis* (9th ed.). St. Louis: Mosby.

Johnson, M., Maas, M., & Moorhead, S. (2000). *Nursing outcomes classification* (2nd ed.). St. Louis: Mosby.

McCloskey, J.C., & Bulechek, G.M. (2000). *Nursing interventions classification* (3rd ed.). St. Louis: Mosby.

Staley, M., Richard, R., Warden, G.D., Miller S., & Shuster, D.B. (1996). Functional outcomes for the patient with burn injuries. *Journal of Burn Care and Rehabilitation, 17,* 362-368.

Vierling, L. (1999). Four components for an improved return to work program. *Case Manager, 10,* 52-54.

Appendix 32A Fire and Burn Safety Checklist for the Older Adult or Mobility Impaired

Is your home fire and burn proof? A few single steps can save your life and the lives of those you love.

Home Safety Checklist

Go through your home weekly and ensure that the following points are covered:

- ☐ Is there a smoke detector in every room? Are the batteries working?
  Batteries replaced ☐ January ☐ April ☐ July ☐ October
  - ☐ If you are hearing impaired, do you have a smoke detector with visual indicators?
  - ☐ If vision impaired, do you have a vibrating smoke detector under your pillow or another appropriate detector?
- ☐ Are all space heaters at least 3 feet from everything, including you?
- ☐ Are all electrical cords and plugs in good condition?
- ☐ Is the water heater set at 120° F (49° C) or lower?
- ☐ Have you installed thermostatically controlled faucet and shower heads?
- ☐ Are all newspapers, empty boxes, paints, and gasoline cans stored away from heaters and outlets?
- ☐ Have you practiced your escape plan? From every room of the house?
  - ☐ Are all windows and doors from which you may need to escape easily opened?
  - ☐ If you use a wheelchair or a walker, have you checked each possible exit route carefully?
- ☐ Does the fire department know about your physical impairment in the event of a fire emergency?
- ☐ Do you have a single box with all important papers within easy access of your bed or the exit?
- ☐ Have you cataloged and updated your household inventory list for insurance claims?

Kitchen

- ☐ Is there a fire extinguisher within easy access of the cooking area?
  - ☐ Do you know how to use it?
- ☐ Is the cooking area grease free?

Bedroom

- ☐ Is there a flashlight near your bed?
  - ☐ Are the batteries working?
- ☐ Is there a whistle by your bed to warn others of a fire and to alert rescuers of your location?

Before You Go to Bed Each Night

- ☐ Did you unplug the coffee pot?
- ☐ Are any candles or oil lamps burning?
- ☐ Is your heating pad turned off?
- ☐ Did you turn the oven and burners off?
- ☐ Are the space heaters turned off?
- ☐ Did you put out your cigarette or cigar?
- ☐ Are your doors locked?
- ☐ Are the lights turned out, leaving one on in the event you need to get up?
- ☐ Are your glasses near your bedside so you can see to escape and avoid injury?
- ☐ Are your house keys and car keys near your bedside so they are easily accessible?

If Exiting the Home during a Fire Emergency

Read these points often and remember:

- Remain calm and keep low.
- Blow your whistle to alert others in the home and rescue personnel.
- Do not stop to call the fire department until you are safely outside unless you absolutely cannot exit!
- If there is no exit possible from the window, shine your flashlight out the window, moving it slowly. Hang a white or light colored sheet or blanket out the window.

Adapted with permission from Burn Awareness Coalition, Encina, CA.

Appendix 32B Burn Prevention for Families

Did You Know . . .

- Fire and burn injuries are the second leading cause of accidental death in children ages one to four
- 75-80% of burn injuries occur in and around the home
- Children's skin is thinner so they burn faster and deeper than adults
- Hot liquids are a major concern of burn injury to children
- Temperatures greater than 140° F cause a burn in 3 seconds that requires surgery!
- Most fatal house fires occur between midnight and 6 AM
- Working smoke detectors throughout your home decreases your chance of injury

Home Precautions

- Do turn hot water heater temperature to less than 120° F
- Don't cook with children underfoot
- Do turn pot handles in on the store
- Don't pour hot liquids around children
- Do make sure microwave food is cooled inside and out
- Don't serve hot food or liquid from a pan with children sitting at the table
- Do keep coffee pots, crockpots, and deep fat fryers pushed to the back of the counter
- Don't leave electrical cords dangling where children may pull
- Don't leave your children alone, even for a "quick trip to the neighbors"
- Never hold an infant while pouring hot liquid
- Small children often use their teeth to pull apart plugs. Keep electrical cords out of reach and teach safety
- Teach children to stay away from high voltage utilities
- Teach older children how to use appliances safely and the dangers of electricity with water
- Do not overload outlets
- Use only UAL-approved portable space heaters and keep 3 feet from everything, including yourself. Do not use extension cords
- Use safety while smoking. Use large, deep ashtrays and dispose of ashes in the toilet
- There is only one acceptable use for gasoline—fueling an engine
- Put sunscreen on you and your children
- Practice escape routes in case of fire with your children and your babysitter. Small children can be frightened and may hide
- Teach children the **stop, drop, and roll** procedure

Adapted with permission from Burn Awareness Coalition, Encino, CA.

Appendix 32C Burn Awareness and Fire Safety Calendar

January

Learn CPR and first aid for burns
Prepare and practice exit drills; learn "Two Ways Out"
Check for improperly discarded smoking materials
Check smoke detector batteries

February

National Burn Awareness Week is the first full week of February beginning with a Sunday
Check your home for fire safety
Check smoke detector batteries and clean detector as per manufacturer's instructions

March

Learn first aid for burns
Spring cleaning for safety
Check chimneys, wood stoves, and fireplaces

April

Store flammable liquids safely
Use gasoline safely—lawnmowers, cars, machinery
Change your clock, change your battery, check and clean your smoke detectors
Practice exit drills—know "Two Ways Out"

May

Electrical safety—check wiring
Fire safety on boats—gasoline awareness
Childproof the house for summer

June

Summer safety with vacation fun
Barbecue caution; camping/campfire safety
Caution—prevent a sunburn
Check smoke detector batteries
Lawnmowers/gasoline precautions

July

Fireworks safety—go to a professional display
Supervise children near fireworks
Practice exit drills; know "Two Ways Out"
Review summer precaution list

August

Poison and chemical alert
Check for improperly discarded smoking materials
Prevent forest fires
Check smoke detector batteries
Travelers—learn hotel/motel safety rules

September

Back to school burn and fire safety
Clean chimneys and fireplaces
Have furnace maintenance done

October

National Fire Prevention Week is the first full week
Halloween safety—flameproof or flame-retardant costumes, use flashlights, not candles
Change you clock, change your batteries, and clean your smoke detector
Heating equipment safety

November

Practice exit drills; know "Two Ways Out"
Fall cleanup for safety

December

Holiday Safety Survey:
- Check tree lights and decorations
- Check candles
- Keep trees well-watered
- Don't block exit ways
- Don't overload electrical outlets
- Check smoke detector batteries

Adapted with permission from Burn Awareness Coalition, Encino, CA.

The Regulatory and Immune Systems and the Client with HIV

33

Deborah J. Konkle-Parker, MSN, FNP, ACRN

"You have saved my life." This is a comment heard often from a young woman with acquired immunodeficiency syndrome (AIDS) who comes to see me in the outpatient infectious diseases clinic where I am a nurse practitioner. This particular young woman told me, "When I found out about my human immunodeficiency virus (HIV) diagnosis, I thought I was going to die; I just couldn't bear to think about it. There was no one I could talk to, and I didn't know what was going to happen to me. I didn't know anyone else who ever had AIDS, and I felt very alone. After I started coming to see you, I started to feel like I was coming back to life."

This woman had been feeling well before her diagnosis, and found out about her HIV disease when she went to the health department for a Pap smear. "I didn't feel that I could tell anyone about this disease, because I was afraid that the word would get spread all around town. I thought I would get sick and die, and I was so afraid." After much active listening, education about HIV disease, and discussions about the changes that would be needed in her life as well as things that would not need to change, this woman became less anxious, less depressed, and able to cope with the transformations that were needed in her self-image. "I don't like taking the medicines, but I know what I need to do to stay alive and healthy, so I keep it up, even while I am waiting for God to take this disease away from me."

Regulation is central to most physiological function. For the body to remain healthy and function adequately, homeostasis and freedom from foreign invasion are essential.

Regulation using negative (or occasionally positive) feedback loops are essential to life. Negative feedback inhibits the release of a biochemical substance when the blood level of another substance reaches a certain threshold. There are multiple examples of this in the body, including hormonal regulation, temperature regulation, and renal regulation. An example of a negative feedback loop is diagrammed in Figure 33-1 (McCance & Huether, 1998). Accurate regulation through these feedback loops are critical to homeostasis, and if these loops do not operate correctly, compensation must occur.

The human body also has several mechanisms to prevent invasion by foreign substances and subsequent development of disease. The skin is the first line of defense; an intact skin tissue serves to protect the internal environment from harmful organisms that flourish in the external environment. If invasion by microorganisms does take place, however, the body responds by activating the inflammatory process to render these agents incapable of altering homeostasis. If this secondary mechanism fails, the body relies on the complexity of the immune response to neutralize or destroy the invading organisms.

Included in this chapter will be physiological description of the body's protective functions, as well as specific alterations in the immune system, especially human immunodeficiency disease (HIV). Regulation of temperature will be discussed briefly, as well as alterations of other regulatory systems. Renal regulation is discussed in Chapter 34, and endocrine regulation, briefly later.

Common to all of these conditions is the inability of the body to regulate or protect itself, leading to chronic illness and a need for lifelong adaptation. This adaptation necessitates lifestyle change of many varieties. Because chronic diseases are so prevalent at this time, nurses can be instrumental in assisting a large number of individuals to make the necessary changes and live life to the maximal level possible.

The bulk of this chapter will focus on protective mechanisms of the body. Alterations of protective mechanisms will be discussed, focusing on HIV disease, including nursing assessment, intervention, and outcomes related to the rehabilitation of individuals with HIV disease.

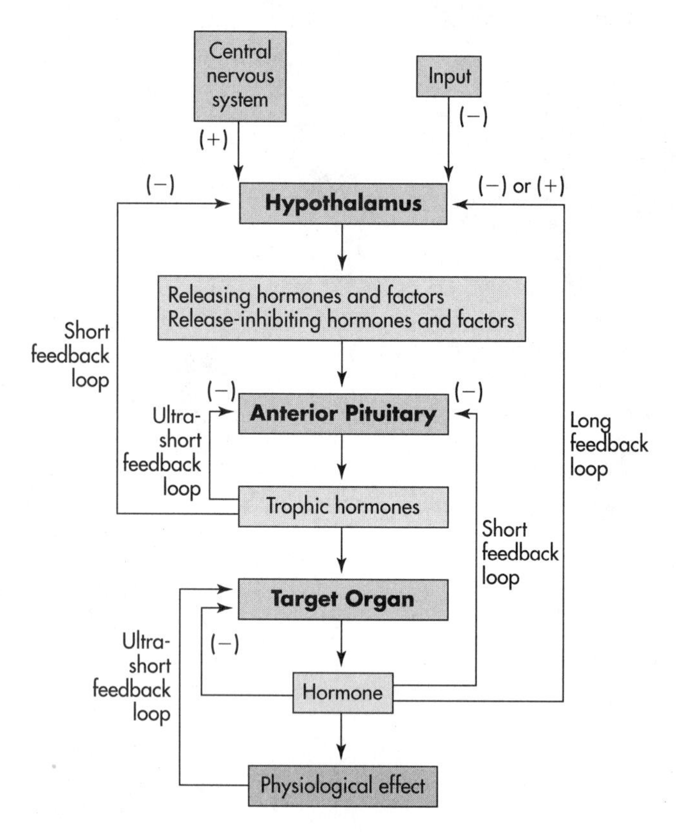

Figure 33-1 Example of negative feedback loop: This shows a general model for release of hormones as directed by the central nervous system, or by input from the environment. The hypothalamus is the intermediary organ, providing direction about release of hormones or releasing factors. The releasing glands or target organs then provide feedback to inhibit the continued release of hormones to control hormone and physiological effect to the desired level. (From Phipps, W.J., Sands, J.K., & Marek, J F. [1999]. *Medical-surgical nursing: Concepts and clinical practice* [6th ed.]. St. Louis: Mosby.)

TEMPERATURE REGULATION

The maintenance of normal body temperature is vital to life. Normal body temperatures vary and may range from 96.4° F to 100° F (35.8° C to 37.8° C). For every degree of elevation in body temperature, the demand for oxygen and nutrients increases; likewise, decreased body temperatures, decreases the demand. Internal body temperature remains relatively constant; even in altered circumstances, internal defense mechanisms and feedback systems strive to maintain constant body temperature.

Mechanisms of Body Temperature Control

The autonomic nervous system controls body temperature, as well as other visceral functions (Guyton & Hall, 1996). The hypothalamus in the brain is the body temperature control center; its function is regulated by neural feedback. Central thermoreceptors in the hypothalamus, spinal cord, abdominal organs, and other central locations as well as peripheral thermoreceptors in the skin provide the hypothalamus with information about skin and core temperatures. When temperatures are low, the hypothalamus responds by triggering heat production and heat conservation mechanisms. When high, heat reduction mechanisms are stimulated. Figure 33-2 describes these mechanisms. Heat production occurs with an increase in metabolic rates, vasoconstriction, and increased glycolysis, all produced by epinephrine. Heat conservation accompanies heat production, stimulated by the sympathetic nervous system (SNS) and producing an increase in muscle tone, vasoconstriction, and shivering. Conscious motor functions include voluntary measures to produce heat and conserve heat loss.

High core temperatures stimulate measures of heat loss. Those under control of the autonomic nervous system include sweating, causing heat loss by evaporation; vasodilation and increased respiration leading to greater heat lost through conduction to the cooler outside air; and reduced muscle tone to decrease heat production.

Elevated Body Temperature

Fever

When body temperature elevates, the body is responding to an injury and the hypothalamus is set at a higher level to maintain normal body temperature. The resulting fever may have a known or an unknown etiology. When the precipitator is an infection, fever may result from the inflammatory response. Fever results from the effects of pyrogenic substances secreted by injured cells. The exudate formed contains endogenous or exogenous pyrogens that cause the set point of the hypothalamic thermostat to rise and within hours, the body temperature elevates.

When fever occurs from a disease state, the controlling mechanisms of the hypothalamus fail and the temperature continues to rise unless interventions promote heat loss. Neurogenic fever, caused by injury to the anterior hypothalamus, results when the ability to promote heat loss is impaired, such as for individuals with severe closed head injuries and basilar skull fractures.

Clients with spinal cord injury often demonstrate a fever related to the interruption of autonomic nervous system communication with the hypothalamus during the acute phase after injury. When local reflex activity resumes, the severity of this problem subsides. Other known causes of fever are infections, deep vein thrombosis, tumor fever, pulmonary embolus, and drug hypersensitivities. Some medications, such as phenothiazides, anticholinergics, diuretics, and certain antihypertensives can interfere with heat loss. In those situations when no clear reason for elevated body temperature is apparent, malignancies or collagen-vascular diseases may be underlying causes.

Specific Conditions Accompanied by Altered Body Temperature

Several pathological states are unique in that they predispose clients to altered ability to maintain normal body temperatures. Examples discussed below are spinal cord injury,

A HEAT PRODUCTION MECHANISMS

HYPOTHALAMUS

TSH-RH → Anterior pituitary → TSH → Thyroid gland → T_4 → Adrenal medulla → Epinephrine → Chemical thermogenesis: Raises BMR, vasoconstriction, glycolysis

SNS → Adrenal cortex → Increase in muscle tone, shivering

Central cortex → BUNDLE UP!

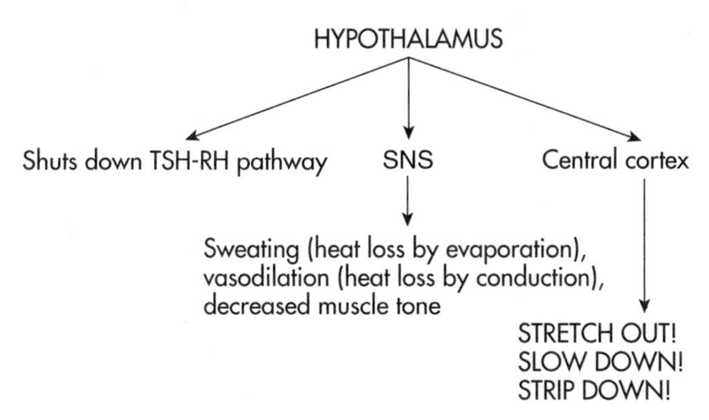

Figure 33-2 Feedback loop involved in temperature regulation. The hypothalamus, having been fed input by peripheral receptors, directs changes in temperature through hormonal pathways, through the sympathetic nervous system, and through the central nervous system. **A,** Heat production mechanisms. **B,** Heat reduction mechanisms.

head trauma, cerebral vascular accidents, and multiple sclerosis.

Spinal Cord Injury

After a spinal cord injury, every body system may be involved in attempts to maintain homeostasis. Fever is common with cervical spinal cord injuries. The disturbed thermoregulatory control in these clients results from loss of autonomic control over vasomotor activity and the sweating mechanism. The problem is prominent in clients with quadriplegia who are unable to maintain a desirable central temperature without protection from environmental temperature changes. After injury, individuals with cord damage above the thoracolumbar outflow of the SNS lose function in the hypothalamic thermoregulatory mechanisms. They are unable to internally control temperature below the level of the lesion because of absent vasoconstriction, inability to shiver to conserve body heat, and lack of thermoregulatory sweating to dissipate heat. With chronic loss of vasomotor tone and passive vasodilation, body heat tends to continual loss.

Clients with complete spinal cord lesions sweat only above the level of the lesion. Those with incomplete lesions can sweat both above and below the level of the lesion. When sweating becomes excessive in people with lesions above the T6 spinal cord level, suspect autonomic dysreflexia, a syndrome associated with a massive uncompensated cardiovascular response to stimulation of the SNS (Boss, 1998). Triggered by stimulation, such as bowel or bladder distension or stimulation of pain receptors below the level of the spinal cord injury, the SNS responds because the lesion prevents the brain from interpreting signals or resolving problems. Symptoms include severe hypertension, bradycardia, dilation, flushing, sweating, and a pounding headache. Trigger problems must be removed or resolved; the situation is life-threatening. See Appendix 19A for full information about this syndrome.

Because controlling body temperature is difficult in clients with high cervical injuries and possible damage to the hypothalamus and brainstem, monitor these individuals closely. Altered body temperature may be a sign of brainstem or medullary dysfunction. Fever in clients with spinal cord injuries is associated with infection, deep vein thrombosis, and emboli.

Head Trauma

Hyperthermia during the acute phase of head trauma is an indicator of damage to the hypothalamus or brainstem and possibly dehydration and infection. When temperature is elevated, metabolic demands grow and more carbon dioxide (CO_2) moves to the cells. CO_2 acts as a vasodilator that increases intracranial pressure. If the client already has increased intracranial pressure, hyperthermia will lead to further damage. Insufficient supply of oxygen to the cerebral tissue develops cerebral ischemia. It is imperative to treat hyperthermia rapidly and effectively in the client with head injury.

Cerebrovascular Accidents

A cerebrovascular accident (CVA) is caused by interruption of blood flow to an area of the brain, resulting in ischemia, necrosis, and often permanent damage to neurons and neural pathways. Hyperthermia in the acute phase of a CVA can result from damage to the brainstem or hypothalamus. Substantial temperature elevations seen in clients with hemorrhagic stroke or subarachnoid hemorrhage may be the result of blood in the cerebrospinal fluid contributing to hypothalamic dysfunction or early aseptic meningitis—or as before, caused by dehydration and infection.

Multiple Sclerosis

Multiple sclerosis, a disease of the central nervous system, characteristically has plaques forming in the spinal cord, cerebellum, cerebrum, brainstem, and optic nerve. The plaques cause demyelination of the myelin sheaths, subsequently causing destruction of the nerves traveling to the lower limbs, eyes, and, to a lesser extent, the upper limbs. Although the reason is unknown, there is increased thermosensitivity in clients with demyelinating disease. This is a critical problem, because increased core body temperature exacerbates neurological symptoms.

Client and Family Education

Major goals in the rehabilitation of all clients are to prevent complications and maintain functions. Formal and informal education programs are effective for clients to learn about preventing and treating complications and information about changes in body temperature. Facility-based programs stress ways to prevent infections and fever. Consider that the majority of clients with spinal cord injury readmitted to hospitals are there because of infected pressure sores, urinary tract infections, respiratory tract infections, and generalized septicemia. These clients have impaired sense of hot and cold and must avoid temperature extremes. Clients with cerebrovascular accidents and spinal cord injuries must beware of hot surfaces including stoves, hot water in bathtubs, and overexposure to the sun; they burn severely with short sun exposure. Excessive heat, such as hot baths, can exacerbate symptoms of multiple sclerosis. Prevention strategies are critical to regulate temperature in people vulnerable to hypo- or hyperthermia.

ENDOCRINE REGULATION

The endocrine system is composed of several glands that secrete hormones to carry out specific body functions. Functions include growth and development, coordinating reproduction, maintaining optimal internal body environment, and initiating adaptive responses when needed (Piano & Huether, 1998).

Hormones operate in a negative or positive feedback system. A negative feedback system turns *off* the release of a chemical substance as it reaches a critical threshold in the blood level, although a positive feedback system turns *on* to release a chemical substance for the same reason. Hormone release occurs either as a response to a change in the cellular environment or as the result of feedback designed to maintain the optimal level of hormone or related substances. In this way, hormone release is influenced not only by levels of the hormones, but also by levels of other chemical factors and by neural control. An example of hormonal regulation earlier in this chapter was the thyroid hormone negative feedback loop. An example of neural regulation is release of epinephrine from the adrenal medulla in response to stress. Insulin regulation by blood glucose levels describes regulation by other chemical substances; increased blood glucose levels promotes insulin secretion, insulin diminishes when glucose levels decrease.

Altered endocrine regulation disturbs the internal cellular environment. The result may be persistently altered levels of the actual hormone as well as of the chemical substance the hormone controls. A ready example is the process of diabetes mellitus (Huether & Tomky, 1998). To discuss diabetes mellitus is beyond the scope of this chapter; however, the section following discusses related endocrine regulation and rehabilitation issues.

Diabetes Mellitus

In 1998, it was estimated that approximately 10.5 million people in the United States had a diagnosis of diabetes mellitus (Harris, 1998). Populations particularly at risk include African Americans, Hispanics, and Native Americans.

Diabetes mellitus is a syndrome characterized by chronic hyperglycemia and other disturbances of carbohydrate, fat, and protein metabolism (Huether & Tomky, 1998). It is caused by inadequate production of insulin by the beta cells in the pancreas, or otherwise by cellular resistance to the effect of insulin. The beta cells secrete insulin, and, when functioning properly, are regulated by chemical, hormonal, and neural control. The level of blood glucose and blood insulin, as well as sympathetic activation of alpha cells in the pancreas in response to stress, all regulate insulin secretion. Insulin affects the rate of glucose uptake by the cells and the synthesis of proteins, carbohydrates, lipids, and nucleic acids. The main classifications are type 1 and type 2, summarized below, and other categories of glucose intolerance.

Type 1

Type 1 diabetes mellitus results from the destruction or defect of the beta cells in the pancreas. Two versions of type 1 diabetes are identified (Huether & Tomky, 1998): immune or nonimmune. In immune diabetes mellitus, destruction of the beta cells is mediated by the immune system, whereas a variety of genetic defects of the beta cells that inhibit insulin secretion depict nonimmune-related.

Symptoms of type 1 diabetes mellitus include those in Box 33-1. External control of blood sugar can manage these symptoms, as well as the complications of ketoacidosis, diabetic neuropathy, retinopathy, nephropathy, and atherosclerosis. Treatment of type 1 diabetes is insulin administration in combination with regulation of glucose supply by intensive diet, drug, and activity programs. Damage to the internal regulation of insulin requires external regulation to maintain euglycemia, and an optimal cellular environment.

Type 2

The etiology of *type 2 diabetes mellitus* is unclear, although the pathophysiology suggests increased cellular resistance to the effect of insulin, as well as a decreased secretion of insulin by the beta cells. As compared to type 1 diabetes, the clinical symptoms of this type of diabetes are nonspecific,

Box 33-1 Acute Symptoms of Type 1 Diabetes Mellitus

Polydypsea: excessive thirst, caused by elevated blood sugar levels and the resulting cellular dehydration as water is osmotically attracted into extracellular fluid
Polyuria: excessive urination, as the amount of glucose in the urine is greater than that which can be reabsorbed by the renal tubules, requiring the dilution of urine for excretion, and the resultant loss of large amounts of water
Polyphagia: excessive hunger, as a result of the depletion of carbohydrates, fats, and proteins in the cells
Weight loss: result of fluid loss from diuresis and the loss of body tissue as fats and proteins are used for energy
Fatigue: result of poor energy distribution to cells (Huether & Tomky, 1998)

such as recurrent infections, pruritus, fatigue, visual changes, or paresthesias. Box 33-2 describes these manifestations.

Treatment for type 2 diabetes mellitus has the same goal as for type 1, to keep the blood sugar as near to normal ranges as possible. Insulin replacement is not indicated in all instances. Management begins with meal planning and restricting total caloric intake. If this is inadequate to reach optimum blood glucose levels, medications may be added either to supplement the insulin secretion from the beta cells or to improve cellular insulin sensitivity. These methods encourage the insulin produced naturally to approach a level of efficacy where the cells access full use of the glucose.

Rehabilitation Issues Related to Endocrine Regulation

Health Risks Associated with Diabetes Mellitus

Health risks related to diabetes include microvascular complications, including retinopathy, nephropathy, and peripheral neuropathies. Other macrovascular complications include ischemic heart disease, stroke, and peripheral vascular disease (Harris, 1998). To prevent or reduce complications, the client and the nurse must become partners. The goals are to maximize glycemic control and limit risk factors, such as hypertension, hyperlipidemia, obesity, and cigarette smoking. Maximizing glycemic control is complex; however, and involves strict adherence to medications, diet, and exercise.

Adherence to Treatment

In conditions with altered endocrine regulation, external regulation must replace the impaired internal regulation. Diabetes requires either administration of external insulin or external control of the amount of sugar ingested. External regulation is required in other hormonal disorders, such as hypothyroidism and diabetes insipidus, where the appropriate regulatory hormone is deficient. Although the concept of external administration is simple to discuss, the lifestyle alteration resulting from dependence on external sources of hormonal control is quite complex. The construct of adherence is central in the mandatory lifelong changes in each client's lifestyle.

Box 33-2 Typical Clinical Manifestations of Type 2 Diabetes Mellitus

Recurrent infections and impaired wound healing
Genital pruritus: vulvovaginal candidiasis is common in women because hyperglycemia and glycosuria favor fungal growth
Visual changes: blurred vision, diabetic retinopathy
Paresthesias: common in diabetic neuropathies
Fatigue: result of poor energy distribution to the cells (Huether & Tomky, 1998)

Many factors influence adherence to a regimen, including client traits, clinician expertise and style, regimen components, and characteristics of the illness (Dowell & Hudson, 1997; Trostle, 1997). Client traits include health status, material resources, cultural beliefs, self-efficacy, social support, personal skills, and knowledge of the disease. Characteristics of the clinician that affect adherence include the clinical and interpersonal style; the clinician's availability and skills with assessment, communication, and clinical expertise. Clients respond to diverse factors involved in medication regimens, including cost, requirements for storing or administering, frequency of dose, the number and size or taste of pills, and medication side effects. They also respond to the perceived effectiveness of medications, as well as accompanying the diet and lifestyle changes. Other factors influencing adherence are actual symptoms of the illness, their duration and severity, and stigma they attach to the condition.

A client-centered approach to adherence begins by identifying issues important to the individual and focusing interventions for the client to cope effectively with the changes required by altered endocrine regulation. Box 33-3 contains a brief case study involving a client with an endocrine disorder. Discussion of the nursing diagnoses, interventions, and outcomes occurs later in this chapter.

THE IMMUNE RESPONSE

Primary functions of the immune system are defense by destroying foreign microorganisms, homeostasis by removing worn out cellular components, and surveillance by the perception of and destruction of mutant cells. The immune system protects the body from foreign invaders, whether disease-producing microorganisms or abnormal cells such as cancer. Actually, the immune system is the third and slowest line of defense against such invasion. An intact skin provides the first line of defense; the inflammatory response is second after an invading organism transgresses beyond the barrier formed by the skin; and finally, the immune response acts.

Box 33-3 Case Study: Endocrine Disorder

Mary W, 52 years old, came to her initial appointment with a report of general malaise, excessive thirst, and frequent urination. These symptoms had lasted for 5 months, with recent exacerbation of malaise and a blurring of her vision. She denied any personal history of diabetes but reported a significant family history of type 2 diabetes mellitus. Other physical characteristics included a weight of 242 pounds, height of 5 feet, 4 inches, and a sedentary lifestyle. She stated that she had gained 50 pounds in the last 5 years, "But nothing I do seems to help." Ms. W worked as a police dispatcher and spent her workday at a desk. "It's so stressful at work that I just want to sit around at home and watch TV to relax." She was taking no medicines, except for short courses of antibiotics for occasional bronchitis. "I always stopped the medicine when I felt better. That way I could save the rest of the doses in case I need them again." Diagnostic tests revealed a blood glucose of 215 mg/dL.

Priority nursing diagnoses for this client will include an altered endocrine function and an education deficit regarding the changes required in her lifestyle, including diet, exercise, and medication administration. To improve her quality of life and duration of a complication-free life, she will require much education, frequent monitoring, and support for the behavior change required.

The inflammatory response consists of cellular components and processes, each with a unique role in maintaining the balance of homeostasis. After annihilating or neutralizing harmful organisms by phagocytosis, the inflammatory process removes the offenders from the site, confines them to limit their effectiveness, stimulates and enhances the immune response, and promotes healing (McCance & Huether, 1998). When this powerful defense is ineffective or fails, the immune system responds.

Immune System

Acting much as a surveillance mechanism, the immune system monitors the internal environment for foreign agents. A complex system of organs and cells capable of distinguishing self from nonself, it can remember previous invaders and react according to needs as they arise. The primary organs of the immune system are the thymus, lymph nodes, spleen, and tonsils. Contributing to the effort of the immune response are lymphoid tissues in nonlymphoid organs and circulating immune cells, such as T cells, B cells, and phagocytes (McCance & Huether, 1998).

The organs responsible for affecting the immune response serve varying roles in this process. The thymus creates T cells; the bone marrow, B cells. Lymphocytes develop in the thymus beginning early in life through puberty. As mature and differentiated lymphocytes release into the bloodstream, they relocate in peripheral lymph tissue such as lymph nodes, tonsils, intestines, and spleen, awaiting a call to action in body defense.

Much like the thymus in T cell maturation, the bursa equivalent in the bone marrow differentiates lymphocytes into B cells. Once released, these immature B cells migrate to the peripheral lymph tissue where they mature and await to defend against foreign agents (McCance & Huether, 1998). Figure 33-3 illustrates the maturation process of immune cells.

The lymph system continuously filters the blood. Lymph nodes distributed throughout the body have large clusters in the axillae, groin, thorax, abdomen, and neck. The nodes filter the lymph fluid and foreign materials and are reservoirs for specialized immunological T and B cells (McCance & Huether, 1998).

Immunity is a normal adaptive response to the external environment that protects the body from disease by resisting and attacking offending organisms. Acquired immunity can be active, developed on exposure to an antigen during which antibodies are programmed to protect the body from illness with future exposures. These antibodies are specific, often providing lifetime immunity against another attack of the same antigen. Lifetime active immunity may develop from exposure to a specific antigen via inoculation. Passive immunity, on the other hand, is temporary immunity involving the transference of antibodies from one person or from another source to the client.

Antigen and Antigen-Antibody Response

The immune system responds to the invasion of the body by foreign material, called antigens. Some antigens are capable of producing disease, whereas others, although not disease-producing, are recognized as foreign and can elicit an immune response. Although capable of differentiating self from nonself, the immune system cannot differentiate harmful organisms from nonharmful ones.

Cells of the Immune Response

At least three types of cells are involved in the immune response to foreign material: the T cell, the B cell, and the macrophage. Each cell has a distinct responsibility and contributes to the integrity of the body as a whole. Sets of cells contain effector cells capable of attacking and destroying a particular antigen, and memory cells that are imprinted with the antigenic code. The memory cells remember and recognize the antigen within minutes of a subsequent exposure (McCance & Huether, 1998). Figure 33-4 summarizes the interconnectedness of the multiple cells of the immune system.

Immune Deficiency

Infection, cancer, and other chronic diseases contribute to a reduced effectiveness of the immune response. Large cancer tumors are able to release antigens into the blood that combine with circulating antibodies to prevent them from attack-

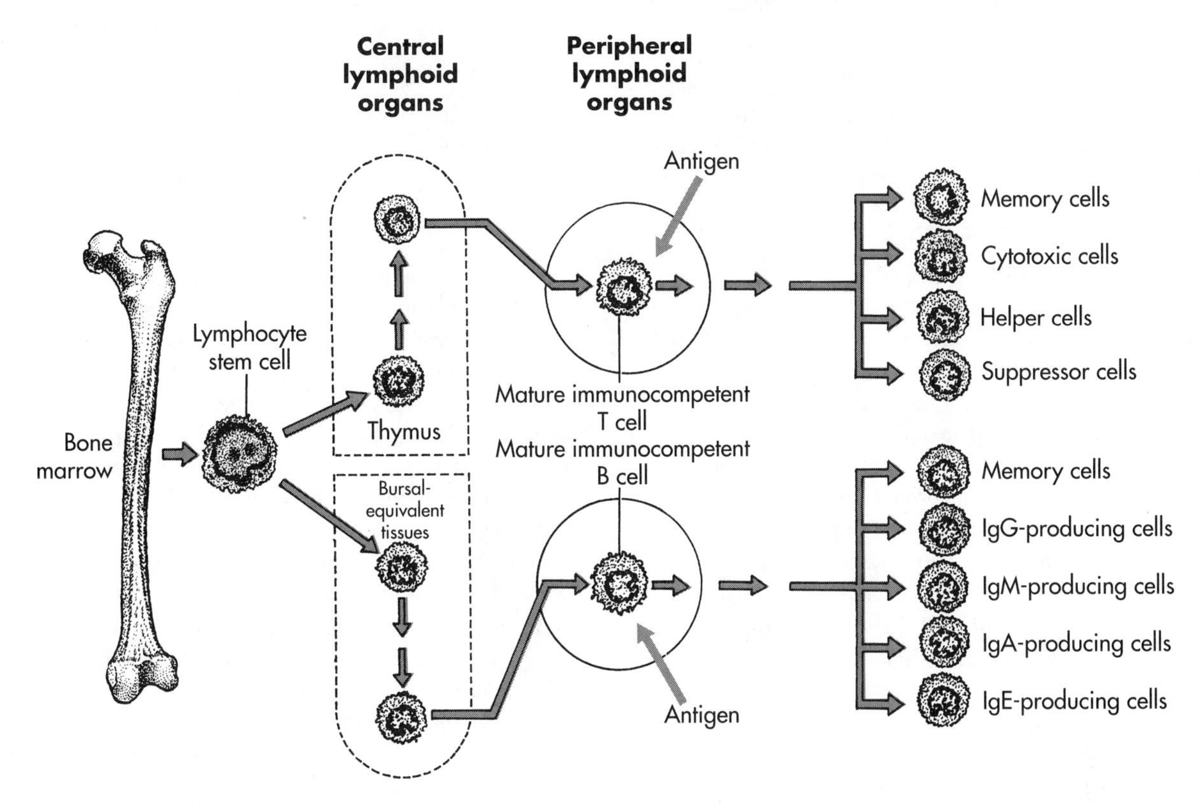

Figure 33-3 Outcomes of lymphocyte maturation. Maturation of lymphocytes through the thymus and bone marrow result in different immune cells that can respond in a variety of ways to foreign invasion. (From McCance, K.L., & Huether, S.E. [1998]. *Pathophysiology: The biologic basis for disease in adults and children* [3rd ed.]. St. Louis: Mosby.)

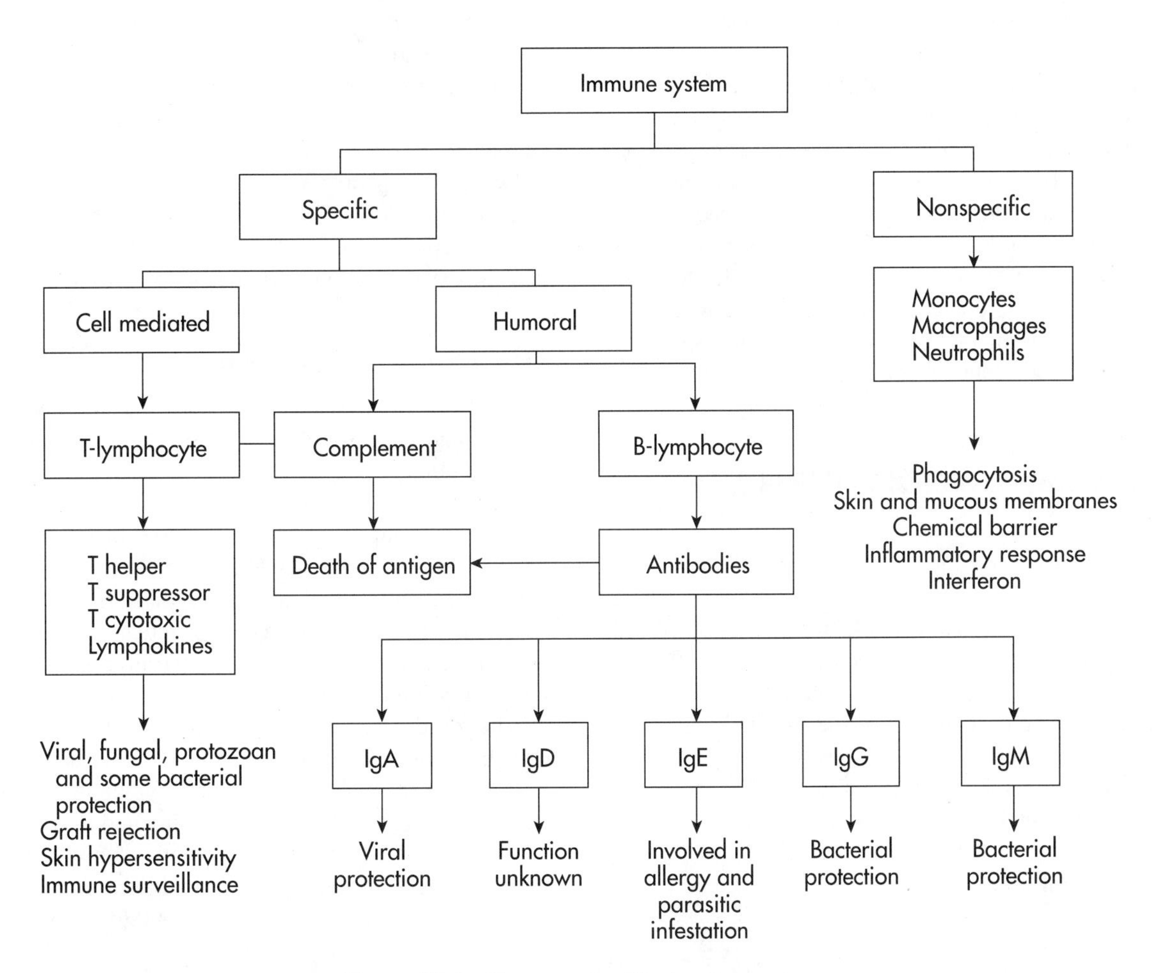

Figure 33-4 Components of the immune system.

ing tumor cells. Furthermore, tumor cells may possess special blocking factors that coat tumor cells and prevent destruction by killer T cells. This understanding is basic to planning care.

Nursing Intervention Related to Immunodeficiency

Nurses are integrally involved in protecting a client with immunodeficiency (Risi & Tomascak, 1998). As primary prevention, the nurse identifies risk factors from the history, such as recent travel, medications that may affect the immune system, drug use, and sexual activity. Educate clients to have invasive procedures, such as venous access devices or dental work completed and chronic conditions of the skin, scalp, or nail beds treated before starting immunosuppression. Updated immunizations help augment the immune system (Risi & Tomascak, 1998) and the nurse may find medial orders to administer granulocyte colony-stimulating factor and granulocyte/macrophage colony-stimulating factor to reduce neutropenia.

Educate clients, family, and significant others about the high risk for infection and teach the skills for infection control (Risi & Tomascak, 1998) with such basics as to clean foods thoroughly and cook meat well. Hand washing is critical for clients and others, including children in proximity to the client. Children pose special risks for infectious disease, as do pets. Emphasize careful hand washing repeatedly. With chronic immunosuppressive conditions, long-term behavior change prevents infection.

Multiple sclerosis, in which long-term steroid therapy is the mainstay of treatment and HIV are examples of precursors chronic immunosuppression. In HIV syndrome, markedly depressed T-lymphocytes function with reduced numbers of T4 cells, impaired killer T-cell capacity, and increased numbers of suppressor T cells. By selectively invading and infecting T cells, the virus damages the very cell whose function it is to orchestrate the identification and destruction of virus as an antigen (Broder, Merigan, & Bolognesi, 1994; Mandell, Bennett, & Dolin; Sande & Volberding, 1999).

HUMAN IMMUNODEFICIENCY VIRUS

HIV is a retrovirus carrying genetic information in ribonucleic acid (RNA) rather than in deoxyribonucleic acid (DNA). It infects the particular T cell known as the CD4 cell by binding to it and inserting its RNA into the CD4 cell. Through the action of reverse transcriptase, HIV is able to reprogram the genetic materials of the infected CD4 cell. When activated to reproduce, the CD4 cell has its genetic information reprogrammed to produce more HIV, instead of viable and functional CD4 lymphocytes. The newly produced virus can then infect other CD4 lymphocytes (Broder et al., 1994; Dolin, Masur, & Saag, 1999; Sande & Volberding, 1999).

Epidemiology

As this chapter is written, new findings are emerging about the epidemiology and etiology of HIV infection and AIDS. HIV infection is a chronic disease manifesting itself in a variety of ways, with AIDS being considered the extreme clinical manifestation. Before the advent of highly active antiretroviral treatment (HAART), the median AIDS-free time was 10 years, with a small subset of HIV-infected people that maintained normal or near normal CD4 lymphocyte counts for many years. Studies of these nonprogressing long-term survivors seek characteristics that may account for their different disease progression (Bartlett, 1999). A new class of antiviral medications called protease inhibitors has slowed the rate of reported AIDS cases in the United States in recent years. Administering this potent suppressive therapy for the first time has greatly lengthen AIDS-free time and decreased rates of conversion to AIDS and AIDS-related mortality rates (Bartlett, 1999).

In states where HIV is a reportable condition, the incidence continues to rise; reported cases are considered only "the tip of the iceberg" related to actual case rates in the United States and globally. AIDS increases exponentially because of the lack of accessible treatment and prevention modalities in many developing countries where anticipated life expectancy will plummet from enormous numbers of AIDS deaths. In the United States incidence is greater in homosexual and bisexual men, and increasingly in their heterosexual partners, particularly in the Southeast. In Africa, South America, and the Caribbean, sexual transmission occurs more often between men and women. Incidence is high among those who have a history of or currently abuse intravenous drugs. Other aggregates at significant risk to develop AIDS include people with hemophilia, sexual partners of high-risk individuals, and children born to high-risk parents because AIDS is transmitted through blood and blood products or sexual intercourse (Sande & Volberding, 1999).

HIV Disease Progression

Rehabilitation nurses may encounter clients in any one of the seven stages of HIV disease. The first three stages—viral transmission, primary HIV infection, and seroconversion—occur close together. After the virus is transmitted, symptomatic primary infection occurs in approximately 80% to 90% of individuals (Bartlett, 1999), followed within 6 months by seroconversion. Until that time a typical HIV antibody test may be negative, although a test for actual viral particles will be positive. The CD4 count is normal (range 650–2500 mm^3), but usually considered to approximate a value of about 1,000.

The fourth stage is asymptomatic infection, when clients may be totally unaware of the HIV virus, but capable of transmitting the disease. Although asymptomatic, the virus is not latent, but is actively replicating and destroying CD4 cells. Individuals may have a variety of mild complaints, such as persistent generalized lymphadenopathy (PGL) or fatigue; the CD4 count ranges from 500 to 750.

The symptomatic stage begins with PGL, weight loss, fatigue, and a multitude of dermatological, musculoskeletal, or gastrointestinal complaints. Fevers or night sweats, weight loss, fatigue, and diarrhea are common. The CD4 count ranges from 200 to 500 with first symptoms, with wide variation. This stage extends into the AIDS stage when opportunistic infections and malignancies that develop as a result of immune system dysfunction become evident. AIDS is a clinical diagnosis assigned to individuals who have opportunistic infections or unusual malignancies, or those with CD4 counts below the threshold of 200; evidence of failed immune response against disease. The sixth or chronic stage evolves with ongoing pathological changes that involve multiple body systems. The end or terminal stage of AIDS presents significant challenges to manage repeated opportunistic infections while preserving the client's self-care and independence. The nurse's role in coordinating the complex interventions and needs for care becomes more difficult (Figure 33-5).

Clinical Manifestations of HIV Disease and Related Opportunistic Infection

Clinical manifestations of AIDS are results of opportunistic infections preying on an impaired immune system. Early in the disease process, opportunistic infections are uncommon. Tuberculosis is a reactivation of latent, encapsulated tuberculosis that flourishes because the immune system is unable to control a formerly inactive bacillus. It becomes problematic midway in HIV disease, with the CD4 count at less than 350 to 400 mm^3.

Candidiasis, a candidal infection of mucous membranes, especially in the oral cavity or the vaginal canal, is a common early clinical feature of HIV infection. Oral candidiasis, or thrush, is a marker of HIV disease progression. Thrush is visualized as white plaques on the buccal mucosa, tongue, and throat that can be removed when scraped with a tongue blade (Johnson & Yu, 1997).

Other opportunistic infections include *Pneumocystis carinii* pneumonia (PCP), cytomegalovirus (CMV), toxoplasmosis, and mycobacterium avium complex (MAC). These tend to occur after immune deterioration (as shown by CD4 count under 200 for PCP; under 50 for CMV), toxoplasmosis, and MAC. PCP is a pneumonia that appears less acute than bacterial pneumonia, but causes significant progressive shortness of breath, weight loss, fatigue, and fevers. CMV frequently affects the retina, starting with blurry vision and leading to blindness. Toxoplasmosis, a lesion in the central nervous system (CNS), produces headache, seizures, fevers, and confusion. MAC is a systemic mycobacterial infection manifested by fever, drenching sweats, weight loss, wasting, fatigue, diarrhea, and abdominal pain. Anogenital simplex herpes (HSV) also occurs with decreasing immune function, and appears

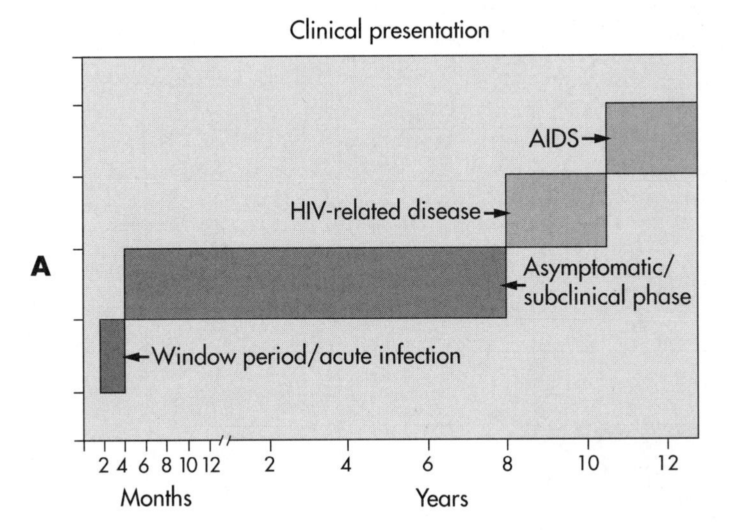

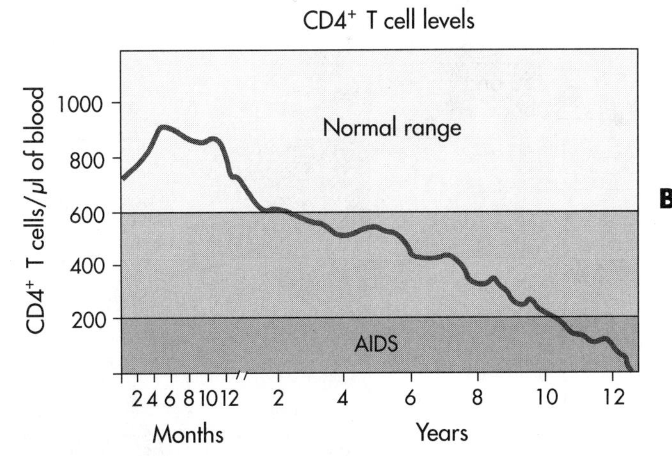

Figure 33-5 Staging of HIV disease. **A,** Typical time frame of progression from HIV infection to AIDS. During the *initial phase* the client may experience flulike symptoms, characterized by fever, lymphadenopathy, and possibly a rash. Antibodies against HIV are not yet detectable (window period), but viral products, including p24 antigen, viral RNA, and infectious virus may be detectable in the blood a few weeks after infection. During the *second phase* of infection the client is generally asymptomatic. Viral replication is active during this phase, antibodies are detectable in the blood, and CD4 T-cell levels are generally decreasing at rates relative to the amount of virus present (viral load). During the *third phase,* the client becomes symptomatic, exhibiting constitutional symptoms and few opportunistic infections. The viral load generally continues to increase and CD4+ T cell levels continue to drop. During the *fourth,* and last, *phase* the client has been diagnosed with AIDS with a CD4+ T-cell count of less than 200, or opportunistic infections or malignancies. **B,** CD4 changes during advancement from human immunodeficiency virus 1 (HIV-1) infection to acquired immunodeficiency syndrome (AIDS). (From McCance, K.L., & Huether, S.E. [1998]. *Pathophysiology: The biologic basis for disease in adults and children* [3rd ed.]. St. Louis: Mosby.)

with persistent, chronic ulcerations over the penis, vulva, or buttocks.

Neoplasias also appear; for example, Kaposi's sarcoma presents with purplish, hemorrhagic patches, plaques, and nodules (Dolin et al., 1999). Lymphomas occur, particularly in the CNS and as cervical cancer. Figure 33-6 illustrates the relationship of opportunistic infections with stages of HIV disease.

ISSUES ACROSS THE LIFE SPAN

Pediatric HIV

Although children represent only 1.3% of the total United States AIDS population, their number is growing to the point that AIDS is among the 10 leading causes of death in children (CDC, 1999). As of June 1991, children infected during the perinatal period accounted for 91% of cases up to 13 years of age; these children and adolescents infected as a result of high-risk sexual behaviors are a majority of the growing aggregate. The previously high percentage of children with hemophilia has declined.

Epidemiology

In the United States, approximately 1,400 to 2,200 infants infected with HIV are born each year. Internationally, the number is vastly larger, with 90% from developing countries; in sub-Saharan Africa, approximately 1,000 infants are born daily with HIV infection (Nielsen, 1999). In 1994, a landmark multicenter clinical trial showed the use of zidovudine (AZT) reduced perinatal HIV infection from 25% to 30% to 8% to 9% of all births to HIV-positive mothers. The drug is given during pregnancy, labor, and delivery, and to the neonate for 6 weeks. High cost and poor distribution infrastructure have been barriers to making AZT available in developing countries where increased prevalence and incidence affects women of child-bearing age. Short-term tests of low-cost alternative antiviral medications are effective, but less so than the gold standard.

Pregnant HIV-infected women must be identified and offered treatment to halt perinatal transmission of HIV disease. In many cultures, identification leads to ostracism, and without finances and infrastructure for treatment of the mother, as well as preventive interventions for the baby, outcomes are limited.

CD4	Tuberculosis	Oral candidiasis	Pneumocystis pneumonia, herpes simplex virus	Non-Hodgkin's lymphoma, cytomegalovirus, toxoplasmosis, systemic fungal infections	Kaposi's sarcoma, *Mycobacterium avium* complex
350 and above					
350					
300					
250					
200					
150					
100					
50					
0					

Figure 33-6 Risk of opportunistic infections related to CD4 count: As immune function worsens, the risk of opportunistic infections increases.

Clinical Manifestations

At least two thirds of children who vertically contract HIV disease are believed to do so during labor and delivery. Those with a positive HIV test at birth are believed to have contracted the disease in utero, whereas those who are HIV negative at birth but seroconvert at a later test (2 to 4 weeks after birth) are believed to have contracted the disease during labor and delivery (Nielsen, 1999). Children with in utero infection tend to have a more rapid disease course and fare less well. Failure to thrive, recurrent diarrhea, and enlarged lymph nodes, liver, and spleen are constitutional symptoms that may go unrecognized early in the disease. Oral candidiasis and diaper dermatitis, chronic nasal discharge, and recurrent otitis media that are unresponsive to the usual therapies may occur. Frequent bacterial infections are a common complication of HIV disease in children. The progression of the disease may cause damage and dysfunction to one or multiple organs including the central nervous system, heart, lungs, and gastrointestinal systems. Encephalopathy manifests along with delays in developmental milestones, impaired cognition and expressive language, spastic paraparesis, ataxia, and hyperirritability (Wong et al., 2000).

Rehabilitation Issues

Rehabilitation efforts are directed to minimizing the deficits caused by the progressive neurological problems, emphasizing the maintenance of existing cognitive skills and facilitating developmental achievement with infant stimulation and speech-language therapy. Antiviral treatment lessens the viral load and allows for immune reconstitution. Treatment with triple antiviral treatment is recommended in children as in adults, but dosing, pharmacokinetics, and side effects are less well known in children and must be monitored carefully (Nielsen, 1999).

Referral for physical and occupational therapy assists children to compensate for motor deficits. Rehabilitation programs also address problems and issues generated by the demographic profile of perinatally infected children who are from socially and economically disadvantaged families. The social structure of these families often is stressed and not a framework for optimal care and management of the complex problems of a child with AIDS. Referrals to social services and home health care nurses, as well as community resources are highly appropriate to incorporate into the rehabilitation plan (Nielsen, 1999).

Young Adult Chronic Illness

Psychosocial Challenges

Psychosocial problems are among the most common difficulties associated with HIV disease in the young adult population. O'Brien and Pheifer (1993) examined physical and psychological problems and needs of people living with HIV infection. Psychosocial issues most frequently identified by the study participants were loneliness and disturbed self-concept resulting from changes in body image and self-esteem. The experience of loneliness and the increased need for social supports offer a serious challenge to clients and their caregivers. Isolation may be self-induced because of apathy or changes in personal appearance, or to the stigma associated with this diagnosis. Disclosure to family and friends is an additional psychological situation. Other psychosocial concerns included maintaining sexual integrity, independent function for activities of daily living, impaired communication (often related to involvement of the CNS), and spiritual distress. Young adults face not being able to parent a child for risk of infecting a partner and the child.

A goal is to promote optimal levels of independent functioning in the community within the limitations imposed by this chronic disease. Educating the client and caregivers about the nature of the disease and necessary life style changes, includes importance of adhering to the plan of care and making changes in sexual and/or drug use practices.

Physical Systems Affected by HIV

Multiple systems affected by the HIV virus, depicted in Figure 33-7, predicts the wide range of clinical manifestations possible in the disease process.

Gastrointestinal Disorders

Clients with HIV faced a number of infections that affect every organ system. The gastrointestinal system is highly vulnerable to the many pathogens capable of invading the immunocompromised client, thus creating some of the most frustrating problems for both the client and the nurse (Gallagher, 1993). The physiological sequelae in the gastrointestinal tract are an important cause of morbidity and mortality. The pathophysiology of intestinal infection is not understood; however, two mechanisms have been postulated. The first is reduced intestinal immunity, resulting in chronic opportunistic infections, that cause altered intestinal functioning. The second is that HIV itself affects the intestinal mucosa and causes malfunctioning. Extensive diarrhea can be seen in people infected with HIV; this may be caused by bacterial overgrowth, decreased mucosal immune function, and abnormal neural and endocrine function of the intestines (Talal & Dieterich, 1999).

Nervous System Disorders

Advancing AIDS involves diffuse and focal central nervous system disorders as well as peripheral neuropathies. People diagnosed with AIDS dementia complex (ADC) may exhibit signs of cognitive, behavioral, and motor disturbances, and each will have a variety of early and late symptoms. A significant number of people with AIDS eventually develop a degree of cognitive, motor, or emotional impairment that responds favorably to counseling and therapeutics, such as zidovudine. Later manifestations of central neurological in-

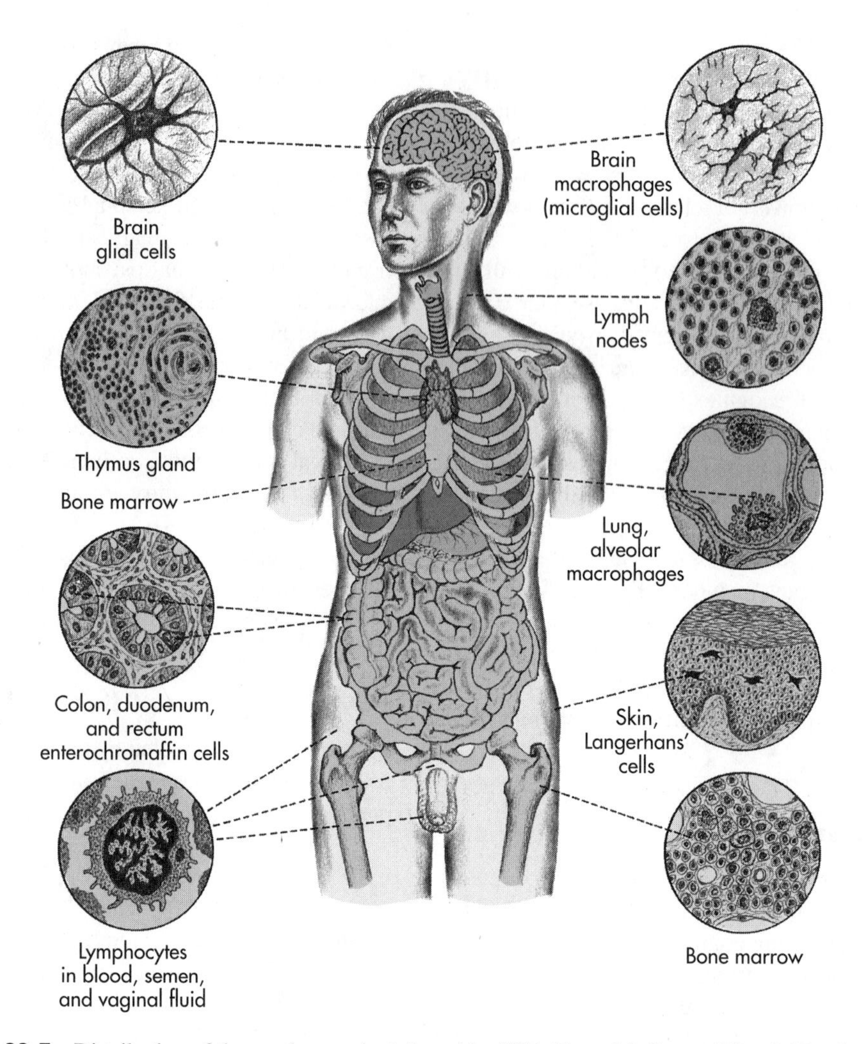

Figure 33-7 Distribution of tissues that can be infected by HIV. (From McCance, K.L., & Huether, S.E. [1998]. *Pathophysiology: The biologic basis for disease in adults and children* [3rd ed.]. St. Louis: Mosby.)

volvement include severe memory loss, speech disturbances, and abnormal reflexes and tone. Gait disturbances from an associated myelopathy are common, as are bowel and bladder deficits, also strokes and visual impairment (Price, 1999).

Peripheral involvement may manifest in four distinct clinical patterns of neuropathy: distal sensorimotor polyneuropathy, inflammatory demyelinating polyneuropathy, mononeuropathy multiplex, and progressive polyradiculopathy (Price, 1999). Outcomes may relate to progressive disease or side effects of medication. Viruses, such as varicella-zoster also may cause neuropathies. With neuromuscular complications, lower extremity wasting eventually extends to the upper with proximal muscle weakness and tenderness. Sensory polyneuropathy is a painful paresthesia of the soles of the feet thought to result from HIV infection of the neurons. Chronic and disabling, clients attempt temporary measures to relieve the pain. Although extremely debilitating, few interventions alleviate the pain and distress effectively; too often providers ignore this symptom (O'Dell, 1996).

Nutritional Status in HIV Disease

Compromised nutritional status exacerbates the complicated clinical picture presented by AIDS. Painful oral and esophageal inflammations cause difficulty with swallowing. Complex drug regimens, fraught with adverse interactions and stress of chronicity contribute to persistent anorexia. Diarrhea, malabsorption, and weight loss frustrate efforts to achieve or maintain adequate nutrition. Nurses have an important challenge to assess and implement appropriate interventions to improve the nutritional status of their clients and to understand the relationship among nutrition, HIV infection, and the immune system. So important that, an epidemiological study found micronutrients including iron, vitamin E, and riboflavin reduced risk of AIDS by 30% for HIV-positive people (Abrams, Duncan, & Hertz-Picciotto, 1993).

Progressive weight loss is a clinical sentinel resulting from reduced intake, malabsorption, hormone abnormalities, or metabolic abnormalities. Malnutrition with weight loss may adversely affect the function of the immune system and further impair the person's ability to avoid or recover from repeated infections and to manage stressors (Ungvarski & Flaskerud, 1999). Need for nutritional support in HIV arises in early asymptomatic stages, continuing to AIDS. People with asymptomatic HIV-positive people benefit from a balanced diet with protein and nutrients. When symptoms develop, progressive, involuntary weight loss commonly ensues with reduced food intake, malabsorption, and altered metabolism; causes include anorexia, conditioned nausea, infection, chronic diarrhea, malabsorption, and poor food availability (O'Brien & Pheifer, 1993). Refer for dietary counseling and home health care services to provide symptom relief and prevent further weight loss. A nutritional assessment must include the following factors:

- Anthropometrics: height, weight, body mass index
- Biochemical tests: albumin, lipids, liver enzymes, renal panel, hemoglobin
- Clinical exam: identifying opportunistic infections
- Dietary history
- Economic and social factors

A cohesive team approach is imperative in planning comprehensive care with clients and families. Goals are to maintain body mass and promote self-concept (Ungvarski & Flaskerud, 1999).

Fatigue and Energy Problems Related to HIV Disease

Although fatigue is common among people with HIV/AIDS, its etiology is unknown. A generalized malaise and loss of motivation unrelated to activity and sleep patterns, generalized fatigue may relate to specific muscle fatigue. Initial complaints are of tiredness, but it persists as a prominent, unexplained symptom. The many physical and psychosocial conditions experienced by immunocompromised people may have profound negative effects on functional level and quality of life (O'Brien & Pheifer, 1993). Fatigue has an economic impact as the overriding symptom that leads people with HIV infection to discontinue employment. Unable to work, they lose health insurance in most instances and turn to public funds throughout the prolonged, slowly progressive deterioration of their illness (Remien, Satriano, & Berkman, 1999).

Elderly and HIV

In the United States, 1% of men and 2% of women older than age 65 years have AIDS. HIV first threatened in the early 1970s before education about safer sex and condoms for birth control. HIV disease is a surprising threat to that generation, now aging. In another view, older adults continuing sexual activity later in life have created an epidemic, particularly within desirable retirement communities. HIV is more difficult to treat and has a faster course in the elderly, perhaps owing to underlying deficiencies in the immune system (Grossman, 1999). Antiviral medicines are untested with the elderly, so that pharmacokinetics are unclear. The stigma associated with the disease may mean fear and social isolation. Research is needed regarding HIV disease and aging.

Box 33-4 Nursing Assessment

History

- Risk factors, date of diagnosis, coping, history of opportunistic infections, history of concomitant illnesses, medication history, normal weight before illness
- Laboratory tests specific to diagnosis

Systems Review

- Neurological
- Integumentary
- Gastrointestinal
- Musculoskeletal
- Constitutional symptoms
- Psychiatric, focusing on presence of depression, inability to cope

Physical Assessment

- Functional limitations, current opportunistic infections, wasting

Psychosocial Assessment

- Assess readiness to change lifestyle: adherence to medications, sexuality, substance abuse
- Family acceptance, coping, social support

Nursing Assessment

Clients with HIV or AIDS can present a variety of conditions, from early asymptomatic HIV to advanced AIDS with multiple, complicated problems or multiple system failure. AIDS care requires knowledge from infection control, neurology, oncology, psychiatry, and pediatrics among others. Early in the disease, nurses educate clients about interventions and assist them to cope effectively. With advanced AIDS and malnourished clients hospitalized for uncontrollable infection, debilitation, feverish illness, and pain nursing roles are more intensive. Box 33-4 lists assessment parameters.

Medical History

A history includes risk factors for transmission of HIV and date of diagnosis; as well as data about previous illnesses, treatments, or chronic illness. Preventive interventions are to reduce spread of HIV and offer strategies to cope effectively with denial and morbidity. Those who have adequate immunity have less morbidity, advanced stages mean significant morbidity. The medication history is connected to past opportunistic illness (OI) history as many OIs are chronic and maintenance medications control infections. Assess weight to understand the status of wasting. A nonpurposeful loss of 10% of normal indicates wasting regardless of current weight.

Systems Review

A multiple systems review determines the extent of damage in this all encompassing disease; assess the following systems in particular:

- Neurological—extent of cognitive deficit or peripheral neuropathy
- Integumentary—rashes or lesions
- Gastrointestinal—diarrhea or other malabsorption or appetite problems, nutritional deficit, oral or esophageal candidiasis
- Musculoskeletal—weakness, inability to perform activities of daily living
- Constitutional symptoms—fevers, night sweats, lymphadenopathy, generalized weakness or fatigue, wasting, and pain
- Psychiatric—depression or inability to cope

Diagnostic Tests

Laboratory tests specific for HIV are useful for disease staging and treatment decisions; clients need to understand the tests and their significance. Specific diagnostic tests are the enzyme-linked immunosorbent assay and the Western Blot to confirm HIV infection. The major test for staging the disease is the CD4 count (T-cell count) that indicates the competence of the immune system and shows the extent of destruction of CD4 cells by the HIV virus. Another key test is the HIV viral load that reports the virulence of infection by the HIV RNA polymerase chain reaction (PCR) or by branched chain DNA (bDNA). Quantitative PCR or bDNA predicts clinical progression or survival and frequently determines treatment efficacy. Laboratory tests in the future will be genotyping or phenotyping of the infecting HIV virus to reveal mutations that will confer resistance to antiviral medications.

Physical Assessment

A full physical assessment is important to identify current opportunistic infections with particular focus on the following:

- Cardiorespiratory system for tuberculosis, PCP, and other respiratory illnesses
- Integumentary system for HSV, Kaposi's sarcoma, and subcutaneous fungal infections
- Gastrointestinal system, including the oral mucosa, for oral or esophageal candidiasis, MAC, CMV, and other malabsorption problems
- Neurological system including visual changes, for CMV retinitis, HIV-encephalopathy, toxoplasmosis, cryptococcal meningitis, ADC, peripheral neuropathy, or other peripheral or CNS problems
- Musculoskeletal system for HIV wasting, HIV-related peripheral neuropathies and other myopathies
- Lymphatic system for lymphomas or HIV-related lymphadenopathy

Psychosocial Assessment

Adaptation to HIV disease as a chronic, rather than terminal, disease is critical to successful living. Assess the client's adjustment, specifically adherence to treatment and modification of sexual lifestyle or drug use. Treatment for HIV disease is complex and must be consistent to prevent resistant mutations of the HIV virus. Treatment involves a minimum of three HIV medications and others to control or prevent OIs.

Nurses have influence in the primarily young adult population where privacy about a stigmatizing illness is paramount. Assessment tools include the Transtheoretical Model of Change, Health Belief Model, and selected screening tests for drug and alcohol misuse. Nonjudgmental questioning is important because many barriers make adherence to medication and lifestyle regimens difficult. Sample questions in Table 33-1 foster frank discussions and interventions based on the Transtheoretical Model of Change. Questions concerning the source of HIV and beliefs about the efficacy of medicines or other therapy reflect the Health Belief Model. The CAGE questionnaire (Table 33-2) is an example of a drug and alcohol assessment tool.

Social support is critical with any chronic condition that requires lifestyle change. Assessing how well the client, family, and others understand the disease, accept changes, and use effective coping strategies helps to reveal both spoken and unspoken needs that the nurse may be able to help them meet.

Nursing Diagnoses

Nursing diagnoses are related to the assessment. Nursing diagnoses with a psychosocial component include: Risk for Ineffective Management of Therapeutic Regimen as seen by poor adherence to medications or other lifestyle change; Hopelessness; Altered Sexuality Patterns; and Ineffective Coping, Individual or Family (Gordon, 2000). Other diagnoses are related to compromised immune status and opportunistic infections. These include: Risk for Infection related to Immune Deficiency Leading to Opportunistic Infections; Altered Nutrition: Less than Body Requirements Related to AIDS Wasting; Diarrhea, related to HIV or to Medication Therapy; Fatigue; Chronic Pain; or Risk for Cognitive Impairment (Gordon, 2000). Box 33-5 lists nursing diagnoses.

Nursing Goals

The nursing care plan will depend greatly on the disease status and extent of disability. The nurse working with those hospitalized for an acute condition concentrate on acute

TABLE 33-1 Assessment of Medication Adherence

Assessment	Rationale
"I know that it is hard for a lot of people taking medicines every day. What are *your* particular difficulties with them?"	Establishing "cons" to adherent taking of medicines. Gives the client permission to admit to nonadherence, which establishes honesty and acceptance in your relationship. Cons to the behavior generally diminish with time when active in engaging in the behavior.
"Because it is difficult for you to take your medicines every day, why are you taking them? What are the benefits to you in taking your medicines?"	Establish the "pros" to adherent taking of medicines, to increase the individual's investment in the behavior. Pros generally increase as the individual knows more about the purpose and becomes more committed to medicine-taking behavior.
"A lot of people have trouble taking their medicines every day, or sometimes they even stop them completely. There are a lot of medicines, and a lot of people find that very hard to get used to. Side effects can also be a problem. Do you take your medicines regularly every day?"	
If no . . .	Accept individual's concerns/difficulties with the medicines as rational explanations to the client that are appropriate for discussion. Give feedback about health status. Establish personalized pros and cons, and educate/reinforce about consequences of not taking medicines.
If not now but is thinking about it . . .	Encourage expression of negative emotions about taking medicines. Give feedback about health status. Establish personalized pros and cons, and educate/reinforce about consequences of not taking medicines.
If yes, I have recently started . . .	Discuss actual or perceived barriers to regular medicine-taking: access problems, forgetfulness, side effects, etc., and present options for addressing those barriers. Support self-efficacy: provide encouragement and feedback. Plan for disruptions in schedule, and for relapses in the future in order to limit the length of time of the relapse.

TABLE 33-2 CAGE Alcohol Screening Questionnaire

Question	Response	
1. Have you ever felt you should *C*ut down on your drinking?	Yes	No
2. Have people *A*nnoyed you by criticizing your drinking?	Yes	No
3. Have you ever felt bad or *G*uilty about your drinking?	Yes	No
4. Have you ever taken a drink first thing in the morning to steady your nerves or get rid of a hangover? (*E*ye-opener)	Yes	No

From Ewing, J.A. (1984). Detecting alcoholism: The CAGE questionnaire. *Journal of the American Medical Association, 252,* 1905-1907. Scoring: Two or more positive answers suggest that the existence of alcohol-related problems is very probable, currently or in the past.

Box 33-5 Nursing Diagnoses for HIV

- Risk for ineffective management of therapeutic regimen
  - Poor adherence to medications, other lifestyle changes
- Hopelessness
- Altered sexuality patterns
- Ineffective coping, individual or family
- Risk for infection
  - Immune deficiency leading to opportunistic infections (OTs)
- Imbalanced nutrition: less than body requirements
  - AIDS wasting
- Diarrhea
  - Related to HIV or to medication therapy
- Fatigue
- Chronic pain
- Risk for cognitive impairment

nursing goals for physiological conditions with underlying psychosocial goals. Home health care nurses may consider setting long-term goals with clients toward acceptance and treatment.

Community Health Goals

Goals in community health include regular health care for continued viral suppression, health maintenance, and case management. The nurse is critical in case management to assess holistic health needs. Ensuring access and removing barriers to care take many forms. Finances or transportation may affect access to health care or medications; situations at home may create problems with adherence; further education may be needed about HIV or treatments; or isolation may call for connecting with support groups.

Goals in home health care, restricted to those who are

homebound and need skilled nursing care, are limited to physical problems associated with AIDS. Goals include administering intravenous medications as treatment or for maintenance for OIs, enhancing optimal independence, and holistic case management for the individual.

Acute Care Goals

Goals in the hospital include resolving acute OIs, initiating education about maintenance therapy, and assuring case management. Effective discharge planning ensures long-term goals are addressed.

Regardless of the setting, partnership with the client is essential in making permanent adaptation to the disease process and effective health care management, including prevention of further complications. Case management involving referrals to resources is critical to maintaining health. Many communities have local AIDS service organizations and support groups. Table 33-3 contains a list of national resources for those with HIV and AIDS. Sites on the World Wide Web are shown in Table 33-4.

Hospice goals are for those with advanced AIDS when antiviral treatment is no longer effective or clients choose not to participate. The goals include comfort with pain management, control of diarrhea, pacing activities to reduce fatigue, and family support.

Apart from the specific treatments to combat OIs and malignancies, no effective cure exists for AIDS. Treatment goals are to preserve and enhance the immune system; although some approaches are symptomatic, others are highly experimental. The mortality rate for individuals with documented AIDS, at one time 95% at 2 years, has improved, but the rate and extent of change remain unclear.

NURSING INTERVENTIONS SPECIFIC TO HIV DISEASE

Rehabilitation interventions for HIV occur throughout all levels of prevention. Primary prevention of infection with HIV in the community, secondary for early screening and diagnosis before extensive immune compromise, and tertiary for reducing severity of disability. A critical role for rehabilitation nurses, HIV care ranges from asymptomatic clients, to adaptation to the disease, to hospice for advanced AIDS.

Primary Prevention

Healthy People 2000 goals pertain to prevention of HIV in the community, the only option a decade ago. Improved medication treatment has not brought a cure or preventive vaccine; thus, education about reducing risks remains the best means to contain the epidemic in the United States. Preventive behaviors include ceasing intravenous (IV) drug use, maintaining monogamous sexual relationships, and eliminating vertical transmission from mother to baby. Behaviors

TABLE 33-3 National Resources for Clients with HIV

Resource	Contact Information	Content
National AIDS Hotline	(800) 342-2437	Hotline for information, counseling
Centers for Disease Control and Prevention National AIDS Clearinghouse	(800) 458-5231	Publications, epidemiology
National Association of People with AIDS	(202) 898-0414	Advocacy information, treatment information
AIDS Treatment Data Network	(800) 734-7104	Record of research data
HIV-AIDS Treatment Information Service	(800) HIV-0440	Treatment information
Project Inform	(800) 822-7422	Linking with HIV services
National Clinical Trials Hotline	(800) TRIALS-A	Listing of AIDS clinical trials

TABLE 33-4 Active Websites for Information about HIV Disease and AIDS

Web Address	Subject Matter
http://hopkins-aids.edu	Johns Hopkins AIDS service—professional education
http://hiv.medscape.com	Current medical professional information. Requires registration
http://hivinsite.ucsf.edu	Medical information, prevention and public education, epidemiology, social issues, links to other sites
http://hivatis.org	HIV/AIDS Treatment Information Service—treatment guidelines, clinical trial information
http://thebody.com	The Body: An AIDS and HIV information resource—public and client-oriented information
http://www.amfar.org	American Foundation for AIDS Research—data derived from AIDS research

to reduce risk include drug use without needle sharing, bleach cleaning needles, and condom use.

HIV is transmitted during sexual contact, sharing IV needles or drug paraphernalia, with exposure to infected blood, blood products, or body fluids, and from mother to newborn perinatally. The Centers for Disease Control and Prevention developed standard precautions for all professionals who have a high probability of exposure to HIV consider blood and body fluids of all clients potentially infectious for HIV, hepatitis B virus, and other blood-borne pathogens. Standard precautions prevent providers from parenteral, mucous membrane, and nonintact skin exposure to clients' blood; other body fluids containing visible blood, semen, and vaginal secretions; and body tissues as well as cerebrospinal, synovial, pleural, peritoneal, pericardial, and amniotic fluids. They do not apply to feces, nasal secretions, sputum, sweat, tears, urine, and vomit unless they contain visible blood. Standard precautions are not optional; apply them consistently. Nurses must know the standards mandated by the Occupational Safety and Health Administration and organizational policies regarding blood-borne pathogens, as well as environmental or special precautions required during invasive procedures.

Secondary Prevention

Early screening identifies people with HIV before clinical symptoms and the onset of AIDS. State Departments of Health mandates to control transmission and secondary prevention should be included in every community health plan.

Tertiary Prevention

For those with HIV, nursing goals have three levels. *Short-term goals* for disease control are medication treatment, suppressing viral replication, and preventing OIs. *Long-term goals* are to control the disease, provide regular health care, and plan for lifestyle changes and adherence. *Lifelong planning* includes clients' recognition of future complications and back to work issues, preparing advanced directives, and regarding a second chance at life or hospice care. Multiple and complex interventions will differ with client needs and situation and with disease progression. Interventions in Box 33-6 apply in various health settings (McCloskey & Bulechek, 2000).

Another goal, to control replication and progression of HIV, involves ongoing coordination to assure efficacious care, assist with lifestyle changes, assess nutrition, con-

Box 33-6 Nursing Interventions in Various Health Care Settings

Community Health
- Active listening
- Behavior modification—reinforcing maintenance of health care
- Case management
- Coping enhancement
- Diarrhea management
- Energy management
- Family involvement promotion
- Health education
- Health system guidance
- Mutual goal setting
- Nutrition management
- Oral health restoration
- Pain management
- Support system enhancement

Home Setting
- Active listening
- Caregiver support
- Case management
- Coping enhancement
- Dementia management
- Diarrhea management
- Electrolyte management
- Energy management
- Family involvement promotion
- Family support
- Health education
- Mutual goal setting
- Nutrition management
- Pain management

Hospital
- Acid-base monitoring
- Case management
- Diarrhea management
- Electrolyte management
- Family involvement promotion
- Health education
- Infection protection
- Nutrition management

Hospice
- Active listening
- Coping enhancement
- Dementia management
- Diarrhea management
- Nutrition management
- Oral health restoration
- Pain management

McCloskey, J.C., & Bulechek, G.M. (Eds.). (2000). *Nursing interventions classifications (NIC)* (3rd ed.). St. Louis: Mosby.

trol symptoms, monitor prognosis, provide education (including websites), and make referrals, such as for social services.

Physiological Interventions

Physiological interventions are to control disease progression, symptoms, and OIs. With *late-stage AIDS,* OIs occur alongside diarrhea, fevers, weight loss, and skin breakdown. Monitor and replace electrolytes and fluid volume, use diet and medications for diarrhea and fever, and attend to restoring oral health. Nutrition may be compromised if candidiasis or mouth sores reduce intake (McCloskey & Bulechek, 2000). As more becomes known of long-term side effects of HIV treatment and HIV disease, nurses can expect to manage hyperlipidemia and hyperglycemia alongside HIV disease (McCloskey & Bulechek, 2000).

Hurley and Ungvarski (1994) surveyed home health care requirements of people with HIV/AIDS. They found the most common physiological symptoms were dyspnea, weakness, fatigue and lethargy, pain, and ataxia. Memory deficit, depression, anxiety, impaired judgment, substance abuse, and insomnia occurred most frequently. Other needs were assistance with cleaning the home, preparing meals, doing laundry, and shopping.

AIDS-related dementia requires assessment of the type and extent of cognitive deficits. Clients, families, and others need education about this situation. Use written materials, visual cues, and assistive equipment to boost poor memory or concentration. These clients need reminders to adhere to treatment. Medication management of OIs and HIV disease helps combat the *fatigue* that becomes part of the situation. Interventions include counseling about nutrition, reducing pace of activities and environmental stimuli, adequate rest, and adjustment to life changes (McCloskey & Bulechek, 2000). Control of *chronic pain,* usually peripheral neuropathy associated with HIV disease or with medication therapy, is essential to quality of life. Interventions include assessing and monitoring pain and identifying sources of exacerbation using both alternative and complementary or pharmacological interventions (McCloskey & Bulechek, 2000). Chapter 24 discusses pain management in more detail.

Terminal Phase of AIDS

Eventually, in the trajectory of the disease, physiological and emotional problems accompanying AIDS will affect an individual's ability to function independently. Continuing rehabilitation appropriately supports caregivers that may become depressed. AIDS networks and groups help in support and information. Nurses help caregivers make informed decisions about care options as the client enters the terminal phase.

Hospice services are appropriate option for comfort without active curative measures or invasive or diagnostic procedures. An array of services based on a holistic health care philosophy, hospice provides the dying person and family with comfort, autonomy, and emotional and physical support. An interdisciplinary team supports the nurse, who coordinates and supervises all hospice services 7 days a week, 24 hours a day from a hospital or in the home setting or other community programs. Chapter 34 discusses hospice care for clients with end-stage renal diseases.

Psychosocial Intervention

Active listening as clients express denial, anger, and depression regarding the diagnosis assists clients to work through their feelings. Encouragement to express feelings with full acceptance of the person is a nursing intervention they may not receive from anyone in their lives; it may help them adjust and form strategies to cope effectively. Clients adjust more if they can assess realistically the impact of the disease, and have facts about their diagnosis, treatment, and prognosis. Other interventions are to promote decision-making and encourage spiritual resources. When clients and their families agree to support one another, clients experience less isolation and fewer concerns that a caregiver will be available when needed (McCloskey & Bulechek, 2000).

Medical Treatment

Currently approved antiviral drugs included in Table 33-5 change rapidly with additions of new drugs identified through research and older drugs that work in entirely new ways. Nucleoside reverse transcriptase inhibitors (NRTI) are the oldest class of antiviral drugs, used until 1995, when a new class, protease inhibitors (PI), emerged with improved suppressive power. Another class—nonnucleoside reverse transcriptase inhibitors (NNRTIs)—inhibit the reverse transcriptase enzyme in a slightly different pathway. Figure 33-8 illustrates the drug actions in the HIV trajectory. Drug combinations, such as two NRTIs and one PI or one NNRTI, create potent suppression of viral replication. Possible combinations are one NRTI with two PIs, or three NRTIs. Several new drugs and classes have entered the FDA approval process.

OUTCOMES

Nursing outcomes for clients with HIV disease include physiological and psychosocial outcomes that vary according to the stage of disease and the client's stage of life. Rehabilitation nurses evaluate the entire range of outcomes to assure holistic care. Box 33-7 contains sample outcomes important when planning care throughout the disease trajectory with clients who have HIV.

TABLE 33-5 Adult Antiretroviral Medications

Chemical	Generic	Brand	Dose	Side Effects
Nucleoside Analog Reverse Transcriptase Inhibitors (Nucleoside Analogs, NRTIs)				
AZT (ZDV)	Zidovudine	Retrovir	300 mg twice daily	Initial nausea, headache, fatigue, anemia neutropenia
3TC	Lamivudine	Epivir	150 mg twice daily	Generally well tolerated
AZT + 3TC	Zidovudine Lamivudine	Combivir	1 tablet twice daily	Combination tablet (see components)
ddI	Didanosine	Videx	400 mg once daily or 200 mg twice daily on empty stomach, may use 250 mg packets of powder as equivalent of 200 mg chewable tablets	Peripheral neuropathy, pancreatitis. Contains antacid.
ddC	Zalcitabine	Hivid	0.375–0.75 mg 3 times daily	Peripheral neuropathy
d4T	Stavudine	Zerit	20–40 mg twice daily	Peripheral neuropathy
ABC	Abacavir	Ziagen	300 mg twice daily	About 3% hypersensitivity reaction: fever, malaise, possible rash, GI, respiratory
AZT, 3TC, and ABC	Zidovudine, lamivudine, and abacavir	Trizivir	1 pill 2 times daily	Combination pill (see components)
Protease Inhibitors (PIs)				
Saquinavir hard gel cap	Invirase		600 mg (3 capsules) 3 times daily with meals	Well tolerated; poor bioavailability
Saquinavir soft gel cap	Fortovase		1600 mg (8 capsules) twice daily or 1200 mg (6 capsules) 3 times daily with food	Well tolerated; improved absorption
Ritonavir	Norvir		600 mg (6 capsules) twice daily, start with 300 mg twice daily and increase to full dose over 10 days	Nausea, diarrhea, numb lips
Indinavir	Crixivan		800 mg (2 capsules) every 8 hours on empty stomach	Kidney stones, nausea, GI upset
Nelfinavir	Viracept		1200 mg (5 tablets) twice daily or 750 mg (3 capsules) 3 times daily with food	Diarrhea
Amprenavir	Agenerase		1200 mg (8 capsules) twice daily	Nausea, diarrhea
Lopinavir and ritonavir	Kaletra		3 pills twice daily or 5 ml twice daily	Diarrhea, gastrointestinal upset
Nonnucleoside Reverse Transcriptase Inhibitors (NNRTIs)				
Nevirapine	Viramune		200 mg (1 tablet) once daily for 14 days, then 200 mg twice daily	Transient rash, hepatitis
Delavirdine	Rescriptor		400 mg (4 tablets) 3 times daily	Transient rash Multiple drug-drug and drug-food interactions
Efavirenz	Sustiva		600 mg (3 capsules) 1 daily initially at bedtime	Initial dizziness, insomnia, transient rash; occasionally hallucinations
Nucleotide Reverse Transcriptase Inhibitors (Experimental Use)				
Adefovir (not Food and Drug Administration approved)			60 mg once daily	Common renal dysfunction
Ribonucleotide Reductase Inhibitors				
Hydroxy-urea (not Food and Drug Administration approved for HIV therapy)	Hydrea		500 mg twice daily	Bone marrow suppressions, aphthous ulcers, peripheral hallucinations neuropathy, hair loss (No direct antiviral effects; Augments action of some NRTIs)

Data from Schutz, M., & Wendrow, A. (2000). *Quick reference guide to antiretrovirals* [On-line]. Available: http://hiv.medscape.com/updates/quickguide.

Stages of HIV reproduction

1. HIV enters a CD4+ cell.
2. HIV is a retrovirus, meaning that its genetic information is stored on single-stranded RNA instead of the double-stranded DNA found in most organisms. To replicate, HIV uses an enzyme known as reverse transcriptase to convert its RNA into DNA.
3. HIV DNA enters the nucleus of the CD4+ cell and inserts itself into the cell's DNA. HIV DNA then instructs the cell to make many copies of the original virus.
4. New virus particles are assembled and leave the cell, ready to infect other CD4+ cells.

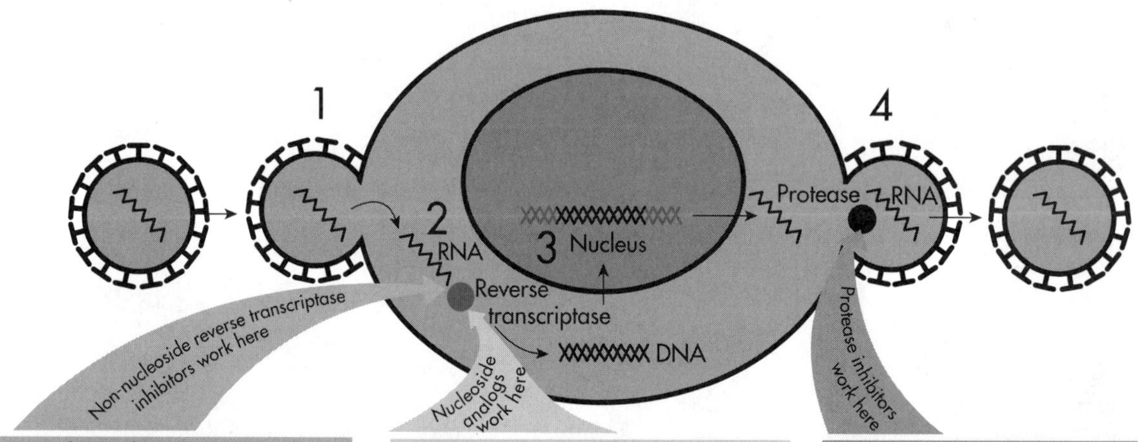

Non-nucleoside reverse transcriptase inhibitors

The newest class of antiretroviral agents, non-nucleoside reverse transcriptase inhibitors (NNRTIs) stop HIV production by binding directly onto reverse transcriptase and preventing the conversion of RNA to DNA. These drugs are called "non-nucleoside" inhibitors because even though they work at the same stage as nucleoside analogs, they act in a completely different way.
VIRAMUNE (nevirapine)
Rescriptor (delavirdine mesylate)
Sustiva (efavirenz)

Nucleoside analogs

The first effective class of antiretroviral drugs was the nucleoside analogs. They act by incorporating themselves into the DNA of the virus, thereby stopping the building process. The resulting DNA is incomplete and cannot create new virus.
Ziagen (abacavir sulfate)
Retrovir (zidovudine; also known as ZDV or AZT)
Epivir (lamivudine; also known as 3TC)
Videx (didanosine; also known as ddI)
Hivid (zalcitabine; also known as ddC)
Zerit (stavudine; also known as d4T)
Combivir (lamivudine/zidovudine)

Protease inhibitors

Protease inhibitors work at the last stage of the virus reproduction cycle. They prevent HIV from being successfully assembled and released from the infected CD4+ cell.
Invirase (saquinavir mesylate)
Crixivan (indinavir)
Norvir (ritonavir)
Viracept (nelfinavir mesylate)
Fortovase (saquinavir)

Note: This information is provided for background only.

Figure 33-8 Areas of impact of antiretroviral medications. A combination of medications that affect different processes in HIV replication can suppress replication to a greater degree. Thus nucleoside or nonnucleoside reverse transcriptase inhibitors are combined with protease inhibitors, to effectively inhibit the process of transcription of RNA to DNA, and to inhibit the process of combining proteins together to form the basis of a replicated HIV virus. (Courtesy Roxane Laboratories, Inc., Columbus, OH.)

Box 33-7 Related Outcomes: Nursing Outcomes Classification

- Acceptance: health status
- Adherence behavior
- Depression control
- Hope
- Pain: psychological response
- Participation: health care decisions
- Quality of life
- Self-care: instrumental activities of daily living
- Symptom control

From Johnson, M., Maas, M., & Moorhead, S. (Eds.). (2000). *Nursing outcomes classification (NOC)* (2nd ed.). St. Louis: Mosby.

A high CD4, an undetectable viral load, improved or lack of symptoms, and no OIs indicate physiological control of HIV disease progression. With wasting, outcomes include improved nutrition and weight, especially with more lean body mass that may help resolve diarrhea or mucosa and skin integrity problems (Johnson, Maas, & Moorhead, 2000).

With fatigue, improved outcomes include endurance in performing activities of daily living and instrumental activities of daily living, rested appearance and interest in activities as opposed to exhaustion and lethargy and at times, reduced chronic pain from peripheral neuropathy. Pain control may reduce impairments in concentration, mobility, and self-care. Cognitive impairment occurs in up to 75% of those with HIV disease and AIDS. Outcomes include early identification and treatment of cognitive deficits and adapting the environment to compensate for permanent deficits. Support systems and interventions are added to maximize cognition as deficits are known (Johnson et al., 2000).

Adequate nutrition as evidenced by weight and body mass because body fat may increase independent of mass, which is an important outcome. Fatigue and activity intolerance and physical changes, such as thinner extremities with increased abdominal girth, are cautions.

Psychosocial Outcomes

Psychosocial outcomes for long-term adjustment to HIV disease are similar to those with other life-threatening chronic illnesses. Education to minimize complications and facilitate coping, as well as to prevent transmission is appropriate in the short-term. Outcomes evaluate the client's ability to describe prevention to others, to avoid contracting OIs, and to demonstrate understanding about *non*transmission to avoid self-imposed isolation. Clients demonstrate learning about the disease when they are able to describe the medication regimen and side effects, sources for medications, and purposes of continual monitoring of CD4s and viral loads. Those who engage in active partnership with health professionals usually understand the importance of adherence to the regimen (Johnson et al., 2000). Clients also need to know what signs or symptoms are concerns for medical attention.

Outcomes of adequate coping vary with comfort, pain level, level of independence, support system, and coping strategies; denial and substance use are nonproductive (Johnson et al., 2000). Functional coping includes acceptance of changes in lifestyle, body image, and spiritual meaning to life. Social stigma is a difficult issue because clients are isolated and feel actively persecution in some communities. Although the community is less changeable, interventions involving active listening, support groups, and environmental changes may help clients accept their reality and cope with the loss of relationships. Certainly some clients will be losing friends and partners to the disease creating further isolation and loss. Changes in sexuality are similar. Education to prevent transmission, such as protected sexual intercourse and other ways to establish intimacy between partners can help acceptance.

Outcomes Related to Stage of Disease

Outcomes in early HIV disease differ from advanced AIDS, where the focus is on short-term symptom relief and OI management and optimal function. Those resistant to antiviral medications no longer obtain a good suppressive response. Clients with advanced disease who have started on new antiviral medications may begin with a short-term focus, but find their immune system reconstituted. Instead of terminal planning, they also must change, but by envisioning a longer life. With early HIV disease, clients focus on long-term adaptation to chronic illness by accepting the disease and the resulting changes in life as the highest priority. Refer to Chapter 12 for a more complete discussion about coping and family caregivers.

Outcomes Related to Life Stage

Children

Children infected with HIV need to live as normal a life as possible. Early identification of developmental difficulties with appropriate interventions involves activities in school. Families choose whether they inform the school, stigma may be problematic; however, a school nurse provides medication during the day, understands absences resulting from sickness or treatments, and facilitates acceptance from children and teachers. Medication therapy for children is complex, perhaps more so than for adults. Parents are responsible for young children adhering to the regimen that can be a burden with frequent dosing and unpleasant medications the child does not like. Active problem solving around these difficulties aids in adherence and supports parent in managing their responsibilities.

Adolescents

Issues important for adolescents involve their desire for peer group acceptance, tasks to accept self, and tendency for taking risks. Outcomes for adolescents are to express self-acceptance, belong to an accepting peer group, and limit risky behaviors, as well as to adhere to the medical regimen. The composition and orientation of peer and support groups directs behaviors in this population.

Young Adults

For young adults psychosocial issues are acceptance of a chronic illness, the resulting altered body image and lifestyle, and the inability to bear children, which is a difficult hurdle. At a time when they envision a career path and partnerships, young adults with AIDS must accept their disability and inability to work. This is especially difficult for those who were once disabled, but who now can return to work because of the effectiveness of new medications. This psychosocial conflict has been called the "Lazarus phenomenon." Many who prepared to die (before HAART), must now plan how to reconsider life and all the accompanying stressors. For example, medicaid may deny benefits without disability, and entering the job market without skills or work history is a difficult situation. Nurse case managers will be instrumental in helping clients resolve these issues and referring them for appropriate resources.

Elderly

Those who are elderly and infected with HIV need to address isolation problems. The prevalence of chronic conditions makes adherence less of an issue. However, elders tend to self-imposed isolation, fear of discrimination and ostracism, and loss of age mates from all causes.

Evaluation of Care with HIV Disease

Clinical Endpoints

Laboratory values and clinical health status, such as undetectable viral loads and rising or stable CD4 counts, indicate fully suppressed viral replication. Even in a situation of rising viral loads, a client's health status may remain very good for several years, especially without OIs and if weight is stable, and low levels of fatigue.

Process Outcomes

Evaluation of nursing care includes process outcomes, as well as clinical endpoints. Satisfaction with care encourages clients to seek health care regularly, an important outcome for any chronic illness. Nurse case managers assure clients have full access to services for their needs, whether for housing, transportation, isolation, or financial hardship. Access is necessary for clients to take medications, keep diets, or visit primary care providers. Clients who express improved quality and satisfaction in their lives and who maintain health reflect effective nursing care.

Evaluation Techniques

Ongoing review and evaluation of interdisciplinary care is a means for continual improvement. Laboratory values and missed appointments are indicators readily available to evaluate clinical care and access to care. More complex evaluation includes periodic surveys for satisfaction with care, or about quality of life, or to identify barriers to the therapeutic regimen. Chapter 7 discusses quality improvement in detail.

Implications of Current Trends in Treatment of HIV Disease

Escalating health care costs continue as an economic issue. Initiatives that emphasize community-based care to enhance functional ability in people with AIDS will become more common. No longer an acute, fulminating disease, chronic AIDS affects all bodily systems and musculoskeletal and neurological problems benefit from rehabilitation. Rehabilitation nurses and the team will have central roles in enhancing the quality of life for individuals with AIDS, in minimizing their functional dependence, and in lowering health care costs (Remien, Satriano, & Berkman, 1999). As more people with AIDS are retained in community settings throughout the trajectory of their illness, it becomes imperative for nurses to develop rehabilitation expertise to address the myriad needs presented by these clients. Chapter 9 explains more about community-based rehabilitation.

Access to Care Issues

Society is clamoring for a solution to the AIDS crisis and issues related to funding for the most efficacious treatment and ultimately, for a cure; ongoing and volatile issues. At this time and although expensive, adequate outpatient treatment is cost effective provided it occurs before conversion to AIDS; and is less costly than hospitalization for OIs.

Low income and no or underinsurance have been barriers to outpatient treatment in HIV disease, as well as for other chronic illnesses. Then in 1990, the Ryan White CARE Act became a federal law. Ryan White gained national attention when denied schooling in his hometown after officials discovered he had acquired AIDS through blood transfusions for hemophilia. Ryan, before he died, became a spokesperson for those discriminated against for HIV disease. The federal program mandates the following.

- Improving quality and availability of care for those with financial barriers
- Improving access to medical care
- Providing early intervention care
- Providing antiviral medications and medicines to treat or prevent opportunistic infections
- Providing education for health care providers on treatment of HIV disease

Political-Economic Issues

Other political-economic issues argue definitions of disability and medicaid coverage. Each state provides medicaid for their designated populations, but definitions of disability vary and in some states, clients must have a diagnosis of AIDS and a history of at least two OIs or major limitations to receive benefits. Thus, health care and medications are available for those with advanced disease, but nothing prevents progression to this stage. Recent initiatives in several states are to allow those with *potential* for catastrophic illness to receive medicaid, rather than waiting for catastrophic illness. This change, authorized by federal legal moves, potentially would include many chronic diseases, such as cancer, diabetes, or congestive heart failure, in addition to HIV disease. The initiatives will be monitored for cost-effective outcomes of providing expensive outpatient health care against the hope to decrease costs from hospitalizations and loss of work.

Those, declared disabled because of the severity of their AIDS symptoms, but who now can work because of successful adequate antiviral treatments were mentioned earlier. They face potential loss of disability payments and medicare or medicaid; however, even with a full-time job providing health insurance, they find most insurance policies will not pay for "preexisting conditions." Clients have a lapse in coverage at best and uncertainty for benefits. Nurses can assist clients with information and resources for correct understanding of the issues. Some nurses will choose political action; Chapter 3 discusses this route to advocacy.

Global Health Issues

The HIV/AIDS epidemic is raging unchecked in parts of the developing world, particularly in Africa and Asia. Rehabilitation in developing countries is symptom control and prevention of transmission as expensive antiretroviral medications are not options. Vertical transmission is a serious concern as a large percent of childbearing populations are infected with HIV and funds for medications to prevent perinatal transmission are insufficient. Economic and cultural needs for breast-feeding may infect infants who avoided HIV earlier. Increasing populations of HIV-infected children further strain resources of poor regions of the world. In the next decade, numbers children becoming orphans because of AIDS will increase dramatically, and a large segment of the workforce will be dead or dying from AIDS. This dire future for developing countries is a preview of the grim realities in the world. At the time of this writing, the International AIDS Conference is meeting in Durban, South Africa. The devastation and despair in some parts of the world are being brought to the attention of scientists from all over the world in the hope for help to change the devastation.

Continued Need for Knowledge of HIV Disease

Information about HIV disease and treatments is changing with multiple implications for practice, research, administration, and professional education. The research agenda about HIV and its treatment and prevention is very active, causing rapid changes in guidelines. Many clients also are active in seeking information so that they may have more recent data than the nurse or other providers. Education updates about medications, clinical guidelines, and behavioral aspects can be a focus of therapeutic partnerships between client and professional.

Clearly, rehabilitation nurses need support for continuing education so they are prepared to meet the needs of these clients. Education should include content about providing emotional support for clients and providers in a field where loss of life is still all too common. Selected websites with updated information are listed in Table 33-4.

Ethical Issues

Our existing knowledge base provides an adequate foundation for designing delivery strategies and for planning interventions to meet the complex physiological and psychosocial needs of the person with HIV/AIDS. Professional nurses are responsible for keeping fully informed of changes in the epidemiology of and treatment approaches for this disease and to modify their care accordingly. Nurses have challenges to define critical pathways and initiate case management approaches that will direct holistic, yet cost-effective, care for clients. Ethical dilemmas will continue about disclosure and confidentiality with HIV disease. As client advocates, nurses must be diligent in their efforts to respect the client's rights. Chapter 4 discusses ethics in rehabilitation in more detail.

CRITICAL THINKING

Ms. W visits for the third time in outpatient care. In the early stages of HIV disease, her laboratory results are monitored for the stage where medication treatment may be indicated. As her level of trust in you has increased, she shares her dilemma. Ms. W thinks she must have been infected by a man who was the only sexual partner she had in the last 5 years. He is married and a professional in the church, a situation that would increase his silence about his HIV disease. Ms. W states that this man told her that his wife does not know about his HIV disease. The health department contacted his wife by mail after he was tested, presumably suggesting she be tested, but he discarded the letter before she could read it.

Ms. W does not want to break this man's confidentiality, nor does she want it known that she was his sexual partner. She is concerned for the wife's safety because she is sure that this man is sexually active with his wife. You do not know the man, and he lives in another state. What do you do?

Options include:

1. You can report the issue to the health department in the district where your client and the man were tested. You must give the name of the man to the health department, so they will be able to contact the wife again. The health department is strict about confidentiality, and would not reveal the name to anyone, including the wife.
2. You could encourage your client to speak with the man, and impress on him the importance of telling his wife.
3. Other?

Case Study

Initial Visit

Thomas L., 38 years old, came to his initial appointment at the infectious diseases clinic at the public hospital with a recent diagnosis of HIV disease. He has lost a bit of weight in the last year, experienced significant fatigue and exertional dyspnea for the last 4 months, and had frequent night sweats. He went to the local health department for an exam and received an HIV test. His only risk factor was unprotected heterosexual sex, with no history of IV drug use, homosexual sex, or blood transfusions before 1985. The test was positive for HIV infection. Still in a state of shock about his HIV diagnosis, he was more distressed because his brother died from AIDS 2 years previously.

Thomas revealed that he was afraid of taking AZT (zidovudine) as a treatment for HIV. His brother had taken it early in his

Continued

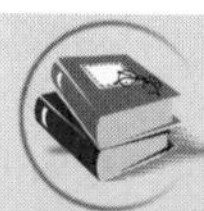

Case Study—cont'd

disease and was very sick. Thomas felt sure that he would be dying of AIDS in the near future "since there's nothing you can do anyway." Anxious about his weight loss and distressed about his emaciated appearance, he thought, "everyone will know what is wrong with me." He was interested in taking medicine if it would help how he felt, but hoped that the medicines would not make him feel bad. "I hate taking medicines."

His medical history revealed intact health with no prior hospitalizations and no previous medications except for "pain pills when I get a headache, or something for a cold when I feel bad." Vital signs were: weight, 126 lb., normally, 175; temperature 99.9° F; pulse 106; respiration 24 breaths per minute; and blood pressure 112/78. Physical assessment was normal except for cachectic appearance and scattered white removable patches on his tongue and buccal mucosa. Laboratory and diagnostic data revealed the following:

- Blood urea nitrogen: 11 mg/dl
- Creatinine: 1.1 mg/dl
- Hemoglobin: 11.8 mg/dl
- Hematocrit: 34.6 g/dl
- White blood count: 4500/mm^3
- Lymphocytes: 45%
- CD4 absolute: 134
- HIV RNA viral load by PCR: > 750,000

Thomas was prescribed an antiviral regimen consisting of zidovudine 300 mg BID and lamivudine 150 mg BID (both of these in a combination pill) and nelfinavir 250 mg, three pills TID. Recommendations included sulfamethoxazole/trimethoprim (Bactrim DS) once a day for prophylaxis for Pneumocystis pneumonia and a prescription for clotrimazole troches, to be dissolved in his mouth 5 times per day for oral candidiasis, as needed.

Priority Nursing Diagnoses, Interventions, and Outcome Criteria

I. Diagnosis 1
  A. Altered Nutrition: Less than Body Requirements as manifested by > 10% weight loss.
    1. Interventions:
      a. Assess nutritional intake
      b. Assess difficulty eating or drinking related to oral candidiasis
      c. Assess self-care ability, in relation to ability to prepare meals of adequate nutritional content
      d. Educate that treatment with effective antiretroviral medications will reverse wasting in most cases
      e. Encourage high-protein, high-carbohydrate meals, with frequent small meals if fatigue impairs ability to eat a full meal
      f. Encourage dietary supplement
      g. Encourage monitoring weight at home every week on the same scale
      h. Monitor weight at each clinic visit
      i. Encourage resistance exercise
    2. Outcomes
      a. Thomas will gain weight, back to baseline normal weight, with trends of increasing weight each week at home and at each clinic visit.
      b. Increased weight will be primarily muscle mass, rather than fat tissue, as measured by bioelectrical impedance analysis.

II. Diagnosis 2
  A. Fatigue, as evidenced by expressions of feeling tired, and limited activity during average day.
    1. Interventions
      a. Encourage pacing of activity throughout the day to maximize self-care ability
      b. Instruct that adequate antiretroviral medications will improve fatigue, and increase activity tolerance
      c. Allow for expressions of frustration related to decreased activity levels
      d. Assess sleep pattern and number of sleeping hours
    2. Outcomes
      a. Thomas gradually increases activity tolerance as evidenced by decreased lethargy, decreased sensations of fatigue, and decreased exertional dyspnea.
      b. Thomas expresses improved quality of life related to increased ability to perform necessary and desired activities.

III. Diagnosis 3
  A. Ineffective coping, as evidenced by expressions of distress about HIV diagnosis.
    1. Interventions
      a. Appraise the client's understanding of the disease process
      b. Provide an atmosphere of acceptance
      c. Use a calm, reassuring approach
      d. Instruct client about disease process, efficacy of medical treatment
      e. Use active listening about personal concerns and fears about HIV disease and its treatment
      f. Encourage questioning of medical provider about treatment options, side effects, and efficacy of treatment
      g. Encourage the client to develop social support structures, such as family members, friends, or support groups
      h. Encourage verbalization of feelings, perceptions, and fears
      i. Assist the client in identifying appropriate short- and long-term goals
    2. Outcomes
      a. Client will verbalize acceptance of the diagnosis and resultant changes in self-image and lifestyle.
      b. Client will use available social support.
      c. Client will report decrease in negative feelings.

IV. Diagnosis 4
  A. Risk for Ineffective Management of Therapeutic Regimen, as evidenced by statement that "I hate to take medicines," history of previous health, and ineffective coping with diagnosis.
    1. Interventions
      a. Assess perceptions and feelings about antiretroviral medications and readiness to start taking them on a regular basis

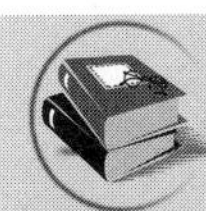

Case Study—cont'd

b. Assess perceptions about efficacy of medications and about chronic nature of treatment
c. Instruct about purpose of medication therapy and realistic outcomes of effective medication therapy
d. Instruct about potential for viral resistance with inconsistent medicine administration and assess readiness for alliance with treatment plan
e. Instruct about side effects and symptomatic treatment as needed
f. Instill realistic hope of suppression of viral replication, with resulting control of disease process, and relief of symptoms

2. Outcomes
   a. Client will participate in health care decisions and attend appointments as scheduled.
   b. Client will report taking medications according to schedule, thus reducing the risk of viral resistance.
   c. Client will verbalize understanding of disease process, and chronic nature of disease.

Next Visit, One Month Later

Thomas returned 1 month later with a 20-pound weight gain, increased energy levels, resolution of oral candidiasis, and expressions of gratitude for his returning feelings of health. He had experienced significant gastrointestinal distress and diarrhea with nelfinavir, so he began by taking only one pill 3 times a day "because it was too strong." He stated that he had only one pill left of the other medicine, but couldn't refill it because of the cost: "They told me that it would cost $500, and I can't pay that!" He has filed for disability because of his inability to work, but has not received a response about the decision. He has not been able to tell family or friends about his diagnosis, because he fears the stigma will affect his six children, whom he is raising alone because his wife left him several years ago. He fears for their well-being in the future because he thinks about his own future and the possibility of his dying before they are grown. Despite the difficulties, however, he feels a burgeoning hope, which accompanies his improved feelings of well-being.

Priority Nursing Diagnoses, Interventions, and Outcome Criteria

I. Diagnosis 1
   A. Ineffective Management of Therapeutic Regimen, as evidenced by subtherapeutic medication dosing.
      1. Interventions
         a. Instruct client about importance of full dosage of antiretroviral medications to prevent viral resistance
         b. Assess tolerance of side effects and willingness to return to full dose of medications
         c. Assess feelings about taking medications and perceptions about the benefits and difficulties in taking the medications on a regular basis
         d. Assist in problem-solving about the expressed difficulties of taking medications
         e. Reinforce importance of expressed benefits of taking medications
         f. Refer client to social services to obtain access to medication programs that will facilitate a continual supply of medications
      2. Outcomes
         a. Client will verbalize understanding about medicine schedule, and will report readiness to adhere to this schedule.
         b. Client will report decreased barriers to taking medications.

II. Diagnosis 2
   A. Diarrhea, related to medication therapy
      1. Interventions
         a. Teach client appropriate use of antidiarrhea medications
         b. Encourage adequate fluid intake to prevent dehydration
         c. Reassure that diarrhea is generally a short-term side effect to medication therapy and instill feelings of confidence that client will learn to cope with changes in life
      2. Outcomes
         a. Client will report decrease of diarrhea by 80%
         b. Client will report willingness to continue taking the offending medication

Next Visit, Three Months Later

In the intervening period, it became apparent that Thomas would not be able to tolerate this particular medication therapy because of intractable diarrhea. For this reason, nelfinavir was discontinued, and hard-gel saquinavir was substituted in its place, which required six pills 3 times per day. Additionally, the initial medication therapy did not suppress viral replication to the desired endpoint of an undetectable viral load. An additional antiretroviral medication was added to those already prescribed: nevirapine 200 mg BID. This brought his medication regimen to 23 pills per day: nine in the morning, six in the afternoon, and eight in the evening. At this visit to clinic, he complained about the pill burden; it filled him up to the point that he felt that he couldn't eat. He had gained 10 more pounds but was still well below his normal weight and he continued to be dissatisfied with his appearance. He began to feel more hopeless about his treatment, and his self-imposed lack of social support made him feel isolated. He had been declared disabled, but now received a disability check that was high enough that he could not received medicaid, which would have supplied health insurance and payment for prescription medications. His disability check was low enough, however, that financial stress added to his other stresses, exacerbating his feelings of hopelessness.

Priority Nursing Diagnoses, Interventions, and Outcome Criteria

I. Diagnosis 1
   A. Hopelessness, as evidenced by expressions of hopelessness and depressed mood.
      1. Interventions
         a. Assist client to identify areas of hope in life
         b. Assist client to devise and revise goals related to health outcome

Continued

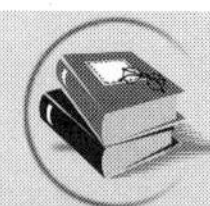

Case Study—cont'd

c. Facilitate client's incorporating change of self-perception into his body image
d. Encourage mutual goal-setting and involvement in decision-making about health care
e. Facilitate the development of a social support network
f. Refer to social services for access to financial assistance programs that may be able to decrease financial stress

2. Outcomes
   a. Client will express realistic optimism, and a sense of self-control
   b. Client will set realistic short- and long-term goals for his health outcome and for his family situation
   c. Client will engage social support structures to improve coping

Two Years Later

Two years later, after two further medication changes resulting from intolerance of side effects and viral resistance, Thomas has lost 15 pounds and reports increased fatigue. Laboratory values indicate a decreasing CD4 count and a high viral load despite consistent medication administration. Thomas has told his family about his diagnosis and they are supportive of him, providing the assistance that he needs at home for care of his children as well as meal preparation. His mother, who had previously lost a child to AIDS, is providing the bulk of the help at home. Thomas complains of poor appetite: "I get hungry, and then after my mother fixes what I want, I don't want it anymore. I can only eat about two bites and then I can't eat any more." Thomas has started having numbness and pain in his legs, which inhibits his ability to get around. Thomas has accepted that he will not live much longer, and has decided to stop taking his medicines "since they make me feel so bad." He expresses gratitude for the extra years he had to live because of the medical treatment he has been receiving, but recognizes that it is no longer working and no longer wants to continue with it.

Priority Nursing Diagnoses, Interventions, and Outcome Criteria

I. Diagnosis 1
   A. Chronic pain related to HIV-induced peripheral neuropathy.
      1. Interventions
         a. Assess pain: location, onset/duration, characteristics, frequency, quality, intensity, and precipitating and relieving factors
         b. Discuss with health care provider the need for adequate pain management to maximize activity tolerance and quality of life
         c. Evaluate current pain control and intervene as needed to improve pain control
         d. Encourage pain medicine administration before desired activity
         e. Promote adequate rest/sleep to facilitate pain relief
         f. Encourage pharmacological, nonpharmacological, and interpersonal pain relief measures, as appropriate
      2. Outcomes
         a. Client will express ability to perform desired activities unlimited by pain
         b. Client will recognize symptoms of pain, and will intervene appropriately
         c. Client will report improved quality of life

II. Diagnosis 2
   A. Risk for Ineffective Coping, Family, as evidenced by mother being primary caretaker in second death of a child from AIDS.
      2. Interventions
         a. Request that mother come with client to clinic appointments to facilitate supportive communication
         b. Use active listening, encouragement of expression of positive and negative feelings about caregiver role
         c. Refer for supportive services as indicated, including home health, hospice, support groups, and respite services
         d. Encourage caregiver to seek help from other family members, as appropriate and needed
         e. Teach caregiver stress management techniques
         f. Support caregiver through anticipated grieving process, and encourage expression of grief
      2. Outcomes
         a. Caregiver will report manageable levels of stress
         b. Caregiver will have support through the anticipated and actual grieving process
         c. Available family members will provide support for the caregiver and client
         d. Appropriate community support services will be engaged

REFERENCES

Abrams, B., Duncan, D., & Hertz-Picciotto, I. (1993). A prospective study of dietary intake and acquired immune deficiency syndrome in HIV-seropositive homosexual men. *Journal of Acquired Immune Deficiency Syndrome, 6,* 949-958.

Bartlett, J.G. (1999). *Medical management of HIV infection.* Baltimore, MD: Johns Hopkins University, Department of Infectious Diseases.

Boss, B.J. (1998). Alterations of neurologic function. In K.L. McCance & S.E. Huether (Eds), *Pathophysiology: The biologic basis for disease in adults and children.* (3rd ed., pp. 510-573). St. Louis: Mosby.

Broder, S., Merigan, T.C., & Bolognesi, D. (1994). *Textbook of AIDS medicine.* Baltimore: Williams & Wilkins.

Centers for Disease Control and Prevention. (1999). http://www.CDC.gov.

Dolin, R., Masur, H., Saag, M.S. (1999). *AIDS therapy.* New York: Churchill Livingstone.

Dowell, J., & Hudson, H. (1997). A qualitative study of medication-taking behaviour in primary care. *Family Practice, 14,* 369-375.

Ewing, J.A. (1984). Detecting alcoholism: The CAGE questionnaire. *Journal of the American Medical Association, 252,* 1905-1907.

Gallagher, D.M. (1993). Gastrointestinal manifestations of HIV/AIDS. *Critical Care Nursing Clinics of North America, 5,* 121-126.
Gordon, M. (2000). *Manual of nursing diagnosis* (9th Ed.). St. Louis: Mosby.
Grossman, A.H. (1999). The needs of special populations: Older adults. In P.J. Ungvarski & J.H Flaskerud (Eds.). *HIV/AIDS: A guide to primary care management* (4th ed., pp. 296-297). Philadelphia: WB Saunders.
Guyton, A.C. & Hall, J.E. (1996). *Textbook and medical physiology* (9th ed.). Philadelphia: WB Saunders.
Harris, M.I. (1998). Diabetes in America: Epidemiology and scope of the problem. Diabetes Care, 21 (Suppl. 3), C11-C14.
Huether, S.E. & Tomky, D. (1998). Alterations of hormonal regulation. In K.L. McCance & S. E. Huether (Eds.) *Pathophysiology: The biologic basis for disease in adults and children.* (3rd ed., pp. 656-706). St. Louis: Mosby.
Hurley, P., & Ungvarski, P. (1994). Home healthcare needs of adults living with HIV disease/AIDS in New York City. *Journal of Association of Nurses in AIDS Care, 5,* 33-40.
Johnson, M., Maas, M., & Moorhead, S. (Eds.). (2000). *Nursing outcomes classification (NOC)* (2nd ed.). St. Louis: Mosby.
Johnson, J.T. & Yu, V.L. (Eds.) (1997). *Infectious disease and antimicrobial therapy of the ears, nose, and throat.* Philadelphia: WB Saunders.
Mandell, G.L., Bennett, J.E., & Dolin, R. (1995). *Principles and practice of infectious diseases* (4th ed.). New York: Churchill Livingstone.
McCance, K.L. & Huether, S.E. (1998). *Pathophysiology: The biologic basis for disease in adults and children* (3rd ed.). St. Louis: Mosby.
McCloskey, J.C. & Bulechek, G.M. (Eds.). (2000). *Nursing interventions classifications (NIC)* (3rd ed.). St. Louis: Mosby.
Morris, L.S., & Schulz, R.M. (1993). Medication compliance: The client's perspective. *Clinical Therapeutics, 15,* 593-606.
Nielsen, K. (1999). Pediatric HIV infection. *Medscape, HIV Clinical Management Series, Vol. 12.* http://www.medscape.com/medscape/HIV/ClinicalMgmt/CM.v12/public/index-CM.v12.html
O'Brien, M., & Pheifer, W.G. (1993). Physical and psychosocial nursing care for patients with HIV infection. *Nursing Clinics of North America, 28,* 303-316.
O'Dell, M.W. (1996). HIV-related neurological disability and prospects for rehabilitation. *Disability and Rehabilitation, 18,* 285-292.
Piano, M.R. & Huether, S.E. (1998). Mechanisms of hormonal regulation. In K.L. McCance & S.E. Huether (Eds.) *Pathophysiology: The biologic basis for disease in adults and children* (3rd ed., pp. 625-655). St. Louis: Mosby.
Price, R.W. (1999). Neurologic disease. In R. Dolin, H. Masur, & M.S. Saag (Eds.), *AIDS Therapy* (pp. 620-638). New York: Churchill Livingstone.
Remien, R.H., Satriano, J., & Berkman, A. (1999). Acquired immune deficiency syndrome and human immunodeficiency virus. In M.G. Eisenberg, R.L. Glueckauf, & H.H. Zaretsky (Eds.) *Medical aspects of disability* (pp. 53-67). New York: Springer.
Risi, G.F. & Tomascak, V. (1998). Prevention of infection in the immunocompromised host. *American Journal of infection Control, 26,* 594-603.
Sande, M.A. & Volberding, P.A. (1999). *The medical management of AIDS* (6th ed.). Philadelphia: WB Saunders.
Schutz, M., & Wendrow, A. (2000). *Quick reference guide to antiretrovirals* [On-line]. Available: http://hiv.medscape.com/updates/quickguide.
Talal, A.H. & Dieterich, D.T. (1999). Gastrointestinal and hepatic manifestations of HIV infection. In M.A. Sande & P.A. Volberding (Eds.). *The medical management of AIDS* (6th ed., pp. 195-216). Philadelphia: WB Saunders.
Trostle, J.A. (1997). The history and meaning of patient compliance as an ideology. In D.S. Gochman (Ed.), *Handbook of health behavior research* (vol. 2, pp. 109-124). New York: Plenum Press.
Wong, D.L., Hockenberry-Eaton, M., Wilson, D., Winkelstein, M.L., Ahmann, E., & DiVito-Thomas, P.A. (2000). *Whaley & Wong's nursing care of infants and children* (6th ed.). St. Louis: Mosby.

34 Renal Rehabilitation

Christy A. Price, MSN, RN, NP

Here is a couple in their late 70s who have shared 40-plus years of life together. As with many aging Americans, they have had various aches and pains, but these never inhibited their active lifestyle in retirement years. Previously, the husband had been self-employed, and the wife was a homemaker caring for their five children. After the children married, she increased her voluntary community activities, in addition to helping with the grandchildren.

At 75 years of age and after many years of adult onset diabetes mellitus, the wife's condition advanced to the well known complication of end stage renal disease (ESRD). Not one to sit for long periods, the client and her husband chose peritoneal dialysis (PD) as the treatment of choice. The couple learned about her disease process and management and successfully completed training for home care. They willingly incorporated continuous ambulatory peritoneal dialysis (CAPD) into their active lifestyle. They assisted each other in performing her peritoneal exchanges four times per day. They learned to regulate her insulin dosing, giving consideration to the extra glucose she received with the high dextrose peritoneal solutions. On a couple of occasions during her 3 years of CAPD treatment, the client experienced peritonitis and required intraperitoneal antibiotic therapy. For brief periods it became medically necessary to undergo hemodialysis (HD) to remove excessive fluid and edema that had accumulated. Overall, CAPD was tremendously successful as her chronic renal replacement therapy. The couple continued to travel cross-country in their mobile recreational vehicle, visiting family and friends and exploring new territories. Her hearty laugh and his loving assistance allowed this couple to fully participate in activities of daily living and age-appropriate experiences. Eventually, because of the chronicity of the diabetes and ESRD with the inherent clinical side effects and complications, the client made the decision to withdraw from her life-sustaining treatment, and with her family at her side she died a death with dignity at home.

Acute renal failure is the abrupt decline of normal renal function, usually within a period of 3 days to 3 weeks. The primary causes are obstruction, exposure to nephrotoxic drugs, and ischemia after prolonged hypotension, leading to acute tubular necrosis (ATN). Elderly persons who undergo extensive cardiac and vascular surgeries and critically ill clients with multiple system failure are representative of most individuals affected by acute renal failure. Some survive their acute renal insult, only to suffer ESRD because of the injury resulting to kidney function. Humans lose 1 ml/min of glomerular filtration rate (GFR) for every year after age 40 (Mathers, 1998). Along with the natural aging process, concurrent events or conditions, such as surgeries, infections, hemorrhaging, cardiomyopathy, hypertension, and diabetes mellitus, directly influence or compromise renal function in the acutely ill and elderly.

Chronic renal failure (ESRD) often has an insidious onset over 3 months to 20 years or results from complications of acute renal failure that is unresolved within 3 months. ESRD means cessation of normal renal function at a level in which the client cannot sustain life without dialysis or kidney transplantation. In the United States the primary causes of ESRD in 1997 were diabetes mellitus (41%), hypertension (27%), and glomerulonephritis (11%) (U.S. Renal Data System [USRDS], 1999). Clients with adult onset diabetes account for 29% of the total population with ESRD. Clients with diabetes and hypertension account for the majority of persons with ESRD; however, this condition is associated with other diseases, including polycystic kidney disease, secondary vasculitis, hereditary nephritis, drug-induced nephropathy, and pyelonephritis.

Clients have potential for multiple metabolic disturbances, such as electrolyte imbalances, fluid imbalance, bone disease, anemia, uremia, risk for infections, risk for bleeding, skin disorders, altered glycemic control, and hypertension. All of these diagnoses are accepted by the North American Nursing Diagnosis Association (NANDA) (Gordon, 2000). In addition, persons with ESRD are confronted with significant dietary restrictions, extensive medication regimens, individualized dialysis prescriptions, frequent comorbid conditions, and procedural complications from their dialysis treatments and/or renal transplantation. The nursing interventions are covered under the Nursing Interventions Classification (NIC), although specific interventions necessary for the renal client may be modified from the NIC (McCloskey & Bulechek, 2000).

REHABILITATION OF THE CLIENT WITH ESRD

Successful rehabilitation of clients with ESRD has long been recognized as one of the failures of the medicare ESRD program. With passage of PL92-603 in 1972, which assured persons who are eligible for medicare coverage of renal dialysis and transplantation regardless of age, with as few as about 10,000 persons with ESRD receiving dialysis treatment in the United States, estimates were for roughly 70% of these individuals to receive kidney transplants and most to return to gainful employment (Evans, Blagg, & Bryan, 1981; Iglehart, 1993). These objectives have never been realized, primarily because the providers shifted the focus of dialysis and transplantation to technology and pharmaceutical advances. The biochemical and physiological concerns overshadowed clients' psychosocial and emotional concerns; financial and scientific agenda arbitraged clients' longevity and took precedence over their quality of life. Table 34-1 shows the growth in the number of clients with ESRD from 1970 to 1998 (USRDS, 1999; Maxwell & Sapolsky, 1987). Table 34-2 shows the distribution of clients with ESRD among dialysis settings as well as the percentage of clients receiving in-center hemodialysis treatment compared with home dialysis therapy and those who received a renal transplant (*Nephrology News & Issues,* 2000). In the early years of dialysis, nearly 75% of clients were treated with home dialysis, which emphasized independence, self-care, and rehabilitation for age-appropriate tasks.

The most controversial issue in ESRD treatment today is selection of individuals for chronic renal replacement therapy and identification of those to be withdrawn from therapy. Who decides when the burden of disease and necessary treatment outweigh benefits (McCormick, 1993)? In the 1960s, client selection committees decided who would be offered dialysis. Often referred to as "Death Committees," their selection criteria are listed in Box 34-1 (Price, 1992; Fox & Swazey, 1974; Alexander, 1962). By 1999, exclusionary criteria were eliminated, granting universal access to services so that merely the discovery of ESRD ensures treatment, regardless of defined benefit to the client. A lack of appropriate evaluation of clients created an inequity in medicare funding; that is to say, chronic care for 0.05% of those eligible for medicare engulf nearly 5% of the entire medicare budget, amounting to a covered amount of approximately $42,000 per person per year for dialysis only (USRDS, 1999). Since medicare pays 80% of expenses, remaining funds are obtained from medicaid, private insurance, or self-payment. As the largest financier of dialysis services, medicare allocates more than $18 billion annually to care for 93% of clients with ESRD. In 1999, a work group with physicians specializing in nephrology, nurses, social workers, clients, ethicists, federal government employees, and primary and critical care physicians met to develop a clinical guideline: the Shared Decision Making for the Appropriate Initiation and Withdrawal of Dialysis for Clients

TABLE 34-1 Growth of ESRD (Dialysis and Renal Transplant) Population

Year	No. of Clients
1970	2,398 (dialysis only)
1972	4,981 (dialysis only)
1973	7,498 (dialysis only)
1974	10,306 (dialysis only)
1975	13,417 (dialysis only)
1978	48,000
1981	68,200
1983	90,000
1988	145,000
1990	160,000
1992	190,000
1995	250,000
1996	270,000
1997	307,967
1998	344,863
2000	+500,000 (estimate)

Before and after enforcement of PL92-603.

TABLE 34-2 Distribution of ESRD Clients in the United States in 1998

Dialysis Setting	No. of Clients	Percent of Total Receiving Dialysis
Incenter hemodialysis	215,960	88%
Freestanding clinics	2,970	
Hospital-based units	914	
Home peritoneal dialysis	27,793	11%
Home hemodialysis	1,607	0.6%
Clients with kidney transplant	99,503	
Total ESRD clients	344,863	

Data from the Health Care Finance Administration (HCFA), Office of Clinical Standards and Quality. Washington, DC: U.S. Department of Health and Human Services. www.hcfa.gov/quality.

Box 34-1 Selection Criteria for Dialysis in the United States Before 1972

- Usually younger than 50 years and older than 6 years; average age: 42 years
- Medical suitability—single organ failure, absence of diabetes mellitus and other disabling disease or comorbidities
- Willingness to cooperate with the treatment regimen; no noncompliant or disruptive behaviors
- Intelligence and understanding of disease and treatment; no dementia, mental retardation, or vegetative state
- Likelihood of vocational rehabilitation, essentially gainful employment
- Availability of vacancy for treatment and finances; few centers and self-pay or insurance
- Psychiatric evaluation for suitability (very subjective)

Data from Alexander, S. (1962). They decide who lives, who dies. *Life Magazine,* 102-125; and Fox, R., & Swazey, J. (1974). *The courage to fail: A social view of organ transplantation and dialysis.* Chicago: University of Chicago Press.

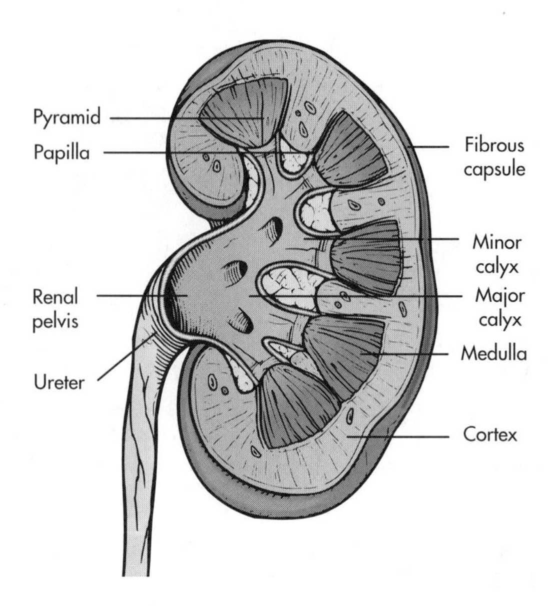

Figure 34-1 Frontal section of the kidney. (From Phipps, W.J., Sands, J.K., & Marek, J.F. [1999]. *Medical-surgical nursing: Concepts and clinical practice* [6th ed.]. St. Louis: Mosby.)

with ARF and ESRD (*Nephrology News & Issues,* 2000). The group proposed nine recommendations for consideration of appropriate dialysis therapy and/or withdrawal. The goals of the guideline are to promote shared decision making between professionals and clients and to promote sound ethical and medical decision making in light of the person's condition.

COMPREHENSIVE CARE OF THE CLIENT WITH ESRD

Care of clients with renal failure requires the specialty knowledge and practice skills of multiple professionals. Every person with this condition has, at a minimum, a primary care provider, nephrologist, nephrology nurse, social worker, and renal dietitian involved in the care. As in other health services, an advanced practice registered nurse greatly enhances the care and outcomes for clients. Unfortunately, most dialysis centers no longer provide the services of a rehabilitation counselor. Apart from hospitalization, in which acutely ill persons have numerous providers, clients with ESRD need varying levels and kinds of services and providers at certain periods in the course of their illness. Many clients with ESRD lead very active, productive lives and are fully engaged in family and community activities, whereas some clients require occasional home health care, physical or occupational therapy, or other rehabilitative services.

At one time, when the average age of clients with renal disease was 42 years, rehabilitation meant returning the client to gainful employment. With a current average age of clients with renal disease close to 64 years, rehabilitation goals have shifted to having clients with ESRD achieve age-appropriate developmental tasks that are comparable with those of their age-mates in the general population. Clients who are debilitated or deconditioned need extended and extensive community services. However, whether services are provided is regulated by insurance or other reimbursement sources, rather than client needs. For some, rehabilitation consists of referral to specific community services for transportation, grocery and pharmacy delivery, and information about opportunities for peer interaction or socialization. Finally, hospice or end of life care is available to those who decide to forego or withdraw dialysis therapy. Hospice or other professionals specializing in terminal care must be involved to ensure death with dignity.

OVERVIEW OF RENAL ANATOMY

Macroanatomy

Most humans (more than 90%) have two kidneys at birth. Since one kidney is sufficient for proper physiological functioning, a person may not discover until later in life that he or she has only one kidney. The gross anatomy is not complex; the kidneys sit retroperitoneal and between T12 and L3. An adult kidney weighs about 300 g, is 10 to 13 cm long, and 5 to 7 cm wide. Kidneys have one or more renal arteries and veins that receive blood from the heart and return it back into the vascular circulation. The kidneys are profused with approximately 25% of the cardiac output, or 1 to 2 L/min, processed at the glomerulus. A single ureter delivers urine to the bladder at a rate of 1½ to 2 L/24 hours. The kidney is surround by a protective cover called the *cortex.* Figures 34-1 and 34-2 illustrate the gross anatomy of the kidney and components of the urinary system.

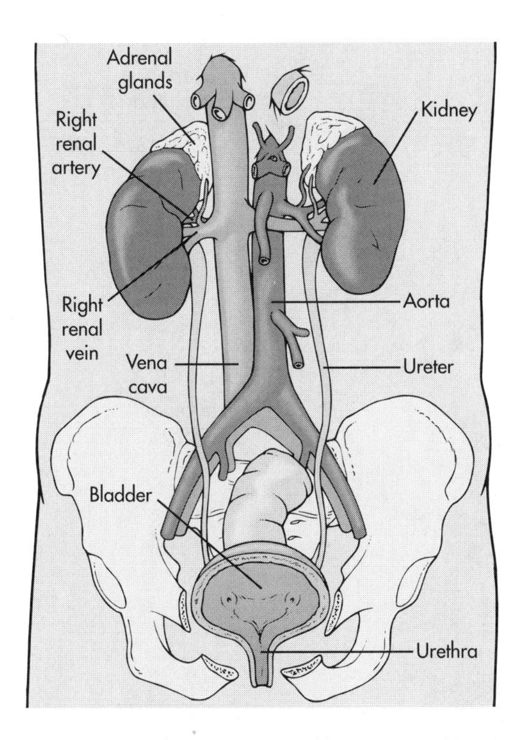

Figure 34-2 Organs and structures of the urinary system. (From Lewis, S.L., Collier, I.C., Heitkemper, M.M., & Dirksen, S.R. [2000]. *Medical-surgical nursing: Assessment and management of clinical problems.* [5th ed.]. St. Louis: Mosby.)

Microanatomy

The microanatomy of the kidney is very complex in structure and function. The kidney is separated into the outer cortical region and the inner medullary region. Within the cortex and juxtamedullary section, each kidney has nearly 1 million nephrons, or functional units. Each nephron is comprised of a glomerulus; Bowman's capsule; proximal convoluted tubule; loop of Henle; distal convoluted tubule; collecting duct; and a peritubular capillary system, or vasa recta. Figure 34-3 depicts the microscopic renal anatomy.

OVERVIEW OF RENAL PHYSIOLOGY

Functionally, the kidneys are responsible for maintaining the body's internal milieu or homeostasis, acid-base balance, electrolytes and fluid balance, removal of toxins or waste products, and production or regulation of certain hormones or biochemical factors (Lancaster, 2001). To achieve the balance and precision of maintaining physiology, the processes controlled by the kidneys must occur without interruption. As outlined in Table 34-3, each segment of the nephron performs a special task toward normal kidney function.

Glomerulus

The renal processes begin at the glomerulus where an ultrafiltrate of whole blood is created. Ultrafiltrate consists of formed cells that are protein free and isotonic with plasma, which helps explain why hematuria and proteinuria are abnormal (Whelan & Whelan, 1999). Creatinine is freely filtered at the glomerulus across the Bowman's capsule and not appreciably reabsorbed or secreted in the remainder of the tubule system. This process makes creatinine clearance the gold standard for assessing kidney function or GFR. Normal GFR for adults is 100 to 125 ml/min for males and is 85% less than this amount for females, or 85 to 110 ml/min. Recalling that kidney function begins to decline at age 40 years, it is extremely important to consider overall health status in estimates of kidney function. Table 34-4 provides the clearance ranges for level of kidney dysfunction.

TABLE 34-3 Description of Functions of the Nephron by Segments

Segment of Nephron	Functions
Glomerulus	Creates an ultrafiltrate of plasma (formed cells that are protein free)
Proximal tubule	Reabsorbs two thirds of filtered Na^+, Cl^-, and H_2O
	Reabsorbs HCO_3^-, glucose, K^+, PO_4, proteins, uric acid, amino acids
	Secretes H^+, NH_4^+, organic acids, and bases
Loop of Henle	Reabsorbs NaCl
Distal tubule	Reabsorbs Na^+, Cl^-, and H_2O
	Secretes H^+, K^+, and NH_4^+
Collecting duct	Reabsorbs Na^+, Cl^-, and H_2O
	Secretes H^+, K^+, and NH_4

TABLE 34-4 Distribution of Renal Dysfunction

Classification of Renal Failure	Lost Function (%)	Creatinine Clearance (ml/min)	Serum Creatinine (mg/dl)
Normal renal function	0	80-125	0.7-1.2
Diminished renal reserve (DRR)	50	>50	1.8-2.5
Chronic renal insufficiency (CRI)	75	>20	2.8-6.5
End stage renal failure (ESRD)	85-90	<10-15	4.0-10+

NOTE: Estimate of renal function is dependent on age, lean body weight, and sex and will be altered by these variables.

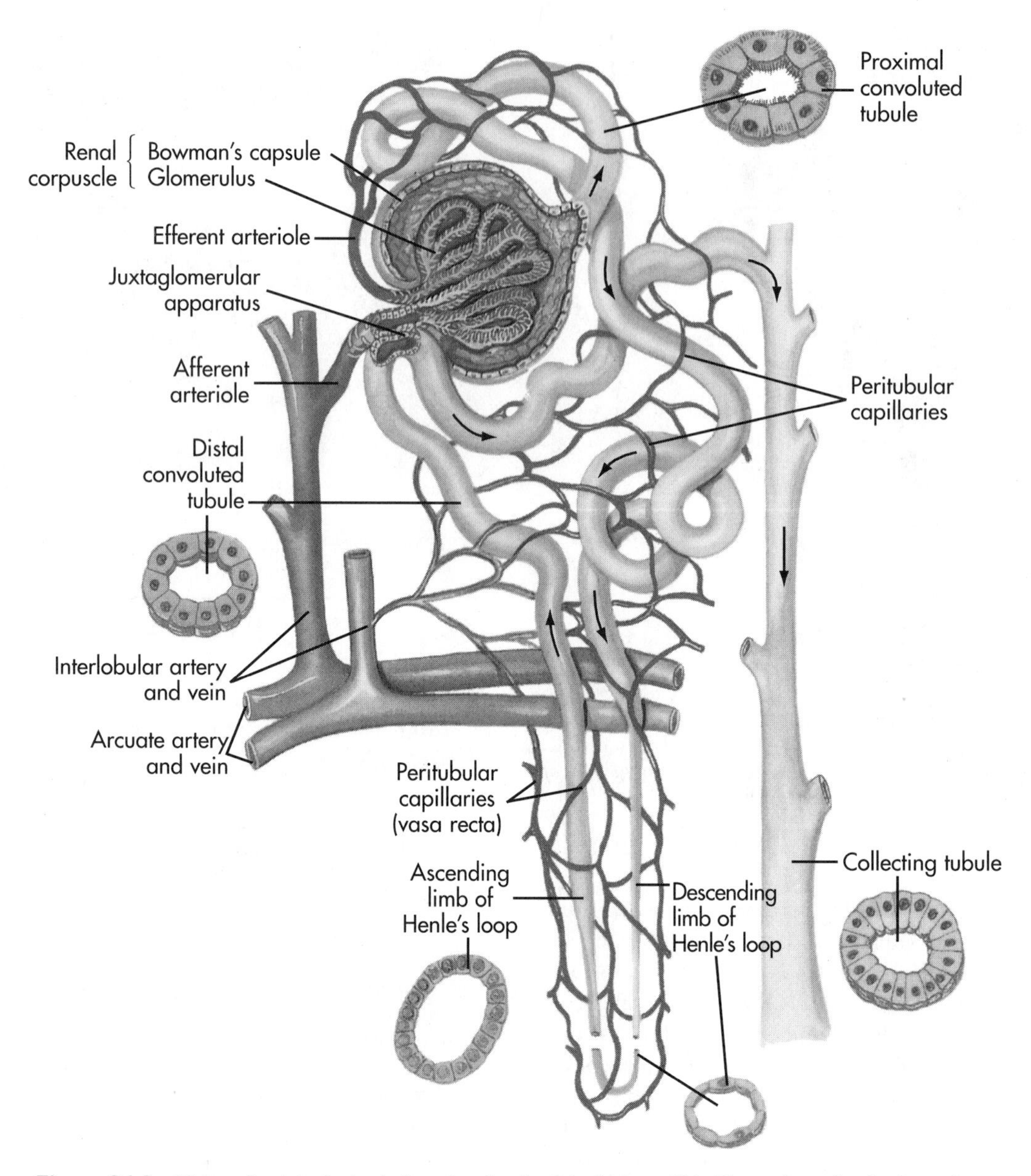

Figure 34-3 The nephron is the basic functional unit of the kidney. This illustration of a single nephron unit also shows the surrounding peritubular blood vessels. (From Thibodeau, G.A., & Patton, K.T. [1999]. *Anatomy & physiology* [4th ed.]. St. Louis: Mosby.)

The Cockcroft and Gault formula is commonly used to calculate creatinine clearance (Zawada, 1994).

$$\text{Creatinine clearance} = (140 - \text{Age in years}) \times \text{Weight in kilograms} \div 72 \times \text{Serum creatinine}$$

A systemic infection, radiographic procedure, prolonged hypotension, or aggressive surgical intervention may add insult to function of an already deteriorating kidney. Equally important is the protein binding status of drugs (e.g., heparin, warfarin, antibiotics, and digoxin) that should not be filtered at the glomerulus. Therefore, drug monitoring for therapeutic levels is essential for anyone with kidney dysfunction. The natural aging process and its relationship to kidney function and drug metabolism must also be factored into interventions and pharmacological management.

Similar to all solid organs, the kidney depends on sufficient pressure to function. It has an amazing ability to autoregulate effectively within mean arterial blood pressures between 80 and 180 mm Hg. The afferent and efferent arterioles are capable of dilating or constricting as necessary to accommodate high or low pressures. However, autoregulation stops at a systolic blood pressure of about 70 mm Hg, or mean arterial pressure of 60 mm Hg. This phenomenon explains the damage incurred to kidney function when clients remain in a state of prolonged hypotension. Damage may begin if hypoperfusion states exist beyond 30 minutes.

Proximal Convoluted Tubule

The processing of the ultrafiltrate begins immediately in the proximal tubule. The body essentially takes back the electrolytes and nutrients necessary to maintain the proper internal milieu. Namely, sodium, potassium, urea, bicarbonate, glucose, phosphates, amino acids, water, and so forth are reabsorbed in sufficient quantity into the peritubular system for return to the general circulation. The reabsorption of bicarbonate is the primary renal component that contributes to proper acid-base balance of the body. The pulmonary system contributes by regulating carbon dioxide blood content. Together they maintain proper blood pH between 7.35 and 7.45. The kidneys also process the ammonia ion and titrated acids to contribute to proper acid-base balance.

If the transmembrane potential, or necessary amount of a particular factor, is exceeded, then the excessive amount will remain in the filtrate and be eliminated in the urine. This phenomenon can be seen in a person with diabetes whose blood glucose level is elevated or in a person under stress after surgery with glucose found in the urine (if the serum glucose level exceeds 180 mg/ml, the transmembrane potential for glucose has been reached).

Loop of Henle

The loop of Henle is primarily responsible for the processing of sodium, chloride, and water. Through a complex system of countercurrent multipliers and an exchange mechanism and a sodium chloride pump, the kidney concentrates and dilutes urine. The thin descending loop is permeable to water, concentrating the filtrate as water moves out into the peritubular capillary system, or vasa recta. The thick ascending loop is impermeable to water, having a diluting effect when sodium and chloride move out as the filtrate moves along the loop up to the distal convoluted tubule.

Distal Convoluted Tubule

The distal convoluted tubule receives this hypo-osomotic, very dilute urine from the loop of Henle. A major function of this segment of the nephron is to reabsorb the water and sodium depending on current physiological needs. The distal tubule operates in part under the influence of renin and aldosterone. Renin stimulates the liver and lungs to produce angiotensin I and angiotensin II, respectively. Angiotensin, a very potent vasoconstrictor, elevates blood pressure; renin also stimulates the secretion of aldosterone from the adrenal medulla, allowing the kidneys to hold on to sodium in exchange for potassium.

The initial section of the distal tubule has a region of very specialized cells called the *juxtaglomerular apparatus,* or *macula densa* (see Figure 34-3). The macula densa borders a segment of the afferent arteriole that eventually receives the blood from the renal artery. The afferent arteriole pushes against the macula densa only when the circulatory volume and pressure of the blood inside the arteriole are high. The volume reflects the hydration status; hypervolumemia results in a high pressure, and hypovolumemia results in a low pressure. High pressure and volume are interpreted as a need to relieve the volume, and therefore the macula densa does not secrete renin and the adrenal glands do not secrete aldosterone. Alternatively, in a low pressure state the macula densa secretes renin, leading to secretion of angiotensin and aldosterone. The distal tubule responds by reabsorbing sodium and water. This mechanism operates consistently and assists the body in maintaining a normal circulatory volume and blood pressure. This is the same mechanism of action exerted by a class of drugs prescribed for hypertension—angiotensin-converting enzyme (ACE) inhibitors and a relatively new class of antihypertensive drugs called angiotensin receptor blockers (ARBs). On the other hand, some clients take potassium sparing diuretics, such as spironolactone, amiloride, and triamterene to prevent the excessive loss of potassium in the distal tubule.

Collecting Duct

The distal tubule and collecting duct are the sites of action of antidiuretic hormone (ADH). As its name implies, ADH halts removal of water in this final segment of the nephron. ADH is secreted by the posterior pituitary gland in response to osmotic receptors in the carotid bodies and right atrium of the heart. The collecting duct of the nephron operates under the influence of ADH to assist in maintaining normal blood volume and osomolarity. Caffeine, alcohol, and cold temperature trigger ADH secretion, explaining the increased need to urinate.

Secretion, another important process, takes place throughout the nephron but mainly in the distal tubule. Secretion is a process whereby the body removes, or eliminates, unnecessary or unneeded elements, such as potassium, antibiotics, acids, phosphates, and a small amount of creatinine. It transfers electrolytes, drugs, ammonia, and other elements from the peritubular capillary system into the tubule to be excreted in the urine.

Hormone Production

The kidney, particularly the nephrons and peritubular capillary system, act to maintain the harmony and balance in the body. When homeostasis is disrupted, life cannot be sustained apart from pharmacological, nutritional, and renal replacement therapy supports. The kidneys also are a site of action and responsible for production of proteins and the hormones erythropoietin and prostaglandins. Erythropoietin stimulates the bone marrow to produce red blood cells; without this stimulus individuals eventually become severely anemic. Prostaglandins play a role in blood pressure control and filtration at the glomerulus.

FACTORS ASSOCIATED WITH FUNCTIONAL HEALTH STATUS

Epidemiology of Renal Disease

ESRD may present as a single system or a multi-organ failure disease; in either case, all aspects of life are affected. Not only are clients subject to restrictions or barriers to their lifestyle, they have many questions and fears. This population of clients has had sufficient exposure to dialysis therapy and transplantation to dread lifelong reliance on machines, dietary restrictions, frequent infections and morbidity, repeated hospitalizations, and constant confrontation with the high mortality associated with ESRD. Once dialysis begins, life expectancy shortens significantly, averaging less than 8 years for clients older than 40 (USRDS, 1999). Mortality rates vary with age at onset, ethnicity, and renal diagnosis and range from fewer than 2 years to 18 years (USRDS, 1999). When an individual decides to withdraw from dialysis voluntarily, life expectancy can be less than 1, to perhaps 3, weeks.

Approximately 70% of those with ESRD have a comorbid diagnosis of diabetes mellitus and/or hypertension, both of which are known to place undue stress on the body and its functions. Similarly, too many adults and children are overweight and lead sedentary lives. These conditions eventually may damage the kidneys, although they may be managed through lifestyle changes. In 1997, the incidence of ESRD in the United States was 287 per 1 million persons, with a prevalence of 1105 per 1 million persons (USRDS, 1999). The incidence and prevalence of chronic kidney failure continues to rise but could be curtailed under the recommendations of *Healthy People 2002* and *Healthy People 2010.* In particular, *Health People 2010* identifies chronic kidney disease as a target area because of the psychosocial impact and the clinical and financial resources involved in treatment.

Ethnic Variables

Chronic renal disease does not discriminate among socioeconomic, ethnic, or cultural variables. Whether related to genetics, access to adequate health care, nutrition, education, or other factors, African Americans have a high incidence of hypertension. African Americans, followed by Native Americans, have a greater incidence of chronic renal disease and diabetes mellitus than do Caucasian, Asian, or Pacific Island peoples (USRDS 1999 Annual Data Report, 1999). Age increases likelihood of ESRD; it is uncommon in individuals younger than 18 years. Use of illegal and/or certain legal drugs, such as nonsteroidal anti-inflammatory drugs (NSAIDs), are implicated as a cause in the United States.

NURSING PROCESS

Nursing Assessment

The nursing assessment begins with the initial history and physical examination for gathering objective and subjective data. The complete history includes chief complaint, present medical illnesses, past medical history, family history, social history, medications, allergies, lifestyle activities, and a review of systems. Collect data in light of the client's renal function (e.g., diminished renal reserve, chronic renal insufficiency [CRI], or ESRD). The client's renal function will dictate nursing interventions and planning for total health care needs.

When obtaining the history, the nurse pays particular attention to and documents risk factors for kidney dysfunction, such as hypertension, obesity, diabetes, smoking, prescription and nonprescription drug history, and hereditary diseases. Excessive intake of NSAIDs can have a negative effect on function of both normal and compromised kidneys. Document use of herbal medicines or dietary supplements. Ask questions about predisposing factors, concurrent illnesses, lifestyle practices, and environmental stimuli that have the potential for worsening the renal dysfunction or complicating the treatment modality. For the acutely ill person, include data about recent surgeries, infections, hemorrhaging, or prolonged illness.

Physical Examination

In addition to conducting a comprehensive physical examination, the nurse assesses for conditions and nursing diagnoses that relate to chronic renal failure (Staney, 1996). Assessment components specifically related to ESRD and potential findings and nursing diagnoses are presented in Table 34-5.

Nursing Diagnoses

The potential medical and nursing diagnoses related to clients with ESRD are numerous because of the complex nature of kidney dysfunction, the etiology of the individual's disease, the secondarily involved organ systems, and the need for aggressive dialytic and/or transplant therapies. Clients are at risk for hyperkalemia and hypokalemia, hypercalcemia and hypocalcemia, azotemia, anemia, chronic cough, fluid overload, peripheral edema, pulmonary edema, dehydration, systemic and local infections, malnutrition, cerebral atrophy, muscle atrophy, cardiomyopathy, left ventricular hypertrophy, congestive heart failure, bleeding and clotting abnormalities, peripheral neuropathy, bone disease, diarrhea, fatigue, sexual dysfunction, sleep disturbances, and pain. Clients may have difficulty with coping effectively; fear and anxiety; mild to severe depression; dealing with anger, loss of independence, social isolation, and reliance on intricate life-sustaining technology; family role changes; and decreased life expectancy. Palliative and end of life care are essential for those who decide to forego or withdraw from dialysis. (All these diagnoses are classified in NANDA.)

The rehabilitation nurse is unlikely to find every problem in this huge spectrum of potential nursing and medical diagnoses in a client. However, the key to appropriate care of clients with ESRD is using the nursing process completely so that potential problems and unusual situations will be discovered and interventions will be timely and therapeutic. The goal for every client must be safe, effective therapy in a

TABLE 34-5 Physical Assessment Related to a Client with Renal Disease

System	Finding	Rationale
Neurological	Dizziness, lightheadedness	Uremia, hypotension, anemia
	Slow thought processes	Uremia, anemia, cerebral atrophy
	Decreased sensation	Peripheral neuropathy
Cardiac	Hypertension/hypotension	Fluid overload or dehydration
		Noncompliance of medication regimen
		Cardiomyopathy, CHF
	Irregular pulse	Hyperkalemia/hypokalemia, hypocalcemia
	S3, rub	Fluid overload, uremic pericarditis
Pulmonary	Cough, congestion,	CHF, fluid overload, medications side effect
	Decreased oxygenation	Fluid overload, pulmonary edema
	Decreased breath sounds	Rales, rhonchi, crackles
	Cyanosis, decreased capillary refill	Anemia
Gastrointestinal	Diarrhea	Uremia, dietary factors
	Constipation	Side effect of medications
	Epigastric pain/discomfort	Uremia, peritoneal fluid pressure
	Impaired gastric mobility	Side effect of diabetes
	Nausea/vomiting	Uremia, inadequate dialysis
	Occult blood in stool	Uremia, heparin dosing for HD or PD
Skin	Dryness, scaling	Dehydration, uremia
	Ulcerations	Hyperphosphatemia
	Erythema, induration	Hematoma over vascular access
	Erythema, drainage	HD or PD catheter site infection
	No bruit or thrill	Clotted vascular access
	Pruritus	Uremia, hyperphosphoremia
	Ecchymosis	Heparin dosing, hematoma
Musculoskeletal	Decreased DTRs	Hypokalemia
	Muscle weakness	Hyperkalemia/hypokalemia
	Muscle atrophy	Malnutrition
	Fatigue/poor endurance	Anemia
Reproductive	Decreased sexual function	Anemia, uremia
	Decreased libido	Anemia, depression
	Irregular menses	Uremia, hormone imbalance

NOTE: Client may have same or similar findings with different etiological factors. *CHF,* Congestive heart failure; *DTRs,* deep tendon reflexes; *PD,* peritoneal dialysis; *HD,* hemodialysis.

supportive, partially compensatory or fully compensatory approach that is individualized to his or her specific needs or death with dignity on the client's own terms. These goals are congruent with the Nursing Outcomes Classification (NOC) expectations (Johnson, Maas, & Moorhead, 2000).

Nursing Interventions for the Client Receiving Hemodialysis

More than half (62%) of clients with ESRD in the United States use in-center hemodialysis (HD) as their chronic renal replacement therapy (USRDS, 1999). Currently, fewer than 1% of clients use HD at home compared with nearly 70% in the 1970s. The rehabilitation nurse coordinates client therapies with the HD center treatment schedule. The NIC interventions may need to be adapted for individualized treatment.

Schedules

Information about the location of the dialysis center, hours of operation, and telephone and pager numbers for the physicians, nurses, social worker, and renal dietitian should be posted. The routine treatment schedule is 3 to 4 hours of HD on alternate days, 3 times per week. This means that the client will be away from home for 5 to 6 hours each treatment day; children are not scheduled during normal school hours.

Planning for care at home or in a rehabilitation center should not be done immediately before or after a client's HD treatment because the client will be the most biochemically imbalanced before dialysis and generally physically fatigued after dialysis. Clients receiving HD rarely feel completely well, partially because of the accumulation of uremic toxins resulting from their kidneys unable to function normally, which includes the processing of fluid, electrolytes, and toxins 24 hours per day. Furthermore, clients who are

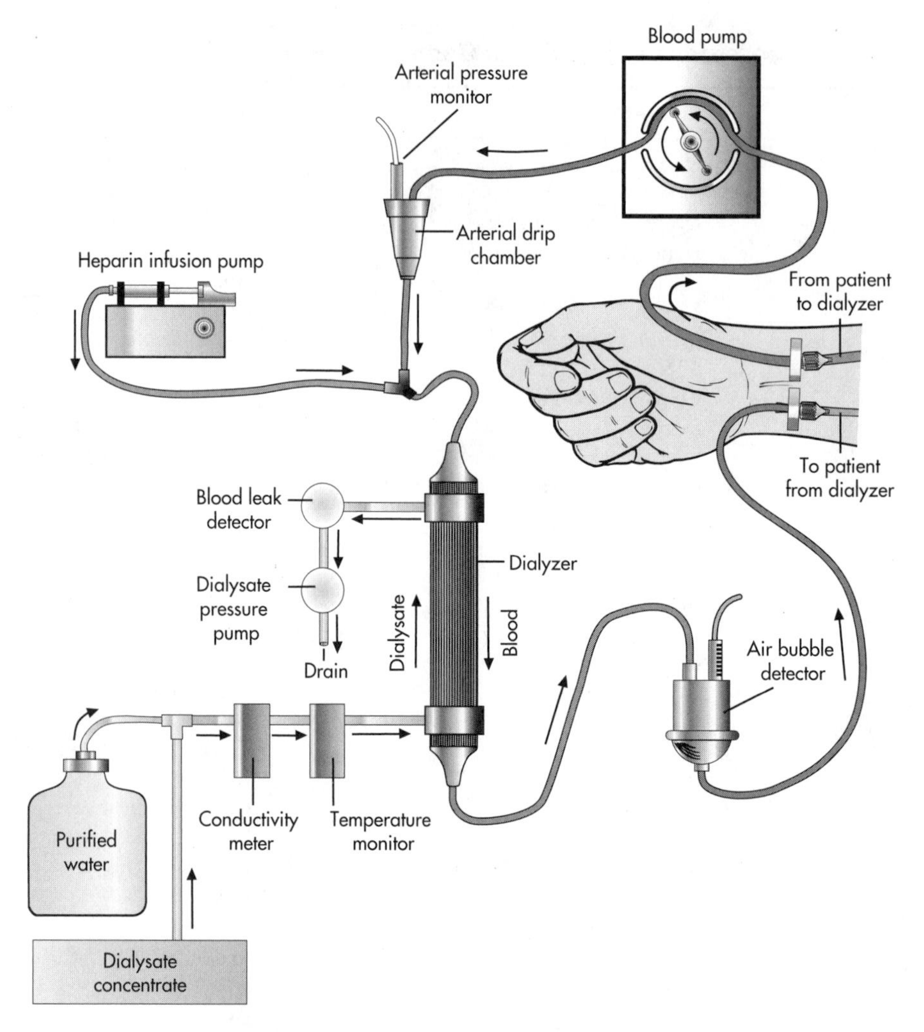

Figure 34-4 Components of a hemodialysis system. (From Lewis, S.L., Collier, I.C., Heitkemper, M.M., & Dirksen, S. R., [2000]. *Medical surgical nursing: Assessment and management of clinical problems* [5th ed.]. St. Louis: Mosby.)

noncompliant with the total HD regimen (i.e., including diet modifications and a medication regimen) have more health-related problems with higher morbidity and mortality.

Treatment

Hemodialysis is a very aggressive life maintenance therapy that processes a client's total blood volume many times through an artificial kidney. Figure 34-4 demonstrates the components of an HD system; Figure 34-5 shows a hemodialysis machine. The HD process restores fluid balance; normalizes electrolytes; and removes uremic toxins through a complex system of pumps, pressures, concentration gradients, blood flow rates, dialysate flow rates, and ultrafiltration. Although HD maintains life, it falls far short as a facsimile of native renal function. Each month the dialysis prescription changes according to laboratory analyses of a comprehensive metabolic profile, complete blood count, and dialysis adequacy. Iron indices are obtained every 3 months, and aluminum and parathyroid hormone levels are measured semiannually.

Vascular Access

Each client has vascular access for the blood to process through the HD system. Figure 34-6 shows a native arteriovenous fistula (AVF) and a synthetic arteriovenous graft (AVG). These blood accesses are placed in the lower or upper arm, usually in the nondominant arm, or in the thigh area. Should problems occur or a clot form in the access, the other arm or leg remains an option. Unfortunately, most accesses do not last the same amount of time that the client receives dialysis, especially grafts that last less than 2 years; a native fistula lasts longer. Home care must include daily cleansing of the extremity, auscultating the bruit, feeling for the thrill, and observing for signs and symptoms of infection. The client cannot wear tight clothing or jewelry. The vascular access extremity is not used for measuring

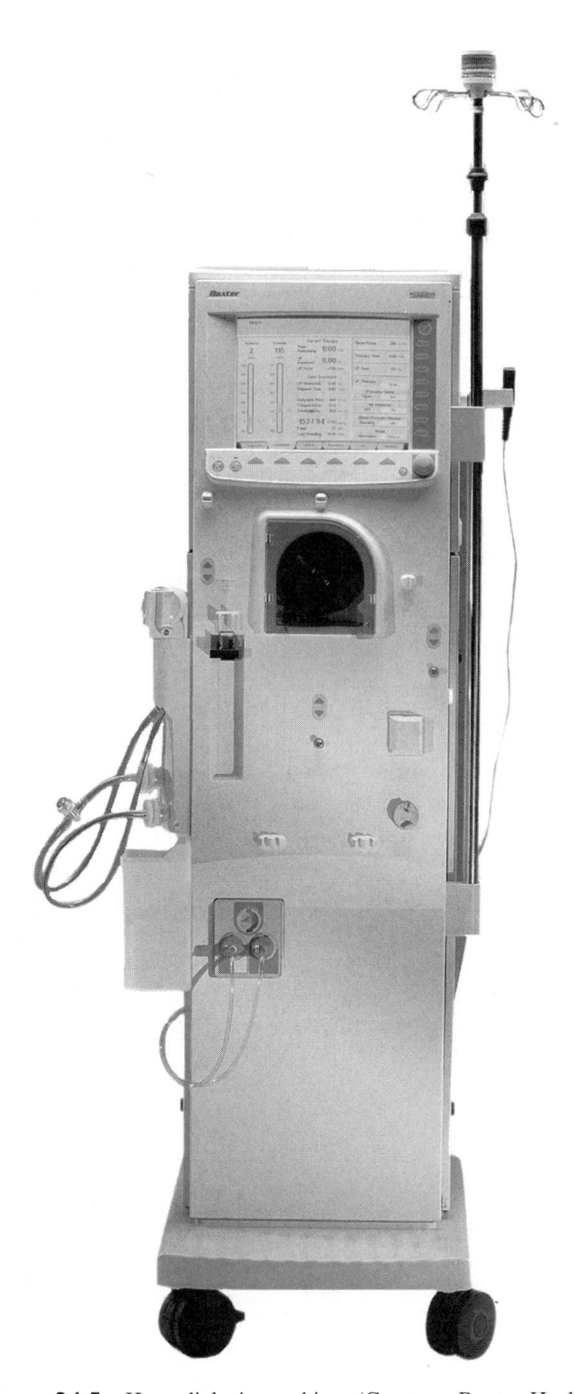

Figure 34-5 Hemodialysis machine. (Courtesy Baxter Healthcare Corp., McGaw Park, IL.)

blood pressures, drawing blood, or placing an intravenous catheter.

The bruit on a vascular access is the sound created as the blood is redirected from the high-pressure artery to a low-pressure vein; it sounds like a passing train. The thrill is the sensation created by the blood being redirected from an arterial inlet through a thin-walled vein or synthetic graft to a venous outlet; it has a vibrating feeling. If either the bruit or thrill is not evident, suspect a clot. The client or family or nurse must telephone the vascular surgeon, the nephrologist, nephrology nurse practitioner, or dialysis unit staff member.

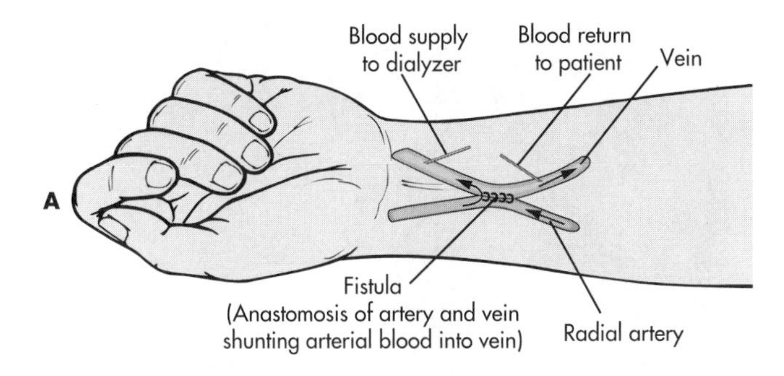

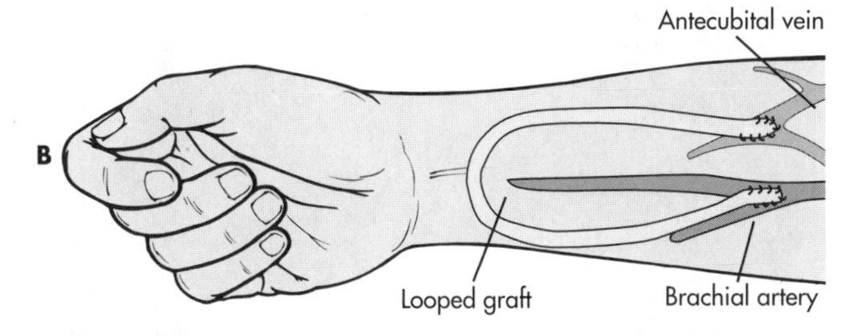

Figure 34-6 Methods of vascular access for hemodialysis. **A,** Internal arteriovenous fistula. **B,** Looped graft in forearm. (From Lewis, S.L., Collier, I.C., Heitkemper, M.M., & Dirksen, S.R., [2000]. *Medical surgical nursing: Assessment and management of clinical problems* [5th ed.]. St. Louis: Mosby.)

An access can be declotted through interventional radiology or surgery if the procedure is attempted within 24 to 48 hours of clot formation in an AVF and less than 2 weeks in an AVG. When the vascular access appears infected or the client has signs and symptoms of systemic infection, evaluate the vascular access and initiate antibiotic therapy. A dialysis catheter or cannula of a fistula or graft is an opening into the circulatory system that is at high risk for infection. Sterile technique and proper flushing are essential to prevent local infection or bacteremia.

Figure 34-7 illustrates the positioning of intrajugular and subclavian catheters that often are the only vascular access clients may have in place when their circulatory systems are unable to support an AVF or AVG.

Diet

Renal dietary restrictions are essential with HD. Although composition varies with nutritional status, age, and diagnosis, the client is limited in protein, potassium, sodium, glucose, phosphorus, and fluid intake. A renal dietitian performs a thorough dietary history and helps the client plan meals. A rule of thumb is 1 to 1½ g/kg of protein, 2 to 3 g of sodium, 60 to 90 mEq of potassium, and 600 to 800 mg of phosphorus per day. Fluid restriction is 1000 to 1200 ml plus urine output. Fluid restrictions may vary depending on the individual's energy expending activities, insensible losses, and seasonal or environmental temperatures. During a home assessment the nurse learns the client's food habits and preferences and ascertains his or her understanding of the renal diet. Education in light of the client's beliefs and values may assist

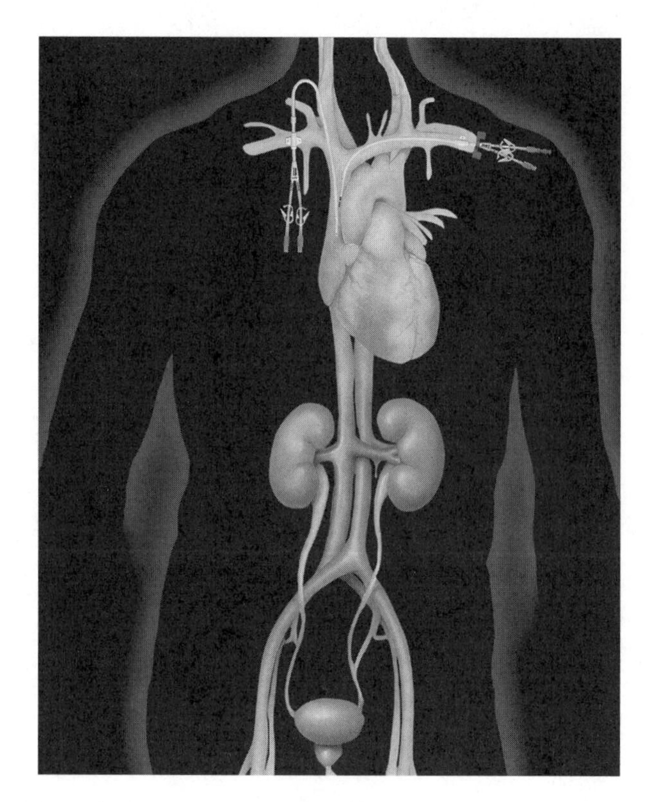

Figure 34-7 Intrajugular and subclavian hemodialysis catheters. (Courtesy Bard Access Systems, Salt Lake City, UT.)

him or her to adhere to dietary restrictions (Wilson, 1995). Written guides for the renal diet, special renal diet recipe books, and fast food or other restaurant listings for food content are convenient aids to ease the meal selection process. Clients who do not adhere to the diet are at risk for hyperkalemia, hyperphosphatemia, fluid overload, bone disease, worsening hypertension, hyperparathyroidism, skin problems, and death. The goal is for clients to make lifestyle choices that are conducive to a healthy life and help prevent complications resulting from noncompliance.

Medications

With ESRD, clients can expect a host of medications to control their disease process. For instance, clients take vitamins, iron supplements, antihypertensive agents, insulin, phosphate binders, calcium carbonate, antidepressants, and potentially many other medications. Children may take human growth hormone to promote near normal stature. Individualized insulin or oral hypoglycemic agent regimens are prescribed for diabetes but must be changed at the stage of renal replacement therapy to accommodate for the increased insulin resistance that coincides with advancing renal dysfunction. Diabetic clients may need less insulin or oral hypoglycemic agents as their renal failures advances, but with a standard 200 mg/dl concentration of glucose in dialysate fluid, they can experience more fluctuations in the blood glucose level between days on and off dialysis treatment. Thus, home blood glucose testing becomes an important measure for the client with diabetes and ESRD.

Hypertension control will wax and wane with HD treatments; blood pressure may be elevated before dialysis, then low afterwards. Blood pressure management is very individualized, and not all clients need pharmaceutical interventions. All classes of drugs have a place in the armamentarium of treatment for hypertension. Antihypertensive drugs have no set regimen; however, they often are not given before HD to prevent hypotension during therapy.

What is critical is a regimen that works for the person, and most clients benefit from supportive counseling to maintain compliance with their medication regimens and dietary and fluid restrictions. Lobley (1997) describes a multidisciplinary approach shown to be effective in achieving the desired outcome of reasonable well controlled hypertension. As with many approaches to preventive or restorative health care, the emphasis is on client education.

Phosphate binders, most often calcium carbonate or calcium acetate, are prescribed with meals to promote the binding of dietary phosphorous and elimination in the stool. If calcium carbonate is used as a calcium supplement, it is ingested between meals. Water-soluble vitamins are taken after hemodialysis. Prolonged imbalance of calcium and phosphorous will result in elevated parathyroid hormone levels and eventually bone disease. Clients must avoid foods and medications containing magnesium and aluminum because these elements are excreted via the kidney. Client education includes information about medications that interact and food-medication combinations. Chapters 17 and 35 contain tables illustrating these interactions.

Activity

These clients with ESRD do not produce sufficient erythropoietin and are anemic. Since 1987, epoetin alpha has benefited clients by stimulating the production of red blood cells. Epoetin alpha is administered either intravenously (IV) or subcutaneously (SQ) during the dialysis treatment. Data from a monthly complete blood count are used to regulate the dose. For the epoetin alpha to be more effective, IV iron preparation may be administered during dialysis therapy to replete lost iron stores. Under the medicare ESRD program in accordance with the Dialysis Outcomes Quality Initiatives (DOQI), the goal for administration of this drug is to maintain the client's hematocrit level between 33% and 36% (*American Journal of Kidney Disease,* 1997a, 1997b). Thus, clients with ESRD remain anemic with the inherent side effects of fatigue, shortness of breath, dyspnea on exertion, and poor exercise tolerance, although regular exercise within limitations is extremely important in rehabilitation of these clients (Colangelo, Stillman, Kessler-Fogil, & Kessler-Hartnett, 1997; Karmiel, 1996; Pianta & Kutner, 1999; Sabath, 1999). The deconditioned state of clients with ESRD has renewed interest in mild to moderate regular exercise, a multidisciplinary approach, physical therapy, and

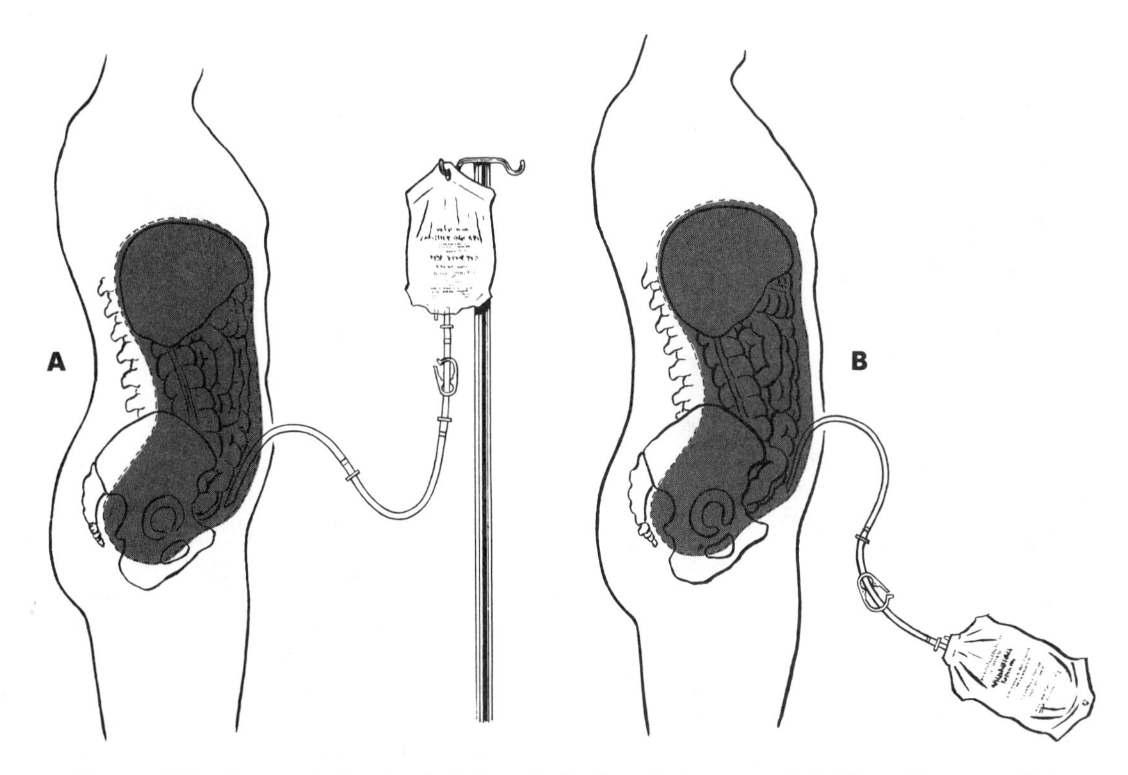

Figure 34-8 Peritoneal dialysis. **A,** Inflow. **B,** Outflow (drains to gravity). (From Thompson, J.M., McFarland, G.K., Hirsch, J.E., & Tucker, S.M. [1997]. *Mosby's clinical nursing* [4th ed.]. St. Louis: Mosby.)

encouraging children to participate in all school activities and organized sports (Schrag, Campbell, Ewert, Hartley, Niemann, & Ross, 1999; Solomon, 1999). Sexual dysfunction, either related to decreased libido or impotence secondary to uremia and anemia, is a major inhibitor to involvement and maintenance in relationships.

In rehabilitation nursing the assessment includes the client's ability to participate in regular exercise, sexuality concerns, and lifestyle behaviors. Interventions must cover all areas of activity.

Psychosocial/Emotional

Clients with ESRD receiving HD as their chronic renal replacement therapy often struggle to cope effectively with their disease and technology; denial and depression are prominent. Children have developmental, growth, and maturation issues that can result in maladaptive behaviors. Rehabilitation nurses are prepared to meet clients along their continuum of adaptation and recommend strategies to improve outcomes.

NURSING INTERVENTIONS FOR THE CLIENT RECEIVING PERITONEAL DIALYSIS

Although home PD continues to be an option for clients with ESRD, only 12% receive this therapy. The procedures and equipment for two standard clinical practices, continuous ambulatory peritoneal dialysis (CAPD) and continuous cycling peritoneal dialysis (CCPD), are illustrated in Figures 34-8 and 34-9. PD is a self-care treatment. The client connects tubing to a peritoneal catheter that is surgically implanted in the peritoneal cavity (Figure 34-10). The semipermeable peritoneal membrane exchanges fluid, electrolytes, and toxins via the concentration gradient between the client's vascular supply and the dialysate solution. Fluid, potassium, phosphorus, amino acids, glucose, and other substances are exchanged and eliminated from the body. PD may not be an option for clients with impaired sight or manual dexterity or who have had extensive abdominal surgeries with residual scar tissue.

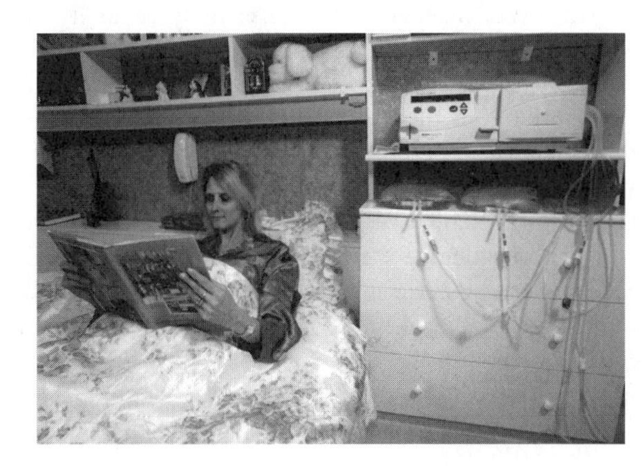

Figure 34-9 Continuous cycling peritoneal dialysis (CCPD). (Courtesy Baxter Healthcare Corp., McGaw Park, IL.)

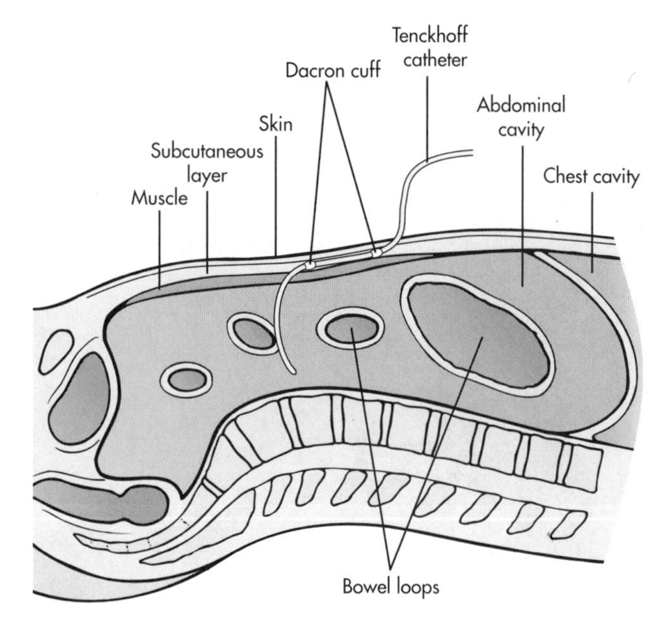

Figure 34-10 Tenckhoff catheter used in peritoneal dialysis. (From Lewis, S.L., Collier, I.C., Heitkemper, M.M., & Dirksen, S.R., [2000]. *Medical surgical nursing: Assessment and management of clinical problems* [5th ed.]. St. Louis: Mosby.)

Schedules

CAPD involves manual performance of three to five exchange procedures—draining, infusing, and dwelling—during the day. The same procedures are performed in CCPD with the use of a peritoneal machine and usually during the night. Either way, peritoneal effluent is disposed of every day. Ideally, children use CAPD or CCPD to avert pain associated with vascular access cannulation, to improve nutrition, and to encourage their involvement in activities. PD procedures can be performed in the home, school, or office daily and generally can accommodate the client's schedule, preferences, and needs.

Client Training

The renal rehabilitation team evaluates the client and situation for opportunities to promote shared decision making. The nephrology nurse and social worker make home visits to identify barriers. Structurally, the client needs a separate area or room to perform CAPD or a table at bed height for the cycler machine for CCPD. Most clients and family quickly grasp essential points, but learning the principles and techniques and "trouble shooting" for complications requires 3 to 5 days of training. With experience, they become proficient. Various pedagogy, such as charts, videos, demonstrations, and written materials positively influence the outcomes (Szczepanik, 1995). Rehabilitation nurses who learn the techniques themselves improve their understanding of the therapy and better assist clients.

The client being treated with CAPD must perform daily exchanges with 1500 to 3000 ml of peritoneal solution using strict sterile technique; each exchanges takes about 30 to 45 minutes. The fill volume, prescribed by the nephrologist or nephrology nurse practitioner, requires 10 to 15 minutes to complete. The drain time also varies, generally 30 to 45 minutes, and the dwell period ranges from 4 to 6 hours and overnight. For ease in remembering, the prescribed schedule is before breakfast, lunch, dinner, and retiring for the evening. For CCPD, every evening the client must set up the cycler machine using strict sterile technique and then in the morning disconnect the machine at completion of therapy, again with sterile technique. Parameters for drain time, fill volume and time, and dwell time are programmed into the machine.

Diet

Clients using CAPD or CCPD have fewer dietary restrictions than clients using HD since PD is performed daily. Clients learn to assess their weight and fluid status daily and how to choose 1.5%, 2.5%, or 4.25% dextrose peritoneal solution to control fluid removal. The higher the dextrose in the solution, the greater the osmotic gradient and therefore the more fluid removed from the intravascular and interstitial spaces. Since fluid removal occurs daily, most of what is consumed is removed within 24 hours. Little fluid accumulates when the correct plan for exchanges is followed and the peritoneal membrane operates properly, and since urea, creatinine, potassium, and sodium are removed daily, there is little chance of them building in the blood. However, more albumin is lost in the peritoneal effluent than in HD so clients must increase their protein intake. In general, clients receiving PD feel better and have a better nutritional status than clients receiving HD, provided the clients receiving PD follow procedures and the prescribed regimen. Monthly laboratory analyses of the comprehensive metabolic panel and complete blood count direct the dialysis prescription. Increased potassium may be needed to prevent hypokalemia.

Medications

Clients receiving PD often use the same medications prescribed to clients with HD but in lower doses. Again, because PD is administered every day, blood pressure management may be remarkably improved and the antihypertension regimens can be simplified. Supplements, such as vitamins, iron, or calcium have no special consideration. Phosphate binders must be consumed with meals.

Diabetic clients receiving PD must incorporate a new regimen for insulin or oral agents because the peritoneal solutions have a heavy dextrose content that adds calories to the diet. Usually the insulin requirements increase, or insulin may be needed to control hyperglycemia. Once clients recognize their unique requirements, management becomes routine. One advantage for persons with ESRD using PD is their ability to add regular insulin to the peritoneal solution, thereby avoiding insulin injections 2 to 4 times a day. Home health care nurses need to learn techniques for adding medication into the peritoneal solution should a client require this.

Clients at home self-administer epoetin alpha via SQ, 2 to 3 three times a week much like an insulin injection. When diet is improved and less blood lost, these clients do not require the medication. Monthly complete blood counts are used to regulate epoetin alpha.

Infection Risks

Clients receiving PD are taught proper techniques for care and cleaning of the catheter exit site and to observe for erythema, drainage, tenderness, leaking, or bleeding. They have responsibility for monitoring for infection or complications and notifying the clinic to obtain cultures and oral antibiotics. Antibiotic ointment or povidone iodine may be applied around the exit site with daily dressing changes. A more serious risk is peritonitis should an infectious agent gain entry into the peritoneal cavity during an exchange or when the catheter becomes disconnected. Clients learn to monitor for cloudy effluent, abdominal pain, fever, and chills. If peritonitis is apparent, they save the first cloudy bag of effluent, then perform two or three rapid flushes for 30 to 60 minutes. Depending on facility protocols, some clients inject antibiotics into the next exchange solution. The first cloudy bag is submitted for cultures and cell count. Generally, clients are not hospitalized, and home health care nurses are instrumental in assisting these often frightened and uncomfortable persons. Intraperitoneal antibiotics are continued for 10 to 14 days.

Activity

Clients with ESRD who are using CAPD or CCPD are extremely independent and proficient in self-care. Since they have no activity restrictions, they play sports and function as energy permits, although those receiving HD report more sexual inactivity than clients receiving PD. Some dialysis centers discourage swimming, soaking in a hot tub, or bathing in a bathtub; all discourage football. As the equipment, catheters, and training have improved, many centers set special precautions such as showering and changing the exit site dressing immediately after participating in these activities. Some recommend enclosing the end of the catheter in a plastic baggy for protection; others modify colostomy bags around the site and end of the catheter. These techniques may be helpful to home health care nurses who plan to assist clients with physical therapy or bathing.

Psychosocial/Emotional

Home self-care is superior to HD in fostering independence since clients can adapt their daily activities around their need for dialysis. Most studies suggest or confirm that clients performing home self-care have a more positive outlook on life and therefore more effective coping with the disease and chronic renal replacement therapy. Clients tend to remain fully involved in age-appropriate activities and to less often reverse roles or interfere with family norms. However, those receiving PD are at risk for fatigue with their chronic treatment and need support, education, and counseling, as well as encouragement and reinforcement of their self-care agency.

NURSING INTERVENTIONS FOR THE CLIENT WITH A RENAL TRANSPLANT

Clients with kidney transplant comprise 28% of the ESRD population (USRDS, 1999). Renal transplantation is the treatment of choice for children. In the past, eligibility ended at 60 years; however some transplant centers perform renal transplants for clients 72 years old or in older clients with excellent health. Donations from cadavers have leveled at 9000 per year, but more donations are arriving and being accepted from living persons who are relatives and nonbiological or emotional related donors. The system of organ distribution is problematic, and policy is in a state of flux in the United States. Discussion is ongoing about the most efficient, practical, and fair way of distributing organs for transplantation. Medical rationing of health care does exist when solid organs are involved. Approximately 50,000 people in the United States await a kidney transplant, and more than 70,000 wait for any solid organ transplant.

Typical clients who receive a kidney transplant are fully involved in age-appropriate activities and require little extra assistance—a scene that may change as more people survive longer with a kidney transplant. These persons manage their immunosuppressive medications and other health care needs and have no dietary restrictions. The only concern is avoiding activities that put the client at risk for any blunt trauma to the abdomen, the donor kidney site (Figure 34-11). Clients are discouraged from activities such as horseback or motorcycle riding and playing contact sports.

Recipients live with an ever-present awareness of potential organ rejection. The signs and symptoms are similar to those experienced by anyone advancing toward ESRD and renal replacement therapy. Clients also must remain alert to their increased risk for opportunistic infections secondary to immunosuppression management; less obvious, they have increased risk for malignancy after years of immunosuppressive therapy.

NURSING OUTCOMES AND GOALS FOR RENAL CLIENTS

The complex nature of ESRD and renal replacement therapies requires partnership between the client and family; the nephrology providers; and when appropriate, the rehabilitation nurses (Kutner, 1998). As noted earlier, the greatest flaw in the ESRD program in the United States is the lack of

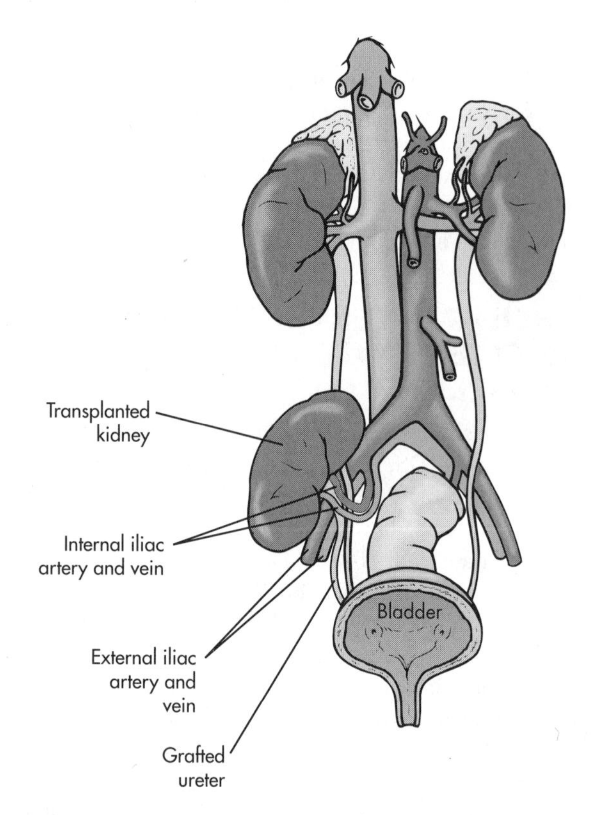

Figure 34-11 Surgical placement of transplanted kidney. (From Lewis, S.L., Collier, I.C., Heitkemper, M.M., & Dirksen, S.R., [2000]. *Medical surgical nursing: Assessment and management of clinical problems* [5th ed.]. St. Louis: Mosby.)

planning for successful rehabilitation of a growing aggregate. When the program began, the client's social worth, gainful employment, and contribution as member of society were factors in the decision process for future care. Rehabilitation with return to independence and active community participation set treatment goals. When the federal government passed PL92-603, ensuring dialysis or kidney transplant, the nephrology community rejoiced at being relieved of the rationing of a then scarce resource. The anticipation in the early 1970s was sound medical assessment and evaluation to ensure the appropriate initiation and withdrawal of renal replacement therapies. While rehabilitation remained a concern, funds were directed to enhance opportunities for clients to meet expected outcomes. Within a few years, after it became evident that the idealistic goals would not be met, funding became less abundant. Rehabilitation nurses and counselors were eliminated. Nephrology nurses have largely been replaced with unlicensed assistive personnel who function as dialysis technicians. Many nephrologists retired or left the field, and fewer new physicians select nephrology as a career path. Finally, the clients with ESRD are older, sicker, more dependent, and often less involved in age-appropriate activities.

In summary, outcomes for the client with renal disease are within biochemical, cognitive, and affective domains. Biochemical goals are to remain in complete fluid, electrolytes, and acid-base balance. Essentially, the body's internal milieu is maintained within the limits of established norms for all plasma and tissue components. Cognitively, clients must comprehend the disease process, prescribed regimen, potential complications of the disease and/or dialytic therapy, and health promotion and resources. Affective goals are to develop effective coping and adherence, family normalization, and personal quality of life. When the disease process and treatment result in a very compromised quality of life, then client and family goals shift to palliative care and a comfortable death with dignity. Clients, families, and providers must participate in a coordinated effort toward individualized goals for unique needs of the person.

The success in achieving these expected outcomes rest on the following three steps:

1. Establish practices of appropriate initiation and withdrawal of dialysis based on weighing benefits versus burdens to the client and family.
2. Reinstitute appropriate levels of funding and professional manpower (i.e., primary care physicians, nephrologists, nephrology nurses, renal dietitians, social workers, and rehabilitation and home health care nurses).
3. Enhance efforts to promote clients' self-care and independence with their full participation in shared decision making and health care planning. Clients with ESRD must identify resources in the community and develop a network and system for support. Rehabilitation nurse advocates can address these issues, and facilitate partnership between the local community and the family.

CRITICAL THINKING

The nature of renal disease and the client care required are complex. The rehabilitation nurse needs to remain mindful of the etiologies for ESRD and the inherent complications, both physiological and psychosocial. The interests of the clients are best served if the nurse questions them about their understanding or knowledge of their disease process and prescribed medical and nursing regimens. Does the client know and/or comprehend the disease and necessary treatments? The nurse could ascertain clients' knowledge about care of their dialysis access, their renal dietary restrictions, and their prescribed medications. Can the client identify a vascular access bruit and a thrill? Does the client know high-potassium, high-phosphorous, and high-protein foods? Can the client relate the medications and their intended expected outcomes?

While in the home, the rehabilitation nurse would have the opportunity to observe and discuss quality-of-life concerns with the client and family. Does the benefit of dialysis outweigh the burdens? Has the client completed advance care planning for end of life? Is the family aware of the desires of the client? Have the family members incorporated their own health belief modal of values, goals, expectations, and potential barriers to success?

Finally the rehabilitation staff should have a list of resources with telephone numbers readily available. Who are the client's doctors? The name and contact numbers for the nurses, social worker, and renal dietitian associated with the client's outpatient dialysis clinic should be conveniently posted. What community agencies will provide services and on what schedule? Who is responsible for client transportation?

Rehabilitation nurses may welcome the challenge of identifying the needs of the ESRD clients and designing a care plan. There are numerous questions be to asked and answers sought. Nurses should develop their own individualized approach to client care. The objective is quality, comprehensive client care and achievement of professional satisfaction in meeting the needs of the clients.

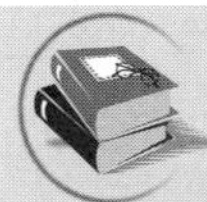

Case Study

A 27-year-old athletic man of Hispanic background entered the hospital emergency room complaining of extreme fatigue, abdominal pain, easy bruising, muscle weakness, and nausea and vomiting. His vital signs were stable; he weighed 78 kg (171.6 lb) at 5 feet, 9 inches tall; and he had no history of medical problems. He was diagnosed with *Helicobacter pylori* gastritis and was sent home. Within 1 week he returned with worsening symptoms, plus a rash and jaundice. Laboratory results revealed normal hematocrit and hemoglobin levels of 48% and 13.8 g/dl, thrombocytopenia with a platelet count of 33,000, and a white blood count within normal range. His serum creatinine level on admission was 1 mg/dl. He was diagnosed with hemolytic uremic syndrome (HUS). Over the next 2 months, his condition deteriorated despite a treatment regimen, blood transfusions, platelet transfusions, antibiotics, and eventually hemodialysis. He was transferred to a teaching hospital, and complications ensued, including sepsis, hypotension, adult respiratory distress syndrome, aspiration pneumonia, and ischemic bowel, which led to splenectomy, right hemicolectomy, ileostomy, and colostomy. Subsequently, he suffered quadriparesis secondary to critical polyneuropathy. The client remained alert and oriented throughout much of his hospitalization, and his wife remained dedicated to assisting with his health care needs. Miraculously the client survived his 5-month hospitalization, probably secondary to being transferred to a major nonuniversity teaching center and his previously excellent health. On discharge he continued to require hemodialysis 3 times a week and nursing supervision of home health care, including speech, physical, and occupational therapy and extensive rehabilitation services.

Expected Outcomes

The discharge plan of care included the following outcomes:

1. Client would be able to return to age-appropriate independent activities of daily living (ADL) and instrumental activities of daily living (IADL).
2. He would regain normal renal function and not require dialytic therapy.
3. The client and his wife would benefit from rehabilitation resources as long as needed.

Discussion

The young couple were delighted to return home together but were well aware of the long road ahead. He was unable to ambulate, required assistance for transfers, had a functioning colostomy, and now weighed 60 kg (132 lb). Three times a week he required hemodialysis, for which he had an indwelling tunneled left intrajugular dialysis catheter. All home services were arranged before discharge so the family was met with considerable support as they tackled the challenges of the client in achieving independent ADLs and IADLs. Each specialty nurse contributed to the total plan of care, as appropriate. Short- and long-term goals were established with family participation.

Basic physiological needs were addressed and included a high-quality protein and caloric diet within the restrictions of renal failure (1.5 g/kg potassium, 2 g sodium, and 800 mg phosphorous; fluid limited to 1000 ml, plus urine output; 30 to 35 calories per kg). The speech, physical, and occupational therapists coordinated their schedules in consideration of the hemodialysis treatments on Monday, Wednesday, and Friday between 8 AM and 12 PM. Assistance was provided for transfer to and from the dialysis unit; the client's wife performed colostomy care and administered medications, with assistance as necessary. The nephrology nurses took responsibility for obtaining all laboratory tests to limit visits and prevent the pain associated with needles.

Resources within the community provided financial support, and the wife took a few weeks of unpaid family medical leave. Coordinating services arranged for help with obtaining supplies, groceries, medial ancillary supplies, and medications. A dietitian reviewed and monitored the daily food intake and recommended meals within the nutritional prescription and what the wife could manage.

As the client gained strength and ability for self-care, the home services were curtailed. Physical therapy continued, but the client also used his home gym equipment to exercise, as his energy and stamina permitted. As his uremia resolved and his appetite improved, he slowly began gaining lean body mass. Eventually, he required another dialysis catheter because after several weeks, his tunneled catheter became dysfunctional.

After 3 months of outpatient hemodialysis treatment, the client's urine output slowly began to increase and renal function improved. The dialysis regimen was reduced to twice weekly, and his appetite and strength continued to improve. Once antihypertensive medications were not needed, the medication regimen was simplified. The wife returned to full-time employment, and family and friends stayed with him on days he did not receive dialysis. Eventually, he could spend longer periods alone because he could ambulate independently. After 2 additional weeks, hemodialysis was no longer necessary, which is extremely unusual after approximately 6 months of necessary treatment.

Summary

After a horrific, prolonged hospital and outpatient experience, this client gained the ability for self-care in all ADLs and IADLs. His wife continued to provide emotional and loving support. His renal function returned to about 25 ml/min by the time of this report. These successful outcomes could never have been realized without the collaborative efforts of many experienced professionals working diligently with the client and his wife.

REFERENCES

Alexander, S. (1962). They decide who lives, who dies. *Life Magazine,* 102-125.

American Journal of Kidney Disease. (1997a). Clinical practice guidelines for hemodialysis adequacy and peritoneal adequacy. *American Journal of Kidney Disease, 30*(3 Suppl. 2).

American Journal of Kidney Disease. (1997b). Clinical practice guidelines for vascular access and anemia of chronic renal failure. *American Journal of Kidney Disease, 304*(4 Suppl. 3).

Colangelo, R., Stillman, M., Kessler-Fogil, D., & Kessler-Hartnett, D. (1997). *Rehabilitation Nursing, 22*(6), 288-292, 302.

Evans, R., Blagg, C., & Bryan, F. (1981). Implications for health care policy. *Journal of the American Medical Association, 245*(5), 487-492.

Fox, R., & Swazey, J. (1974). *The courage to fail: A social view of organ transplantation and dialysis.* Chicago: University of Chicago Press.

Gordon, M. (2000) *Manual of nursing diagnosis* (9th ed.). St. Louis: Mosby.

Iglehart, J. (1993). Health policy report: The end stage renal disease program. *New England Journal of Medicine, 328*(5), 366-371.

Johnson, M., Maas, M., & Moorhead, S. (2000). *Nursing outcomes classification (NOC)* (2nd ed.). St. Louis: Mosby.

Karmiel, J. (1996). The easy bike program: An exercise during dialysis program. *Topics in Clinical Nutrition, 12*(1), 74-78.

Kutner, N. (1998). Rehabilitation of the renal patient. In J. Parker (Ed.), *Contemporary nephrology nursing* (pp. 405-431). Pitman, NJ: AJ Jannetti.

Lancaster, L. (2001). *ANNA core curriculum for nephrology nursing* (3rd ed.). Pitman, NJ: AJ Jannetti.

Lobley, L. (2001) Using nursing diagnosis to achieve desired outcomes for hemodialysis clients. *Advances in Renal Replacement Therapy, 4*(2), 112-124.

Mathers, T. (1998). The geriatric patient. In J. Parker (Ed.), *Contemporary nephrology nursing* (pp. 481–513). Pitman, NJ: AJ Jannetti.

Maxwell, J., & Sapolsky, H. (1987). The first DRG: Lessons from the end stage renal disease program for the prospective payment system. *Contemporary Dialysis & Nephrology, June,* 26-34.

McCloskey, J., & Bulechek, G. (2000). *Nursing interventions classification (NIC)* (3rd ed.). St. Louis: Mosby.

McCormick, T. (1993). Ethical issues in caring for patients wit renal failure. *American Nephrology Nurses Association Journal, 20*(5), 549-555.

Nephrology News & Issues. (2000). RPA/ASN guidelines aimed at helping nephrologists make difficult decisions on initiation, withdrawing dialysis therapy. *Nephrology News & Issues, January,* 14-16.

Pianta, T., & Kutner, N. (1999). Improving physical functioning in the elderly dialysis patient: Relevance of physical therapy. *American Nephrology Nurses Association Journal, 26*(1), 11-14.

Price, C. (1992). Is it time again for patient selection criteria ? *Nephrology News & Issues, February,* 18-20.

Sabath, R. (1999) Exercise evaluation of children with end stage renal disease. *Advances in Renal Replacement Therapy, 6*(2), 189-194.

Schrag, W., Campbell, M., Ewert, J., Hartley, S., & Ross, D. (1999). Multidisciplinary team renal rehabilitation: Interventions and outcomes. *Advances in Renal Replacement Therapy, 6*(3), 282-288.

Solomon, D. (1999). Focus on rehabilitation: Teamwork that works. *Advances in Renal Replacement Therapy, 6*(3), 278-281.

Staney, S. (1996). Caring for a rehabilitation patient with chronic renal failure and end stage renal disease. *Rehabilitation Nursing, 21*(6), 303–306, 325.

Szczepanik, M. (1995). Assessment and selection considerations: ESRD patient materials and media. *Advances in Renal Replacement Therapy, 2*(3), 207-216.

U.S. Renal Data System (USRDS). (1999). 1999 Annual data report. *American Journal of Kidney Diseases, 34*(2 Suppl. 1).

Whelan, C., & Whelan, W. (1999). The management of hematuria and proteinuria in the adult primary care setting. *The American Journal for Nurse Practitioners, September/October,* 29-34.

Wilson, B. (1995). Promoting compliance: The patient-provider partnership. *Advances in Renal Replacement Therapy, 2*(3), 199-206.

Zawada, E. (1994). Indications for dialysis. In J. Daugirdas & T. Ing (Eds.), *Handbook of dialysis* (2nd ed., pp. 3-9). Boston: Little, Brown.

BIBLIOGRAPHY

Burton, B., & Hirschman, G. (1976). Demographic analysis: End stage renal disease and its treatment in the United States. *Journal of Dialysis, 11*(2), 47-51.

Cancer Rehabilitation 35

Patricia L. McCollom, MS, RN, CRRN, CDMS, CCM, CLCP

Pain, anguish—a profound change in my life ... that cold February day, finding a lump in my breast.
Surgery, recovery—a loss of femininity ... changes that were never dreamed or imagined.
Chemotherapy—a loss of dignity! Six months to life—a harsh sentence, for no reason.
Survival—knowing and appreciating each day as a gift!
To honor life, love and family ... to experience joy in every moment. The lesson of breast cancer.

PLM—October 1999

Cancer is the second most common cause of death in the United States; an estimated 7.5 million persons have or have had the disease (American Cancer Society, 1998). The number of survivors increases annually because of advances in client education, early detection, and new treatment and technology. Cancer is now considered a chronic condition, with associated functional, physical, emotional, and spiritual sequelae. The Association of Rehabilitation Nurses (ARN) and the Oncology Nurses Society (ONS) collaborated to develop the following statement published in February 2000:

> The sequelae of cancer are best addressed through a comprehensive oncology rehabilitation program. The focus of the program must be collaborative and interdisciplinary, whether based in acute, sub-acute, or home care.

It is the position of ARN and ONS that oncology rehabilitation has the following characteristics:

- Is a part of quality cancer care, which is a right of all citizens
- Is an option for all clients at any stage of cancer
- Incorporates the individual with cancer and the family as fully informed partners and decision makers
- Includes timely access to and reimbursement for a coordinated, comprehensive, and interdisciplinary approach
- Is coordinated and delivered by competent rehabilitative cancer care providers

Accountability and coordination of quality oncology rehabilitation care are best accomplished by registered nurses who have been educated and certified in oncology or rehabilitation specialties.

Collaboration by these professional organizations represents a foundation for the advancement of rehabilitation care for clients with cancer.

CANCER TREATMENT BASICS

Surgical intervention in cancer treatment is designed to resect the tumor tissue from the space-occupying area. Tumor control surgery ranges from breast conservation surgery for breast cancer to highly complex surgical procedures for pancreatic, bowel, and brain cancer.

Adjuvant therapy, such as chemotherapy or hormonal therapy, has been demonstrated to improve longevity and quality of life for clients with cancer. Using breast cancer as an example, tamoxifen trials have shown promise. In a 5-year follow-up of one trial conducted by the National Surgical Adjuvant Breast and Bowel Project (NSABP), women treated with chemotherapy and tamoxifen demonstrated a 91% disease-free survival and a 96% overall survival.

Radiation treatment for cancer uses ionizing radiation to deposit energy that injures or destroys cells in the area treated. Radiation damages normal cells as well; however, they are able to regenerate. Radiotherapy may be used to treat solid tumors or diseases of the blood-forming and lymphatic systems.

Other treatments showing promise for cancer are angiogenesis inhibitors, biological therapies, lasers, photodynamic therapy, and vaccines.

CANCER AND REHABILITATION

With the prevalence of newly diagnosed and existing clients with cancer, it is apparent that rehabilitation interventions will play an increasing role in cancer care. The outcomes of rehabilitation and restorative care in cancer treatment are described in the following:

1. *Quality of care:* Improved clinical outcomes related to body image enhancement, bowel management, emotional support, family support, health education, mutual goal setting, pain management, self-care, and elimination.
2. *Service:* Improved process outcomes resulting in increased client and family satisfaction, provider satisfaction, and payer understanding of the treatment plan.
3. *Cost management:* Improved functional abilities and perceived control by the client results in decreased inpatient stays and improved response to treatment.

ISSUES IN CANCER TREATMENT

Medical treatment for cancer is continually changing as a result of research, clinical trials, and new discoveries. Recent research has contributed to outpatient chemotherapy, supportive therapy to address nausea and fatigue, and potential cures for various types of cancer.

Clinical Trials

Clinical trials represent research in which clients participate in the clinical evaluation of methods to prevent, diagnose, and treat cancer. A clinical trial occurs only after extensive research and serves to identify safe and effective outcomes.

Screening trials examine options for early diagnosis for cancer. Prevention trials research new approaches, such as diet, supplements, vitamins or other medications, with the aim of lowering the risk of development of specific types of cancer.

Treatment trials test new drugs, surgical intervention, and radiation therapy. Quality-of-life trials study methods to improve comfort and quality of life for clients with cancer (National Cancer Institute, 2000).

Clinical trials represent the current methodology for monitoring and comparing treatment protocols for cancer care and treatment. It is through clinical trials that objective evaluations of new treatment can be completed. Institutions participating in clinical trials must adhere to rigid guidelines established by the Food and Drug Administration (FDA) and the Office of Protection from Research Risk (OPRR). Further, all clinical trials must be approved and maintain standards established by institutional review boards. Clients are closely monitored, and reports of patient responses are submitted to the FDA for evaluation of safety and treatment efficacy.

Reimbursement

The goal of oncology care is to provide timely, appropriate, and cost-effective treatment and care to clients diagnosed with cancer (Mellody, Owen, & Klein, 1998). In the world of changing health care paradigms, the rules for reimbursement under managed care may represent a major issue in cancer treatment.

Communication with payers to approve cancer treatment becomes a critical component of achieving the oncology care goals. Barriers to effective communication may be identified in two sectors.

First, oncology providers often have limited knowledge of the types of health plans and their legal impact on care. Providers may have little understanding of the plan's contractual financial agreements or requirements and may have difficulty in articulating the treatment plan to the payer.

Conversely the payer may have little clinical knowledge about the needs and treatment of clients with cancer. The payer also may have difficulty in translating the language of cancer care into the language of managed care, as the United States transitions into new paradigms of health care delivery.

Recommendations for resolution of reimbursement issues for cancer care by providers are described in the following:

- Obtain preauthorization for care as outlined in the treatment plan by submitting requests in writing, outlining expected outcomes.
- Supply a rationale for treatment, specifying objective information to support requested procedures and protocols. Evidence-based practice guidelines are valuable tools in developing a rationale for treatment.
- Provide a detailed treatment plan.
- Know the payer's appeal process after denial of authorization.

Reimbursement conflicts are a direct result of external efforts to control client care costs. Approval and denial issues are at the heart of growing litigation in health care. Improved communication that promotes collaboration may be the single tool for resolution of these issues.

GOALS FOR CANCER REHABILITATION

Treatment goals for cancer rehabilitation are collaboration, communication, coordination of care, client education, consistency of information across the continuum, and support for the client-family unit. Rehabilitation philosophy promotes these treatment goals.

Psychosocial support is one outcome of the treatment goals. Research of the literature demonstrates that cancer care results in decreased physiological, psychological, and social functioning, which develops into severe distress for the client and caregivers. Treatment plans for clients with cancer must address these issues, from a rehabilitation perspective, to achieve outcomes of increased function and positive health change.

NURSING INTERVENTIONS

In June 1995, the ONS and ARN participated in a survey by the developers of the third edition of Nursing Interventions Classification (NIC) to identify core interventions for their specialties. Comparison of the core interventions allows for a perspective of how providers in each specialty practice view their roles in health care delivery and how integration of rehabilitation principles into cancer care can promote achievement of cancer treatment goals (Table 35-1).

A comparison of the three common oncology nursing and rehabilitation nursing diagnoses and major interventions with associated nursing outcomes demonstrates the potential for positive health care results in cancer care (Table 35-2).

It is interesting to note that both specialty nursing practices identified "energy management" as a core intervention. Rehabilitation nurses noted the need for body image enhancement and specified many interventions directed at client empowerment. This chapter focuses on fatigue and body image because practitioners identified these as intervention areas. The principles of rehabilitation nursing, described throughout this text and directed toward client empowerment, may be applied in care delivery for clients with cancer.

FATIGUE

"The feeling cannot even be described! It is as if all of life is in slow motion—no even worse—still frames, connected to one another and going on around me, not a part of me. Sounds are processed in syllables, not words. And, oh the effort to even move across the room.... I would have chemotherapy on Fridays. Saturday the slowness would begin and by the afternoon, sleep was my only refuge. I would sleep, often without turning for hours. Some weeks I would sleep until Tuesday mornings, only getting out of bed to go to the bathroom—and of course to drink the gallons of fluid to help wash the poison from my soul."

These are the words of a client with breast cancer sharing the response she had to chemotherapy. *Fatigue* is defined as "an overwhelming sustained sense of exhaustion and decreased capacity for physical and mental work at usual levels" (McCloskey & Bulechek, 2000). Fatigue is one of the most prevalent complications for clients with cancer and contributes to quality of life and to outcomes of treatment. Vogelzang, Breitbard, Cella, and others found in a 1997 survey that fatigue affected 78% of cancer clients during the course of their disease, and 61% reported that their everyday lives were affected *more* by fatigue than pain.

There is no known cause for fatigue in clients with cancer. It is currently believed that multiple variables interact. Physiological factors include anemia, metabolic disturbances, and nutritional deficits. The client with cancer may be experiencing depression, lack of sleep, fear, and stress. As these factors combine, the human body seems to respond with a retreat into the need for a state of rest (Wolfe, 1998).

TABLE 35-1 Identification of Core Interventions

Oncology Nursing Society	Association of Rehabilitation Nurses
Analgesic administration	Amputation care
Anxiety reduction	Behavior management
Bleeding precautions	Body image enhancement
Caregiver support	Body mechanics promotion
Chemotherapy management	Bowel management
Dying care	Communication enhancement: speech deficits
Energy management	Coping enhancement
Environmental management: comfort	Decision-making support
Fever treatment	Discharge planning
Infection control	Embolus precautions
Infection protection	Emotional support
Nutrition management	**Energy management**
Nutrition monitoring	Environmental management: safety
Pain management	Family support
Peripheral sensation management	Health education
Preparatory sensory information	Learning facilitation
Radiation therapy management	Memory training
Support group	Multidisciplinary care conference
Teaching: disease process	Mutual goal setting
Teaching: procedure/ treatment	Normalization promotion
Therapeutic touch	**Pain management**
Urinary elimination management	Positioning
Venous access devices maintenance	Pressure ulcer care
	Pressure ulcer prevention
	Self-care assistance
	Self responsibility facilitation
	Socialization enhancement
	Swallowing therapy
	Teaching: individual
	Unilateral neglect management
	Urinary elimination management

Assessment of Fatigue

To specify appropriate nursing interventions, a comprehensive nursing assessment must be completed. Understanding of the diagnosis and treatment plan is critical for the nurse as a basis for assessment of fatigue.

Nursing assessment must rely on the client's self-report. It is important to ask the client his or her definition of fatigue. The words exhaustion, lethargy, tiredness, or lack of energy are most commonly used to describe fatigue. Symptoms may vary, and each client's perception of fatigue is unique. See Chapter 21 (Table 21-4) for additional information on energy conservation.

When the presence of fatigue has been stated by the client, an in-depth approach to gather information is needed. Questions must be directed to determining the onset, dura-

TABLE 35-2 Common Oncology and Rehabilitation Nursing Interventions and Outcomes

Diagnosis	Definition	Outcomes	Major Interventions
Activity intolerance	A state in which an individual has insufficient physiological or psychological energy to endure or complete required or desired daily activities	Activity tolerance (responses to energy-consuming body movements involved in required or desired daily activities)	Activity therapy Energy management Exercise promotion: strength training
		Endurance (extent that energy enables a person to sustain activity)	Activity therapy Energy management Exercise promotion: strength training
		Energy conservation (extent of active management of energy to initiate and sustain activity)	Energy management Nutrition management
Pain	An unpleasant sensory and emotional experience arising from actual or potential tissue damage or described in terms of such damage (International Association for the Study of Pain); sudden or slow onset of any intensity from mild to severe with an anticipated or predictable end and a duration of <6 mo	Comfort level (feelings of physical and psychological ease)	Medication management Pain management
		Pain control (personal actions to control pain)	Medication management Pain management Patient-controlled analgesia assistance
Urinary urge incontinence, risk for	Risk for involuntary loss of urine associated with a sudden, strong sensation or urinary urgency	Urinary elimination (ability of the urinary system to filter wastes, conserve solutes, and collect and discharge urine in a healthy pattern)	Urinary elimination management

Data from Johnson, M., Bulechek, G., Dochterman, J.M., Maas, M., & Moorhead, S. (2001). *Nursing diagnoses, outcomes and interventions: NANDA, NOC, and NIC linkages.* St. Louis: Mosby.

tion, and patterns of fatigue. The nurse must inquire about methods used to alleviate fatigue or factors that exacerbate the fatigue experience.

Since fatigue has a major effect on quality of life, assessment includes gathering information about how the fatigue is affecting physical, emotional, and mental well-being. Questions may include the following:

- Do you have problems remembering?
- Are you able to complete projects start to finish?
- Are you involved in social situations?
- Do you feel sad or depressed?

To assess the physiological impact of fatigue, note anemia and hemoglobin and hematocrit levels. Review laboratory studies for metabolic changes and the chemotherapy or radiation treatment plan. Nutritional status may be assessed by monitoring weight and recording intake. To determine the physiological effect, inquire about the following:

- Are you able to participate in your usual daily activities?
- Describe your exercise program.
- How do you think fatigue is affecting your life?

Assessment of fatigue is imperative to define interventions to manage it. Management of fatigue promotes the client's ability to participate in healing.

Interventions

Once assessment is complete, specific interventions can be identified to assist the individual to manage fatigue. Interventions should address sleep and rest, depression, anxiety, and inactivity. Physiological interventions should address anemia, nutrition, infection, and pain (Table 35-3).

Fatigue associated with cancer may be seen before, during, and after treatment. Clients, in follow-up after treatment, report ongoing fatigue for months or longer. Rehabilitation nurses involved in providing care must be aware of this response to develop appropriate plans to assist survivors and promote quality of life.

BODY IMAGE

"At first I could deal with loss of my breast. But my hair . . . that was my dignity! For the year I was bald, I cried every time I looked into the mirror. After awhile, there were no more tears. . . ."

TABLE 35-3 Nursing Interventions and Outcomes for Nursing Diagnosis: Fatigue

Nursing Interventions	Outcomes
Sleep enhancement	Hours of sleep documented Sleep patterns identified Sleep quality identified Sleep routine specified Feelings of rejuvenation after sleep Wakeful at appropriate times Energy maintained at consistent levels
Counseling/emotional support	Fear control Depression control Health beliefs clarified Uses relaxation techniques Remains productive Maintains a sense of purpose
Energy management	Performance of usual routine Rested appearance Concentration Exhaustion not present Lethargy not present Libido

Data from Johnson, M., Maas, M.L., & Moorhead, S. (2000). *Nursing outcomes classification (NOC)* (2nd ed.). St. Louis: Mosby; McCloskey, J.C., & Bulechek, G.M. (2000). *Nursing interventions classification (NIC)* (3rd ed.). St. Louis: Mosby; and North American Nursing Diagnosis Association. (2001). *Nursing diagnosis: Definitions and classification 2001-2002* (4th ed.). Philadelphia: Author.

One of man's earliest self-states to evolve is that of the body image concept. This concept involves the individual's perception of his or her physique, body symmetry, boundaries of the body, agility, and the aesthetics of the total appearance. Our sense of body image is acquired from verbal and nonverbal input from the environment. Any change in the perception of one's body image results in a significant effect in emotional health.

Assessment of Body Image Disturbance

Individuals diagnosed with cancer will have a change in appearance or loss or limits of a body part. The result is negative feelings or perceptions about the changes, which may affect response to treatment and quality of life.

Nurses again must rely on self-report from the client. Nurses must be alert to client's verbalizations regarding the change in body structure or feelings of fear of rejection or the reaction of others. Clients may repeat negative responses to body changes or dwell on past appearance.

During the assessment, questions that may provide data to formulate a nursing diagnosis of *body image disturbance* (Gordon, 2000) include the following:

- What do you see as the changes in your body?
- Are there lifestyle changes you are experiencing since your diagnosis?
- Do you continue your usual social activities?

In addition, during assessment the rehabilitation nurse must note the client's body language. Is the body part hidden or overexposed? Does the client touch or decline to look at the changed body part?

Management of response to body image change is critical to promote quality of life and to prevent long-term emotional complications for the client. It is through assessment of response to body image change that a clear plan for interventions may be identified.

TABLE 35-4 Nursing Interventions and Outcomes for Body Image Change

Nursing Interventions	Outcomes
Body image enhancement	Indicators: • Positive perception of own appearance and body functions • Congruence between body perception and reality • Description of affected body part • Willingness to touch affected body part • Satisfaction with body appearance • Satisfaction with body function • Adjustment to change in appearance • Willingness to use strategies to enhance appearance and function

Data from Johnson, M., Maas, M.L., & Moorhead, S. (2000). *Nursing outcomes classification (NOC)* (2nd ed.). St. Louis: Mosby; McCloskey, J.C., & Bulechek, G.M. (2000). *Nursing interventions classification (NIC)* (3rd ed.). St. Louis: Mosby; and North American Nursing Diagnosis Association. (2001). *Nursing diagnosis: Definitions and classification 2001-2002* (4th ed.). Philadelphia: Author.

Interventions

Body image enhancement is defined as improving a client's conscious and unconscious perceptions and attitudes toward his or her body (McCloskey & Bulechek, 2000). In dealing with the implementation of interventions, the nurse may function as a counselor to provide effective coping behaviors and to assist the client and family in constructing a positive attitude toward treatment and ongoing requirements for care. Table 35-4 identifies nursing interventions and correlating outcomes

It may require months or years for a client to become adjusted to an altered body image and for associated problems to resolve. Support groups for clients, family members, and friends are active in most community settings and can be an important adjunct in implementing interventions to promote positive outcomes.

SUMMARY

With improved outcomes for individuals with cancer, this medical diagnosis has now been identified as a chronic and/or disabling condition. Furthermore, an individual with a disability may have a dual diagnosis of a cancer. Clients who are expected to improve after diagnosis and treatment for cancer may require therapeutic and preventative interventions, adaptive equipment, or assistive devices that are common in rehabilitation settings. Clients seeking oncology rehabilitation include those with breast or bone reconstruction, grafts, amputations, surgical removal of muscle or tissues, sectioning or removal of functional parts, altered sensory function, or chronic pain.

Oncology rehabilitation may be preventative, restorative, supportive, or palliative. Clients with cancer have a clear need for the rehabilitation process, which addresses a health-oriented approach to promote maximum functioning. In dealing with oncology in rehabilitation, the nurse and other team members, client, and family comprise a sociocultural, psychoemotional, holistically interactive unit dedicated to identifying and mobilizing the client's internal and external coping resources. Rehabilitation outcomes improve when a client has an active support system and professional support for appropriate referrals and care.

CRITICAL THINKING

PLM is a 52-year-old woman who has had a right radical mastectomy. She expresses a great deal of anxiety regarding chemotherapy. Ms. M is a newlywed in a second marriage and is self-employed.

1. What are the potential side effects of chemotherapy that will affect this woman's quality of life?
2. What are rehabilitation nursing interventions to address these side effects?
3. How will Ms. M's anxiety regarding chemotherapy affect the treatment plan?
4. What potential nursing diagnosis relates to Ms. M's marital status?
5. What nursing interventions may be implemented to deal with this woman's work situation?

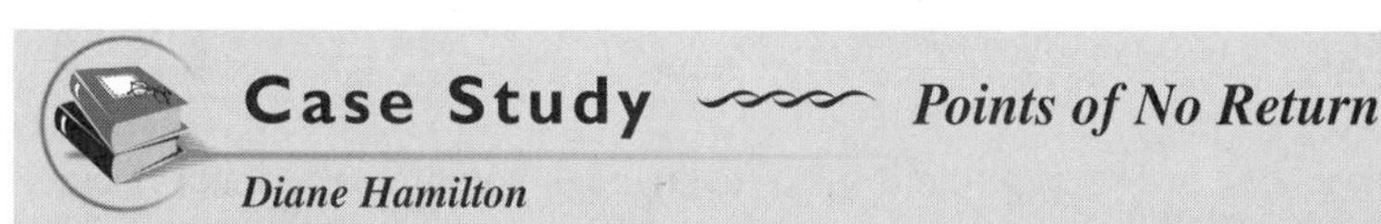

Case Study ~ *Points of No Return*

Diane Hamilton

Kalamazoo, Mich., June 1999—

The diagnosis of breast cancer hung in the air, a palpable barrier between us.

The physician stood blandly by the bed, as I lay frozen in solemn dread. Addressing the virtues of chemotherapy, radiation and mastectomy, she did not seem aware of the truisms that I was to learn later from master patients. First, breast cancer relentlessly demands movement, creative effort and performance from patients. Second, breast cancer—without a bit of remorse—forces patients to points-of-no-return that forevermore govern life choices.

Experts suggest that a breast cancer diagnosis generates a fear of death—initially. Indeed, cancer is neither innocent nor hesitant when it boldly validates the finiteness of existence. Knowing that the diagnosis brings seismic tremors in which linear time (chronos) stops, the professionals try to relieve a patient's fear with teaching; to reintegrate time with kindness; and to offer hope. Despite their efforts, it is the wise master-patients who divulge to novice-patients a great secret: It is creation which is the solution to the fear of death.

In creating a prayer, a garden, a poem or a journal, the patient-artist sculpts something immortal, and the fear of death is overcome by simply loving the act of creation more. Through the process of creation, intuition and cognition mysteriously unite. The union allows the cancer patient to swing between suffering and production, order and disorder, child and adult, inner and outer freedom. Being free, wise cancer patients are perpetually driven toward life and creativity. It is a point-of-no-return.

Paradoxically, the master-patients caution novices that the fear of life may also be exceptionally powerful. The risks and dangers of life, as well as the laughter, intimacy, and discovery involved with trying to survive cancer is quite astonishing. Rather than the obituarist's idea of "waging a fight with cancer," one is forced to wholeheartedly enter into a dance with life. The novice-patient learns not to escape from struggle, but to go straight into it, because she cannot do otherwise. It is a point-of-no-return.

As you penetrate the struggle deep enough, you touch your core of vulnerability, enter into it, share it, and taste it—in so far as that is possible. The person-one-has-been, whose goal was happiness, is replaced by the person-to-be, whose goal is living. The dance of life is not about avoiding suffering. It is not about making nice. It is not about the power of positive thinking. It is about being real and authentic, about understanding that life's joy and suffering are somehow two sides of the same thing.

Points-of-no-return are not simply part of emotional recovery. They reawaken. While distinctive among patients, they are real. Patients frequently tell nurses, "Cancer was a blessing in disguise," or "I learned so much." Nurses nod knowingly but often do not understand. Forevermore, points of no return give patients new markers for what nourishes the soul, what provides interconnections, what reconnects split-off parts of themselves, and what is right for them.

Before embarking on any experience, master-patients ask these questions: Is this path creative? Does it give wonder and healing? Does it have joy?

From Hamilton, D. (1999). Points of no return. *Reflections.* Reprinted with permission from Sigma Theta Tau.

Diane Hamilton, RN, PhD, a historian of ideas within nursing, is an associate professor at Western Michigan University School of Nursing in Kalamazoo, Mich., and a breast cancer survivor.

RESOURCES

American Association for Cancer Education (AACE)
P.O. Box 601
Snellville, GA 30278-0601
http://rpci.med.buffalo.edu/departments/education/aace2.html

American Cancer Society
1599 Clifton Road N.E.
Atlanta, GA 30329
(404) 320-3333
http://www.cancer.org

American Institute of Cancer Research
1759 R St. N.W.
Washington, DC 20009
(202) 328-7744; (800) 843-8114
Fax: (202) 328-7226
http://www:aicr.org

American Society of Clinical Oncology (ASCO)
435 N. Michigan Ave., Suite 1717
Chicago, IL 60611
(312) 644-0828

Association of Community Cancer Centers (ACCC)
11600 Nebel St., Suite 201
Rockville, MD 20852
(301) 984-9496

Canadian Cancer Society
10 Alcorn Ave., Suite 200
Toronto, Canada M4V 1E4
Canada
(416) 961-7223
http://www.cancer.ca

Cancer Archives
http://cure.medinfo.org/lists/cancer/index.html

Cancer Care, Inc.
1180 Avenue of the Americans
New York, NY 10036
(800) 813-HOPE

Cancer Federation, Inc.
21250 Box Spring Road
Morena Valley, CA 92388
(714) 682-7989

Cancer Guide
http://cancerguide.org/

Cancer Hotline
(800) 525-3777; (800) 638-6070 (Alaska); (800) 636-5700 (District of Columbia)
(808) 524-1234 (Hawaii, call collect)

Cancer Information Service (CIS)
NIH Building 32, Room 10A 24
Bethesda, MD 20892
(800) 4-CANCER; (800) 638-6070 (Alaska)
(808) 524-1234 (Hawaii; in Oahu, dial direct; call collect from neighboring islands)

Cancer News on the Net
http://www.cancernews.com

International Society of Nurses in Cancer Care
Mulberry House, The Royal Marsden Hospital
Fulham Road
London SW3 6JJ
England
(071) 252-8171, ext. 2123

International Union Against Cancer
3 rue du Conseil General
1205 Geneva
Switzerland
http://www.uicc.ch/

Memorial Sloan-Kettering Cancer Center
1275 York Ave.
New York, NY 10021
(212) 639-2000
http://www.mskcc.org/

National Cancer Institute–International Cancer Information Center
(CancerNet and CancerFax)
Building 82, Room 123
Bethesda, MD 20892
(800) 4-CANCER; (301) 496-4907
Fax: (301) 402-0212
http://www.nci.nih.gov/

National Coalition for Cancer Survivorship (NCCS)
1010 Wayne Ave., 5th Floor
Silver Spring, MD 20910
(301) 650-8868; (301) 565-9670

National Foundation for Cancer Research
7315 Wisconsin Ave., Suite 500-W
Bethesda, MD 20814
(301) 654-1250
Fax: (301) 654-5824

OncoLink (cancer information site)
http://www.oncolink.upenn.edu

Oncology Nursing Society
501 Holiday Drive
Pittsburgh, PA 15220
(412) 921-7373
http://www.ons.org

Society of Gynecologic Oncologists
401 N. Michigan Ave.
Chicago, IL 60611
(312) 644-6610
http://www.sgo.org/

REFERENCES

American Cancer Society (1998). *Cancer facts and figures—1998.* Atlanta: American Cancer Society.

Gordon, M. (2000). *Manual of nursing diagnosis* (9th ed.). St. Louis: Mosby.

Johnson, M., Maas, M., & Moorhead, S. (2000). *Nursing outcomes classification (NOC)* (2nd ed.). St. Louis: Mosby.

McCloskey, J., & Bulechek, G. (2000). *Nursing interventions classifications (NIC)* (3rd ed.). St. Louis: Mosby.

Mellody, P., Owen, M., & Klein, P. (1998). Timely solutions for improving oncology provider case manager communications. Pittsburgh, PA: Oncology Education Services.

National Cancer Institute. (2000).*Understanding trials* [On-line]. Available: http://cancertrials.nci.nih.gov.

Vogelzang, N.J., Breitbard, W., Cella D., et al. (1997). Patient, caregiver and oncologist perceptions of cancer-related fatigue: Results of a tripart assessment survey. *Seminars in Hematology, 34* (Suppl. 2), 4–12.

Wolfe, G. (1998). Recognizing the impact of anemia-related fatigue in oncology patients. *Journal of Care Management, November,* 27–32 [Special Edition].

RECOMMENDED READING

Bender, C., Vasko, J., & Strohl, R. (2000). Cancer. In S. Lewis, et al. (Eds), *Medical-surgical nursing: Assessment and management of clinical problems* (5th ed.). St. Louis: Mosby.

Coluzzi, P.H., Grant, M., Doroshow, J.H., et al. (1995). Survey of the provision of supportive care services at National Cancer Institute—designated cancer centers. *Journal of Clinical Oncology 13,* 756-764.

Deters, G. (2000). Cancer. In W. Phipps et al. (Eds), *Medical surgical nursing concepts and clinical practice* (6th ed.). St. Louis: Mosby.

Dodd, M., Miakowski, C., & Paul, S. (2001). Symptom clusters and their effect on the functional status of patients with cancer. *Oncology Nursing Forum, 28*(3), 465-470.

Edwards, P., Hertzberg, D., Hays, S., & Youngblood, N. (1999). *Pediatric rehabilitation nursing.* Philadelphia: WB Saunders.

Fisher, B., Dignam J., Wolmark, N., et al. (1997). Tamoxifen and chemotherapy for lymph node negative, estrogen receptor positive breast cancer. *Journal of the National Cancer Institute, 89*(22), 1673-1682.

Glaspy, J., Bukowski, R., & Steinberg, D., et al. (1997). Impact of therapy with epoetin alpha on clinical outcomes in patients with nonmyeloid malignancies during cancer chemotherapy in community oncology practice. *Journal of Clinical Oncology, 3*(15), 1218-1234.

Gotay, C.C., & Muraoka, M.Y. (1998). Quality of life in long-term survivors of adult-onset cancers. *Journal of the National Cancer Institute, 90,* 656-667.

Mandelblatt, J.S., Ganz, P., & Kahn, K.L. (1999). Proposed agenda for the measurement of quality of care outcomes in oncology practice. *Journal of Clinical Oncology, 17,* 2614.

Mock, V., et al. (1997). Effects of exercise on fatigue, physical functioning and emotional distress during radiation for breast cancer. *Oncology Nurses Forum, 24,* 991.

Oncology Nursing Society. (1996). *Cancer chemotherapy guidelines and recommendations for practice.* Pittsburgh: Oncology Nursing Society Press.

Schaefer, K., Ladd, E., Gergits, M., & Gyauch, L. (2001). Backing and forthing: The process of decision making by women considering participation in a breast cancer prevention trial. *Oncology Nursing Forum, 28*(4), 703-709.

Appendix A

Pharmacology for Rehabilitation Nursing

Nicole Brandt, PharmD, CGP

This appendix is intended to assist rehabilitation nurses in pharmacological management for clients. This is not a complete presentation of the issues of pharmacology in rehabilitation medicine; it is not intended to replace comprehensive pharmacology texts or drug references. Objectives for this appendix are to define terminology, explain principles of drug action, describe pharmacokinetic functions and principles of pharmacodynamics, identify adverse drug reactions, and to apply this knowledge to decisions in clinical practice.

Appropriate prescribing, administering, and monitoring are instrumental in minimizing medication adverse effects and errors.

PHARMACEUTICS

Pharmaceutics evaluates the physical and chemical principles involved in the designing, formulating, manufacturing, and stability of drug delivery systems and the application of this knowledge to the bioavailability of medications in various routes of administration.

A medication is a chemical that interacts with a living organism to produce a biological response. In general medications have the following characteristics:

1. Medications do not bestow any new function on a tissue or organ in the body—they only modify existing functions. *Example:* Enzyme inhibition with angiotensin-converting enzyme (ACE) inhibitors for blood pressure or congestive heart failure.
2. Medications generally exhibit multiple actions rather than a single effect. Consequently, medications have incidence of side effects in addition to therapeutic effects. Therefore choosing an agent that is more selective for a particular receptor could minimize this. *Example:* antihistamines (e.g., first generations such as diphenhydramine [Benadryl]) have more anticholinergic side effects (e.g., dry mouth, blurred vision, confusion and sedation) versus the newer antihistamines, such as loratadine (Claritin), which are more selective.
3. Medication action results from a physiochemical interaction between the drug and an important molecule in the body. This molecule could be a receptor or a component of a membrane structure.

ROUTES OF ADMINISTRATION

Medications are ranked from the quickest to the slowest in terms of gastrointestinal absorption rate of preparations: liquids → suspensions → powders → capsules → tablets → coated tables (Table A-1).

PHARMACOKINETICS

Pharmacokinetics (PK) evaluates the absorption, distribution, metabolism, and elimination of medication. In essence, it is what the body does to the medication. Many variables affect PK and are discussed throughout this section. Different models offer explanations for the concentration of a medication over a time period. The First Order Kinetics model states that the rate of change of drug concentration by any process is directly proportional to the drug concentration remaining to undertake that process. First Order Kinetics is an assumption of a linear model, not a one-compartment model. In a linear model, doubling a dose will cause the concentration to double at each point in time.

The Non-Linear Kinetics model does not describe a proportional relationship; rather, it states that serum drug concentrations change more or less than expected. Examples include the following:

- Michaelis-Menten equation: This refers to the greater-than-expected increase in serum drug concentration based on the saturation of the enzymes that metabolize or eliminate a certain medication. The classic example of this is phenytoin. Phenytoin has a constant (K_m) of 4 mg/ml, yet the therapeutic range is 10-20 mg/ml. At

TABLE A-1 Routes of Administration

Route	Bioavailability	Comments
Intravenous (IV) • Bolus • Infusion	Complete 100% systemic drug absorption	Advantages: Good for large molecules, drugs with poor lipid solubility, and/or irritating medications Disadvantage: Evaluate for tissue damage at injection site
Intramuscular injection (IM)	Rapid absorption from aqueous solution, and slow absorption from nonaqueous solution	Advantage: Larger volume than subcutaneous Disadvantage: Different rates of absorption based on blood flow
Subcutaneous (SQ)	Absorption slow but usually complete	Advantage: Can be administered by client, (e.g., insulin) Disadvantages: Can be painful Irritant drugs can cause local tissue damage Maximum of 2 ml injection, thus small doses often limit use
Oral (PO)	Absorption may vary	Advantage: Safest and easiest route of drug administration Disadvantage: Erratic absorption
Rectal (PR)	Absorption may vary	Advantage: Useful when individual cannot swallow medications Disadvantage: Some client discomfort
Transdermal	Slow absorption rate; may be enhanced with client variables and/or occlusive dressing	Advantage: Easy to use Beneficial with low dose and low molecular weight Disadvantage: Variability and often skin irritation
Inhalation	Rapid absorption	Advantage: Local or systemic effects Disadvantage: Particle size affects deposition in the respiratory tract

low concentration the apparent half-life is about 12 hours, whereas at higher concentration, the half-life may be much greater than 24 hours.

- Non-linear protein binding: In the case of a low clearance medication, such as valproic acid which is highly protein bound (approximately 98%), the steady state concentration increases less than the dose secondary to the saturation of protein binding sites and the increased clearance.

Understanding these models sets the stage for understanding the various distinct but related processes that ultimately affect the concentrations available. The first process is absorption.

Absorption

Medications have 100% absorption when administered intravenously. All other forms of administration are dependent on the physiochemical properties of the drug, dosage form, and anatomy and physiology of the absorption site. For instance, older individuals have thinner skin with a reduced amount of fat in the subcutaneous layer; ultimately, this affects the absorption of hydrophilic medications, such as nitroglycerin patches.

Bioavailability

Bioavailability measures the rate and extent of therapeutically active medication that reaches the systemic circulation. When the bioavailability is rated less than 1, this means that either the dosage form did not release all of the medication or that some of the medication was eliminated or destroyed by stomach acid or other means before it reached the systemic circulation.

Some medications have very low bioavailability, such as alendronate (Fosamax). Administering these drugs correctly is very important. Check references for any drug-food interactions and to determine whether the medications must be taken with food to increase bioavailability. Just as important, some medications must be taken on an empty stomach (Table A-2).

Clinicians need to understand the meaning of the term *bioequivalence* when explaining brand-name versus generic medications. A medication is deemed bioequivalent when the area under the curve (AUC), maximum of serum or blood concentrations (C_{max}), and the times that C_{max} occur (T_{max}) are neither clinically nor statistically different. When this occurs, the serum concentration versus time curves for the two dosage forms could be superimposed and therefore identical. The United States Pharmacopeia (USP) publishes the *Orange Book* that contains lists of agents that are bioequivalent. This information is crucial when a client changes from a brand-name medication to a generic form, especially with narrow therapeutic agents.

Distribution

The next process to understand is distribution. When a medication is absorbed, the drug molecules are carried through-

TABLE A-2 Medications and Nutrient Interactions

Drug Category	Medication	Interaction	Recommendations
Psychotropics	Lithium carbonate	Food may enhance absorption, decrease irritation	Take with food
		Excessive sodium chloride (salt) intake will decrease lithium levels	Sodium chloride (salt) use in the diet should be consistent
		Low salt intake may increase lithium levels	Drink 8-12, 8-ounce glasses of water/day
		Lithium can predispose a person to dehydration and salt loss	
	Antipsychotics (e.g., haloperidol)	Coffee or tea may decrease absorption	Avoid caffeinated beverages
	Zolpidem (Ambien)	Food decreases absorption and delays onset of action	Do not take with or immediately after a meal
Anticonvulsants	Phenytoin (Dilantin)	Food and tube feedings alter absorption	Take at the same time in relation to meals Flush feeding tubes well with water; wait 1 hr to administer phenytoin, then 2 hr to resume tube feedings
Anticoagulants	Warfarin (Coumadin)	Food and supplements that contain Vitamin K	Consistent daily intake of food high in vitamin K (e.g., green leafy vegetables, potatoes, animal livers, dairy products)

NOTE: This table is not all-inclusive, but it does address the more common interactions. It is best to check with your pharmacist, health care provider, or the product label to minimize adverse effects and optimize therapeutic efficacy.

out the body by the systemic circulation, which carries them to the target site of action (receptor) as well as other tissues and organs. The passage of a drug molecule across a membrane depends on the chemical make-up of the drug. Small molecules permeate quickly; however, lipophilic medications deposit in fat tissues that release the medication slowly. Medications bound to proteins, such as albumin, may become too large for easy diffusion. The apparent volume of distribution the amount of drug in the body compared to the concentration measured in plasma, serum, or blood.

Metabolism

Metabolism is the process in the body that makes a chemical molecule more polar to hinder its reabsorption and facilitate elimination. The four main processes of drug metabolism are grouped into phase I (oxidation, hydrolysis, and reduction) and Phase II (conjugation). Phase I reactions include the cytochrome P-450 system. Enzymes involved in the biotransformation are located primarily in the liver; however, other tissues, such as the kidney, lung, small intestine, and skin also contain enzymes. New findings about the multiple interactions within these various enzymes are being reported, and a summary of the known information alone would be extensive (Michalets, 1998). One interaction to highlight is that of grapefruit juice because it inhibits intestinal cytochrome P-450. As a result, it increases levels of drugs metabolized by intestinal CYP 3A4, such as alprazolam (Xanax), cyclosporine (Neoral, Sandimmune), felodipine (Plendil), and nifedipine (Procardia).

Elimination

Elimination is the irreversible removal of drug from the body by all routes. The main organ in this process is the kidney. As clinicians, it is important to evaluate an individual's renal function to appropriately prescribe dosages of certain medications. There are various formulas used, but the most common is the Cockcroft-Gault. These formulas are described further in Chapter 34.

Clearance

The rate at which a drug is eliminated by the body is an important parameter that can be affected by many variables. Physiologically, it is determined by the blood flow to the organ that metabolizes (i.e., liver) or eliminates (i.e., kidney) the medication and the efficiency of the organ in extracting the medication from the body (DiPiro, 1999). High clearance medications, such as propranolol, are extensively metabolized by the liver. With low clearance medications, such as warfarin, elimination is equal to the fraction of unbound, "active," medication in the blood and the intrinsic ability of the organ. These issues become important when introducing drugs that increase or decrease the metabolism of certain substrates or displace binding of highly protein bound medications. This is especially the case with anticonvulsants, such as phenytoin and valproic acid.

Half-Life

The half-life ($t_{1/2}$) is the amount of time it takes a medication to decrease by one half after completing absorption and distribution. This is an important parameter because it provides the clinician with an insight into when a medication will reach steady state (approximately 3 to 5 half-lives).

Many factors affect PK principles and need to be taken into consideration, including the following:

- Age (e.g., pediatric and geriatric changes)
- Gender
- Body make-up
- Drug-drug, drug-disease, and drug-food interactions (see Chapter 17)

PHARMACODYNAMICS

Pharmacodynamics (PD) is the study of biochemical and physiological effects of medications and their mechanism of action (i.e., what the drug does to the body). Core definitions and concepts aid in understanding these processes.

Core Components

Protein targets for drug binding include the following:

- Enzymes (e.g., cyclooxygenase)
- Carrier molecules (e.g., Na/K pump)
- Ion channels (e.g., voltage gated calcium channels)
- Receptors (usually proteins designed by nature to confer a response or transduce a signal to a naturally occurring ligand)

Some references group all of the aforemention protein targets as receptors. A specific example is the dopamine receptors.

Medications act selectively on a particular tissue or cell, a process termed *drug specificity.* For example, angiotensin acts selectively on vascular smooth muscle and kidney tubule but has little effect on other smooth muscle. Most drugs do not act with complete specificity, therefore side effects may occur. Medications bind to receptors differently, as described in the following:

1. At equilibrium, binding is related to drug concentration.
2. Higher affinity or selective drugs need lower concentrations to approach saturation of the receptors and clinically can result in fewer adverse side effects.
3. Competitive antagonism occurs when two or more medications compete for the same receptors, and one may reduce the affinity or selectivity of the other.

After binding to the receptor site, the following different responses can occur:

1. *Agonists* initiate changes in cell function, producing various effects. The potency depends on affinity (tendency to bind to receptors) and efficacy (ability once bound to produce an effect). Full agonists produce maximal effect and have high efficacy; partial agonists produce only submaximal effect and intermediate efficacy.
2. *Antagonists* bind to receptors without initiating changes. Types of antagonisms include:
   - Chemical antagonism, such as when a chelating agent binds to a heavy metal.
   - Pharmacokinetic antagonism, such as cytochrome P-450 inducers (e.g., carbamazepine, phenobarbital) that increase the metabolism of a substrate such as warfarin.
   - Noncompetitive antagonism (i.e., blocking a receptor-effector linkage) such as omeprazole (Prilosec), a proton pump inhibitor.
   - Physiological antagonism, wherein two agents balance each other, such as with acetylcholinesterase inhibitors and anticholinergics.

Receptor Level Changes

Receptor level changes describe a change in conformational state or a loss of receptors, such as what happens with beta receptors. Again, knowing the basic pharmacodynamic principles assists clinicians in understanding how long medications require to reach efficacy and what to expect concerning side effects or toxicity.

UNDERSTANDING PHARMACOLOGICAL CHANGES ACROSS THE LIFE SPAN

Pediatric Considerations

A client younger than 18 years old is considered pediatric for purposes of this text. Physiological changes occur with aging and affect the process of drug absorption, distribution, metabolism, and elimination, as described below.

Effects on Absorption

1. Full-term infants have a pH of 6 to 8 at birth that decreases to 1 to 3 within 24 hours. The change in pH increases the bioavailability of acid labile penicillins. Premature infants have an elevated gastric pH level as a result of their immature acid secretion.
2. Gastric emptying is slowed in a premature infant.
3. Intramuscular (IM) injections are rarely used for infants because of the great variability in absorption.
4. An infant's skin has increased permeability secondary to an underdeveloped epidermal barrier (stratum corneum).

Effects on Distribution

1. Total water is 94% in a fetus, 85% in premature infants, 78% in a full-term infant, and 60% in adults. Water-soluble drugs, such as gentamicin and tobramycin, have an increased volume of distribution.

2. Protein binding is decreased in newborns secondary to their decreased plasma concentration, lowered binding capacity, and decreased affinity.
3. Body fat is substantially lower in neonates.

Effects on Metabolism

Glucoronidation (phase II) is not developed at birth; therefore, avoid use of chloramphenicol because it cannot be metabolized.

Effects on Elimination

The processes of glomerular filtration, tubular secretion, and resorption determine the efficiency of renal excretion. These processes may take several weeks of life and fully develop after 1 year of age.

Geriatric Considerations

Elders are the most rapidly growing segment of the U.S. population. All practitioners need to heighten their awareness about medications and the elderly. Many medications are more likely to produce adverse effects and lead to negative outcomes in older persons. The complications with medications and side effects during recovery of a hip fracture are an example. A review of the PK differences in this population helps with understanding the processes.

Effects on Absorption

Absorption is not usually clinically significant. However, older persons have decreased gastric acidity and decreased gastrointestinal tract blood flow. They also have delayed gastric emptying and a reduced lipid content of their skin.

Effects on Distribution

1. Decreased total body water that increases potential dehydration, especially when taking diuretics.
2. Body fat increases from 15% to 30%, and lean body weight decreases in proportion to total body weight. The result is an increase in the volume of distribution and half-life of agents such as diazepam (Valium).
3. There is a decreased serum albumin level leading to an increase in concentrations of highly protein-bound drugs (e.g., phenytoin).
4. There is a decrease in cardiac output resulting in reduced hepatic blood flow, which can lead to a slowed rate of metabolism for medications such as warfarin that increase risk for bleeding.

Effects on Metabolism

1. Decrease in liver mass.
2. Change in phase I oxidative process by the cytochrome P-450 appears to be decreased.
3. No changes have been noted in the phase II coupling of a parent drug or phase by glucoronidation, sulfation, or acetylation

Effects on Elimination

Elimination of medications is affected by a decrease in the size of the kidney (20%) accompanied by reduced renal blood flow, glomerular filtration rate, and tubular excretory capacity.

ADVERSE DRUG REACTIONS

The World Health Organization (WHO) defines an adverse drug reaction (ADR) as "any response to a drug which is noxious and unintended and which occurs at doses normally used in man for prophylaxis, diagnosis or therapy of disease or for modification of physiological function" (American Society of Health System Pharmacists, 1995). It is important to note that ADRs have been reported as the fourth leading cause of death in the United States, following heart disease, cancer, and stroke (Lazarou, Pomeranz, & Corey, 1998).

Health care providers must advocate for a prospective, ongoing, and concurrent surveillance system that mandates reports of suspected ADRs, as well as screening for high-risk indicators. Clients at high risk for ADRs include, but are not limited to, pediatric and geriatric aggregates and persons with hepatic or renal failure. High-risk medications extend beyond aminoglycosides, digoxin, heparin, phenytoin, and warfarin.

Application of the pharmacology principles discussed in this chapter is an initial step to minimize ADRs in rehabilitation practice.

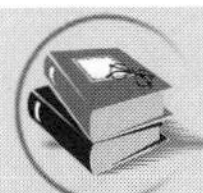

Case Study ⁓ *Rheumatoid Arthritis*

A 32-year-old woman came to the clinic complaining of morning stiffness in the metocarpophalangeal joints in both hands. She has had the problem for several months and is tired. Taking ibuprofen is not relieving the pain; she also has dyspepsia.

A complete blood count, SMA-7 chemistries, iron studies, and a rheumatoid factor are appropriate laboratory studies. The results should confirm a positive rheumatoid factor, low hematocrit and hemoglobin levels, plus a low serum iron level and low iron binding capacity. What are your recommendations?

Guidelines for Pharmacological Management

Table A-3 describes disease modifying antirheumatic drugs (DMARDs). Nonsteroidal anti-inflammatory drugs (NSAIDs) are described in Table A-4 (American College of Rheumatology, 1996). Related variables specific to this client are dyspepsia and low hematocrit and hemoglobin levels; consider conducting iron studies. Choose a cyclooxygenase (COX)-II specific NSAID (e.g., rofecoxib [Vioxx] or celecoxib [Celebrex]), but apply dosing and precautions to lessen secondary GI irritation.

TABLE A-3 Disease-Modifying Antirheumatic Drugs

Medication	Dose	Side Effects	Comments
Methotrexate (Rheumatrex)	Oral or IM: 7.5-15 mg q wk	Myelosuppression, proteinuria, rash, stomatitis, worsening liver function	The DMARD of choice, but not used in pregnant or nursing clients Give additional folic acid since methotrexate is a folic acid antagonist
Hydroxychloroquine (Plaquenil)	PO: 200-300 mg bid	Macular damage, rash, diarrhea	Main benefit is lack of myelosuppression Take with food
Sulfasalazine (Azulfidine)	500 mg bid, then increase to 1 g bid max	Myelosuppression, rash, nausea, vomiting, diarrhea and anorexia	Can cause urine and skin to turn yellow-orange
Leflunomide (Arava)	100 mg qd for 3 days, then 10-20 mg qd	Diarrhea, hepatotoxicity, alopecia, rash	Comparable efficacy to sulfasalazine and methotrexate Costs about $3000/yr
Etanercept (Enbrel)	25 mg SQ twice weekly	Injection site irritation, upper respiratory infections	Second-line treatment option Costs $5000-8000/yr

NOTE: Take client variables, administration, comorbid conditions, and cost into account when planning. The client may initially begin taking methotrexate 7.5 mg po q weekly with monitoring.

TABLE A-4 Medications Commonly Used in Rehabilitation Practice

NOTE: This table is not comprehensive, but it does include information about medications from different classes common to practice. Individual chapters contain other information about applications of medications and treatments specific to their content.

Generic Name (Selected Trade Name)	Normal Adult Dosage	Therapeutic Uses	Major Adverse Effects/Cautions	Comments
Anticonvulsants				
Phenytoin (Dilantin)	Individualized therapeutic levels: 10-20 μg/ml	Tonic-clonic (grand mal), simple, complex, or partial seizures	CNS toxicities (e.g., ataxia, blood dyscrasias, gingival hyperplasia)	Check albumin levels in individual who is poorly nourished secondary to increased likelihood for increased free levels and toxicities
Carbamazepine (Tegretol)	Up to 1.6 g/day Level for seizures: 6-12 μg/ml	Partial seizures with simple or complex symptoms, generalized tonic-clonic seizures, mixed, trigeminal neuralgia, bipolar disorder	CNS toxicity, blood dyscrasias, hyponatremia, diarrhea, GI irritation, increase in liver function, hypocalcemia	Numerous drug interactions, autoinduction of metabolism Take with food to minimize irritation If using liquid via G-tube must be spaced out from other medications
Valproic acid (divalproex, Depakote, Depekene)	Up to 60 mg/kg body weight/day (50-100 μg/ml)	Simple and complex absence (petit mal), mixed, and tonic-clonic seizures; bipolar disorder, migraine headaches (prophylactic)	CNS toxicity, blood dyscrasias, GI irritation, worsening liver function, sedation	Highly protein bound May use higher levels in clients bipolar disorder Assess for drug interactions
Newer Agents				
Oxcarbazepine (Trileptal)	Initial in adults 600 mg/day Recommended 1200 mg/day as adjunct and 2400 mg/day as monotherapy	Monotherapy or adjunctive therapy of partial seizures in adults with epilepsy Adjunct of partial seizures in children ages 4-16 yr	Dizziness, drowsiness, abnormal vision, fatigue, nausea, vomiting, ataxia, tremor, dyspepsia and gait abnormalities, hyponatremia	Appears to be better tolerated than carbamazepine and does not induce its own metabolism, which is seen with carabamazepine Monitoring serum level not normally required
Levetiracetam (Keppra)	Initial 1000 mg/day Increase to 3000 mg/day	Adjunct treatment for partial onset seizures	Somnolence, weakness, infection, dizziness	Little drug interactions secondary to not being a substrate or inhibitor of cytochrome P-450 Renally excreted Monitor for blood dyscrasias Not necessary to monitor serum levels
Zonisamide (Zonegran)	Up to 600 mg/day	Adjunct in treatment of partial seizures No safety profile in clients younger than 16 yr	Somnolence, anorexia, dizziness, headache, nausea, agitation and irritability Commonly associated with CNS side effects such as psychiatric symptoms, including depression and psychosis, psychomotor slowing, and cognitive effect About 4% incidence of kidney stones	Do *not* use in individuals with sulfa allergy Metabolized by liver and renally eliminated Increasing fluid intake and urine output can help reduce risk of kidney stones

Data from American Society of Health System Pharmacists. (2000). *AHFS drug information.* Bethesda, MD: Author; and Lackner, T.E. (1999). Urinary health management in the long-term care setting. *Consultant Pharmacist, 14* (Suppl B), 3-16.

Continued

TABLE A-4 Medications Commonly Used in Rehabilitation Practice—cont'd

Generic Name (Selected Trade Name)	Normal Adult Dosage	Therapeutic Uses	Major Adverse Effects/Cautions	Comments
Tiagabine (Gabatril)	32-64 mg/day	Adjunct therapy in adults and children older than 12 yr for the treatment of partial seizures	Common: Dizziness, nervousness, tremor, abnormal thinking Serious/rare: Depression	Do not need to monitor serum levels
Topiramate (Topamax)	Up to 400 mg/day	Adjunct therapy in adults and children 2 yr and older with partial onset seizures	Common: Fatigue, dizziness, somnolence, impaired concentration, ataxia, weight loss Serious/rare: Nephrolithiasis	Topiramate clearance increased by phenytoin and carbamazepine Topiramate may increase phenytoin levels Monitoring serum levels not necessary Use lower doses in individuals with renal impairment *Start with low doses*
Gabapentin (Neurontin)	Up to 3600 mg/day	Adjunct in treatment of partial seizures with or without secondary generalization in adults and adolescents older than 12 yr	Common: Dizziness, fatigue, somnolence, ataxia, tremor	Titrate slowly to minimize CNS toxicities Renally eliminated Do not need to monitor serum levels Little potential for drug interactions
Antidepressants				
Tricyclic Antidepressants			All agents, some more than others, produce anticholinergic side effects such as blurred vision, confusion, delirium (especially in the elderly), irregular heartbeat	Numerous agents in this class Look at PK and PD difference plus indication for use when choosing a tricyclic antidepressant
Nortriptyline (Pamelor)	Up to 150 mg/day	Depression Numerous other uses for this class such as peripheral neuropathy, enuresis		
Selective Serotonin Reuptake Inhibitors (SSRIs)		Major depressive disorder, obsessive compulsive disorder, panic disorder	Sexual dysfunction, hyponatremia, confusion, dizziness, drowsiness, serotonin syndrome, anorexia, stomach or abdominal cramps, agitation or nervousness, abnormal movements—tremor Some side effects are dose related	Takes 2-4 wk to see the full benefit of an antidepressant *Do not* abruptly stop treatment
Sertraline (Zoloft)	Up to 200 mg/day			
Others				
Mirtazapine (Remeron)	Up to 45 mg/day	Major depressive disorder	Constipation, dizziness, drowsiness, dryness of mouth, increased appetite and weight gain	Good for clients needing help with sleep At lower doses has more antihistaminic properties and causes sedation
Venlafaxine (Effexor)	Up to 375 mg/day	Major depressive disorder	Headache, sexual dysfunction, abnormal dreams, anorexia, weight loss, dizziness, increase in blood pressure	Available in extended release as well; do not break these tablets Dosage adjustments needed for renal or hepatic impairment

Data from American Society of Health System Pharmacists. (2000). *AHFS drug information.* Bethesda, MD: Author; and Lackner, T.E. (1999). Urinary health management in the long-term care setting. *Consultant Pharmacist, 14* (Suppl B), 3-16.

TABLE A-4 Medications Commonly Used in Rehabilitation Practice—cont'd

Generic Name (Selected Trade Name)	Normal Adult Dosage	Therapeutic Uses	Major Adverse Effects/Cautions	Comments
Bupropion (Wellbutrin)	Up to 450 mg/day, with no single dose exceeding 150 mg	Major depressive disorder, nicotine dependence	Agitation, anxiety, headache, abdominal pain, decrease in appetite, nausea or vomiting, dryness of mouth, insomnia	Note importance of no single dose greater than 150 mg secondary to decreased seizure threshold Also available in extended release
Antianxiety				
Benzodiazepines				Important to assess active metabolites as well as elimination (e.g., avoid diazepam in an elderly person because it goes through the cytochrome P-450 system and has an active metabolite that accumulates)
LONG HALF-LIFE		Anxiety, alcohol withdrawal, insomnia, epilepsy, panic disorders, skeletal muscle spasm	CNS side effects: Confusion, fatigue, mental depression High fall risk medication	
Diazepam (Valium)	4-40 mg/day			
SHORT-INTERMEDIATE HALF-LIFE				
Alprazolam (Xanax)	0.75-4 mg/day			
Clonazepam (Klonopin)	1.5-20 mg/day			
Lorazepam (Ativan)	2-4 mg/day			
Oxazepam (Serax)	30-120 mg/day			
Buspirone (BuSpar)	Up to 60 mg/day	Anxiety Not indicated but may be used as adjunct for depression plus for aggressive behavior	Causes less sedation or confusion compared with benzodiazepines Incidence of dizziness, lightheadedness, headache, nausea	Takes 1-2 wk before antianxiety effects are noticed Less efficacious if used after benzodiazepines
Common Cardiac Medications				
Angiotensin-Converting Enzyme (ACE) Inhibitors		Hypertension congestive heart failure, postmyocardial infarction (MI), diabetic nephropathy	Hypotension, hyperkalemia, cough	Numerous agents from which to choose Look at PK differences in labeling of products to evaluate for frequency of dosing
Lisinopril (Zestril, Prinivil)	5-40 mg/day			
Beta Blockers				
B1 SELECTIVE				Note: More beta-1 selective at doses less than 100 mg qd
Atenolol (Tenormin)	25-100 mg/day	Hypertension, angina, MI and postmyocardial infarction post-MI, atrial and ventricular tachycardia, congestive heart failure	Bradycardia CNS: Dizziness, fatigue, confusion GI: Nausea, vomiting	Increased half-life in individuals with creatinine clearance (CrCl) of 15-35 ml/min (half-life = 16- 27 hr) vs normal CrCl half-life 6-7 hr Shorter half life (4.6 hr) in children 5-16 yr
NONSELECTIVE B-ADRENERGIC WITH SELECTIVE ALPHA-1 ADRENERGIC BLOCKING ACTIVITY		Hypertension, congestive heart failure	Bradycardia CNS: Dizziness, fatigue, confusion GI: Nausea, vomiting	
Carvedilol (Coreg)	6.25-50 mg/day			

Continued

TABLE A-4 Medications Commonly Used in Rehabilitation Practice—cont'd

Generic Name (Selected Trade Name)	Normal Adult Dosage	Therapeutic Uses	Major Adverse Effects/Cautions	Comments
Calcium Channel Blockers		Hypertension, angina		Note: Calcium channel blockers act differently secondary to their specificity to certain receptors that are prevalent in different tissues (PD)
FIRST GENERATION (DIHYDROPYRIDNE)			Peripheral edema, dizziness, tachycardia	
Nifedipine (Procardia)	Up to 90 mg/day of extended release tablets		Do *not* use short acting–immediate release nifedipine	
SECOND GENERATION (DIHYDROPYRIDINE)				No dose adjustment needed in renal impairment, yet start at 2.5 mg in clients with hepatic impairment
Amlodipine (Norvasc)	2.5-10 mg/day		Hypotension	Note: Available in combination formulation with ACE inhibitor (benazepril)
BENZOTHIAZEPINE DERIVATIVE				
Diltiazem (Cardizem)	Up to 360 mg/day		Bradycardia	Depresses sinoatrial and atrioventricular nodes
Diuretics				
THIAZIDE				
Hydrochlorothiazide (HydroDiuril)	Up to 25-100 mg/day	Edema, hypertension	Increased sensitivity to the sun, orthostatic hypotension, electrolyte imbalance	Note: No additional antihypertensive benefit at doses greater than 25 mg/day
LOOP				
Furosemide (Lasix)	Up to 600 mg/day	Edema, hypertension, hypercalcemia,	Skin rash, electrolyte imbalance, increased sensitivity to the sun, orthostatic hypotension	Various agents in this class Look at PK and PD
POTASSIUM SPARING				
Spirinolactone (Aldactone)	Up to 400 mg/day	Edema, hypertension, hyperaldosteronism, hypokalemia	Hyperkalemia, antiandrogenic or endocrine effects, headache, dizziness, GI irritation	
Angiotensin Receptor Blockers (ARBs)		Hypertension, congestive heart failure	Dizziness, headache	Great agent for clients who cannot tolerate ACE inhibitors secondary to cough Note numerous agents in this class; some available in combinations
Losartan (Cozaar)	Up to 100 mg/day			
Anti-Inflammatory				
Nonsteroidal Anti-inflammatory Drugs (NSAIDs)		Various per agent: Rheumatoid arthritis and osteoarthritis, pain, gouty arthritis or acute gouty attacks, inflammation, fever, dysmenorrhea	GI upset/bleeds, worsening renal function; some cause blood dyscrasias	Numerous agents in this class Look at PK differences for information on dosing. Available over the counter Some concomitant illnesses can worsen hypertension and congestive heart failure
Naproxen (Naprosyn)	Up to 1.25 g/day			
Nabumetone (Relafen)	Up to 2 g/day			
Indomethacin (Indocin)	Up to 200 mg/day			

Data from American Society of Health System Pharmacists. (2000). *AHFS drug information.* Bethesda, MD: Author; and Lackner, T.E. (1999). Urinary health management in the long-term care setting. *Consultant Pharmacist, 14* (Suppl B), 3-16.

TABLE A-4 Medications Commonly Used in Rehabilitation Practice—cont'd

Generic Name (Selected Trade Name)	Normal Adult Dosage	Therapeutic Uses	Major Adverse Effects/Cautions	Comments
COX II Inhibitors				
Rofecoxib (Vioxx)	12.5-25 mg qd	Osteoarthritis, rheumatoid arthritis	Less GI upset and bleeds vs NSAIDs	Note: Do *not* use Celecoxib in clients sensitive to sulfa
Celecoxib (Celebrex)	100-200 mg bid	Acute short-term pain	Still can affect renal function	
Analgesics				
Acetaminophen (Tylenol)	325-650 mg q4hr or 650 mg-1 g q6hr prn (up to 4 g/day)	Analgesic, antipyretic		First-line agent for osteoarthritis
Morphine	PO 10-30 mg q3-4hr IM 5-10 mg q3-4hr IV 1-2.5 mg q5min prn SR 15-30 mg q12hr (q8hr may be needed in some clients) Rectal 10-20 mg q3-4hr	Drug of choice for acute severe pain Use immediate-release product with SR product to control breakthrough pain in clients with cancer		
Hydromorphone	PO 2-4 mg q3-4hr IM 0.5-1 mg q3-4hr Rectal 2-4 mg q3-4hr	Severe pain More potent than morphine, otherwise no advantages		
Oxymorphone	IM 1-1.5 mg q4-6hr IV 0.5 mg initially Rectal 5 mg q3-4hr	No advantages over morphine		
Levorphanol	PO 2-4 mg q6-8hr IM 2 mg q6-8hr IV 2 mg q6-8hr	Severe pain Extended half-life Useful in clients with cancer		
Codeine	PO 15-60 mg q3-4hr IM 15-60 mg q3-4hr IV 2 mg q6-8hr	Moderate pain Weak analgesic; use with NSAIDs, aspirin, or acetaminophen		
Hydrocodone	PO 5-10 mg q3-4hr	Moderate or severe pain Most effective when used with NSAIDs, aspirin, or acetaminophen		
Oxycodone	PO 5-10 mg q3-4hr Controlled release 10-20 mg q12hr	Moderate or severe pain Most effective when used with NSAIDs, aspirin, or acetaminophen Use immediate-release product with controlled-release product to control breakthrough pain in clients with cancer		
Fentanyl	IM 0.05-0.1 mg q1-2hr Transdermal 25 μg/hr q72hr Transmucosal (investigational)	Severe pain Do not use transdermal for acute pain Takes up to 72 hr to see full benefit		

Continued

TABLE A-4 Medications Commonly Used in Rehabilitation Practice—cont'd

Generic Name (Selected Trade Name)	Normal Adult Dosage	Therapeutic Uses	Major Adverse Effects/Cautions	Comments
Propoxyphene	PO 65-100 mg q3-4hr	Moderate pain Weak analgesic; most effective when used with NSAIDs, aspirin, or acetaminophen Will cause carbamazepine level to increase		
Tramadol (Ultram)	PO 50-100 mg q4-6hr Maximum dose 400 mg/24hr			
Parkinson's Disease				
Carbidopa-Levodopa	Initially: 50/200 mg controlled release bid (should wait 3 days before dosage adjustments) Up to 1 g/day	Controversial as to when to start Assess client; if younger client may want to start with a dopamine agonist secondary to motor complications associated with levodopa	GI: Nausea CV: Postural hypotension Neurological: Dyskinesias, dystonias, myoclonus, akathisia CNS: Nightmares, hallucinations—usually visual, confusion, insomnia	Food-drug interactions: High-protein meals can interfere with absorption of levodopa across GI endothelium and across blood-brain barrier; timing of meals may be clinically important as disease progresses Symptoms unresponsive to levodopa: Motor: Postural instability, freezing, speech abnormalities Mental changes: Dementia, depression, sensory phenomena, olfactory changes Autonomic: Constipation, sexual dysfunction, urinary problems, sweating
Anticholinergics		Tremor-predominant disease Adjunct to levodopa if tremor not well controlled	Impair cognitive function; constipation, dry mouth, sedation, urinary retention, blurred vision	Not recommended in clients older than 60 yr All equally effective Benztropine can be given once or twice/day Inexpensive
Benztropine (Cogentin)	0.5, 1, 2 mg tablets; 1 mg/ml inj			
Trihexyphenidyl (Artane)	2, 5 mg tablets; 5 mg sustained release capsule; 2 mg/5 ml elixir			
Amantadine				
Symmetrel	Available in 100 mg capsules; 50 mg/5 ml syrup Monotherapy: 100 mg bid Adjunctive therapy: 100 mg qd to start, titrate to total daily dose of 400 mg Requires dose adjustment in renal	Mild bradykinesia, tremor, rigidity May be used as initial therapy to delay starting levodopa	Confusion, hallucinations, nightmares, insomnia, ankle edema, worsening congestive heart failure, peripheral anticholinergic effects	Not recommended in clients older than 60 yr because of cognitive effects; however, there is increasing use in older clients, but dose adjustment required because of renal impairment Tolerance may develop: stop, then restart; sensitivity may be restored Do not abruptly stop because

Data from American Society of Health System Pharmacists. (2000). *AHFS drug information.* Bethesda, MD: Author; and Lackner, T.E. (1999). Urinary health management in the long-term care setting. *Consultant Pharmacist, 14* (Suppl B), 3-16.

Table A-4 Medications Commonly Used in Rehabilitation Practice—cont'd

Generic Name (Selected Trade Name)	Normal Adult Dosage	Therapeutic Uses	Major Adverse Effects/Cautions	Comments
	dysfunction (80% to 90% excreted unchanged in the kidneys) Half-life = 2-7 hr in healthy adults, 7-10 days in clients with end stage renal diseaes			of possibility of rebound parkinsonian symptoms Modestly effective Used in early therapy or adjunctive later in treatment
Selegiline (SD-Deprenyl, Eldepryl)	Available in 5 mg capsules and tablets (generic) 5 mg bid (dose with breakfast and lunch)	Useful in early disease for symptomatic management (possibly neuroprotective) Adjunctive therapy with levodopa later in disease	Augments levodopa toxicities, insomnia (give in morning), confusion, agitation, hypomania, diarrhea, sweating, shivering, serotonin syndrome, hyperreflexia, myoclonus, hypertension incoordination	Drug interactions: Antidepressants, monoamine oxidase inhibitors and selective serotonin reuptake inhibitors, meperidine Half-life 10 hr Metabolized in the liver to amphetamine and methamphetamine Well tolerated
Dopamine Agonists		Monotherapy in early disease to delay starting levodopa	Poorly tolerated by about 30% of clients for following reasons: Allergy, palpitations/ sinus tachycardia, agitation, dizziness/ fainting (especially when initiating treatment of increasing doses)	Bromocriptine and pergolide: Edema (hands, feet, face), erythromyalgia, Raynaud's syndrome, pleural effusions More difficult to use in clients older than 60 because of CNS effects such as confusion, hallucinations, delusions
ERGOT DERIVATIVES				
Pergolide (Permax)	0.05, 0.25, 1 mg tablets	"Levodopa-sparing" and may theoretically delay the development of motor complications; studies under way		
Bromocriptine (Parlodel)	2.5, 5 mg tablets			
NONERGOT DERIVATIVES				
Ropinirole (Requip)	0.25, 0.5, 1,2, 5 mg	Adjunctive therapy with other agents including carbidopa-levodopa When added to carbidopa-levodopa, dopamine agonists may decrease dyskinesias, prolong "on" time, reduce "off" time, and reduce wearing off complications Dopamine agonists are not as effective as carbidopa-levodopa in relieving symptoms of Parkinson's disease	Side effect profile similar to levodopa	
Pramipexole (Mirapex)	0.125, 0.25, 1, and 1.5 mg			Very complex titration schedule; manufacturer starter packs available When dopamine agonists are added to carbidopa-levodopa, the dose of carbidopa-levodopa needs to be reduced
Incontinence				
Anticholinergic Agents				
Oxybutynin (Ditropan)	2.5-5 mg bid-qid	Overactive bladder	Dry mouth,blurred vision, constipation, confusion,	Anticholinergics are the first-line drug therapy

Continued

TABLE A-4 Medications Commonly Used in Rehabilitation Practice—cont'd

Generic Name (Selected Trade Name)	Normal Adult Dosage	Therapeutic Uses	Major Adverse Effects/Cautions	Comments
Oxybutynin XL (Ditropan XL)	5-30 mg once/day		tachycardia, orthostatic hypotension, dizziness, urine retention	(oxybutynin or tolterodine are preferred)
Tolterodine (Detrol)	1-2 mg bid		Interactions: CYP 3A4 inhibitors Increased intraocular pressure with anticholinergics	
Tricyclic Antidepressants (TCAs)		Overactive bladder Stress or combined stress and overactive urinary incontinence (i.e., mixed type)	Anticholinergic effects (as previously described), orthostatic hypotension, cardiac dysrhythmia	TCAs are generally reserved for clients with an additional indication (e.g., depression, neuralgia) at an initial dose of 10-25 mg, 1-3 times/day Do not use in clients with urinary obstruction Interactions: monoamine oxidase inhibitors, sympathomimetic amines
Nortriptyline (Pamelor)	25-100 mg/day (with water or juice)			
Impramine	25-100 mg/day (with water or juice)			
Doxepin (Sinequan)	25-100 mg/day (with water or juice)			
Estrogen		Overactive bladder Stress or combined stress and overactive urinary incontinence (i.e., mixed type), incontinence	Few adverse effects with cream and vaginal insert Adverse effects of systemic therapy are headache, vaginal spotting, edema, breast tenderness, possible depression	Systemic therapy should not be used if there is suspected or confirmed breast or endometrial cancer, or active or past thromboembolism with past oral contraceptive, estrogen, or pregnancy Progestin (e.g., medroxyprogesterone 2.5-10 mg/day) necessary with intact uterus; progestin unnecessary without uterus or short-term topical cream or estrogen vaginal insert Give progestin with systemic estrogen (e.g., Prempro, Combipatch) if uterus intact Pretreatment: Periodic mammogram, gynecologic and breast examinations Interactions: Carbamazepine, phenobarbital, rifampin may decrease effect; may increase cyclosporine level/toxicity; may decrease tamoxifen effect
Conjugated estrogen (Premarin)	0.5 g vaginal cream 3 times/wk, up to 8 mo; repeat course if symptom recurrence Or, estradiol vaginal insert/ring (2 mg [1 ring]) and replaced after 90 days, if needed; if ineffective, start systemic therapy with conjugated estrogens, 0.3-0.625 mg/day orally immediately after food to decrease nausea Or, Estraderm or Combipatch			
Alpha-Adrenergic Agonists		Stress incontinence	Anxiety, insomnia, agitation, palpitations, headache, agina, cardiac dysrhythmia, hypertension, tremor	Pseudoephedrine is first-line therapy for women with no contraindications (notably, hypertension)
Pseudophedrine (Sudafed)	15-60 tid. taken with food, water, or milk			

Data from American Society of Health System Pharmacists. (2000). *AHFS drug information.* Bethesda, MD: Author; and Lackner, T.E. (1999). Urinary health management in the long-term care setting. *Consultant Pharmacist, 14* (Suppl B), 3-16.

TABLE A-4 Medications Commonly Used in Rehabilitation Practice—cont'd

Generic Name (Selected Trade Name)	Normal Adult Dosage	Therapeutic Uses	Major Adverse Effects/Cautions	Comments
			Should not be used in clients with obstructive syndromes and/or hypertension Interactions: Methyldopa may increase pressor response	
Alpha-Adrenergic Antagonists		Overflow (because of enlarged benign prostate)		
Terazosin (Hytrin)	1 mg at bedtime with first dose Increase by 1 mg every 4 days to 5 mg/day, as needed		Postural hypotension, syncope in supine palpitations, edema, headache, dizziness, vertigo, drowsiness, weakness Interactions: Antihypertensives may increase hypotension	Possible benefit in men with obstructive position, heart symptoms of benign prostatic hyperplasia Monitor sitting and standing blood pressures with first dose/each dose increase May worsen female stress incontinence
Doxazosin (Cardura)	1 mg at bedtime, with first dose in supine position Increase by 1 mg every 7-14 days to 5 mg/day, as needed		Same as for terazosin	Same as for terazosin
Tamsulosin (Flumax)	0.4 mg once daily Increase after 2-4 wk, if needed, to 0.8 mg/day		Same as for terazosin	Benefit: Fewer incidences of orthostatic hypotension
Antiandrogens		Overflow (because of enlarged benign prostate)		
Finasteride (Proscar)	5 mg/day Can crush but don't handle if possibly pregnant		Erectile impotence, decreased libido, gynecomastia	Maximum therapeutic effect after 6-12 mo Causes 50% decrease in PSA test Interactions: Falsely decreased prostate specific antigen (PSA) concentration
Phytotherapy		Overflow (because of enlarged benign prostate)		
Serenoa repens (saw palmetto)	160 mg bid		Headache, GI upset, hypertension, decreased libido, erectile dysfunction	Long-term efficacy and safety unknown
Cholinergics		Overflow (because of atonic bladder)		
Bethanechol (Urecholine)	1-30 mg qid		Nausea, vomiting, abdominal cramps, diarrhea, bradycardia, bronchoconstriction, hypotension Interactions: Decreased effect by anticholinergics	Avoid use in clients with asthma or heart disease Short-term use only

Continued

TABLE A-4 Medications Commonly Used in Rehabilitation Practice—cont'd

Generic Name (Selected Trade Name)	Normal Adult Dosage	Therapeutic Uses	Major Adverse Effects/Cautions	Comments
Stimulants				
Bisacodyl (Dulcolax)	Tablet: 10-15 mg in a single dose once/day Up to 30 mg has been used for preparation of lower GI tract for special procedures	Constipation	Chronic use can lead to electrolyte imbalance or abdominal cramping	Should be used intermittently
Senna (Senokot)	Tablets (187 and 217 mg): 2 tablets (up to 8/day) Tablets (374 mg): 1 tablet at bedtime (up to 4/day) Granules: 1 tsp (up to 4 tsp/day) Suppositories: 1 at bedtime; repeat in 2 hr, if necessary Liquid: 15-30 ml with or after meals or at bedtime Syrup: 10-15 ml at bedtime (up to 30 ml/day)			
Hyperosmolar				
Glycerin	Suppositories: Insert 1 suppository high in the rectum and retain 15 min; it need not melt to produce laxative action Rectal liquid: With gentle, steady pressure, insert stem with tip pointing toward navel; Squeeze unit until nearly all the liquid is expelled, then remove; a small amount of liquid will remain in unit	Constipation		
Lactulose (Chrorulac, Constilac, Duphalac)	15-30 ml (10-20 g lactulose)/day, increase to 60 ml/day if necessary			Sorbitol is as effective as lactulose yet less expensive
Saline Products Magnesium citrate (Citrate of Magnesia)	1 glassful (approximately 250 ml/day), as needed	Acute evacuation of the bowel	Fluid and electrolyte imbalance	

Data from American Society of Health System Pharmacists. (2000). *AHFS drug information.* Bethesda, MD: Author; and Lackner, T.E. (1999). Urinary health management in the long-term care setting. *Consultant Pharmacist, 14* (Suppl B), 3-16.

TABLE A-4 Medications Commonly Used in Rehabilitation Practice—cont'd

Generic Name (Selected Trade Name)	Normal Adult Dosage	Therapeutic Uses	Major Adverse Effects/Cautions	Comments
Diabetes Medications				
Oral Sulfonylureas	10-20 mg once or in split doses (divided)	Type 2 diabetes	Hypoglycemia, weight gain, rash	Assess for sulfa allergy
Glipizide (Glucotrol, Glucontrol XL [sustained-release tablets])	5 mg once			
Glyburide (DiaBeta, Micronase)				
Glynase [micronized tablets])	5-20 mg once or divided 3-12 mg once or divided			
Alpha-Glucosidase Inhibitors			Flatulence, abdominal discomfort	Take with first bite of meal to reduce postprandial blood glucose level
Acarbose (Precose)	50-100 mg tid with meals			
Miglitol (Glyset)	50-100 mg tid with meals			
Thiazolidinediones (Glitazones)			GI upset	Monitor liver function
Rosiglitazone (Avandia)	4-8 mg once per day or 2-4 mg bid			
Pioglitazone (Actos)	15-45 mg once per day			
Metformin (glucophage)	500-2550 mg/day		GI upset, lactic acidosis	Do *not* use with creatinine clearance greater than 1.4 in women or greater than 1.5 in men

REFERENCES

American College of Rheumatology Ad Hoc Committee on Clinical Guidelines. (1996). Guidelines for monitoring drug therapy in rheumatoid arthritis. *Arthritis and Rheumatism 39,* 723-731.

American Society of Health System Pharmacists. (1995). ASHP guideline on adverse drug reaction monitoring and reporting. *American Journal of Health-System Pharmacy, 52,* 417-419.

Crockgroft, D.W., & Gault, M.H. (1976). Prediction of creatinine clearance from serum creatinine. *Nephron, 16,* 31.

DiPiro, J., Talbert, R., Yee, G., Matzke, G., Wells, B., & Posey, L. (1999). *Pharmacotherapy: A pathophysiologic approach* (4th ed.). Norwalk, CT: Appleton and Lange.

Lazarou, J., Pomeranz, B.H., & Corey, P. (1998). Incidence of adverse drug reactions in hospitalized patients. A meta-analysis of prospective patients. *Journal of the American Medical Association, 279,* 1200-1205.

Michalets, E.L. (1998). Update: Clinically significant cytochrome P-450 drug interactions. *Pharmacotherapy, 18*(1), 84-112.

BIBLIOGRAPHY

Allen, J. (1999). New treatments for rheumatoid arthritis. *Pharmacist's Letter, November.*

American Society of Health System Pharmacists (2000). *AHFS drug information.* Bethesda, MD: Author.

Katzung, B.G. (1995). *Basic and clinical pharmacology* (6th ed.). Norwalk, CT: Appleton and Lange.

Kompoliti, K., & Goetz, C. (1998). Neuropharmacology in the elderly. *Neurology Clinics of North America, 16*(3), 599-610.

Lackner, T.E. (1999). Urinary health management in the long-term care setting. *Consultant Pharmacist, 14*(Suppl B), 3-16.

Levien, T.L., & Baker, D.E. (1999). Selected interactions caused by cytochrome P450 enzymes. *Pharmacist's Letter, April.*

Pratt, W.B., & Taylor, P. (1990). *Principals of drug action: The basis of pharmacology* (3rd ed.). New York: Churchill Livingstone.

Rang, H.P., Dale, M.M., Ritter, J.M., & Gardner, P. (1995). *Pharmacology.* New York: Churchill Livingstone.

Shargel, L., & Yu A.B.C. (1993). *Applied biopharmaceutics and pharmacokinetics* (3rd ed.). Norwalk, CT: Appleton and Lange.

Index

A

B

C

D

F

G

H

I

J

K

L

M

N

O

P

Q

R

S

T

U

X

Z